Nursing Outcomes Classification (NOC)

Measurement of Health Outcomes

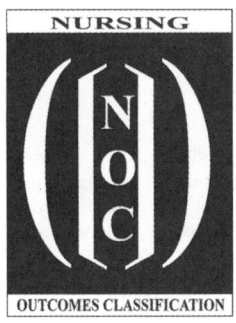

Fifth Edition

Editors

Sue Moorhead, PhD, RN

Marion Johnson, PhD, RN

Meridean L. Maas, PhD, RN, FAAN

Elizabeth Swanson, PhD, RN

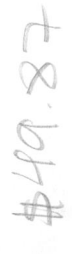

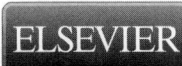

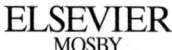

3251 Riverport Lane
St. Louis, Missouri 63043

NURSING OUTCOMES CLASSIFICATION (NOC)　　　　ISBN: 978-0-323-10010-6

Notices

Knowledge and best practice in this field are constantly changing. As new research and experience broaden our understanding, changes in research methods, professional practices, or medical treatment may become necessary.

Practitioners and researchers must always rely on their own experience and knowledge in evaluating and using any information, methods, compounds, or experiments described herein. In using such information or methods they should be mindful of their own safety and the safety of others, including parties for whom they have a professional responsibility.

With respect to any drug or pharmaceutical products identified, readers are advised to check the most current information provided (i) on procedures featured or (ii) by the manufacturer of each product to be administered, to verify the recommended dose or formula, the method and duration of administration, and contraindications. It is the responsibility of practitioners, relying on their own experience and knowledge of their patients, to make diagnoses, to determine dosages and the best treatment for each individual patient, and to take all appropriate safety precautions.

To the fullest extent of the law, neither the Publisher nor the authors, contributors, or editors, assume any liability for any injury and/or damage to persons or property as a matter of products liability, negligence or otherwise, or from any use or operation of any methods, products, instructions, or ideas contained in the material herein.

Library of Congress Cataloging-in-Publication Data
Nursing outcomes classification (NOC) : measurement of health outcomes / editors, Sue Moorhead . . . [et al.]. — 5th ed.
　　p. ; cm.
　Includes bibliographical references and index.
　ISBN 978-0-323-10010-6 (pbk. : alk. paper)
　I. Moorhead, Sue.
　[DNLM: 1. Nursing Process—standards. 2. Outcome Assessment (Health Care)—standards. WY 100.1]

　610.73012—dc23

　　　　　　　　　　　　　　　　　　　　　　　　201203

Senior Content Strategist: Sandra Clark
Senior Content Development Specialist: Karen C. Turner
Publishing Services Manager: Jeff Patterson
Senior Project Manager: Clay S. Broeker
Designer: Amy Buxton

Printed in the United States of America

Last digit is the print number:　9　8　7　6　5　4　3　2　1

Recognition List, Fifth Edition

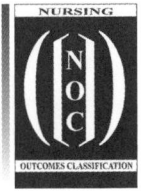

We wish to thank the following individuals who have shared their expertise by reviewing or developing specific outcomes or contributing in other ways to this edition.

Sandra L. Bellinger, EdD, RN, Retired, Trinity College of Nursing & Health Sciences, Rock Island, IL

Veronica Brighton, MA, ARNP, CS, Assistant Professor (Clinical), The University of Iowa, College of Nursing, Iowa City, IA

Jane Brokel, PhD, RN, Assistant Professor, The University of Iowa, College of Nursing, Iowa City, IA

Judy Carlson, EdD, APRN, FNP, Senior Nurse Scientist, Tripler Army Medical Center, Honolulu, HI

Mary Clarke, PhD, RN, BC, Director of Nursing Practice, Research and Innovation, Magnet Project Director, Genesis Medical Center, Davenport, IA

Janice Denehy, PhD, RN, Associate Professor Emerita, The University of Iowa, College of Nursing, Iowa City, IA

Janet Enslein, PhD, RN, Nursing Faculty, St. Ambrose University, Davenport, IA

İsmet Eşer, PhD, RN, Professor, Fundamentals of Nursing Department, Ege University Faculty of Nursing, Bornova, İzmir, Turkey

Mary Ann Fahrenkrug, MSN, RN, Nursing Faculty, St. Ambrose University, Davenport, IA

Elem Kocaçal Güler, MS(c), Research Assistant, Fundamentals of Nursing Department, Ege University School of Nursing, Bornova İzmir, Turkey

Susan R. Johnson, MD, MS, Professor of Obstetrics & Gynecology and Epidemiology, The University of Iowa, Carver College of Medicine, Iowa City, IA

Peg Kerr, MS, PhD, RN, Associate Professor, Nursing Department Head, University of Dubuque, Dubuque, IA

Joan Klehr, RNC, MPH, Information Systems Analyst, Aspirus Wausau Hospital, Wausau, WI

Cathy Konrad PhD, RNC, Faculty, Trinity College of Nursing & Health Sciences, Rock Island, IL

Regina Holly Lange, MS, RN, Faculty, Trinity College of Nursing & Health Sciences, Rock Island, IL

Sue Lehman, MSN, RN, Assistant Professor (Clinical), The University of Iowa, College of Nursing, Iowa City, IA

Kathleen Lenaghan MSN, RN-BC, Nursing Outcomes Specialist, Genesis Medical Center, Davenport, IA

Kathryn McKnight, PhD(c), MSN, PNP, MPH, Nursing Faculty, St. Ambrose University, Davenport, IA

Juleann Miller, PhD, RN, Nursing Faculty, St. Ambrose University, Davenport, IA

Shelley-Rae Pehler, PhD, RN, Associate Professor, University of Wisconsin-Eau Claire, Eau Claire, WI

Kelly Smith, MSN, RN, Instructor (Clinical), The University of Iowa, College of Nursing, Iowa City, IA

Cheryl Wagner, PhD, MSN, MBA, RN, Associate Dean, American Sentinel University, MSN Programs, Aurora, CO

Bonnie Wakefield, PhD, RN, FAAN, Associate Research Professor, Sinclair School of Nursing, University of Missouri, Columbia, MO

Students

Noriko Abe, Doctoral student, The University of Iowa, College of Nursing, Iowa City, IA

Elaine Cook, Doctoral student, The University of Iowa, College of Nursing, Iowa City, IA

Renata Pereira de Melo, Doctoral student, Universidade Federal do Ceará, Brazil

Mikyoung Lee, Doctoral student, The University of Iowa, College of Nursing, Iowa City, IA

Mikyung Moon, Doctoral student, The University of Iowa, College of Nursing, Iowa City, IA

Hyunkyoung Oh, Doctoral student, The University of Iowa, College of Nursing, Iowa City, IA

Hye Jin Park, Doctoral student, The University of Iowa, College of Nursing, Iowa City, IA

Hui-Chen Tseng, Doctoral student, The University of Iowa, College of Nursing, Iowa City, IA

Visiting Professors

Prisca Olabisi Adejumo, RN, PhD, FWACN, Senior Lecturer, Department of Nursing, University of Ibadan, Ibadan, Nigeria

Adenike Olaogun, PhD, RN, RM, RPHN, Department of Nursing Science, Ile Ife, Nigeria

Staff

Sharon Sweeney, BSB, Coordinator, Center for Nursing Classification & Clinical Effectiveness, University of Iowa, College of Nursing, Iowa City, IA

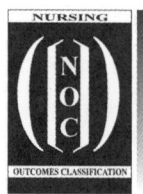

Fellows—Center for Nursing Classification & Clinical Effectiveness

The Center for Nursing Classification & Clinical Effectiveness (CNC) at the College of Nursing, The University of Iowa, has a fellows program. *Fellow, Center for Nursing Classification & Clinical Effectiveness* is designated for individuals who contribute significantly to the ongoing upkeep and implementation of NIC and NOC. These individuals are actively contributing to the Center and may include research team members, staff at cooperating agencies, retired professors, and visiting scholars. Students who are within a year of finishing their doctoral dissertations and who have made substantial contributions to the work of the CNC are eligible.

Fellows donate a portion of their time to some work activity of the Center. They are available as resource persons for such activities as providing ad hoc reviews of proposed new interventions and outcomes, participating in team or other meetings, serving on a planning committee for a conference, reviewing drafts of monographs, participating in grant writing activities, and advising the board of current developments related to classification work. An appointment of a fellow is for a 3-year period, or for a shorter time depending on need (e.g. Visiting Scholar).

The following individuals are serving as Fellows as of July 1, 2012:

Mary Ann Anderson, Associate Professor, University of Illinois, College of Nursing, Quad Cities Regional Program, Moline, IL

Ida Androwich, Professor, Loyola University, School of Nursing, Chicago, IL

Sandra Bellinger, Retired, Trinity College of Nursing & Health Sciences, Rock Island, IL

Sharon Eck Birmingham, Chief Nursing Executive, Clairvia Business Unit, Cerner Corporation, Durham, NC

Veronica Brighton, Assistant Professor (Clinical), University of Iowa, College of Nursing

Jane Brokel, Assistant Professor, University of Iowa, College of Nursing

Gloria Bulechek, Professor Emerita, University of Iowa, College of Nursing

Lisa Burkhart, Associate Professor, Loyola University, School of Nursing, Chicago, IL

Howard Butcher, Associate Professor, University of Iowa, College of Nursing

Teresa Clark, Advance Practice Nurse, Informatics, University of Iowa Hospitals and Clinics

Mary Clarke, Director of Nursing Practice, Research, and Innovation, Genesis Medical Center, Davenport, IA

Deborah Conley, Gerontological Clinical Nurse Specialist, Nebraska Methodist Hospital, Omaha, NE

Elaine Cook, Assistant Professor, Mount Mercy University, Cedar Rapids, IA

Sister Ruth Cox, Faculty, Kirkwood Community College, Cedar Rapids, IA

Martha Craft-Rosenberg, Professor Emerita, University of Iowa, College of Nursing, IA

Jeanette Daly, Associate Research Scientist, University of Iowa Hospitals and Clinics

Connie Delaney, Dean and Professor, University of Minnesota, School of Nursing, Minneapolis, MN

Janice Denehy, Associate Professor Emerita, University of Iowa, College of Nursing

Joanne Dochterman, Professor Emerita, College of Nursing, University of Iowa

Gloria Dorr, Advance Practice Nurse, Informatics, University of Iowa Hospitals and Clinics

Mary Ann Fahrenkrug, Adjunct Faculty, Ambrose University, Davenport, IA

Joe Greiner, Advanced Practice Nurse, University of Iowa Hospitals and Clinics

Barbara Head, Assistant Professor Emerita, University of Nebraska Medical Center, College of Nursing, Omaha, NE

Todd Ingram, Assistant Professor (Clinical), University of Iowa, College of Nursing

Gwenneth Jensen, Clinical Nurse Specialist, Sandford Health, Sioux Falls, SD

Marion Johnson, Professor Emerita, University of Iowa, College of Nursing

Tess Judge-Ellis, Associate Professor (Clinical), University of Iowa, College of Nursing

Gail Keenan, Associate Professor, Director of Nursing Informatics Initiative, University of Illinois, College of Nursing, Chicago, IL

Peg Kerr, Associate Professor, Nursing Department Head, University of Dubuque, Dubuque, IA

Cathy Konrad, Faculty, Trinity College of Nursing & Health Sciences, Rock Island, IL

Marie Kozel, CARE Project Lead, Methodist Health System, Omaha, NE

Mikyoung Lee, Assistant Professor, Indiana University, School of Nursing, Indianapolis, IN

Sue Lehmann, Assistant Professor (Clinical), University of Iowa, College of Nursing

Der-Fa Lu, Assistant Professor, University of Iowa, College of Nursing

Meridean L. Maas, Professor Emerita, University of Iowa, College of Nursing

Paula Mobily, Associate Professor, University of Iowa, College of Nursing

Lou Ann Montgomery, Director of Nursing Administration, Co-Director of Nursing Clinical Education Center, University of Iowa Hospitals and Clinics

Sue Moorhead, Associate Professor and Director, Center for Nursing Classification & Clinical Effectiveness, University of Iowa, College of Nursing

Hye Jin Park, Assistant Professor, Florida State University, College of Nursing, Tallahassee, FL

Shelley-Rae Pehler, Associate Professor, University of Wisconsin—Eau Claire, Eau Claire, WI

Aleta Porcella, Clinical Nurse Specialist—Informatics, University of Iowa Hospitals and Clinics

Barb Rakel, Assistant Professor, College of Nursing, University of Iowa

David Reed, Research Associate, University of North Carolina, Cecil G. Sheps Center for Health Services Research, Chapel Hill, NC

K. Reeder, Assistant Professor, Goldfarb School of Nursing, Barnes-Jewish College, St. Louis, MO

Cindy Scherb, Professor, Winona State University, Graduate Programs in Nursing University Center Rochester, Winona, MN

Debra Schutte, Associate Professor, Michigan State University, College of Nursing, East Lansing, MI

Jill Scott-Cawiezell, Professor and Associate Dean for Academic Affairs, University of Iowa, College of Nursing

Lisa Segre, Assistant Professor, University of Iowa, College of Nursing

Margaret Simons, Diabetes Nurse Specialist, Iowa City VA Medical Center

Kelly Smith, Instructor (Clinical), University of Iowa, College of Nursing

Janet Specht, Professor, University of Iowa, College of Nursing

Anita Stineman, Associate Professor (Clinical), College of Nursing, University of Iowa

Elizabeth Swanson, Associate Professor, University of Iowa, College of Nursing

Mary Tarbox, Professor and Chair, Department of Nursing, Mount Mercy University, Cedar Rapids, IA

Toni Tripp-Reimer, Professor, University of Iowa, College of Nursing

Hui-Chen Tseng, Postdoctoral Fellow, University of Utah, College of Nursing, Salt Lake City, UT

Sharon Tucker, Director, Nursing Research and Evidence-Based Practice, University of Iowa Hospitals and Clinics

Cheryl Wagner, Associate Dean, American Sentinel University, MSN Programs, Aurora, CO

Bonnie Wakefield, Associate Research Professor, University of Missouri, Sinclair School of Nursing, Columbia, MO

Ann Williamson, Associate Vice President for Nursing, UI Health Care, and Chief Nursing Officer, University of Iowa Hospitals and Clinics

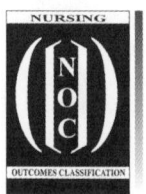

Preface

The fifth edition of *Nursing Outcomes Classification (NOC)* contains 490 outcomes and represents over 20 years of work by the Iowa Outcomes team. The classification standardizes the outcome names and definitions for use in practice, education, and research. Each outcome includes a label name; a definition; a set of indicators that describe specific states, perceptions, or behaviors related to the outcome; a 5-point Likert measurement scale or scales; and selected references used in the development of the outcome. The outcomes assist nurses and other health care providers to evaluate and quantify the status of the patient, caregiver, family, or community. The classification focuses on the measurement of outcomes across a variety of specialties and settings and has outcomes for use across the lifespan. Nurses incorporating NOC in their practice are able to quantify the change in patient status after interventions and monitor progress. Feedback from clinicians using the outcome measures in clinical settings has been positive, and their suggestions have helped improve the classification.

This edition contains 490 outcomes and includes 107 new outcomes. A complete list of new outcomes and changes in previously published outcomes can be found in Appendix A. We have added a new class to the taxonomy focused on self-management of acute and chronic health conditions. This edition provides practical guidance on how to use NOC in clinical practice. Chapter 1 describes the current classification presented in this edition. Definition of terms, frequently asked questions, and new features are highlighted. Chapter 2 discusses how to use NOC in clinical practice, education, and research. Linkages between the NANDA-I diagnoses and the NOC outcomes are included in the book. The reader will note that the NANDA-I diagnoses are listed by key concept, in alphabetical order, and consistent with the terminology used in the 2012-2014 edition of the NANDA International Classification. Also included in this section are linkages to Gordon's Functional Patterns. It is important to note that these linkages are not prescriptive and need to be validated with clinical data

across settings and populations. They are suggested to assist nurses with identifying possible outcomes when a diagnosis is made or to develop a framework for clinical information systems. The nurse's clinical judgment remains the most important factor in selecting outcomes.

The need for nursing to define the patient outcomes that are responsive to nursing care has continued to increase since the first edition of this book was published. The growth of managed care, the emphasis on cost containment and safety, and the need for evidence-based practice continue to bring concerns about effectiveness of nursing interventions and health care quality to the attention of nurses, consumers, health care organizations, payers, and policy makers. Nursing plays a key role in the delivery of safe, cost-effective care in every health care setting; therefore it is imperative that nursing data be included in the evaluation of health care effectiveness. The NOC completes the nursing process elements of the Nursing Minimum Data Set (NMDS). NOC is a companion language to the NIC interventions and the NANDA International diagnoses. Standardized nursing languages are required to ensure that the nursing elements identified in the NMDS are included in electronic patient databases. They also facilitate the study and teaching of diagnostic reasoning and the development of mid-range theory as linkages between patient characteristics, nursing diagnoses, nursing interventions, and nursing-sensitive outcomes are tested.

The editors of this book thank the many nurses who have contributed to the development of NOC. The team has worked diligently to continue to expand and evaluate the NOC outcomes. Many individuals have shared their knowledge and work with us or have agreed to review an outcome related to their specialty. Without them, this edition would not be possible.

Sue Moorhead
Marion Johnson
Meridean L. Maas
Elizabeth Swanson

Strengths of the Nursing-Sensitive Outcomes Classification

Comprehensive. The NOC contains outcomes for individuals, caregivers, families, and communities that can be used with all clinical specialties in numerous settings. Although there are still outcomes to develop, the outcomes in this fifth edition are useful for the entire scope of nursing practice.

Research-based. The research, conducted by a large team of University of Iowa College of Nursing faculty and students in conjunction with clinicians from a variety of settings, began in 1991. Both qualitative and quantitative strategies were used to develop the classification. Methods included content analysis, concept analysis, survey of experts, similarity analysis, hierarchical clustering analysis, multidimensional scaling, and clinical field site testing. The outcomes were evaluated for inter-rater reliability, validity, and usefulness in 10 clinical sites representing the care continuum.

Developed inductively and deductively. Sources of data for the initial development of outcomes and indicators were nursing textbooks, care plan guides, nursing clinical information systems, standards of practice, and research instruments. Research team focus groups reviewed outcomes in eight broad categories that were drawn from the Medical Outcomes Study and nursing literature. Based on a review of literature, outcomes were grouped in broad categories and refined through concept analysis.

Grounded in clinical practice and research. Developed initially from nursing texts, care plan guides, and clinical information systems, the outcomes were reviewed by clinical experts, and many were tested in clinical field sites. Feedback from clinicians and educators was solicited through a defined feedback process. Beginning work on core NOC outcomes for specialty practice was first included in the third edition. This grounding in clinical practice continues with this edition as numerous outcomes were developed by clinical experts and forwarded to the authors.

Has an easy-to-use organizing structure. The taxonomy has five levels: domains, classes, outcomes, indicators, and measurement scales. All five levels have been coded for use in practice. New outcomes are added to the taxonomy as the classification is further developed. This structure aids nurses in identifying outcomes to use in their clinical practice and provides a framework for teaching NOC to students in educational settings.

Allows outcomes to be shared by all disciplines. Although the NOC emphasizes outcomes that are most responsive to nursing interventions, the outcomes describe patient, family, or community states at a conceptual level. Thus the NOC provides a classification of patient outcomes that are potentially influenced by all health care disciplines. Use of the outcomes by all members of the interdisciplinary team provides standardization yet allows the selection of indicators that are most responsive to each discipline. Field testing demonstrated that the outcomes were useful to interdisciplinary teams in practice.

Optimizes information used for the evaluation of effectiveness. The outcomes and indicators are variable concepts. They allow for measurement of the patient, family, or community outcome at any point on a continuum from most negative to most positive and at different points in time. Rather than the limited information of whether a goal is met or unmet, NOC outcomes can be used to monitor the extent of progress, or lack of progress, throughout an episode of care and across different care settings. Changes in outcome ratings can be reported and recorded as a result of nursing interventions instituted across time and care setting.

Funded by extramural grants. To date, the NOC research has received 9 years of peer-reviewed grant funding: 1 year from Sigma Theta Tau International and 8 years from the National Institute of Nursing Research (NINR).

Tested in clinical field sites. Testing of the NOC has been conducted in a variety of clinical field sites, including tertiary-care hospitals, intermediate-care hospitals, a nursing home, home health care settings, nurse-managed clinics, and a parish nursing organization. The field tests have provided important information about the clinical usefulness of the outcomes and indicators; linkages between nursing diagnoses, interventions, and outcomes; and the process of implementing the outcomes in clinical nursing information systems.

Dissemination emphasized. Information about the classification, its development, and its use is available in this book (published by Elsevier every 4 to 5 years) and in numerous journal articles and book chapters. The NOC research is described on a University of Iowa College of Nursing website (http://www.nursing.uiowa.edu/cnc/), and a listserv is maintained to share information about the NOC and for dialogue with interested users. The NOC work has been disseminated in numerous national and international presentations. Although developed in the United States, nurses in other countries are finding the classification useful. Translations are available for the following languages: Chinese (simplified and traditional), Dutch, French, German, Italian, Japanese, Korean, Norwegian, Portuguese, and Spanish. The English editions and the translations are listed in Appendix C.

Linked to other nursing languages. Linkages have been developed by the NIC and NOC research teams to assist nurses with the use of the classifications and to facilitate use in clinical information systems. Linkages with NANDA International diagnoses and Gordon's Functional Health Care Patterns are included in the book. Linkages among NANDA-I diagnoses, NOC outcomes, and NIC interventions are available in the book *NOC and NIC Linkages to NANDA-I and Clinical Conditions: Supporting Critical Reasoning and Quality Care,* published by Elsevier in 2012. In addition, linkages have been developed between the International Classification of Functioning, Disability and Health (ICF) and NOC in an attempt to explore the components of ICF and identify the relevant concepts to promote language development in nursing. In addition, ICF was chosen due to its international and interdisciplinary use.

Included in initiatives for electronic clinical records. Concepts for NOC are included in SNOMED Clinical Terms, a reference terminology for use in clinical information systems. NOC has been registered with Health Level 7,

a U.S. standards organization dedicated to simplifying the exchange, management, and integration of clinical and administrative data in health records. A growing number of vendors have licensed NOC for inclusion in their software.

Developed as companion to the NIC. Experience with the NIC at Iowa has aided the NOC research. Both classifications are comprehensive and research-based and reflect current clinical nursing practice. They are both housed in the Center for Nursing Classification & Clinical Effectiveness.

Recipient of national recognition. NOC is recognized by the American Nurses Association (ANA), included in the Metathesaurus for a Unified Medical Language at the National Library of Medicine, included in the CINAHL index, and listed as one of the languages that meets the standards set by ANA's Nursing Information and Data Set Evaluation Center (NIDSEC).

Structured for continued development and refinement. The classification continues to be evaluated, developed, and refined by the NOC research team. Continued refinement will be facilitated through the Center for Nursing Classification & Clinical Effectiveness, the College of Nursing, and the University of Iowa. In addition to seeking continued grant support, a $1 million endowment is being raised to ensure a solid financial foundation for supporting further development of both NIC and NOC. Revenue from the sales of the book and licensing are used to support the staff and work of the Center for Nursing Classification & Clinical Effectiveness.

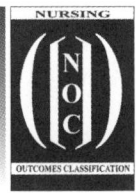

Nursing-Sensitive Patient Outcome

An individual, family, or community state, behavior, or perception that is measured along a continuum in response to a nursing intervention or interventions. Each outcome has an associated group of indicators that are used to determine patient status in relation to the outcome. In order to be measured, the outcome requires identification of a series of more specific indicators.

Outcome Indicator

A more concrete individual, family, or community state, behavior, or perception that serves as a cue for measuring an outcome. Nursing-sensitive patient outcome indicators characterize a patient, family, or community state at the concrete level. Some examples of indicators include "Uses strategies to maximize health," "Maintains usual family routines," and "Intake of adequate fluid."

Measure

A 5-point Likert-type scale that quantifies a patient outcome or indicator status on a continuum from least to most desirable and provides a rating at a point in time. Measurement will reflect a continuum, such as 1 = Severely compromised, 2 = Substantially compromised, 3 = Moderately compromised, 4 = Mildly compromised, and 5 = Not compromised.

Change Score

The difference between a baseline rating of the outcome and the post-intervention rating(s) of the outcome. This change score can be positive (the outcome rating increased) or negative (the outcome rating decreased), or there can be no change (the outcome rating stayed the same). This change in rating score represents the outcome achieved following a health care intervention or interventions.

NOC Taxonomy

A systematic organization of outcomes into groups or categories based upon similarities, dissimilarities, and relationships among the outcomes. The NOC taxonomy structure has five levels: domains, classes, outcomes, indicators, and measures.

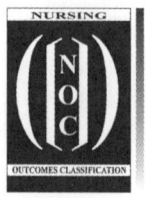

Acknowledgments

Continual development of the Nursing Outcomes Classification (NOC) and this publication would not have been possible without the work and support of numerous individuals and organizations. We are indebted to the many individuals who have supported our work and encouraged us along the way. We would like to acknowledge and thank the following individuals and organizations for their efforts:

- *Sigma Theta Tau International* for a 1-year grant (1992-1993) and the Office of Nursing Research, University of Iowa, for seed grants (1992-1993). These grants partially funded the pilot work and beginning development of the NOC.
- *The National Institute of Nursing Research, National Institutes of Health,* for a 4-year grant (1993-1997) to continue the development of the classification, construct the taxonomy, and field test the outcomes, and for a 4-year continuation grant (1998-2001) entitled "Evaluation of Nursing-Sensitive Patient Outcome Measures" to pilot the outcomes and evaluate the measurement scales in clinical sites.
- The *College of Nursing* at the *University of Iowa* for support of this work by *past Deans Geraldene Felton and Melanie Dreher, Interim Dean Martha Craft-Rosenberg, and current dean Rita Frantz.* This support for the Center for Nursing Classification & Clinical Effectiveness since it was founded in 1995 has been instrumental in the continuing development and refinement of both NIC and NOC and our work on linkages among diagnoses, interventions, and outcomes.
- The *team members, clinicians, educators, fellows, and students* who have devoted hours of work to develop, review, and refine the outcomes, associated indicators, and measurement scales that appear in the NOC.
- The *NANDA International* organization for its partnership through the Alliance that links NANDA-I, NIC, and NOC in efforts such as the NNN taxonomy structure development and NANDA-I, NIC, and NOC national conferences.
- *Nurses from a variety of nursing specialty organizations* who shared their expertise by completing validation surveys and core surveys to further this effort.
- The many *patients and their families* who were willing to participate in our research and complete both outcome ratings and criterion tool measures as we tested our outcomes in clinical settings.
- *Contributors to our endowment fund* to support the efforts of the Center for Nursing Classification & Clinical Effectiveness.
- The great staff we work with at Elsevier, *Sandra Clark and Karen Delany,* for their diligent work on our behalf.
- Our very competent staff member, *Sharon Sweeney,* who shares in our vision and manages the data and details of this classification to make this edition possible.

Contents

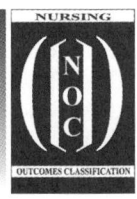

PART ONE Overview and Use of Nursing Outcomes Classification (NOC), 1

1 The Current Classification, 2
The Nursing Outcomes Classification (NOC): What Is It?, 2
Definition of an Outcome, 2
Measurement of an Outcome, 3
Use of a Reference Person for Comparison, 3
Level of Abstraction of NOC Outcomes, 3
Sensitivity of the Outcomes, 4
Use by Other Disciplines, 4
The Nursing Outcomes Classification: What It Is Not, 4
The Classification Is Not Complete, 4
NOC Outcomes Are Not Prescriptive, 5
NOC Outcomes Are Not Nursing Diagnoses, 5
Outcomes Are Not Assessments, 5
Frequently Asked Questions, 6
Who Is the Patient?, 6
What Do Patient Outcomes Describe?, 6
At What Levels of Abstraction Should Outcomes Be Developed?, 6
How Should Outcomes Be Stated?, 8
Why Are the Outcomes Not Stated as Goals?, 8
What Are Nursing-Sensitive Patient Outcomes?, 9
Are Nursing-Sensitive Patient Outcomes the Resolution of Nursing Diagnoses?, 9
How Are the Outcomes Different from Nursing Diagnoses?, 9
When Should Patient Outcomes Be Measured?, 10
At What Intervals Should the Outcomes Be Assessed and Documented?, 10
How Are the Outcomes Used in Standardized Care Plans/Critical Paths?, 10
Why Is It Necessary for Nurses to Have Their Own List of Outcomes?, 10
Why Is It Important to Assess Outcomes Across Care Settings?, 10
Why Is It Necessary to Use the Outcome Labels When the Indicators May Be More Useful?, 11
Why Is the Standardization of Outcomes Advocated When Each Patient, Caregiver, Family, or Community/Population is Unique?, 11
How Do I Identify Outcomes for Use in my Practice?, 11
When Is a New Outcome Developed and How Is It Done?, 11
Why Are There So Many Different Measurement Scales?, 11
Why Do Some Outcomes Have Two Scales?, 18
Refinement of the Classification: Ongoing and Future Development, 22
Summary, 31

2 Using NOC in Clinical, Research, and Educational Settings, 32
Considerations When Using NOC in Practice, 32
Selecting Outcomes, 32
After Outcome Selection, 34
Implementing NOC in Clinical Settings, 36
Implementation Planning, 36
Implementing NOC in Electronic Systems, 37
Implementing NOC in Educational Programs, 38
Implemention Strategies, 38
Aids for Curriculum Development and Teaching, 38
Using NOC in Research, 39
Evaluating Nursing Quality and Effectiveness, 39
Licensing NOC Outcomes, 40
Summary, 40

PART TWO NOC Taxonomy, 43

Overview of the NOC Taxonomy, 44
Historical Development of the NOC Taxonomy, 44
Revisions Made in the Taxonomy Since Its Creation. 44
Second Edition, 44
Third Edition, 45
Fourth Edition, 45
Fifth Edition, 45
Coding of the Classification, 47

PART THREE Outcomes, 69

Abstract Thinking, 70
Abuse Cessation, 71
Abuse Protection, 71

Abuse Recovery, 72
Abuse Recovery: Emotional, 73
Abuse Recovery: Financial, 74
Abuse Recovery: Physical, 75
Abuse Recovery: Sexual, 76
Abusive Behavior Self-Restraint, 77
Acceptance: Health Status, 78
Activity Tolerance, 79
Acute Respiratory Acidosis Severity, 80
Acute Respiratory Alkalosis Severity, 81
Adaptation to Physical Disability, 82
Adherence Behavior, 83
Adherence Behavior: Healthy Diet, 84
Aggression Self-Restraint, 85
Agitation Level, 86
Alcohol Abuse Cessation Behavior, 87
Allergic Response: Localized, 88
Allergic Response: Systemic, 89
Ambulation, 90
Ambulation: Wheelchair, 91
Anger Self-Restraint, 91
Anxiety Level, 93
Anxiety Self-Control, 94
Appetite, 95
Aspiration Prevention, 95
Balance, 97
Blood Coagulation, 98
Blood Glucose Level, 99
Blood Loss Severity, 99
Blood Transfusion Reaction, 100
Body Image, 101
Body Mechanics Performance, 102
Body Positioning: Self-Initiated, 103
Bone Healing, 104
Bottle Feeding Establishment: Infant, 106
Bottle Feeding Performance, 106
Bowel Continence, 107
Bowel Elimination, 108
Breastfeeding Establishment: Infant, 109
Breastfeeding Establishment: Maternal, 110
Breastfeeding Maintenance, 111
Breastfeeding Weaning, 112
Burn Healing, 113
Burn Recovery, 114
Cardiac Pump Effectiveness, 115
Cardiopulmonary Status, 116
Caregiver Adaptation to Patient Institutionalization, 117
Caregiver Emotional Health, 118
Caregiver Home Care Readiness, 119
Caregiver Lifestyle Disruption, 120
Caregiver-Patient Relationship, 121
Caregiver Performance: Direct Care, 121
Caregiver Performance: Indirect Care, 123

Caregiver Physical Health, 124
Caregiver Role Endurance, 125
Caregiver Stressors, 126
Caregiver Well-Being, 127
Child Adaptation to Hospitalization, 128
Child Development: 1 Month, 129
Child Development: 2 Months, 130
Child Development: 4 Months, 130
Child Development: 6 Months, 131
Child Development: 12 Months, 132
Child Development: 2 Years, 133
Child Development: 3 Years, 134
Child Development: 4 Years, 134
Child Development: 5 Years, 135
Child Development: Middle Childhood, 136
Child Development: Adolescence, 137
Circulation Status, 138
Client Satisfaction, 139
Client Satisfaction: Access to Care Resources, 140
Client Satisfaction: Caring, 141
Client Satisfaction: Case Management, 142
Client Satisfaction: Communication, 143
Client Satisfaction: Continuity of Care, 144
Client Satisfaction: Cultural Needs Fulfillment, 145
Client Satisfaction: Functional Assistance, 146
Client Satisfaction: Pain Management, 147
Client Satisfaction: Physical Care, 148
Client Satisfaction: Physical Environment, 149
Client Satisfaction: Protection of Rights, 150
Client Satisfaction: Psychological Care, 151
Client Satisfaction: Safety, 152
Client Satisfaction: Symptom Control, 153
Client Satisfaction: Teaching, 154
Client Satisfaction: Technical Aspects of Care, 155
Cognition, 156
Cognitive Orientation, 157
Comfort Status, 158
Comfort Status: Environment, 158
Comfort Status: Physical, 159
Comfort Status: Psychospiritual, 160
Comfort Status: Sociocultural, 161
Comfortable Death, 162
Communication, 163
Communication: Expressive, 164
Communication: Receptive, 164
Community Competence, 165
Community Disaster Readiness, 166
Community Disaster Response, 167
Community Grief Response, 168
Community Health Screening Effectiveness, 169
Community Health Status, 170
Community Immune Status, 172
Community Program Effectiveness, 173

Community Resiliency, 174
Community Risk Control: Chronic Disease, 175
Community Risk Control: Communicable Disease, 176
Community Risk Control: Lead Exposure, 177
Community Risk Control: Obesity, 178
Community Risk Control: Unhealthy Cultural
   Traditions, 179
Community Risk Control: Violence, 180
Community Violence Level, 180
Compliance Behavior, 181
Compliance Behavior: Prescribed Activity, 182
Compliance Behavior: Prescribed Diet, 183
Compliance Behavior: Prescribed Medication, 185
Concentration, 186
Coordinated Movement, 187
Coping, 188
Cup Feeding Establishment: Infant, 189
Cup Feeding Performance, 190
Decision-Making, 191
Delirium Level, 192
Dementia Level, 193
Depression Level, 194
Depression Self-Control, 195
Development: Late Adulthood, 196
Development: Middle Adulthood, 198
Development: Young Adulthood, 199
Dignified Life Closure, 201
Discharge Readiness: Independent Living, 202
Discharge Readiness: Supported Living, 203
Discomfort Level, 203
Distorted Thought Self-Control, 204
Drug Abuse Cessation Behavior, 205
Dry Eye Severity, 207
Eating Disorder Self-Control, 208
Electrolyte & Acid/Base Balance, 209
Electrolyte Balance, 211
Elopement Occurrence, 211
Elopement Propensity Risk, 212
Endurance, 213
Energy Conservation, 214
Exercise Participation, 214
Fall Prevention Behavior, 216
Falls Occurrence, 217
Family Coping, 217
Family Functioning, 218
Family Health Status, 219
Family Integrity, 221
Family Normalization, 222
Family Participation in Professional Care, 223
Family Resiliency, 224
Family Risk Control: Obesity, 225
Family Social Climate, 227
Family Support During Treatment, 228

Fatigue: Disruptive Effects, 229
Fatigue Level, 230
Fear Level, 231
Fear Level: Child, 232
Fear Self-Control, 233
Fetal Status: Antepartum, 234
Fetal Status: Intrapartum, 235
Fluid Balance, 236
Fluid Overload Severity, 237
Gait, 238
Gastrointestinal Function, 239
Grief Resolution, 240
Growth, 241
Guilt Resolution, 241
Health Beliefs, 243
Health Beliefs: Perceived Ability to Perform, 243
Health Beliefs: Perceived Control, 244
Health Beliefs: Perceived Resources, 245
Health Beliefs: Perceived Threat, 245
Health Orientation, 246
Health Promoting Behavior, 247
Health Seeking Behavior, 248
Hearing Compensation Behavior, 249
Heedfulness of Affected Side, 250
Hemodialysis Access, 251
Hope, 252
Hydration, 253
Hyperactivity Level, 254
Hypercalcemia Severity, 255
Hyperchloremia Severity, 256
Hyperglycemia Severity, 256
Hyperkalemia Severity, 257
Hypermagnesemia Severity, 258
Hypernatremia Severity, 258
Hyperphosphatemia Severity, 259
Hypertension Severity, 260
Hypocalcemia Severity, 261
Hypochloremia Severity, 262
Hypoglycemia Severity, 262
Hypokalemia Severity, 263
Hypomagnesemia Severity, 264
Hyponatremia Severity, 265
Hypophosphatemia Severity, 266
Hypotension Severity, 266
Identity, 268
Immobility Consequences: Physiological, 269
Immobility Consequences: Psycho-Cognitive, 270
Immune Hypersensitivity Response, 270
Immune Status, 271
Immunization Behavior, 272
Impulse Self-Control, 274
Infant Nutritional Status, 275
Infection Severity, 276

Infection Severity: Newborn, 277
Information Processing, 278
Joint Movement, 279
Joint Movement: Ankle, 279
Joint Movement: Elbow, 280
Joint Movement: Fingers, 281
Joint Movement: Hip, 282
Joint Movement: Knee, 283
Joint Movement: Neck, 283
Joint Movement: Passive, 284
Joint Movement: Shoulder, 284
Joint Movement: Spine, 285
Joint Movement: Wrist, 286
Kidney Function, 287
Knowledge: Acute Illness Management, 288
Knowledge: Anticoagulation Therapy Management, 289
Knowledge: Arthritis Management, 290
Knowledge: Asthma Management, 292
Knowledge: Body Mechanics, 293
Knowledge: Bottle Feeding, 294
Knowledge: Breastfeeding, 295
Knowledge: Cancer Management, 296
Knowledge: Cancer Threat Reduction, 297
Knowledge: Cardiac Disease Management, 298
Knowledge: Child Physical Safety, 299
Knowledge: Chronic Disease Management, 300
Knowledge: Chronic Obstructive Pulmonary Disease
   Management, 301
Knowledge: Conception Prevention, 302
Knowledge: Coronary Artery Disease Management, 303
Knowledge: Cup Feeding, 304
Knowledge: Dementia Management, 305
Knowledge: Depression Management, 306
Knowledge: Diabetes Management, 307
Knowledge: Disease Process, 308
Knowledge: Dysrhythmia Management, 309
Knowledge: Eating Disorder Management, 310
Knowledge: Energy Conservation, 311
Knowledge: Fall Prevention, 312
Knowledge: Fertility Promotion, 313
Knowledge: Health Behavior, 314
Knowledge: Health Promotion, 315
Knowledge: Health Resources, 316
Knowledge: Healthy Diet, 316
Knowledge: Healthy Lifestyle, 317
Knowledge: Heart Failure Management, 319
Knowledge: Hypertension Management, 320
Knowledge: Infant Care, 322
Knowledge: Infection Management, 323
Knowledge: Inflammatory Bowel Disease
   Management, 324
Knowledge: Kidney Disease Management, 325
Knowledge: Labor & Delivery, 326

Knowledge: Lipid Disorder Management, 327
Knowledge: Medication, 328
Knowledge: Multiple Sclerosis Management, 329
Knowledge: Osteoporosis Management, 330
Knowledge: Ostomy Care, 331
Knowledge: Pain Management, 331
Knowledge: Parenting, 333
Knowledge: Peripheral Artery Disease Management, 334
Knowledge: Personal Safety, 335
Knowledge: Pneumonia Management, 336
Knowledge: Postpartum Maternal Health, 337
Knowledge: Preconception Maternal Health, 338
Knowledge: Pregnancy, 338
Knowledge: Pregnancy & Postpartum Sexual
   Functioning, 340
Knowledge: Prescribed Activity, 341
Knowledge: Prescribed Diet, 342
Knowledge: Preterm Infant Care, 343
Knowledge: Sexual Functioning, 344
Knowledge: Stress Management, 344
Knowledge: Stroke Management, 345
Knowledge: Stroke Prevention, 347
Knowledge: Substance Use Control, 348
Knowledge: Thrombus Prevention, 349
Knowledge: Time Management, 350
Knowledge: Treatment Procedure, 350
Knowledge: Treatment Regimen, 351
Knowledge: Weight Management, 352
Leisure Participation, 353
Lifestyle Balance, 354
Liver Function, 355
Loneliness Severity, 356
Maternal Status: Antepartum, 357
Maternal Status: Intrapartum, 358
Maternal Status: Postpartum, 359
Mechanical Ventilation Response: Adult, 360
Mechanical Ventilation Weaning Response: Adult, 361
Medication Response, 363
Memory, 364
Metabolic Acidosis Severity, 364
Metabolic Alkalosis Severity, 365
Mobility, 366
Mood Equilibrium, 367
Motivation, 368
Mutilation Self-Restraint, 369
Nausea & Vomiting Control, 371
Nausea & Vomiting: Disruptive Effects, 372
Nausea & Vomiting Severity, 373
Neglect Cessation, 374
Neglect Recovery, 374
Neurological Status, 376
Neurological Status: Autonomic, 377
Neurological Status: Central Motor Control, 378

Neurological Status: Consciousness, 378
Neurological Status: Cranial Sensory/Motor Function, 379
Neurological Status: Peripheral, 380
Neurological Status: Spinal Sensory/Motor Function, 382
Newborn Adaptation, 383
Nutritional Status, 384
Nutritional Status: Biochemical Measures, 384
Nutritional Status: Energy, 385
Nutritional Status: Food & Fluid Intake, 386
Nutritional Status: Nutrient Intake, 386
Oral Health, 387
Ostomy Self-Care, 388
Pain: Adverse Psychological Response, 389
Pain Control, 390
Pain: Disruptive Effects, 391
Pain Level, 392
Parent-Infant Attachment, 393
Parenting Performance, 394
Parenting Performance: Adolescent, 395
Parenting Performance: Adolescent Physical Safety, 397
Parenting Performance: Early/Middle Childhood
    Physical Safety, 398
Parenting Performance: Infant, 399
Parenting Performance: Infant/Toddler Physical Safety, 400
Parenting Performance: Middle Childhood, 402
Parenting Performance: Preschooler, 403
Parenting Performance: Psychosocial Safety, 405
Parenting Performance: Toddler, 406
Participation in Health Care Decisions, 407
Perimenopause Symptom Severity, 408
Peripheral Artery Disease Severity, 408
Personal Autonomy, 409
Personal Health Screening Behavior, 410
Personal Health Status, 411
Personal Resiliency, 413
Personal Safety Behavior, 414
Personal Time Management, 415
Personal Well-Being, 416
Physical Aging, 417
Physical Fitness, 418
Physical Injury Severity, 418
Physical Maturation: Female, 419
Physical Maturation: Male, 420
Play Participation, 420
Postpartum Maternal Health Behavior, 421
Post-Procedure Recovery, 422
Premenstrual Syndrome (PMS) Severity, 423
Prenatal Health Behavior, 424
Pre-Procedure Readiness, 425
Preterm Infant Organization, 426
Psychomotor Energy, 427
Psychosocial Adjustment: Life Change, 427
Quality of Life, 429

Relocation Adaptation, 430
Respiratory Status, 431
Respiratory Status: Airway Patency, 432
Respiratory Status: Gas Exchange, 433
Respiratory Status: Ventilation, 434
Rest, 435
Risk Control, 435
Risk Control: Alcohol Use, 436
Risk Control: Cancer, 438
Risk Control: Cardiovascular Disease, 439
Risk Control: Drug Use, 440
Risk Control: Dry Eye, 441
Risk Control: Hearing Impairment, 442
Risk Control: Hypertension, 443
Risk Control: Hyperthermia, 444
Risk Control: Hypotension, 445
Risk Control: Hypothermia, 446
Risk Control: Infectious Process, 447
Risk Control: Lipid Disorder, 448
Risk Control: Osteoporosis, 448
Risk Control: Sexually Transmitted
    Diseases (STD), 450
Risk Control: Stroke, 451
Risk Control: Sun Exposure, 452
Risk Control: Thrombus, 453
Risk Control: Tobacco Use, 454
Risk Control: Unintended Pregnancy, 455
Risk Control: Visual Impairment, 456
Risk Detection, 457
Role Performance, 458
Safe Health Care Environment, 459
Safe Home Environment, 460
Safe Wandering, 461
Seizure Self-Control, 462
Self-Awareness, 463
Self-Care Status, 464
Self-Care: Activities of Daily Living (ADL), 465
Self-Care: Bathing, 465
Self-Care: Dressing, 466
Self-Care: Eating, 467
Self-Care: Hygiene, 468
Self-Care: Instrumental Activities of Daily Living
    (IADL), 469
Self-Care: Non-Parenteral Medication, 470
Self-Care: Oral Hygiene, 471
Self-Care: Parenteral Medication, 471
Self-Care: Toileting, 472
Self-Direction of Care, 473
Self-Esteem, 474
Self-Management: Acute Illness, 475
Self-Management: Anticoagulation Therapy, 476
Self-Management: Asthma, 477
Self-Management: Cardiac Disease, 479

Self-Management: Chronic Disease, 481
Self-Management: Chronic Obstructive Pulmonary Disease, 483
Self-Management: Coronary Artery Disease, 484
Self-Management: Diabetes, 486
Self-Management: Dysrhythmia, 488
Self-Management: Heart Failure, 489
Self-Management: Hypertension, 491
Self-Management: Kidney Disease, 493
Self-Management: Lipid Disorder, 494
Self-Management: Multiple Sclerosis, 496
Self-Management: Osteoporosis, 497
Self-Management: Peripheral Artery Disease, 498
Sensory Function, 500
Sensory Function: Hearing, 500
Sensory Function: Proprioception, 501
Sensory Function: Tactile, 502
Sensory Function: Taste & Smell, 503
Sensory Function: Vision, 503
Sexual Functioning, 504
Sexual Identity, 506
Shock Severity: Anaphylactic, 507
Shock Severity: Cardiogenic, 508
Shock Severity: Hypovolemic, 509
Shock Severity: Neurogenic, 510
Shock Severity: Septic, 510
Skeletal Function, 511
Sleep, 512
Smoking Cessation Behavior, 513
Social Anxiety Level, 515
Social Interaction Skills, 516
Social Involvement, 517
Social Support, 518
Spiritual Health, 519
Stress Level, 520
Student Health Status, 521
Substance Addiction Consequences, 522
Substance Withdrawal Severity, 523
Suffering Severity, 524
Suicide Self-Restraint, 525
Surgical Recovery: Convalescence, 526
Surgical Recovery: Immediate Post-Operative, 528
Swallowing Status, 529
Swallowing Status: Esophageal Phase, 530
Swallowing Status: Oral Phase, 531
Swallowing Status: Pharyngeal Phase, 532
Symptom Control, 533
Symptom Severity, 534
Systemic Toxin Clearance: Dialysis, 535
Thermoregulation, 536
Thermoregulation: Newborn, 537
Tissue Integrity: Skin & Mucous Membranes, 538

Tissue Perfusion, 539
Tissue Perfusion: Abdominal Organs, 540
Tissue Perfusion: Cardiac, 541
Tissue Perfusion: Cellular, 542
Tissue Perfusion: Cerebral, 543
Tissue Perfusion: Peripheral, 544
Tissue Perfusion: Pulmonary, 545
Transfer Performance, 546
Urinary Continence, 547
Urinary Elimination, 548
Vision Compensation Behavior, 549
Vital Signs, 550
Weight: Body Mass, 551
Weight Gain Behavior, 552
Weight Loss Behavior, 553
Weight Maintenance Behavior, 555
Will to Live, 556
Wound Healing: Primary Intention, 557
Wound Healing: Secondary Intention, 558

PART FOUR NOC Linkages: Health Patterns and NANDA International, 561

NOC Linkages—Health Patterns, 562
Nursing Outcomes Classification (NOC) Organized by the Eleven Health Patterns, 563
NOC Linkages—NANDA International Diagnoses, 571
Actual Nursing Diagnoses, 572
Activity Intolerance, 572
Activity Planning, Ineffective, 572
Airway Clearance, Ineffective, 573
Anxiety, 573
Autonomic Dysreflexia, 574
Body Image, Disturbed, 575
Bowel Incontinence, 575
Breast Milk, Insufficient, 576
Breastfeeding, Ineffective, 576
Breastfeeding, Interrupted, 577
Breathing Pattern, Ineffective, 577
Cardiac Output, Decreased, 578
Caregiver Role Strain, 578
Childbearing Process, Ineffective, 579
Comfort, Impaired, 580
Communication, Impaired Verbal, 580
Community Coping, Ineffective, 581
Community Health, Deficient, 581
Confusion, Acute, 582
Confusion, Chronic, 582
Constipation, 583
Constipation, Perceived, 583
Contamination, 584

Coping, Defensive, 584
Coping, Ineffective, 585
Death Anxiety, 586
Decisional Conflict, 586
Denial, Ineffective, 587
Dentition, Impaired, 587
Diarrhea, 588
Diversional Activity, Deficient, 588
Energy Field, Disturbed, 589
Environmental Interpretation Syndrome, Impaired, 589
Failure to Thrive, Adult, 590
Family Coping, Compromised, 590
Family Coping, Disabled, 591
Family Processes, Dysfunctional, 592
Family Processes, Interrupted, 593
Family Therapeutic Regimen Management,
    Ineffective, 593
Fatigue, 594
Fear, 594
Fluid Volume, Deficient, 595
Fluid Volume, Excess, 595
Gas Exchange, Impaired, 596
Gastrointestinal Motility, Dysfunctional, 596
Grieving, 597
Grieving, Complicated, 597
Growth and Development, Delayed, 598
Health Behavior, Risk-Prone, 599
Health Maintenance, Ineffective, 600
Home Maintenance, Impaired, 601
Hopelessness, 601
Hyperthermia, 602
Hypothermia, 602
Impulse Control, Ineffective, 603
Infant Behavior, Disorganized, 603
Infant Feeding Pattern, Ineffective, 604
Insomnia, 604
Intracranial Adaptive Capacity, Decreased, 605
Knowledge, Deficient, 606
Latex Allergy Response, 607
Lifestyle, Sedentary, 607
Memory, Impaired, 608
Mobility: Bed, Impaired, 608
Mobility: Physical, Impaired, 609
Mobility: Wheelchair, Impaired, 609
Moral Distress, 610
Nausea, 611
Neonatal Jaundice, 611
Noncompliance, 611
Nutrition: Imbalanced, Less than Body
    Requirements, 613
Nutrition: Imbalanced, More than Body
    Requirements, 613
Oral Mucous Membrane, Impaired, 614

Pain, Acute, 615
Pain, Chronic, 615
Parental Role Conflict, 616
Parenting, Impaired, 617
Personal Identity, Disturbed, 618
Post-Trauma Syndrome, 618
Powerlessness, 619
Protection, Ineffective, 620
Rape-Trauma Syndrome, 621
Relationship, Ineffective, 621
Religiosity, Impaired, 622
Relocation Stress Syndrome, 623
Resilience, Impaired Individual, 623
Role Performance, Ineffective, 624
Self-Care Deficit: Bathing, 625
Self-Care Deficit: Dressing, 625
Self-Care Deficit: Feeding, 626
Self-Care Deficit: Toileting, 626
Self-Esteem: Chronic Low, 627
Self-Esteem: Situational Low, 627
Self-Health Management, Ineffective, 628
Self-Mutilation, 629
Self-Neglect, 629
Sexual Dysfunction, 630
Sexuality Pattern, Ineffective, 630
Skin Integrity, Impaired, 631
Sleep Deprivation, 631
Sleep Pattern, Disturbed, 632
Social Interaction, Impaired, 632
Social Isolation, 633
Sorrow: Chronic, 633
Spiritual Distress, 634
Stress Overload, 634
Surgical Recovery, Delayed, 635
Swallowing, Impaired, 635
Thermoregulation, Ineffective, 636
Tissue Integrity, Impaired, 636
Tissue Perfusion: Peripheral, Ineffective, 637
Transfer Ability, Impaired, 637
Unilateral Neglect, 638
Urinary Elimination, Impaired, 638
Urinary Incontinence: Functional, 639
Urinary Incontinence: Overflow, 639
Urinary Incontinence: Reflex, 639
Urinary Incontinence: Stress, 640
Urinary Incontinence: Urge, 640
Urinary Retention, 640
Ventilation, Impaired Spontaneous, 641
Ventilatory Weaning Response, Dysfunctional, 641
Walking, Impaired, 642
Wandering, 642
Risk Nursing Diagnoses, 643
Activity Intolerance, Risk for, 643

Activity Planning, Risk for Ineffective, 643

Adverse Reaction to Iodinated Contrast Media, Risk for, 644

Allergy Response, Risk for, 644

Aspiration, Risk for, 644

Attachment, Risk for Impaired, 645

Autonomic Dysreflexia, Risk for, 645

Bleeding, Risk for, 646

Blood Glucose Level, Risk for Unstable, 646

Body Temperature, Risk for Imbalanced, 647

Caregiver Role Strain, Risk for, 648

Childbearing Process, Risk for Ineffective, 649

Confusion, Risk for Acute, 649

Constipation, Risk for, 650

Contamination, Risk for, 650

Development, Risk for Delayed, 651

Disuse Syndrome, Risk for, 652

Dry Eye, Risk for, 652

Electrolyte, Risk for Imbalance, 653

Falls, Risk for, 654

Fluid Volume, Risk for Deficient, 655

Fluid Volume, Risk for Imbalanced, 655

Gastrointestinal Motility, Risk for Dysfunctional, 656

Gastrointestinal Perfusion, Risk for Ineffective, 656

Grieving, Complicated, Risk for, 657

Growth, Risk for Disproportionate, 657

Human Dignity, Risk for Compromised, 658

Infant Behavior, Risk for Disorganized, 659

Infection, Risk for, 659

Injury, Risk for, 660

Latex Allergy Response, Risk for, 661

Liver Function, Risk for Impaired, 661

Loneliness, Risk for, 661

Maternal-Fetal Dyad, Risk for Disturbed, 662

Neonatal Jaundice, Risk for, 663

Nutrition: Imbalanced, Risk for More than Body Requirements, 663

Parenting, Risk for Impaired, 664

Perioperative Positioning Injury, Risk for, 665

Peripheral Neurovascular Dysfunction, Risk for, 665

Personal Identity, Risk for Disturbed, 666

Poisoning, Risk for, 666

Post-Trauma Syndrome, Risk for, 667

Powerlessness, Risk for, 667

Relationship, Risk for Ineffective, 668

Religiosity, Risk for Impaired, 668

Relocation Stress Syndrome, Risk for, 669

Renal Perfusion, Risk for Ineffective, 669

Resilience, Risk for Compromised, 670

Self-Esteem: Chronic Low, Risk for, 671

Self-Esteem: Situational Low, Risk for, 671

Self-Mutilation, Risk for, 672

Shock, Risk for, 672

Skin Integrity, Risk for Impaired, 673

Spiritual Distress, Risk for, 673

Sudden Infant Death Syndrome, Risk for, 674

Suffocation, Risk for, 674

Suicide, Risk for, 675

Thermal Injury, Risk for, 676

Tissue Perfusion: Cardiac, Risk for Decreased, 676

Tissue Perfusion: Cerebral, Risk for Ineffective, 677

Tissue Perfusion: Peripheral, Risk for Ineffective, 677

Trauma, Risk for, 678

Urinary Incontinence: Urge, Risk for, 679

Vascular Trauma, Risk for, 680

Violence: Other-Directed, Risk for, 680

Violence: Self-Directed, Risk for, 681

Health-Promotion Nursing Diagnoses, 682

Breastfeeding, Readiness for Enhanced, 682

Childbearing Process, Readiness for Enhanced, 683

Comfort, Readiness for Enhanced, 683

Communication, Readiness for Enhanced, 684

Community Coping, Readiness for Enhanced, 684

Coping, Readiness for Enhanced, 684

Decision-Making, Readiness for Enhanced, 685

Family Coping, Readiness for Enhanced, 686

Family Processes, Readiness for Enhanced, 686

Fluid Balance, Readiness for Enhanced, 686

Hope, Readiness for Enhanced, 687

Immunization Status, Readiness for Enhanced, 688

Infant Behavior, Organized, Readiness for Enhanced, 688

Knowledge, Readiness for Enhanced, 689

Nutrition, Readiness for Enhanced, 691

Parenting, Readiness for Enhanced, 692

Power, Readiness for Enhanced, 692

Relationship, Readiness for Enhanced, 693

Religiosity, Readiness for Enhanced, 693

Resilience, Readiness for Enhanced, 694

Self-Care, Readiness for Enhanced, 695

Self-Concept, Readiness for Enhanced, 696

Self-Health Management, Readiness for Enhanced, 696

Sleep, Readiness for Enhanced, 697

Spiritual Well-Being, Readiness for Enhanced, 697

Urinary Elimination, Readiness for Enhanced, 698

PART FIVE   Core Outcomes for Nursing Specialties, 699

Core Outcomes for Nursing Specialities, 700

Efforts to Identify Core Outcomes, 700

Air & Surface Transport, 701

Ambulatory Care, 701

Anesthesia, 702

Cardiac Rehabilitation, 702

Chemical Dependency, 703

Community Health, 703
Critical Care, 704
Dermatology, 705
Diabetes, 705
Emergency Care, 705
Gastroenterology, 706
Genetics, 706
Gerontology, 707
HIV/AIDS, 707
Home Healthcare, 708
Hospice & Palliative Care, 709
Infection Control & Epidemiological, 710
Intravenous Therapy, 711
Medical-Surgical, 711
Neonatology, 712
Nephrology, 713
Neuroscience, 713
Nurse Practitioner, 714
Occupational Health, 715
Oncology, 716
Operating Room, 717
Ophthalmology, 717
Orthopedics, 718
Otorhinolaryngology & Head-Neck, 718
Pain Management, 719
Parish Nursing, 719
Pediatrics, 720
Pediatric Oncology, 721

Perianesthesia, 722
Perioperative Care, 722
Psychiatric–Mental Health, 723
Plastic Surgery, 724
Radiology, 724
Rehabilitation, 725
School Health, 725
Spinal Cord Injury, 726
Transplant, 726
Urology, 727
Vascular, 728
Women's Health, Obstetrics, & Neonatology, 728

PART SIX Appendixes, 731

Appendix A Outcomes: New, Revised, and Retired Since the Fourth Edition, 732

Appendix B Guidelines for Submission of a New or Revised Outcome, 735

Appendix C Previous Editions and Translations, 736

Index, 737

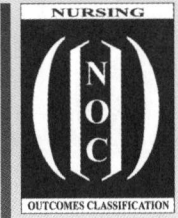

PART ONE

Overview and Use of Nursing Outcomes Classification (NOC)

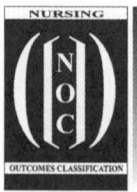

CHAPTER ONE

The Current Classification

Identifying patient outcomes responsive to nursing care is critical work as nurses face the challenge of implementing electronic health records and continue to focus on cost, safety, and effectiveness of care in the changing health care system. Evidence-based practice is an essential requirement for our professional practice. Efforts by nurses to measure outcomes and capture changes in the status of patients over time provide a way to improve the quality of patient care and add to the knowledge base of nursing. In the past nursing has been dependent on the use of interdisciplinary outcomes developed primarily for physician practice. Consensus among nurses on standardized nursing-sensitive patient outcomes allows them to study the effects of nursing interventions over time and across care settings. This is a very important component of measuring outcomes since patients move quickly across a variety of care settings and frequently spend the majority of time convalescing at home. Measurement of outcomes validates whether patients are positively responding to nursing interventions and helps determine if changes in care are needed. The use of standardized outcomes provides the data needed to (1) elucidate nursing knowledge, (2) advance theory development, (3) determine the effectiveness of nursing care, and (4) showcase the contributions of nursing to patients, families, and communities. Nurses have documented the outcomes of their interventions for decades, but the lack of a common language and associated outcome measures has impeded data aggregation, analysis, and synthesis of information focused on the effects of nursing interventions on patient outcomes.

The Nursing Outcomes Classification (NOC) is complementary to the NANDA International (NANDA-I)[2] and the Nursing Interventions Classification (NIC).[1] The NOC provides language for the outcome identification and evaluation steps of the nursing process and the content for the outcomes element of the Nursing Minimum Data Set (NMDS).[8] NOC can also be used as an important component of the Outcome-Present State-Test Model (OPT) for clinical reasoning developed by Pesut and Herman.[6] In addition, the documentation of outcomes has been encouraged by the work of NANDA-I,[2,5] the recommendations of the NMDS,[7,8] the Nursing Intervention Classification work,[1,5] the development of computerized information systems in health care and the associated large uniform databases, and the emphasis on demonstrating health care effectiveness. The definition and classification of clinically useful nursing-sensitive patient outcomes, however, was not accomplished until the first edition of NOC was published in 1997. Further, there are few conceptual frameworks of nursing-sensitive patient outcomes, and existing ones tend to describe broad categories of outcomes that are not validated. The NOC is especially significant because standardized languages for computerized nursing diagnoses, interventions, and outcomes are needed for the study of linkages among these patient phenomena using actual patient data. Further, the standardized languages represent concepts that describe the basic phenomena for which the nursing discipline is accountable and, together with the linkages among the concepts, represent an important stage of nursing theory development.

THE NURSING OUTCOMES CLASSIFICATION (NOC): WHAT IS IT?

This book presents standardized terminology for nursing-sensitive outcomes for use by nurses across specialties and practice settings to capture changes in patient status after intervention. Each outcome represents a concept that can be used to measure the state of a patient, caregiver, family, or community before and after intervention. In some clinical situations outcomes from a variety of these perspectives may be used for a patient situation. The outcomes have been developed for use by nurses, but other disciplines may find them helpful for evaluating the effectiveness of the interventions they provide independently or in collaboration with nurses. Each outcome has a definition, a measurement scale(s), a list of associated indicators for the concept, and supporting references. The outcomes are organized in a taxonomy that facilitates the identification of outcomes for use in practice. The three levels of the taxonomy help nurses and others quickly identify outcomes useful for their practice. The current classification contains 490 outcomes, including 107 new outcomes developed after the publication of the fourth edition in 2008.

Definition of an Outcome

A nursing-sensitive patient outcome is an individual, family, or community state, behavior, or perception that is measured along a continuum in response to nursing intervention(s). The outcomes are variable concepts that can be measured along a continuum using a measurement scale(s). The outcomes are stated as concepts that reflect a patient, caregiver, family, or community state, behavior, or perception rather than as expected goals.

Measurement of an Outcome

A five-point Likert type scale is used with all outcomes and indicators providing an adequate number of options to demonstrate variability in the state, behavior, or perception described by the outcome. For example, the outcome *Cognition* is measured on a five-point scale from "severely compromised" to "not compromised" and *Caregiver Performance: Direct Care* is measured on a five-point scale from "not adequate" to "totally adequate." The measurement scales are standardized, so a rating of "5" is always the best possible score, and a rating of "1" is the worst possible score. Each scale provides anchors for the scores from "1" to "5." There is an option to rate an indicator as "not applicable" for the patient by selecting the NA column. This scale structure does not demand the degree of precision required for a 10-point scale format yet has been successful in capturing incremental changes for short acute care hospitalizations.

By measuring the outcome prior to intervention, the nurse establishes a baseline score on the selected outcome and can then rate the outcome after the intervention is provided. This allows nurses to follow changes in patient status or maintenance of outcome states over time and across settings. For example, if a patient is rated a "2" prior to intervention and a "4" after intervention, the change score is +2. The true outcome is the change seen in the outcome rating after nursing interventions. This change score can be positive (the outcome rating increased), negative (the outcome rating decreased), or there can be no change (the outcome rating stayed the same). In some cases a change score of zero is the goal. This may be the case in situations where the nurse does not expect the patient to improve but wants to maintain the current status of the patient and provides interventions to accomplish this. This is a common situation when working with elderly or terminally ill patients.

Use of a Reference Person for Comparison

When measuring outcomes we advocate the use of a "reference person" for comparison to the patient the nurse is caring for. The reference person is defined as a *healthy* person of the same age and gender. For example, the nurse compares a 60-year-old male patient to a *healthy* 60-year-old male, implying that the nurse uses personal experience with other patients in this age group for the comparison. This is an important step in ensuring that the measurement of outcomes is comparable across populations. When the patient has a chronic condition, such as arthritis, and the nurse is trying to improve the patient's mobility, the comparison person is *not* a 60-year-old male with arthritis but a healthy male of the same age. This comparison maintains the rating of "5" on the measurement scales as the healthy rating. The "5" rating should not be undermined by conditions that reflect the normal best state for the population of patients the

nurse works with in a specialty practice. This is especially true for populations of patients with serious conditions, such as renal failure or congestive heart failure, so the highest rating that a patient with a chronic condition may be able to achieve is a "3." Since nursing is working toward benchmarking outcomes of care, this is an important requirement for measuring patient outcomes.

Level of Abstraction of NOC Outcomes

Outcomes in the classification are at a higher level of abstraction than a typical goal statement written by a nurse. The indicators used to determine patient condition in relation to an outcome represent the more specific outcomes often reflected in goal statements. For example, a few of the indicators used in the outcome *Cognition* are "immediate memory," "remote memory," "communication clear for age," and "information processing." While these may serve as intermediate outcomes or indicators of cognition, they do not measure the multidimensional aspects of the concept cognition when used alone. The use of midlevel concepts like cognition facilitates the use of outcomes in computerized systems and the aggregation of data for effectiveness research and policy formulation. The midlevel concept also may be useful in efficacy research. For example, a researcher evaluating an intervention to improve memory can use outcome indicators to determine the effects of the intervention on memory and on other factors that determine cognition. Whereas the outcomes currently do not provide tested measures for assessing the effects of an intervention on memory, they do suggest other factors to consider and can be used in conjunction with tested measures to arrive at a determination of how improvement of memory influences cognition. Further, if outcome measurement scales are found to be psychometrically sound, there is potential for the use of outcomes to measure impact variables in efficacy research. Development and testing of outcome measures that have practical use in clinical settings, and are valid for use in research, have important implications for documenting the nursing profession's contributions to health care and providing data to influence health care policy. These advantages also apply for family and community level outcomes.

The outcomes, while representative of broad, midlevel concepts, are at varied levels of abstraction. For example, *Risk Control* is a broad outcome defined as "personal actions to understand, prevent, eliminate, or reduce modifiable health threats" that can be used with any nursing intervention directed at assisting patients to identify and control risks; however, more specific outcomes for risks of common concern to nurses such as *Risk Control: Alcohol Use* and *Risk Control: Drug Use* are found in the classification. As additional outcomes are developed and refined, we expect that greater homogeneity of the level of abstraction among outcomes will evolve or that multiple levels of abstraction may be seen as useful. Decisions regarding the inclusion of broad vs. specific outcomes, however, will depend upon what is useful to nurses. Our experience to date is that nurses in different settings may need different levels of abstraction based on their specialty and health care setting. The best example of this is that nurses working in intensive-care units prefer more specific outcomes for use in their practice. In the taxonomic structure, level of abstraction also is reflected in the domain, class, and outcome structure.

The classification structure uses colons to separate broad from specific outcome terms. As much as possible, the first term in the outcome reflects the word that practitioners might select when looking for the outcome. For example, recovery from abuse is found under the broad category *Abuse Recovery* but is further specified by *Abuse Recovery: Emotional*, *Abuse Recovery: Financial*, *Abuse Recovery: Physical*, and *Abuse Recovery: Sexual*. This pattern of creating more global outcomes, in addition to more specific outcomes using colons, has been helpful in the development of this classification. Nurses can choose between the specific outcomes or use the more global outcome that contains the more specific content as indicators. This may result in nurses' selecting fewer outcomes for some patients.

Sensitivity of the Outcomes

Each concept represents a patient, caregiver, family, or community state that is sensitive in varying degrees to nursing interventions. Originally, the research team assessed sensitivity to nursing interventions by (1) selecting the concepts from outcomes in nursing literature and clinical information systems, (2) determining that the outcomes have been used to measure the effects of nursing interventions, and (3) surveying expert nurses about the importance of the outcomes as measures of the effects of nursing interventions. The ultimate test of sensitivity will be the widespread selection and use of outcomes in practice and research with careful analyses that isolate the effects of interventions on the outcomes. Because the outcomes have been developed for use in all settings where nurses provide care, some of the outcome indicators may be more applicable in one setting than another. For example, blood values and other diagnostic results used as indicators may be pertinent in an intensive or acute care setting, but they may be less useful in a home or nursing home setting. When in doubt we have included indicators that we believe are still used in practice globally, such as urine testing for diabetes, even though the standard in the United States has been focused on blood samples. These indicators allow outcomes in this classification to have value for nurses in other countries. Community-level outcomes are most likely useful in community health settings or in the evaluation of community actions. This continues to be the least-developed area of the classification although six additional community-focused outcomes are included in the fifth edition.

Use by Other Disciplines

Many of the nursing-sensitive outcomes developed to date are not specific to just the nursing profession; thus, they could be used to evaluate the care provided by other health care disciplines since the focus is on the patient. For example, physical therapists may greatly influence a patient's overall outcome rating for *Mobility* and *Activity Tolerance.* In this situation these outcomes measure the collaborative results of nursing care and physical therapy and would be an example of how the NOC can increase opportunities for collaboration. While the outcomes may be used in other disciplines, the indicators used to assess patient condition in relation to the outcome may vary from discipline to discipline. For example, physical therapists may use indicators that measure progress with the use of equipment not routinely used by nursing. In this case additional indicators may be added to the outcome by care providers to address these specific needs for measuring an outcome.

THE NURSING OUTCOMES CLASSIFICATION: WHAT IT IS NOT

The previous section highlighted key points about the NOC. This section highlights what it is not: complete, prescriptive, focused on nursing diagnoses, or focused on nursing assessments.

The Classification Is Not Complete

Although the NOC contains outcomes frequently used by nurses, at this stage of development the classification does not include all outcomes that might be important for nursing. This edition includes 107 new outcomes available for use by nurses and other care providers. As nurses review the outcomes and use them in practice and research, the need for additional outcomes will be identified, and published outcomes may require modification. Because the classification of outcomes must be modified to reflect changes in nursing practice and health care delivery, the classification will be continually evolving. The testing of the outcomes in clinical sites resulted in many revisions to the third edition based on feedback from nurses in practice. Changes in the fourth edition of the classification were made to better position the classification for use in electronic health records to ensure that the contributions of nurses can be accurately represented in the future. The fifth edition refined the taxonomy and added a class. Efforts of this type enhance the classification, build nursing knowledge, and improve the care nurses provide to patients, families and communities.

The outcomes published in this volume do not include all outcomes for individuals, families, and communities for which nurses provide interventions. Family and community level outcomes are included in this edition, building on previous work, but more outcomes are needed in these areas. However, many individual-level outcomes can be aggregated to characterize families, communities, and populations (e.g., a nursing or medical diagnosis, a diagnostic related group [DRG], the unit or geographic location in which care is provided, or the nurse providing the care). Additional family and community level outcomes will be developed to assess the effectiveness of nursing interventions aimed at these units of analysis. It is possible that some of the individual-level outcomes can be modified for use with aggregates, and feedback about such modifications from users will be extremely helpful for future editions. The outcome classification also does not contain outcomes of organizational performance or the cost of health care. These outcomes are important in effectiveness research but do not reflect the effects of interventions on a patient. Rather, organizational and cost outcomes are more often useful for evaluating the effectiveness of nursing management or health services delivery interventions.

NOC Outcomes Are Not Prescriptive

NOC outcomes are not goals for individual patients or patient populations although they can be translated into goals by identifying the desired state on the measurement scale and setting a target rating for the patient. Individual-level outcomes are not prescribed for a particular nursing diagnosis or nursing intervention. They can be selected for a diagnosis or intervention based on the clinical judgment of the nurse responsible for the care of an individual patient or based on the collective judgment of the health care providers responsible for developing a critical path or standardized care plan for a patient population. Possible linkages to NANDA-I nursing diagnoses are suggested in this book and are found in Part Four. These linkages assist nurses to select outcomes and to conduct research for validation of suggested linkages. Additional linkages among diagnoses, interventions, and outcomes can be found in other publications.[3,4] NOC outcomes linked to some frequent, high-cost medical conditions are available in the book focused on linkages published in 2012.[3]

NOC Outcomes Are Not Nursing Diagnoses

Many of the outcomes rate the same states addressed by nursing diagnoses. A diagnosis identifies a state that is altered, has the potential to be altered, or has the potential to be improved, whereas an outcome assesses the actual state at a given point in time using a five-point measurement scale. Table 1-1 illustrates some of the differences in diagnostic and outcome language using NANDA-I diagnoses and NOC outcomes.

The comparisons in Table 1-1 illustrate the difference between the language used to identify a state for which a diagnosis is made and the state that is measured as an outcome. They also illustrate that some outcomes are more specific than a related diagnosis (e.g., knowledge outcomes) while some diagnoses are more specific than the related

Table 1-1	COMPARISONS OF NANDA-I DIAGNOSES AND NOC OUTCOMES
NANDA-I Diagnosis	**NOC Outcome**
Impaired Physical Mobility	Mobility
Hopelessness	Hope
Deficient Knowledge	Knowledge: Disease Process Knowledge: Medication Knowledge: Diabetes Management Knowledge: Health Behavior Knowledge: Treatment Regimen
Constipation	Bowel Continence
Diarrhea	Bowel Elimination
Stress Urinary Incontinence	Urinary Elimination
Reflex Urinary Incontinence	Urinary Continence Tissue Integrity: Skin & Mucous Membranes
Interrupted Family Processes	Family Functioning Family Coping Family Social Climate
Comfort, Readiness for Enhanced	Comfort Status Comfort Status: Environment Comfort Status: Physical Comfort Status: Psychospiritual Comfort Status: Sociocultural Discomfort Level

outcome (e.g., diagnosis of constipation). There also are some global outcomes for which similar language is not used in the NANDA-I diagnoses; however, these outcomes might be selected for a number of the diagnoses.

Outcomes Are Not Assessments

Outcomes are not focused on the assessment phase of the nursing process although indicators may represent patient states, behaviors, or perceptions evaluated during a patient assessment. No outcome represents the total range of individual, family, or community states that comprise a comprehensive assessment. An assessment provides the database for clinical reasoning and decisions, including the selection of nursing diagnoses, outcomes, and interventions. Although the defining assessment data for a diagnosis should correspond with outcome indicators that refer to the same patient state, the validation of nursing diagnoses and nursing-sensitive patient outcomes needed to achieve complete correspondence has not yet been done. NOC outcomes can be used as focused assessment tools when determining the baseline rating. When an outcome is selected, the individual, family, or community state, behavior, or perception needs to be evaluated and rated on the measurement scale to provide a baseline measure for comparison with post-intervention measures. It is the baseline measure of a variable outcome state that should correspond to the diagnosis.

FREQUENTLY ASKED QUESTIONS

Initial work on the NOC identified conceptual questions that have formed the foundation on which this work is built. The original research team reviewed the literature on patient outcomes, information systems, taxonomic classification science, effectiveness research, and relevant qualitative and quantitative methods to address these issues. Team members reviewed multiple sources of patient outcomes used by nurses (textbooks, nursing information systems, critical pathways and care plans, outcome studies, standards of practice, conceptual frameworks, and outcome classifications). As nurses use standardized outcomes rather than goals in their practices, many of these initial issues and other key questions need to be addressed. The most frequently asked questions about the classification are included here, and each question is briefly addressed.

Who Is the Patient?

Patient outcomes focus on the recipient of care, but the traditional use of the term *patient* is too limiting. *Patient* traditionally is defined as an individual recipient of care; however, family caregivers and significant others often are involved integrally with patients and also are recipients of nursing care. The term *patient* is used in many of the outcomes even though the care recipient may be called *client* or *resident* in some settings. The first two editions used the term patient consistently. When the satisfaction outcomes were added to the third edition, the term *patient satisfaction* as the label name was considered by the research team to be too limiting, so the term *client satisfaction* is used to describe these outcomes. This issue has continued in nursing with some health care organizations wanting to use the term *consumer* for their patients. Regardless of what they are called, individuals are the focus of most of the outcomes in this classification. Data ordinarily are collected on individuals and aggregated to characterize other units of analysis (e.g., patient groups, organizations, communities), but some outcomes require data to be collected at a group level. The research team decided to use individuals as the focal unit for the initial development of the NOC, with family caregivers included to assess the impact of nursing on the family members as individuals. The development and testing of outcomes for other units, such as family and community, were included in previous editions and characterize family and community units as a whole. Additional

outcomes will be developed in these areas as the classification expands and is revised.

What Do Patient Outcomes Describe?

Like nursing diagnoses, the phenomena of concern with nursing-sensitive patient outcomes are individual patient or caregiver states or behaviors, including perceptions or subjective states. These phenomena are in contrast to nursing interventions that describe nurse behaviors.[1] The phenomena of concern for outcomes also are in contrast to nursing diagnoses, where the phenomena of concern are patient states identified because an improvement is desired. Outcomes define a patient status at a particular point in time and may indicate improvement or deterioration of the state compared to a previous evaluation of the patient. The defining data for a diagnosis typically correspond to outcomes and indicators at an undesirable point on the status continuum. Patient states that are assessed but are not the focus of nursing interventions of a patient (do not follow an intervention) are not outcomes as typically defined. Outcomes describe patient states that follow and are expected to be influenced by an intervention. A *nursing-sensitive patient outcome* is defined as an individual, family, or community state, behavior, or perception that is measured along a continuum in response to nursing intervention(s). Each outcome has an associated group of indicators that are used to determine patient status in relation to the outcome. *Nursing-sensitive patient outcome indicators* are defined as a more concrete individual, family, or community state, behavior, or perception that serves as a cue for measuring an outcome. The definitions and indicators acknowledge that nurses, family caregivers, and patients supply outcome data and that both the patient and family caregiver are the focus of outcomes. Some outcomes can be measured only by the patient, some only by the nurse, and some by the patient (or family) and the nurse or other health provider. Definitions of some common terms used in the classification are listed in Box 1-1.

At What Levels of Abstraction Should Outcomes Be Developed?

The NOC contains patient outcomes and indicators at four general levels of abstraction with measurement procedures at the empirical level (Table 1-2). At the highest levels outcome categories and classes were derived from the results of hierarchical clustering and qualitative strategies used in the development of the taxonomy. The least abstract level of the taxonomy contains indicator statements for each outcome label. Outcomes are at middle levels of abstraction, and in some instances indicators for more abstract, global outcomes are developed as more specific, less abstract outcomes. For example, an indicator for the outcome *Mobility* is "joint movement" while "flexion 45 degrees" is an indicator for the outcome *Joint Movement: Neck*. The empirical

Box 1-1

Selected Terms and Definitions

Ability
Power or capacity to perform actions.
Adequate
Sufficient in quantity or quality to meet a need or function.
Adherence
To hold fast to a selected action to improve health.
Adolescence
The period of time in a child's life from 12 years through 17 years.
Appropriate
Suitable to meet requirements, demands, or needs.
Avoid
Withdrawing from something; to keep away from.
Behavior
The observable or reported response of an individual, family, or community to its environment.
Caregiver
A family member, significant other, friend, or other person who cares for or acts on behalf of the patient.
Care Recipient
The person, such as patient, caregiver (specify), parent (specify), family (specify),or community (specify), receiving services from a professional.
Change in Rating Score
The difference between a baseline rating of the outcome and the post-intervention rating(s) of the outcome. This change score can be positive (the outcome rating increased) or negative (the outcome rating decreased) or there can be no change (the outcome rating stayed the same).
This change in rating score represents the outcome achieved following a health care intervention(s).
Child
Overall term for childhood from one year through 17 years old.
Childcare Provider
Family caregiver or an individual who is paid to provide childcare.
Community
An interactive population with relationships that emerge as members develop and use, in common, some agencies and institutions.
Compliance
To hold fast to a recommendation from a health professional.
Confidence
Belief that one can act to achieve a desired goal.
Core Outcomes
A concise set of outcomes that captures the essence of an area of specialty practice.
Data Source
Documentation of where data are obtained from, such as the patient, family member, caregiver, direct observation by health care provider, clinical record, or other sources.
Decreased
Lesser in size, degree, or amount.
Disease
A specific pathological process defined by a set of signs and symptoms that affects a body part or the whole body where the etiology, pathology, and prognosis may be known or unknown.
Early Childhood
The period of time in a child's life from one year through five years (includes Toddler and Preschool).

Effective
Producing desired health-related results.
Family
Two or more people who are related biologically, legally, or by choice that has a societal expectation to socialize, enculturate, and care for its members.
Function
Special action or physiologic property of an organ or other part of the body to perform its specific work.
Functioning
To carry out a set of actions in the expression or performance of a role.
Health
A state of physical, psychological, social, and spiritual functioning.
Health Professionals
Individuals with advanced education and licensure that are reimbursed for providing health care services.
Health Providers
Professional and assistive personnel who are reimbursed for providing health care services.
Inappropriate
Not suitable for meeting requirements, demands, or needs.
Increased
Greater in amount, degree, or size.
Infant
The term used for a baby from birth to first birthday.
Late Adulthood
Period of time in an adult's life from 65 and older.
Measure
A five-point Likert-type scale that quantifies a patient outcome or indicator status on a continuum from least-to-most desirable and provides a rating at a point in time.
Mental
Total emotional and intellectual response.
Middle Adulthood
Period of time in an adult's life from 40 years through 64 years.
Middle Childhood
The period of time in a child's life from six years through 11 years.
Newborn
The term used for a baby the first 28 days of life.
NOC Taxonomy
A systematic organization of outcomes into groups or categories based upon similarities, dissimilarities, and relationships among the outcomes. The NOC taxonomy structure has five levels: domains, classes, outcomes, indicators, and measures.
Nursing-Sensitive Patient Outcome
An individual, family, or community state, behavior, or perception that is measured along a continuum in response to a nursing intervention(s). Each outcome has an associated group of indicators that are used to determine patient status in relation to the outcome.
Obtains
To gain or attain by planned effort or action.
Outcome Indicator
A more concrete individual, family, or community state, behavior, or perception that serves as a cue for measuring an outcome.
Parent
Mother, father, or individual assuming the childrearing role.

Continued

Selected Terms and Definitions—cont'd

Perception
A conscious mental thought or an image or sensation from a sensory stimulus.
Personal Actions
Actions taken by the individual, caregiver, significant other, or family member.
Population
A collection of individuals who have one or more personal (e.g., gender, age, illness) or environmental (e.g., country, worksite) characteristics in common.
Preschool
The term used for a child from three years through five years.
Recommended
Presented as worthy of confidence, acceptance, or use.
Reference Person
A healthy person of the same age and gender used for comparison when rating an outcome or indicator.

Refrains
Keeps oneself from following a passing impulse.
Reputable
Recognized as positive by health providers or experts in the field.
Resources
Source of supply, support, or information.
Status
State of health of the focus of the outcome. This may be at the individual, family, or community level or a function of a system or state of the body.
Toddler
The term used for a child from one year through two years.
Well-Being
Extent of positive perception of one's own health status.
Young Adulthood
Period of time in adult's life from 18 years through 39 years.

Table 1-2	**LEVELS OF ABSTRACTION IN THE TAXONOMY**
Most Abstract	Nursing-Sensitive Outcome Domain
High Middle Level Abstraction	Nursing-Sensitive Outcome Classes
Middle Level Abstraction	Nursing-Sensitive Outcome
Low Level Abstraction	Nursing-Sensitive Outcome Indicators
Empirical Level	Measurement Activities for Outcomes

level includes measurement activities for each outcome and its indicators.

How Should Outcomes Be Stated?

Because outcomes and indicators are conceptualized as variable patient, caregiver, family, or community states, behaviors, or perceptions, they are given labels representing concepts that can be measured along a continuum as negative or positive states. Whenever possible the team avoids labels that describe an undesirable state; however, because of the common use of some labels or difficulty identifying an antonym, some do describe an undesirable state. Examples are *Infection Severity, Discomfort Level, Fear Level,* and *Pain Level.* These types of outcomes are used frequently by nurses to help patients validate the severity of the symptoms they experience. From the patient

viewpoint these symptoms are their perceptions of the extent to which they are experiencing the indicators present in an outcome. Conceptualization of the outcomes as variables allows measurement of negative or positive changes, as well as no change, resulting from nursing interventions. Box 1-2 summarizes the basic rules used in the development of the outcomes for this classification.

Why Are the Outcomes Not Stated as Goals?

The outcomes were developed as variable concepts for several reasons. First, NOC outcomes are variable concepts so that the response of the patient, caregiver, family, or community to nursing interventions can be documented and monitored over time and across settings and then compared. A goal statement developed for each patient does not allow for this cross comparison. Second, variable outcomes yield more information than just whether or not a goal is met. For clinical and research purposes, either/or type data provide very limited information and constrain nurses' abilities to adequately evaluate the effectiveness of their interventions. If goals are not met, it is important to know whether any progress was made or to what extent the outcome status deteriorated, if at all. Third, with the current short length of stays in acute care settings, it has become very important to be able to document even slight increases in outcome scores at discharge. Goals for short timeframes become meaningless for monitoring progress across time. NOC outcomes can be used to state a goal for a patient, family, or community, but this should be in addition to the measurement of status on the outcome at baseline and over time. Fourth, in many cases the goal of nursing care may be

Rules for Standardization of Nursing-Sensitive Outcomes

- Outcome labels should be concise (stated in five words or less).
- Outcome labels should be stated in nonevaluative terms rather than as a decreased, increased, or improved state.
- Outcome labels should use common nursing terms as much as possible.
- Outcomes should *not* describe a nurse behavior or intervention.
- Outcome labels should *not* be stated as a nursing diagnosis.
- Outcomes should describe a state, behavior, or perception that is inherently variable and can be measured and quantified.
- Outcome labels should be conceptualized and stated at a middle level of abstraction.
- Outcomes may be developed using one or two measurement scales.
- Definitions for outcomes should be defined consistent with the measurement scale.
- Wording of indicators should be standardized as much as possible for outcomes using the same measurement scale.
- Colons should be used to make broader concept labels more specific; however, the broader label is stated first, with the colon and more specific label following (e.g., Nutritional Status: Nutrient Intake, Self Care: Bathing).

Criteria for Evaluating Nursing Sensitivity

- A nursing intervention produced a positive outcome.
- A nursing intervention influenced a positive outcome.
- A nursing intervention was carried out with the intent to produce or influence the outcome.
- A nursing intervention produced improvement or maintenance of the outcome or prevented deterioration or occurrence of a negative outcome.
- The nursing intervention occurred before observation of the outcome.
- A failure to provide nursing intervention resulted in failure to achieve a positive outcome or to prevent a negative outcome.
- The interventions that produced or influenced the outcome are within nursing's scope of practice.

to maintain a patient at a particular outcome rating when an improvement in status is not possible. For example, the goal for a patient with self-care issues may be to maintain their outcome status at a "3" for the outcome *Self-Care: Bathing*. Finally, the strength of using outcomes rather than goals is that a change score can be determined after nursing care is provided. This change score is not possible with goals and is important for evaluating the effectiveness of nursing treatments and comparing outcomes for specific patient populations over time.

What Are Nursing-Sensitive Patient Outcomes?

To be useful for assessing the effectiveness of nursing, outcomes and indicators must be identified that are influenced by nursing and comprehensive enough to assess all aspects of nursing practice. The majority of patient outcomes, including those traditionally used to evaluate physician care, are not influenced by any one discipline alone. For nursing to monitor and improve its practice, however, it is important to identify the outcomes that are responsive to nursing care. The more abstract and global the outcome, the more likely its achievement will be the result of interventions from several health care disciplines. Specific disciplines will have more influence on certain intermediate outcomes than

others. For example, at different times nursing, medicine, and physical therapy have the most impact on the outcome *Mobility* although all share influence on the outcome. Specific indicators of an outcome are more likely to be sensitive to the interventions of a single discipline; therefore, it is essential to identify the indicators most sensitive to nursing interventions. This identification enables nurses to document the effects of their interventions and to be held individually and collectively accountable for care delivered to patients. A set of criteria for evaluating the evidence of nursing sensitivity or responsiveness has been developed. These criteria are listed in Box 1-3.

Are Nursing-Sensitive Patient Outcomes the Resolution of Nursing Diagnoses?

The majority of nursing-sensitive patient outcomes represent the resolution of nursing diagnoses although some outcomes are more generic and not necessarily related to specific diagnoses. Clearly, client satisfaction and the financial charges to patients that are attributable to nursing care are not diagnosis-specific and cannot be conceived as the resolution of a diagnosis. At this time it appears that the more general (abstract) the outcome, such as *Quality of Life*, the less likely it will be diagnosis-specific. Conversely, the less abstract the outcome concept, such as *Self-Care: Toileting*, the more likely it will be diagnosis-specific.

How Are the Outcomes Different from Nursing Diagnoses?

NOC outcomes describe a variable state, behavior, or perception. The outcome state at a particular time can be at any point on a negative-to-positive continuum. The outcomes can be used to measure nursing diagnoses stated as problems, risk states, or potential-for-enhancement diagnoses with the same measure. Nursing diagnoses, on the other hand, generally describe states that are in some way less positive than what is desired. Nursing diagnoses describe problems, actual or potential, that the nurse seeks to resolve through intervention. More recently nursing diagnoses focused on wellness have been developed. The relationship between these diagnoses and outcomes needs further discussion and evaluation.

When Should Patient Outcomes Be Measured?

The appropriate time to measure patient outcomes will vary because some patients respond very quickly to interventions, and others respond over a longer period. The outcomes of health promotion interventions, for example, are likely to occur over a considerable time period while the response to interventions to improve nutritional intake could be immediate. There also are outcomes such as *Transfer Performance* where the full response may take several weeks. One problem is to select a time for measurement close enough to the intervention to be assured that change is due to the intervention but far enough removed to be able to measure a change. Medicine has begun to place more emphasis on intermediate outcomes. Nurses need to be able to follow the patient across settings to evaluate the effectiveness of interventions for some outcomes.

At What Intervals Should the Outcomes Be Assessed and Documented?

More research is needed to definitively answer this question. At present the nurse determines the intervals for measurement and documentation of the outcome based on clinical judgment as to when the effects of interventions need to be assessed. This is greatly influenced by the setting and characteristics of the patient. Organizational policies also determine the intervals for measurement and documentation in some situations. Frequent rating of outcomes can become a workload burden for the nurse, so the decision of how often to measure an outcome is a critical one. At minimum the outcomes selected should be rated and documented when: (1) the patient or family is admitted to a care setting or makes an initial visit to a nurse for care, (2) the patient or family is discharged, transferred, or referred to another setting or clinician for care, or (3) there is a significant change in status for an outcome. Time intervals for measurement of outcomes should vary based on the characteristics of the concept. For example, the nurse might want to measure *Pain Level* at least every 4 hours but would not measure the patient's *Quality of Life* on the same timeframe. The nurse and/or interdisciplinary health care team should determine the measurement timeframes for family and community level outcomes.

How Are the Outcomes Used in Standardized Care Plans/Critical Paths?

NOC outcomes are very useful in clinical pathways because they allow quantification of the patient state, behavior, or perception that is expected to occur at specific points in time for a desired pathway of an episode of care. Major advantages of their use are (1) the ability to monitor variance from the pathway and (2) the ability to compare the achievement of specific patient states across settings and providers. Use of standardized outcomes greatly facilitates the development of large databases across settings and providers, rather than the more limited, unique databases that result when setting or provider-specific outcomes are used in critical pathways and care planning.

Why Is It Necessary for Nurses to Have Their Own List of Outcomes?

The NOC includes patient, caregiver, family, and community level outcomes that are responsive to nursing interventions. These outcomes are not intended to be unique to nursing. Most, if not all, patient outcomes are influenced by multiple health care providers; by environmental factors; and by other patient, caregiver, family, and community characteristics. However, it is critically important for nurses to measure the effects of their interventions on patient outcomes. The NOC provides a set of indicators for each outcome that is considered to be sensitive to nursing interventions. When used with interdisciplinary teams, different indicators may be the focus of interventions for various disciplines. Without discipline-specific indicators for shared outcomes, it will be impossible to monitor the accountability of each discipline for its contribution to outcome improvement or deterioration. To ensure that the contributions of nursing interventions to patient, caregiver, family, and community level outcomes are not credited to other health care providers, standardized nursing data elements must be included in clinical databases. Large data sets that include these data along with other salient system, patient, caregiver, family, or community characteristics, along with provider characteristics, are necessary to isolate the independent effects of nursing interventions on patient outcomes.

Why Is It Important to Assess Outcomes Across Care Settings?

Continuity of care always is an important value for the nursing profession, yet communication among settings and nurse providers is constrained. A major obstacle is the lack of standardized nomenclatures to describe the problems that nurses treat, the interventions used, and the resulting outcome states. The inability to optimize continuity of care is costly to patients, families, and the health care system. In the current resource-constrained environment, more emphasis is placed on continuity of care to reduce costs. Further, networks that include providers and settings across the continuum of care are being developed to enhance continuity and optimize care in the most cost-efficient environment. The effort to reduce costs has prompted a corresponding emphasis on the demonstration of outcomes effectiveness. The NOC provides a standardized language for outcomes that can be measured across the entire continuum of care, providing essential information that clinicians need to achieve continuity and to assess the cost-effectiveness of care.

Why Is It Necessary to Use the Outcome Labels When the Indicators May Be More Useful?

Along with medicine the nursing profession is a key member of the interdisciplinary health care team. The profession's contribution to interdisciplinary outcomes must be documented, and the effectiveness of nursing interventions must be evaluated. Large, standardized databases contain outcomes, such as those provided by NOC, but likely not discipline-specific indicators in all cases because of space limitations. It is therefore essential that the nursing profession use standardized outcomes that are included in large databases so that the profession's influence on outcomes will be used to determine nursing effectiveness and influence health policy.

Why Is the Standardization of Outcomes Advocated When Each Patient, Caregiver, Family, or Community/Population Is Unique?

Standardizing the language used to describe outcomes in no way interferes with assessing the unique response of each patient, caregiver, family, or community/population. Use of the NOC outcomes enables nurses to measure each outcome state for each individual, caregiver, family, and community and provides more information for monitoring the progress of each. Specific, quantified goals can be set for each, and the extent that the goals are or are not met can be documented over time and compared across settings. In other words standardized nursing diagnoses, interventions, and outcomes actually increase the ability of nurses to identify and document the diagnoses that are unique for each patient, prescribe interventions that are specific for the patient, and document the patient outcomes in response to the interventions for each individual across time and settings.

How Do I Identify Outcomes for Use in my Practice?

With 490 outcomes in the fifth edition of NOC, this task may seem difficult at first. The scope of the classification is to identify all outcomes needed by nurses to evaluate the outcomes of nursing interventions, but most nurses will focus on a limited set of outcomes based on their specialty and practice setting. Beginning efforts to identify core outcomes

for specialty practice have supported this belief that nurses can identify a list of outcomes they use daily with their patients. The easiest way to identify outcomes for use in clinical practice is to review the NOC Taxonomy where similar outcomes are grouped under key concepts in nursing. A second way is to review the list of outcomes identified by a nursing specialty to see if the outcomes identified match those needed to evaluate the effectiveness of interventions. It is important that specialty practice is adequately reflected in this classification. A third way to identify NOC outcomes is to examine the NOC linkages provided to NANDA-I diagnoses and to Gordon's Health Patterns in Part Four.

When Is a New Outcome Developed and How Is It Done?

New outcomes are identified by the developers, by nurses from clinical practice, and through the linkage with other classifications. The NOC team maintains a list of potential concepts for development. A nurse or group of nurses conducts a concept analysis, defines the outcome, identifies indicators, and chooses a measurement scale(s) for use with the outcome. Part of the review process involves ensuring that the outcome is useful and clinically accurate for patients across the life span. If it is not, then a target population is identified in the concept label. Many of the outcomes are sent to additional experts for further review. Once the outcome is accepted for inclusion in the NOC, it is placed in the taxonomy and coded. Instructions on how to submit an outcome can be found in Appendix B.

Why Are There So Many Different Measurement Scales?

Although we have tried to limit the number of measurement scales used in the classification, there are currently outcomes with one or two scales used in the 490 outcomes in the fifth edition. There are 398 outcomes that use one scale. The same scale has been used to measure similar concepts as more outcomes are developed. Since the outcomes focus on states, behaviors, or perceptions, it is not surprising that different measurement scales are needed to fit the focus of the outcome. After a careful review of field testing results in 10 clinical settings, an effort was made to solve some of the problems encountered by nurses using NOC in practice. In the third edition, the measurement scales for each outcome and the corresponding outcome definition were carefully reviewed and resulted in a reduction in the number of scales and a standard format for definitions based on the specific measurement scale. The evaluation of the anchors for each of the scales resulted in modifications, and some outcomes had a change in measurement scale. A more detailed description of this review is available in the third edition. Table 1-3 identifies the primary measurement scales with anchors, a definition of the focus of each scale, and a list of the outcomes using the scale.

Text continued on p. 18

Table 1-3	SINGLE MEASUREMENT SCALES USED IN NOC

Scale Code		Scales and Associated Outcomes

01

Severely compromised	*Substantially compromised*	*Moderately compromised*

DEFINITION: Extent of impairment of health or well-being

Abstract Thinking	Communication: Receptive
Activity Tolerance	Concentration
Ambulation	Coordinated Movement
Ambulation: Wheelchair	Decision-Making
Appetite	Information Processing
Body Positioning: Self-Initiated	Memory
Caregiver Physical Health	Mobility
Cognition	Personal Health Status
Cognitive Orientation	Physical Fitness
Comfort Status	Preterm Infant Organization
Comfort Status: Environment	Rest
Comfort Status: Sociocultural	Self-Care Status
Communication	Self-Care: Activities of Daily Living (ADL)
Communication: Expressive	Self-Care: Bathing

02

Severe deviation from normal range	*Substantial deviation from normal range*	*Moderate deviation from normal range*

DEFINITION: Extent of departure from an established norm or standard

Blood Glucose Level	Joint Movement: Hip
Electrolyte Balance	Joint Movement: Knee
Fetal Status: Antepartum	Joint Movement: Neck
Fetal Status: Intrapartum	Joint Movement: Passive
Growth	Joint Movement: Shoulder
Joint Movement	Joint Movement: Spine
Joint Movement: Ankle	Joint Movement: Wrist
Joint Movement: Elbow	Newborn Adaptation
Joint Movement: Fingers	Nutritional Status

06

Not adequate	*Slightly adequate*	*Moderately adequate*

DEFINITION: Extent of sufficiency in quantity or quality to achieve a desired state

Abuse Protection	Caregiver Performance: Indirect Care
Bottle Feeding Establishment: Infant	Caregiver Role Endurance
Breastfeeding Establishment: Infant	Community Disaster Readiness
Breastfeeding Establishment: Maternal	Community Disaster Response
Breastfeeding Maintenance	Community Grief Response
Breastfeeding Weaning	Cup Feeding Establishment: Infant
Caregiver Home Care Readiness	Infant Nutritional Status
Caregiver Performance: Direct Care	

07

10 and over	*7-9*	*4-6*

DEFINITION: Number of occurrences

Elopement Occurrence	Falls Occurrence

Mildly compromised	*Not compromised*

Self-Care: Dressing
Self-Care: Eating
Self-Care: Hygiene
Self-Care: Instrumental Activities of Daily Living (IADL)
Self-Care: Non-Parenteral Medication
Self-Care: Oral Hygiene
Self-Care: Parenteral Medication
Self-Care: Toileting
Sensory Function
Skeletal Function
Spiritual Health
Transfer Performance

N=40

Mild deviation from normal range	*No deviation from normal range*

Nutritional Status: Biochemical
      Measures
Nutritional Status: Energy
Physical Aging
Physical Maturation: Female
Physical Maturation: Male
Tissue Perfusion
Vital Signs
Weight: Body Mass

N=26

Substantially adequate	*Totally adequate*

Nutritional Status: Food & Fluid Intake
Nutritional Status: Nutrient Intake
Pre-Procedure Readiness
Role Performance
Safe Health Care Environment
Safe Home Environment
Social Support

N=22

1-3	*None*

N=2

Continued

Table 1-3	SINGLE MEASUREMENT SCALES USED IN NOC—cont'd

Scale Code			Scales and Associated Outcomes
09	*None*	*Limited*	*Moderate*

DEFINITION: Range over which an entity extends

Abuse Cessation		Abuse Recovery: Financial
Abuse Recovery		Abuse Recovery: Physical

Scale Code			
11	*Never positive*	*Rarely positive*	*Sometimes positive*

DEFINITION: Frequency of an affirmative and accepting perception or characteristics

Body Image		Caregiver-Patient Relationship

Scale Code			
12	*Very weak*	*Weak*	*Moderate*

DEFINITION: Extent of intensity

Health Beliefs		Health Beliefs: Perceived Control
Health Beliefs: Perceived Ability to Perform		Health Beliefs: Perceived Resources

Scale Code			
13	*Never demonstrated*	*Rarely demonstrated*	*Sometimes demonstrated*

DEFINITION: Frequency of making clear by report or behavior

Abusive Behavior Self-Restraint	Compliance Behavior: Prescribed Diet
Acceptance: Health Status	Compliance Behavior: Prescribed Medication
Adaptation to Physical Disability	Coping
Adherence Behavior	Cup Feeding Performance
Adherence Behavior: Healthy Diet	Depression Self-Control
Aggression Self-Restraint	Dignified Life Closure
Alcohol Abuse Cessation Behavior	Discharge Readiness: Supported Living
Anger Self-Restraint	Distorted Thought Self-Control
Anxiety Self-Control	Drug Abuse Cessation Behavior
Aspiration Prevention	Energy Conservation
Body Mechanics Performance	Exercise Participation
Bottle Feeding Performance	Fall Prevention Behavior
Caregiver Adaptation to Patient Institutionalization	Family Coping
	Family Functioning
Child Development: 1 Month	Family Integrity
Child Development: 2 Months	Family Normalization
Child Development: 4 Months	Family Participation in Professional Care
Child Development: 6 Months	Family Resiliency
Child Development: 12 Months	Family Risk Control: Obesity
Child Development: 2 Years	Family Social Climate
Child Development: 3 Years	Family Support During Treatment
Child Development: 4 Years	Fear Self-Control
Child Development: 5 Years	Grief Resolution
Child Development: Middle Childhood	Guilt Resolution
Child Development: Adolescence	Health Promoting Behavior
Compliance Behavior	Health Seeking Behavior
Compliance Behavior: Prescribed Activity	Hearing Compensation Behavior

Substantial	*Extensive*
Neglect Cessation	N=5

Often positive	*Consistently positive*
Self-Esteem	N=3

Strong	*Very strong*
Health Beliefs: Perceived Threat Health Orientation	N=6

Often demonstrated	*Consistently demonstrated*
Heedfulness of Affected Side	
Hope	
Identity	
Immunization Behavior	
Impulse Self-Control	
Leisure Participation	
Lifestyle Balance	
Motivation	
Mutilation Self-Restraint	
Nausea & Vomiting Control	
Ostomy Self-Care	
Pain Control	
Parent-Infant Attachment	
Parenting Performance	
Parenting Performance: Adolescent	
Parenting Performance: Adolescent Physical Safety	
Parenting Performance: Early/Middle Childhood Physical Safety	
Parenting Performance: Infant	
Parenting Performance: Infant/ Toddler Physical Safety	
Parenting Performance: Middle Childhood	
Parenting Performance: Preschooler	
Parenting Performance: Psychosocial Safety	
Parenting Performance: Toddler	
Participation in Health Care Decisions	
Personal Autonomy	

Continued

Table 1-3	SINGLE MEASUREMENT SCALES USED IN NOC—cont'd

Scale Code		Scales and Associated Outcomes
13—cont'd	Personal Health Screening Behavior	Risk Control: Lipid Disorder
	Personal Resiliency	Risk Control: Osteoporosis
	Personal Safety Behavior	Risk Control: Sexually Transmitted Diseases (STD)
	Personal Time Management	Risk Control: Stroke
	Play Participation	Risk Control: Sun Exposure
	Postpartum Maternal Health Behavior	Risk Control: Thrombus
	Prenatal Health Behavior	Risk Control: Tobacco Use
	Psychosocial Adjustment: Life Change	Risk Control: Unintended Pregnancy
	Risk Control	Risk Control: Visual Impairment
	Risk Control: Alcohol Use	Risk Detection
	Risk Control: Cancer	Seizure Self-Control
	Risk Control: Cardiovascular Disease	Self-Awareness
	Risk Control: Drug Use	Self-Direction of Care
	Risk Control: Dry Eye	Self-Management: Acute Illness
	Risk Control: Hearing Impairment	Self-Management: Anticoagulation Therapy
	Risk Control: Hypertension	Self-Management: Cardiac Disease
	Risk Control: Hyperthermia	Self-Management: Chronic Disease
	Risk Control: Hypotension	Self-Management: Chronic Obstructive
	Risk Control: Hypothermia	Pulmonary Disease
	Risk Control: Infectious Process	Self-Management: Coronary Artery Disease

14	*Severe*	*Substantial*	*Moderate*

DEFINITION: Extent of a negative or adverse state or response

Acute Respiratory Acidosis Severity		Hyperchloremia Severity
Acute Respiratory Alkalosis Severity		Hyperglycemia Severity
Agitation Level		Hyperkalemia Severity
Allergic Response: Localized		Hypermagnesemia Severity
Allergic Response: Systemic		Hypernatremia Severity
Anxiety Level		Hyperphosphatemia Severity
Blood Loss Severity		Hypertension Severity
Blood Transfusion Reaction		Hypocalcemia Severity
Caregiver Stressors		Hypochloremia Severity
Delirium Level		Hypoglycemia Severity
Dementia Level		Hypokalemia Severity
Depression Level		Hypomagnesemia Severity
Discomfort Level		Hyponatremia Severity
Dry Eye Severity		Hypophosphatemia Severity
Fatigue: Disruptive Effects		Hypotension Severity
Fear Level		Infection Severity
Fear Level: Child		Infection Severity: Newborn
Fluid Overload Severity		Loneliness Severity
Hyperactivity Level		Metabolic Acidosis Severity
Hypercalcemia Severity		Metabolic Alkalosis Severity

17	*Poor*	*Fair*	*Good*

DEFINITION: Extent of proximity to a desired state

Community Competence	Community Resiliency
Community Health Screening Effectiveness	Community Risk Control: Chronic Disease
Community Health Status	Community Risk Control: Communicable Disease
Community Immune Status	Community Risk Control: Lead Exposure
Community Program Effectiveness	

Self-Management: Diabetes
Self-Management: Dysrhythmia
Self-Management: Heart Failure
Self-Management: Hypertension
Self-Management: Kidney Disease
Self-Management: Lipid Disorder
Self-Management: Multiple Sclerosis
Self-Management: Osteoporosis
Self-Management: Peripheral Artery Disease
Sexual Functioning
Sexual Identity
Smoking Cessation Behavior
Social Interaction Skills
Social Involvement
Suicide Self-Restraint
Symptom Control
Vision Compensation Behavior
Weight Gain Behavior
Weight Loss Behavior
Weight Maintenance Behavior   N=137

Mild   *None*

Nausea & Vomiting: Disruptive Effects
Nausea & Vomiting Severity
Pain: Adverse Psychological Response
Pain: Disruptive Effects
Perimenopause Symptom Severity
Peripheral Artery Disease Severity
Physical Injury Severity
Premenstrual Syndrome (PMS) Severity
Shock Severity: Anaphylactic
Shock Severity: Cardiogenic
Shock Severity: Hypovolemic
Shock Severity: Neurogenic
Shock Severity: Septic
Social Anxiety Level
Stress Level
Substance Addiction Consequences
Substance Withdrawal Severity
Suffering Severity
Symptom Severity   N=59

Very good   *Excellent*

Community Risk Control: Obesity
Community Risk Control: Unhealthy Cultural Traditions
Community Risk Control: Violence
Community Violence Level   N=13

Continued

Table 1-3	SINGLE MEASUREMENT SCALES USED IN NOC—cont'd

Scale Code			Scales and Associated Outcomes
18	*Not at all satisfied*	*Somewhat satisfied*	*Moderately satisfied*

DEFINITION: Extent of perception of positive expectations

Caregiver Well-Being	Client Satisfaction: Cultural Needs Fulfillment
Client Satisfaction	Client Satisfaction: Functional Assistance
Client Satisfaction: Access to Care	Client Satisfaction: Pain Management
Resources	Client Satisfaction: Physical Care
Client Satisfaction: Caring	Client Satisfaction: Physical Environment
Client Satisfaction: Case Management	Client Satisfaction: Protection of Rights
Client Satisfaction: Communication	Client Satisfaction: Psychological Care
Client Satisfaction: Continuity of Care	

Scale Code			
19	*Consistently demonstrated*	*Often demonstrated*	*Sometimes demonstrated*

DEFINITION: Frequency of making clear by report or behavior

Elopement Propensity Risk

Scale Code			
20	*No knowledge*	*Limited knowledge*	*Moderate knowledge*

DEFINITION: Extent of cognitive information that is understood

Knowledge: Acute Illness Management	Knowledge: Eating Disorder Management
Knowledge: Anticoagulation Therapy	Knowledge: Energy Conservation
Knowledge: Arthritis Management	Knowledge: Fall Prevention
Knowledge: Asthma Management	Knowledge: Fertility Promotion
Knowledge: Body Mechanics	Knowledge: Health Behavior
Knowledge: Bottle Feeding	Knowledge: Health Promotion
Knowledge: Breastfeeding	Knowledge: Health Resources
Knowledge: Cancer Management	Knowledge: Healthy Diet
Knowledge: Cancer Threat Reduction	Knowledge: Healthy Lifestyle
Knowledge: Cardiac Disease Management	Knowledge: Heart Failure Management
Knowledge: Child Physical Safety	Knowledge: Hypertension Management
Knowledge: Chronic Disease Management	Knowledge: Infant Care
Knowledge: Chronic Obstructive	Knowledge: Infection Management
Pulmonary Disease Management	Knowledge: Inflammatory Bowel Disease
Knowledge: Conception Prevention	Management
Knowledge: Coronary Artery Disease	Knowledge: Kidney Disease Management
Management	Knowledge: Labor & Delivery
Knowledge: Cup Feeding	Knowledge: Lipid Disorder Management
Knowledge: Dementia Management	Knowledge: Medication
Knowledge: Depression Management	Knowledge: Multiple Sclerosis Management
Knowledge: Diabetes Management	Knowledge: Osteoporosis Management
Knowledge: Disease Process	Knowledge: Ostomy Care
Knowledge: Dysrhythmia Management	Knowledge: Pain Management

Why Do Some Outcomes Have Two Scales?

An issue identified from the testing of the NOC in clinical sites was that some indicators were difficult to use because they contained double negatives to fit the measurement scale. Nurses felt the negative indicators were important to document because they focused on symptoms indicating complications of the patient's condition and were monitored frequently by nurses in practice. As a solution to this problem, a second scale for measuring the negative states was added to 72 outcomes in the third edition. This was an important revision to the classification as it allowed for better

Very satisfied	*Completely satisfied*
Client Satisfaction: Safety	
Client Satisfaction: Symptom Control	
Client Satisfaction: Teaching	
Client Satisfaction: Technical Aspects of Care	
Personal Well-Being	
Quality of Life	
	N=20

Rarely demonstrated	*Never demonstrated*
	N=1

Substantial knowledge	*Extensive knowledge*
Knowledge: Parenting	
Knowledge: Peripheral Artery Disease Management	
Knowledge: Personal Safety	
Knowledge: Pneumonia Management	
Knowledge: Postpartum Maternal Health	
Knowledge: Preconception Maternal Health	
Knowledge: Pregnancy	
Knowledge: Pregnancy & Postpartum Sexual Functioning	
Knowledge: Prescribed Activity	
Knowledge: Prescribed Diet	
Knowledge: Preterm Infant Care	
Knowledge: Sexual Functioning	
Knowledge: Stress Management	
Knowledge: Stroke Management	
Knowledge: Stroke Prevention	
Knowledge: Substance Use Control	
Knowledge: Thrombus Prevention	
Knowledge: Time Management	
Knowledge: Treatment Procedure	
Knowledge: Treatment Regimen	
Knowledge: Weight Management	
	N=64

documentation of complications associated with the outcome. A second problem that made the indicators difficult to use was the wording of indicators as "free of" (e.g. "free of bleeding"). A second scale allowed the nurse to rate the severity of bleeding experienced by the patient, rather than whether bleeding was present or absent in the outcome *Oral Health*. This provided better data and more information on a change in the status of the patient. In the fifth edition there are 92 outcomes with two scales. This change in format makes these outcomes easier to use for nurses, and the change has resulted in positive feedback. Table 1-4 lists the outcomes using two scales in combination.

Table 1-4	Combination Measurement Scales Used in NOC

Scale Code / **Scales and Associated Outcomes**

21	*Severely compromised*	*Substantially compromised*	*Moderately compromised*
	Severe	*Substantial*	*Moderate*
	Balance	Liver Function	
	Bowel Elimination	Medication Response	
	Caregiver Emotional Health	Neurological Status	
	Comfort Status: Physical	Neurological Status: Autonomic	
	Comfort Status: Psychospiritual	Neurological Status: Central Motor Control	
	Comfortable Death	Neurological Status: Consciousness	
	Endurance	Neurological Status: Cranial Sensory/Motor Function	
	Family Health Status	Neurological Status: Peripheral	
	Fluid Balance	Neurological Status: Spinal Sensory/Motor Function	
	Gait	Oral Health	
	Gastrointestinal Function	Sensory Function: Hearing	
	Hemodialysis Access	Sensory Function: Proprioception	
	Hydration	Sensory Function: Tactile	
	Immune Status		
	Kidney Function		

22	*Severe deviation from normal range*	*Substantial deviation from normal range*	*Moderate deviation from normal range*
	Severe	*Substantial*	*Moderate*
	Blood Coagulation	Mechanical Ventilation Weaning Response: Adult	
	Cardiac Pump Effectiveness	Post-Procedure Recovery	
	Cardiopulmonary Status	Respiratory Status	
	Circulation Status	Respiratory Status: Airway Patency	
	Electrolyte & Acid/Base Balance	Respiratory Status: Gas Exchange	
	Maternal Status: Antepartum	Respiratory Status: Ventilation	
	Maternal Status: Intrapartum	Surgical Recovery: Convalescence	
	Maternal Status: Postpartum		
	Mechanical Ventilation Response: Adult		

23	*None*	*Limited*	*Moderate*
	Extensive	*Substantial*	*Moderate*
	Abuse Recovery: Emotional	Burn Healing	
	Abuse Recovery: Sexual	Burn Recovery	
	Bone Healing	Neglect Recovery	

24	*Never demonstrated*	*Rarely demonstrated*	*Sometimes demonstrated*
	Consistently demonstrated	*Often demonstrated*	*Sometimes demonstrated*
	Bowel Continence	Discharge Readiness: Independent Living	
	Child Adaptation to Hospitalization	Eating Disorder Self-Control	
	Development: Late Adulthood	Mood Equilibrium	
	Development: Middle Adulthood	Psychomotor Energy	
	Development: Young Adulthood	Relocation Adaptation	

25	*Severe*	*Substantial*	*Moderate*
	Severely compromised	*Substantially compromised*	*Moderately compromised*
	Caregiver Lifestyle Disruption	Immobility Consequences: Psycho-Cognitive	
	Fatigue Level		
	Immobility Consequences: Physiological		

26	*Severe*	*Substantial*	*Moderate*
	Severe deviation from normal range	*Substantial deviation from normal range*	*Moderate deviation from normal range*
	Pain Level		

Mildly compromised   *Not compromised*

    Mild   *None*

Sensory Function: Taste & Smell
Sensory Function: Vision
Sleep
Student Health Status
Swallowing Status
Swallowing Status: Esophageal Phase
Swallowing Status: Oral Phase
Swallowing Status: Pharyngeal Phase
Thermoregulation
Thermoregulation: Newborn
Tissue Integrity: Skin & Mucous Membranes
Urinary Elimination
Will to Live

                                                   N=41

Mild deviation   *No deviation*
from normal range   *from normal range*

    Mild   *None*

Surgical Recovery: Immediate Post-Operative
Systemic Toxin Clearance: Dialysis
Tissue Perfusion: Abdominal Organs
Tissue Perfusion: Cardiac
Tissue Perfusion: Cellular
Tissue Perfusion: Cerebral
Tissue Perfusion: Peripheral
Tissue Perfusion: Pulmonary

                                                   N=24

Substantial   *Extensive*

    Limited   *None*

Wound Healing: Primary Intention
Wound Healing: Secondary Intention

                                                   N=8

Often demonstrated   *Consistently demonstrated*

Rarely demonstrated   *Never demonstrated*

    Safe Wandering
    Self-Management: Asthma
    Urinary Continence

                                                   N=13

    Mild   *None*

Mildly compromised   *Not compromised*

    Immune Hypersensitivity Response

                                                   N=5

    Mild   *None*

Mild deviation   *No deviation*
from normal range   *from normal range*

                                                   N=1

REFINEMENT OF THE CLASSIFICATION: ONGOING AND FUTURE DEVELOPMENT

The current classification represents the completion of over 20 years of research to develop and test a classification and taxonomy of nursing-sensitive patient outcomes. The classification contains 490 outcomes designed for measuring the impact of nursing treatments on individual, caregiver, family, and community outcomes. The outcomes are classified in the NOC taxonomy under 7 domains and 32 classes. This taxonomic structure has served the classification well. As the classification grows, each new outcome must be evaluated to see how it "fits" with the current outcomes in the classification. Sometimes, this involves the modification of an existing outcome or outcomes, as the new outcome may focus on a different age group or patient population. This work is ongoing, and continual updating of the classification is needed to keep it relevant for clinical practice. This is crucial to having valid and reliable standardized language for outcome measurement in nursing. The fifth edition added 107 new outcomes, and the number of outcomes developed for use with teaching interventions continues to increase with each edition. The fifth edition added 23 new knowledge outcomes and created a new class in the taxonomy for the 16 outcomes focused on self-management. The knowledge and self-management outcomes can easily be used by other disciplines providing care to patients. This is important additional content for NOC because of the current focus on health and patient involvement in the care process. Table 1-5 proves linkages of knowledge outcomes with behavioral outcomes in NOC. These are important to identify if teaching interventions and knowledge lead to behavioral changes that enhance health.

Domains and classes for family and community level outcomes were added to the NOC taxonomy in the second edition. Additional outcome submissions are needed to develop and refine family and community level outcomes. Input from specialty organizations is also helpful in these areas.

Text continued on page 31

Table 1-5   NOC Performance Outcomes Related to NOC Knowledge Outcomes

Knowledge Outcomes	Primary Behavioral Outcomes	Secondary Behavioral Outcomes
All Knowledge Outcomes	1600 Adherence Behavior 1601 Compliance Behavior 1602 Health Promoting Behavior 1603 Health Seeking Behavior 1606 Participation in Health Care Decisions 1908 Risk Detection 3100 Self-Management: Acute Illness 3102 Self-Management: Chronic Disease	2013 Lifestyle Balance 1209 Motivation 1614 Personal Autonomy 1634 Personal Health Screening Behavior 1635 Personal Time Management 1902 Risk Control
1844 Knowledge: Acute Illness Management	1600 Adherence Behavior 1601 Compliance Behavior 0313 Self-Care Status 3100 Self-Management: Acute Illness	1603 Health Seeking Behavior 1634 Personal Health Screening Behavior 1902 Risk Control 1924 Risk Control: Infectious Process 1608 Symptom Control
1845 Knowledge: Anticoagulation Therapy Management	1623 Compliance Behavior: Prescribed Medication 1909 Fall Prevention Behavior 1932 Risk Control: Thrombus 3101 Self-Management: Anticoagulation Therapy	1602 Health Promoting Behavior 1634 Personal Health Screening Behavior 1911 Personal Safety Behavior 1902 Risk Control 1931 Risk Control: Stroke
1831 Knowledge: Arthritis Management	1308 Adaptation to Physical Disability 0200 Ambulation 1632 Compliance Behavior: Prescribed Activity 1623 Compliance Behavior: Prescribed Medication 1633 Exercise Participation 1605 Pain Control 0300 Self-Care: Activities of Daily Living (ADL) 0306 Self-Care: Instrumental Activities of Daily Living (IADL) 3102 Self-Management: Chronic Disease	0002 Energy Conservation 1909 Fall Prevention Behavior 1602 Health Promoting Behavior 1634 Personal Health Screening Behavior 1309 Personal Resiliency 1305 Psychosocial Adjustment: Life Change 1902 Risk Control 0313 Self-Care Status 1627 Weight Loss Behavior

Table 1-5	NOC PERFORMANCE OUTCOMES RELATED TO NOC KNOWLEDGE OUTCOMES—cont'd	
Knowledge Outcomes	**Primary Behavioral Outcomes**	**Secondary Behavioral Outcomes**
1832 Knowledge: Asthma Management	1632 Compliance Behavior: Prescribed Activity 1623 Compliance Behavior: Prescribed Medication 0002 Energy Conservation 1603 Health Seeking Behavior 1924 Risk Control: Infectious Process 0704 Self-Management: Asthma 1608 Symptom Control	2605 Family Participation in Professional Care 1602 Health Promoting Behavior 1634 Personal Health Screening Behavior 0313 Self-Care Status 1625 Smoking Cessation Behavior
1827 Knowledge: Body Mechanics	1616 Body Mechanics Performance 1909 Fall Prevention Behavior	0200 Ambulation 0201 Ambulation: Wheelchair 1602 Health Promoting Behavior 0210 Transfer Performance
1846 Knowledge: Bottle Feeding	1918 Aspiration Prevention 1017 Bottle Feeding Performance	2904 Parenting Performance: Infant
1800 Knowledge: Breastfeeding	1000 Breastfeeding Establishment: Infant 1001 Breastfeeding Establishment: Maternal 1002 Breastfeeding Maintenance 1003 Breastfeeding Weaning	1634 Personal Health Screening Behavior 1500 Parent-Infant Attachment
1833 Knowledge: Cancer Management	1623 Compliance Behavior: Prescribed Medication 1603 Health Seeking Behavior 1618 Nausea & Vomiting Control 1605 Pain Control 1606 Participation in Health Care Decisions 1634 Personal Health Screening Behavior 3102 Self-Management: Chronic Disease 1608 Symptom Control	1302 Coping 1409 Depression Self-Control 2609 Family Support During Treatment 1309 Personal Resiliency 1305 Psychosocial Adjustment: Life Change 0313 Self-Care Status 1917 Risk Control: Cancer 1924 Risk Control: Infectious Process 1925 Risk Control: Sun Exposure
1834 Knowledge: Cancer Threat Reduction	1602 Health Promoting Behavior 1634 Personal Health Screening Behavior 1917 Risk Control: Cancer 1906 Risk Control: Tobacco Use 1908 Risk Detection	1625 Smoking Cessation Behavior
1830 Knowledge: Cardiac Disease Management	1632 Compliance Behavior: Prescribed Activity 1623 Compliance Behavior: Prescribed Medication 1622 Compliance Behavior: Prescribed Diet 1603 Health Seeking Behavior 1605 Pain Control 1914 Risk Control: Cardiovascular Disease 1928 Risk Control: Hypertension 1929 Risk Control: Lipid Disorder 1617 Self-Management: Cardiac Disease 1608 Symptom Control	1308 Adaptation to Physical Disability 0002 Energy Conservation 2605 Family Participation in Professional Care 2609 Family Support During Treatment 1606 Participation in Health Care Decisions 1634 Personal Health Screening Behavior 1305 Psychosocial Adjustment: Life Change 1902 Risk Control 0313 Self-Care Status 1625 Smoking Cessation Behavior 1628 Weight Maintenance Behavior
1801 Knowledge: Child Physical Safety	2211 Parenting Performance 2902 Parenting Performance: Adolescent Physical Safety 2901 Parenting Performance: Early/Middle Childhood Physical Safety 2900 Parenting Performance: Infant/Toddler Physical Safety	2501 Abuse Protection 1630 Drug Abuse Cessation Behavior 1901 Parenting Performance: Psychosocial Safety 1625 Smoking Cessation Behavior

Continued

Table 1-5	NOC Performance Outcomes Related to NOC Knowledge Outcomes—cont'd	
Knowledge Outcomes	**Primary Behavioral Outcomes**	**Secondary Behavioral Outcomes**
1847 Knowledge: Chronic Disease Management	1632 Compliance Behavior: Prescribed Activity 1622 Compliance Behavior: Prescribed Diet 1623 Compliance Behavior: Prescribed Medication 1603 Health Seeking Behavior 1605 Pain Control 1305 Psychosocial Adjustment: Life Change 3102 Self-Management: Chronic Disease 1608 Symptom Control	1302 Coping 1606 Participation in Health Care Decisions 1634 Personal Health Screening Behavior 1924 Risk Control: Infectious Process 0313 Self-Care Status
1848 Knowledge: Chronic Obstructive Pulmonary Disease Management	0002 Energy Conservation 1632 Compliance Behavior: Prescribed Activity 1623 Compliance Behavior: Prescribed Medication 1603 Health Seeking Behavior 1605 Pain Control 3103 Self-Management: Chronic Obstructive Pulmonary Disease 1625 Smoking Cessation Behavior 1608 Symptom Control	1302 Coping 1606 Participation in Health Care Decisions 1634 Personal Health Screening Behavior 1924 Risk Control: Infectious Process 1914 Risk Control: Cardiovascular Disease 1906 Risk Control: Tobacco Use 0313 Self-Care Status
1821 Knowledge: Conception Prevention	1907 Risk Control: Unintended Pregnancy	1606 Participation in Health Care Decisions 1634 Personal Health Screening Behavior 1902 Risk Control 1905 Risk Control: Sexually Transmitted Diseases (STD)
1849 Knowledge: Coronary Artery Disease Management	1632 Compliance Behavior: Prescribed Activity 1622 Compliance Behavior: Prescribed Diet 1623 Compliance Behavior: Prescribed Medication 3104 Self-Management: Coronary Artery Disease 1625 Smoking Cessation Behavior	1606 Participation in Health Care Decisions 1634 Personal Health Screening Behavior 1914 Risk Control: Cardiovascular Disease 1906 Risk Control: Tobacco Use
1850 Knowledge: Cup Feeding	1018 Cup Feeding Establishment: Infant 1019 Cup Feeding Performance	1918 Aspiration Prevention 1500 Parent-Infant Attachment 2904 Parenting Performance: Infant
1851 Knowledge: Dementia Management	1902 Risk Control 1608 Symptom Control	1302 Coping 1920 Elopement Propensity Risk 1926 Safe Wandering 0313 Self-Care Status 1613 Self-Direction of Care
1836 Knowledge: Depression Management	1623 Compliance Behavior: Prescribed Medication 1409 Depression Self-Control 1603 Health Seeking Behavior 1634 Personal Health Screening Behavior 1408 Suicide Self-Restraint	1302 Coping 2013 Lifestyle Balance 1606 Participation in Health Care Decisions 0313 Self-Care Status 1503 Social Involvement 1608 Symptom Control 1628 Weight Maintenance Behavior

Table 1-5	NOC Performance Outcomes Related to NOC Knowledge Outcomes—cont'd	

Knowledge Outcomes	Primary Behavioral Outcomes	Secondary Behavioral Outcomes
1820 Knowledge: Diabetes Management	1622 Compliance Behavior: Prescribed Diet 1623 Compliance Behavior: Prescribed Medication 1632 Compliance Behavior: Prescribed Activity 1633 Exercise Participation 1603 Health Seeking Behavior 1619 Self-Management: Diabetes 1608 Symptom Control 1628 Weight Maintenance Behavior	1302 Coping 1634 Personal Health Screening Behavior 1902 Risk Control 1916 Risk Control: Visual Impairment 3107 Self Management: Hypertension 3109 Self-Management: Lipid Disorder 1611 Vision Compensation Behavior 1627 Weight Loss Behavior 1628 Weight Maintenance Behavior
1803 Knowledge: Disease Process	1302 Coping 1409 Depression Self-Control 1603 Health Seeking Behavior 1605 Pain Control 1911 Personal Safety Behavior 1608 Symptom Control	1402 Anxiety Self-Control 1918 Aspiration Prevention 1616 Body Mechanics Performance 1403 Distorted Thought Self-Control 1610 Hearing Compensation Behavior 0918 Heedfulness of Affected Side 1405 Impulse Self-Control 1618 Nausea & Vomiting Control 1615 Ostomy Self-Care 1620 Seizure Self-Control 1406 Mutilation Self-Restraint 1408 Suicide Self-Restraint 1611 Vision Compensation Behavior
1852 Knowledge: Dysrhythmia Management	1632 Compliance Behavior: Prescribed Activity 1623 Compliance Behavior: Prescribed Medication 1605 Pain Control 3105 Self-Management: Dysrhythmia	1402 Anxiety Self-Control 1302 Coping 1606 Participation in Health Care Decisions 1634 Personal Health Screening Behavior 1914 Risk Control: Cardiovascular Disease 1931 Risk Control: Stroke 0313 Self-Care Status
1853 Knowledge: Eating Disorder Management	1302 Coping 1411 Eating Disorder Self-Control 1602 Health Promoting Behavior	1402 Anxiety Self-Control 1622 Compliance Behavior: Prescribed Diet 1409 Depression Self-Control 1634 Personal Health Screening Behavior 1914 Risk Control: Cardiovascular Disease 1626 Weight Gain Behavior 1627 Weight Loss Behavior
1804 Knowledge: Energy Conservation	0002 Energy Conservation 1602 Health Promoting Behavior	0200 Ambulation 1616 Body Mechanics Performance 1302 Coping 0313 Self-Care Status
1828 Knowledge: Fall Prevention	1632 Compliance Behavior: Prescribed Activity 1909 Fall Prevention Behavior	0200 Ambulation 0201 Ambulation: Wheelchair 0918 Heedfulness of Affected Side 0313 Self-Care Status
1816 Knowledge: Fertility Promotion	1607 Prenatal Health Behavior 0119 Sexual Functioning	1302 Coping 1905 Risk Control: Sexually Transmitted Diseases (STD) 1908 Risk Detection

Continued

Table 1-5	NOC PERFORMANCE OUTCOMES RELATED TO NOC KNOWLEDGE OUTCOMES—cont'd	
Knowledge Outcomes	**Primary Behavioral Outcomes**	**Secondary Behavioral Outcomes**
1805 Knowledge: Health Behavior	1602 Health Promoting Behavior 1900 Immunization Behavior 1605 Pain Control 1634 Personal Health Screening Behavior 1911 Personal Safety Behavior 1902 Risk Control 1903 Risk Control: Alcohol Use 1917 Risk Control: Cancer 1914 Risk Control: Cardiovascular Disease 1927 Risk Control: Dry Eye 1904 Risk Control: Drug Use 1915 Risk Control: Hearing Impairment 1928 Risk Control: Hypertension 1922 Risk Control: Hyperthermia 1923 Risk Control: Hypothermia 1924 Risk Control: Infectious Process 1929 Risk Control: Lipid Disorder 1930 Risk Control: Osteoporosis 1905 Risk Control: Sexually Transmitted Diseases (STD) 1931 Risk Control: Stroke 1925 Risk Control: Sun Exposure 1932 Risk Control: Thrombus 1906 Risk Control: Tobacco Use 1907 Risk Control: Unintended Pregnancy 1916 Risk Control: Visual Impairment 1908 Risk Detection	1600 Adherence Behavior 1621 Adherence Behavior: Healthy Diet 1629 Alcohol Abuse Cessation Behavior 1402 Anxiety Self-Control 1616 Body Mechanics Performance 2807 Community Health Screening Effectiveness 2808 Community Program Effectiveness 2801 Community Risk Control: Chronic Disease 2802 Community Risk Control: Communicable Disease 2803 Community Risk Control: Lead Exposure 2809 Community Risk Control: Obesity 2810 Community Risk Control: Unhealthy Cultural Traditions 2805 Community Risk Control: Violence 1302 Coping 1630 Drug Abuse Cessation Behavior 0002 Energy Conservation 1909 Fall Prevention Behavior 2610 Family Risk Control: Obesity 1405 Impulse Self-Control 1604 Leisure Participation 1635 Personal Time Management 1607 Prenatal Health Behavior 1625 Smoking Cessation Behavior 1628 Weight Maintenance Behavior
1823 Knowledge: Health Promotion	1602 Health Promoting Behavior 1900 Immunization Behavior 1911 Personal Safety Behavior 1634 Personal Health Screening Behavior 1908 Risk Detection 1628 Weight Maintenance Behavior	2809 Community Risk Control: Obesity 2810 Community Risk Control: Unhealthy Cultural Traditions 2610 Family Risk Control: Obesity 1903 Risk Control: Alcohol Use 1904 Risk Control: Drug Use 1927 Risk Control: Dry Eye 1928 Risk Control: Hypertension 1929 Risk Control: Lipid Disorder 1930 Risk Control: Osteoporosis 1905 Risk Control: Sexually Transmitted Diseases (STD) 1931 Risk Control: Stroke 1932 Risk Control: Thrombus 1906 Risk Control: Tobacco Use
1806 Knowledge: Health Resources	2206 Caregiver Performance: Indirect Care 1613 Self-Direction of Care	1308 Adaptation to Physical Disability 2700 Community Competence 2602 Family Functioning
1854 Knowledge: Healthy Diet	1621 Adherence Behavior: Healthy Diet	1602 Health Promoting Behavior 1603 Health Seeking Behavior
1855 Knowledge: Healthy Lifestyle	1621 Adherence Behavior: Healthy Diet 1633 Exercise Participation 1634 Personal Health Screening Behavior 1902 Risk Control 1908 Risk Detection	1602 Health Promoting Behavior 1603 Health Seeking Behavior 2013 Lifestyle Balance 1635 Personal Time Management

Knowledge Outcomes	Primary Behavioral Outcomes	Secondary Behavioral Outcomes
1835 Knowledge: Heart Failure Management	1632 Compliance Behavior: Prescribed Activity 1622 Compliance Behavior: Prescribed Diet 1623 Compliance Behavior: Prescribed Medication 0002 Energy Conservation 1603 Health Seeking Behavior 1605 Pain Control 3106 Self-Management: Heart Failure 3107 Self-Management: Hypertension 1608 Symptom Control	1308 Adaptation to Physical Disability 1629 Alcohol Abuse Cessation Behavior 2605 Family Participation in Professional Care 1634 Personal Health Screening Behavior 1305 Psychosocial Adjustment: Life Change 1902 Risk Control 1914 Risk Control: Cardiovascular Disease 1908 Risk Detection 0313 Self-Care Status 1625 Smoking Cessation Behavior 1628 Weight Maintenance Behavior
1837 Knowledge: Hypertension Management	1622 Compliance Behavior: Prescribed Diet 1623 Compliance Behavior: Prescribed Medication 1603 Health Seeking Behavior 3107 Self-Management: Hypertension 1608 Symptom Control	1302 Coping 1634 Personal Health Screening Behavior 1908 Risk Detection 1625 Smoking Cessation Behavior 1628 Weight Maintenance Behavior
1819 Knowledge: Infant Care	1500 Parent-Infant Attachment 2211 Parenting Performance 2904 Parenting Performance: Infant 2900 Parenting Performance: Infant/Toddler Physical Safety 1901 Parenting Performance: Psychosocial Safety 1908 Risk Detection	2501 Abuse Protection 1400 Abusive Behavior Self-Restraint 1017 Bottle Feeding Performance 1001 Breastfeeding Establishment: Maternal 1019 Cup Feeding Performance 2608 Family Resiliency 1900 Immunization Behavior
1842 Knowledge: Infection Management	1623 Compliance Behavior: Prescribed Medication 1900 Immunization Behavior 1634 Personal Health Screening Behavior 1924 Risk Control: Infectious Process 1905 Risk Control: Sexually Transmitted Diseases (STD)	2800 Community Immune Status 2802 Community Risk Control: Communicable Disease 1607 Prenatal Health Behavior 1902 Risk Control 1908 Risk Detection 0313 Self-Care Status
1856 Knowledge: Inflammatory Bowel Disease Management	1632 Compliance Behavior: Prescribed Activity 1622 Compliance Behavior: Prescribed Diet 1623 Compliance Behavior: Prescribed Medication 1605 Pain Control 1608 Symptom Control	1302 Coping 1634 Personal Health Screening Behavior 1902 Risk Control 1626 Weight Gain Behavior 1628 Weight Maintenance Behavior
1857 Knowledge: Kidney Disease Management	1623 Compliance Behavior: Prescribed Medication 1622 Compliance Behavior: Prescribed Diet 1603 Health Seeking Behavior 1928 Risk Control: Hypertension 3108 Self-Management: Kidney Disease 1608 Symptom Control	1634 Personal Health Screening Behavior 1914 Risk Control: Cardiovascular Disease Risk Control: Infectious Process 1619 Self-Management: Diabetes 3107 Self-Management: Hypertension 3109 Self-Management: Lipid Disorder
1817 Knowledge: Labor & Delivery	2605 Family Participation in Professional Care 1608 Symptom Control	1302 Coping 0002 Energy Conservation 1605 Pain Control 1928 Risk Control: Hypertension
1858 Knowledge: Lipid Disorder Management	1632 Compliance Behavior: Prescribed Activity 1622 Compliance Behavior: Prescribed Diet 1623 Compliance Behavior: Prescribed Medication 1608 Symptom Control	1634 Personal Health Screening Behavior 1914 Risk Control: Cardiovascular Disease 1928 Risk Control: Hypertension 1931 Risk Control: Stroke 1908 Risk Detection 1628 Weight Maintenance Behavior

Continued

Table 1-5	NOC Performance Outcomes Related to NOC Knowledge Outcomes—cont'd	

Knowledge Outcomes	Primary Behavioral Outcomes	Secondary Behavioral Outcomes
1808 Knowledge: Medication	2205 Caregiver Performance: Direct Care 1623 Compliance Behavior: Prescribed Medication 0307 Self-Care: Non-Parenteral Medication 0309 Self-Care: Parenteral Medication	1911 Personal Safety Behavior 1908 Risk Detection 1613 Self-Direction of Care
1838 Knowledge: Multiple Sclerosis Management	1623 Compliance Behavior: Prescribed Medication 1603 Health Seeking Behavior 1631 Self-Management: Multiple Sclerosis 1608 Symptom Control	1632 Compliance Behavior: Prescribed Activity 1622 Compliance Behavior: Prescribed Diet 1909 Fall Prevention Behavior 1606 Participation in Health Care Decisions 1908 Risk Detection 0307 Self-Care: Non-Parenteral Medication 0313 Self-Care Status
1859 Knowledge: Osteoporosis Management	1623 Compliance Behavior: Prescribed Medication 1305 Psychosocial Adjustment: Life Change	1909 Fall Prevention Behavior 1902 Risk Control 1908 Risk Detection
1829 Knowledge: Ostomy Care	1615 Ostomy Self-Care 1305 Psychosocial Adjustment: Life Change 1608 Symptom Control	1908 Risk Detection 0305 Self-Care: Hygiene
1843 Knowledge: Pain Management	1623 Compliance Behavior: Prescribed Medication 1618 Nausea & Vomiting Control 1605 Pain Control 1608 Symptom Control	1302 Coping 1606 Participation in Health Care Decisions 1902 Risk Control 0307 Self-Care: Non-Parenteral Medication 0309 Self-Care: Parenteral Medication
1826 Knowledge: Parenting	1500 Parent-Infant Attachment 2211 Parenting Performance 2904 Parenting Performance: Infant 2903 Parenting Performance: Adolescent 2902 Parenting Performance: Adolescent Physical Safety 2905 Parenting Performance: Middle Childhood 2906 Parenting Performance: Preschooler 2907 Parenting Performance: Toddler 2901 Parenting Performance: Early/Middle Childhood Physical Safety 2900 Parenting Performance: Infant/Toddler Physical Safety 1901 Parenting Performance: Psychosocial Safety	2501 Abuse Protection 1017 Bottle Feeding Performance 1001 Breastfeeding Establishment: Maternal 1019 Cup Feeding Performance 2602 Family Functioning 2605 Family Participation in Professional Care 2608 Family Resiliency 2610 Family Risk Control: Obesity 0116 Play Participation 1501 Role Performance
1860 Knowledge: Peripheral Artery Disease Management	1623 Compliance Behavior: Prescribed Medication 1632 Compliance Behavior: Prescribed Activity 1605 Pain Control 1305 Psychosocial Adjustment: Life Change	1902 Risk Control 1906 Risk Control: Tobacco Use 1908 Risk Detection 0313 Self-Care Status
1809 Knowledge: Personal Safety	1909 Fall Prevention Behavior 1911 Personal Safety Behavior	1616 Body Mechanics Performance 1405 Impulse Self-Control 1902 Risk Control 1903 Risk Control: Alcohol Use 1904 Risk Control: Drug Use 1922 Risk Control: Hyperthermia 1923 Risk Control: Hypothermia 1908 Risk Detection

Table 1-5	NOC PERFORMANCE OUTCOMES RELATED TO NOC KNOWLEDGE OUTCOMES—cont'd	
Knowledge Outcomes	**Primary Behavioral Outcomes**	**Secondary Behavioral Outcomes**
1861 Knowledge: Pneumonia Management	1623 Compliance Behavior: Prescribed Medication 1605 Pain Control 1608 Symptom Control	0002 Energy Conservation 1902 Risk Control 1906 Risk Control: Tobacco Use 0313 Self-Care Status
1818 Knowledge: Postpartum Maternal Health	1302 Coping 1605 Pain Control 1624 Postpartum Maternal Health Behavior 1305 Psychosocial Adjustment: Life Change	1001 Breastfeeding Establishment: Maternal 0002 Energy Conservation 2605 Family Participation in Professional Care 1907 Risk Control: Unintended Pregnancy 1908 Risk Detection
1822 Knowledge: Preconception Maternal Health	1602 Health Promoting Behavior 1607 Prenatal Health Behavior	1911 Personal Safety Behavior 1905 Risk Control: Sexually Transmitted Diseases (STD) 1908 Risk Detection 1628 Weight Maintenance Behavior
1810 Knowledge: Pregnancy	1602 Health Promoting Behavior 1607 Prenatal Health Behavior 1903 Risk Control: Alcohol Use 1904 Risk Control: Drug Use 1906 Risk Control: Tobacco Use	2501 Abuse Protection 1616 Body Mechanics Performance 1622 Compliance Behavior: Prescribed Diet 0002 Energy Conservation 1618 Nausea & Vomiting Control 1902 Risk Control 1908 Risk Detection 1628 Weight Maintenance Behavior
1839 Knowledge: Pregnancy & Postpartum Sexual Functioning	1624 Postpartum Maternal Health Behavior 1907 Risk Control: Unintended Pregnancy	2501 Abuse Protection 1607 Prenatal Health Behavior 1602 Health Promoting Behavior 1905 Risk Control: Sexually Transmitted Diseases (STD) 0119 Sexual Functioning
1811 Knowledge: Prescribed Activity	0200 Ambulation 1632 Compliance Behavior: Prescribed Activity 1633 Exercise Participation	1308 Adaptation to Physical Disability 0200 Ambulation 0201 Ambulation: Wheelchair 1616 Body Mechanics Performance 1602 Health Promoting Behavior 1908 Risk Detection 1607 Prenatal Health Behavior
1802 Knowledge: Prescribed Diet	1622 Compliance Behavior: Prescribed Diet 1626 Weight Gain Behavior 1627 Weight Loss Behavior 1628 Weight Maintenance Behavior	1603 Health Seeking Behavior 1607 Prenatal Health Behavior
1840 Knowledge: Preterm Infant Care	1302 Coping 1500 Parent-Infant Attachment 2211 Parenting Performance 2605 Family Participation in Professional Care	2202 Caregiver Home Care Readiness 2205 Caregiver Performance: Direct Care 2206 Caregiver Performance: Indirect Care 1305 Psychosocial Adjustment: Life Change 1908 Risk Detection

Continued

Table 1-5	NOC PERFORMANCE OUTCOMES RELATED TO NOC KNOWLEDGE OUTCOMES—cont'd	

Knowledge Outcomes	Primary Behavioral Outcomes	Secondary Behavioral Outcomes
1815 Knowledge: Sexual Functioning	0119 Sexual Functioning	1602 Health Promoting Behavior 1905 Risk Control: Sexually Transmitted Diseases (STD) 1907 Risk Control: Unintended Pregnancy
1862 Knowledge: Stress Management	1302 Coping 2013 Lifestyle Balance 1305 Psychosocial Adjustment: Life Change 1613 Self-Direction of Care	1602 Health Promoting Behavior 1634 Personal Health Screening Behavior 1635 Personal Time Management 1902 Risk Control 1908 Risk Detection
1863 Knowledge: Stroke Management	1308 Adaptation to Physical Disability 1632 Compliance Behavior: Prescribed Activity 1622 Compliance Behavior: Prescribed Diet 1623 Compliance Behavior: Prescribed Medication 0918 Heedfulness of Affected Side	0200 Ambulation 1633 Exercise Participation 1602 Health Promoting Behavior 1931 Risk Control: Stroke 1932 Risk Control: Thrombus 1906 Risk Control: Tobacco Use 1908 Risk Detection 0313 Self-Care Status
1864 Knowledge: Stroke Prevention	1622 Compliance Behavior: Prescribed Diet 1623 Compliance Behavior: Prescribed Medication 1928 Risk Control: Hypertension 1931 Risk Control: Stroke 3107 Self-Management: Hypertension 3109 Self-Management: Lipid Disorder	1602 Health Promoting Behavior 1906 Risk Control: Tobacco Use 1908 Risk Detection
1812 Knowledge: Substance Use Control	1903 Risk Control: Alcohol Use 1904 Risk Control: Drug Use 1906 Risk Control: Tobacco Use	1602 Health Promoting Behavior 1405 Impulse Self-Control 1911 Personal Safety Behavior 1908 Risk Detection
1865 Knowledge: Thrombus Prevention	1632 Compliance Behavior: Prescribed Activity 1623 Compliance Behavior: Prescribed Medication	0200 Ambulation 1602 Health Promoting Behavior 1932 Risk Control: Thrombus 1908 Risk Detection
1866 Knowledge: Time Management	1635 Personal Time Management 1613 Self-Direction of Care	1302 Coping 1602 Health Promoting Behavior
1814 Knowledge: Treatment Procedure	2205 Caregiver Performance: Direct Care 1921 Pre-Procedure Readiness 1613 Self-Direction of Care	1918 Aspiration Prevention 2609 Family Support During Treatment 1615 Ostomy Self-Care 1908 Risk Detection
1813 Knowledge: Treatment Regimen	2205 Caregiver Performance: Direct Care 1632 Compliance Behavior: Prescribed Activity 1622 Compliance Behavior: Prescribed Diet 1623 Compliance Behavior: Prescribed Medication 1605 Pain Control 0309 Self-Care: Parenteral Medication 1613 Self-Direction of Care 3100 Self Management: Acute Illness 3102 Self Management: Chronic Disease 1608 Symptom Control	1308 Adaptation to Physical Disability 2206 Caregiver Performance: Indirect Care 1908 Risk Detection 0704 Self-Management: Asthma 1617 Self-Management: Cardiac Disease 3103 Self-Management: Chronic Obstructive Pulmonary Disease 1619 Self-Management: Diabetes 3106 Self-Management: Heart Failure 3107 Self-Management: Hypertension 3109 Self-Management: Lipid Disorder 1631 Self-Management: Multiple Sclerosis

Table 1-5	NOC Performance Outcomes Related to NOC Knowledge Outcomes—cont'd	

Knowledge Outcomes	Primary Behavioral Outcomes	Secondary Behavioral Outcomes
1841 Knowledge: Weight Management	1632 Compliance Behavior: Prescribed Activity 1622 Compliance Behavior: Prescribed Diet 1626 Weight Gain Behavior 1627 Weight Loss Behavior 1628 Weight Maintenance Behavior 1633 Exercise Participation	2809 Community Risk Control: Obesity 2610 Family Risk Control: Obesity 1602 Health Promoting Behavior 1908 Risk Detection

SUMMARY

This chapter provided an overview of the current outcomes classification and changes made to this edition based on current work. Common questions about NOC were posed and answered. This edition added 107 new outcomes. A classification of nursing-sensitive patient, family, and community level outcomes will never be complete but will continue to expand and improve with further knowledge of the discipline and testing in practice. Readers and users of the classification are encouraged to provide feedback to the editors of NOC.

Although there is increasing interest in outcomes management, quality assessment and improvement, and effectiveness research, nursing remains largely invisible in large data sets, and little nursing effectiveness research is being conducted. Those nursing studies completed often are done in a single health care system, and most are not reported. The use of NOC provides data so that contributions made by the nursing profession to health care are documented and made visible. The health care organizations that adopt NOC are able to demonstrate nursing's accountability and contributions to health care and are able to compare the achievement of outcomes of care across time and settings. Use of NOC over the last decade has demonstrated that nurses can make dramatic improvements in outcomes in a short period of time. With shorter lengths of stay in acute care institutions, it is critical that nurses choose interventions that are effective in improving outcomes. Nurses also need to identify ineffective or poorly timed interventions in current practice. Nurses need to identify outcomes that are essential to care delivery and key outcomes for specialty practice. Organizations beyond acute care hospitals should use outcomes in evaluating the care provided as the ability to evaluate NOC outcomes across settings is one of its strengths.

Classification work of this kind is essential to the future of the profession. All nurses can join in the effort to include standardized nursing languages in all clinical information systems so that nursing data will be available in large local, national, and international data sets. Our colleagues are invited to assist with further testing of the psychometric integrity and clinical usefulness of the NOC outcomes. Research by nurse scientists, clinicians, and graduate students that is published and shared with the NOC research team will greatly advance the nursing profession and benefit the clients that nurses serve. Armed with data that demonstrate nursing effectiveness, nurses will influence health policy to optimally benefit the individuals, families, and communities to whom they provide care.

References

1. Bulechek, G., Butcher, H., Dochterman, J., & Wagner, C. (Eds.). (2013). *Nursing interventions classification (NIC)* (6th ed.). St. Louis: Elsevier.
2. Herdman, T. H. (Ed.). (2012). *NANDA International nursing diagnoses: Definitions & classification 2012-2014*. Oxford: Wiley-Blackwell.
3. Johnson, M., Bulechek, G., Butcher, H., Maas, M., McCloskey Dochterman, J., Moorhead, S., & Swanson, E. (2006). *NANDA, NOC, and NIC linkages: Nursing diagnoses, outcomes and interventions* (2nd ed.). St. Louis: Mosby.
4. Johnson, M., Moorhead, S., Bulechek, G., Butcher, H., Maas, M., & Swanson, E. (2012). *NOC and NIC linkages to NANDA-I and clinical conditions: Supporting critical reasoning and quality care* (3rd ed.). St. Louis: Elsevier Mosby.
5. McCloskey, J., & Bulechek, G. (1994). Standardizing the language for nursing treatments: An overview of the issues. *Nursing Outlook, 42*(2), 56–63.
6. Pesut, D. J., & Herman, J. (1999). *Clinical reasoning: The art & science of critical & creative thinking*. Albany, NY: Delmar.
7. Werley, H. H., & Devine, E. C. (1987). The Nursing Minimum Data Set: Status and implications. In K. J. Hanna, M. Reimer, W. C. Mills, & S. Letourneau (Eds.), *Clinical judgment and decision-making: The future of nursing diagnosis* (pp. 540–551). New York: John Wiley.
8. Werley, H. H., & Lang, N. M. (Eds.). (1988). *Identification of the Nursing Minimum Data Set*. New York: Springer.

CHAPTER TWO

Using NOC in Clinical, Research, and Educational Settings

The value of using the Nursing Outcomes Classification (NOC) and other standardized languages is based on the contribution they make to delineate professional nursing practice.[14] To be successful in implementing NOC, strong leadership, administrative commitment, detailed planning, and educational sessions are required. Organizational leaders and staff need to be educated about the importance of using standardized languages for nursing practice. In addition, it is critical that persons working with NOC in clinical practice, research, and education possess knowledge of the taxonomic structure and the outcome labels, definitions, indicators, scales, and methods to rate patient outcomes. This knowledge of the components of the classification will be extremely helpful in addressing application issues and questions that arise.

Standardized outcomes are important for evaluating the effectiveness of nursing interventions, facilitating the continuity of care in integrated health systems, and assuring nursing accountability.[30] In addition, The Institute of Medicine (IOM) report (2010) *The Future of Nursing: Leading Change, Advancing Health*[12] reinforces the importance of nursing and the value of using outcomes to improve patient care in health care settings. The strengths of using a standardized outcomes classification such as NOC need to be communicated to nursing staff and reinforced by organizational leaders. The recognition of the importance of outcomes by the IOM requires sound measurement, tracking of patient outcomes, and delineation of the critical impact nursing has on patient care.[12] It is time for the nursing profession to truly embrace the evaluation of care using standardized outcomes.

CONSIDERATIONS WHEN USING NOC IN PRACTICE

Evaluating the effectiveness of nursing care requires outcomes focused on patient status that can measure both short-term changes following an intervention or episode of care and long-term changes over the course of an illness or disease. NOC was developed to measure both levels of change in patient status. Outcomes were developed for nursing, but other health professionals, including interdisciplinary teams, have found them useful for evaluating the effectiveness of their interventions.

Selecting Outcomes

Selecting patient outcomes for a particular patient or a group of patients is one step in the nurse's clinical decision-making process. The use of standardized terms and measures to evaluate outcomes does not decrease the nurse's responsibility to make an informed assessment and engage in clinical reasoning; selected factors are paramount in the choice of patient outcomes. These factors are (1) the type of health problem, (2) the nursing or medical diagnoses, (3) patient characteristics, (4) available resources, (5) patient preferences, and (6) treatment potential.[1,16]

Type of Health Problem

Health concerns can be categorized as (1) problems for referral that are addressed primarily by other health providers, (2) interdisciplinary problems that are addressed collaboratively with other providers, and (3) nursing diagnoses for which nurses have primary responsibility.[11] When the health concern falls in the first category, the primary responsibility for identifying the desired outcome will usually reside with the responsible health provider. When the health concern falls under the second category, nurses and other responsible providers should work together to identify the outcomes. When the health concern is a nursing diagnosis, nurses should assume primary responsibility for identifying patient outcomes related to the diagnosis. In all three cases the provider of care should include the patient in the decision-making process.

Nursing Diagnosis or Medical Diagnosis

It is important to consider all health-related diagnoses when nurses select an outcome, but many of the outcomes directly relate to an identified nursing diagnosis. When using NANDA International (NANDA-I) diagnoses, consideration in selecting outcomes should be given to the diagnosis definition, the defining characteristics, and related factors or the risk factors for a risk diagnosis. For example, *Activity Intolerance* is defined as "Insufficient physiological or psychological energy to endure or complete required or desired daily activities" (p. 231).[11] Based on this definition, nurses might select *Activity Tolerance, Endurance, Psychomotor Energy,* or *Self-Care Status* as outcomes. In the NOC outcomes, *Activity Tolerance* and *Endurance* are related to insufficient physiological energy while *Psychomotor Energy* is related to insufficient psychological energy. When considering the defining characteristics (e.g., blood pressure, cardiac response to activity, dyspnea, or fatigue) of the same diagnosis, the outcomes *Vital Signs* or *Cardiopulmonary*

Status might be selected. These could serve as intermediate outcome measures to signify improvement in the outcome *Activity Tolerance* over time.

When outcome selection is based on the medical diagnoses, nurses should consider the signs and symptoms of the medical diagnosis as well as the causative and other related factors. For example, if the medical diagnosis is Diabetes Mellitus, blood glucose control is critical, and a nurse may select a specific NOC outcome such as *Blood Glucose Level*. Another example is the symptom of pulmonary edema associated with the medical diagnosis of Congestive Heart Failure; appropriate NOC outcomes may be *Cardiac Pump Effectiveness*, *Fluid Overload Severity*, or *Respiratory Status*. Part Four contains a list of outcomes commonly associated with each NANDA-I nursing diagnosis based primarily on expert opinion.

Patient Characteristics

Patient characteristics to be considered include demographic factors, psychological and cognitive processes, illness and health-related factors, and personal health beliefs or values. A few examples will be provided but are not intended to be all-inclusive. First, in considering demographic factors, the child and adult development NOCs are age-specific while others such as *Self-Management: Cardiac Disease* may not be appropriate for children due to the focus of self-care of the disease state. Age and gender are both relevant in *Breastfeeding Establishment: Maternal* since this outcome is obviously for females of childbearing age. Race and ethnicity relate to one's predisposition and response to illness and indicate cultural beliefs. All of these factors may affect the acceptance of outcomes by the patient or family. Education level is important when selecting outcomes related to knowledge and participation in health care.

Psychological and cognitive variables such as depression or anxiety and processes such as concentration, memory, information processing, and decision-making can influence the patient's response to illness, ability to learn, and motivation, and they need to be considered. Knowledge outcomes should not be selected for the patient who has short-term memory loss or the inability to process information while *Anxiety Self-Control* may be the most important outcome for the severely anxious patient.

Illness or health-related variables such as initial severity of illness have a strong influence on outcome selection. For example, *Mobility* is generally not selected for a terminally ill patient while *Comfortable Death* would be quite appropriate. Functional status and ability to perform activities of daily living also influence outcome selection. While *Ambulation* is not an appropriate outcome for the quadriplegic patient, *Transfer Performance* may be a significant outcome.

Available Resources

All available resources that influence patient outcomes need to be considered. These can be financial, social, family, and health resources that influence lifestyle, living conditions, and access to health care. These resources can influence outcome achievement negatively or positively or limit outcomes that are selected in some cases. For example, improvement in *Compliance Behavior* or *Self-Management: Diabetes* is not likely to occur if patients do not have the financial resources to purchase the medications, equipment, or food required to manage the disease. Social factors include social support, social relationships, and the availability of someone to assist the patient as needed. *Loneliness Severity* or *Caregiver Performance: Direct Care* may be important outcomes if social support is absent or if a caregiver needs to learn multiple procedures and activities to provide care in the home.

Patient Preferences

Preferences are influenced by the patient's personal perceptions of health, desired health goals and preferences in relation to treatment, religious and cultural beliefs. If patients believe their health is satisfactory, they may be less inclined to accept outcomes aimed at measuring improvements in overall health such as *Physical Fitness*. If patients are unable to accept emotional or psychological diagnoses because of their religious or cultural beliefs, they are not likely to find outcomes such as *Mood Equilibrium* or *Depression Level* acceptable. Patients should collaborate on selecting the outcome and participate in determining how much change they want to achieve. It may become very important for nurses to assist patients in identifying realistic outcome scores. For example, the nurse may have to set realistic expectations for a patient with pulmonary emphysema who wants to achieve a "5" (no deviation) on the outcome *Respiratory Status: Ventilation* when it may be physiologically impossible.

Treatment Potential

When considering this factor, the first step is to determine if an intervention exists to achieve a designated outcome. If the diagnosis for a patient with Alzheimer's disease is *Chronic Confusion*, nursing interventions may be able to assist patients to maintain their current cognitive status for a period of time, but even with these interventions, an eventual cognitive decline can be expected. When further decline occurs, nurses would likely select outcomes related to nutrition, safety, and hygiene in lieu of cognitive outcomes. Secondly, one must consider whether the nursing personnel required to implement the intervention are available. For example, teaching patients and their families requires a professional nurse possessing appropriate knowledge and skills if a knowledge outcome is selected. The *Nursing Interventions Classification*

(NIC)[4,5] includes nursing interventions and recommendations for the level of nursing personnel to provide the intervention.

After Outcome Selection

Once a problem has been established and an appropriate outcome or set of outcomes is identified, the nurse further identifies how the outcomes will be used to facilitate and evaluate the care of the patient for each problem.

Using the Outcome Indicators

After selecting the outcomes for an individual patient, nurses select the indicators that will be used to determine patient status and the overall outcome rating. To increase the ease of use of NOC on patient care units, nursing staff as a group may designate important indicators they view as representative of the outcome concept and relevant to their patient population prior to implementation of NOC. Upon completing this review, some users have selected four to seven indicators of each outcome to determine patient status while other users select more indicators. In both situations the selected indicators can be used to determine the patient status for the outcome. With the indicators selected, the nurses evaluate the indicators and outcome on the accompanying measurement scale.

Selecting Additional Information

After outcomes and/or indicators have been identified, the nursing staff collects additional information from the care recipient, and other data sources are identified. The care recipient can be the patient, caregiver, parent (mother, father, or both), family, or community, and the source of the data can be the patient, a family member, a caregiver, the direct observation by a health care provider, or the clinical record. The source of data to evaluate the indicators and the outcome will vary. Data may be obtained from the patient record (e.g., biochemical measures or vital signs) or from direct observation or physical assessments (e.g., a patient's ability to carry out treatments or the presence of certain signs and symptoms). Other indicators may require soliciting information or perceptions from the patient or family (e.g., knowledge about the disease process or treatment, perceptions of health, and satisfaction with care). Providers may wish to identify additional care recipients or data sources unique to their practice or situation and include that information in the documentation.

Using the Measurement Scales

Currently outcomes have one or two scales used to measure the outcome, and selected indicators are evaluated using these scales. It is critical to use the measurement scales published with their respective outcome as the scales have been chosen to semantically align with the outcome and

indicators. In addition, each of the indicators has been reviewed in conjunction with the scales to ensure that data reflective of the indicator can be collected using the measurement scale. For example, the behavior outcomes measurement scale is based on the demonstration scale to enable the nurses to actually evaluate the behavior of patients in meeting the outcome. A scale based on the "severe to none" scale would be difficult and ineffective in measuring the behavior of patients.

In each 5-point scale "1" is the "least desirable" and "5" is the "most desirable" patient condition on the outcome. Nurses can make a judgment about the outcome rating on the measurement scale for patients without using the indicators; however, most nurses find selected indicators helpful for evaluating the patient status on the measurement scale. When rating the indicators of the outcome, nurses evaluate the indicators by comparing the patient's current status on each indicator to the indicator status of a healthy individual of the same age and gender. When using a healthy person, that individual's score will result in the rating of a "5," the most desirable condition on the indicator. This comparison to a healthy individual or "reference person" assists nurses to determine the patient's rating for those indicators and the overall outcome. If an indicator selected for the patient population is not applicable to the patient, the Not Applicable or "NA" column can be checked and is not included in the evaluation. With experience using NOC, it may not be necessary to rate the patient status on each indicator because nurses will automatically consider the most important indicators to determine the patient's outcome rating; however, it must be recognized that valuable indicator data reflecting the patient's status will be lost when indicator ratings on the measurement scale are not retained. Outcomes focused on the patient's perceptions are always rated by the patient (e.g. *Nausea and Vomiting Severity, Fatigue Level, Client Satisfaction: Physical Care,* and *Quality of Life*).

Establishing an Outcome Rating

The indicator ratings provide the evidence to assist in determining the patient's overall rating on the outcome although indicators currently are not weighted to provide a mean or summated rating. It is recommended that practitioners use both the range of scores on the indicators (i.e., 1-5) and the frequency of scores of indicator ratings as an aid in arriving at the overall outcome rating. In general, ratings on the scale of "1" and "2" on important indicators will mean that the patient has a "1" or "2" rating on the outcome. For example, Patient Q had indicator ratings of 1s and 2s on all of the indicators of the outcome *Activity Tolerance*. This evaluation would suggest that *Activity Tolerance* should be rated overall as "severely compromised" since a number of the indicators are rated as severely compromised. Data from

Patient M may present a different situation. In this scenario the selected indicators range from "severely compromised" on the single indicator *ability to speak with physical activity* to "mildly compromised" and "not compromised" for all the remaining indicators. Since one indicator is "severely compromised" and is not consistent with the rating of the other indicators, the nurse may want to determine if the "severely compromised" rating is correct. Specifically, does this patient rating on this indicator occur only with intense activity? If the patient is having difficulty only with intense activity, the nurse may rate the patient as "mildly compromised" on the outcome instead of "severely compromised." If this is a new symptom and occurs with minimal activity, the nurse may adjust the indicator and outcome rating to "moderately compromised."

Using the Outcome Rating to Evaluate Care

Once the initial rating of the patient on the outcome and indicators is completed prior to the implementation of care, the target outcome rating to be achieved is determined with the patient and/or family members when possible. For example, initially a patient may have "extremely compromised" *Endurance* because of a condition such as congestive heart failure (CHF) or pneumonia, and the nurse in discussion with the patient may arrive at a post-treatment target outcome rating of "moderately compromised" or "slightly compromised." This rating may be very achievable by implementing care and controlling (CHF) or eliminating (pneumonia) the condition(s). In a different scenario a patient may enter the care situation with the outcome *Endurance* rated as "substantially compromised" and want to be at a post-treatment target rating of "slightly compromised." This may be very unrealistic as a target rating since the medical origin of the decreased endurance (e.g., myocardial myopathy) cannot be eliminated. With this patient the target rating of the outcome may be to maintain the rating of "substantially compromised" for as long as possible. In both of these care situations, the overall target rating of the outcome enables nurses to indicate either increased capacity or maintenance of the patient's functioning. In either case the effectiveness of the nursing care provided has been demonstrated and documented through the use of ratings on the outcomes.

Using the Outcomes to Evaluate Care in Short-Term Stays

The outcomes within NOC are variable concepts and can be measured along a continuum. Even in situations where patients do not have the opportunity to achieve the designated outcome associated with a complete recovery due to shortened hospital stays, outcomes can be individualized for each patient while maintaining standardized outcome language and measures. The use of intermediate outcomes along the continuum of the outcome concept enables nurses to use outcomes to document improvement in the patients' statuses even when it is not possible for patients to achieve the most desirable outcome. For example, the patient may have a NANDA-I diagnosis of *Insomnia*, and the outcome that would measure the resolution of the diagnosis is *Sleep*. The patient may not be able to achieve that desired outcome; thus, intermediate outcomes of *Discomfort Level*, *Depression Level*, or *Comfort Status: Environment* may be used and measured to enable nurses to determine the impact of the nursing interventions implemented.

Using the Indicator Rating to Evaluate Care

While it is the expectation that outcomes be used to measure the impact interventions have on patient status in care situations, the use of specific indicators may be more appropriate. If an indicator is considered an important measure of patient progress, nurses may choose to collect data on a particular indicator and on the outcome overall rating at designated points in care. An example may be selected indicators of the outcome *Social Involvement*. The individual may have an initial outcome rating of "2" and "3" on all of the indicators of the outcome, but upon receiving nursing interventions of *Mood Management* or *Therapy Group*, some subtle changes may occur. The individual experiencing depression on evaluation may demonstrate changes in the rating of the designated indicator of "Interacts with close friends" or "Interacts with family members" with an increase in the rating to a "3" on both indicators when the rating previously was a "2." If the individual indicators had not been reviewed and measured, these changes would not have been identified due to the negligible impact these changes had on the rating of the entire outcome. This approach may be very appropriate for patients with short episodes of care, patients of a unique population, or treatments over extended periods of time with no progress in relation to the outcome. It is also a viable approach to examine the individual indicators before discontinuing selected interventions and initiating new interventions. Critical to this evaluative process is what Jones and colleagues[14] identify as a unique benefit of using NOC outcomes, that both the patient and nurses can evaluate the impact of the interventions.

Timing of the rating of the patient status on the selected outcomes and indicators is completed as a baseline measure or during the nurses' first contact with the patient, and the outcome should be rated when care is completed (i.e., the discharge measure). This may be sufficient in acute care settings if the patient has a short stay; however, some acute care settings have chosen to evaluate patient status once a day or once a shift depending on how rapidly changes in the outcome status are expected. The frequency of the evaluation may differ for a variety of reasons (e.g., acuity level of the patient, therapeutic response of the intervention, or the length of time in care setting). Community agencies may elect to evaluate patient status at each visit or at every other visit if the patient is seen frequently.[30] Measurement times are not standardized, so it is important for making comparisons between populations and among units to report the date and time when measures were obtained. This information will support recommended time intervals for the various outcomes and for varied patient populations.

It is crucial that nurses have a minimum of two outcome ratings to determine if change in the outcome has occurred and to what level or degree it has occurred. As was mentioned previously, this type of data will be valuable in evaluating how nursing interventions, other aspects of the patient's care, and the patient characteristics affect outcome achievement. If the desired change is not occurring in patients, data will allow nurses to determine what differences exist between those who achieve the outcome target rating and those who do not. In addition, it enables nurses to identify if the type of intervention or care program needs to be or can be changed. If it is a patient characteristic that cannot be changed, such as age, gender, or initial severity of illness, then the target rating of the outcome may need reevaluation and adjustment.

Using the Measurement Scales

As previously discussed, the scales are rated on a 1- to 5-point scale. The indicators have been provided to assist nurses in determining the patient's status and to serve as evidence for the outcome rating, but the presence of the indicators does not eliminate the need for a nursing judgment. Because the scale anchors are not specifically defined for each indicator and outcome, the nurse must make a nursing judgment about the patient status for the indicators used and for the overall outcome. Although the accuracy of this judgment becomes more important when assigning the target rating, it requires the same judgment process when determining if the patient has achieved a "5" on the rating of the outcome. To assist the nursing staff, some organizations have elected to provide more specific anchors for each of the outcome ratings used in the respective facilities. Examples of this work are documented in the fourth edition of NOC.[21] This approach is especially useful when using the outcomes in a standard plan, when the number of outcomes is limited for a particular population, or in a research study.

The NOC outcome also can be used in conjunction with published measurement scales. The scales could be used for assessment purposes to identify nursing problems or diagnoses, and the NOC outcomes can be chosen to measure the impact of the interventions. For an example, there are recognized patient assessment tools to assess pain, neurological status, pedal pulses, and edema or to grade pressure ulcers and burns. These scales tend to measure a more specific or limited concept while the NOC outcome may be at a more abstract level, but it will be critical in this exercise to ensure that the concepts of both the published measurement scales and the NOC are conceptually aligned with one another. Another recommendation would be that users determine what they want to measure and if the published measurement scale serves their need more appropriately; they may elect to use that scale instead of a NOC outcome. For example, the 10-point pain scale that measures the patient's report of pain may be more appropriate for the practice situation than using the NOC outcome *Pain Level*, particularly if the patient's verbal report of pain is the only measure desired.

While the process described for using the outcomes in practice is important, the processes associated with preparing to implement NOC in a clinical setting and in an electronic patient record are equally important. With a shrinking workforce, increased requirements for documentation, higher patient acuity, and concerns over patient safety, administrators need tools or strategies to meet these challenges.[12,22] The next section gives a brief overview of these aspects of implementation.

Implementing NOC in Clinical Settings

Organizational leaders and staff may need to be educated about the importance of using standardized languages for nursing practice. A key person or "champion" is one who is committed to the project and able to articulate the advantages of using standardized languages. This person needs to be responsible for the planning as well as the implementation process. The nurse in charge of nursing informatics or outcome management is often one of the persons most appropriate for this role.

In addition, the "champion" staff members who use NOC need to be identified and educated about the classification. Education of the staff is one of the most important factors for the successful implementation of NOC, and it should include the process for using NOC outcomes and the issues and concerns that arise as nurses begin to use them. Staff should not have to become familiar with the use of NOC and a new computer system at the same time. If an organization is going to select a new computer system, the time used for evaluation and selection of the system should be used to orient nurses to using NOC outcomes and to piloting written forms.

Implementation Planning

A set of representatives from key areas and pilot units should be established to assist the "champions" with the implementation process. The representatives can assist with the development of the plan and with staff education during the implementation process. Components of the plan include goals, timelines, evaluation plans, and cost projections. The implementation plan for the respective units should include at least the following considerations: (1) Which patient populations or designated units are part of the implementation? (2) Who are the nurses to be involved? (3) How is the data source and care recipient to be identified? (4) What are the selected outcomes, and how many will be evaluated? (5) Are four to seven specific indicators chosen for each outcome, or will all indicators be considered relevant? (6) What are the most critical indicators to be used for each outcome? (7) How are the target ratings determined for each patient? (8) Will the outcome ratings be measured at admission and discharge only or also at critical stages of the patients' stays? (9) How are the outcomes, indicators, and ratings incorporated into the care planning document? (10) How are the ratings to evaluate the outcomes documented within the record of the patients? (11) Will the care plan incorporate timing reminders for evaluating the rating on the outcomes? (12) Will the care plan collect linked data on the nursing diagnoses, interventions, and outcomes that have been used in the care? (13) Will paper documentation forms be needed to implement NOC, when will they be used in the process, how will they be tested, and how will the forms be incorporated in the patients' records?

Once these questions are addressed, the educational programs can be designed to build clinician competency in the use of NANDA-I, NOC, and NIC (NNN) among the nurses with limited knowledge of standardized language. Lunney[20] offers different educational strategies in the intellectual, interpersonal, and technical domains to enhance the expertise of nurses at varying levels to acquire the needed knowledge of NNN for the implementation of the electronic health record. Another resource is a detailed example of an educational strategy for NANDA-I, NOC, and NIC presented by Keenan, Falan, Heath, and Treder.[17] The authors encourage the reader to refer to both of these articles for assistance in developing their own unique educational programs.

Planning should include the identification of other data that need to be collected in conjunction with the outcome data for clinical and administrative analyses. For example, patient characteristics, staff mix, nursing costs, nursing diagnoses, and interventions may need to be linked with outcome data to answer clinical and administrative questions. During this phase the ability or inability of the electronic information system to link patient outcomes with other data should be evaluated, and plans to establish the necessary linkages to other databases should be developed if needed.

IMPLEMENTING NOC IN ELECTRONIC SYSTEMS

There is increased recognition in clinical settings that standardized languages are a necessary component for the implementation of electronic health records (EHR). The use of these languages can lead to improved decision-making, improved documentation, and more accurate measurement of outcomes that impact care.[14] Without standardization, however, information within the EHR cannot be identified, analyzed, or compared to assess whether patient care meets the standards of quality-based care. This is what is currently being defined as meaningful use.[6,23]

Analyzing data requires that the system be developed in such a way that the information and linkages are available to answer the questions posed. One way to begin is by determining what such a system should do. An important step for nursing is to determine the data sets that are needed, the elements of the data sets, and the types of linkages nurses want among the data sets.[6] Data sets that are of interest to nursing include clinical data sets, provider data sets, fiscal data sets, and utilization data sets. Nurses involved in the development of the electronic nursing system should know the data sets available in the organization and whether the sets can be linked with nursing data. The system should contain information about the patient necessary for nursing practice and the relevant nursing diagnoses, interventions, and outcomes. Nurses need to give careful consideration to the type of information they want retained. If NANDA-I diagnoses are used, retaining information about the defining characteristics and related factors or risk factors will increase the types of analyses that can be done. Likewise, obtaining information about the outcomes, such as indicators selected and the data source, will facilitate analysis. For the intervention adequate information to capture intensity of the activities should be maintained.[6,26] The dose and frequency of the treatment will provide information about the strength of the treatment. The time of day the treatment is administered and the staff providing the treatment can be important information when analyzing the effectiveness of interventions. Perhaps one of the most important factors to consider in the nursing data sets is how linkages between the diagnoses, interventions, and outcomes will be provided.

While many of the questions about patient care that clinical nurses want answered require links among clinical databases, many of the questions that nurse administrators want answered require links among the clinical, provider, fiscal, and utilization databases. Nurses have a major opportunity to plan for data sets with the required links when new electronic systems are being put in place. Provider data sets include information about the nurse, such as age, education, and skill level, and information about the setting, such as unit size, staffing, and type of care delivery system, in addition to the type of organization. Fiscal data sets include information about costs and charges that are necessary to compute the cost of nursing and the income generated. The American Nurses Association (ANA)–recognized terminologies and data element sets include methods, content, and designated setting components for measuring many of these elements.[6,30] Utilization data sets are available in most organizations that provide health care services; they are measures of the care provided[6,30] and will vary with the type of organization. In hospital settings they will include patient days, hospital admissions, and discharges. In community settings they will include number of visits, number of admissions, and discharges from the service.

For standardized nursing languages such as NOC to become consistently used in nursing, they must be incorporated into nursing education and research.[20] The use of standardized languages in education is becoming more prevalent as nursing textbooks are using the languages and faculties are becoming more familiar with the languages. The validation of standardized languages and their use in nursing research are in their beginning stages, but the implementation of evidence-based practice and the electronic medical record will offer more opportunities to test the use of standardized languages in practice settings.

IMPLEMENTING NOC IN EDUCATIONAL PROGRAMS

All facets of the curriculum—the philosophy, program goals, and individual course objectives—need to reflect this commitment to the use of NOC within nursing educational programs. Frequently, one or more faculty members become interested in piloting a standardized language in a course, using the language in the course, and then encouraging its adoption throughout the curriculum. They can act as the project leaders in educating other faculty and demonstrating how course content can be adapted to include NOC and other standardized languages.

Many programs have been using NANDA-I diagnoses, thereby making it easier to incorporate Nursing Interventions Classification (NIC) and NOC. Use of NANDA-I, NIC, and NOC (NNN) as the standardized languages in a curriculum has a number of advantages. The languages can be used across all clinical settings to enhance the students' clinical thinking skills in their learning experiences. Standardized languages can be used as an organizing thread, and their use will better prepare students for the future as electronic records become routine.

Implementation Strategies

A number of strategies can be used when planning how NOC will be implemented throughout the undergraduate curriculum. In each of these steps, the decisions can be made by an individual faculty member, the faculty of a course, or the faculty as a whole. The process is all very dependent on the faculty governance of the respective department or program of nursing. One strategy assumes the implementation of NANDA-I diagnoses, NIC, and NOC and includes the following steps.

1. Determine which diagnoses are used in each course and clinical area.
2. Identify nursing diagnoses used in more than one course and those not used in any of the courses. Determine how these will be incorporated in more than one course, assigned to one course, or not included in the curriculum.
3. Select the NOC outcomes that are frequently linked to the nursing diagnoses. This can be done by using some of the linkage work or selecting the outcomes used in care plans of the facility.
4. Identify the NIC interventions to be taught in each course.
5. Remove those interventions that are not being taught in the undergraduate curriculum.
6. Match all of the interventions that will be used to one of the diagnoses and the associated outcomes. You may find some disparity, most likely some interventions that do not fit a diagnosis. Decide whether these interventions will remain in the curriculum or be deleted.

The end result should be a list of diagnoses matched to outcomes and interventions that will comprise the curriculum and reflect the goals of the program. The last step is to decide in which course each of the diagnoses and associated interventions and outcomes will be taught. This is a time-consuming strategy but preserves critical thinking and allows nursing diagnoses, outcomes, and interventions appropriate for the student level to drive the system.

Another strategy is to begin with the core interventions used by the clinical specialties[5] and to determine which of these are appropriate for the undergraduate program. These interventions can be mapped to respective courses within the curriculum, and then steps can be taken to add or eliminate some of the interventions previously taught. Upon completing this exercise, faculty members can link the selected interventions with the appropriate nursing diagnoses and patient outcomes. The end result is a practice-based curriculum incorporating the nursing languages.

Aids for Curriculum Development and Teaching

Smith and Craft-Rosenberg[28] suggest additional sources to use in educating students to gain knowledge of NANDA-I, NOC, and NIC. In addition, they identify "a Step-by-Step NNN Teaching Strategy" that could be adopted by nursing faculty members across the curricula. The linkages provided in this book, in the Nursing Interventions Classification book,[5] and in the linkage book[13] can assist with the process. These linkages can be used as a teaching tool when students are learning to become familiar with the languages and beginning to plan care.

USING NOC IN RESEARCH

Using NOC in research studies is a most effective method of providing the evidence needed to align nursing knowledge with quality outcomes, which truly measure the impact of the profession of nursing in patient care. "The evaluation of research to support the development, use, and continued refinement of nursing language is critical to research and the transformation of patient care by nurses on a global level (p. 286)."[14]

There are a number of reported studies that define and use nursing-sensitive patient outcomes to assess the adequacy of staffing and effects of other work environment variables, analyze adverse effects of nurses' overtime work, develop quality assessment benchmarks and databases, and measure quality and the effects of nursing interventions in specific patient populations.[2, 3, 7, 8, 9, 10, 14, 18, 19, 24, 25, 27] These studies and others illustrate intensifying interest in using patient outcomes to document the effects of nursing structures and processes. In addition, other research studies examining the impact of standardized language are presented in the work of Jones and colleagues in the chapter entitled *Standardized Nursing Languages Essential for the Nursing Workforce* in the *Annual Review of Nursing Research.*[14]

Evaluating Nursing Quality and Effectiveness

Outcomes are the triggers for the evaluation of quality and effectiveness since they answer the question "Did the patient benefit or not benefit from the care provided?"[26] It also enables nurses to address the questions of what interventions or combination of interventions are most effective in achieving desired outcomes for patients. Using outcomes in the evaluation of care enables researchers to account for the individual differences in outcome achievement attributed to patient characteristics, such as age, gender, or functional status. Determining how patient characteristics affect outcome achievement is an important area for further research; data from this type of research will provide outcomes which can be realistically achieved with varied patient populations. It is important to be able to identify an outcome that is achievable, or resources may be used and the impact patients and nurses expect will not be achieved.[16]

Clinical innovations initially are evaluated through controlled clinical studies with attention given to the measurement of desired or expected outcomes. Many clinical studies in nursing are conducted in one site and with relatively small samples; subsequently, nursing cannot demonstrate or evaluate the difference or the impact of these clinical interventions. By using outcomes and standardized language, comparable studies across settings could be conducted. Teams of researchers could develop specific research questions examining the effect of an intervention (e.g., patient education on diabetes) on patients' self-management of diabetes and define the specific data to be collected as well as the method for implementing the intervention. As a part of the team's work, research methods would need to be developed to ensure consistency in the selection of patients, in the implementation of data collection, and in the implementation of the educational programming. The outcomes of *Blood Glucose Level* and *Self-Management: Diabetes* then could be used to examine the impact of the educational intervention. Timing of the data collection on the outcomes of *Blood Glucose Level* and *Self-Management: Diabetes* also would need to be standardized across the sites. In addition, this work would also enable the researchers to examine the impact of other variables (e.g., staff mix, selected patient characteristics) on the quality of care being provided.

As the previous basic example was presented to demonstrate how outcomes could be used in a specific research project, there are many other research questions regarding the use of standardized languages such as NANDA-I, NOC, and NIC to be addressed. The following section will identify some of the research work that could advance the use of standardized languages within nursing.

Clinical evaluation and testing of NANDA-I, NOC, and NIC linkages are needed. The linkages provide a discipline-specific "conceptual roadmap" or blueprint for linking diagnoses, interventions, and outcomes that prepare nurses for the "big picture," but evidence is needed based on clinical studies to document their grounding within the profession. The linkages can be used for designing evidence-based care for patient populations or for individual patients.

The development of nursing knowledge requires evaluation of the effectiveness of various nursing interventions and the appropriateness of the decision-making process in selecting interventions to resolve a diagnosis or to achieve a particular outcome. Kautz and Van Horn[15] have clearly illustrated how NNN languages can be used in developing evidence-based practice guidelines for guiding practice and conducting research. They conclude by asserting that "the use and continued development of uniform, standardized language capture the essence of nursing practice and help advance nursing knowledge in addition to providing the appropriate framework for evidence based practice (p. 18)."

Coherence among diagnoses, interventions, and outcomes displayed as evidence-based linkages is crucial to ensuring quality improvement and safety. The linkage work contains numerous relationships that require testing and evaluation in a clinical setting. Questions about which of the suggested interventions achieve the best outcome for a particular diagnosis, which of the outcomes are most achievable for a particular patient population, and which diagnoses and interventions are associated with specific medical diagnoses are just a sample of the questions that can be addressed. Studies should also be testing the use of the outcomes and interventions with specific patient populations and add to the body of knowledge.

As well as studying the relationships between interventions and outcomes, the relationships among the environment, the structure of the health care organization, the processes of care, and patient outcomes need to be studied. Without these types of data, organizations have little information that supports the adjustment of staff mix or determination of the cost-effectiveness of structural or process changes in the nursing care delivery system. Issues related to the study of organizational factors that influence patient outcomes have gained increased emphasis in recent years.

Identification of patient factors that influence outcome attainment, referred to as risk factors, is another area that needs to be studied to carry out effectiveness research related to nursing interventions. Personal factors need to be identified to reduce or remove the effects of confounding factors in studies where the cases are not randomly assigned to different treatments, as is typical in most effectiveness research. Identification of the personal factors that influence outcome achievement for a particular diagnosis or the effectiveness of an intervention for patients with varying personal characteristics and life circumstances will add to the body of nursing knowledge and allow nurses to provide the highest quality care possible. As effectiveness research and evidence-based practice gain momentum in nursing, both organizational and personal factors that need to be considered in the analysis of data are being identified in the literature.[29]

In addition to these other examples, the rating scales for the indicators of the outcomes need to be developed more completely. An example of this work is presented by Brokel and Hoffman[3] in the refinement of indicators and the scale and subsequent retirement of an outcome label. It is critical that patients who are evaluated on an outcome present the different levels of the scale ratings of "1" through "5." For example, if the indicator for an outcome is "appears calm" and your observations after reviewing numerous charts help you to base the ratings in certain behaviors, you may come up with the following rating example:

Rating of 1: Continuous crying out, moaning, groaning, thrashing

Rating of 2: Three fourths of the day crying out, moaning, groaning, thrashing

Rating of 3: Half of the day crying out, moaning, groaning, thrashing

Rating of 4: One fourth of the day crying out, moaning, groaning, thrashing

Rating of 5: Restful, sleeping throughout the entire day[3]

With this example a large amount of patient data was used to base (or operationalize) the ratings in the behavior of the specific indicator.[3]

Other projects that need to be completed relate to these following questions: (1) Are some outcomes selected more frequently for a particular nursing diagnosis? (2) What is the difference in the selection of outcomes for a particular nursing diagnosis across settings of care? (3) How do the outcomes selected for a particular nursing diagnosis vary with patient age, gender, education, or social and economic status? (4) Are there particular interventions or combinations of nursing interventions that produce the best nursing outcomes? This type of information will be invaluable in designing protocols for novice nurses to make judgments and decisions about care. It is also important to examine the diagnoses, interventions, and outcomes linkages or selected components of the NNN that reflect the core specialty content of our colleagues in specialty areas of practice.

LICENSING NOC OUTCOMES

A license is needed to use NOC if you use it in an electronic information system or if you use more than a few outcomes in a product for commercial gain. Mosby, now a part of Elsevier, holds the copyright on NOC. Requests for permission to use or license NOC should be sent to Elsevier. The inside front cover contains information about whom to contact to use NOC or to obtain a license.

The use of NOC in an electronic system requires a license because significant portions of the book will be available to multiple users. Fees for the use of NOC in an organization's electronic system depend upon the number of users. If the user purchases a software product that uses NOC, the license fees often will be included as part of the product cost. In addition, a license is required if a significant portion of the classification in a book is used or products using portions of the book are being sold. Many requests are consistent with fair use and do not require fees. Fees are not required if the organization uses the outcomes in a paper format; however, the organization should purchase sufficient books so that it does not have to make multiple copies of the classification. Fees are generally not required for schools of nursing that want to use NOC in educational products for their own students; however, if the school is using a significant portion of NOC, it is expected that students will have the books to use with the products produced by the schools. Fees are generally not required for research using NOC, and fees for use in another publication will depend on the number of outcomes used.

SUMMARY

The use of NOC in practice, education, and research is increasing as more of the nurses, clinicians, faculty members, and scholars move toward the use of standardized languages. These are important steps for the nursing profession and will ensure that future nurses are better equipped to deal with the changes that will take place with the implementation of electronic records and electronic documentation. Research studies using NOC are beginning to appear in the literature, and it is hoped that research studies and evaluations making use of the classification will increase. It is only through research that evaluates patient outcomes related to practice that nurses will have the data required to demonstrate the quality and effectiveness of our practice. The potential and importance of the contribution that studies using NOC outcomes will make to quality health care worldwide cannot be overestimated as the electronic health record is implemented containing standardized nursing nomenclatures.

References

1. Benner, P. (2004). Designing formal classification systems to better articulate knowledge, skills, and meanings in nursing practice. *American Journal of Critical Care, 13*(3), 426–430.
2. Berney, B., & Needleman, J. (2006). Impact of nursing overtime on nurse-sensitive patient outcomes in New York hospitals. *Policy, Politics, & Nursing Practice, 7*(2), 87–100.
3. Brokel, J., & Hoffman, F. (2005). Hospice methods to measure and analyze nursing-sensitive patient outcomes. *Journal of Hospice and Palliative Nursing, 7*(1), 37–44.
4. Bulechek, G., Butcher, H., & Dochterman, J. (Eds.). (2008). *Nursing interventions classification (NIC)* (5th ed.). St. Louis: Elsevier Mosby.
5. Bulechek, G., Butcher, H., Dochterman, J., & Wagner, C. (Eds.). (2013). *Nursing interventions classification (NIC)* (6th ed.). St. Louis: Elsevier.
6. Conrad, D., & Schneider, J. (2011). Enhancing the visibility of NP practice in electronic health records. *The Journal for Nurse Practitioners, 7*(10), 832–838.
7. Deaton, C., & Grady, K. (2004). State of the science for cardiovascular nursing outcomes. *Journal of Cardiovascular Nursing, 19*(5), 329–338.
8. Fairley, D., & Closs, S. (2006). Evaluation of a nurse consultant's clinical activities and the search for patient outcomes in critical care. *Journal of Clinical Nursing, 15*(9), 1106–1114.
9. Head, B., Scherb, C., Maas, M., Swanson, E., Moorhead, S., Reed, D., Conley, D., & Kozel, M. (2011). Clinical documentation data retrieval for hospitalized older adults with heart failure: Part 2. *International Journal of Nursing Terminologies and Classifications, 22*(2), 68–76.
10. Head, B., Scherb, C., Reed, D., Conley, D., Weinberg, B., Kozel, M., Gillette, S., Clarke, M., & Moorhead, S. (2011). Nursing diagnoses, interventions, and patient outcomes for hospitalized older adults with pneumonia. *Research in Gerontological Nursing, 4*(2), 95–105.
11. Herdman, T. H. (Ed.). (2012). *NANDA International nursing diagnoses: Definitions & classification 2012-2014.* Oxford: Wiley-Blackwell.
12. Institute of Medicine. (2010). *The future of nursing: Leading change, advancing health.* Washington, DC: National Academies Press.
13. Johnson, M., Moorhead, S., Bulechek, G., Butcher, H., Maas, M., & Swanson, E. (2012). *NOC and NIC linkages to NANDA-I and clinical conditions: Supporting critical reasoning and quality care* (3rd ed.). St. Louis: Elsevier Mosby.
14. Jones, D., Lunney, M., Keenan, G., & Moorhead, S. (2010). Standardized nursing languages: Essential for the nursing workforce. In A.T. Debisette & J.A. Vessey (Eds.). *Annual review of nursing research: Vol. 28. Nursing workforce issues* (pp. 253–304). New York: Springer.
15. Kautz, D., & Van Horn, E. (2008). An exemplar of the use of NNN language in developing evidence-based practice guidelines. *International Journal of Nursing Terminologies and Classifications, 19*(1), 14–19.
16. Keenan, G., & Aquilino, M. (1998). Standardized nomenclatures: Keys to continuity of care, nursing accountability, and nursing effectiveness. *Outcomes Management for Nursing, 2*(2), 81–86.
17. Keenan, G., Falan, S., Heath, C., & Treder, M. (2003). Establishing competency in the use of North American Nursing Diagnosis Association, Nursing Outcomes Classification, and Nursing Interventions Classification terminology. *Journal of Nursing Measurement, 11*(2), 183–198.
18. Lacey, S., Klaus, S., Smith, J., Cox, K., & Dunton, N. (2006). Developing measures of pediatric nursing quality. *Journal of Nursing Care Quality, 21*(3), 210–222.
19. Lake, E., & Cheung, R. (2006). Are patient falls and pressure ulcers sensitive to nurse staffing. *Western Journal of Nursing Research, 28*(6), 654–657.
20. Lunney, M. (2006). Helping nurses use NANDA, NOC, and NIC: Novice to expert. *Nurse Educator, 31*(1), 40–46.
21. Moorhead, S., Johnson, M., Maas, M., & Swanson, E. (Eds.). (2008). *Nursing outcomes classification (NOC)* (4th ed.) St. Louis: Elsevier Mosby.
22. Myny, D., Van Goubergen, D., Limère, V., Gobert, M., Verhaeghe, S., & Defloor, T. (2009). Determination of standard times of nursing activities based on a nursing minimum dataset. *Journal of Advanced Nursing, 66*(1), 92–102.
23. National Committee on Vital and Health Statistics. (2010). *Toward enhanced information capacities for health: An NCVHS concept paper.* Retrieved from http://www.ncvhs.hhs.gov/100526concept.pdf
24. Scherb, C., Head, B., Hertzog, M., Swanson, E., Reed, D., Maas, M., Moorhead, S., Conley, D., Clarke, M., Gillette, S., & Weinberg, B. (2011). Evaluation of outcome change scores for patients with pneumonia or heart failure [online version]. *Western Journal of Nursing Research.*
25. Scherb, C., Head, B., Maas, M., Swanson, E., & Moorhead, S., Reed, D., Conley, D., & Kozel, M. (2011). Most frequent nursing diagnoses, nursing interventions, and nursing-sensitive patient outcomes of hospitalized older adults with heart failure: Part 1. *International Journal of Nursing Terminologies and Classifications, 22*(1), 13–22.
26. Scherb, C., & Weydt, A. (2009). Work complexity assessment, nursing interventions classification, and nursing outcomes classification: Making connections. *Creative Nursing, 15*(1), 16–22.
27. Schoenfelder, D., Swanson, E., Specht, J., Johnson, M., & Maas, M. (2000). Outcome indicators for direct and indirect caregiving. *Clinical Nursing Research, 9*(1), 47–69.
28. Smith, K., & Craft-Rosenberg, M. (2010). Using NANDA, NIC, and NOC in an undergraduate nursing practicum. *Nurse Educator, 35*(4), 162–166.
29. Titler, M., Dochterman, J., & Reed, D. (2004). *Guidelines for conducting effectiveness research in nursing & other health care services.* Iowa City, IA: Center for Nursing Classification & Clinical Effectiveness.
30. Westra, B., Delaney, C., Konicek, D., & Keenan, G. (2008). Nursing standards to support the electronic health record. *Nursing Outlook, 56*(5), 258–266.

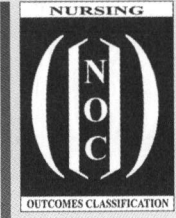

PART TWO

NOC Taxonomy

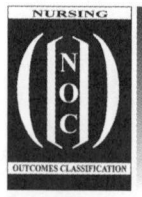

Overview of the NOC Taxonomy

The following section of this book contains the three-level taxonomy for the NOC. The NOC taxonomy was created to (1) organize the key concepts in the taxonomy into domains, classes, and outcomes, (2) provide a stable structure for outcome placement over time, (3) allow for the addition of new outcomes, (4) identify missing outcomes needed for future editions, and (5) assist nurses and other health care providers in identifying and selecting outcomes for the diagnoses they treat for patients, families, and communities. Use of the taxonomy makes identification of possible outcomes for use in practice easier than an alphabetical list of outcomes. The domain and class levels in the taxonomy have become even more important as the classification has grown over time.

HISTORICAL DEVELOPMENT OF THE NOC TAXONOMY

The taxonomic structure was developed during the second phase of the original research and was first distributed in a publication from the Center[3] and then published in an article overviewing the methods in 1998.[5] The NOC taxonomic structure was developed using strategies refined by the Iowa Intervention Project.[1] The goal was to create a three-level taxonomic structure similar to the one developed for the Nursing Interventions Classification (NIC).[2] This required an inductive approach using qualitative similarity-dissimilarity analysis with many participants sorting outcomes into clusters. Each participant identified a concept label that he or she felt captured the essence of the cluster of outcomes. In the first sort, 175 outcomes were grouped in this manner and the participants were asked to create 15 to 25 clusters based on the sorting process. Hierarchical cluster analysis was then applied to combine the results of each participant's individual sort. This process created the class level of the NOC taxonomy which when finalized created 24 classes: *Energy Maintenance, Growth and Development, Mobility, Self-Care, Cardiopulmonary, Elimination, Fluid and Electrolytes, Immune Response, Metabolic Regulation, Neurocognitive, Nutrition, Tissue Integrity, Psychological Well-Being, Psychological Adaptation, Self-Control, Social Interaction, Health Behavior, Health Beliefs, Health Knowledge, Risk Control and Safety, Health and Life Quality, Symptom Status, Family Caregiver Status*, and *Maltreatment Resolution*. Each outcome is listed in only one class in the taxonomy.

In the second phase of the development of the taxonomy, the 24 classes were sorted by participants to create the top level of the taxonomy using the same methods used to create the concept labels for each class. The results of this process identified 6 domains: *Functional Health, Physiologic Health, Psychosocial Health, Health Knowledge and Behavior, Perceived Health,* and *Family Health*. By the time the first publication was available, 197 outcomes had been placed in the taxonomy including several outcomes that were included for the first time in the second edition of NOC. A more detailed description of the process used to create the taxonomy is available elsewhere.[5]

REVISIONS MADE IN THE TAXONOMY SINCE ITS CREATION

The following sections highlight the changes made in the NOC taxonomy by edition. The reader can review a more complete list of new and revised outcomes in the appendix of previous editions. In general, new classes are added to the taxonomy when outcomes are identified that do not fit easily into the current classes in the taxonomy or when a substantial number of outcomes focused on a concept are added to the classification.

Second Edition

The NOC taxonomy was first published within the classification in the second edition[4] in 2000. At that time there were 7 domains, 29 classes, and 260 outcomes. The revisions to the taxonomy for the second edition included 5 new classes: *Therapeutic Response* and *Sensory Function* in the *Functional Health Domain, Family Member Health Status* in the *Family Health Domain,* and *Community Well-Being and Community Health Protection* in the new Domain *Community Health. Community Health* was added as a domain to the taxonomy to allow for the inclusion of outcomes focused on the community as the recipient of care. This domain contains outcomes that describe the health, well-being, and functioning of a community or population. Like the *Family Domain* the focus of care is on a group rather than an individual. In this case the population might be an entire community, a neighborhood, or a population of patients with the same health concern (e.g., diabetes). The addition of another domain enlarged the taxonomy to 7 domains, 29 classes, and 260 outcomes. In addition, the definitions for 4 classes, *Nutrition, Symptom Status, Family Care Status,* and *Family*

Well-Being, were modified, and the class *Maltreatment Resolution* was changed to *Family Well-Being.*

Third Edition

The addition of 2 new classes to the NOC taxonomy in the third edition[6] resulted in some changes in the placement of outcomes within the taxonomy. A class called *Satisfaction with Care* was added, and it includes outcomes that describe an individual's perceptions of the quality and adequacy of health care provided. Due to this addition the definition of the class *Health and Life Quality* was modified. Several changes were made in Domain VI, *Family Health*. A second class was added called *Parenting,* containing outcomes that describe behaviors of parents that promote growth and development. The class *Family Care Status* was renamed *Family Caregiver Performance* to better reflect the outcomes in this class. This enlarged the taxonomy to 7 domains, 31 classes, and 330 outcomes. Overall the definitions for 3 classes, *Health Knowledge, Health and Life Quality,* and

Family Well-Being, were modified along with the *Perceived Health* domain.

Fourth Edition

The NOC taxonomy in the fourth edition[7] contained 7 domains, 31 classes, and 385 outcomes. In this edition the class *Nutrition* was changed to *Digestion and Nutrition,* and the definition was modified to define this broader class. Three other class definitions, *Satisfaction with Care, Family Member Health Status*, and *Family Well-Being,* were modified.

Fifth Edition

The fifth edition of NOC has 7 domains, 32 classes, and 490 outcomes. The class *Health Management* was added to include outcomes that describe the individual's role in the management of an acute or chronic condition. Definition changes to the *Psychological Well-Being* and *Health Behavior* classes were also made in this edition. Table II-1

Table II-1 DEVELOPMENT OF THE NOC TAXONOMY ACROSS EDITIONS

NOC Taxonomy	Original [‡]	2nd Edition	3rd Edition	4th Edition	5th Edition
Energy Maintenance	4	6	6	7	8
Growth & Development	18	20	21	24	24
Mobility	11	12	20	21	22
Self-Care	11	11	13	13	13
Functional Health	**44**	**49**	**60**	**65**	**67**
Cardiopulmonary	9	11	14	17	23
Elimination	4	4	5	5	5
Fluid and Electrolytes	3	3	4	4	21
Immune Response	4	5	7	7	7
Metabolic Regulation	3	3	4	4	5
Neurocognitive	15	15	16	19	21
Digestion and Nutrition	10	14[†]	14	15[*†]	20
Therapeutic Response	-	3	4	4	6
Tissue Integrity	5	6	6	8	8
Sensory Function	-	5	6	6	6
Physiologic Health	**53**	**69**	**80**	**89**	**122**

Continued

Table II-1 DEVELOPMENT OF THE NOC TAXONOMY ACROSS EDITIONS—cont'd

NOC Taxonomy	Original [‡]	2nd Edition	3rd Edition	4th Edition	5th Edition
Psychological Well-Being	7	9	14	15	17[†]
Psychosocial Adaptation	7	7	7	8	10
Self-Control	9	10	10	9	11
Social Interaction	5	5	5	5	5
Psychosocial Health	**28**	**31**	**36**	**37**	**43**
Health Behavior	10	14	22	32	31[†]
Health Beliefs	6	6	6	6	6
Health Knowledge	15	26	30[†]	42	64
Health Management	-	-	-	-	16
Risk Control and Safety	14	19	18	26	34
Health Knowledge & Behavior	**45**	**65**	**76**	**106**	**151**
Health and Life Quality	3	5	8[†]	12	13
Symptom Status	5	6[†]	9	12	18
Satisfaction with Care	-	-	14	17[†]	17
Perceived Health	**8**	**11**	**31**[#]	**41**	**48**
Family Caregiver Performance	12	9[†]	8[*]	8	8
Family Member Health Status	-	13	15	15[†]	15
Family Well-Being	7	7[*†]	10[†]	9[†]	10
Parenting	-	-	5	5	10
Family Health	**19**	**29**	**38**	**37**	**43**
Community Well-Being	-	2	4	4	6
Community Health Protection	-	4	5	6	10
Community Health	**-**	**6**	**9**	**10**	**16**
	6 domains	7 domains	7 domains	7 domains	7 domains
	24 classes	29 classes	31 classes	31 classes	32 classes
	197 outcomes	260 outcomes	330 outcomes	385 outcomes	490 outcomes

*Change in class label.
[†]Change in definition.
[‡]Source: Iowa Outcomes Project. (1997). *Taxonomy of nursing outcomes classification (NOC)*. Iowa City, IA: Author; Moorhead, S., Head, B., Johnson, M., & Maas, M. (1998). The nursing outcomes taxonomy: Development and coding. *Journal of Nursing Care Quality, 12*(6), 56–63.

summarizes the changes made to the NOC taxonomy for the second through the fifth editions. Details of these changes can be found by comparing previous editions of the taxonomy.

CODING OF THE CLASSIFICATION

Once the taxonomic structure was created, coding of the NOC became a high priority and was first included in the second edition of the classification. Coding is important since it creates a way to (1) represent each of the taxonomic elements, (2) facilitate use of NOC in computer systems, (3) create nursing data sets that can be linked with large regional and national health care databases, and (4) facilitate client outcome evaluation to improve the quality of patient care. The coding structure for NOC includes the domains, classes, outcomes and their indicators, measurement scales, and actual outcome scores recorded by users.

Every effort has been made to retain codes used in the previous editions of this classification. With classification work it is important to keep coding of the outcomes consistent across editions. When changes were made, careful decisions had to be made on whether the outcome was new or a revision, and any outcome that was just updated or revised retained its original code. In a few cases, revisions resulted in the creation of new outcomes from a previous outcome in the classification. In this case the old outcome was retired (along with its code) and each new outcome was given a new code. Codes for any indicator retired from the outcome resulted in the retiring of the code assigned to that indicator. In many outcomes the indicators were reordered, but the indicators retained their original code in spite of placement in the outcome.

The addition of a second scale to some outcomes in the third edition resulted in the need to modify the coding scheme for the scale data. Scales in the second edition were coded with a letter of the alphabet. We now have moved to assigning numbers to each scale or combination of scales. This is a change in the coding schema since the third edition. The coding uses a number to reflect the scale or scale combinations used for that outcome, and because there are more than nine scales, the codes for the scales require two spaces in the structure. In the second edition numbers were used for the original set of measurement scales. If a scale was previously attached to a number, that number was reinstituted as the code for the scale. This means that numbers for scales previously retired have not been used in the recoding for the fifth edition. In addition, the code for the classes now uses all uppercase letters and started using double letters, such as AA, because the use of uppercase and lowercase letters was confusing in database entries. This also requires two spaces (Table II-2).

This coding structure allows for expansion of the NOC at every level of the taxonomy and creates a unique identifier for each outcome, indicator, and measurement scale. For example, two additional domains can be added to the NOC taxonomy and 21 new classes can be added, each containing up to 99 outcomes. This structure allows for substantial additions to the classifications without changing the coding structure. Since the first draft of the taxonomy was created, new outcomes have been developed and easily placed in the taxonomy. Few changes in the structure have been needed to accomplish this. Changes in the outcomes for this edition are summarized in Appendix A.

Table II-2   CODING STRUCTURE OF NOC

Domain (1-9)	Class (A-Z) or (AA-ZZ)	Outcome (4 numbers)	Indicator (01-99)	Scale (01-99)	Scale Value (1-5)
#	##	####	##	##	#

THE NOC TAXONOMY

	Domain I	Domain II	Domain III
Level 1 Domains	**Functional Health** Outcomes that describe the capacity for and performance of basic tasks of life	**Physiologic Health** Outcomes that describe organic functioning	**Psychosocial Health** Outcomes that describe psychological and social functioning
Level 2 Classes	**Energy Maintenance** Outcomes that describe an individual's energy rejuvenation, conservation, and expenditure **Growth & Development** Outcomes that describe an individual's physical, emotional, and social maturation **Mobility** Outcomes that describe an individual's physical mobility and the sequelae of restricted movement **Self-Care** Outcomes that describe an individual's ability to accomplish basic and instrumental activities of daily living	**Cardiopulmonary** Outcomes that describe an individual's cardiac, pulmonary, circulatory, or tissue perfusion status **Elimination** Outcomes that describe an individual's waste excretion, elimination patterns, and status **Fluid & Electrolytes** Outcomes that describe an individual's fluid and electrolyte status **Immune Response** Outcomes that describe an individual's physiological reaction to substances that are foreign or interpreted by the body as foreign **Metabolic Regulation** Outcomes that describe an individual's ability to regulate body metabolism **Neurocognitive** Outcomes that describe an individual's neurological and cognitive status **Digestion & Nutrition** Outcomes that describe an individual's digestion and nutritional patterns **Therapeutic Response** Outcomes that describe an individual's systemic reaction to a remedial health treatment, agent, or method **Tissue Integrity** Outcomes that describe the condition and function of an individual's body tissues **Sensory Function** Outcomes that describe an individual's perception and use of sensory information	**Psychological Well-Being** Outcomes that describe an individual's emotional health and related self-perception **Psychosocial Adaptation** Outcomes that describe an individual's psychological and/or social adaptation to altered health or life circumstances **Self-Control** Outcomes that describe an individual's ability to restrain behavior that may be emotionally or physically harmful to self or others **Social Interaction** Outcomes that describe an individual's relationships with others

Domain IV	Domain V	Domain VI	Domain VII
Health Knowledge & Behavior Outcomes that describe attitudes, comprehension, and actions with respect to health and illness	**Perceived Health** Outcomes that describe impressions of an individual's health and health care	**Family Health** Outcomes that describe health status, behavior, or functioning of the family as a whole or of an individual as a family member	**Community Health** Outcomes that describe the health, well-being, and functioning of a community or population
Health Behavior Outcomes that describe an individual's actions to promote or restore health	**Health & Life Quality** Outcomes that describe an individual's perceived health status and related life circumstances	**Family Caregiver Performance** Outcomes that describe the adaptation and performance of a family member caring for a dependent child or adult	**Community Health Protection** Outcomes that describe the structures and programs of a community to eliminate or reduce health risks and increase community resistance to health threats
Health Beliefs Outcomes that describe an individual's ideas and perceptions that influence health behavior	**Satisfaction with Care** Outcomes that describe an individual's perceptions of the quality and adequacy of health care provided	**Family Member Health Status** Outcomes that describe the physical, psychological, social, and spiritual health of an individual family member	**Community Well- Being** Outcomes that describe the overall health status and social competence of a community or population
Health Knowledge Outcomes that describe an individual's understanding in applying information to promote, maintain, and restore health	**Symptom Status** Outcomes that describe an individual's indications of a disease, injury, or loss	**Family Well-Being** Outcomes that describe the family environment, overall health status, and social competence of a family as a unit	
Health Management Outcomes that describe an individual's actions to manage an acute or chronic condition		**Parenting** Outcomes that describe behaviors of parents that promote optimum growth and development of a child	
Risk Control & Safety Outcomes that describe an individual's safety status and/or actions to avoid, limit, or control identifiable health threats			

Level 1 *Domain*	**(1) Domain I—Functional Health** **Outcomes that describe the capacity for and performance of basic tasks of life**	
Level 2 *Classes*	**A-Energy Maintenance** Outcomes that describe an individual's energy rejuvenation, conservation, and expenditure	**B-Growth & Development** Outcomes that describe an individual's physical, emotional, and social maturation
Level 3 *Outcomes*	0005-Activity Tolerance 0001-Endurance 0002-Energy Conservation 0008-Fatigue: Disruptive Effects 0007-Fatigue Level 0006-Psychomotor Energy 0003-Rest 0004-Sleep	0120-Child Development: 1 Month 0100-Child Development: 2 Months 0101-Child Development: 4 Months 0102-Child Development: 6 Months 0103-Child Development: 12 Months 0104-Child Development: 2 Years 0105-Child Development: 3 Years 0106-Child Development: 4 Years 0107-Child Development: 5 Years 0108-Child Development: Middle Childhood 0109-Child Development: Adolescence 0121-Development: Late Adulthood 0122-Development: Middle Adulthood 0123-Development: Young Adulthood 0111-Fetal Status: Antepartum 0112-Fetal Status: Intrapartum 0110-Growth 0118-Newborn Adaptation 0113-Physical Aging 0114-Physical Maturation: Female 0115-Physical Maturation: Male 0116-Play Participation 0117-Preterm Infant Organization 0119-Sexual Functioning

C-Mobility

Outcomes that describe an individual's physical mobility and the sequelae of restricted movement

0200-Ambulation
0201-Ambulation: Wheelchair
0202-Balance
0203-Body Positioning: Self-Initiated
0212-Coordinated Movement
0222-Gait
0204-Immobility Consequences: Physiological
0205-Immobility Consequences: Psycho-Cognitive
0206-Joint Movement
0213-Joint Movement: Ankle
0214-Joint Movement: Elbow
0215-Joint Movement: Fingers
0216-Joint Movement: Hip
0217-Joint Movement: Knee
0218-Joint Movement: Neck
0207-Joint Movement: Passive
0219-Joint Movement: Shoulder
0220-Joint Movement: Spine
0221-Joint Movement: Wrist
0208-Mobility
0211-Skeletal Function
0210-Transfer Performance

D-Self-Care

Outcomes that describe an individual's ability to accomplish basic and instrumental activities of daily living

0311-Discharge Readiness: Independent Living
0312-Discharge Readiness: Supported Living
0313-Self-Care Status
0300-Self-Care: Activities of Daily Living (ADL)
0301-Self-Care: Bathing
0302-Self-Care: Dressing
0303-Self-Care: Eating
0305-Self-Care: Hygiene
0306-Self-Care: Instrumental Activities of Daily Living (IADL)
0307-Self-Care: Non-Parenteral Medication
0308-Self-Care: Oral Hygiene
0309-Self-Care: Parenteral Medication
0310-Self-Care: Toileting

Level 1
Domain

Level 2
Classes

Level 3
Outcomes

(2) Domain II—Physiologic Health
Outcomes that describe organic functioning

E-Cardiopulmonary
Outcomes that describe an individual's cardiac, pulmonary,
circulatory, or tissue perfusion status

F-Elimination
Outcomes that describe an individual's waste
excretion, elimination patterns, and status

0409-Blood Coagulation
0413-Blood Loss Severity
0400-Cardiac Pump Effectiveness
0414-Cardiopulmonary Status
0401-Circulation Status
0411-Mechanical Ventilation Response: Adult
0412-Mechanical Ventilation Weaning Response: Adult
0415-Respiratory Status
0410-Respiratory Status: Airway Patency
0402-Respiratory Status: Gas Exchange
0403-Respiratory Status: Ventilation
0417-Shock Severity: Anaphylactic
0418-Shock Severity: Cardiogenic
0419-Shock Severity: Hypovolemic
0420-Shock Severity: Neurogenic
0421-Shock Severity: Septic
0422-Tissue Perfusion
0404-Tissue Perfusion: Abdominal Organs
0405-Tissue Perfusion: Cardiac
0416-Tissue Perfusion: Cellular
0406-Tissue Perfusion: Cerebral
0407-Tissue Perfusion: Peripheral
0408-Tissue Perfusion: Pulmonary

0500-Bowel Continence
0501-Bowel Elimination
0504-Kidney Function
0502-Urinary Continence
0503-Urinary Elimination

G-Fluid & Electrolytes	H-Immune Response	I-Metabolic Regulation
Outcomes that describe an individual's fluid and electrolyte status	Outcomes that describe an individual's physiological reaction to substances that are foreign or interpreted by the body as foreign	Outcomes that describe an individual's ability to regulate body metabolism

G-Fluid & Electrolytes

0604-Acute Respiratory Acidosis Severity
0605-Acute Respiratory Alkalosis Severity
0600-Electrolyte & Acid/Base Balance
0606-Electrolyte Balance
0601-Fluid Balance
0603-Fluid Overload Severity
0602-Hydration
0607-Hypercalcemia Severity
0608-Hyperchloremia Severity
0609-Hyperkalemia Severity
0610-Hypermagnesemia Severity
0611-Hypernatremia Severity
0612-Hyperphosphatemia Severity
0613-Hypocalcemia Severity
0614-Hypochloremia Severity
0615-Hypokalemia Severity
0616-Hypomagnesemia Severity
0617-Hyponatremia Severity
0618-Hypophosphatemia Severity
0619-Metabolic Acidosis Severity
0620-Metabolic Alkalosis Severity

H-Immune Response

0705-Allergic Response: Localized
0706-Allergic Response: Systemic
0700-Blood Transfusion Reaction
0707-Immune Hypersensitivity Response
0702-Immune Status
0703-Infection Severity
0708-Infection Severity: Newborn

I-Metabolic Regulation

0803-Liver Function
0800-Thermoregulation
0801-Thermoregulation: Newborn
0802-Vital Signs
1006-Weight: Body Mass

Level 1 Domain	(2) Domain II—Physiologic Health—cont'd	

Level 2 Classes

J-Neurocognitive
Outcomes that describe an individual's neurological and cognitive status

K-Digestion & Nutrition
Outcomes that describe an individual's digestion and nutritional patterns

Level 3 Outcomes

0919-Abstract Thinking
0900-Cognition
0901-Cognitive Orientation
0902-Communication
0903-Communication: Expressive
0904-Communication: Receptive
0905-Concentration
0906-Decision-Making
0916-Delirium Level
0920-Dementia Level
0918-Heedfulness of Affected Side
0915-Hyperactivity Level
0907-Information Processing
0908-Memory
0909-Neurological Status
0910-Neurological Status: Autonomic
0911-Neurological Status: Central Motor Control
0912-Neurological Status: Consciousness
0913-Neurological Status: Cranial Sensory/Motor Function
0917-Neurological Status: Peripheral
0914-Neurological Status: Spinal Sensory/Motor Function

1014-Appetite
1016-Bottle Feeding Establishment: Infant
1017-Bottle Feeding Performance
1000-Breastfeeding Establishment: Infant
1001-Breastfeeding Establishment: Maternal
1002-Breastfeeding Maintenance
1003-Breastfeeding Weaning
1018-Cup Feeding Establishment: Infant
1019-Cup Feeding Performance
1015-Gastrointestinal Function
1020-Infant Nutritional Status
1004-Nutritional Status
1005-Nutritional Status: Biochemical Measures
1007-Nutritional Status: Energy
1008-Nutritional Status: Food & Fluid Intake
1009-Nutritional Status: Nutrient Intake
1010-Swallowing Status
1011-Swallowing Status: Esophageal Phase
1012-Swallowing Status: Oral Phase
1013-Swallowing Status: Pharyngeal Phase

AA-Therapeutic Response
Outcomes that describe an individual's systemic reaction to a remedial health treatment, agent, or method

2300-Blood Glucose Level
2301-Medication Response
2303-Post-Procedure Recovery
2304-Surgical Recovery: Convalescence
2305-Surgical Recovery: Immediate
    Post-Operative
2302-Systemic Toxin Clearance: Dialysis

L-Tissue Integrity
Outcomes that describe the condition and function of an individual's body tissues

1104-Bone Healing
1106-Burn Healing
1107-Burn Recovery
1105-Hemodialysis Access
1100-Oral Health
1101-Tissue Integrity: Skin & Mucous Membranes
1102-Wound Healing: Primary Intention
1103-Wound Healing: Secondary Intention

Y-Sensory Function
Outcomes that describe an individual's perception and use of sensory information

2405-Sensory Function
2401-Sensory Function: Hearing
2402-Sensory Function: Proprioception
2400-Sensory Function: Tactile
2403-Sensory Function: Taste & Smell
2404-Sensory Function: Vision

Level 1 Domain		
	(3) Domain III—Psychosocial Health	
	Outcomes that describe psychological and social functioning	

Level 2 Classes	**M-Psychological Well-Being**	**N-Psychosocial Adaptation**
	Outcomes that describe an individual's emotional health and related self-perception	Outcomes that describe an individual's psychological and/or social adaptation to altered health or life circumstances

Level 3 Outcomes		
	1214-Agitation Level	1300-Acceptance: Health Status
	1211-Anxiety Level	1308-Adaptation to Physical Disability
	1200-Body Image	1301-Child Adaptation to Hospitalization
	1208-Depression Level	1302-Coping
	1210-Fear Level	1307-Dignified Life Closure
	1213-Fear Level: Child	1304-Grief Resolution
	1201-Hope	1310-Guilt Resolution
	1202-Identity	1309-Personal Resiliency
	1203-Loneliness Severity	1305-Psychosocial Adjustment: Life Change
	1204-Mood Equilibrium	1311-Relocation Adaptation
	1209-Motivation	
	1215-Self-Awareness	
	1205-Self-Esteem	
	1207-Sexual Identity	
	1216-Social Anxiety Level	
	1212-Stress Level	
	1206-Will to Live	

O-Self-Control

Outcomes that describe an individual's
ability to restrain behavior that may be emotionally or physically
harmful to self or others

1400-Abusive Behavior Self-Restraint
1401-Aggression Self-Restraint
1410-Anger Self-Restraint
1402-Anxiety Self-Control
1409-Depression Self-Control
1403-Distorted Thought Self-Control
1411-Eating Disorder Self-Control
1404-Fear Self-Control
1405-Impulse Self-Control
1406-Mutilation Self-Restraint
1408-Suicide Self-Restraint

P-Social Interaction

Outcomes that describe an individual's relationships with others

1500-Parent-Infant Attachment
1501-Role Performance
1502-Social Interaction Skills
1503-Social Involvement
1504-Social Support

Level 1 Domain	**(4) Domain IV—Health Knowledge & Behavior**
	Outcomes that describe attitudes, comprehension, and actions with respect to health and illness

Level 2 Classes	**Q-Health Behavior**	**R-Health Beliefs**
	Outcomes that describe an individual's actions to promote or restore health	Outcomes that describe an individual's ideas and perceptions that influence health behavior

Level 3 Outcomes	
1600-Adherence Behavior	1700-Health Beliefs
1621-Adherence Behavior: Healthy Diet	1701-Health Beliefs: Perceived Ability to Perform
1629-Alcohol Abuse Cessation Behavior	1702-Health Beliefs: Perceived Control
1616-Body Mechanics Performance	1703-Health Beliefs: Perceived Resources
1601-Compliance Behavior	1704-Health Beliefs: Perceived Threat
1632-Compliance Behavior: Prescribed Activity	1705-Health Orientation
1622-Compliance Behavior: Prescribed Diet	
1623-Compliance Behavior: Prescribed Medication	
1630-Drug Abuse Cessation Behavior	
1633-Exercise Participation	
1602-Health Promoting Behavior	
1603-Health Seeking Behavior	
1610-Hearing Compensation Behavior	
1604-Leisure Participation	
1618-Nausea & Vomiting Control	
1615-Ostomy Self-Care	
1605-Pain Control	
1606-Participation in Health Care Decisions	
1614-Personal Autonomy	
1634-Personal Health Screening Behavior	
1635-Personal Time Management	
1624-Postpartum Maternal Health Behavior	
1607-Prenatal Health Behavior	
1620-Seizure Self-Control	
1613-Self-Direction of Care	
1625-Smoking Cessation Behavior	
1608-Symptom Control	
1611-Vision Compensation Behavior	
1626-Weight Gain Behavior	
1627-Weight Loss Behavior	
1628-Weight Maintenance Behavior	

FF-Health Management
Outcomes that describe an individual's actions to manage an acute or chronic condition

3100-Self-Management: Acute Illness
3101-Self-Management: Anticoagulation Therapy
0704-Self-Management: Asthma
1617-Self-Management: Cardiac Disease
3102-Self-Management: Chronic Disease
3103-Self-Management: Chronic Obstructive Pulmonary Disease
3104-Self-Management: Coronary Artery Disease
1619-Self-Management: Diabetes
3105-Self-Management: Dysrhythmia
3106-Self-Management: Heart Failure
3107-Self-Management: Hypertension
3108-Self-Management: Kidney Disease
3109-Self-Management: Lipid Disorder
1631-Self-Management: Multiple Sclerosis
3110-Self-Management: Osteoporosis
3111-Self-Management: Peripheral Artery Disease

Level 1 *Domain*	**(4) Domain IV—Health Knowledge & Behavior—cont'd**

Level 2
Classes

S-Health Knowledge
Outcomes that describe an individual's understanding in applying information to promote, maintain, and restore health

Level 3
Outcomes

1844-Knowledge: Acute Illness Management
1845-Knowledge: Anticoagulation Therapy Management
1831-Knowledge: Arthritis Management
1832-Knowledge: Asthma Management
1827-Knowledge: Body Mechanics
1846-Knowledge: Bottle Feeding
1800-Knowledge: Breastfeeding
1833-Knowledge: Cancer Management
1834-Knowledge: Cancer Threat Reduction
1830-Knowledge: Cardiac Disease Management
1801-Knowledge: Child Physical Safety
1847-Knowledge: Chronic Disease Management
1848-Knowledge: Chronic Obstructive Pulmonary Disease
    Management
1821-Knowledge: Conception Prevention
1849-Knowledge: Coronary Artery Disease Management
1850-Knowledge: Cup Feeding
1851-Knowledge: Dementia Management
1836-Knowledge: Depression Management
1820-Knowledge: Diabetes Management
1803-Knowledge: Disease Process
1852-Knowledge: Dysrhythmia Management
1853-Knowledge: Eating Disorder Management
1804-Knowledge: Energy Conservation
1828-Knowledge: Fall Prevention
1816-Knowledge: Fertility Promotion
1805-Knowledge: Health Behavior
1823-Knowledge: Health Promotion
1806-Knowledge: Health Resources
1854-Knowledge: Healthy Diet
1855-Knowledge: Healthy Lifestyle
1835-Knowledge: Heart Failure Management
1837-Knowledge: Hypertension Management

1819-Knowledge: Infant Care
1842-Knowledge: Infection Management
1856-Knowledge: Inflammatory Bowel Disease Management
1857-Knowledge: Kidney Disease Management
1817-Knowledge: Labor & Delivery
1858-Knowledge: Lipid Disorder Management
1808-Knowledge: Medication
1838-Knowledge: Multiple Sclerosis Management
1859-Knowledge: Osteoporosis Management
1829-Knowledge: Ostomy Care
1843-Knowledge: Pain Management
1826-Knowledge: Parenting
1860-Knowledge: Peripheral Artery Disease Management
1809-Knowledge: Personal Safety
1861-Knowledge: Pneumonia Management
1818-Knowledge: Postpartum Maternal Health
1822-Knowledge: Preconception Maternal Health
1810-Knowledge: Pregnancy
1839-Knowledge: Pregnancy & Postpartum Sexual
    Functioning
1811-Knowledge: Prescribed Activity
1802-Knowledge: Prescribed Diet
1840-Knowledge: Preterm Infant Care
1815-Knowledge: Sexual Functioning
1862-Knowledge: Stress Management
1863-Knowledge: Stroke Management
1864-Knowledge: Stroke Prevention
1812-Knowledge: Substance Use Control
1865-Knowledge: Thrombus Prevention
1866-Knowledge: Time Management
1814-Knowledge: Treatment Procedure
1813-Knowledge: Treatment Regimen
1841-Knowledge: Weight Management

T-Risk Control & Safety
Outcomes that describe an individual's safety status and/or actions to avoid, limit, or control identifiable health threats

1918-Aspiration Prevention
1919-Elopement Occurrence
1920-Elopement Propensity Risk
1909-Fall Prevention Behavior
1912-Falls Occurrence
1900-Immunization Behavior
1911-Personal Safety Behavior
1913-Physical Injury Severity
1921-Pre-Procedure Readiness
1902-Risk Control
1903-Risk Control: Alcohol Use
1917-Risk Control: Cancer
1914-Risk Control: Cardiovascular Disease
1904-Risk Control: Drug Use
1927-Risk Control: Dry Eye
1915-Risk Control: Hearing Impairment
1928-Risk Control: Hypertension
1922-Risk Control: Hyperthermia
1933-Risk Control: Hypotension
1923-Risk Control: Hypothermia
1924-Risk Control: Infectious Process
1929-Risk Control: Lipid Disorder
1930-Risk Control: Osteoporosis
1905-Risk Control: Sexually Transmitted Diseases (STD)
1931-Risk Control: Stroke
1925-Risk Control: Sun Exposure
1932-Risk Control: Thrombus
1906-Risk Control: Tobacco Use
1907-Risk Control: Unintended Pregnancy
1916-Risk Control: Visual Impairment
1908-Risk Detection
1934-Safe Health Care Environment
1910-Safe Home Environment
1926-Safe Wandering

Level 1 Domain	(5) Domain V—Perceived Health Outcomes that describe impressions of an individual's health and health care	
Level 2 Classes	**U-Health & Life Quality** Outcomes that describe an individual's perceived health status and related life circumstances	**V-Symptom Status** Outcomes that describe an individual's indications of a disease, injury, or loss
Level 3 Outcomes	2008-Comfort Status 2009-Comfort Status: Environment 2010-Comfort Status: Physical 2011-Comfort Status: Psychospiritual 2012-Comfort Status: Sociocultural 2007-Comfortable Death 2013-Lifestyle Balance 2006-Personal Health Status 2002-Personal Well-Being 2004-Physical Fitness 2000-Quality of Life 2001-Spiritual Health 2005-Student Health Status	2109-Discomfort Level 2110-Dry Eye Severity 2111-Hyperglycemia Severity 2112-Hypertension Severity 2113-Hypoglycemia Severity 2114-Hypotension Severity 2106-Nausea & Vomiting: Disruptive Effects 2107-Nausea & Vomiting Severity 1306-Pain: Adverse Psychological Response 2101-Pain: Disruptive Effects 2102-Pain Level 2104-Perimenopause Symptom Severity 2115-Peripheral Artery Disease Severity 2105-Premenstrual Syndrome (PMS) Severity 1407-Substance Addiction Consequences 2108-Substance Withdrawal Severity 2003-Suffering Severity 2103-Symptom Severity

EE-Satisfaction with Care

Outcomes that describe an individual's perceptions of the quality and adequacy of health care provided

3014-Client Satisfaction
3000-Client Satisfaction: Access to Care Resources
3001-Client Satisfaction: Caring
3015-Client Satisfaction: Case Management
3002-Client Satisfaction: Communication
3003-Client Satisfaction: Continuity of Care
3004-Client Satisfaction: Cultural Needs Fulfillment
3005-Client Satisfaction: Functional Assistance
3016-Client Satisfaction: Pain Management
3006-Client Satisfaction: Physical Care
3007-Client Satisfaction: Physical Environment
3008-Client Satisfaction: Protection of Rights
3009-Client Satisfaction: Psychological Care
3010-Client Satisfaction: Safety
3011-Client Satisfaction: Symptom Control
3012-Client Satisfaction: Teaching
3013-Client Satisfaction: Technical Aspects of Care

Level 1 Domain	(6) Domain VI—Family Health	
	Outcomes that describe health status, behavior, or functioning of the family as a whole or of an individual as a family member	
Level 2 Classes	**W-Family Caregiver Performance** Outcomes that describe the adaptation and performance of a family member caring for a dependent child or adult	**Z-Family Member Health Status** Outcomes that describe the physical, psychological, social, and spiritual health of an individual family member
Level 3 outcomes	2200-Caregiver Adaptation to Patient Institutionalization 2202-Caregiver Home Care Readiness 2203-Caregiver Lifestyle Disruption 2204-Caregiver-Patient Relationship 2205-Caregiver Performance: Direct Care 2206-Caregiver Performance: Indirect Care 2210-Caregiver Role Endurance 2208-Caregiver Stressors	2500-Abuse Cessation 2501-Abuse Protection 2514-Abuse Recovery 2502-Abuse Recovery: Emotional 2503-Abuse Recovery: Financial 2504-Abuse Recovery: Physical 2505-Abuse Recovery: Sexual 2506-Caregiver Emotional Health 2507-Caregiver Physical Health 2508-Caregiver Well-Being 2509-Maternal Status: Antepartum 2510-Maternal Status: Intrapartum 2511-Maternal Status: Postpartum 2513-Neglect Cessation 2512-Neglect Recovery

X-Family Well-Being
Outcomes that describe the family environment, overall health status, and social competence of a family as a unit

2600-Family Coping
2602-Family Functioning
2606-Family Health Status
2603-Family Integrity
2604-Family Normalization
2605-Family Participation in Professional Care
2608-Family Resiliency
2610-Family Risk Control: Obesity
2601-Family Social Climate
2609-Family Support During Treatment

DD-Parenting
Outcomes that describe behaviors of parents that promote optimum growth and development of a child

2211-Parenting Performance
2903-Parenting Performance: Adolescent
2902-Parenting Performance: Adolescent Physical Safety
2901-Parenting Performance: Early/Middle Childhood Physical Safety
2904-Parenting Performance: Infant
2900-Parenting Performance: Infant/Toddler Physical Safety
2905-Parenting Performance: Middle Childhood
2906-Parenting Performance: Preschooler
1901-Parenting Performance: Psychosocial Safety
2907-Parenting Performance: Toddler

Level 1
Domain

(7) **Domain VII—Community Health**
Outcomes that describe the health, well-being, and functioning of a community or population

Level 2
Classes

BB-Community Well-Being
Outcomes that describe the overall health status and social competence of a community or population

Level 3
Outcomes

2700-Community Competence
2703-Community Grief Response
2701-Community Health Status
2800-Community Immune Status
2704-Community Resiliency
2702-Community Violence Level

CC-Community Health Protection

Outcomes that describe the structures and programs of a community to eliminate or reduce health risks and increase community resistance to health threats

2804-Community Disaster Readiness
2806-Community Disaster Response
2807-Community Health Screening Effectiveness
2808-Community Program Effectiveness
2801-Community Risk Control: Chronic Disease
2802-Community Risk Control: Communicable Disease
2803-Community Risk Control: Lead Exposure
2809-Community Risk Control: Obesity
2810-Community Risk Control: Unhealthy Cultural Traditions
2805-Community Risk Control: Violence

References

1. Iowa Intervention Project. (1993). The NIC taxonomy structure. *Image: Journal of Nursing Scholarship, 25*(3), 187–192.
2. Iowa Intervention Project, McCloskey, J. C., & Bulechek, G. M. (Eds.). (1996). *Nursing interventions classification (NIC)* (2nd ed.). St. Louis: Mosby.
3. Iowa Outcomes Project. (1997). *Taxonomy of nursing outcomes classification (NOC).* Iowa City, IA: Author.
4. Iowa Outcomes Project, Johnson, M., Maas, M., & Moorhead, S. (Eds.). (2000). *Nursing outcomes classification (NOC)* (2nd ed.). St. Louis: Mosby.
5. Moorhead, S., Head, B., Johnson, M., & Maas, M. (1998). The nursing outcomes taxonomy: Development and coding. *Journal of Nursing Care Quality, 12*(6), 56–63.
6. Moorhead, S., Johnson, M., & Maas, M. (Eds.). (2004). *Nursing outcomes classification (NOC)* (3rd ed.). St. Louis: Mosby.
7. Moorhead, S., Johnson, M., Maas, M., & Swanson, E. (Eds.). (2008). *Nursing outcomes classification (NOC)* (4th ed.). St. Louis: Elsevier Mosby.

PART THREE

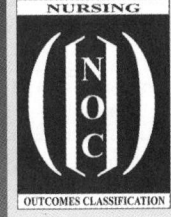

Outcomes

A

Abstract Thinking

0919

Definition: Ability to recognize multiple meanings and patterns of concepts and generalize to new meanings, ideas, or contexts

OUTCOME TARGET RATING: Maintain at_____   Increase to_____

OUTCOME OVERALL RATING		Severely compromised 1	Substantially compromised 2	Moderately compromised 3	Mildly compromised 4	Not compromised 5	
Indicators:							
091901	Identification of separate components of a concept	1	2	3	4	5	NA
091902	Identification of multiple meanings of a concept	1	2	3	4	5	NA
091903	Use of concrete thinking	1	2	3	4	5	NA
091904	Comparison of unfamiliar experiences to familiar ones	1	2	3	4	5	NA
091905	Use of memories to retrieve patterns of similar situations	1	2	3	4	5	NA
091906	Use of memories to assist in solving problems	1	2	3	4	5	NA
091907	Use of visual representations to accelerate understanding of concepts and relationships	1	2	3	4	5	NA
091908	Identification of missing concepts in abstract patterns	1	2	3	4	5	NA
091909	Integration of previously understood concept relationships into judgments	1	2	3	4	5	NA
091910	Use of creative thinking	1	2	3	4	5	NA
091911	Complex problem solving	1	2	3	4	5	NA
091912	Application of concepts to new contexts	1	2	3	4	5	NA
091913	Description of thought process	1	2	3	4	5	NA
091914	Use of reasonable assertions or conclusions from inferences	1	2	3	4	5	NA
091915	Use of imagery as an abstract form of visual input	1	2	3	4	5	NA

Domain-Physiologic Health (II)   *Class*-Neurocognitive (J)   5th edition 2013

OUTCOME CONTENT REFERENCES:

Butler, S. M., & McMunn, N. D. (2006). *A teacher's guide to classroom assessment: Understanding and using assessment to improve student learning.* San Francisco, CA: Jossey-Bass.

Donald, J. (2002). *Learning to think: Disciplinary perspectives.* San Francisco, CA: Jossey-Bass.

Leh, S. K. (2007). Preconceptions: A concept analysis for nursing. *Nursing Forum, 42*(3), 109–122.

Ormrod, J. E. (1999). *Human learning* (3rd ed.). Upper Saddle River, NJ: Prentice Hall.

Pohlman, C. (2008). *Revealing minds: Assessing to understand and support struggling learning.* San Francisco, CA: Jossey Bass.

Willingham, D. (2009). *Why don't students like school? A cognitive scientist answers questions about how the mind works and what it means for your classroom.* San Francisco, CA: Jossey-Bass.

NOTE: The + sign on a content reference identifies the instrument used as a criterion tool in our research using 10 clinical field sites.

Abuse Cessation   2500

Definition: Evidence that the victim is no longer hurt or exploited

OUTCOME TARGET RATING: Maintain at_____ Increase to_____

		None	Limited	Moderate	Substantial	Extensive	
OUTCOME OVERALL RATING		1	2	3	4	5	
Indicators:							
250002	Evidence that physical abuse has ceased	1	2	3	4	5	NA
250003	Evidence that emotional abuse has ceased	1	2	3	4	5	NA
250004	Evidence that sexual abuse has ceased	1	2	3	4	5	NA
250006	Evidence that financial exploitation has ceased	1	2	3	4	5	NA

Domain-Family Health (VI) *Class*-Family Member Health Status (Z) *1st edition 1997; revised 2004*

OUTCOME CONTENT REFERENCES:
Amundson, M. J. (1989). Family crisis care: A home-based intervention program for child abuse. *Issues in Mental Health Nursing, 10*(3–4), 285–296.
Cowen, P. (1991). *The Iowa crisis nursery project as a factor in the prevention of abuse.* Unpublished doctoral dissertation, University of Iowa, Iowa City, IA.
Marshall, E., Buckner, E., Perkins, J., Lowry, J., Hyatt, C., Campbell, C., & Helms, D. (1996). Effects of a child abuse prevention unit in health classes in four schools. *Journal of Community Health Nursing, 13*(2), 107–122.
Olds, D. L., Henderson, C. R., Chamberlin, R., & Tatelbaum, R. (1986). Preventing child abuse and neglect: A randomized trial of nurse home visitation. *Pediatrics, 78*(1), 65–78.
Pressel, D. M. (2000). Evaluation of physical abuse in children. *American Family Physician, 61*(10), 3057–3064.
Reuter, M. M. (1988). Parenting needs of abusing parents: Development of a tool for evaluation of parent education class. *Journal of Community Health Nursing, 5*(2), 129–140.
+Shepard, M., & Campbell, J. A. (1992). The abusive behavior inventory: A measure of psychological and physical abuse. *Journal of Interpersonal Violence, 7*(3), 291–305.
Silverman, J., & Hudson, M. F. (2000). Elder mistreatment: A guide for medical professionals. *North Carolina Medical Journal, 61*(5), 291–296.
Wang, J. J., Lin, J. N., & Lee, F. P. (2006). Psychologically abusive behaviors by those caring for the elderly in a domestic context. *Geriatric Nursing, 27*(5), 284–291.

Abuse Protection   2501

Definition: Protection of self and/or dependent others from abuse

OUTCOME TARGET RATING: Maintain at_____ Increase to_____

		Not adequate	Slightly adequate	Moderately adequate	Substantially adequate	Totally adequate	
OUTCOME OVERALL RATING		1	2	3	4	5	
Indicators:							
250101	Plan for leaving situation	1	2	3	4	5	NA
250102	Safety of residence	1	2	3	4	5	NA
250103	Plan for avoiding abuse	1	2	3	4	5	NA
250104	Implementation of plan to avoid abuse	1	2	3	4	5	NA
250105	Safety of self	1	2	3	4	5	NA
250106	Safety of children	1	2	3	4	5	NA
250112	Limitation of contact with abuser	1	2	3	4	5	NA
250108	Self-advocacy	1	2	3	4	5	NA
250113	Facilitation of counseling for abused person	1	2	3	4	5	NA
250110	Withdrawal when relationship is unsafe	1	2	3	4	5	NA
250111	Severance of relationship	1	2	3	4	5	NA
250114	Safety of dependent adult	1	2	3	4	5	NA
250115	Use of restraining order	1	2	3	4	5	NA
250116	Social support	1	2	3	4	5	NA

Domain-Family Health (VI) *Class*-Family Member Health Status (Z) *1st edition 1997; revised 2004, 2008*

A

OUTCOME CONTENT REFERENCES:

Brendtro, M., & Bowker, L. H. (1989). Battered women: How can nurses help? *Issues in Mental Health Nursing, 10*(2), 169–180.

+Dutton, M. A. (1992). *Empowering and healing the battered woman: A model for assessment and intervention.* New York: Springer.

Helton, A., McFarlane, J., & Anderson, E. (1987). Prevention of battering during pregnancy: Focus on nurse behavioral change. *Public Health Nursing, 4*(3), 166–174.

Hoff, L. A. (1992). Battered woman: Understanding, identification, and assessment. A psychosocial perspective, Part 1. *Journal of the American Academy of Nurse Practitioners, 4,* 148–155.

Hoff, L. A. (1993). Battered women: Intervention and prevention. A psychosocial cultural perspective, Part 2. *Journal of the American Academy of Nurse Practitioners, 5*(1), 34–39.

Schiamberg, L. B., & Gans, D. (2000). Elder abuse by adult children: An applied ecological framework for understanding contextual risk factors and the intergenerational character of quality of life. *International Aging & Human Development, 50*(4), 329–359.

Theran, S. A., Sullivan, C. M., Bogat, G. A., Stewart, C. S. (2006). Abusive partners and ex-partners: Understanding the effects of relationship to the abuser on women's well-being. *Violence Against Women, 12*(10), 950–969.

Abuse Recovery   2514

Definition: Extent of healing following physical or psychological abuse that may include sexual or financial exploitation

OUTCOME TARGET RATING: Maintain at_____   Increase to_____

		None	Limited	Moderate	Substantial	Extensive	
OUTCOME OVERALL RATING		1	2	3	4	5	
Indicators:							
251401	Recognition of abusive relationship(s)	1	2	3	4	5	NA
251402	Healing of psychological injuries	1	2	3	4	5	NA
251403	Healing of physical injuries	1	2	3	4	5	NA
251404	Healing of physical injuries due to sexual abuse	1	2	3	4	5	NA
251405	Healing of psychological injuries due to sexual abuse	1	2	3	4	5	NA
251406	Control of personal finances following financial exploitation	1	2	3	4	5	NA
251407	Control of legal matters following financial exploitation	1	2	3	4	5	NA
251408	Self-esteem	1	2	3	4	5	NA
251409	Feelings of empowerment	1	2	3	4	5	NA
251410	Positive interpersonal relationships	1	2	3	4	5	NA

Domain-Family Health (VI)   **Class**-Family Member Health Status (Z)   *3rd edition 2004; revised 2008*

OUTCOME CONTENT REFERENCES:

Bass, E., & Davis, L. (1994). *The courage to heal: A guide for women survivors of child sexual abuse* (3rd ed.). New York: Harper & Row.

Campbell, J., McKenna, L. S., Torres, S., Sheridan, D., & Landenburger, K. (1993). Nursing care of abused women. In J. Campbell & J. Humphreys (Eds.), *Nursing care of survivors of family violence* (pp. 248–289). St. Louis: Mosby.

Hudson, M. F., & Johnson, T. F. (1986). Elder neglect and abuse: A review of the literature. *Annual Review of Nursing Research, 6*(3), 81–134.

Kaplan, S. J., Pelcovitz, D., & Labruna, V. (1999). Child and adolescent abuse and neglect research: A review of the past 10 years. Part I: Physical and emotional abuse and neglect. *Journal of the American Academy of Child & Adolescent Psychiatry, 38*(10), 1214–1222.

Reed, K. (2005). When elders lose their cents: Financial abuse of the elderly. *Clinics in Geriatric Medicine, 21*(2), 365–382.

Smith, M. E., & Kelly, L. M. (2001). The journey of recovery after a rape experience. *Issues in Mental Health Nursing, 22*(4), 337–352.

Taylor, J. Y. (2000). Sisters of the Yam: African American women's healing and self-recovery from intimate male partner violence. *Issues in Mental Health Nursing, 21*(5), 515–531.

Walsh, K., & Bennett, G. (2000). Financial abuse of older people. *Journal of Adult Protection, 2*(1), 21–29.

Wang, J. J., Lin, J. N., & Lee, F. P. (2006). Psychologically abusive behaviors by those caring for the elderly in a domestic context. *Geriatric Nursing, 27*(5), 284–291.

Abuse Recovery: Emotional   2502   A

Definition: Extent of healing of psychological injuries due to abuse

OUTCOME TARGET RATING: Maintain at_____   Increase to_____

		None	Limited	Moderate	Substantial	Extensive	
OUTCOME OVERALL RATING		1	2	3	4	5	
Indicators:							
250202	Self-confidence	1	2	3	4	5	NA
250203	Self-esteem	1	2	3	4	5	NA
250204	Affect appropriate for situation	1	2	3	4	5	NA
250212	Impulse control	1	2	3	4	5	NA
250213	Self-advocacy	1	2	3	4	5	NA
250214	Feelings of empowerment	1	2	3	4	5	NA
250215	Recognition of abusive relationship	1	2	3	4	5	NA
250217	Expressions of comfort with returning to the abusive environment	1	2	3	4	5	NA
250218	Insight into abusive relationship	1	2	3	4	5	NA
250219	Positive social interactions	1	2	3	4	5	NA
250220	Positive interpersonal relationships	1	2	3	4	5	NA
250221	Positive adjustment to change in living arrangements	1	2	3	4	5	NA

		Extensive	Substantial	Moderate	Limited	None	
250201	Depression	1	2	3	4	5	NA
250223	Suicide ideation	1	2	3	4	5	NA
250205	Suicide attempts	1	2	3	4	5	NA
250206	Trauma-induced psychoneurotic behaviors	1	2	3	4	5	NA
250207	Inappropriate attention-seeking behaviors	1	2	3	4	5	NA
250208	Trauma-induced conduct disorders	1	2	3	4	5	NA
250209	Trauma-induced learning difficulties	1	2	3	4	5	NA
250210	Self-injurious behaviors	1	2	3	4	5	NA
250211	Neurotic behaviors	1	2	3	4	5	NA

Domain-*Family Health (VI)*   **Class**-*Family Member Health Status (Z)*   *1st edition 1997; revised 2004, 2013*

OUTCOME CONTENT REFERENCES:
+Briere, J., & Runtz, . (1989). The trauma symptom checklist (TSC-33): Early data on a new scale. *Journal of Interpersonal Violence, 4*(2), 151–163.
Campbell, J., McKenna, L. S., Torres, S., Sheridan, D., & Landenburger, K. (1993). Nursing care of abused women. In J. Campbell & J. Humphreys (Eds.), *Nursing care of survivors of family violence* (pp. 248–289). St. Louis: Mosby.
Campbell, J., & Fishwick, N. (1993). Abuse of female partners. In J. Campbell & J. Humphreys (Eds.), *Nursing care of survivors of family violence* (pp. 68–104). St. Louis: Mosby.
Humphreys, J., Lee, K., Neylan, T., & Marmar, C. (2001). Psychological and physical distress of sheltered battered women. *Health Care for Women International, 22*(4), 401–414.
Kaplan, S. J., Pelcovitz, D., & Labruna, V. (1999). Child and adolescent abuse and neglect research: A review of the past 10 years. Part I: Physical and emotional abuse and neglect. *Journal of the American Academy of Child & Adolescent Psychiatry, 38*(10), 1214–1222.
Rosen, L. N., & Martin, L. (1998). Long-term effects of childhood maltreatment history on gender-related personality characteristics. *Child Abuse & Neglect, 22*(3), 197–211.
Taylor, J. Y. (2000). Sisters of the Yam: African American women's healing and self-recovery from intimate male partner violence. *Issues in Mental Health Nursing, 21*(5), 515–531.

A

Abuse Recovery: Financial   2503

Definition: Extent of control of monetary and legal matters following financial exploitation

OUTCOME TARGET RATING: Maintain at_____   Increase to_____

		None	Limited	Moderate	Substantial	Extensive	
OUTCOME OVERALL RATING		1	2	3	4	5	
Indicators:							
250301	Control of personal possessions	1	2	3	4	5	NA
250303	Control of personal finances	1	2	3	4	5	NA
250306	Control of withdrawal of money from account(s)	1	2	3	4	5	NA
250302	Control of Social Security and pension income	1	2	3	4	5	NA
250311	Control of earned income	1	2	3	4	5	NA
250313	Control of court-ordered benefits	1	2	3	4	5	NA
250304	Control of legal matters	1	2	3	4	5	NA
250305	Exercise of legal rights	1	2	3	4	5	NA
250315	Knowledge about financial resources	1	2	3	4	5	NA
250308	Knowledge about legal matters	1	2	3	4	5	NA
250309	Participation in financial planning	1	2	3	4	5	NA
250316	Involvement in occupation	1	2	3	4	5	NA
250312	Protection in financial resources	1	2	3	4	5	NA

Domain-*Family Health (VI)*   **Class**-*Family Member Health Status (Z)*   *1st edition 1997; revised 2004, 2008, 2013*

OUTCOME CONTENT REFERENCES:

Anetzberger, G. J. (1987). *The etiology of elder abuse of adult offspring.* Springfield, IL: Charles C. Thomas.

Baumhover, L. A., Beall, S. C., & Pieroni, R. E. (1990). Elder abuse: An overview of social and medical indicators. *Journal of Health and Human Resources Administration, 12*(4), 414–443.

Hudson, M. F., & Johnson, T. F. (1986). Elder neglect and abuse: A review of the literature. *Annual Review of Nursing Research, 6*(3), 81–134.

Lavrisha, M. (1997). What can nurses do about financial exploitation of elders? *Journal of Gerontological Nursing, 23*(7), 49–50.

Reed, K. (2005). When elders lose their cents: Financial abuse of the elderly. *Clinics in Geriatric Medicine, 21*(2), 365–382.

+Sullivan, C., Campbell, R., Angelique, H., Eby, K., & Davidson, W. (1994). An advocacy intervention program for women with abusive partners: Six-month follow-up. *American Journal of Community Psychology, 22*(1), 101–122.

Walsh, K., & Bennett, G. (2000). Financial abuse of older people. *Journal of Adult Protection, 2*(1), 21–29.

Weiler, K. (1989). Financial abuse of the elderly: Recognizing and acting on it. *Journal of Gerontological Nursing, 15*(8), 10–15.

Abuse Recovery: Physical 2504

Definition: Extent of healing of physical injuries due to abuse

OUTCOME TARGET RATING: Maintain at_____   Increase to_____

		None	Limited	Moderate	Substantial	Extensive	
OUTCOME OVERALL RATING		1	2	3	4	5	
Indicators:							
250403	Timely treatment of injuries	1	2	3	4	5	NA
250401	Healing of physical injuries	1	2	3	4	5	NA
250407	Resolution of physical health problems	1	2	3	4	5	NA
250404	Use of therapeutic health care as needed	1	2	3	4	5	NA
250405	Use of preventive health care	1	2	3	4	5	NA
250411	Evidence of expected response to treatment	1	2	3	4	5	NA
250408	Maintenance of nutritional requirements	1	2	3	4	5	NA
250409	Urinary continence	1	2	3	4	5	NA
250402	Regular bowel elimination	1	2	3	4	5	NA

Domain-Family Health (VI)   *Class*-Family Member Health Status (Z)   *1st edition 1997; revised 2004, 2008*

OUTCOME CONTENT REFERENCES:

+Briere, J., & Runtz, M. (1989). The trauma symptom checklist (TSC-33): Early data on a new scale. *Journal of Interpersonal Violence, 4*(2), 151–163.

Campbell, J., & Fishwick, N. (1993). Abuse of female partners. In J. Campbell & J. Humphreys (Eds.), *Nursing care of survivors of family violence* (pp. 68–104). St. Louis: Mosby.

Campbell, J., McKenna, L. S., Torres, S., Sheridan, D., & Landenburger, K. (1993). Nursing care of abused women. In J. Campbell & J. Humphreys (Eds.), *Nursing care of survivors of family violence* (pp. 248–289). St. Louis: Mosby.

Humphreys, J., Lee, K., Neylan, T., & Marmar, C. (2001). Psychological and physical distress of sheltered battered women. *Health Care for Women International, 22*(4), 401–414.

Kaplan, S. J., Pelcovitz, D., & Labruna, V. (1999). Child and adolescent abuse and neglect research: A review of the past 10 years. Part I: Physical and emotional abuse and neglect. *Journal of the American Academy of Child & Adolescent Psychiatry, 38*(10), 1214–1222.

Marshall, C. E., Benton, D., & Brazier, J. M. (2000). Elder abuse: Using clinical tools to identify clues of mistreatment. *Geriatrics, 55*(2), 42–44.

McFarlane, J., Parker, B., & Soeken, K. (1996). Abuse during pregnancy: Associations with maternal health and infant birth weight. *Nursing Research, 45*(1), 37–42.

Abuse Recovery: Sexual 2505

Definition: Extent of healing of physical and psychological injuries due to sexual abuse or exploitation

OUTCOME TARGET RATING: Maintain at_____ Increase to_____

OUTCOME OVERALL RATING		None 1	Limited 2	Moderate 3	Substantial 4	Extensive 5	
Indicators:							
250502	Acknowledgment of right to disclose abusive situation	1	2	3	4	5	NA
250505	Expressions of right to have been protected from abuse	1	2	3	4	5	NA
250523	Healing of physical injuries	1	2	3	4	5	NA
250509	Relief of anger in non-destructive ways	1	2	3	4	5	NA
250510	Self-advocacy	1	2	3	4	5	NA
250511	Feelings of empowerment	1	2	3	4	5	NA
250512	Expressions of hope	1	2	3	4	5	NA
250513	Consistency of behavior with social norms	1	2	3	4	5	NA
250514	Evidence of non-abusive same-sex relationships	1	2	3	4	5	NA
250515	Evidence of non-abusive opposite-sex relationships	1	2	3	4	5	NA
250524	Expressions of comfort with gender identity	1	2	3	4	5	NA
250525	Expressions of comfort with sexual orientation	1	2	3	4	5	NA
250521	Verbalization of accurate information about sexual functioning	1	2	3	4	5	NA
250526	Resolution of feelings about abuse	1	2	3	4	5	NA
250527	Resolution of guilt	1	2	3	4	5	NA

		Extensive	Substantial	Moderate	Limited	None	
250501	Verbalization of details of abuse	1	2	3	4	5	NA
250507	Sleep disturbance	1	2	3	4	5	NA
250508	Depression	1	2	3	4	5	NA
250518	Eating disorders	1	2	3	4	5	NA
250519	Self-mutilation	1	2	3	4	5	NA
250520	Suicide attempts	1	2	3	4	5	NA

Domain-Family Health (VI)   **Class**-Family Member Health Status (Z)   *1st edition 1997; revised 2004, 2013*

OUTCOME CONTENT REFERENCES:

Bass, E., & Davis, L. (1994). *The courage to heal: A guide for women survivors of child sexual abuse* (3rd ed.). New York: Harper & Row.

+Briere, J., & Runtz, M. (1989). The trauma symptom checklist (TSC-33): Early data on a new scale. *Journal of Interpersonal Violence, 4*(2), 151–163.

DePanfilis, D. (1986). *Literature review of sexual abuse* (DHHS Publication No. [OHDSA] 87-30530). Washington, DC: USDHHS, National Center on Child Abuse & Neglect.

Gries, L. T., Goh, D. S., Andrews, M. B., Gilbert, J., Praver, F., & Stelzer, D. N. (2000). Positive reaction to disclosure and recovery from child sexual abuse. *Journal of Child Sexual Abuse, 9*(1), 29–51.

Hill, E. L., Gold, S. N., & Bornstein, R. F. (2000). Interpersonal dependency among adult survivors of childhood sexual abuse in therapy. *Journal of Child Sexual Abuse, 9*(2), 71–86.

Sgroi, S. M. (1982). *Handbook of clinical intervention in child sexual abuse.* Lexington, MA: Lexington Books.

Sgroi, S. M. (Ed.) (1988). *Vulnerable populations: Evaluation and treatment of sexually abused children and adult survivors* (Vol. 1). Lexington, MA: Lexington Books.

Sgroi, S. M. (Ed.) (1988). *Vulnerable populations: Sexual abuse treatment for children, adult survivors, offenders, and persons with mental retardation* (Vol. 2). Lexington, MA: Lexington Books.

Smith, M. E., & Kelly, L. M. (2001). The journey of recovery after a rape experience. *Issues in Mental Health Nursing, 22*(4), 337–352.

Symes, L. (2000). Arriving at readiness to recover emotionally after sexual assault. *Archives of Psychiatric Nursing, 14*(1), 30–38.

Tremblay, C., Hebért, M., & Piché, C. (2000). Type I and type II posttraumatic stress disorder in sexually abused children. *Journal of Child Sexual Abuse, 9*(1), 65–90.

A

Abusive Behavior Self-Restraint   1400

Definition: Personal actions to refrain from abusive and neglectful behaviors toward others

OUTCOME TARGET RATING: Maintain at_____   Increase to_____

	Never demonstrated	Rarely demonstrated	Sometimes demonstrated	Often demonstrated	Consistently demonstrated	
OUTCOME OVERALL RATING	1	2	3	4	5	
Indicators:						
140022 Obtains needed treatment	1	2	3	4	5	NA
140020 Participates in required treatment regimen	1	2	3	4	5	NA
140006 Discusses the abusive behavior	1	2	3	4	5	NA
140007 Identifies factors contributing to abusive behavior	1	2	3	4	5	NA
140010 Expresses frustrations	1	2	3	4	5	NA
140013 States expectations congruent with developmental level	1	2	3	4	5	NA
140012 Exhibits self-esteem	1	2	3	4	5	NA
140005 Uses alternative coping mechanisms for stress	1	2	3	4	5	NA
140023 Uses personal support system	1	2	3	4	5	NA
140017 Controls impulses	1	2	3	4	5	NA
140018 Uses correct role behaviors	1	2	3	4	5	NA
140024 Uses appropriate caregiving techniques	1	2	3	4	5	NA
140025 Refrains from physically abusive behavior	1	2	3	4	5	NA
140026 Refrains from emotionally abusive behavior	1	2	3	4	5	NA
140027 Refrains from sexually abusive behavior	1	2	3	4	5	NA
140028 Refrains from neglect of dependent's basic needs	1	2	3	4	5	NA
140008 Expresses feelings about victim	1	2	3	4	5	NA
140016 Expresses empathy for victim	1	2	3	4	5	NA
140011 Uses nurturing behavior toward victim	1	2	3	4	5	NA
140009 Identifies available community resources	1	2	3	4	5	NA

*Domain-Psychosocial Health (III)   **Class**-Self-Control (O)   1st edition 1997; revised 2000, 2004, 2008, 2013*

OUTCOME CONTENT REFERENCES:

Amundson, M. J. (1989). Family crisis care: A home-based intervention program for child abuse. *Issues in Mental Health Nursing, 10*(3–4), 285–296.

Anderson, C. L. (1987). Assessing parenting potential for child abuse risk. *Pediatric Nursing, 13*(5), 323–327.

+Buss, A. H., & Perry, M. (1992). The Aggression Questionnaire. *Journal of Personality and Social Psychology, 63*(3), 452–459.

Cowen, P. (1991). *The Iowa crisis nursery project as a factor in the prevention of child abuse.* Unpublished doctoral dissertation, University of Iowa, Iowa City, IA.

Olds, D. L., Henderson, C. R., Chamberlin, R., & Tatelbaum, R. (1986). Preventing child abuse and neglect: A randomized trial of nurse home visitation. *Pediatrics, 78*(1), 65–78.

Marshall, E., Buckner, E., & Powell, K. (1991). Evaluation of a teen parent program designed to reduce child abuse and neglect and to strengthen families. *Journal of Child and Adolescent Psychiatric and Mental Health Nursing, 4*(3), 96–100.

Reuter, M. M. (1988). Parenting needs of abusing parents: Development of a tool for evaluation of parent education class. *Journal of Community Health Nursing, 5*(2), 129–140.

Taylor, D. K., & Beauchamp, C. (1988). Hospital-based primary prevention strategy in child abuse: A multi-level needs assessment. *Child Abuse and Neglect, 12*(3), 343–354.

Tolman, R. M., Edleson, J. L., & Fendrich, M. (1996). The applicability of the theory of planned behavior to abusive men's cessation of violent behavior. *Violence & Victims, 11*(4), 341–354.

A

Acceptance: Health Status

1300

Definition: Personal actions to reconcile significant changes in health circumstances

OUTCOME TARGET RATING: Maintain at_____ Increase to_____

OUTCOME OVERALL RATING	Never demonstrated 1	Rarely demonstrated 2	Sometimes demonstrated 3	Often demonstrated 4	Consistently demonstrated 5	
Indicators:						
130002 Relinquishes previous concept of personal health	1	2	3	4	5	NA
130008 Recognizes reality of health situation	1	2	3	4	5	NA
130020 Reports positive self-regard	1	2	3	4	5	NA
130016 Maintains relationships	1	2	3	4	5	NA
130007 Reports decreased need to verbalize feelings about health	1	2	3	4	5	NA
130017 Adjusts to change in health status	1	2	3	4	5	NA
130021 Expresses inner peace	1	2	3	4	5	NA
130018 Exhibits resiliency	1	2	3	4	5	NA
130009 Pursues information about health	1	2	3	4	5	NA
130010 Copes with health situation	1	2	3	4	5	NA
130011 Makes decisions about health	1	2	3	4	5	NA
130012 Clarifies personal values	1	2	3	4	5	NA
130019 Clarifies life priorities	1	2	3	4	5	NA
130013 Reports sense of life being worth living	1	2	3	4	5	NA
130014 Performs self-care tasks	1	2	3	4	5	NA

Domain-*Psychosocial Health (III)*   **Class**-*Psychosocial Adaptation (N)*   *1st edition 1997; revised 2000, 2004, 2008, 2013*

OUTCOME CONTENT REFERENCES:

Clayton, J. W. (1993). Paving the way to acceptance: Psychological adaptation to death and dying in cancer. *Professional Nurse, 8*(4), 206–211.

Kelley, M. P., & Henry, P. (1993). Open discussion can lead to acceptance: The psychosocial effects of stoma surgery. *Professional Nurse, 9*(2), 101–110.

Kubler-Ross, E. (1977). *On death and dying.* London: Tavistock Press.

Lazarus, R. S., & Folkman, S. (1984). *Stress, appraisal, and coping.* New York: Springer.

Longo, M. B. (1993). Facilitating acceptance of a patient's decision to stop treatment. *Clinical Nurse Specialist, 7*(3), 233–243.

Melamed, S., Groswasser, Z., & Stern, M. (1992). Acceptance of disability, work involvement and subjective rehabilitation status of traumatic brain-injured (TBI) patients. *Brain Injury, 6*(3), 233–243.

Reynaud, S. N., & Meeker, B. J. (2002). Coping styles of older adults with ostomies. *Journal of Gerontological Nursing, 28*(5), 30–36.

+Wagnild, G. M., & Young, H. M. (1993). Development and psychometric evaluation of the resilience scale. *Journal of Nursing Measurement, 1*(2), 165–178.

Activity Tolerance 0005

A

Definition: Physiologic response to energy-consuming movements with daily activities

OUTCOME TARGET RATING: Maintain at_____ Increase to_____

	Severely compromised	Substantially compromised	Moderately compromised	Mildly compromised	Not compromised	
OUTCOME OVERALL RATING	1	2	3	4	5	

Indicators:

000501	Oxygen saturation with activity	1	2	3	4	5	NA
000502	Pulse rate with activity	1	2	3	4	5	NA
000503	Respiratory rate with activity	1	2	3	4	5	NA
000508	Ease of breathing with activity	1	2	3	4	5	NA
000504	Systolic blood pressure with activity	1	2	3	4	5	NA
000505	Diastolic blood pressure with activity	1	2	3	4	5	NA
000506	Electrocardiogram findings	1	2	3	4	5	NA
000507	Skin color	1	2	3	4	5	NA
000509	Walking pace	1	2	3	4	5	NA
000510	Walking distance	1	2	3	4	5	NA
000511	Stair-climbing tolerance	1	2	3	4	5	NA
000516	Upper body strength	1	2	3	4	5	NA
000517	Lower body strength	1	2	3	4	5	NA
000518	Ease of performing activities of daily living (ADL)	1	2	3	4	5	NA
000514	Ability to speak with physical activity	1	2	3	4	5	NA

Domain-*Functional Health (I)*   **Class**-*Energy Maintenance (A)*   *2nd edition 2000; revised 2004*

OUTCOME CONTENT REFERENCES:

Barnett-Damewood, M., & Carlson-Catalano, J. (2000). Physical activity deficit: A proposed nursing diagnosis. *Nursing Diagnosis, 11*(1), 24–31.

Buchner, D. M. (1995). Clinical assessments of physical activity in older adults. In L. Z. Rubenstein, D. Wieland, & R. Bernabei (Eds.), *Geriatric assessment technology: The state of the art* (pp. 147–159). New York: Springer.

Hosking, R., & Hiller, G. (1989). Using nursing diagnosis in a cardiovascular clinical nurse specialist practice. *Journal of Advanced Medical-Surgical Nursing, 1*(3), 33–41.

Larson, J. L., & Leidy, N. K. (1998). Chronic obstructive pulmonary disease: Strategies to improve functional status. *Annual Review of Nursing Research, 16*, 253–286.

Melillo, K. D., Houde, S. C., Williamson, E., & Futrell, M. (2000). Perceptions of nurse practitioners regarding their role in physical activity and exercise prescription for older adults. *Clinical Excellence for Nurse Practitioners, 4*(2), 108–116.

Mol, V. J., & Baker, C. A. (1991). Activity intolerance in the geriatric stroke patient. *Rehabilitation Nursing, 16*(6), 337–344.

Roberts, S. L., & White, B. (1992). Common nursing diagnoses for pulmonary alveolar edema patients. *Dimensions of Critical Care Nursing, 11*(1), 13–27.

Tack, B. B., & Gilliss, C. L. (1990). Nurse-monitored cardiac recovery: A description of the first 8 weeks. *Heart & Lung, 19*(5), 491–499.

Wieseke, A., Twibell, R., Bennett, S., Marine, M., & Schoger, J. (1994). A content validation study of five nursing diagnoses by critical care nurses. *Heart & Lung, 23*(4), 345–351.

A

Acute Respiratory Acidosis Severity   0604

Definition: Severity of signs and symptoms of decreased blood pH and increased partial arterial carbon dioxide pressure due to hypoventilation and retention of carbon dioxide

OUTCOME TARGET RATING: Maintain at_____   Increase to_____

OUTCOME OVERALL RATING	Severe 1	Substantial 2	Moderate 3	Mild 4	None 5	
Indicators:						
060401 Decrease in blood plasma pH	1	2	3	4	5	NA
060402 Increase in serum hydrogen ions	1	2	3	4	5	NA
060403 Increase in serum partial arterial carbon dioxide pressure	1	2	3	4	5	NA
060404 Decrease in serum partial arterial oxygen pressure	1	2	3	4	5	NA
060405 Hypoxia	1	2	3	4	5	NA
060406 Increased apical heart rate	1	2	3	4	5	NA
060407 Arrhythmias	1	2	3	4	5	NA
060408 Increased respiratory rate	1	2	3	4	5	NA
060409 Increased blood pressure	1	2	3	4	5	NA
060410 Muscle twitching	1	2	3	4	5	NA
060411 Drowsiness	1	2	3	4	5	NA
060412 Decreased level of consciousness	1	2	3	4	5	NA
060413 Confusion	1	2	3	4	5	NA
060414 Slowed verbal response	1	2	3	4	5	NA
060415 Dizziness	1	2	3	4	5	NA
060416 Dilated conjunctival blood vessels	1	2	3	4	5	NA
060417 Headache	1	2	3	4	5	NA
060418 Diaphoresis	1	2	3	4	5	NA

Domain-*Physiologic Health (II)*   **Class-***Fluid & Electrolytes (G)*   *5th edition 2013*

OUTCOME CONTENT REFERENCES:

Appel, S. J., & Downs, C. A. (2007). Steady a disturbed equilibrium: Accurately interpret the acid-base balance of acutely ill patients. *Nursing Critical Care, 2*(4), 45–53.

Clancy, J., & McVicar, A. (2007). Intermediate and long-term regulation of acid-base homeostasis. *British Journal of Nursing, 16*(17), 1076–1079.

Isenhour, J. L., & Slovis, C. M. (2008). Arterial blood gas analysis: A 3-step approach to acid-base disorders. *The Journal of Respiratory Diseases, 29*(2), 74–82.

Kraut, J. A., & Madeas, N. E. (2001). Approach to patients with acid-base disorders. *Respiratory Care, 46*(4), 392–402.

Lian, J. X. (2010). Interpreting and using the arterial blood gas analysis. *Nursing Critical Care, 5*(3), 26–36.

Lynch, F. (2009). Arterial blood gas analysis: Implications for nursing. *Paediatric Nursing, 21*(1), 41–44.

Porth, C. M. (2007). *Essentials of pathophysiology* (2nd ed.). Philadelphia: Lippincott Williams & Wilkins.

Priestly, M. A., & Litman, R. (2009). Acidosis, respiratory. In *Emedicine*. Retrieved from http://emedicine.medscape.com/article/906545-overview

Ruholl, L. (2006). Arterial blood gases: Analysis and nursing responses. *MEDSURG Nursing, 15*(6), 343–351.

Acute Respiratory Alkalosis Severity   0605   A

Definition: Severity of signs and symptoms of increased blood pH and decreased partial arterial carbon dioxide pressure due to hyperventilation and increased elimination of carbon dioxide

OUTCOME TARGET RATING: Maintain at_____   Increase to_____

	Severe	Substantial	Moderate	Mild	None	
OUTCOME OVERALL RATING	1	2	3	4	5	
Indicators:						
060501 Increase in blood plasma pH	1	2	3	4	5	NA
060502 Decrease in serum hydrogen ions	1	2	3	4	5	NA
060503 Decrease in serum bicarbonate	1	2	3	4	5	NA
060504 Decrease in partial pressure of carbon dioxide in arterial blood (PaCO$_2$)	1	2	3	4	5	NA
060505 Decrease in partial pressure of oxygen in arterial blood (PaO$_2$)	1	2	3	4	5	NA
060506 Decrease in serum potassium	1	2	3	4	5	NA
060507 Decrease in ionized serum calcium	1	2	3	4	5	NA
060508 Decrease in serum phosphate	1	2	3	4	5	NA
060509 Increased apical heart rate	1	2	3	4	5	NA
060510 Arrhythmias	1	2	3	4	5	NA
060511 Heart palpitations	1	2	3	4	5	NA
060512 Increased respiratory rate	1	2	3	4	5	NA
060513 Increased respiratory depth	1	2	3	4	5	NA
060514 Tinnitus	1	2	3	4	5	NA
060515 Dizziness	1	2	3	4	5	NA
060516 Lightheadedness	1	2	3	4	5	NA
060517 Decreased level of consciousness	1	2	3	4	5	NA
060518 Tingling in extremities	1	2	3	4	5	NA
060519 Hyperactive reflexes	1	2	3	4	5	NA
060520 Hypertonic muscles	1	2	3	4	5	NA
060521 Paresthesias	1	2	3	4	5	NA

Domain-*Physiologic Health (II)*   **Class**-*Fluid & Electrolytes (G)*   *5th edition 2013*

OUTCOME CONTENT REFERENCES:

Appel, S. J., & Downs, C. A. (2007). Steady a disturbed equilibrium: Accurately interpret the acid-base balance of acutely ill patients. *Nursing Critical Care, 2*(4), 45–53.

Clancy, J., & McVicar, A. (2007). Intermediate and long-term regulation of acid-base homeostasis. *British Journal of Nursing, 16*(17), 1076–1079.

Foster, G. T., Vaziri, N. D., & Sassoon, C. S. (2001). Respiratory alkalosis. *Respiratory Care, 46*(4), 384–391.

Isenhour, J. L., & Slovis, C. M. (2008). Arterial blood gas analysis: A 3-step approach to acid-base disorders. *The Journal of Respiratory Diseases, 29*(2), 74–82.

Kraut, J. A., & Madeas, N. E. (2001). Approach to patients with acid-base disorders. *Respiratory Care, 46*(4), 392–402.

Lian, J. X. (2010). Interpreting and using the arterial blood gas analysis. *Nursing Critical Care, 5*(3), 26–36.

Lynch, F. (2009). Arterial blood gas analysis: Implications for nursing. *Paediatric Nursing, 21*(1), 41–44.

Ruholl, L. (2006). Arterial blood gases: Analysis and nursing responses. *MEDSURG Nursing, 15*(6), 343–351.

A

Adaptation to Physical Disability   1308

Definition: Personal actions to adapt to a significant functional challenge due to a physical disability

OUTCOME TARGET RATING: Maintain at_____   Increase to_____

OUTCOME OVERALL RATING	Never demonstrated 1	Rarely demonstrated 2	Sometimes demonstrated 3	Often demonstrated 4	Consistently demonstrated 5	
Indicators:						
130801 Verbalizes ability to adjust to disability	1	2	3	4	5	NA
130802 Verbalizes reconciliation to disability	1	2	3	4	5	NA
130803 Adapts to functional limitations	1	2	3	4	5	NA
130804 Modifies lifestyle to accommodate disability	1	2	3	4	5	NA
130805 Modifies career goals to accommodate disability	1	2	3	4	5	NA
130806 Uses strategies to reduce stress related to disability	1	2	3	4	5	NA
130807 Identifies ways to increase sense of control	1	2	3	4	5	NA
130808 Identifies ways to cope with life changes	1	2	3	4	5	NA
130809 Identifies risk of complications associated with disability	1	2	3	4	5	NA
130810 Identifies plan to meet activities of daily living	1	2	3	4	5	NA
130811 Identifies plan to meet instrumental activities of daily living	1	2	3	4	5	NA
130812 Accepts need for physical assistance	1	2	3	4	5	NA
130821 Obtains information about disability	1	2	3	4	5	NA
130822 Uses community resources	1	2	3	4	5	NA
130823 Obtains assistance from health professional	1	2	3	4	5	NA
130824 Uses personal support system	1	2	3	4	5	NA
130817 Reports decrease in stress related to disability	1	2	3	4	5	NA
130818 Reports decrease in negative feelings	1	2	3	4	5	NA
130819 Reports decrease in negative body image	1	2	3	4	5	NA
130820 Reports increase in psychological comfort	1	2	3	4	5	NA

Domain-*Psychosocial Health (III)*   **Class**-*Psychosocial Adaptation (N)*   *3rd edition 2004; revised 2008, 2013*

OUTCOME CONTENT REFERENCES:

Carlsson, E., Berglund, B., & Norgren, S. (2001). Living with an ostomy and short bowel syndrome: Practical aspects and impact on daily life. *Journal of WOCN: Wound, Ostomy, and Continence Nursing, 28*(2), 96–105.

Gignac, M. A., Cott, C., & Badley, E. M. (2000). Adaptation to chronic illness and disability and its relationship to perceptions of independence and dependence. *Journal of Gerontology Series B—Psychological Sciences, 55*(6), P362–P372.

Livneh, H., Antonak, R. F., & Gerhardt, J. (1999). Psychosocial adaptation to amputation: The role of sociodemographic variables, disability-related factors and coping strategies. *International Journal of Rehabilitation Research, 22*(1), 21–31.

Wingate, S. J. (1986). Levels of pacemaker acceptance by patients. *Heart & Lung, 15*(1), 93–100.

Adherence Behavior   1600   A

Definition: Self-initiated actions to promote optimal wellness, recovery, and rehabilitation

OUTCOME TARGET RATING: Maintain at_____   Increase to_____

	Never demonstrated	Rarely demonstrated	Sometimes demonstrated	Often demonstrated	Consistently demonstrated	
OUTCOME OVERALL RATING	1	2	3	4	5	

Indicators:

		Never	Rarely	Sometimes	Often	Consistently	
160001	Asks health-related questions	1	2	3	4	5	NA
160002	Seeks health information from a variety of sources	1	2	3	4	5	NA
160016	Evaluates accuracy of health information obtained	1	2	3	4	5	NA
160003	Uses reputable health information to develop strategies	1	2	3	4	5	NA
160004	Weighs risks/benefits of health behavior	1	2	3	4	5	NA
160007	Provides rationale for adopting a health behavior	1	2	3	4	5	NA
160008	Uses strategies to eliminate unhealthy behavior	1	2	3	4	5	NA
160009	Uses strategies to optimize health	1	2	3	4	5	NA
160010	Uses health care services congruent with need	1	2	3	4	5	NA
160011	Performs activities of daily living consistent with energy and tolerance	1	2	3	4	5	NA
160012	Performs self-screening	1	2	3	4	5	NA
160013	Describes rationale for deviating from a health regimen	1	2	3	4	5	NA
160014	Performs self-monitoring of health status	1	2	3	4	5	NA

Domain-Health Knowledge & Behavior (IV)   **Class**-Health Behavior (Q)   *1st edition 1997; revised 2004, 2008*

OUTCOME CONTENT REFERENCES:

Burkhart, P. V., Dunbar-Jacob, J. M., & Rohay, J. M. (2001). Accuracy of children's self-reported adherence to treatment. *Journal of Nursing Scholarship, 33*(1), 27–32.

Epstein, L., & Cluss, P. A. (1982). A behavioral perspective on adherence to long-term medical regimens. *Journal of Consulting and Clinical Psychology, 50*(6), 950–971.

Folden, S. L. (1993). Definitions of health and health goals of participants in a community-based pulmonary rehabilitation program. *Public Health Nursing, 10*(1), 31–35.

+Hettler, B. (1982). Wellness promotion and risk reduction on a university campus. In M. Faber & A. Reinhardt (Eds.), *Promoting health through risk reduction.* New York: Macmillan.

Jensen, L., & Allen, M. (1993). Wellness: The dialect of illness. *Image—The Journal of Nursing Scholarship, 25*(3), 220–224.

Konradi, D. B., & Lyon, B. L. (2000). Measuring adherence to a self-care fitness walking routine. *Journal of Community Health Nursing, 17*(3), 159–169.

Kravits, R., Hays, R. D., Sherbourne, C. D., DiMatteo, M. R., Rogers, W. H., Ordway, L., & Greenfield, S. (1993). Recall of recommendations and adherence to advice among patients with chronic medical conditions. *Archives of Internal Medicine, 153*(16), 1869–1878.

Miller, P., Wikoff, R., & Hiatt, A. (1972). Fishbein's Model of measured behavior of hypertensive patients. *Nursing Research, 41*(2), 104–109.

Pender, N. J. (1990). Expressing health through lifestyle patterns. *Nursing Science Quarterly, 3*(3), 115–122.

Pender, N. J., & Pender, A. R. (1986). Attitudes, subjective norms, and intentions of engagement in health behaviors. *Nursing Research, 35*(1), 15–18.

Shumaker, S. A., Schron, E. B., & Ockene, J. K. (1998). *The handbook of health behavior change* (2nd ed.). New York: Springer.

Toljamo, M., & Hentinen, M. (2001). Adherence to self-care and social support. *Journal of Clinical Nursing, 10*(5), 618–627.

Woods, N. (1989). Conceptualizations of self-care: Toward health-oriented models. *Advances in Nursing Science, 12*(1), 1–13.

Adherence Behavior: Healthy Diet   1621

Definition: Self-initiated actions to monitor and optimize a balanced nutritional dietary regimen

OUTCOME TARGET RATING: Maintain at_____   Increase to_____

		Never demonstrated	Rarely demonstrated	Sometimes demonstrated	Often demonstrated	Consistently demonstrated	
OUTCOME OVERALL RATING		1	2	3	4	5	
Indicators:							
162101	Sets achievable dietary goals	1	2	3	4	5	NA
162102	Balances caloric intake and caloric requirements	1	2	3	4	5	NA
162103	Seeks information about established nutritional guidelines	1	2	3	4	5	NA
162104	Uses recommended nutritional guidelines to plan meals	1	2	3	4	5	NA
162105	Selects foods consistent with recommended nutritional guidelines	1	2	3	4	5	NA
162106	Selects portions consistent with recommended nutritional guidelines	1	2	3	4	5	NA
162107	Selects foods based on nutritional information on food labels	1	2	3	4	5	NA
162108	Washes fresh fruits and vegetables before eating	1	2	3	4	5	NA
162109	Prepares foods following dietary recommendations for fat, sodium, and carbohydrates	1	2	3	4	5	NA
162110	Cooks meat, poultry, fish, and eggs based on safety recommendations	1	2	3	4	5	NA
162111	Eats recommended servings of fruits per day	1	2	3	4	5	NA
162112	Eats recommended servings of vegetables per day	1	2	3	4	5	NA
162113	Eats more whole-grain products than refined-grain products	1	2	3	4	5	NA
162114	Minimizes foods with high caloric value and little nutritional value	1	2	3	4	5	NA
162115	Balances fluid intake and fluid loss	1	2	3	4	5	NA
162116	Maintains hydration	1	2	3	4	5	NA
162117	Selects foods that provide calcium to meet requirements	1	2	3	4	5	NA
162118	Supplements with vitamins/minerals within suggested guidelines	1	2	3	4	5	NA
162119	Chooses foods consistent with cultural religious beliefs	1	2	3	4	5	NA
162120	Discusses use of herbal remedies with health provider	1	2	3	4	5	NA
162121	Avoids foods that interact with medications	1	2	3	4	5	NA
162122	Avoids foods that interact with herbal remedies	1	2	3	4	5	NA
162123	Avoids foods that trigger allergic reactions	1	2	3	4	5	NA

Domain-*Health Knowledge & Behavior (IV)*   **Class**-*Health Behavior (Q)*   *4th edition 2008; revised 2013*

OUTCOME CONTENT REFERENCES:
Brownell, K. D., & Cohen, L. R. (1995). Adherence to dietary regimen 2: Components of effective intervention. *Behavioral Medicine, 20*(4), 155–164.
Dudek, S. G. (2007). *Nutrition essentials for nursing practice* (5th rev. ed.). Philadelphia: Lippincott Williams & Wilkins.
Marotz, L. R., Rush, J. M., & Cross, M. Z. (2001). *Health, safety, and nutrition for the young child*. Albany, NY: Thomson Delmar Learning.
U.S. Department of Agriculture and U.S. Department of Health and Humans Services. (2010). *Dietary guidelines for Americans 2010* (7th ed.). Washington, DC: U.S. Government Printing Office.

Aggression Self-Restraint 1401

Definition: Personal actions to refrain from assaultive, combative, or destructive behaviors toward others

OUTCOME TARGET RATING: Maintain at_____   Increase to_____

OUTCOME OVERALL RATING	Never demonstrated 1	Rarely demonstrated 2	Sometimes demonstrated 3	Often demonstrated 4	Consistently demonstrated 5	
Indicators:						
140110 Identifies when angry	1	2	3	4	5	NA
140111 Identifies when frustrated	1	2	3	4	5	NA
140112 Identifies situations that precipitate hostility	1	2	3	4	5	NA
140113 Identifies responsibility to maintain control	1	2	3	4	5	NA
140114 Identifies when feeling aggressive	1	2	3	4	5	NA
140115 Identifies alternatives to aggression	1	2	3	4	5	NA
140116 Identifies alternatives to verbal outbursts	1	2	3	4	5	NA
140124 Uses effective conflict resolution skills	1	2	3	4	5	NA
140125 Expresses needs in a non-destructive manner	1	2	3	4	5	NA
140117 Vents negative feelings in a non-destructive manner	1	2	3	4	5	NA
140101 Refrains from verbal outbursts	1	2	3	4	5	NA
140126 Avoids violating others' personal space	1	2	3	4	5	NA
140103 Refrains from striking others	1	2	3	4	5	NA
140104 Refrains from harming others	1	2	3	4	5	NA
140105 Refrains from harming animals	1	2	3	4	5	NA
140106 Refrains from destroying property	1	2	3	4	5	NA
140109 Controls impulses	1	2	3	4	5	NA
140121 Uses physical activity to reduce pent-up energy	1	2	3	4	5	NA
140122 Uses techniques to control anger	1	2	3	4	5	NA
140123 Uses techniques to control frustration	1	2	3	4	5	NA
140118 Upholds contract to restrain aggressive behaviors	1	2	3	4	5	NA
140119 Maintains self-control without supervision	1	2	3	4	5	NA

Domain-Psychosocial Health (III) *Class*-Self-Control (O) *1st edition 1997; revised 2000, 2004, 2008, 2013*

OUTCOME CONTENT REFERENCES:
Berkowitz, L. (1993). *Aggression: Its causes, consequences, and control.* New York: McGraw-Hill.
+Buss, A. H., & Perry, M. (1992). The aggression questionnaire. *Journal of Personality and Social Psychology, 63*(3), 452–459.
Crowell, D. H., Evans, I. M., & O'Donnell, C. R. (Eds.). (1987). *Childhood aggression and violence.* New York: Plenum.
Grancola, P. R., & Zeichner, A. (1993). Aggressive behavior in the elderly: A critical review. *Clinical Gerontologist, 13*(2), 3–22.
Ingram, T. N. (2001). Risk for violence: Self-directed or directed at others. In M. Maas, K. Buckwalter, M. Hardy, T. Tripp-Reimer, M. Titler & J. Specht (Eds.), *Nursing care of older adults: Diagnoses, outcomes & interventions* (pp. 696–705). St. Louis: Mosby.
Mason, T., Chandley, M. (1999). *Managing violence and aggression: A manual for nurses and health care workers.* Edinburgh: Churchill Livingstone.
Maxfield, M. C., Lewis, R. E., & Connor, S. (1996). Training staff to prevent aggressive behavior of cognitively impaired elderly patients during bathing and grooming. *Journal of Gerontological Nursing, 22*(1), 37–43.
Pepler, D. J., & Rubin, K. H. (Eds.). (1991). *The development and treatment of childhood aggression.* Hillsdale, NJ: Erlbaum.
Rantz, M. J., & McShane, R. E. (1995). Nursing interventions for chronically confused nursing home residents. *Geriatric Nursing, 16*(1), 22–27.
Ryden, M. B. (1992). Aggressive behavior in persons with dementia who live in the community. *Alzheimer Disease and Associated Disorders, 2*(4), 342–355.

A

Agitation Level

1214

Definition: Severity of disruptive physiologic and behavioral manifestations of stress or biochemical triggers

OUTCOME TARGET RATING: Maintain at_____   Increase to_____

OUTCOME OVERALL RATING	Severe 1	Substantial 2	Moderate 3	Mild 4	None 5	
Indicators:						
121401 Difficulty processing information	1	2	3	4	5	NA
121402 Restlessness	1	2	3	4	5	NA
121403 Frustration	1	2	3	4	5	NA
121404 Irritability	1	2	3	4	5	NA
121405 Pacing	1	2	3	4	5	NA
121406 Repetitious movements	1	2	3	4	5	NA
121407 Inability to remain seated	1	2	3	4	5	NA
121408 Difficulty staying on tasks	1	2	3	4	5	NA
121409 Resists assistance	1	2	3	4	5	NA
121410 Combativeness	1	2	3	4	5	NA
121411 Thrashing in bed	1	2	3	4	5	NA
121432 Insomnia	1	2	3	4	5	NA
121412 Pulling at tubes or restraints	1	2	3	4	5	NA
121413 Repetitious mannerisms	1	2	3	4	5	NA
121414 Grabbing	1	2	3	4	5	NA
121415 Hoarding	1	2	3	4	5	NA
121416 Hitting	1	2	3	4	5	NA
121417 Kicking	1	2	3	4	5	NA
121418 Throwing	1	2	3	4	5	NA
121419 Spitting	1	2	3	4	5	NA
121420 Biting	1	2	3	4	5	NA
121421 Emotional lability	1	2	3	4	5	NA
121422 Verbal outbursts	1	2	3	4	5	NA
121423 Inappropriate verbalizations	1	2	3	4	5	NA
121424 Inappropriate gestures	1	2	3	4	5	NA
121425 Disinhibition	1	2	3	4	5	NA
121426 Interrupted sleep	1	2	3	4	5	NA
121427 Weight loss	1	2	3	4	5	NA
121428 Dehydration	1	2	3	4	5	NA
121429 Increased blood pressure	1	2	3	4	5	NA
121430 Increased radial pulse rate	1	2	3	4	5	NA
121431 Increased respiratory rate	1	2	3	4	5	NA

Domain-Psychosocial Health (III)   *Class-Psychological Well-Being (M)*   *4th edition 2008; revised 2013*

OUTCOME CONTENT REFERENCES:

Cohen-Mansfield, J. (1996). Behavioral and mood evaluations: Assessment of agitation. *International Psychogeriatrics, 8*(2), 233–245.

Gray, K. F. (2004). Managing agitation and difficult behavior in dementia. *Clinics in Geriatric Medicine, 20*(1), 69–82.

Hamill-Ruth, R. J. (2006). Managing pain and agitation in the critically ill—are we there yet? *Critical Care Medicine, 34*(6), 1838–1839.

Jaber, S., Chanques, G., Altairac, C., Sebbane, M., Vergne, C., Perrigault, P., Eledjam, J. (2005). A prospective study of agitation in a medical-surgical ICU: Incidence, risk factors, and outcomes. *Chest, 128*(4), 2749–2757.

Nott, M. T., Chapparo, C., & Baguley, I. J. (2006). Agitation following traumatic brain injury: An Australian sample. *Brain Injury, 20*(11), 1175–1182.

Sessler, C. N., Gosnell, M. S., Grap, M. J., Brophy, G. M., O'Neal, P. V., Keane, K. A., Tesoro, E. P., & Elswick, R. K. (2002). The Richmond agitation-sedation scale: Validity and reliability in adult intensive care unit patients. *American Journal of Respiratory Critical Care Medicine, 166*(10), 1338–1344.

Alcohol Abuse Cessation Behavior   1629   **A**

Definition: Personal actions to eliminate alcohol use that poses a threat to health

OUTCOME TARGET RATING: Maintain at_____   Increase to_____

		Never demonstrated	Rarely demonstrated	Sometimes demonstrated	Often demonstrated	Consistently demonstrated	
OUTCOME OVERALL RATING		1	2	3	4	5	
Indicators:							
162901	Expresses willingness to stop alcohol use	1	2	3	4	5	NA
162902	Expresses belief in the ability to stop alcohol use	1	2	3	4	5	NA
162903	Identifies benefits of eliminating alcohol use	1	2	3	4	5	NA
162904	Identifies negative consequences of alcohol use	1	2	3	4	5	NA
162905	Develops effective strategies to eliminate alcohol use	1	2	3	4	5	NA
162906	Identifies barriers to alcohol elimination	1	2	3	4	5	NA
162907	Identifies emotional states that trigger alcohol use	1	2	3	4	5	NA
162908	Adjusts alcohol elimination strategies as needed	1	2	3	4	5	NA
162909	Commits to alcohol elimination strategies	1	2	3	4	5	NA
162910	Follows selected alcohol elimination strategies	1	2	3	4	5	NA
162911	Participates in screening for associated health problems	1	2	3	4	5	NA
162912	Uses strategies to cope with withdrawal symptoms	1	2	3	4	5	NA
162913	Uses behavior modification strategies	1	2	3	4	5	NA
162914	Uses effective coping strategies	1	2	3	4	5	NA
162915	Obtains assistance from health professional	1	2	3	4	5	NA
162916	Uses personal support system	1	2	3	4	5	NA
162917	Uses reputable sources of information	1	2	3	4	5	NA
162918	Participates in Alcoholics Anonymous	1	2	3	4	5	NA
162919	Contacts sponsor for cessation support	1	2	3	4	5	NA
162920	Encourages family to participate in Al-Anon	1	2	3	4	5	NA
162921	Uses alternative therapy	1	2	3	4	5	NA
162922	Adjusts lifestyle to promote alcohol elimination	1	2	3	4	5	NA
162923	Uses prescribed medication as recommended	1	2	3	4	5	NA
162924	Uses non-prescription medication as recommended	1	2	3	4	5	NA
162925	Avoids situations that encourage alcohol use	1	2	3	4	5	NA
162926	Uses available support groups	1	2	3	4	5	NA
162927	Uses available community resources	1	2	3	4	5	NA
162928	Participates in counseling	1	2	3	4	5	NA
162929	Monitors for signs of depression	1	2	3	4	5	NA
162930	Eliminates alcohol use	1	2	3	4	5	NA

Domain-Health Knowledge & Behavior (IV)   **Class**-Health Behavior (Q)   4th edition 2008

A

OUTCOME CONTENT REFERENCES:

Fox, H. C., Bergquist, K. L., Hong, K., & Sinha, R. (2007). Stress-induced and alcohol cue-induced craving in recently abstinent alcohol-dependent individuals. *Alcoholism: Clinical and Experimental Research, 31*(3), 395–403

Graham, K., Massak, A., Demers, A., & Rehm, J. (2007). Does the association between alcohol consumption and depression depend on how they are measured? *Alcoholism: Clinical and Experimental Research, 31*(1), 78–88.

Grucza, R. A., & Bierut, L. J. (2006). Cigarette smoking and the risk for alcohol use disorders among adolescent drinkers. *Alcoholism: Clinical and Experimental Research, 30*(12), 2046–2054.

Humphreys, K., & Moos, R. H. (2007). Encouraging posttreatment self-help group involvement to reduce demand for continuing care services: Two-year clinical and utilization outcomes. *Alcoholism: Clinical and Experimental Research, 31*(1), 64–68.

Williams, E. C., Horton, N. J., Samet, J. H., & Saitz, R. (2007). Do brief measures of readiness to change predict alcohol consumption and consequences in primary care patients with unhealthy alcohol use? *Alcoholism: Clinical and Experimental Research, 31*(3), 428–435.

Allergic Response: Localized   0705

Definition: Severity of localized hypersensitive immune response to a specific environmental (exogenous) antigen

OUTCOME TARGET RATING: Maintain at_____ Increase to_____

OUTCOME OVERALL RATING	Severe 1	Substantial 2	Moderate 3	Mild 4	None 5	
Indicators:						
070501 Sinus pain	1	2	3	4	5	NA
070502 Headache	1	2	3	4	5	NA
070503 Conjunctivitis	1	2	3	4	5	NA
070504 Lacrimation	1	2	3	4	5	NA
070505 Rhinitis	1	2	3	4	5	NA
070506 Sneezing	1	2	3	4	5	NA
070507 Mucous secretions	1	2	3	4	5	NA
070508 Circumoral edema	1	2	3	4	5	NA
070509 Periorbital edema	1	2	3	4	5	NA
070510 Dark circles under eyes	1	2	3	4	5	NA
070511 Burning sensation of eyes	1	2	3	4	5	NA
070512 Localized itching	1	2	3	4	5	NA
070513 Localized rash	1	2	3	4	5	NA
070514 Localized erythema	1	2	3	4	5	NA
070515 Increased localized skin temperature	1	2	3	4	5	NA
070516 Localized edema	1	2	3	4	5	NA
070517 Localized pain	1	2	3	4	5	NA
070518 Localized granuloma	1	2	3	4	5	NA
070519 Localized necrotizing vasculitis	1	2	3	4	5	NA

Domain-*Physiologic Health (II)*   **Class**-*Immune Response (H)*   *3rd edition 2004*

OUTCOME CONTENT REFERENCES:

Altman, G. B., Buchsel, P., & Coxon, V. (2000). *Delmar's fundamental & advanced nursing skills.* Albany, NY: Thomson Delmar Learning.

Beltrani, V. S. (2004). Dermatologic allergy. *Pediatric Asthma Allergy and Immunology, 17*(1), 97–99.

Huether, S. E., & McCance, K. L. (2000). *Understanding pathophysiology* (2nd ed.). St. Louis: Mosby.

Krause, H. F. (2003). Allergy and chronic rhinosinusitis. *Otolaryngological Head Neck Surgery, 128*(1), 14–16.

Ledgerwood, G. L., & D'Arienzo, P. A. (2004). Allergic eye disorders: Identification—and alleviation. *Consultant 44*(6), 781–786, 788–789.

Lewis, S., Heitkemper, M., & Dirksen, S. (2000). *Medical-surgical nursing: Assessment and management of clinical problems* (5th ed.). St. Louis: Mosby.

McCance, K. L., & Huether, S. E. (2001). *Pathophysiology: The biological basis for disease in adults and children* (4th ed.). St. Louis: Mosby.

Morris, A. J. (2004). Allergy explained: The new definitive terminology. *Nurse, 4*(2), 40–41.

Mudge-Grout, C., (1992). *Immunologic disorders: Mosby's clinical nursing series.* St. Louis: Mosby.

Opperwall, B. (2003). Asthma, allergy, and upper airway disease. *Nursing Clinics of North America, 38*(4), 697–711.

Scally, R. (2003). Living with latex allergies. *Nursezone, 2*(1), 5–7.

Smeltzer, S. C., & Bare, B. G. (Eds.). (2003). *Brunner and Suddarth's textbook of medical-surgical nursing* (10th ed.). Philadelphia: Lippincott Williams & Wilkins.

Thelan, L., Urden, L., Lough, M., & Stacy, K. (1998). *Critical care nursing: Diagnosis and management* (3rd ed.). St. Louis: Mosby.

Tortora, G., & Grabowski, S. (1996). *Principles of anatomy and physiology* (8th ed.). New York: Harper Collins.

Allergic Response: Systemic 0706

A

Definition: Severity of systemic hypersensitive immune response to a specific environmental (exogenous) antigen

OUTCOME TARGET RATING: Maintain at_____   Increase to_____

OUTCOME OVERALL RATING		Severe	Substantial	Moderate	Mild	None	
		1	2	3	4	5	
Indicators:							
070601	Laryngeal edema	1	2	3	4	5	NA
070602	Dyspnea at rest	1	2	3	4	5	NA
070603	Wheezing	1	2	3	4	5	NA
070604	Stridor	1	2	3	4	5	NA
070605	Adventitious breath sounds	1	2	3	4	5	NA
070606	Tachycardia	1	2	3	4	5	NA
070607	Decreased blood pressure	1	2	3	4	5	NA
070608	Dysrhythmia(s)	1	2	3	4	5	NA
070609	Pulmonary edema	1	2	3	4	5	NA
070610	Decreased level of consciousness	1	2	3	4	5	NA
070611	Mucous secretions	1	2	3	4	5	NA
070612	Facial edema	1	2	3	4	5	NA
070613	Generalized itching	1	2	3	4	5	NA
070614	Hives	1	2	3	4	5	NA
070615	Body exfoliation	1	2	3	4	5	NA
070616	Petechiae	1	2	3	4	5	NA
070617	Erythema	1	2	3	4	5	NA
070618	Increased skin temperature	1	2	3	4	5	NA
070619	Fever	1	2	3	4	5	NA
070620	Chills	1	2	3	4	5	NA
070621	Nausea	1	2	3	4	5	NA
070622	Vomiting	1	2	3	4	5	NA
070623	Diarrhea	1	2	3	4	5	NA
070624	Abdominal cramping	1	2	3	4	5	NA
070625	Red blood cell hemolysis	1	2	3	4	5	NA
070626	Increased bilirubin	1	2	3	4	5	NA
070627	Enlarged spleen	1	2	3	4	5	NA
070628	Enlarged lymph nodes	1	2	3	4	5	NA
070629	Joint pain	1	2	3	4	5	NA
070630	Muscle pain	1	2	3	4	5	NA
070631	Anaphylactic shock	1	2	3	4	5	NA

Domain-*Physiologic Health (II)*   **Class**-*Immune Response (H)*   *3rd edition 2004*

OUTCOME CONTENT REFERENCES:
Altman, G. B., Buchsel, P., & Coxon, V. (2000). *Delmar's fundamental & advanced nursing skills.* Albany, NY: Thomson Delmar Learning.
Gupta, R., Sheikh, A., Strachan, D., & Anderson, H. R. (2003). Increasing hospital admissions for systemic allergic disorders in England: Analysis of national admissions data. *British Medical Journal, 327*(7424), 1142–1143
Huether, S. E., & McCance, K. L. (2000). *Understanding pathophysiology* (2nd ed.). St. Louis: Mosby.
Lewis, S., Heitkemper, M., & Dirksen, S. (2000). *Medical-surgical nursing: Assessment and management of clinical problems* (5th ed.). St. Louis: Mosby.
McCance, K., & Huether, S., (2001). *Pathophysiology: The biological basis for disease in adults and children* (4th ed.). St. Louis: Mosby.
Mudge-Grout, C. (1992). *Immunologic disorders: Mosby's clinical nursing series.* St. Louis: Mosby.
Reading, D. (2004). Managing anaphylaxis. *Practicing Nurse, 28*(3), 28, 30–31.
Ryder, S., & Waldmann, C. (2003). Anaphylaxis. *Care for Critical Illness, 19*(6), 174–176.
Smeltzer, S. C., & Bare, B. G. (Eds.). (2003). *Brunner and Suddarth's textbook of medical-surgical nursing* (10th ed.). Philadelphia: Lippincott Williams & Wilkins.
Thelan, L., Urden, L., Lough, M., & Stacy, K., (1998). *Critical care nursing: Diagnosis and management* (3rd ed.). St. Louis: Mosby.
Tortora, G., & Grabowski, S. (1996). *Principles of anatomy and physiology* (8th ed.). New York: Harper Collins.

A

Ambulation 0200

Definition: Personal actions to walk from place to place independently with or without assistive device

OUTCOME TARGET RATING: Maintain at_____ Increase to_____

OUTCOME OVERALL RATING	Severely compromised 1	Substantially compromised 2	Moderately compromised 3	Mildly compromised 4	Not compromised 5	
Indicators:						
020001 Bears weight	1	2	3	4	5	NA
020002 Walks with effective gait	1	2	3	4	5	NA
020003 Walks at slow pace	1	2	3	4	5	NA
020004 Walks at moderate pace	1	2	3	4	5	NA
020005 Walks at fast pace	1	2	3	4	5	NA
020006 Walks up steps	1	2	3	4	5	NA
020007 Walks down steps	1	2	3	4	5	NA
020008 Walks up inclines	1	2	3	4	5	NA
020009 Walks down inclines	1	2	3	4	5	NA
020010 Walks short distance (< 1 block)	1	2	3	4	5	NA
020011 Walks moderate distance (> 1 block < 5 blocks)	1	2	3	4	5	NA
020012 Walks long distance (5 blocks or >)	1	2	3	4	5	NA
020014 Walks around room	1	2	3	4	5	NA
020015 Walks around dwelling	1	2	3	4	5	NA
020016 Adjusts to different surface textures	1	2	3	4	5	NA
020017 Walks around obstacles	1	2	3	4	5	NA

Domain-*Functional Health (I)* **Class**-*Mobility (C)* *1st edition 1997; revised 2004, 2008, 2013*

OUTCOME CONTENT REFERENCES:

Green, J., Forster, A., & Young, J. (2002). Reliability of gait speed measured by a timed walking test in patients one year after stroke. *Clinical Rehabilitation, 16*(3), 306–314.

Hoeman, S. (2002). *Rehabilitation nursing: Process, application, and outcomes* (3rd ed.). St. Louis: Mosby.

Jirovec, M. M. (1991). The impact of daily exercise on the mobility, balance, and urine control of cognitively impaired nursing home residents. *International Journal of Nursing Studies, 28*(2), 145–151.

Lord, S. R., & Menz, H. B. (2002). Physiologic, psychologic, and health predictors of 6-minute walk performance in older people. *Archives of Physical Medicine & Rehabilitation, 83*(7), 907–911.

Mikulic, M. A., Griffith, E. R., & Jebsen, R. H. (1976). Clinical application of a standardized mobility test. *Archives of Physical Medicine and Rehabilitation, 57*(3), 143–146.

Pomeroy, V. (1990). Development of an ADL-oriented assessment-of-mobility scale suitable for use for elderly people with dementia. *Physiotherapy, 76*(8), 446–448.

Tinetti, M. E. (1986). Performance-oriented assessment of mobility problems in elderly patients. *Journal of the American Geriatric Society, 34*(2), 119–126.

+Uniform Data System for Medical Rehabilitation. (1997). *Guide for the Uniform Data Set for Medical Rehabilitation* (including the FIM™ instrument) (version 5.1). Buffalo, NY: Author.

A

Ambulation: Wheelchair 0201

Definition: Personal actions to move from place to place in a wheelchair

OUTCOME TARGET RATING: Maintain at_____ Increase to_____

OUTCOME OVERALL RATING	Severely compromised 1	Substantially compromised 2	Moderately compromised 3	Mildly compromised 4	Not compromised 5	
Indicators:						
020101 Transfers to and from wheelchair	1	2	3	4	5	NA
020102 Propels wheelchair safely	1	2	3	4	5	NA
020103 Propels wheelchair short distance	1	2	3	4	5	NA
020104 Propels wheelchair moderate distance	1	2	3	4	5	NA
020105 Propels wheelchair long distance	1	2	3	4	5	NA
020106 Maneuvers curbs	1	2	3	4	5	NA
020107 Maneuvers doorways	1	2	3	4	5	NA
020108 Maneuvers ramps	1	2	3	4	5	NA

Domain-Functional Health (I) **Class**-Mobility (C) 1st edition 1997; revised 2004, 2013

OUTCOME CONTENT REFERENCES:

Hoeman, S. (2002). *Rehabilitation nursing: Process, application, and outcomes* (3rd ed.). St. Louis: Mosby.

Kane, R. L., & Kane, R. A. (2000). *Assessing older persons: Measures, meaning, and practical applications.* New York: Oxford University Press.

Lan, T. Y., Melzer, D., Tom, B. D., & Guralnik, J. M. (2002). Performance tests and disability: Developing an objective index of mobility-related limitation in older populations. *Journals of Gerontology. Series A, Biological Sciences & Medical Sciences, 57*(5), M294–M301.

Mikulic, M. A., Griffith, E. R., & Jebsen, R. H. (1976). Clinical application of a standardized mobility test. *Archives of Physical Medicine and Rehabilitation, 57*(3), 143–146.

+Uniform Data System for Medical Rehabilitation. (1997). *Guide for the Uniform Data Set for Medical Rehabilitation* (including the FIM™ instrument) (version 5.1). Buffalo, NY: Author.

Anger Self-Restraint 1410

Definition: Personal actions to eliminate or reduce intense hostile thoughts, feelings, and behaviors

OUTCOME TARGET RATING: Maintain at_____ Increase to_____

OUTCOME OVERALL RATING	Never demonstrated 1	Rarely demonstrated 2	Sometimes demonstrated 3	Often demonstrated 4	Consistently demonstrated 5	
Indicators:						
141001 Identifies when angry	1	2	3	4	5	NA
141002 Identifies when frustrated	1	2	3	4	5	NA
141003 Identifies early signs of anger	1	2	3	4	5	NA
141004 Identifies situations that precipitate anger	1	2	3	4	5	NA
141005 Approaches unpredictable situation with an open mind	1	2	3	4	5	NA
141006 Identifies the basis of angry feelings	1	2	3	4	5	NA
141007 Assumes responsibility for personal behaviors	1	2	3	4	5	NA

Continued

A

Anger Self-Restraint—cont'd

		Never demonstrated	Rarely demonstrated	Sometimes demonstrated	Often demonstrated	Consistently demonstrated	
141008	Uses effective conflict resolution skills	1	2	3	4	5	NA
141009	Expresses needs in a constructive manner	1	2	3	4	5	NA
141010	Vents negative feelings in a non-threatening manner	1	2	3	4	5	NA
141011	Monitors behavioral manifestations of anger	1	2	3	4	5	NA
141012	Monitors physical manifestations of anger	1	2	3	4	5	NA
141013	Uses physical activity to reduce repressed anger	1	2	3	4	5	NA
141014	Refrains from vacillating between outbursts of anger and passivity	1	2	3	4	5	NA
141015	Avoids imposing one's values on others	1	2	3	4	5	NA
141016	Shares feelings of anger with others	1	2	3	4	5	NA
141017	Uses strategies to control anger	1	2	3	4	5	NA
141018	Uses strategies to control frustration	1	2	3	4	5	NA
141019	Obtains counseling as needed	1	2	3	4	5	NA
141020	Maintains self-control without supervision	1	2	3	4	5	NA

Domain-Psychosocial Health (III)   **Class**-Self-Control(O)   5th edition 2013

OUTCOME CONTENT REFERENCES:

Dunbar, B. (2004). Anger management: A holistic approach. *Journal of the American Psychiatric Nurses Association, 10*(1), 16–23.

Howells, K., & Day, A. (2003). Readiness for anger management: Clinical and theoretical issues. *Clinical Psychology Review, 23*(2), 319–337.

Park, Y., Ryu, H., Han, K., Kwon, J., Kyeom-Kim, H., Kang, H., Yoon, J., Cheon, S., Shin, H. (2010). Anger, anger expression, and suicidal ideation in Korean adolescents. *Archives of Psychiatric Nursing, 24*(3), 168–177.

Puskar, K., Stark, K., Northcut, T., Williams, R., & Haley, T. (2010). Teaching kids to cope with anger: Peer education. *Journal of Child Health Care, 15*(1), 5–13.

Walker, A., Nott, M., Doyle, M., Onus, M., McCarthy, K., & Baguley, I. (2010). Effectiveness of a group anger management programme after severe traumatic brain injury. *Brain Injury, 24*(3), 517–524.

Anxiety Level   1211   A

Definition: Severity of manifested apprehension, tension, or uneasiness arising from an unidentifiable source

OUTCOME TARGET RATING: Maintain at_____   Increase to_____

	Severe	Substantial	Moderate	Mild	None	
OUTCOME OVERALL RATING	1	2	3	4	5	

Indicators:

		Severe	Substantial	Moderate	Mild	None	
121101	Restlessness	1	2	3	4	5	NA
121102	Pacing	1	2	3	4	5	NA
121103	Hand wringing	1	2	3	4	5	NA
121104	Distress	1	2	3	4	5	NA
121105	Uneasiness	1	2	3	4	5	NA
121106	Muscle tension	1	2	3	4	5	NA
121107	Facial tension	1	2	3	4	5	NA
121108	Irritability	1	2	3	4	5	NA
121109	Indecisiveness	1	2	3	4	5	NA
121110	Outbursts of anger	1	2	3	4	5	NA
121111	Problem behavior	1	2	3	4	5	NA
121112	Difficulty concentrating	1	2	3	4	5	NA
121113	Difficulty learning	1	2	3	4	5	NA
121114	Difficulty problem solving	1	2	3	4	5	NA
121115	Panic attack	1	2	3	4	5	NA
121116	Verbalized apprehension	1	2	3	4	5	NA
121117	Verbalized anxiety	1	2	3	4	5	NA
121118	Exaggerated concern about life events	1	2	3	4	5	NA
121119	Increased blood pressure	1	2	3	4	5	NA
121120	Increased pulse rate	1	2	3	4	5	NA
121121	Increased respiratory rate	1	2	3	4	5	NA
121122	Dilated pupils	1	2	3	4	5	NA
121123	Sweating	1	2	3	4	5	NA
121124	Dizziness	1	2	3	4	5	NA
121125	Fatigue	1	2	3	4	5	NA
121126	Decreased productivity	1	2	3	4	5	NA
121127	Decreased school achievement	1	2	3	4	5	NA
121128	Withdrawal	1	2	3	4	5	NA
121129	Sleep disturbance	1	2	3	4	5	NA
121130	Change in bowel pattern	1	2	3	4	5	NA
121131	Change in eating pattern	1	2	3	4	5	NA

Domain-Psychosocial Health (III)   *Class-Psychological Well-Being (M)*   *3rd edition 2004*

OUTCOME CONTENT REFERENCES:

American Psychiatric Association. (2000). *Diagnostic and statistical manual of mental disorders* (4th ed. text rev.). Washington, DC: Author.

Byrne, B. (2000). Relationships between anxiety, fear, self-esteem, and coping strategies in adolescence. *Adolescence, 35*(137), 201–216.

Charron, H. S. (1998). Anxiety disorders. In E. M. Varcarolis (Ed.), *Foundations of psychiatric mental health nursing* (3rd ed., pp. 443–477). Philadelphia: W. B. Saunders.

Kim, M., Sertella, R., Gulanick, M., Moyer, K., Parsons, E., Scherbel, J., Stafford, M., Suhayada, R., & Yocum, C. (1984). Clinical validation of cardiovascular nursing diagnoses. In M. Kim, G. McFarland, & A. McLane (Eds.), *Classification of nursing diagnoses: Proceedings of the fifth national conference* (pp. 128–137). St. Louis: Mosby.

Shuldham, C. M., Cunningham, G., Hiscock, M., & Luscombe, P. (1995). Assessment of anxiety in hospital patients. *Journal of Advanced Nursing, 22*(1), 87–93.

Taylor-Loughran, A. E., O'Brien, M. E., LaChapelle, R., & Rangel, S. (1989). Defining characteristics of the nursing diagnoses fear and anxiety: A validation study. *Applied Nursing Research, 2*(4), 178–186.

Whitley, G. G., & Tousman, S. A. (1996). A multivariate approach for validation of anxiety and fear. *Nursing Diagnosis, 7*(3), 116–124.

A

Anxiety Self-Control 1402

Definition: Personal actions to eliminate or reduce feelings of apprehension, tension, or uneasiness from an unidentifiable source

OUTCOME TARGET RATING: Maintain at_____ Increase to_____

	Never demonstrated	Rarely demonstrated	Sometimes demonstrated	Often demonstrated	Consistently demonstrated	
OUTCOME OVERALL RATING	1	2	3	4	5	
Indicators:						
140201 Monitors intensity of anxiety	1	2	3	4	5	NA
140202 Eliminates precursors of anxiety	1	2	3	4	5	NA
140203 Decreases environmental stimuli when anxious	1	2	3	4	5	NA
140204 Seeks information to reduce anxiety	1	2	3	4	5	NA
140205 Plans coping strategies for stressful situations	1	2	3	4	5	NA
140206 Uses effective coping strategies	1	2	3	4	5	NA
140207 Uses relaxation techniques to reduce anxiety	1	2	3	4	5	NA
140208 Monitors duration of episodes	1	2	3	4	5	NA
140209 Monitors length of time between episodes	1	2	3	4	5	NA
140210 Maintains role performance	1	2	3	4	5	NA
140211 Maintains social relationships	1	2	3	4	5	NA
140212 Maintains concentration	1	2	3	4	5	NA
140213 Monitors sensory perceptual distortions	1	2	3	4	5	NA
140214 Maintains adequate sleep	1	2	3	4	5	NA
140215 Monitors physical manifestations of anxiety	1	2	3	4	5	NA
140216 Monitors behavioral manifestations of anxiety	1	2	3	4	5	NA
140217 Controls anxiety response	1	2	3	4	5	NA

Domain-*Psychosocial Health (III)* **Class**-*Self-Control (O)* *1st edition 1997; revised 2000, 2004*

OUTCOME CONTENT REFERENCES:

+Hudson, W. W. (1992). *The WALMYR assessment scales scoring manual.* Tempe, AZ: WALMYR.

Laraia, M. T., Stuart, G. W., & Best, C. L. (1989). Behavioral treatment of panic-related disorders: A review. *Archives of Psychiatric Nursing, 3*(3), 125–133.

Moorhead, S. A., & Brighton, V. A. (2001). Anxiety and fear. In M. Maas, K. Buckwalter, M. Hardy, T. Tripp-Reimer, M. Titler, & J. Specht (Eds.), *Nursing care of older adults: Diagnoses, outcomes & interventions* (pp. 571–592). St. Louis: Mosby.

Stuart, G. W., & Laraia, M. T. (2001). *Principles and practice of psychiatric nursing* (7th ed.). St. Louis: Mosby.

Tucker, S., Moore, W., & Luedtke, C. (2000). Outcomes of a brief inpatient treatment program for mood and anxiety disorders. *Outcomes Management for Nursing Practice, 4*(3), 117–123.

Waddell, K. L., & Demi, A. S. (1993). Effectiveness of an intensive partial hospitalization program for treatment of anxiety disorders. *Archives of Psychiatric Nursing, 7*(1), 2–10.

A

Appetite 1014

Definition: Desire to eat

OUTCOME TARGET RATING: Maintain at_____ Increase to_____

	Severely compromised	Substantially compromised	Moderately compromised	Mildly compromised	Not compromised	
OUTCOME OVERALL RATING	1	2	3	4	5	
Indicators:						
101401 Desire to eat	1	2	3	4	5	NA
101402 Craving for food	1	2	3	4	5	NA
101403 Enjoyment of food	1	2	3	4	5	NA
101404 Taste of food	1	2	3	4	5	NA
101405 Energy to eat	1	2	3	4	5	NA
101406 Food intake	1	2	3	4	5	NA
101407 Nutrient intake	1	2	3	4	5	NA
101408 Fluid intake	1	2	3	4	5	NA
101409 Stimulus to eat	1	2	3	4	5	NA

Domain-Physiologic Health (II)   **Class**-Digestion & Nutrition (K)   *3rd edition 2004; revised 2013*

OUTCOME CONTENT REFERENCES:
Anderson, K. N., Anderson, L. E., & Glanze, W. D. (2002). *Mosby's medical, nursing, & allied health dictionary* (6th ed.). St. Louis: Mosby.
Dudek, S. G. (2001). *Nutrition essentials for nursing practice.* Philadelphia: Lippincott Williams & Wilkins.
Lewis, S. M., Heitkemper, M. M., & Dirksen, S. R. (2000). *Medical-surgical nursing: Assessment and management of clinical problems.* St. Louis: Mosby.
McCanse, K. L., & Huether, S. E. (2002). *Pathophysiology: The biological basis for disease in adults and children.* St. Louis: Mosby.
Potter, P. A., & Perry, A. G. (2001). *Fundamentals of nursing* (5th ed.). St. Louis: Mosby.
Thomas, C. L. (Ed.). (1993). *Taber's cyclopedic medical dictionary* (17th ed.). Philadelphia: F. A. Davis.

Aspiration Prevention 1918

Definition: Personal actions to prevent the passage of fluid and solid particles into the lung

OUTCOME TARGET RATING: Maintain at_____ Increase to_____

	Never demonstrated	Rarely demonstrated	Sometimes demonstrated	Often demonstrated	Consistently demonstrated	
OUTCOME OVERALL RATING	1	2	3	4	5	
Indicators:						
191801 Identifies risk factors	1	2	3	4	5	NA
191802 Avoids risk factors	1	2	3	4	5	NA
191809 Maintains oral hygiene	1	2	3	4	5	NA
191803 Positions self upright for eating and drinking	1	2	3	4	5	NA
191805 Positions self on side for eating and drinking as needed	1	2	3	4	5	NA
191804 Selects foods according to swallowing ability	1	2	3	4	5	NA
191806 Selects food and fluid of proper consistency	1	2	3	4	5	NA

Continued

A

Aspiration Prevention—cont'd

	Never demonstrated	Rarely demonstrated	Sometimes demonstrated	Often demonstrated	Consistently demonstrated	
191808 Uses liquid thickeners as needed	1	2	3	4	5	NA
191810 Remains upright for 30 minutes after eating	1	2	3	4	5	NA

Domain-*Health Knowledge & Behavior (IV)*   ***Class-****Risk Control & Safety (T)*   *2nd edition 2000; revised 2004, 2008*

OUTCOME CONTENT REFERENCES:

Fellows, L. S., Miller, E. H., Frederickson, M., Bly, B., & Felt, P. (2000). Evidence-based practice for enteral feedings: Aspiration prevention strategies, bedside detection, and practice change. *Medsurg Nursing, 9*(1), 27–31.

The Joanna Briggs Institute for Evidence Based Nursing and Midwifery. (2000). Identification and nursing management of dysphagia in adults with neurological impairment. *Best Practice, 4*(2), Blackwell Science-Asia, Australia.

Johnson, J. L., & Hirsch, C. S. (2003). Aspiration pneumonia. *Postgraduate Medicine, 113*(3), 99–107.

Lewis, S. M., Collier, I. C., Heitkemper, M. M., & Dirksen, S. R. (2000). *Medical-surgical nursing: Assessment & management of clinical problems* (5th ed.). St. Louis: Mosby.

McCance, K. L., & Huether, S. E. (2002). *Pathophysiology: The biologic basis for disease in adults and children* (4th ed.). St. Louis: Mosby.

Oh, E., Weintraub, N., & Dhanai, S. (2004). Can we prevent aspiration pneumonia in the nursing home? *Journal of the American Medical Directors Association, 6*(3, Suppl. 1), S76–S80.

Smeltzer, S. C., & Bare, B. G. (Eds.). (2003). *Brunner and Suddarth's textbook of medical-surgical nursing* (10th ed.). Philadelphia: Lippincott Williams &Wilkins.

Balance 0202

B

Definition: Ability to maintain body equilibrium

OUTCOME TARGET RATING: Maintain at_____ Increase to_____

	Severely compromised	Substantially compromised	Moderately compromised	Mildly compromised	Not compromised	
OUTCOME OVERALL RATING	1	2	3	4	5	
Indicators:						
020202 Maintains balance while sitting without back support	1	2	3	4	5	NA
020212 Maintains balance while rising from sitting position	1	2	3	4	5	NA
020201 Maintains balance while standing	1	2	3	4	5	NA
020203 Maintains balance while walking	1	2	3	4	5	NA
020209 Maintains balance while standing on one foot	1	2	3	4	5	NA
020210 Maintains balance while shifting weight from one foot to another	1	2	3	4	5	NA
020213 Maintains balance while turning 360 degrees	1	2	3	4	5	NA
020211 Posture	1	2	3	4	5	NA
	Severe	Substantial	Moderate	Mild	None	
020205 Weaving	1	2	3	4	5	NA
020206 Dizziness	1	2	3	4	5	NA
020207 Shakiness	1	2	3	4	5	NA
020208 Stumbling	1	2	3	4	5	NA

Domain-*Functional Health (I)* **Class**-*Mobility (C)* *1st edition 1997; revised 2004, 2008, 2013*

OUTCOME CONTENT REFERENCES:
+Berg, K., Wood-Dauphinee, S., Williams, J. I., & Gayton, D. (1989). Measuring balance in the elderly: Preliminary development of an instrument. *Physiotherapy Canada, 41*(6), 304–311.
Dittmar, S. (1989). *Rehabilitation nursing: Process and application.* St. Louis: Mosby.
Our balancing act. (2006). *Harvard Health Letter, 31*(10), 1–3.
Pettersson, A. F., Engardt, M., & Wahlund, L. O. (2002). Activity level and balance in subjects with mild Alzheimer's disease. *Dementia & Geriatric Cognitive Disorders, 13*(4), 213–216.
Pomeroy, V. (1990). Development of an ADL-oriented assessment-of-mobility scale suitable for use with elderly people with dementia. *Physiotherapy, 76*(8), 446–448.
Roberts, B. L. (1989). Effects of walking on balance among elders. *Nursing Research, 38*(3), 180–182.
Tinetti, M. E. (1986). Performance-oriented assessment of mobility problems in elderly patients. *Journal of the American Geriatric Society, 34*(2), 119–126.

B

Blood Coagulation

0409

Definition: Extent to which blood clots within normal period of time

OUTCOME TARGET RATING: Maintain at_____   Increase to_____

		Severe deviation from normal range	Substantial deviation from normal range	Moderate deviation from normal range	Mild deviation from normal range	No deviation from normal range	
OUTCOME OVERALL RATING		1	2	3	4	5	
Indicators:							
040901	Clot formation	1	2	3	4	5	NA
040912	Prothrombin time (PT)	1	2	3	4	5	NA
040905	Prothrombin time - international normalized ratio (PT-INR)	1	2	3	4	5	NA
040907	Partial thromboplastin time (PTT)	1	2	3	4	5	NA
040913	Hemoglobin (Hgb)	1	2	3	4	5	NA
040908	Platelet count	1	2	3	4	5	NA
040909	Plasma fibrinogen	1	2	3	4	5	NA
040914	Fibrin split products (FSP)	1	2	3	4	5	NA
040910	Hematocrit (Hct)	1	2	3	4	5	NA
040915	Activated clotting time (ACT)	1	2	3	4	5	NA

		Severe	Substantial	Moderate	Mild	None	
040902	Bleeding	1	2	3	4	5	NA
040903	Bruising	1	2	3	4	5	NA
040904	Petechiae	1	2	3	4	5	NA
040916	Ecchymosis	1	2	3	4	5	NA
040917	Purpura	1	2	3	4	5	NA
040918	Hematuria	1	2	3	4	5	NA
040919	Blood in stool	1	2	3	4	5	NA
040920	Hemoptysis	1	2	3	4	5	NA
040921	Hematemesis	1	2	3	4	5	NA
040922	Bleeding gums	1	2	3	4	5	NA

Domain-Physiologic Health (II)   *Class-Cardiopulmonary (E)*   *2nd edition 2000; revised 2004*

OUTCOME CONTENT REFERENCES:

Arnett, C. (1998). Thrombocytopenia in the newborn. *Neonatal Network—Journal of Neonatal Nursing, 17*(8), 27–37.

Beyth, R. J. (2001). Thromboembolic disease and anticoagulation in the elderly: Hemorrhagic complications of oral anticoagulant therapy (electronic version). *Clinics in Geriatric Medicine, 17*(1), 49–56.

Clochesy, J. M., Brey, C., Cardin, S., Whittaker, A. A., & Rudy, E. B. (1996). *Critical care nursing* (2nd ed.). Philadelphia: W. B. Saunders.

Fahey, V. A. (Ed.). (1999). *Vascular nursing* (3rd ed.). Philadelphia: W. B. Saunders.

Fihn, S. D., Callahan, C. M., Martin, D., McDonell, M. B., Henikoff, J. G., & White, R. H. (1996). The risk for and severity of bleeding complications in elderly patients treated with warfarin. *Annals of Internal Medicine, 124*(11), 970–979.

Lewis, S. M., Collier, I. C., Heitkemper, M. M., & Dirksen, S. R. (2000). *Medical-surgical nursing: Assessment & management of clinical problems* (5th ed.). St. Louis: Mosby.

McCance, K. L., & Huether, S. E. (2002). *Pathophysiology: The biologic basis for disease in adults and children* (4th ed.). St. Louis: Mosby.

Smeltzer, S. C., & Bare, B. G. (Eds.). (2003). *Brunner and Suddarth's textbook of medical-surgical nursing* (10th ed.). Philadelphia: Lippincott Williams & Wilkins.

Blood Glucose Level 2300

Definition: Extent to which glucose levels in plasma and urine are maintained in normal range

OUTCOME TARGET RATING: Maintain at_____ Increase to_____

		Severe deviation from normal range	Substantial deviation from normal range	Moderate deviation from normal range	Mild deviation from normal range	No deviation from normal range	
OUTCOME OVERALL RATING		1	2	3	4	5	
Indicators:							
230001	Blood glucose	1	2	3	4	5	NA
230004	Glycosylated hemoglobin	1	2	3	4	5	NA
230005	Fructosamine	1	2	3	4	5	NA
230007	Urine glucose	1	2	3	4	5	NA
230008	Urine ketones	1	2	3	4	5	NA

Domain-Physiologic Health (II) **Class**-Therapeutic Response (AA) *2nd edition 2000; revised 2004*

OUTCOME CONTENT REFERENCES:

American Diabetes Association. (1998). Standards of medical care for patients with diabetes mellitus. *Diabetes Care, 21*(Suppl. 1), S23–S31.
American Diabetes Association. (1998). Testing of glycemia in diabetes. *Diabetes Care, 21*(Suppl. 1), S69–S71.
Cryer, P. E. (2001). Hypoglycemia risk reduction in type 1 diabetes. *Experimental & Clinical Endocrinology & Diabetes, 109*(Suppl. 2), S412–S423.
Dalewitz, J., Khan, N., & Hershey, C. (2000). Barriers to control of blood glucose in diabetes mellitus. *American Journal of Medical Quality, 15*(1), 16–25.
Funnell, M. M., Hunt, C., Kulkarni, K., Rubin, R. R., & Yarborough, P. C. (Eds.). (1998). *A core curriculum for Association of Diabetes Educators.* Chicago: American Association of Diabetes Educators.
Kelley, D. B. (Ed.). (1998). *Intensive diabetes management* (2nd ed.). Alexandria, VA: American Diabetes Association.
Lebovitz, H. E. (Ed.). (1998). *Therapy for diabetes mellitus and related disorders* (3rd ed.). Alexandria, VA: American Diabetes Association.
Lewis, S. M., Collier, I. C., Heitkemper, M. M., & Dirksen, S. R. (2000). *Medical-surgical nursing: Assessment & management of clinical problems* (5th ed.). St. Louis: Mosby.
McCance, K. L., & Huether, S. E. (2002). *Pathophysiology: The biologic basis for disease in adults and children* (4th ed.). St. Louis: Mosby.
Zgibor, J. C., & Simmons, D. (2002). Barriers to blood glucose monitoring in a multiethnic community. *Diabetes Care, 25*(10), 1772–1777.

Blood Loss Severity 0413

Definition: Severity of signs and symptoms of internal or external bleeding

OUTCOME TARGET RATING: Maintain at_____ Increase to_____

		Severe	Substantial	Moderate	Mild	None	
OUTCOME OVERALL RATING		1	2	3	4	5	
Indicators:							
041301	Visible blood loss	1	2	3	4	5	NA
041302	Hematuria	1	2	3	4	5	NA
041303	Frank blood from anus	1	2	3	4	5	NA
041304	Hemoptysis	1	2	3	4	5	NA
041305	Hematemesis	1	2	3	4	5	NA
041306	Abdominal distention	1	2	3	4	5	NA
041307	Vaginal bleeding	1	2	3	4	5	NA
041308	Post surgical bleeding	1	2	3	4	5	NA
041309	Decreased systolic blood pressure	1	2	3	4	5	NA
041310	Decreased diastolic blood pressure	1	2	3	4	5	NA
041311	Increased apical heart rate	1	2	3	4	5	NA
041312	Loss of body heat	1	2	3	4	5	NA
041313	Skin and mucous membrane pallor	1	2	3	4	5	NA
041314	Anxiety	1	2	3	4	5	NA
041315	Decreased cognition	1	2	3	4	5	NA

Continued

Blood Loss Severity—cont'd

		Severe	Substantial	Moderate	Mild	None	
041316	Decreased hemoglobin (Hgb)	1	2	3	4	5	NA
041317	Decreased hematocrit (Hct)	1	2	3	4	5	NA

Estimated blood loss: _____(cc)

Domain-Physiologic Health (II)   **Class**-Cardiopulmonary (E)   3rd edition 2004; revised 2013

OUTCOME CONTENT REFERENCES:
American College of Surgeons Committee on Trauma. (1997). *Advanced trauma life support for doctors*. Chicago: American College of Surgeons.
Baron, B. J., Sinert, R., Zehtabchi, S., Stavile, K. L., & Scalea, T. M. (2004). Diagnostic utility of sublingual PCO2 for detecting hemorrhage in penetrating trauma patients. *Journal of Trauma, 57*(1), 69–74.
Blankenship, J. C. (1999). Bleeding complications of glycoprotein IIb-IIIa receptor inhibitors. *American Heart Journal, 138*(4 Pt 2), 287–296.
Bose, P., Regan, F., & Paterson-Brown, S. (2006). Improving the accuracy of estimated blood loss at obstetric haemorrhage using clinical reconstructions. *BJOG: An International Journal of Obstetrics & Gynaecology, 113*(8), 919–924.
deGuzman, E., Shankar, M. N., & Mattox, K. L. (1999). Limited volume resuscitation in penetrating thoracoabdominal trauma. *AACN Clinical Issues, 10*(1), 61–68.
Fihn, S. D., Callahan, C. M., Martin, D., McDonell, M. B., Henikoff, J. G., & White, R. H. (1996). The risk for and severity of bleeding complications in elderly patients treated with warfarin. *Annals of Internal Medicine, 124*(11), 970–979.
Maxson, J. H. (2000). Management of disseminated intravascular coagulation. *Critical Care Nursing Clinics of North America, 12*(3), 341–352.
Sims, C., Seigne, P., Menconi, M., Monarca, J., Barlow, C., Pettit, J., & Puyana, J. C. (2001). Skeletal muscle acidosis correlates with the severity of blood volume loss during shock and resuscitation. *Journal of Trauma, 51*(6), 1137–1146.
Swearington, P. L., & Keen, J. H. (2001). *Manual of critical care nursing: Nursing interventions and collaborative management* (4th ed.). St. Louis: Mosby.

Blood Transfusion Reaction
0700

Definition: Severity of complications with blood transfusion reaction

OUTCOME TARGET RATING: Maintain at_____   Increase to_____

		Severe	Substantial	Moderate	Mild	None	
OUTCOME OVERALL RATING		1	2	3	4	5	
Indicators:							
070020	Shortness of breath	1	2	3	4	5	NA
070003	Decreased urine output	1	2	3	4	5	NA
070004	Increased apical heart rate	1	2	3	4	5	NA
070022	Decreased blood pressure	1	2	3	4	5	NA
070007	Fever	1	2	3	4	5	NA
070008	Chills	1	2	3	4	5	NA
070009	Itching	1	2	3	4	5	NA
070010	Rash	1	2	3	4	5	NA
070011	Restlessness	1	2	3	4	5	NA
070012	Anxiety	1	2	3	4	5	NA
070013	Malaise	1	2	3	4	5	NA
070021	Nausea	1	2	3	4	5	NA
070014	Chest pain	1	2	3	4	5	NA
070015	Lumbar pain	1	2	3	4	5	NA
070017	Hemoglobinuria	1	2	3	4	5	NA
070023	Muscle spasms	1	2	3	4	5	NA
070024	Twitching	1	2	3	4	5	NA

Domain-Physiologic Health (II)   **Class**-Immune Response (H)   1st edition 1997; revised 2004, 2008

OUTCOME CONTENT REFERENCES:
McCance, K. L., & Huether, S. E. (2002). *Pathophysiology: The biologic basis for disease in adults and children* (4th ed.). St. Louis: Mosby.
Raife, T. J. (1997). Adverse effects of transfusions caused by leukocytes. *Journal of Intravenous Nursing, 20*(5), 238–244.
Smeltzer, S. C., & Bare, B. G. (Eds.). (2003). *Brunner and Suddarth's textbook of medical-surgical nursing* (10th ed.). Philadelphia: Lippincott Williams & Wilkins.

Body Image

1200

Definition: Perception of own appearance and body functions

OUTCOME TARGET RATING: Maintain at_____   Increase to_____

		Never positive	Rarely positive	Sometimes positive	Often positive	Consistently positive	
OUTCOME OVERALL RATING		1	2	3	4	5	
Indicators:							
120001	Internal picture of self	1	2	3	4	5	NA
120002	Congruence between body reality, body ideal, and body presentation	1	2	3	4	5	NA
120003	Description of affected body part	1	2	3	4	5	NA
120016	Attitude toward touching affected body part	1	2	3	4	5	NA
120017	Attitude toward using strategies to enhance appearance	1	2	3	4	5	NA
120005	Satisfaction with body appearance	1	2	3	4	5	NA
120018	Attitude toward using strategies to enhance function	1	2	3	4	5	NA
120006	Satisfaction with body function	1	2	3	4	5	NA
120007	Adjustment to changes in physical appearance	1	2	3	4	5	NA
120008	Adjustment to changes in body function	1	2	3	4	5	NA
120009	Adjustment to changes in health status	1	2	3	4	5	NA
120013	Adjustment to body changes due to injury	1	2	3	4	5	NA
120014	Adjustment to body changes due to surgery	1	2	3	4	5	NA
120015	Adjustment to body changes due to aging	1	2	3	4	5	NA

Domain-Psychosocial Health (III)   **Class**-Psychological Well-Being (M)   1st edition 1997; revised 2004, 2008

OUTCOME CONTENT REFERENCES:

Fritz, G. K. (Ed.). (2004). Body image—tips for parents. *The Brown University Child and Adolescent Behavior Letter.* Providence, RI: Manisses Communications.

Comunale, D. L. (1992). Collaborative care planning with the arthritic client at home. *Journal of Home Health Care Practice, 4*(2), 8–15.

Dixon, J. B., Dixon, M. E., & O'Brien, P. E. (2002). Body image: Appearance orientation and evaluation in the severely obese. Changes with weight loss. *Obesity Surgery, 12*(1), 65–71.

Kater, K. J., Rohwer, J., & Londre, K. (2002). Evaluation of an upper elementary school program to prevent body image, eating, and weight concerns. *Journal of School Health, 72*(5), 199–204.

Key, A., George, C. L., Beattie, D., Stammers, K., Lacey, H., & Waller, G. (2002). Body image treatment within an inpatient program for anorexia nervosa: The role of mirror exposure in the desensitization process. *International Journal of Eating Disorders, 31*(2), 185–190.

LeMone, P. (1991). Analysis of human phenomenon: Self-concept. *Nursing Diagnosis, 2*(3), 129–130.

Low, M. B. (1993). Women's body image: The nurse's role in promotion of self-acceptance. *AWONN's Clinical Issues, 4*(2), 213–219.

MacGinley, K. J. (1993). Nursing care of the patient with altered body image. *British Journal of Nursing, 2*(22), 1098–1102.

Martin, H., & Ammerman, S. D. (2002). Adolescents with eating disorders: Primary care screening, identification, and early intervention. *Nursing Clinics of North America, 37*(3), 537–551.

Newell, R. (1991). Body-image disturbance: Cognitive behavioral formulation and intervention. *Journal of Advanced Nursing, 16*(12), 1400–1405.

Price, B. (1990). A model for body image care. *Journal of Advanced Nursing, 15*(5), 585–593.

Price, B. (1992). Living with altered body image: The cancer experience. *British Journal of Nursing, 1*(13), 641–645.

Price, B. (1993). Profiling the high-risk altered body image patient. *Senior Nurse, 13*(4), 17–21.

+Rosen, J. C., Srebnik, D., Saltzberg, E., & Wendt, S. (1991). Development of a body image avoidance questionnaire. *Psychological Assessment: A Journal of Consulting and Clinical Psychology, 3*(1), 32–37.

Van Deusen, J., Harlowe, D., & Baker, L. (1989). Body image perceptions of the community-based elderly. *The Occupational Therapy Journal of Research, 9*(4), 243–248.

Wasson, D., & Anderson, M. A. (1995). Chemical dependency and adolescent self-esteem. *Clinical Nursing Research, 4*(3), 274–289.

B

Body Mechanics Performance   1616

Definition: Personal actions to maintain proper body alignment and to prevent musculoskeletal strain

OUTCOME TARGET RATING: Maintain at_____   Increase to_____

		Never demonstrated	Rarely demonstrated	Sometimes demonstrated	Often demonstrated	Consistently demonstrated	
OUTCOME OVERALL RATING		1	2	3	4	5	
Indicators:							
161601	Uses correct standing posture	1	2	3	4	5	NA
161602	Uses correct sitting posture	1	2	3	4	5	NA
161603	Uses correct lying posture	1	2	3	4	5	NA
161604	Uses correct lifting techniques	1	2	3	4	5	NA
161605	Uses correct carrying techniques	1	2	3	4	5	NA
161612	Uses correct pushing technique	1	2	3	4	5	NA
161607	Uses supportive devices correctly	1	2	3	4	5	NA
161608	Obtains assistance with heavy load	1	2	3	4	5	NA
161613	Maintains muscle strength	1	2	3	4	5	NA
161614	Maintains joint flexibility	1	2	3	4	5	NA
161611	Uses prescribed exercises to prevent injury	1	2	3	4	5	NA
161615	Uses proper body mechanics	1	2	3	4	5	NA

Domain-Health Knowledge & Behavior (IV)   *Class*-Health Behavior (Q)   *3rd edition 2004; revised 2008*

OUTCOME CONTENT REFERENCES:

Chan, D., Laporte, D. M., & Sveistrup, H. (1999). Rising from sitting in elderly people, Part 2: Strategies to facilitate rising. *British Journal of Occupational Therapy, 62*(2), 64–68.

Laporte, D. M., Chan, D., & Sveistrup, H. (1999). Rising from sitting in elderly people, Part 1: Implications of biomechanics and physiology. *British Journal of Occupational Therapy, 62*(1), 36–42.

Potter, P. A., & Perry, A. G. (2001). *Fundamentals of nursing* (5th ed.). St. Louis: Mosby.

Body Positioning: Self-Initiated   0203

B

Definition: Personal actions to change own body position independently with or without assistive device

OUTCOME TARGET RATING: Maintain at_____   Increase to_____

OUTCOME OVERALL RATING	Severely compromised 1	Substantially compromised 2	Moderately compromised 3	Mildly compromised 4	Not compromised 5	

Indicators:

		Severely compromised	Substantially compromised	Moderately compromised	Mildly compromised	Not compromised	
020302	Moves from lying to sitting	1	2	3	4	5	NA
020303	Moves from sitting to lying	1	2	3	4	5	NA
020304	Moves from sitting to standing	1	2	3	4	5	NA
020305	Moves from standing to sitting	1	2	3	4	5	NA
020306	Moves from standing to kneeling	1	2	3	4	5	NA
020307	Moves from kneeling to standing	1	2	3	4	5	NA
020308	Moves from standing to squatting	1	2	3	4	5	NA
020309	Moves from squatting to standing	1	2	3	4	5	NA
020310	Bends at waist while standing	1	2	3	4	5	NA
020311	Moves from side to side while lying	1	2	3	4	5	NA
020301	Moves from front to back while lying	1	2	3	4	5	NA
020313	Moves from back to front while lying	1	2	3	4	5	NA

Domain-Functional Health (I)   *Class*-Mobility (C)   *1st edition 1997; revised 2000, 2004, 2013*

OUTCOME CONTENT REFERENCES:

+Berg, K., Wood-Dauphinee, S., Williams, J. I., & Gayton, D. (1989). Measuring balance in the elderly: Preliminary development of an instrument. *Physiotherapy Canada, 41*(6), 304–311.

Melzer, I., Benjuya, N., & Kaplanski, J. (2000). Age related changes in muscle strength and fatigue. *Isokinetics & Exercise Science, 8*(2), 73–83.

Mikulic, M. A., Griffith, E. R., & Jebsen, R. H. (1976). Clinical application of a standardized mobility test. *Archives of Physical Medicine and Rehabilitation, 57*(3), 143–146.

Bone Healing

B

Definition: Extent of regeneration of cells and tissues following bone injury

OUTCOME TARGET RATING: Maintain at_____   Increase to_____

		None	Limited	Moderate	Substantial	Extensive	
OUTCOME OVERALL RATING		1	2	3	4	5	
Indicators:							
110402	Cellular proliferation	1	2	3	4	5	NA
110403	Callus formation	1	2	3	4	5	NA
110404	Ossification, consolidation, and remodeling	1	2	3	4	5	NA
110405	Intact peripheral circulation	1	2	3	4	5	NA
110406	Return of skeletal function	1	2	3	4	5	NA

		Extensive	Substantial	Moderate	Limited	None	
110401	Hematoma	1	2	3	4	5	NA
110407	Pain	1	2	3	4	5	NA
110408	Edema	1	2	3	4	5	NA
110410	Infection in surrounding tissue	1	2	3	4	5	NA
110411	Infection in bone	1	2	3	4	5	NA

Site of fracture (# from skeleton): _____

Domain-*Physiologic Health (II)*   **Class**-*Tissue Integrity (L)*   *1st edition 1997; revised 2004*

OUTCOME CONTENT REFERENCES:
Abdullah, D., Ford, T. R., Papaioannou, S., Nicholson, J., & McDonald, F. (2002). An evaluation of accelerated Portland cement as a restorative material. *Biomaterials, 23*(19), 4001–4010.
Mandracchia, V. J., Nelson, S. C., & Barp, E. A. (2001). Current concepts of bone healing. *Clinics in Podiatric Medicine & Surgery, 18*(1), 55–77.
Porth, C. M. (2002). *Pathophysiology: Concepts of altered health states* (6th ed.). Philadelphia: Lippincott Williams & Wilkins.
Potter, P. A., & Perry, A. G. (2001). *Fundamentals of nursing* (5th ed.). St. Louis: Mosby.
Wade, R., & Richardson, J. (2001). Outcome in fracture healing: A review. *Injury, 32*(2), 109–114.

B

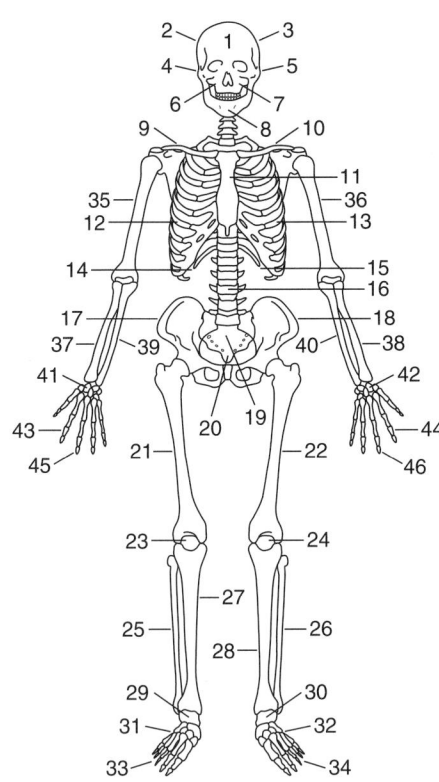
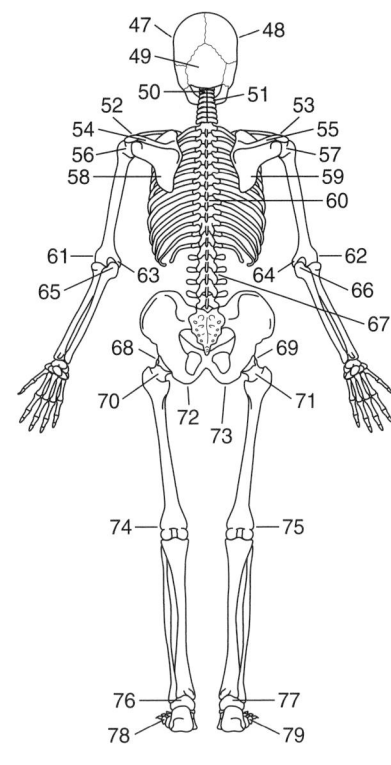

Bones of the head
1. Frontal
2. Right temporal
3. Left temporal
4. Right zygomatic
5. Left zygomatic
6. Right maxilla
7. Left maxilla
8. Mandible
47. Left parietal
48. Right parietal
49. Occipital

Bones of the neck and chest
9. Right clavicle
10. Left clavicle
11. Sternum
12. Right ribs
13. Left ribs
14. Right floating rib
15. Left floating rib
16. Vertebral column
50. Atlas
51. Cervical vertebra(e) specify _____
52. Left acromion
53. Right acromion
54. Left spine of scapula
55. Right spine of scapula
58. Left scapula
59. Right scapula
60. Thoracic vertebra(e) specify _____

Bones of the abdomen
16. Vertebral column
17. Right ilium
18. Left ilium
19. Sacrum
20. Coccyx
72. Left ischium
73. Right ischium
67. Lumbar vertebra(e) specify _____

Bones of the arm
35. Right humerus
36. Left humerus
37. Right radius
38. Left radius
39. Right ulna
40. Left ulna
41. Right carpals
42. Left carpals
43. Right metacarpals
44. Left metacarpals
45. Right phalanges
46. Left phalanges
56. Right head of humerus
57. Left head of humerus
61. Left epicondyle
62. Right epicondyle
63. Left epitrochlea
64. Right epitrochlea
65. Left olecranon
66. Right olecranon

Bones of the leg
21. Right femur
22. Left femur
23. Right patella
24. Left patella
25. Right fibula
26. Left fibula
27. Right tibia
28. Left tibia
29. Right tarsals
30. Left tarsals
31. Right metatarsals
32. Left metatarsals
33. Right phalanges
34. Left phalanges
68. Left head of femur
69. Right head of femur
70. Left neck of femur
71. Right neck of femur
74. Left condyle of femur
75. Right condyle of femur
76. Left talus
77. Right talus
78. Left calcaneus
79. Right calcaneus

Bottle Feeding Establishment: Infant 1016

Definition: Establishment of bottle feeding for hydration and nourishment of an infant

OUTCOME TARGET RATING: Maintain at_____ Increase to_____

	Not adequate	Slightly adequate	Moderately adequate	Substantially adequate	Totally adequate	
OUTCOME OVERALL RATING	1	2	3	4	5	
Indicators:						
101601 Proper grasp of nipple	1	2	3	4	5	NA
101602 Suck reflex	1	2	3	4	5	NA
101603 Ability to consume milk or formula from bottle	1	2	3	4	5	NA
101604 Formula flow rate tolerance	1	2	3	4	5	NA
101605 Audible swallow	1	2	3	4	5	NA
101606 Periodic burping	1	2	3	4	5	NA
101607 Feeding tolerance	1	2	3	4	5	NA
101608 Feedings per day	1	2	3	4	5	NA
101609 Contentment after feeding	1	2	3	4	5	NA
101610 Urine output appropriate for age	1	2	3	4	5	NA
101611 Stools appropriate for age	1	2	3	4	5	NA
101612 Weight gain appropriate for age	1	2	3	4	5	NA

Domain-*Physiologic Health (II)* **Class**-*Digestion & Nutrition (K)* *5th edition 2013*

OUTCOME CONTENT REFERENCES:

Hancock, M. E., & Brown, J. (2010). Formula feeding safety: What nurses need to teach parents who choose to formula-feed. *Nursing for Women's Health, 14*(4), 302–309.
Hockenberry, M. J., & Wilson, D. (2011). Wong's nursing care of infants and children (9th ed.). St. Louis: Elsevier Mosby.

Bottle Feeding Performance 1017

Definition: Caregiver actions to provide fluids to an infant using a bottle

OUTCOME TARGET RATING: Maintain at_____ Increase to_____

	Never demonstrated	Rarely demonstrated	Sometimes demonstrated	Often demonstrated	Consistently demonstrated	
OUTCOME OVERALL RATING	1	2	3	4	5	
Indicators:						
101701 Washes hands prior to preparation of formula	1	2	3	4	5	NA
101702 Prepares formula according to directions	1	2	3	4	5	NA
101703 Uses clean bottles and nipples	1	2	3	4	5	NA
101704 Uses correct size of nipple to regulate fluid flow	1	2	3	4	5	NA
101705 Uses formula before expiration date	1	2	3	4	5	NA
101706 Stores mixed formula correctly	1	2	3	4	5	NA
101707 Stores breast milk correctly	1	2	3	4	5	NA

Bottle Feeding Performance—*cont'd*

		Never demonstrated	Rarely demonstrated	Sometimes demonstrated	Often demonstrated	Consistently demonstrated	
101708	Warms bottle in warm water	1	2	3	4	5	NA
101709	Tests temperature of formula prior to feeding	1	2	3	4	5	NA
101710	Responds to infant hunger cues	1	2	3	4	5	NA
101711	Positions infant correctly while feeding	1	2	3	4	5	NA
101712	Positions bottle correctly while feeding	1	2	3	4	5	NA
101713	Burps infant at frequent intervals	1	2	3	4	5	NA
101714	Responds to infant cues to stop feeding	1	2	3	4	5	NA
101715	Repositions infant in response to choking	1	2	3	4	5	NA

Domain-*Physiologic Health (II)*   **Class-***Digestion & Nutrition (K)*   *5th edition 2013*

OUTCOME CONTENT REFERENCES:
Lowdermilk, D., & Perry, S. (2007). *Maternity & women's health care* (9th ed.). Philadelphia: Elsevier.
Hockenberry, M. J., & Wilson, D. (2011). *Wong's nursing care of infants and children* (9th ed.). St. Louis: Elsevier Mosby.

Bowel Continence   0500

Definition: Control of passage of stool from the bowel

OUTCOME TARGET RATING: Maintain at_____   Increase to_____

		Never demonstrated	Rarely demonstrated	Sometimes demonstrated	Often demonstrated	Consistently demonstrated	
	OUTCOME OVERALL RATING	1	2	3	4	5	
Indicators:							
050008	Recognizes urge to defecate	1	2	3	4	5	NA
050001	Maintains predictable pattern of stool evacuation	1	2	3	4	5	NA
050002	Maintains control of stool passage	1	2	3	4	5	NA
050003	Evacuates stool at least q 3 days	1	2	3	4	5	NA
050006	Sphincter tone adequate to control defecation	1	2	3	4	5	NA
050007	Sphincter innervation functional	1	2	3	4	5	NA
050009	Responds to urge in timely manner	1	2	3	4	5	NA
050012	Gets to toilet between urge and evacuation of stool	1	2	3	4	5	NA
050017	Maintains barrier-free environment for independent toileting	1	2	3	4	5	NA
050013	Ingests adequate amount of fluid	1	2	3	4	5	NA
050014	Ingests adequate amount of fiber	1	2	3	4	5	NA

Continued

Bowel Continence—cont'd

		Never demonstrated	Rarely demonstrated	Sometimes demonstrated	Often demonstrated	Consistently demonstrated	
050015	Describes relationship of food intake to stool consistency	1	2	3	4	5	NA
050018	Monitors amount and consistency of stool	1	2	3	4	5	NA
050019	Toilets independently	1	2	3	4	5	NA

		Consistently demonstrated	Often demonstrated	Sometimes demonstrated	Rarely demonstrated	Never demonstrated	
050004	Diarrhea	1	2	3	4	5	NA
050005	Constipation	1	2	3	4	5	NA
050020	Overuse of laxatives	1	2	3	4	5	NA
050021	Overuse of enemas	1	2	3	4	5	NA
050022	Soils clothing during day	1	2	3	4	5	NA
050023	Soils clothing or bedding during night	1	2	3	4	5	NA

Domain-*Physiologic Health (II)*   **Class**-*Elimination (F)*   *1st edition 1997; revised 2004, 2008*

OUTCOME CONTENT REFERENCES:

Hogstel, M. O., & Nelson, M. (1992). Anticipation and early detection can reduce bowel elimination complications. *Geriatric Nursing, 13*(1), 28–33.

Maas, M. L., & Specht, J. P. (2001). Bowel incontinence. In M. Maas, K. Buckwalter, M. Hardy, T. Tripp-Reimer, M. Titler, & J. Specht (Eds.), *Nursing care of older adults: Diagnoses, outcomes & interventions* (pp. 238–251). St. Louis: Mosby.

McLane, A. (1987). *Classification of nursing diagnoses: Proceedings of the 7th conference.* St. Louis: Mosby.

+Morris, J. N., Hawes, C., Fries, B. E., Phillips, C. D., Mor, V., Katz, S., Murphy, K., Drugovich, M. L., & Friedlob, A. S. (1990). Designing the national resident assessment instrument for nursing homes. *Gerontologist, 30*(3), 293–307.

Bowel Elimination

0501

Definition: Formation and evacuation of stool

OUTCOME TARGET RATING: Maintain at_____   Increase to_____

		Severely compromised	Substantially compromised	Moderately compromised	Mildly compromised	Not compromised	
OUTCOME OVERALL RATING		1	2	3	4	5	
Indicators:							
050101	Elimination pattern	1	2	3	4	5	NA
050102	Control of bowel movements	1	2	3	4	5	NA
050103	Stool color	1	2	3	4	5	NA
050104	Stool amount for diet	1	2	3	4	5	NA
050105	Stool soft and formed	1	2	3	4	5	NA
050112	Ease of stool passage	1	2	3	4	5	NA
050118	Sphincter tone	1	2	3	4	5	NA
050119	Muscle tone to evacuate stool	1	2	3	4	5	NA
050121	Passage of stool without aids	1	2	3	4	5	NA
050129	Bowel sounds	1	2	3	4	5	NA

		Severe	Substantial	Moderate	Mild	None	
050107	Fat in stool	1	2	3	4	5	NA
050108	Blood in stool	1	2	3	4	5	NA
050109	Mucus in stool	1	2	3	4	5	NA
050110	Constipation	1	2	3	4	5	NA
050111	Diarrhea	1	2	3	4	5	NA

Bowel Elimination—cont'd

		Severe	Substantial	Moderate	Mild	None	
050123	Abuse of elimination aids	1	2	3	4	5	NA
050128	Pain with passage of stool	1	2	3	4	5	NA

Domain-Physiologic Health (II)   **Class**-Elimination (F)   1st edition 1997; revised 2004, 2008

OUTCOME CONTENT REFERENCES:
Heading, C. (1987). Factors affecting bowel functions. *Nursing, 3*(21), 773–783.
Hogstel, M. O., & Nelson, M. (1992). Anticipation and early detection can reduce bowel elimination complications. *Geriatric Nursing, 13*(1), 28–33.
Lepshy, M. S., & Michael, A. (1993). Chronic diarrhea: Evaluation and treatment. *American Family Physician, 48*(8), 1461–1466.
Loening-Baucke, V. (1994). Management of chronic constipation in infants and toddlers. *American Family Physician, 46*(2), 397–406.
McKenna, S., Wallis, M., Brannelly, A., & Cawood, J. (2001). The nursing management of diarrhoea and constipation before and after the implementation of a bowel management protocol. *Australian Critical Care, 14*(1), 10–16.
McLane, A. M., & McShane, R. E. (2001). Constipation. In M. Maas, K. Buckwalter, M. Hardy, T. Tripp-Reimer, M. Titler, & J. Specht (Eds.), *Nursing care of older adults: Diagnoses, outcomes & interventions* (pp. 220–226). St. Louis: Mosby.
McShane, R. E., & McLane, A. M. (1988). Constipation: Impact of etiological factors. *Journal of Gerontological Nursing, 14*(4), 31–34.
Potter, P. A., & Perry, A. G. (2001). *Fundamentals of nursing* (5th ed.). St. Louis: Mosby.
Wadle, K. R. (2001). Diarrhea. In M. Maas, K. Buckwalter, M. Hardy, T. Tripp-Reimer, M. Titler, & J. Specht (Eds.), *Nursing care of older adults: Diagnoses, outcomes & interventions* (pp. 227–237). St. Louis: Mosby.

Breastfeeding Establishment: Infant   1000

Definition: Infant attachment to and sucking from the mother's breast for nourishment during the first 3 weeks of breastfeeding

OUTCOME TARGET RATING: Maintain at_____   Increase to_____

		Not adequate	Slightly adequate	Moderately adequate	Substantially adequate	Totally adequate	
OUTCOME OVERALL RATING		1	2	3	4	5	
Indicators:							
100001	Proper alignment and latch on	1	2	3	4	5	NA
100002	Proper areolar grasp	1	2	3	4	5	NA
100003	Proper areolar compression	1	2	3	4	5	NA
100013	Correct tongue placement	1	2	3	4	5	NA
100014	Suck reflex	1	2	3	4	5	NA
100005	Audible swallow	1	2	3	4	5	NA
100006	Nursing a minimum of 5-10 minutes per breast	1	2	3	4	5	NA
100015	Stop to burp infant at frequent intervals	1	2	3	4	5	NA
100007	Minimum of 8 feedings per day	1	2	3	4	5	NA
100008	Urinations per day appropriate for age	1	2	3	4	5	NA
100009	Loose, yellow, seedy stools per day appropriate for age	1	2	3	4	5	NA
100010	Weight gain appropriate for age	1	2	3	4	5	NA
100011	Infant contentment after feeding	1	2	3	4	5	NA

Domain-Physiologic Health (II)   **Class**-Digestion & Nutrition (K)   1st edition 1997; revised 2004, 2013

OUTCOME CONTENT REFERENCES:
Biancuzzo, M. (2003). *Breastfeeding the newborn* (2nd ed.). St. Louis: Mosby.
Cricco-Lizza, R. (2006). Black non-Hispanic mothers' perceptions about the promotion of infant feeding methods by nurses and physicians. *Journal of Obstetric, Gynecologic, and Neonatal Nursing (JOGNN), 35*(2), 173–180.
Henderson, A. M., Pincombe, J., & Stamp, G. E. (2000). Assisting women to establish breastfeeding: Exploring midwives' practices. *Breastfeeding Review, 8*(3), 11–17.
Lang, S. (2002). *Breastfeeding special care babies* (2nd ed.). London: Bailliere Tindall.

Lawrence, R. A., & Lawrence, R. M. (1999). *Breastfeeding: A guide for the medical profession* (5th ed.). St. Louis: Mosby.
Minchin, M. K. (1989). Positioning for breastfeeding. *Birth, 16*(2), 67–80.
+Muldford, C. (1992). The mother-baby assessment (MBA): An "Apgar Score" for breastfeeding. *Journal of Human Lactation, 8*(2), 79–82.
Neifert, M. R., & Seacat, J. M. (1986). A guide to successful breastfeeding. *Contemporary Pediatrics, 3*, 1–14.
Page-Goertz, S. (1989). Discharge planning for the breastfeeding dyad. *Pediatric Nursing, 15*(5), 543–544.
Righard, L., & Alade, M. O. (1992). Sucking technique and its effect on success of breastfeeding. *Birth, 19*(4), 185–189.
Riordan, J., & Auerbach, K. G. (1999). *Breastfeeding and human lactation* (2nd ed.). Sudbury, MA: Jones and Bartlett.
Shrago, L., & Bocar, D. (1990). The infant's contribution to breastfeeding. *Journal of Obstetric, Gynecologic, & Neonatal Nursing, 19*(3), 209–213.
Walker, M. (1989). Functional assessment of infant breastfeeding patterns. *Birth, 16*(3), 140–147.

Breastfeeding Establishment: Maternal 1001

Definition: Maternal establishment of proper attachment of an infant to and sucking from the breast for nourishment during the first 3 weeks of breastfeeding

OUTCOME TARGET RATING: Maintain at_____ Increase to_____

OUTCOME OVERALL RATING	Not adequate 1	Slightly adequate 2	Moderately adequate 3	Substantially adequate 4	Totally adequate 5	
Indicators:						
100101 Comfort of position during nursing	1	2	3	4	5	NA
100102 Supports breast using "C" hold (cupping)	1	2	3	4	5	NA
100103 Breast fullness prior to feeding	1	2	3	4	5	NA
100104 Milk ejection (let-down) reflex	1	2	3	4	5	NA
100106 Recognition of infant swallowing	1	2	3	4	5	NA
100107 Suction broken before removing infant from breast	1	2	3	4	5	NA
100121 Techniques to prevent nipple tenderness	1	2	3	4	5	NA
100109 Avoidance of artificial nipple use with infant	1	2	3	4	5	NA
100110 Avoidance of giving water to infant	1	2	3	4	5	NA
100122 Supplemental feedings	1	2	3	4	5	NA
100112 Response to infant's temperament	1	2	3	4	5	NA
100113 Recognition of early hunger cues	1	2	3	4	5	NA
100120 Fluid intake of mother	1	2	3	4	5	NA
100123 Pumping of breast	1	2	3	4	5	NA
100115 Safe storage of breastmilk	1	2	3	4	5	NA
100124 Use of family support	1	2	3	4	5	NA
100125 Use of community support	1	2	3	4	5	NA
100118 Satisfaction with breastfeeding process	1	2	3	4	5	NA

Domain-*Physiologic Health (II)* **Class**-*Digestion & Nutrition (K)* *1st edition 1997; revised 2004, 2008*

OUTCOME CONTENT REFERENCES:
Biancuzzo, M. (2003). *Breastfeeding the newborn* (2nd ed.). St. Louis: Mosby.
Cricco-Lizza, R. (2006). Black non-Hispanic mothers' perceptions about the promotion of infant feeding methods by nurses and physicians. *Journal of Obstetric, Gynecologic, and Neonatal Nursing (JOGNN), 35*(2), 173–180.
Henderson, A. M., Pincombe, J., & Stamp, G. E. (2000). Assisting women to establish breastfeeding: Exploring midwives' practices. *Breastfeeding Review, 8*(3), 11–17.
Hill, P., & Aldag, J. (1991). Potential indicators of insufficient milk supply syndrome. *Research in Nursing and Health, 14*(1), 11–19.
Lawrence, R. A., & Lawrence, R. M. (1999). Breastfeeding: A guide for the medical profession (5th ed.). St. Louis: Mosby.
Lowdermilk, D., & Perry, S. (2004). Maternity & women's health care (8th ed.). St. Louis: Mosby.
Minchin, M. K. (1989). Positioning for breastfeeding. *Birth, 16*(2), 67–80.
+Muldford, C. (1992). The mother-baby assessment (MBA): An "Apgar Score" for breastfeeding. *Journal of Human Lactation, 8*(2), 79–82.
Neifert, M. R., & Seacat, J. M. (1986). A guide to successful breastfeeding. *Contemporary Pediatrics, 3*, 1–14.
Page-Goertz, S. (1989). Discharge planning for the breastfeeding dyad. *Pediatric Nursing, 15*(5), 543–544.
Righard, L., & Alade, M. O. (1992). Sucking technique and its effect on success of breastfeeding. *Birth, 19*(4), 185–189.
Riordan, J., & Auerbach, K. G. (1999). *Breastfeeding and human lactation* (2nd ed.). Sudbury, MA: Jones and Bartlett.
Shrago, L., & Bocar, D. (1990). The infant's contribution to breastfeeding. *Journal of Obstetric, Gynecologic, & Neonatal Nursing, 19*(3), 209–213.
Walker, M. (1989). Functional assessment of infant breastfeeding patterns. *Birth, 16*(3), 140–147.

Breastfeeding Maintenance 1002

B

Definition: Continuation of breastfeeding from establishment to weaning for nourishment of an infant/toddler

OUTCOME TARGET RATING: Maintain at_____ Increase to_____

	Not adequate	Slightly adequate	Moderately adequate	Substantially adequate	Totally adequate	
OUTCOME OVERALL RATING	1	2	3	4	5	
Indicators:						
100201 Infant's growth in normal range	1	2	3	4	5	NA
100202 Infant's development in normal range	1	2	3	4	5	NA
100205 Ability to safely collect and store breastmilk	1	2	3	4	5	NA
100217 Ability to safely thaw and warm stored breastmilk	1	2	3	4	5	NA
100218 Techniques to prevent breast tenderness	1	2	3	4	5	NA
100208 Recognition of signs of decreased milk supply	1	2	3	4	5	NA
100219 Recognition of signs of plugged ducts	1	2	3	4	5	NA
100220 Recognition of signs of mastitis	1	2	3	4	5	NA
100221 Awareness that breastfeeding can continue beyond infancy	1	2	3	4	5	NA
100210 Avoidance of self-medication without checking with health professional	1	2	3	4	5	NA
100222 Perceived family support for breastfeeding	1	2	3	4	5	NA
100223 Perceived support for continuation of lactation on return to work	1	2	3	4	5	NA
100224 Perceived support for continuation of lactation on return to school	1	2	3	4	5	NA
100204 Knowledge of benefits from continued breastfeeding	1	2	3	4	5	NA
100225 Knowledge of resources for support	1	2	3	4	5	NA
100215 Satisfaction with breastfeeding process	1	2	3	4	5	NA

Domain-Physiologic Health (II) **Class-***Digestion & Nutrition (K)* *1st edition 1997; revised 2004, 2008*

OUTCOME CONTENT REFERENCES:
Bear, K., & Tigges, B. B. (1993). Management strategies for promoting successful breastfeeding. *Nurse Practitioner, 18*(6), 50, 53–54, 56–58, 60.
Callahan, S., Sejourne, N., & Denis, A. (2006). Fatigue and breastfeeding—an inevitable relationship. *Journal of Human Lactation, 22*(2), 182–187.
Coreil, J., & Murphy, J. E. (1988). Maternal commitment, lactation practices, and breastfeeding duration. *Journal of Obstetric, Gynecologic, & Neonatal Nursing, 17*(4), 273–278.
Cricco-Lizza, R. (2006). Black non-Hispanic mothers' perceptions about the promotion of infant feeding methods by nurses and physicians. *Journal of Obstetric, Gynecologic, and Neonatal Nursing (JOGNN), 35*(2), 173–180.
Dick, M. J., Evans, M. L., Arthurs, J. B., Barnes, J. K., Caldwell, R. S., Hutchins, S. S., & Johnson, L. K. (2002). Predicting early breastfeeding attrition. *Journal of Human Lactation, 18*(1), 21–28.
Hauck, Y., & Reinbold, J. (1996). Criteria for successful breastfeeding: Mothers' perceptions. *Journal—Australian College of Midwives, 9*(1), 21–27.
Lawrence, R. A., & Lawrence, R. M. (1999). *Breastfeeding: A guide for the medical profession* (5th ed.). St. Louis: Mosby.
Rentschler, D. D. (1991). Correlates of successful breastfeeding. *Image—The Journal of Nursing Scholarship, 23*(3), 151–154.
Riordan, J., & Auerbach, K. G. (1999). *Breastfeeding and human lactation* (2nd ed.). Sudbury, MA: Jones and Bartlett.

B

Breastfeeding Weaning 1003

Definition: Progressive discontinuation of breastfeeding of an infant/toddler

OUTCOME TARGET RATING: Maintain at_____   Increase to_____

OUTCOME OVERALL RATING		Not adequate 1	Slightly adequate 2	Moderately adequate 3	Substantially adequate 4	Totally adequate 5	
Indicators:							
100302	Recognition of weaning readiness cues	1	2	3	4	5	NA
100318	Recognition of signs of decreased milk supply	1	2	3	4	5	NA
100304	Knowledge of benefits of gradual weaning	1	2	3	4	5	NA
100305	Knowledge of guidelines for rapid "emergency" weaning	1	2	3	4	5	NA
100319	Knowledge of appropriate methods to reduce breast tenderness	1	2	3	4	5	NA
100320	Mother's freedom from plugged ducts	1	2	3	4	5	NA
100321	Mother's freedom from mastitis	1	2	3	4	5	NA
100322	Introduction of solids as recommended by health professional	1	2	3	4	5	NA
100308	Replacement of one additional breast-feeding with solids every few days	1	2	3	4	5	NA
100323	Replacement of breastmilk with other fluids	1	2	3	4	5	NA
100309	Introduction of solid foods one at a time	1	2	3	4	5	NA
100310	Introduction of solid foods using a spoon	1	2	3	4	5	NA
100311	Additional physical touch during time of weaning	1	2	3	4	5	NA
100313	Knowledge of resources available for support	1	2	3	4	5	NA
100314	Use of available resources	1	2	3	4	5	NA
100316	Satisfaction with weaning process	1	2	3	4	5	NA

Domain-Physiologic Health (II)   **Class**-Digestion & Nutrition (K)   1st edition 1997; revised 2004, 2008

OUTCOME CONTENT REFERENCES:
Castiglia, P. T. (1992). Weaning. *Journal of Pediatric Health Care, 6*(1), 38–39.
Hendricks, K. M., & Badruddin, S. H. (1992). Weaning recommendations: The scientific basis. *Nutrition Reviews, 50*(5), 125–133.
Hervada, A. R. (1992). Weaning: Historical perspectives, practical recommendations, and current controversies. *Current Problems in Pediatrics, 22*(5), 223–241.
Huggins, K., & Ziedrich, L. (1994). *The nursing mother's guide to weaning*. Boston: The Harvard Common Press.
Kleinman, R. E. (Ed.). (1998). *Pediatric nutrition handbook* (4th ed.). Elk Grove Village, IL: American Academy of Pediatrics.
Lawrence, R. A., & Lawrence, R. M. (1999). *Breastfeeding: A guide for the medical profession* (5th ed.). St. Louis: Mosby.
Lewallen, L. P., Dick, M. J., Flowers, J., Powell, W., Zickefoose, K. T., Wall, Y. G., & Price, Z. M. (2006). Breastfeeding support and early cessation. *Journal of Obstetric, Gynecologic, and Neonatal Nursing (JOGNN), 35*(2), 166–172.
Riordan, J., & Auerbach, K. G. (1999). *Breastfeeding and human lactation* (2nd ed.). Sudbury, MA: Jones and Bartlett.
Rogers, C. S., Morris, S., & Taper, L. J. (1987). Weaning from the breast: Influences on maternal decisions. *Pediatric Nursing, 13*(5), 341–345.
Spangler, A. (1992). *Amy Spangler's breastfeeding: A parent's guide*. Atlanta: Abbey Drue.
Walker, C. (1995). When to wean: Whose advice do mothers find helpful? *Health Visitor, 68*(3), 109–111.

Burn Healing   1106

Definition: Extent of healing of a burn site

OUTCOME TARGET RATING: Maintain at_____   Increase to_____

OUTCOME OVERALL RATING	None 1	Limited 2	Moderate 3	Substantial 4	Extensive 5	

Indicators:

		None 1	Limited 2	Moderate 3	Substantial 4	Extensive 5	
110601	Percent of graft site healed	1	2	3	4	5	NA
110602	Percent of burn site healed	1	2	3	4	5	NA
110603	Tissue granulation	1	2	3	4	5	NA
110604	Joint movement of affected extremity	1	2	3	4	5	NA
110605	Tissue perfusion of burn site	1	2	3	4	5	NA

		Extensive 1	Substantial 2	Moderate 3	Limited 4	None 5	
110606	Pain	1	2	3	4	5	NA
110607	Infection	1	2	3	4	5	NA
110608	Blistered skin	1	2	3	4	5	NA
110609	Purulent drainage	1	2	3	4	5	NA
110610	Foul wound odor	1	2	3	4	5	NA
110611	Burn site edema	1	2	3	4	5	NA
110612	Difficulty breathing	1	2	3	4	5	NA
110613	Tissue necrosis	1	2	3	4	5	NA

Grafted: Yes / No
Location of burn:_____

001 Head	007 Right upper arm	013 Right thigh
002 Neck	008 Left upper arm	014 Left thigh
003 Anterior trunk	009 Right lower arm	015 Right leg
004 Posterior trunk	010 Left lower arm	016 Left leg
005 Buttock	011 Right hand	017 Right foot
006 Genitalia	012 Left hand	018 Left foot

Domain-*Physiologic Health (II)*   **Class**-*Tissue Integrity (L)*   4th edition 2008

OUTCOME CONTENT REFERENCES:

American Burn Association. (1990). Hospital and prehospital resources for optimal care of patients with burn injury: Guidelines for development and operation of burn centers. *Journal of Burn Care and Rehabilitation, 11*(2), 98–104.

Black, J., & Hawks, J. (2005). *Medical-surgical nursing: Clinical management for positive outcomes* (7th ed.). St. Louis: Saunders.

Mendez-Eastman, S. (2005). Burn injuries. *Plastic Surgical Nursing 25*(3), 133–139.

Nowlin, A. (2006). The delicate business of burn care. *RN, 69*(1), 52–58.

Osborn, K. (2003). Nursing burn injuries (critical care). *Nursing Management, 34*(5), 49–56.

Regojo, P. (2003). Burn care basics: How to extinguish problems. *Nursing 2003, 3*(3), 50–53.

Burn Recovery 1107

B

Definition: Extent of overall physical and psychological healing following major burn injury

OUTCOME TARGET RATING: Maintain at_____   Increase to_____

	None	Limited	Moderate	Substantial	Extensive	
OUTCOME OVERALL RATING	1	2	3	4	5	

Indicators:

		None	Limited	Moderate	Substantial	Extensive	
110701	Tissue granulation	1	2	3	4	5	NA
110702	Tissue perfusion of burn site	1	2	3	4	5	NA
110703	Percent of burn healed	1	2	3	4	5	NA
110704	Temperature stability	1	2	3	4	5	NA
110705	Electrolyte stability	1	2	3	4	5	NA
110706	Fluid balance	1	2	3	4	5	NA
110707	Self-care ability	1	2	3	4	5	NA
110708	Joint movement of extremities	1	2	3	4	5	NA
110709	Ambulation tolerance	1	2	3	4	5	NA
110710	Positive attitude toward touching affected part	1	2	3	4	5	NA
110711	Psychological adjustment to changes in physical appearance	1	2	3	4	5	NA
110712	Psychological adjustment to changes in body function	1	2	3	4	5	NA

		Extensive	Substantial	Moderate	Limited	None	
110713	Pain	1	2	3	4	5	NA
110714	Decreased cognition	1	2	3	4	5	NA
110715	Pain medication requirements	1	2	3	4	5	NA
110716	Decreased oxygen saturation	1	2	3	4	5	NA
110717	Difficulty breathing	1	2	3	4	5	NA
110718	Weight loss	1	2	3	4	5	NA
110719	Infection	1	2	3	4	5	NA
110720	Blistered skin	1	2	3	4	5	NA
110721	Purulent drainage	1	2	3	4	5	NA
110722	Foul wound odor	1	2	3	4	5	NA
110723	Burn site edema	1	2	3	4	5	NA
110724	Tissue necrosis	1	2	3	4	5	NA
110725	Generalized edema	1	2	3	4	5	NA
110726	Gastrointestinal complications	1	2	3	4	5	NA
110727	Decreased urine output	1	2	3	4	5	NA
110728	Burn site grafting required	1	2	3	4	5	NA

Domain-Physiologic Health (II)   **Class**-Tissue Integrity (L)   4th edition 2008

OUTCOME CONTENT REFERENCES:

American Burn Association. (1990). Hospital and prehospital resources for optimal care of patients with burn injury: Guidelines for development and operation of burn centers. *Journal of Burn Care and Rehabilitation, 11*(2), 98–104.

Black, J., & Hawks, J. (2005). *Medical-surgical nursing: Clinical management for positive outcomes* (7th ed.). St. Louis: Saunders.

Mendez-Eastman, S. (2005). Burn injuries. *Plastic Surgical Nursing 25*(3), 133–139.

Nowlin, A. (2006). The delicate business of burn care. *RN, 69*(1), 52–58.

Osborn, K. (2003). Nursing burn injuries (critical care). *Nursing Management, 34*(5), 49–56.

Regojo, P. (2003). Burn care basics: How to extinguish problems. *Nursing 2003, 3*(3), 50–53.

Cardiac Pump Effectiveness **0400**

Definition: Adequacy of blood volume ejected from the left ventricle to support systemic perfusion pressure

OUTCOME TARGET RATING: Maintain at_____   Increase to_____

	Severe deviation from normal range	Substantial deviation from normal range	Moderate deviation from normal range	Mild deviation from normal range	No deviation from normal range	
OUTCOME OVERALL RATING	1	2	3	4	5	
Indicators:						
040001 Systolic blood pressure	1	2	3	4	5	NA
040019 Diastolic blood pressure	1	2	3	4	5	NA
040002 Apical heart rate	1	2	3	4	5	NA
040003 Cardiac index	1	2	3	4	5	NA
040004 Ejection fraction	1	2	3	4	5	NA
040006 Peripheral pulses	1	2	3	4	5	NA
040007 Heart size	1	2	3	4	5	NA
040020 Urine output	1	2	3	4	5	NA
040022 24-hour intake and output balance	1	2	3	4	5	NA
040025 Central venous pressure	1	2	3	4	5	NA

	Severe	Substantial	Moderate	Mild	None	
040009 Neck vein distension	1	2	3	4	5	NA
040010 Dysrhythmia	1	2	3	4	5	NA
040011 Abnormal heart sounds	1	2	3	4	5	NA
040012 Angina	1	2	3	4	5	NA
040013 Peripheral edema	1	2	3	4	5	NA
040014 Pulmonary edema	1	2	3	4	5	NA
040015 Diaphoresis	1	2	3	4	5	NA
040016 Nausea	1	2	3	4	5	NA
040017 Fatigue	1	2	3	4	5	NA
040023 Dyspnea at rest	1	2	3	4	5	NA
040026 Dyspnea with mild exertion	1	2	3	4	5	NA
040024 Weight gain	1	2	3	4	5	NA
040027 Ascites	1	2	3	4	5	NA
040028 Hepatomegaly	1	2	3	4	5	NA
040029 Impaired cognition	1	2	3	4	5	NA
040030 Activity intolerance	1	2	3	4	5	NA
040031 Pallor	1	2	3	4	5	NA
040032 Cyanosis	1	2	3	4	5	NA
040033 Flushed	1	2	3	4	5	NA

Domain-Physiologic Health (II)   **Class**-Cardiopulmonary (E)   *1st edition 1997; revised 2004, 2008*

OUTCOME CONTENT REFERENCES:

Bumann, R., & Speltz, M. (1989). Decreased cardiac output: A nursing diagnosis. *Dimensions of Critical Care Nursing, 8*(1), 6–15.

Dalton, J. (1985). A descriptive study: Defining characteristics of the nursing diagnosis cardiac output, alterations in: Decreased. *Image—The Journal of Nursing Scholarship, 17*(4), 113–117.

Dougherty, C. (1986). Decreased cardiac output: Validation of a nursing diagnosis. *Dimensions of Critical Care Nursing, 5*(3), 182–188.

Dougherty, C. M. (2001). Decreased cardiac output. In M. Maas, K. Buckwalter, M. Hardy, T. Tripp-Reimer, M. Titler, & J. Specht (Eds.), *Nursing care of older adults: Diagnoses, outcomes & interventions* (pp. 285–297). St. Louis: Mosby.

Futrell, A. (1990). Decreased cardiac output: Case for a collaborative diagnosis. *Dimensions of Critical Care Nursing, 9*(4), 202–209.

C

Cardiopulmonary Status 0414

Definition: Adequacy of blood volume ejected from the ventricles and exchange of carbon dioxide and oxygen at the alveolar level

OUTCOME TARGET RATING: Maintain at_____   Increase to_____

		Severe deviation from normal range	Substantial deviation from normal range	Moderate deviation from normal range	Mild deviation from normal range	No deviation from normal range	
OUTCOME OVERALL RATING		1	2	3	4	5	
Indicators:							
041401	Systolic blood pressure	1	2	3	4	5	NA
041402	Diastolic blood pressure	1	2	3	4	5	NA
041403	Peripheral pulses	1	2	3	4	5	NA
041404	Apical heart rate	1	2	3	4	5	NA
041405	Cardiac rhythm	1	2	3	4	5	NA
041406	Respiratory rate	1	2	3	4	5	NA
041407	Respiratory rhythm	1	2	3	4	5	NA
041408	Depth of inspiration	1	2	3	4	5	NA
041409	Expulsion of air	1	2	3	4	5	NA
041410	Urinary output	1	2	3	4	5	NA
041411	Cardiac index	1	2	3	4	5	NA
041412	Oxygen saturation	1	2	3	4	5	NA
041413	Movement of sputum out of airway	1	2	3	4	5	NA

		Severe	Substantial	Moderate	Mild	None	
041414	Activity intolerance	1	2	3	4	5	NA
041415	Impaired cognition	1	2	3	4	5	NA
041416	Pallor	1	2	3	4	5	NA
041417	Cyanosis	1	2	3	4	5	NA
041418	Flushed	1	2	3	4	5	NA
041419	Neck vein distention	1	2	3	4	5	NA
041420	Chest retraction	1	2	3	4	5	NA
041421	Pursed lip breathing	1	2	3	4	5	NA
041422	Peripheral edema	1	2	3	4	5	NA
041423	Pulmonary edema	1	2	3	4	5	NA
041424	Dyspnea at rest	1	2	3	4	5	NA
041425	Dyspnea with mild exertion	1	2	3	4	5	NA
041426	Fatigue	1	2	3	4	5	NA
041427	Restlessness	1	2	3	4	5	NA
041428	Somnolence	1	2	3	4	5	NA
041429	Weight gain	1	2	3	4	5	NA
041430	Weight loss	1	2	3	4	5	NA
041431	Diaphoresis	1	2	3	4	5	NA

Domain-Physiologic Health (II)   *Class*-Cardiopulmonary (E)   *4th edition 2008*

OUTCOME CONTENT REFERENCES:

Berry, B. E., & Pinard, A. E. (2002). Assessing tissue oxygenation. *Critical Care Nurse, 22*(3), 22–36.

Dougherty, C. M. (2001). Decreased cardiac output. In M. Maas, K. Buckwalter, M. Hardy, T. Tripp-Reimer, M. Titler, & J. Specht (Eds.), *Nursing care of older adults: Diagnoses, outcomes & interventions* (pp. 285–297). St. Louis: Mosby.

Smeltzer, S. C., & Bare, B. G. (2004). *Brunner & Suddarth's textbook of medical surgical nursing* (Vols. 1 & 2) (10th ed.). Philadelphia: Lippincott Williams & Wilkins.

Wakefield, B. (2001). Ineffective breathing pattern. In M. Maas, K. Buckwalter, M. Hardy, T. Tripp-Reimer, M. Titler, & J. Specht (Eds.), *Nursing care of older adults: Diagnoses, outcomes & interventions* (pp. 313–323). St. Louis: Mosby.

Caregiver Adaptation to Patient Institutionalization   2200

Definition: Adaptive response of family caregiver when the care recipient is moved to an institution

OUTCOME TARGET RATING: Maintain at_____   Increase to_____

		Never demonstrated	Rarely demonstrated	Sometimes demonstrated	Often demonstrated	Consistently demonstrated	
OUTCOME OVERALL RATING		1	2	3	4	5	
Indicators:							
220001	Trusts non-family caregiver	1	2	3	4	5	NA
220002	Maintains desired control over care	1	2	3	4	5	NA
220003	Participates in care as desired	1	2	3	4	5	NA
220004	Maintains caregiver-care recipient relationship	1	2	3	4	5	NA
220016	Collaborates with health provider in determining care	1	2	3	4	5	NA
220006	Reports decreased need to verbalize feelings about change	1	2	3	4	5	NA
220007	Resolves feelings of guilt	1	2	3	4	5	NA
220008	Resolves feelings of anger	1	2	3	4	5	NA
220009	Uses conflict resolution strategies	1	2	3	4	5	NA
220017	Reports comfort with role transition	1	2	3	4	5	NA
220011	Provides consent for treatment	1	2	3	4	5	NA
220012	Provides information about patient's routine	1	2	3	4	5	NA
220013	Provides patient's comfort items	1	2	3	4	5	NA
220014	Communicates needs of nonverbal patient	1	2	3	4	5	NA

Domain-Family Health (VI)   *Class*-Family Caregiver Performance (W)   *1st edition 1997; revised 2004, 2008*

OUTCOME CONTENT REFERENCES:

Gaugler, J. E., Pearlin, L. I., Leitsch, S. A., & Davey, A. (2001). Relinquishing in-home dementia care: Difficulties and perceived helpfulness during the nursing home transition. *American Journal of Alzheimer's Disease & Other Dementias, 16*(1), 32–42.

Kaus, K. J. (1990). Fostering family integrity. In M. Craft & J. A. Denehy (Eds.), *Nursing interventions for infants and children* (pp. 181–200). Philadelphia: W. B. Saunders.

Langford, M. (2001). A view from the front lines. Residential treatment: Have I done the right thing? *Premier Outlook, 2*(1), 16, 18.

Lindgren, C. L. (1993). The caregiver career. *Image—The Journal of Nursing Scholarship, 25*(3), 214–219.

Lindsay, J. K., Roman, L., DeWys, M., Eager, M., Levick, J., & Quinn, M. (1993). Creative caring in the NICU: Parent to parent support. *Neonatal Network, 12*(4), 37–44.

Maas, M., Buckwalter, K., Swanson, E., Specht, J., Tripp-Reimer, T., & Hardy, M. (1994). The caring partnership: Staff and families of persons institutionalized with Alzheimer's disease. *The American Journal of Alzheimer's Care and Related Disorders & Research, 9*(6), 21–30.

+Montgomery, R. J. V., Gonyea, J. G., & Hooyman, N. R. (1985). Caregiving and the experience of subjective and objective burden. *Family Relations, 34*(1), 19–26.

Moyle, W., Edwards, H., & Clinton, M. (2002). Living with loss: Dementia and the family caregiver. *Australian Journal of Advanced Nursing, 19*(3), 25–31.

Olson, R. K., Heater, B. S., & Becker, A. M. (1990). A meta-analysis of the effects of nursing interventions on children and parents. *Maternal-Child Nursing, 15*(2), 104–108.

+Picot, S. J., Youngblut, J., & Zeller, R. (1997). Development and testing of a measure of perceived caregiver rewards in adults. *Journal of Nursing Measurement, 5*(1), 33–52.

Stevenson, J. E. (1990). Family stress related to home care of Alzheimer's disease patients and implications for support. *Journal of Neuroscience Nursing, 22*(3), 179–188.

Swanson, E., Jensen, D. P., Specht, J., Saylor, D., Johnson, M., & Maas, M. (1997). Caregiving: Concept analysis and outcomes. *Scholarly Inquiry for Nursing Practice, 11*(1), 65–79.

Wilson, H. S. (1989). Family caregiving for a relative with Alzheimer's dementia: Coping with negative choices. *Nursing Research, 38*(2), 94–98.

Caregiver Emotional Health 2506

Definition: Emotional well-being of a family care provider while caring for a family member

OUTCOME TARGET RATING: Maintain at_____ Increase to_____

OUTCOME OVERALL RATING		Severely compromised	Substantially compromised	Moderately compromised	Mildly compromised	Not compromised	
		1	2	3	4	5	
Indicators:							
250601	Satisfaction with life	1	2	3	4	5	NA
250602	Sense of control	1	2	3	4	5	NA
250603	Self-esteem	1	2	3	4	5	NA
250610	Certainty about future	1	2	3	4	5	NA
250611	Perceived social connectedness	1	2	3	4	5	NA
250612	Perceived spiritual well-being	1	2	3	4	5	NA
250614	Perceived adequacy of resources	1	2	3	4	5	NA
		Severe	Substantial	Moderate	Mild	None	
250604	Anger	1	2	3	4	5	NA
250605	Resentfulness	1	2	3	4	5	NA
250606	Guilt	1	2	3	4	5	NA
250607	Depression	1	2	3	4	5	NA
250608	Frustration	1	2	3	4	5	NA
250609	Ambivalence about situation	1	2	3	4	5	NA
250613	Perceived burden	1	2	3	4	5	NA
250615	Psychotropic medication use	1	2	3	4	5	NA

Domain-*Family Health (VI)*   **Class**-*Family Member Health Status (Z)*   *1st edition 1997; revised 2004*

OUTCOME CONTENT REFERENCES:

Brown, M. A., & Powell-Cope, G. M. (1991). AIDS family caregiving: Transitions through uncertainty. *Nursing Research, 40*(6), 338–345.

Bull, M. J. (1990). Factors influencing family caregiver burden and health. *Western Journal of Nursing Research, 12*(6), 758–776.

Croog, S. H., Sudilovsky, A., Burleson, J. A., & Baume, R. M. (2001). Vulnerability of husband and wife caregivers of Alzheimer disease patients to caregiving stressors. *Alzheimer Disease & Associated Disorders, 15*(4), 201–210.

Ducharme, F., LeVesque, L., Gendron, M., & Legault, A. (2001). Development process and qualitative evaluation of a program to promote the mental health of family caregivers. *Clinical Nursing Research, 10*(2), 182–201.

Fruewirth, S. E. (1989). An application of Johnson's Behavioral Model: A case study. *Journal of Community Health Nursing, 6*(2), 61–71.

Given, B. A., Kozachik, S. L., Collins, C. E., DeVoss, D. N., & Given, C. W. (2001). Caregiver role strain. In M. Maas, K. Buckwalter, M. Hardy, T. Tripp-Reimer, M. Titler, & J. Specht (Eds.), *Nursing care of older adults: Diagnoses, outcomes & interventions* (pp. 679–695). St. Louis: Mosby.

Grant, I., Adler, K. A., Patterson, T. L., Dimsdale, J. E., Ziegler, M. G., & Irwin, M. R. (2002). Health consequences of Alzheimer's caregiving transitions: Effects of placement and bereavement. *Psychosomatic Medicine, 64*(3), 477–486.

Haley, W. E., LaMonde, L. A., Han, B., Narramore, S., & Schonwetter, R. (2001). Family caregiving in hospice: Effects on psychological and health functioning among spousal caregivers of hospice patients with lung cancer or dementia. *Hospice Journal, 15*(4), 1–18.

Lindgren, C. L. (1990). Burnout and social support in family caregivers. *Western Journal of Nursing Research, 12*(4), 469–487.

Ptok, U., Papassotiropoulos, A., & Heun, R. (2001). Mental health in spouses of patients with gerontopsychiatric disorders. *International Journal of Geriatric Psychiatry, 16*(10), 1014–1016.

+Robinson, B. C. (1983). Validation of a caregiver strain index. *Journal of Gerontology, 38*(3), 344–348.

Romeis, J. C. (1989). Caregiver strain. *Journal of Aging and Health, 1*(2), 188–208.

Thompson, E. H., Futterman, A. M., Gallagher-Thompson, D., Rose, J. M., & Lovett, S. B. (1993). Social support and caregiving burden in family caregivers of frail elders. *Journal of Gerontology, 48*(5), S245–S254.

Caregiver Home Care Readiness 2202

Definition: Preparedness of a caregiver to assume responsibility for the health care of a family member in the home

OUTCOME TARGET RATING: Maintain at_____ Increase to_____

C

		Not adequate	Slightly adequate	Moderately adequate	Substantially adequate	Totally adequate	
OUTCOME OVERALL RATING		1	2	3	4	5	
Indicators:							
220201	Willingness to assume caregiving role	1	2	3	4	5	NA
220204	Participation in decisions about home care	1	2	3	4	5	NA
220202	Knowledge about caregiving role	1	2	3	4	5	NA
220203	Demonstration of positive regard for care recipient	1	2	3	4	5	NA
220205	Knowledge of care recipient's disease process	1	2	3	4	5	NA
220206	Knowledge of recommended treatment regimen	1	2	3	4	5	NA
220207	Knowledge of recommended procedures	1	2	3	4	5	NA
220219	Knowledge of equipment and supplies required	1	2	3	4	5	NA
220220	Knowledge of equipment operation	1	2	3	4	5	NA
220208	Knowledge of prescribed activity	1	2	3	4	5	NA
220209	Knowledge of follow-up care	1	2	3	4	5	NA
220210	Knowledge of emergency care	1	2	3	4	5	NA
220211	Knowledge of financial resources	1	2	3	4	5	NA
220212	Financial resources for caregiving	1	2	3	4	5	NA
220213	Knowledge of when to contact health professional	1	2	3	4	5	NA
220214	Perceived social support for caregiving	1	2	3	4	5	NA
220215	Confidence in ability to manage care at home	1	2	3	4	5	NA
220217	Willingness to involve care recipient in planning care	1	2	3	4	5	NA
220218	Evidence of plans for caregiver backup	1	2	3	4	5	NA
220222	Participation in discharge planning	1	2	3	4	5	NA

Domain-*Family Health (VI)* **Class-***Family Caregiver Performance (W)* *1st edition 1997; revised 2004, 2008*

OUTCOME CONTENT REFERENCES:

Axelrod, J., Geismar, L., & Ross, R. (1994). Families of chronically mentally ill patients: Their structure, coping resources, and tolerance for deviant behavior. *Health & Social Work, 19*(4), 271–278.

Baginski, Y. (1994). Roadblocks to home care. *Continuing Care, 13*(8), 16–18, 24, 28–29.

Bull, M. J., Hansen, H. E., & Gross, C. R. (2000). Differences in family caregiver outcomes by their level of involvement in discharge planning. *Applied Nursing Research, 13*(2), 76–82.

Coppa, C., Hepburn, J., Strauss, D., & Yody, B. B. (1999). Return to home after acquired brain injury: Is the family ready? *Brain Injury Source, 3*(2), 18–20, 22.

Gennaro, S., & Bakewell-Sachs, S. (1992). Discharge planning and home care for low-birth-weight infants. *NAACOGS Clinical Issues in Perinatal & Women's Health Nursing, 3*(1), 129–145.

Magilvy, J. K., & Lakomy, J. M. (1991). Transitions of older adults to home care. *Home Health Care Services Quarterly, 12*(4), 59–70.

+Picot, S. J., Youngblut, J., & Zeller, R. (1997). Development and testing of a measure of perceived caregiver rewards in adults. *Journal of Nursing Measurement, 5*(1), 33–52.

Scherbring, M. (2002). Effect of caregiver perception of preparedness of burden in an oncology population. *Oncology Nursing Forum, 29*(6), E70–E76.

Titler, M. G., & Pettit, D. M. (1995). Discharge readiness assessment. *Journal of Cardiovascular Nursing, 9*(4), 64–74.

Caregiver Lifestyle Disruption 2203

Definition: Severity of disturbances in the lifestyle of a family member due to caregiving

OUTCOME TARGET RATING: Maintain at_____ Increase to_____

		Severe	Substantial	Moderate	Mild	None	
OUTCOME OVERALL RATING		1	2	3	4	5	
Indicators:							
220315	Disruption of routine	1	2	3	4	5	NA
220317	Disruption of family dynamics	1	2	3	4	5	NA
220318	Disruption of living environment	1	2	3	4	5	NA
220319	Financial burden from caregiving	1	2	3	4	5	NA

		Severely compromised	Substantially compromised	Moderately compromised	Mildly compromised	Not compromised	
220310	Role responsibilities	1	2	3	4	5	NA
220302	Role performance	1	2	3	4	5	NA
220320	Sleep	1	2	3	4	5	NA
220303	Role flexibility	1	2	3	4	5	NA
220304	Opportunities for privacy	1	2	3	4	5	NA
220305	Relationships with family members	1	2	3	4	5	NA
220306	Social interactions	1	2	3	4	5	NA
220307	Social support	1	2	3	4	5	NA
220308	Diversional activities	1	2	3	4	5	NA
220312	Relationships with friends	1	2	3	4	5	NA
220313	Relationships with pets	1	2	3	4	5	NA
220309	Work productivity	1	2	3	4	5	NA

Domain-Family Health (VI) *Class*-Family Caregiver Performance (W) *1st edition 1997; revised 2004, 2008*

OUTCOME CONTENT REFERENCES:

Baldwin, B. A., Kleeman, K. M., Stevens, G. L., & Rasin, J. (1989). Family caregiver stress: Clinical assessment and management. *International Psychogeriatrics*, *1*(2), 183–193.

Gaynor, S. E. (1990). The long haul: The effects of home care on caregivers. *Image—The Journal of Nursing Scholarship*, *22*(4), 208–212.

Given, B. A., & Given, C. W. (1991). Family caregiving for the elderly. *Annual Review of Nursing Research*, *9*, 77–101.

Hinds, C. (1992). Suffering: A relatively unexplored phenomenon among family caregivers of non-institutionalized patients with cancer. *Journal of Advanced Nursing*, *17*(8), 918–925.

Kuhlman, G. J., Wilson, H. S., Hutchison, S. A., & Wallhagen, M. (1991). Alzheimer's disease and family caregiving: Critical syntheses of the literature and research agenda. *Nursing Research*, *40*(6), 331–337.

Lindgren, C. L. (1990). Burnout and social support in family caregivers. *Western Journal of Nursing Research*, *12*(4), 469–487.

Lindgren, C. L. (1993). The caregiver career. *Image—The Journal of Nursing Scholarship*, *25*(3), 214–219.

Oberst, M. T., Thomas, S. E., Gass, K. A., & Ward, S. E. (1989). Caregiving demands and appraisal of stress among family caregivers. *Cancer Nursing*, *12*(4), 209–215.

+Robinson, B. C. (1983). Validation of a caregiver strain index. *Journal of Gerontology*, *38*(3), 344–348.

Robinson, K. (1990). The relationships between social skills, social support, self-esteem and burden in adult caregivers. *Journal of Advanced Nursing*, *15*(7), 788–795.

Robinson, K. M. (1989). Predictors of depression among wife caregivers. *Nursing Research*, *38*(8), 359–363.

Stern, S., Doolan, M., Staples, E., Szmukler, G. L., & Eisler, I. (1999). Disruption and reconstruction: Narrative insights into the experience of family members caring for a relative diagnosed with serious mental illness. *Family Process*, *38*(3), 353–369.

Stevenson, J. E. (1990). Family stress related to home care of Alzheimer's disease patients and implications for support. *Journal of Neuroscience Nursing*, *22*(3), 179–188.

Thompson, E. H., Futterman, A. M., Gallagher-Thompson, D., Rose, J. M., & Lovette, S. B. (1993). Social support and caregiving burden in family caregivers of frail elders. *Journal of Gerontology*, *48*(5), S245–S254.

Caregiver-Patient Relationship 2204

Definition: Positive interactions and connections between the caregiver and care recipient

OUTCOME TARGET RATING: Maintain at_____ Increase to_____

C

		Never positive	Rarely positive	Sometimes positive	Often positive	Consistently positive	
OUTCOME OVERALL RATING		1	2	3	4	5	
Indicators:							
220401	Effective communication	1	2	3	4	5	NA
220402	Patience	1	2	3	4	5	NA
220404	Calmness	1	2	3	4	5	NA
220405	Nurturance and affirmation	1	2	3	4	5	NA
220406	Companionship	1	2	3	4	5	NA
220407	Caring	1	2	3	4	5	NA
220408	Long-term commitment	1	2	3	4	5	NA
220409	Mutual acceptance	1	2	3	4	5	NA
220410	Mutual respect	1	2	3	4	5	NA
220411	Collaborative problem solving	1	2	3	4	5	NA
220412	Sense of responsibility	1	2	3	4	5	NA
220413	Mutual sense of attachment	1	2	3	4	5	NA

Domain-Family Health (VI) *Class*-Family Caregiver Performance (W) *1st edition 1997; revised 2004, 2008*

OUTCOME CONTENT REFERENCES:
Caldwell, S. M. (1988). Measuring family well-being: Conceptual model, reliability, validity and use. In C. F. Waltz & O. L. Strickland (Eds.), *Measurement of nursing outcomes: Measuring client outcomes* (Vol. 1, pp. 396–422). New York: Springer.
Clemen-Stone, S., McGuire, S., & Eigsti, D. (2002). *Comprehensive community health nursing: Family, aggregate and community practice* (6th ed.). St. Louis: Mosby.
Craft, M. J., & Willadsen, J. A. (1992). Interventions related to family. *Nursing Clinics of North America, 27*(20), 517–540.
Gaynor, S. E. (1990). The long haul: The effects of home care on caregivers. *Image—The Journal of Nursing Scholarship, 22*(4), 208–212.
Hooyman, M., Gonyea, J., & Montgomery, R. (1985). Impact of in-home services termination on family caregivers. *The Gerontologist, 25*(2), 141–145.
O'Neill, C., & Sorenson, E. S. (1991). Home care of the elderly: A family perspective. *Advances in Nursing Science, 13*(4), 28–37.
Phillips, L. R. (1988). The fit of elder abuse with the family violence paradigm, and the implications of a paradigm shift for clinical practice. *Public Health Nursing, 5*(4), 222–229.
+Picot, S. J., Youngblut, J., & Zeller, R. (1997). Development and testing of a measure of perceived caregiver rewards in adults. *Journal of Nursing Measurement, 5*(1), 33–52.
Printz-Feddersen, V. (1990). Group process effect on caregiver burden. *Journal of Neuroscience Nursing, 22*(3), 164–168.
+Vermooij-Dassen, M. J. F. J. (1993). *Dementia and home care: Determinants of the sense of competence of primary caregivers and the effect of professionally guided caregiver support* (in Dutch). Lisse, The Netherlands: Swets & Seitliger.

Caregiver Performance: Direct Care 2205

Definition: Provision by family care provider of appropriate personal and health care for a family member

OUTCOME TARGET RATING: Maintain at_____ Increase to_____

		Not adequate	Slightly adequate	Moderately adequate	Substantially adequate	Totally adequate	
OUTCOME OVERALL RATING		1	2	3	4	5	
Indicators:							
220503	Knowledge of disease process	1	2	3	4	5	NA
220504	Knowledge of treatment regimen	1	2	3	4	5	NA
220505	Adherence to treatment regimen	1	2	3	4	5	NA
220516	Performance of procedures	1	2	3	4	5	NA

Continued

Caregiver Performance: Direct Care—cont'd

		Not adequate	Slightly adequate	Moderately adequate	Substantially adequate	Totally adequate	
220502	Assistance with care recipient's activities of daily living needs	1	2	3	4	5	NA
220506	Assistance with care recipient's instrumental activities of daily living needs	1	2	3	4	5	NA
220501	Provision of emotional support to care recipient	1	2	3	4	5	NA
220508	Surveillance of health status of care recipient	1	2	3	4	5	NA
220509	Surveillance of behavior of care recipient	1	2	3	4	5	NA
220510	Anticipation of care recipient's needs	1	2	3	4	5	NA
220517	Unconditional positive regard for care recipient	1	2	3	4	5	NA
220518	Competence monitoring own caregiving skill level	1	2	3	4	5	NA
220513	Confidence performing needed tasks	1	2	3	4	5	NA
220515	Provision of safe environment	1	2	3	4	5	NA

Domain-Family Health (VI) **Class**-Family Caregiver Performance (W) *1st edition 1997; revised 2004, 2008*

OUTCOME CONTENT REFERENCES:

Given, B. A., & Given, C. W. (1991). Family caregiving for the elderly. *Annual Review of Nursing Research, 9*, 77–101.

Given, B. A., Kozachik, S. L., Collins, C. E., DeVoss, D. N., & Given, C. W. (2001). Caregiver role strain. In M. Maas, K. Buckwalter, M. Hardy, T. Tripp-Reimer, M. Titler, & J. Specht (Eds.), *Nursing care of older adults: Diagnoses, outcomes & interventions* (pp. 679–695). St. Louis: Mosby.

Oberst, M. T., Thomas, S. E., Gass, K. A., & Ward, S. E. (1989). Caregiving demands and appraisal of stress among family caregivers. *Cancer Nursing, 12*(4), 209–215.

+Picot, S. J., Youngblut, J., & Zeller, R. (1997). Development and testing of a measure of perceived caregiver rewards in adults. *Journal of Nursing Measurement, 5*(1), 33–52.

Pierson, M. A., & Irons, K. (1992). Identification of a cluster of nursing diagnoses for a caregiver support group. *Nursing Diagnosis, 3*(1), 36–41.

Printz-Feddersen, V. (1990). Group process effect on caregiver burden. *Journal of Neuroscience Nursing, 22*(3), 164–168.

Thomas, V. M., Ellison, K., Howell, E. V., & Winters, K. (1992). Caring for the person receiving ventilatory support at home: Caregivers' needs and involvement. *Heart & Lung, 21*(2), 180–186.

+Vermooij-Dassen, M. J. F. J. (1993). *Dementia and home care: Determinants of the sense of competence of primary caregivers and the effect of professionally guided caregiver support* (in Dutch). Lisse, The Netherlands: Swets & Seitliger.

Wallhagen, M. I., & Kagan, S. H. (1993). Staying within bounds: Perceived control and the experience of elderly caregivers. *Journal of Aging Studies, 7*(2), 197–213.

Caregiver Performance: Indirect Care 2206

Definition: Arrangement and oversight by family care provider of appropriate care for a family member

OUTCOME TARGET RATING: Maintain at_____ Increase to_____

OUTCOME OVERALL RATING	Not adequate	Slightly adequate	Moderately adequate	Substantially adequate	Totally adequate	
	1	2	3	4	5	
Indicators:						
220601 Confidence in problem solving	1	2	3	4	5	NA
220602 Recognition of changes in health status of care recipient	1	2	3	4	5	NA
220603 Recognition of changes in behavior of care recipient	1	2	3	4	5	NA
220614 Anticipation of care recipient's needs	1	2	3	4	5	NA
220605 Procurement of needed health care services for care recipient	1	2	3	4	5	NA
220611 Procurement of needed transportation for care recipient	1	2	3	4	5	NA
220612 Procurement of needed equipment and supplies for care recipient	1	2	3	4	5	NA
220606 Skill in overseeing provision of care	1	2	3	4	5	NA
220615 Unconditional positive regard for care recipient	1	2	3	4	5	NA
220608 Skill in pursuing care problems with direct care providers	1	2	3	4	5	NA
220609 Confidence in performing needed tasks	1	2	3	4	5	NA
220613 Recognition of requirements for safety	1	2	3	4	5	NA

Domain-Family Health (VI) *Class-Family Caregiver Performance (W)* *1st edition 1997; revised 2004, 2008*

OUTCOME CONTENT REFERENCES:

Bowers, B. J. (1987). Intergenerational caregiving: Adult caregivers and their aging parents. *Advances in Nursing Science, 9*(2), 20–31.

Given, B. A., & Given, C. W. (1991). Family caregiving for the elderly. *Annual Review of Nursing Research, 9,* 77–101.

Given, B. A., Kozachik, S. L., Collins, C. E., DeVoss, D. N., & Given, C. W. (2001). Caregiver role strain. In M. Maas, K. Buckwalter, M. Hardy, T. Tripp-Reimer, M. Titler, & J. Specht (Eds.), *Nursing care of older adults: Diagnoses, outcomes & interventions* (pp. 679–695). St. Louis: Mosby.

Oberst, M. T., Thomas, S. E., Gass, K. A., & Ward, S. E. (1989). Caregiving demands and appraisal of stress among family caregivers. *Cancer Nursing, 12*(4), 209–215.

Pierson, M. A., & Irons, K. (1992). Identification of a cluster of nursing diagnoses for a caregiver support group. *Nursing Diagnosis, 3*(1), 36–41.

Printz-Feddersen, V. (1990). Group process effect on caregiver burden. *Journal of Neuroscience Nursing, 22*(3), 164–168.

Thomas, V. M., Ellison, K., Howell, E. V., & Winters, K. (1992). Caring for the person receiving ventilatory support at home: Caregivers' needs and involvement. *Heart & Lung, 21*(2), 180–186.

+Vermooij-Dassen, M. J. F. J. (1993). *Dementia and home care: Determinants of the sense of competence of primary caregivers and the effect of professionally guided caregiver support* (in Dutch). Lisse, The Netherlands: Swets & Seitliger.

Wallhagen, M. I., & Kagan, S. H. (1993). Staying within bounds: Perceived control and the experience of elderly caregivers. *Journal of Aging Studies, 7*(2), 197–213.

C

Caregiver Physical Health

2507

Definition: Physical well-being of a family care provider while caring for a family member

OUTCOME TARGET RATING: Maintain at_____   Increase to_____

OUTCOME OVERALL RATING	Severely compromised 1	Substantially compromised 2	Moderately compromised 3	Mildly compromised 4	Not compromised 5	
Indicators:						
250715 Physical fitness	1	2	3	4	5	NA
250702 Sleep-rest pattern	1	2	3	4	5	NA
250703 Blood pressure	1	2	3	4	5	NA
250704 Energy level	1	2	3	4	5	NA
250705 Physical comfort	1	2	3	4	5	NA
250706 Mobility level	1	2	3	4	5	NA
250707 Resistance to infection	1	2	3	4	5	NA
250708 Physical function	1	2	3	4	5	NA
250709 Weight	1	2	3	4	5	NA
250710 Gastrointestinal function	1	2	3	4	5	NA
250716 Cardiac function	1	2	3	4	5	NA
250717 Pulmonary function	1	2	3	4	5	NA
250718 Nutritional status	1	2	3	4	5	NA
250719 Cognitive status	1	2	3	4	5	NA
250711 Medication use	1	2	3	4	5	NA
250712 Perceived general health	1	2	3	4	5	NA

Domain-Family Health (VI)   **Class**-Family Member Health Status (Z)   *1st edition 1997; revised 2004, 2008*

OUTCOME CONTENT REFERENCES:

Collins, C. E., Given, B. A., & Given, C. W. (1994). Interventions with family caregivers of persons with Alzheimer's disease. *Nursing Clinics of North America, 29*(1), 127–131.

Given, B. A., & Given, C. W. (1991). Family caregiving for the elderly. *Annual Review of Nursing Research, 9,* 77–101.

Given, B. A., Kozachik, S. L., Collins, C. E., DeVoss, D. N., & Given, C. W. (2001). Caregiver role strain. In M. Maas, K. Buckwalter, M. Hardy, T. Tripp-Reimer, M. Titler, & J. Specht (Eds.), *Nursing care of older adults: Diagnoses, outcomes & interventions* (pp. 679–695). St. Louis: Mosby.

Grant, I., Adler, K. A., Patterson, T. L., Dimsdale, J. E., Ziegler, M. G., & Irwin, M. R. (2002). Health consequences of Alzheimer's caregiving transitions: Effects of placement and bereavement. *Psychosomatic Medicine, 64*(3), 477–486.

Grasel, E. (2002). When home care ends—changes in the physical health of informal caregivers caring for dementia patients: A longitudinal study. *Journal of American Geriatric Society, 50*(5), 843–849.

Haley, W. E., LaMonde, L. A., Han, B., Narramore, S., & Schonwetter, R. (2001). Family caregiving in hospice: Effects on psychological and health functioning among spousal caregivers of hospice patients with lung cancer or dementia. *Hospice Journal, 15*(4), 1–18.

Pepin, J. I. (1992). Family caring and caring in nursing. *Image—The Journal of Nursing Scholarship, 24*(2), 127–131.

+Robinson, B. C. (1983). Validation of a caregiver strain index. *Journal of Gerontology, 38*(3), 344–348.

Springer, D., & Brubaker, T. H. (1984). *Caregiving and the dependent elderly.* Thousand Oaks, CA: Sage.

Winslow, B., & O'Brien, R. (1992). Use of formal community resources by spouse caregivers of chronically ill adults. *Public Health Nursing, 9*(27), 128–132.

Zeisel, J., Hyde, J., & Levkoff, S. (1994). Best practices: An environment-behavior (E-B) model for Alzheimer special care units. *The American Journal of Alzheimer's Care and Related Disorders & Research, 9*(2), 4–21.

Caregiver Role Endurance 2210

Definition: Factors that promote family care provider's capacity to sustain caregiving over an extended period of time

OUTCOME TARGET RATING: Maintain at_____ Increase to_____

OUTCOME OVERALL RATING		Not adequate	Slightly adequate	Moderately adequate	Substantially adequate	Totally adequate	
		1	2	3	4	5	
Indicators:							
221001	Mutually satisfying care recipient-caregiver relationship	1	2	3	4	5	NA
221002	Mastery of direct care activities	1	2	3	4	5	NA
221003	Mastery of indirect care activities	1	2	3	4	5	NA
221004	Supplemental services to assist with care	1	2	3	4	5	NA
221012	Health provider support for caregiver	1	2	3	4	5	NA
221013	Supplies for caregiving	1	2	3	4	5	NA
221011	Financial resources for caregiving	1	2	3	4	5	NA
221005	Social support for caregiver	1	2	3	4	5	NA
221008	Respite for caregiver	1	2	3	4	5	NA
221009	Opportunities for caregiver leisure activities	1	2	3	4	5	NA

Domain-Family Health (VI) **Class-***Family Caregiver Performance (W)* *1st edition 1997; revised 2004, 2008*

OUTCOME CONTENT REFERENCES:

Czaja, S. J., & Rubert, M. P. (2002). Telecommunications technology as an aid to family caregivers of persons with dementia. *Psychosomatic Medicine, 64*(3), 469–476.

Given, B. A., Stommel, M., Collins, C., King, S., & Given, C. W. (1990). Responses of elderly spouse caregivers. *Research in Nursing & Health, 13*(2), 77–85.

Oberst, M. T., Thomas, S. E., Gass, K. A., & Ward, S. E. (1989). Caregiving demands and appraisal of stress among family caregivers. *Cancer Nursing, 12*(4), 209–215.

+Picot, S. J., Youngblut, J., & Zeller, R. (1997). Development and testing of a measure of perceived caregiver rewards in adults. *Journal of Nursing Measurement, 5*(1), 33–52.

Rawlins, S. R. (1991). Using the connecting process to meet family caregiver needs. *Journal of Professional Nursing, 7*(4), 213–220.

Romeis, J. C. (1989). Caregiver strain. *Journal of Aging and Health, 1*(2), 188–208.

Stevenson, J. E. (1990). Family stress related to home care of Alzheimer's disease patients and implications for support. *Journal of Neuroscience Nursing, 22*(3), 179–188.

Thompson, E. H., Futterman, A. M., Gallagher-Thompson, D., Rose, J. M., & Lovett, S. B. (1993). Social support and caregiving burden in family caregivers of frail elders. *Journal of Gerontology, 48*(5), S245–S254.

Wallhagen, M. I. (1992). Caregiving demands: Their difficulty and effects on the well-being of elderly caregivers. *Scholarly Inquiry for Nursing Practice: An International Journal, 6*(2), 111–133.

Winslow, B., & O'Brien, R. (1992). Use of formal community resources by spouse caregivers of chronically ill adults. *Public Health Nursing, 9*(27), 128–132.

C

Caregiver Stressors 2208

Definition: Severity of biopsychosocial pressure on a family care provider caring for another over an extended period of time

OUTCOME TARGET RATING: Maintain at_____ Increase to_____

		Severe	Substantial	Moderate	Mild	None	
OUTCOME OVERALL RATING		1	2	3	4	5	
Indicators:							
220801	Reported stressors of caregiving	1	2	3	4	5	NA
220802	Physical limitations for caregiving	1	2	3	4	5	NA
220803	Psychological limitations for caregiving	1	2	3	4	5	NA
220804	Cognitive limitations	1	2	3	4	5	NA
220805	Role conflict	1	2	3	4	5	NA
220815	Sense of isolation	1	2	3	4	5	NA
220807	Perceived lack of social support	1	2	3	4	5	NA
220818	Perceived lack of health professional support	1	2	3	4	5	NA
220816	Loss of personal time	1	2	3	4	5	NA
220819	Conflict between work and caregiver responsibilities	1	2	3	4	5	NA
220820	Perceived burden of care recipient's progressive health problems	1	2	3	4	5	NA
220813	Impairment of caregiver-patient relationship	1	2	3	4	5	NA
220821	Impairment of family relationships	1	2	3	4	5	NA

Domain-Family Health (VI) *Class*-Family Caregiver Performance (W) *1st edition 1997; revised 2004, 2008*

OUTCOME CONTENT REFERENCES:

Andersson, A., Levin, L.A., Emtinger, B. G. (2002). The economic burden of informal care. *International Journal of Technology Assessment in Health Care, 18*(1), 46–54.

Brown, M. A., & Powell-Cope, G. M. (1991). AIDS family caregiving: Transitions through uncertainty. *Nursing Research, 40*(6), 338–345.

Chambers, M., Ryan, A. A., & Connors, S. L. (2001). Exploring the emotional needs and coping strategies of family careers. *Journal of Psychiatric and Mental Health Nursing, 8*(2), 99–106.

Davis, L. L. (2001). Altered family processes. In M. Maas, K. Buckwalter, M. Hardy, T. Tripp-Reimer, M. Titler, & J. Specht (Eds.), *Nursing care of older adults: Diagnoses, outcomes & interventions* (pp. 719–727). St. Louis: Mosby.

Given, C. W., Given, B., Stommel, M., Collins, C., King, S., & Franklin, S. (1992). The caregiver reaction assessment (CRA) for caregivers to persons with chronic physical and mental impairments. *Research in Nursing & Health, 15*(4), 271–283.

Glasscock, R. (2000). A phenomenological study of the experience of being a mother of a child with cerebral palsy. *Pediatric Nursing, 26*(4), 407–410.

Laidlaw, T. M., Coverdale, J. H., Falloon, I. R., & Kydd, R. R. (2002). Caregivers' stresses when living together or apart from patients with chronic schizophrenia. *Community Mental Health Journal, 38*(4), 303–310.

Levesque, L., Ducharme, F., & Lachance, L. (1999). Is there a difference between family caregiving of institutionalized elders with or without dementia? *Western Journal of Nursing Research, 21*(4), 472–497.

+Robinson, B. C. (1983). Validation of a caregiver strain index. *Journal of Gerontology, 38*(3), 344–348.

Saban, K., Sherwood, P., DeVon, H., & Hynes, D. (2010). Measures of psychological stress and physical health in family caregivers of stroke survivors: A literature review. *Journal of Neuroscience Nursing, 42*(3), 128–138.

Stevenson, J. E. (1990). Family stress related to home care of Alzheimer's disease patients and implications for support. *Journal of Neuroscience Nursing, 22*(3), 179–188.

Thompson, E. H., Futterman, A. M., Gallagher-Thompson, D., Rose, J. M., & Lovett, S. B. (1993). Social support and caregiving burden in family caregivers of frail elders. *Journal of Gerontology, 48*(5), S245–S254.

Wallhagen, M. I. (1992). Caregiving demands: Their difficulty and effects on the well-being of elderly caregivers. *Scholarly Inquiry for Nursing Practice: An International Journal, 6*(2), 111–133.

Caregiver Well-Being   2508

Definition: Extent of positive perception of primary care provider's health status

OUTCOME TARGET RATING: Maintain at_____   Increase to_____

	Not at all satisfied	Somewhat satisfied	Moderately satisfied	Very satisfied	Completely satisfied	
OUTCOME OVERALL RATING	1	2	3	4	5	
Indicators:						
250801 Physical health	1	2	3	4	5	NA
250802 Psychological health	1	2	3	4	5	NA
250803 Lifestyle	1	2	3	4	5	NA
250804 Performance of usual roles	1	2	3	4	5	NA
250805 Social support	1	2	3	4	5	NA
250806 Support for instrumental activities of daily living	1	2	3	4	5	NA
250807 Health professional support	1	2	3	4	5	NA
250808 Social relationships	1	2	3	4	5	NA
250811 Family sharing of responsibilities for caregiving	1	2	3	4	5	NA
250812 Availability for respite	1	2	3	4	5	NA
250813 Ability to cope	1	2	3	4	5	NA
250809 Caregiver role	1	2	3	4	5	NA
250814 Financial resources for caregiving	1	2	3	4	5	NA

Domain-Family Health (VI)   *Class-Family Member Health Status (Z)*   *1st edition 1997; revised 2004, 2008*

OUTCOME CONTENT REFERENCES:

Brown, M. A., & Powell-Cope, G. M. (1991). AIDS family caregiving: Transitions through uncertainty. *Nursing Research, 40*(6), 338–345.

Given, B. A., Kozachik, S. L., Collins, C. E., DeVoss, D. N., & Given, C. W. (2001). Caregiver role strain. In M. Maas, K. Buckwalter, M. Hardy, T. Tripp-Reimer, M. Titler, & J. Specht (Eds.), *Nursing care of older adults: Diagnoses, outcomes & interventions* (pp. 679–695). St. Louis: Mosby.

Given, C. W., Given, B., Stommel, M., Collins, C., King, S., & Franklin, S. (1992). The Caregiver Reaction Assessment (CRA) for caregivers to persons with chronic physical and mental impairments. *Research in Nursing & Health, 15*(4), 271–283.

Jungbauer, J., & Angermeyer, M. C. (2002). Living with a schizophrenic patient: A comparative study of burden as it affects parents and spouses. *Psychiatry, 65*(2), 110–123.

Pender, N., Murdaugh, C., & Parsons, M. A. (2001). *Health promotion in nursing practice* (4th ed.). Upper Saddle River, NJ: Prentice Hall.

+Picot, S. J., Youngblut, J., & Zeller, R. (1997). Development and testing of a measure of perceived caregiver rewards in adults. *Journal of Nursing Measurement, 5*(1), 33–52.

Stevenson, J. E. (1990). Family stress related to home care of Alzheimer's disease patients and implications for support. *Journal of Neuroscience Nursing, 22*(3), 179–188.

Thompson, E. H., Futterman, A. M., Gallagher-Thompson, D., Rose, J. M., & Lovett, S. B. (1993). Social support and caregiving burden in family caregivers of frail elders. *Journal of Gerontology, 48*(5), S245–S254.

Wade, S. L., Taylor, H. G., Drotar, D., Stancin, T., Yeates, K. O., & Minich, N. M. (2002). A prospective study of long-term caregiver and family adaptation following brain injury in children. *Journal of Health Trauma Rehabilitation, 17*(2), 96–111.

Wallhagen, M. I. (1992). Caregiving demands: Their difficulty and effects on the well-being of elderly caregivers. *Scholarly Inquiry for Nursing Practice: An International Journal, 6*(2), 111–133.

Warfield, M. E. (2001). Employment, parenting, and well-being among mothers of children with disabilities. *Mental Retardation, 39*(4), 297–309.

Child Adaptation to Hospitalization   1301

Definition: Adaptive response of a child from 3 years through 17 years of age to hospitalization

OUTCOME TARGET RATING: Maintain at_____   Increase to_____

		Never demonstrated	Rarely demonstrated	Sometimes demonstrated	Often demonstrated	Consistently demonstrated	
OUTCOME OVERALL RATING		1	2	3	4	5	
Indicators:							
130112	Interacts with parent	1	2	3	4	5	NA
130121	Maintains usual routine	1	2	3	4	5	NA
130113	Recognizes reason forhospitalization	1	2	3	4	5	NA
130115	Participates in decision-making	1	2	3	4	5	NA
130123	Asks questions about illness	1	2	3	4	5	NA
130124	Asks questions about treatment	1	2	3	4	5	NA
130125	Describes illness	1	2	3	4	5	NA
130126	Describes prescribed treatment	1	2	3	4	5	NA
130127	Maintains sense of control	1	2	3	4	5	NA
130118	Cooperates with procedures	1	2	3	4	5	NA
130109	Responds to comfort measures	1	2	3	4	5	NA
130110	Responds to diversional therapy	1	2	3	4	5	NA
130111	Participates in social interaction	1	2	3	4	5	NA
130119	Interacts with peers	1	2	3	4	5	NA
130117	Maintains pre-admission self-care behaviors	1	2	3	4	5	NA

		Consistently demonstrated	Often demonstrated	Sometimes demonstrated	Rarely demonstrated	Never demonstrated	
130101	Agitation	1	2	3	4	5	NA
130102	Separation anxiety	1	2	3	4	5	NA
130103	Regressive behaviors	1	2	3	4	5	NA
130104	Anxiety	1	2	3	4	5	NA
130105	Fear	1	2	3	4	5	NA
130106	Anger	1	2	3	4	5	NA
130128	Withdrawal	1	2	3	4	5	NA
130129	Aggressive behaviors	1	2	3	4	5	NA

Domain-Psychosocial Health (III)   **Class**-Psychosocial Adaptation (N)   1st edition 1997; revised 2004, 2008

OUTCOME CONTENT REFERENCES:

Coucouvanis, J. A. (1990). Behavior management. In M. Craft & J. A. Denehy (Eds.), *Nursing interventions for infants and children* (pp. 151–165). Philadelphia: W. B. Saunders.

Hockenberry, M. J., Wilson, D., Winkelstein, M. L., & Kline, N. E. (2003). *Wong's nursing care of infants and children* (7th ed.). St. Louis: Mosby.

Manion, J. (1990). Preparing children for hospitalization, procedures, or surgery. In M. Craft & J. A. Denehy (Eds.), *Nursing interventions for infants and children* (pp. 74–90). Philadelphia: W. B. Saunders.

Olson, R. K., Heater, B. S., & Becker, A. M. (1990). A meta-analysis of the effects of nursing interventions on children and parents. *Maternal-Child Nursing, 15*(2), 104–108.

Shields, L. (2001). A review of the literature from developed and developing countries relating to the effects of hospitalization on children and parents. *International Nursing Review, 48*(1), 29–37.

Wolfer, J. A., & Visintainer, M. A. (1975). Pediatric surgical patients' and parents' stress responses and adjustment as a function of psychologic preparation and stress-point nursing care. *Nursing Research, 24*(4), 244–255.

Ziegler, D. B., & Prior, M. M. (1994). Preparation for surgery and adjustment to hospitalization. *Nursing Clinics of North America, 29*(4), 655–669.

Child Development: 1 Month 0120

Definition: Milestones of physical, cognitive, and psychosocial progression by 1 month of age

OUTCOME TARGET RATING: Maintain at_____   Increase to_____

		Never demonstrated	Rarely demonstrated	Sometimes demonstrated	Often demonstrated	Consistently demonstrated	
OUTCOME OVERALL RATING		1	2	3	4	5	
Indicators:							
012001	Signals hunger	1	2	3	4	5	NA
012002	Signals discomfort	1	2	3	4	5	NA
012003	Responds to sounds	1	2	3	4	5	NA
012004	Responds to voice	1	2	3	4	5	NA
012005	Responds to face	1	2	3	4	5	NA
012006	Coos	1	2	3	4	5	NA
012007	Smiles spontaneously	1	2	3	4	5	NA
012008	Eyes follow to mid-line	1	2	3	4	5	NA
012009	Signals overstimulation	1	2	3	4	5	NA
012010	Exhibits five sleep and alert states	1	2	3	4	5	NA
012011	Flexes extremity	1	2	3	4	5	NA
012012	Holds head erect momentarily	1	2	3	4	5	NA
012013	Turns head side to side when prone	1	2	3	4	5	NA
012014	Holds head in horizontal line with back when prone	1	2	3	4	5	NA
012015	Moro reflex	1	2	3	4	5	NA
012016	Tonic neck reflex	1	2	3	4	5	NA
012017	Dance reflex	1	2	3	4	5	NA
012018	Crawl reflex	1	2	3	4	5	NA
012019	Babinski reflex	1	2	3	4	5	NA
012020	Suck reflex	1	2	3	4	5	NA
012021	Palmer reflex	1	2	3	4	5	NA
012022	Plantar reflex	1	2	3	4	5	NA
012023	Rooting reflex	1	2	3	4	5	NA

Domain-*Functional Health (I)*   **Class**-*Growth & Development (B)*   *3rd edition 2004*

OUTCOME CONTENT REFERENCES:
Berger, K. S. (2001). *The developing person through the life span* (5th ed.). New York: Worth.
Broome, M. E., & Rollins, J. A. (Eds.). (1999). *Core curriculum for the nursing care of children and their families.* Pitman, NJ: Anthony J. Jannetti.
Darrah, J., Redfern, L., Maguire, T. O., Beaulne, A. P., & Watt, J. (1998). Intra-individual stability of rate of gross motor development in full-term infants. *Early Human Development, 52*(2), 169–179.
Hockenberry, M. J., Wilson, D., Winkelstein, M. L., & Kline, N. E. (2003). *Wong's nursing care of infants and children* (7th ed.). St. Louis: Mosby.
Kimmel, S. R., Quinn, E. A., & Phelps, K. A. (1994). Assessing child development. *Primary Care, 21*(4), 673–692.
Piper, M. C., Pinnell, L. E., Darrah, J., Maguire, T., & Byrne, P. J. (1992). Construction and validation of the Alberta Infant Motor Scale (AIMS). *Canadian Journal of Public Health, 83*(Suppl. 2), S46–S50.
Trachtenbarg, D. E., & Golemon, T. B. (1998). Care of the premature infant, part 1: Monitoring growth and development. *American Family Physician, 57*(9), 2123–2131.

Child Development: 2 Months 0100

Definition: Milestones of physical, cognitive, and psychosocial progression by 2 months of age

OUTCOME TARGET RATING: Maintain at_____ Increase to_____

		Never demonstrated	Rarely demonstrated	Sometimes demonstrated	Often demonstrated	Consistently demonstrated	
OUTCOME OVERALL RATING		1	2	3	4	5	
Indicators:							
010002	Crawl reflex disappearance	1	2	3	4	5	NA
010003	Lifts head, neck, and upper chest with support of forearms while in prone position	1	2	3	4	5	NA
010004	Shows some head control in upright position	1	2	3	4	5	NA
010005	Hands frequently open	1	2	3	4	5	NA
010006	Grasp reflex fading	1	2	3	4	5	NA
010007	Coos and vocalizes	1	2	3	4	5	NA
010008	Shows interest in auditory stimuli	1	2	3	4	5	NA
010009	Shows interest in visual stimuli	1	2	3	4	5	NA
010010	Smiles	1	2	3	4	5	NA
010011	Shows pleasure in interactions, especially with primary caregivers	1	2	3	4	5	NA

Domain-*Functional Health (I)*   **Class**-*Growth & Development (B)*   *1st edition 1997; revised 2004*

OUTCOME CONTENT REFERENCES:

Berger, K. S. (2001). *The developing person through the life span* (5th ed.). New York: Worth.

Bricker, D. (Ed.). (2002). *Assessment, evaluation, and programming system for infants and children* (2nd ed.). Baltimore: Paul H. Brookes.

Darrah, J., Redfern, L., Maguire, T. O., Beaulne, A. P., & Watt, J. (1998). Intra-individual stability of rate of gross motor development in full-term infants. *Early Human Development, 52*(2), 169–179.

Green, M., & Palfrey, J. S. (Eds.). (2002). *Bright futures: Guidelines for health supervision of infants, children and adolescents.* Arlington, VA: National Center for Education in Maternal and Child Health.

Hockenberry, M. J., Wilson, D., Winkelstein, M. L., & Kline, N. E. (2003). *Wong's nursing care of infants and children* (7th ed.). St. Louis: Mosby.

Child Development: 4 Months 0101

Definition: Milestones of physical, cognitive, and psychosocial progression by 4 months of age

OUTCOME TARGET RATING: Maintain at_____ Increase to_____

		Never demonstrated	Rarely demonstrated	Sometimes demonstrated	Often demonstrated	Consistently demonstrated	
OUTCOME OVERALL RATING		1	2	3	4	5	
Indicators:							
010101	Holds head erect and raises body on hands while in prone position	1	2	3	4	5	NA
010102	Controls head well	1	2	3	4	5	NA
010103	Rolls over from prone to supine	1	2	3	4	5	NA
010104	Holds own hands	1	2	3	4	5	NA
010105	Grasps rattle	1	2	3	4	5	NA
010106	Reaches for objects	1	2	3	4	5	NA
010107	Bats at objects	1	2	3	4	5	NA
010108	Babbles and coos	1	2	3	4	5	NA
010109	Recognizes parents' voices	1	2	3	4	5	NA

Child Development: 4 Months—*cont'd*

		Never demonstrated	Rarely demonstrated	Sometimes demonstrated	Often demonstrated	Consistently demonstrated	
010110	Recognizes parents' touch	1	2	3	4	5	NA
010111	Looks at and becomes excited by mobile	1	2	3	4	5	NA
010112	Smiles, laughs, and squeals	1	2	3	4	5	NA
010116	Exhibits a nocturnal sleep pattern	1	2	3	4	5	NA
010114	Comforts self	1	2	3	4	5	NA

Domain-*Functional Health (I)*   **Class**-*Growth & Development (B)*   *1st edition 1997; revised 2004, 2008*

OUTCOME CONTENT REFERENCES:
Berger, K. S. (2001). *The developing person through the life span* (5th ed.). New York: Worth.
Green, M., & Palfrey, J. S. (Eds.). (2002). *Bright futures: Guidelines for health supervision of infants, children and adolescents.* Arlington, VA: National Center for Education in Maternal and Child Health.
Hockenberry, M. J., Wilson, D., Winkelstein, M. L., & Kline, N. E. (2003). *Wong's nursing care of infants and children* (7th ed.). St. Louis: Mosby.

Child Development: 6 Months   0102

Definition: Milestones of physical, cognitive, and psychosocial progression by 6 months of age

OUTCOME TARGET RATING: Maintain at_____   Increase to_____

		Never demonstrated	Rarely demonstrated	Sometimes demonstrated	Often demonstrated	Consistently demonstrated	
OUTCOME OVERALL RATING		1	2	3	4	5	
Indicators:							
010201	Supports head when pulled to sit	1	2	3	4	5	NA
010202	Rolls over	1	2	3	4	5	NA
010203	Sits with support	1	2	3	4	5	NA
010204	Stands when placed and bears weight	1	2	3	4	5	NA
010205	Grasps and mouths objects	1	2	3	4	5	NA
010206	Gestures (e.g., points, shakes head)	1	2	3	4	5	NA
010207	Starts to self-feed	1	2	3	4	5	NA
010208	Shows interest in toys	1	2	3	4	5	NA
010209	Transfers small objects from hand to hand	1	2	3	4	5	NA
010210	Vocalizes/sings syllables (dada, baba)	1	2	3	4	5	NA
010211	Babbles reciprocally	1	2	3	4	5	NA
010212	Smiles, laughs, squeals, imitates noise	1	2	3	4	5	NA
010213	Turns to sounds	1	2	3	4	5	NA
010214	Shows beginning signs of stranger anxiety	1	2	3	4	5	NA
010215	Comforts self	1	2	3	4	5	NA

Domain-*Functional Health (I)*   **Class**-*Growth & Development (B)*   *1st edition 1997; revised 2004*

OUTCOME CONTENT REFERENCES:
Berger, K. S. (2001). *The developing person through the life span* (5th ed.). New York: Worth.
Bricker, D. (Ed.). (2002). *Assessment, evaluation, and programming system for infants and children* (2nd ed.). Baltimore: Paul H. Brookes.
Green, M., & Palfrey, J. S. (Eds.). (2002). *Bright futures: Guidelines for health supervision of infants, children and adolescents.* Arlington, VA: National Center for Education in Maternal and Child Health.
Hockenberry, M. J., Wilson, D., Winkelstein, M. L., & Kline, N. E. (2003). *Wong's nursing care of infants and children* (7th ed.). St. Louis: Mosby.
Rossetti, L. M. (1990). *Infant-toddler assessment: An interdisciplinary approach.* Boston: Little, Brown & Company.

C

Child Development: 12 Months

0103

Definition: Milestones of physical, cognitive, and psychosocial progression by 12 months of age

OUTCOME TARGET RATING: Maintain at_____   Increase to_____

OUTCOME OVERALL RATING	Never demonstrated 1	Rarely demonstrated 2	Sometimes demonstrated 3	Often demonstrated 4	Consistently demonstrated 5	
Indicators:						
010301 Pulls to stand	1	2	3	4	5	NA
010302 Cruises around furniture	1	2	3	4	5	NA
010303 Attempts to take steps alone	1	2	3	4	5	NA
010304 Precise pincer grasp	1	2	3	4	5	NA
010305 Points with index fingers	1	2	3	4	5	NA
010306 Bangs blocks together	1	2	3	4	5	NA
010307 Drinks from cup	1	2	3	4	5	NA
010308 Feeds self finger foods	1	2	3	4	5	NA
010309 Feeds self with spoon	1	2	3	4	5	NA
010310 Uses vocabulary of one to three words in addition to mama, dada	1	2	3	4	5	NA
010311 Imitates vocalizations	1	2	3	4	5	NA
010312 Looks for dropped or hidden object	1	2	3	4	5	NA
010313 Plays social games	1	2	3	4	5	NA
010314 Waves bye-bye	1	2	3	4	5	NA

Domain-Functional Health (I)   **Class**-Growth & Development (B)   *1st edition 1997; revised 2004*

OUTCOME CONTENT REFERENCES:
Berger, K. S. (2001). *The developing person through the life span* (5th ed.). New York: Worth.
Bricker, D. (Ed.). (2002). *Assessment, evaluation, and programming system for infants and children* (2nd ed.). Baltimore: Paul H. Brookes.
Green, M., & Palfrey, J. S. (Eds.). (2002). *Bright futures: Guidelines for health supervision of infants, children and adolescents.* Arlington, VA: National Center for Education in Maternal and Child Health.
Hockenberry, M. J., Wilson, D., Winkelstein, M. L., & Kline, N. E. (2003). *Wong's nursing care of infants and children* (7th ed.). St. Louis: Mosby.
Rossetti, L. M. (1990). *Infant-toddler assessment: An interdisciplinary approach.* Boston: Little, Brown & Company.
Santos, D. C., Gabbard, C., & Goncalves, V. M. (2001). Motor development during the first year: A comparative study. *Journal of Genetic Psychology, 162*(2), 143–153.
Vaivre-Douret, L., & Burnod, Y. (2001). Development of a global motor rating scale for young children (0-4 years) including eye-hand grip coordination. *Child Care Health & Development, 27*(6), 515–534.

Child Development: 2 Years 0104

Definition: Milestones of physical, cognitive, and psychosocial progression by 2 years of age

OUTCOME TARGET RATING: Maintain at_____   Increase to_____

		Never demonstrated	Rarely demonstrated	Sometimes demonstrated	Often demonstrated	Consistently demonstrated	
OUTCOME OVERALL RATING		1	2	3	4	5	
Indicators:							
010401	Walks quickly	1	2	3	4	5	NA
010402	Stoops well	1	2	3	4	5	NA
010403	Walks up and down stairs one step at a time	1	2	3	4	5	NA
010404	Walks backwards	1	2	3	4	5	NA
010405	Kicks a ball	1	2	3	4	5	NA
010406	Throws a ball	1	2	3	4	5	NA
010407	Makes circular and horizontal strokes with crayon	1	2	3	4	5	NA
010408	Stacks five to six blocks	1	2	3	4	5	NA
010409	Feeds self with spoon and fork	1	2	3	4	5	NA
010410	Follows two-step commands	1	2	3	4	5	NA
010411	Indicates wants verbally	1	2	3	4	5	NA
010412	Uses phrases of two to three words	1	2	3	4	5	NA
010413	Listens to story looking at pictures	1	2	3	4	5	NA
010414	Points to some body parts	1	2	3	4	5	NA
010415	Begins parallel play	1	2	3	4	5	NA
010416	Imitates adults	1	2	3	4	5	NA
010417	Interacts with adults in simple games	1	2	3	4	5	NA

Domain-Functional Health (I)   *Class*-Growth & Development (B)   *1st edition 1997; revised 2004*

OUTCOME CONTENT REFERENCES:

Berger, K. S. (2001). *The developing person through the life span* (5th ed.). New York: Worth.

Bricker, D. (Ed.). (2002). *Assessment, evaluation, and programming system for infants and children* (2nd ed.). Baltimore: Paul H. Brookes.

Green, M., & Palfrey, J. S. (Eds.). (2002). *Bright futures: Guidelines for health supervision of infants, children and adolescents.* Arlington, VA: National Center for Education in Maternal and Child Health.

Hockenberry, M. J., Wilson, D., Winkelstein, M. L., & Kline, N. E. (2003). *Wong's nursing care of infants and children* (7th ed.). St. Louis: Mosby.

Provost, B., Crowe, T. K., & McClain, C. (2000). Concurrent validity of the Bayley Scales of Infant Development II Motor Scale and the Peabody Developmental Motor Scales in two-year-old children. *Physical & Occupational Therapy in Pediatrics, 20*(1), 5–18.

Rossetti, L. M. (1990). *Infant-toddler assessment: An interdisciplinary approach.* Boston: Little, Brown & Company.

Vaivre-Douret, L., & Burnod, Y. (2001). Development of a global motor rating scale for young children (0-4 years) including eye-hand grip coordination. *Child Care Health & Development, 27*(6), 515–534.

C

Child Development: 3 Years 0105

Definition: Milestones of physical, cognitive, and psychosocial progression by 3 years of age

OUTCOME TARGET RATING: Maintain at_____ Increase to_____

		Never demonstrated	Rarely demonstrated	Sometimes demonstrated	Often demonstrated	Consistently demonstrated	
OUTCOME OVERALL RATING		1	2	3	4	5	
Indicators:							
010501	Balances on one foot	1	2	3	4	5	NA
010502	Pedals a riding toy	1	2	3	4	5	NA
010503	Dresses self	1	2	3	4	5	NA
010504	Manipulates writing/coloring instruments	1	2	3	4	5	NA
010505	Copies a circle	1	2	3	4	5	NA
010506	Copies a cross	1	2	3	4	5	NA
010507	Controls bowel in daytime	1	2	3	4	5	NA
010508	Controls bladder in daytime	1	2	3	4	5	NA
010509	Distinguishes gender differences	1	2	3	4	5	NA
010510	Gives own first name	1	2	3	4	5	NA
010511	Gives own age	1	2	3	4	5	NA
010512	Engages in magical thinking/fantasy	1	2	3	4	5	NA
010513	Plays interactive games with peers	1	2	3	4	5	NA
010514	Begins cooperative group play	1	2	3	4	5	NA
010515	Uses sentences of three or four words	1	2	3	4	5	NA
010516	Speech understood by strangers	1	2	3	4	5	NA

Domain-*Functional Health (I)* **Class**-*Growth & Development (B)* *1st edition 1997; revised 2004*

OUTCOME CONTENT REFERENCES:
Berger, K. S. (2001). *The developing person through the life span* (5th ed.). New York: Worth.
Bricker, D. (Ed.). (2002). *Assessment, evaluation, and programming system for infants and children* (2nd ed.). Baltimore: Paul H. Brookes.
Green, M., & Palfrey, J. S. (Eds.). (2002). *Bright futures: Guidelines for health supervision of infants, children and adolescents.* Arlington, VA: National Center for Education in Maternal and Child Health.
Hemgren, E., & Persson, K. (1999). A model for combined assessment of motor performance and behaviour in 3-year-old children. *Upsala Journal of Medical Sciences, 104*(1), 49–85.
Hockenberry, M. J., Wilson, D., Winkelstein, M. L., & Kline, N. E. (2003). *Wong's nursing care of infants and children* (7th ed.). St. Louis: Mosby.
Vaivre-Douret, L., & Burnod, Y. (2001). Development of a global motor rating scale for young children (0-4 years) including eye-hand grip coordination. *Child Care Health & Development, 27*(6), 515–534.

Child Development: 4 Years 0106

Definition: Milestones of physical, cognitive, and psychosocial progression by 4 years of age

OUTCOME TARGET RATING: Maintain at_____ Increase to_____

		Never demonstrated	Rarely demonstrated	Sometimes demonstrated	Often demonstrated	Consistently demonstrated	
OUTCOME OVERALL RATING		1	2	3	4	5	
Indicators:							
010601	Walks, climbs, runs	1	2	3	4	5	NA
010602	Walks up and down stairs	1	2	3	4	5	NA
010603	Hops and jumps on one foot	1	2	3	4	5	NA
010604	Rides tricycle or bicycle with training wheels	1	2	3	4	5	NA

Child Development: 4 Years—cont'd

		Never demonstrated	Rarely demonstrated	Sometimes demonstrated	Often demonstrated	Consistently demonstrated	
010605	Throws overhand ball	1	2	3	4	5	NA
010606	Builds tower of 10 blocks	1	2	3	4	5	NA
010607	Draws person with three parts	1	2	3	4	5	NA
010608	Gives first and last name	1	2	3	4	5	NA
010609	Uses sentences of four to five words, short paragraphs	1	2	3	4	5	NA
010610	Uses past tense in vocabulary	1	2	3	4	5	NA
010611	Describes a recent experience	1	2	3	4	5	NA
010612	Sings a song	1	2	3	4	5	NA
010613	Distinguishes fantasy from reality	1	2	3	4	5	NA
010614	Describes use of common items in home	1	2	3	4	5	NA
010616	Engages in creative play	1	2	3	4	5	NA

Domain-Functional Health (I)   **Class-**Growth & Development (B)   1st edition 1997; revised 2004

OUTCOME CONTENT REFERENCES:

Berger, K. S. (2001). *The developing person through the life span* (5th ed.). New York: Worth.

Green, M., & Palfrey, J. S. (Eds.). (2002). *Bright futures: Guidelines for health supervision of infants, children and adolescents.* Arlington, VA: National Center for Education in Maternal and Child Health.

Hockenberry, M. J., Wilson, D., Winkelstein, M. L., & Kline, N. E. (2003). *Wong's nursing care of infants and children* (7th ed.). St. Louis: Mosby.

Vaivre-Douret, L., & Burnod, Y. (2001). Development of a global motor rating scale for young children (0-4 years) including eye-hand grip coordination. *Child Care Health & Development, 27*(6), 515–534.

Child Development: 5 Years   0107

Definition: Milestones of physical, cognitive, and psychosocial progression by 5 years of age

OUTCOME TARGET RATING: Maintain at_____   Increase to_____

		Never demonstrated	Rarely demonstrated	Sometimes demonstrated	Often demonstrated	Consistently demonstrated	
OUTCOME OVERALL RATING		1	2	3	4	5	
Indicators:							
010717	Walks	1	2	3	4	5	NA
010718	Climbs	1	2	3	4	5	NA
010719	Runs	1	2	3	4	5	NA
010702	Skips	1	2	3	4	5	NA
010703	Dresses self without assistance	1	2	3	4	5	NA
010704	Draws a person with head, body, arms, and legs	1	2	3	4	5	NA
010705	Copies a triangle or square	1	2	3	4	5	NA
010706	Counts using fingers	1	2	3	4	5	NA
010707	Recognizes most letters of alphabet	1	2	3	4	5	NA
010708	Prints some letters	1	2	3	4	5	NA
010709	Uses complete sentence of five words	1	2	3	4	5	NA
010710	Uses future tense in vocabulary	1	2	3	4	5	NA
010711	Speaks short paragraphs	1	2	3	4	5	NA
010712	Gives own address	1	2	3	4	5	NA
010713	Gives own phone number	1	2	3	4	5	NA

Continued

C

Child Development: 5 Years—cont'd

		Never demonstrated	Rarely demonstrated	Sometimes demonstrated	Often demonstrated	Consistently demonstrated	
010714	Follows simple rules of interactive games with peers	1	2	3	4	5	NA
010716	Engages in creative play	1	2	3	4	5	NA

Domain-Functional Health (I)   **Class**-Growth & Development (B)   1st edition 1997; revised 2004, 2008

OUTCOME CONTENT REFERENCES:
Berger, K. S. (2001). *The developing person through the life span* (5th ed.). New York: Worth.
Boucher, B. H., Doescher, S. M., & Sugawara, A. I. (1993). Preschool children's motor development and self-concept. *Perceptual & Motor Skills, 76*(1), 11–17.
Green, M., & Palfrey, J. S. (Eds.). (2002). *Bright futures: Guidelines for health supervision of infants, children and adolescents*. Arlington, VA: National Center for Education in Maternal and Child Health.
Hockenberry, M. J., Wilson, D., Winkelstein, M. L., & Kline, N. E. (2003). *Wong's nursing care of infants and children* (7th ed.). St. Louis: Mosby.

Child Development: Middle Childhood   0108

Definition: Milestones of physical, cognitive, and psychosocial progression from 6 years through 11 years of age

OUTCOME TARGET RATING: Maintain at_____   Increase to_____

		Never demonstrated	Rarely demonstrated	Sometimes demonstrated	Often demonstrated	Consistently demonstrated	
OUTCOME OVERALL RATING		1	2	3	4	5	
Indicators:							
010801	Practices good health habits	1	2	3	4	5	NA
010802	Plays in groups	1	2	3	4	5	NA
010803	Develops close friendships	1	2	3	4	5	NA
010804	Identifies with same-sex peer group	1	2	3	4	5	NA
010805	Assumes responsibility for selected household tasks	1	2	3	4	5	NA
010806	Follows through with commitments to extracurricular activities	1	2	3	4	5	NA
010807	Expresses feelings constructively	1	2	3	4	5	NA
010808	Displays self-confidence	1	2	3	4	5	NA
010817	Exhibits self-esteem	1	2	3	4	5	NA
010809	Understands right and wrong	1	2	3	4	5	NA
010810	Follows safety rules	1	2	3	4	5	NA
010811	Expresses increasingly complex thoughts	1	2	3	4	5	NA
010812	Shows creativity	1	2	3	4	5	NA
010813	Comprehends increasingly complex ideas	1	2	3	4	5	NA
010814	Assumes responsibility for homework	1	2	3	4	5	NA
010815	Performs in school to level of ability	1	2	3	4	5	NA

Domain-Functional Health (I)   **Class**-Growth & Development (B)   1st edition 1997; revised 2004, 2013

OUTCOME CONTENT REFERENCES:
Berger, K. S. (2001). *The developing person through the life span* (5th ed.). New York: Worth.
Green, M., & Palfrey, J. S. (Eds.). (2002). *Bright futures: Guidelines for health supervision of infants, children and adolescents*. Arlington, VA: National Center for Education in Maternal and Child Health.
Hockenberry, M. J., Wilson, D., Winkelstein, M. L., & Kline, N. E. (2003). *Wong's nursing care of infants and children* (7th ed.). St. Louis: Mosby.

Child Development: Adolescence — 0109

Definition: Milestones of physical, cognitive, and psychosocial progression from 12 years through 17 years of age

OUTCOME TARGET RATING: Maintain at_____ Increase to_____

		Never demonstrated	Rarely demonstrated	Sometimes demonstrated	Often demonstrated	Consistently demonstrated	
OUTCOME OVERALL RATING		1	2	3	4	5	
Indicators:							
010901	Practices good health habits	1	2	3	4	5	NA
010904	Uses effective social interaction skills	1	2	3	4	5	NA
010905	Uses conflict resolution strategies	1	2	3	4	5	NA
010920	Vents negative feelings in a non-destructive manner	1	2	3	4	5	NA
010906	Maintains good peer relationships with same gender	1	2	3	4	5	NA
010907	Maintains good peer relationships with opposite gender	1	2	3	4	5	NA
010921	Respects others	1	2	3	4	5	NA
010911	Uses effective coping strategies	1	2	3	4	5	NA
010922	Discusses feelings of distress with supportive adult	1	2	3	4	5	NA
010912	Displays increasing levels of autonomy	1	2	3	4	5	NA
010913	Describes personal value system	1	2	3	4	5	NA
010914	Uses formal operational thinking	1	2	3	4	5	NA
010930	Uses abstract thinking	1	2	3	4	5	NA
010915	Sets academic goals	1	2	3	4	5	NA
010916	Performs in school to level of ability	1	2	3	4	5	NA
010923	Participates in extracurricular school activities	1	2	3	4	5	NA
010924	Performs in work to level of ability	1	2	3	4	5	NA
010925	Identifies occupational goals	1	2	3	4	5	NA
010926	Observes rules	1	2	3	4	5	NA
010927	Obeys laws	1	2	3	4	5	NA
010908	Shows capacity for intimacy	1	2	3	4	5	NA
010902	Describes sexual development	1	2	3	4	5	NA
010931	Exhibits self-esteem	1	2	3	4	5	NA
010932	Expresses comfort with own body	1	2	3	4	5	NA
010903	Expresses comfort with own sexual identity	1	2	3	4	5	NA
010928	Postpones sexual activity	1	2	3	4	5	NA
010929	Avoids high-risk sexual activity	1	2	3	4	5	NA
010910	Avoids alcohol use	1	2	3	4	5	NA
010918	Avoids tobacco use	1	2	3	4	5	NA
010919	Avoids recreational drug use	1	2	3	4	5	NA

Domain-Functional Health (I)   *Class*-Growth & Development (B)   *1st edition 1997; revised 2004, 2008, 2013*

OUTCOME CONTENT REFERENCES:

Berger, K. S. (2001). *The developing person through the life span* (5th ed.). New York: Worth.

Hockenberry, M. J., Wilson, D., Winkelstein, M. L., & Kline, N. E. (2003). *Wong's nursing care of infants and children* (7th ed.). St. Louis: Mosby.

Green, M., & Palfrey, J. S. (Eds.). (2002). *Bright futures: Guidelines for health supervision of infants, children and adolescents*. Arlington, VA: National Center for Education in Maternal and Child Health.

Krueger, D. W. (2001). Body self. Development, psychopathologies, and psychoanalytic significance. *Psychoanalytic Study of the Child, 56*, 238–259.

Mitchell, J. J. (1996). *Adolescent vulnerability: A sympathetic look at the frailties and limitations of youth*. Calgary, Alberta, Canada: Detselig.

Circulation Status

0401

Definition: Unobstructed, unidirectional blood flow at an appropriate pressure through large vessels of the systemic and pulmonary circuits

C

OUTCOME TARGET RATING: Maintain at_____ Increase to_____

		Severe deviation from normal range	Substantial deviation from normal range	Moderate deviation from normal range	Mild deviation from normal range	No deviation from normal range	
OUTCOME OVERALL RATING		1	2	3	4	5	
Indicators:							
040101	Systolic blood pressure	1	2	3	4	5	NA
040102	Diastolic blood pressure	1	2	3	4	5	NA
040103	Pulse pressure	1	2	3	4	5	NA
040104	Mean blood pressure	1	2	3	4	5	NA
040105	Central venous pressure	1	2	3	4	5	NA
040106	Pulmonary wedge pressure	1	2	3	4	5	NA
040141	Right carotid pulse strength	1	2	3	4	5	NA
040142	Left carotid pulse strength	1	2	3	4	5	NA
040143	Right brachial pulse strength	1	2	3	4	5	NA
040144	Left brachial pulse strength	1	2	3	4	5	NA
040145	Right radial pulse strength	1	2	3	4	5	NA
040146	Left radial pulse strength	1	2	3	4	5	NA
040147	Right femoral pulse strength	1	2	3	4	5	NA
040148	Left femoral pulse strength	1	2	3	4	5	NA
040149	Right pedal pulse strength	1	2	3	4	5	NA
040150	Left pedal pulse strength	1	2	3	4	5	NA
040135	PaO_2 (Partial pressure of oxygen in arterial blood)	1	2	3	4	5	NA
040136	$PaCO_2$ (Partial pressure of carbon dioxide in arterial blood)	1	2	3	4	5	NA
040137	Oxygen saturation	1	2	3	4	5	NA
040112	Arterial-venous oxygen difference	1	2	3	4	5	NA
040140	Urine output	1	2	3	4	5	NA
040151	Capillary refill	1	2	3	4	5	NA

		Severe	Substantial	Moderate	Mild	None	
040107	Orthostatic hypotension	1	2	3	4	5	NA
040113	Adventitious breath sounds	1	2	3	4	5	NA
040118	Large vessel bruits	1	2	3	4	5	NA
040119	Neck vein distention	1	2	3	4	5	NA
040120	Peripheral edema	1	2	3	4	5	NA
040121	Ascites	1	2	3	4	5	NA
040123	Fatigue	1	2	3	4	5	NA
040152	Weight gain	1	2	3	4	5	NA
040153	Impaired cognition	1	2	3	4	5	NA
040154	Pallor	1	2	3	4	5	NA
040155	Dependent rubor	1	2	3	4	5	NA
040156	Intermittent claudication	1	2	3	4	5	NA
040157	Decreased skin temperature	1	2	3	4	5	NA
040158	Paresthesia	1	2	3	4	5	NA
040159	Syncope	1	2	3	4	5	NA
040160	Pitting edema	1	2	3	4	5	NA
040161	Lower extremity ulcers	1	2	3	4	5	NA
040162	Numbness	1	2	3	4	5	NA

Domain-Physiologic Health (II)   *Class-Cardiopulmonary (E)*   *1st edition 1997; revised 2004, 2008*

OUTCOME CONTENT REFERENCES:
Andreoli, K. G., Zipes, D. P., Wallace, A. G., Kinney, M. R., & Fowkes, V. K. (Eds.). (1996). *Comprehensive cardiac care* (8th ed.). St. Louis: Mosby.
Cullen, L. (1992). Interventions related to circulatory care. *Nursing Clinics of North America, 27*(2), 445–477.
Dougherty, C. M. (2001). Decreased cardiac output. In M. Maas, K. Buckwalter, M. Hardy, T. Tripp-Reimer, M. Titler, & J. Specht (Eds.), *Nursing care of older adults: Diagnoses, outcomes & interventions* (pp. 285–297). St. Louis: Mosby.
Fahey, V. A. (Ed.). (1999). *Vascular nursing* (3rd ed.). Philadelphia: W. B. Saunders.
Murphy, T. G., & Bennett, E. J. (1992). Low-tech, high-touch perfusion assessment. *American Journal of Nursing, 92*(5), 36–46.
Reischman, R. R. (2002). Critical care cardiovascular nurse expert and novice diagnostic cue utilization. *Journal of Advanced Nursing, 39*(1), 24–34.
Sheehy, S. B. (1999). *Manual of emergency care* (5th ed.). St. Louis: Mosby.
Smeltzer, S. C., & Bare, B. G. (Eds.). (2003). *Brunner and Suddarth's textbook of medical-surgical nursing* (10th ed.). Philadelphia: Lippincott Williams & Wilkins.
Smith, S. L. (1990). Postoperative perfusion deficits. *Critical Care Nursing Clinics of North America, 2*(4), 567–578.

Client Satisfaction 3014

Definition: Extent of positive perception of care provided by nursing staff

OUTCOME TARGET RATING: Maintain at_____ Increase to_____

OUTCOME OVERALL RATING		Not at all satisfied 1	Somewhat satisfied 2	Moderately satisfied 3	Very satisfied 4	Completely satisfied 5	
Indicators:							
301401	Access to nursing staff	1	2	3	4	5	NA
301402	Access to supplies and equipment needed for care	1	2	3	4	5	NA
301403	Knowledge and expertise of nursing staff	1	2	3	4	5	NA
301404	Competence of nursing staff to perform procedures	1	2	3	4	5	NA
301405	Protection of legal rights by nursing staff	1	2	3	4	5	NA
301406	Protection of human rights by nursing staff	1	2	3	4	5	NA
301407	Concern for the client by nursing staff	1	2	3	4	5	NA
301408	Concern for the family by nursing staff	1	2	3	4	5	NA
301409	Questions answered completely	1	2	3	4	5	NA
301410	Instruction to improve understanding of illness	1	2	3	4	5	NA
301411	Instruction to improve participation in care	1	2	3	4	5	NA
301412	Integration of cultural beliefs into nursing care	1	2	3	4	5	NA
301413	Integration of values into nursing care	1	2	3	4	5	NA
301414	Assistance to achieve mobility	1	2	3	4	5	NA
301415	Assistance to achieve self-care	1	2	3	4	5	NA
301416	Assistance to cope with emotional concerns	1	2	3	4	5	NA
301417	Assistance to address spiritual needs	1	2	3	4	5	NA
301418	Relief of symptoms of illness	1	2	3	4	5	NA
301419	Care to control pain	1	2	3	4	5	NA
301420	Care to prevent harm or injury	1	2	3	4	5	NA
301421	Care to maintain body functions	1	2	3	4	5	NA
301422	Care to maintain cleanliness	1	2	3	4	5	NA
301423	Cleanliness of care environment	1	2	3	4	5	NA
301424	Coordination of care as the client moves from one care setting to another	1	2	3	4	5	NA
301425	Client/family included in discharge planning	1	2	3	4	5	NA

Domain-Perceived Health (V) *Class*-Satisfaction with Care (EE) 4th edition 2008

OUTCOME CONTENT REFERENCES:
Abdellah, F. G., & Levine, E. (1957). Developing a measure of patient and personnel satisfaction with nursing care. *Nursing Research, 5*(3), 100–108.
Abramowitz, S., Cote, A. A., & Berry, E. (1987). Analyzing patient satisfaction: A multianalytic approach. *Quality Review Bulletin, 13*(4), 122–130.

Davis, B. A., & Bush, H. A. (1995). Developing effective measurement tools: A case study of the consumer emergency care satisfaction scale. *Journal of Nursing Care Quality*, 9(2), 26–35.

Davis, J., Davis, M., & Riggs, H. (1999). Taking the measure of patient satisfaction. *Nursing Times*, 95(24), 52–53.

Eriksen, L. (1988). Measuring patient satisfaction with nursing care: A magnitude estimation approach. In C. F. Waltz & O. W. Stickland (Eds.), *Measurement of nursing outcomes* (Vol. 1, pp. 523–527). New York: Springer.

Gesell, S. B., & Gregory, N. (2003). Identifying priority actions for improving patient satisfaction with outpatient cancer care. *Journal of Nursing Care Quality*, 19(3), 226–233.

Hegedus, K. S. (1999). Providers' and consumers' perspective of nurses' caring behaviours. *Journal of Advanced Nursing*, 30(5), 1090–1096.

Hinshaw, A. S., & Atwood, J. R. (1982). A patient satisfaction instrument: Precision by replication. *Nursing Research*, 31(3), 170–175.

LaMonica, E. L., Oberst, M. T., Madea, A. R., & Wolf, R. M. (1986). Development of a patient satisfaction scale. *Research in Nursing and Health*, 9(1), 43–50.

Larrabee, J. H., Ostrow, C. L., Withrow, M. L., Janney, M. A., Hobbs, G. R., Jr., & Burant, C. (2004). Predictors of patient satisfaction with inpatient hospital nursing care. *Research in Nursing & Health*, 27(4), 254–268.

Laschinger, H. S., Hall, L. M., Pedersen, C., & Almost, J. (2004). A psychometric analysis of the patient satisfaction with nursing care quality questionnaire: An actionable approach to measuring patient satisfaction. *Journal of Nursing Care Quality*, 20(3), 220–230.

Mark, B. A., & Wan, T. T. (2005). Testing measurement equivalence in a patient satisfaction instrument. *Western Journal of Nursing Research*, 27(6), 772–787.

Marsh, G. W. (1999). Measuring patient satisfaction outcomes across provider disciplines. *Journal of Nursing Measurement*, 7(1), 47–62.

Nussbaum, G. B. (2003). Spirituality in critical care: Patient comfort and satisfaction. *Critical Care Nursing Quarterly*, 26(3), 214–220.

Risser, N. L. (1975). Development of an instrument to measure patient satisfaction with nurses and nursing care in primary care settings. *Nursing Research*, 24(1), 45–52.

Ryden, M. B., Gross, C. R., Savik, K., Snyder, M., Oh, H. L., Jang, Y., Wang, J., & Krichbaum, K. E. (2000). Development of a measure of resident satisfaction with the nursing home. *Research in Nursing & Health*, 23(3), 237–245.

Walsh, M., & Walsh, A. (1999). Measuring patient satisfaction with nursing care: Experience of using the Newcastle Satisfaction with Nursing Scale. *Journal of Advanced Nursing*, 29(2), 307–315.

Ware, J. E., Davies-Avery, A., & Stewart, A. I. (1978). The measurement and meaning of patient satisfaction. *Health & Medical Care Services Review*, 1(1), 1, 3–14.

Wolf, L. R., Giardino, E. R., Osborne, P. A., & Ambrose, M. S. (1994). Dimensions of nurse caring. *Image—The Journal of Nursing Scholarship*, 26(2), 107–111.

Client Satisfaction: Access to Care Resources   **3000**

Definition: Extent of positive perception of access to nursing staff, supplies, and equipment needed for care

OUTCOME TARGET RATING: Maintain at_____   Increase to_____

OUTCOME OVERALL RATING	Not at all satisfied 1	Somewhat satisfied 2	Moderately satisfied 3	Very satisfied 4	Completely satisfied 5	
Indicators:						
300001 Availability of registered nurses	1	2	3	4	5	NA
300002 Availability of assistive staff	1	2	3	4	5	NA
300003 Availability of supplies needed for care	1	2	3	4	5	NA
300004 Availability of equipment needed for care	1	2	3	4	5	NA
300005 Informed of registered nurse and assistive staff responsible for care	1	2	3	4	5	NA
300006 Access to registered nurse responsible for care	1	2	3	4	5	NA
300007 Assistance with access to health providers	1	2	3	4	5	NA
300008 Assistance with contacting physician	1	2	3	4	5	NA
300009 Coordination of health care resources	1	2	3	4	5	NA
300010 Coordination of health providers	1	2	3	4	5	NA
300011 Wait times for getting an appointment	1	2	3	4	5	NA
300012 Wait times to be seen at appointment	1	2	3	4	5	NA
300013 Access to support group	1	2	3	4	5	NA

Domain-Perceived Health (V)   **Class**-Satisfaction with Care (EE)   3rd edition 2004

OUTCOME CONTENT REFERENCES:

Larrabee, J. H., Ostrow, C. L., Withrow, M. L., Janney, M. A., Hobbs, G. R., Jr., & Burant, C. (2004). Predictors of patient satisfaction with inpatient hospital nursing care. *Research in Nursing & Health*, 27(4), 254–268.

Laschinger, H. S., Hall, L. M., Pedersen, C., & Almost, J. (2004). A psychometric analysis of the patient satisfaction with nursing care quality questionnaire: An actionable approach to measuring patient satisfaction. *Journal of Nursing Care Quality*, 20(3), 220–230.

Linder-Pelz, S. (1982). Toward a theory of patient satisfaction. *Social Science & Medicine*, 16(5), 577–582.

Mark, B. A., & Wan, T. T. (2005). Testing measurement equivalence in a patient satisfaction instrument. *Western Journal of Nursing Research*, 27(6), 772–787.

Marsh, G. W. (1999). Measuring patient satisfaction outcomes across provider disciplines. *Journal of Nursing Measurement*, 7(1), 47–62.

Ware, J. E., Davies-Avery, A., & Stewart, A. I. (1978). The measurement and meaning of patient satisfaction. *Health & Medical Care Services Review*, 1(1), 1, 3–14.

Client Satisfaction: Caring 3001

Definition: Extent of positive perception of nursing staff's concern for the client

OUTCOME TARGET RATING: Maintain at_____   Increase to_____

		Not at all satisfied	Somewhat satisfied	Moderately satisfied	Very satisfied	Completely satisfied	
OUTCOME OVERALL RATING		1	2	3	4	5	
Indicators:							
300101	Courtesy shown by staff	1	2	3	4	5	NA
300102	Compassion shown by staff	1	2	3	4	5	NA
300103	Kindness shown by staff	1	2	3	4	5	NA
300104	Respect shown by staff	1	2	3	4	5	NA
300105	Consideration for feelings	1	2	3	4	5	NA
300106	Consideration for opinions	1	2	3	4	5	NA
300107	Concern shown for individual needs	1	2	3	4	5	NA
300108	Relationship with nursing staff	1	2	3	4	5	NA
300109	Frequency with which checked on by staff	1	2	3	4	5	NA
300110	Promptness answering call light	1	2	3	4	5	NA
300111	Promptness responding to inquiries	1	2	3	4	5	NA
300123	Follow through with client request	1	2	3	4	5	NA
300112	Emotional support provided	1	2	3	4	5	NA
300124	Assistance to address spiritual needs	1	2	3	4	5	NA
300113	Appropriate use of touch	1	2	3	4	5	NA
300114	Orientation to room, equipment, and routines	1	2	3	4	5	NA
300115	Visiting arrangements	1	2	3	4	5	NA
300116	Family and friends made welcome	1	2	3	4	5	NA
300117	Assistance with letter writing	1	2	3	4	5	NA
300118	Leisure activities provided	1	2	3	4	5	NA
300119	Information provided about options of care	1	2	3	4	5	NA
300120	Consideration for cost of care	1	2	3	4	5	NA
300121	Supplies and equipment not wasted	1	2	3	4	5	NA

Domain-*Perceived Health (V)*   **Class**-*Satisfaction with Care (EE)*   *3rd edition 2004; revised 2008*

OUTCOME CONTENT REFERENCES:

Abdellah, F. G., & Levine, E. (1957). Developing a measure of patient and personnel satisfaction with nursing care. *Nursing Research*, 5(3), 100–108.

Davis, B. A., & Bush, H. A. (1995). Developing effective measurement tools: A case study of the consumer emergency care satisfaction scale. *Journal of Nursing Care Quality*, 9(2), 26–35.

Davis, J., Davis, M., & Riggs, H. (1999). Taking the measure of patient satisfaction. *Nursing Times*, 95(24), 52–53.

Deitrick, L., Bokovoy, J., Stern, G., & Panik, A. (2006). Dance of the call bells: Using ethnography to evaluate patient satisfaction with quality of care. *Journal of Nursing Care Quality*, 21(4), 316–324.

Eriksen, L. (1988). Measuring patient satisfaction with nursing care: A magnitude estimation approach. In C. F. Waltz & O. W. Stickland (Eds.), *Measurement of nursing outcomes* (Vol. 1, pp. 523–527). New York: Springer.

Hegedus, K. S. (1999). Providers' and consumers' perspective of nurses' caring behaviours. *Journal of Advanced Nursing*, 30(5), 1090–1096.

Hinshaw, A. S., & Atwood, J. R. (1982). A patient satisfaction instrument: Precision by replication. *Nursing Research*, 31(3), 170–175.

LaMonica, E. L., Oberst, M. T., Madea, A. R., & Wolf, R. M. (1986). Development of a patient satisfaction scale. *Research in Nursing & Health*, 9(1), 43–50.

Larrabee, J. H., Ostrow, C. L., Withrow, M. L., Janney, M. A., Hobbs, G. R., Jr., & Burant, C. (2004). Predictors of patient satisfaction with inpatient hospital nursing care. *Research in Nursing & Health*, 27(4), 254–268.

Laschinger, H. S., Hall, L. M., Pedersen, C., & Almost, J. (2004). A psychometric analysis of the patient satisfaction with nursing care quality questionnaire: An actionable approach to measuring patient satisfaction. *Journal of Nursing Care Quality*, 20(3), 220–230.

Mark, B. A., & Wan, T. T. H. (2005). Testing measurement equivalence in a patient satisfaction instrument. *Western Journal of Nursing Research*, 27(6), 772–787.

Marsh, G. W. (1999). Measuring patient satisfaction outcomes across provider disciplines. *Journal of Nursing Measurement*, 7(1), 47–62.

Nussbaum, G. B. (2003). Spirituality in critical care: Patient comfort and satisfaction. *Critical Care Nursing Quarterly*, 26(3), 214–220.

Risser, N. L. (1975). Development of an instrument to measure patient satisfaction with nurses and nursing care in primary care settings. *Nursing Research*, 24(1), 45–52.

Ryden, M. B., Gross, C. R., Savik, K., Snyder, M., Oh, H. L., Jang, Y., Wang, J., & Krichbaum, K. E. (2000). Development of a measure of resident satisfaction with the nursing home. *Research in Nursing & Health*, 23(3), 237–245.

Walsh, M., & Walsh, A. (1999). Measuring patient satisfaction with nursing care: Experience of using the Newcastle Satisfaction with Nursing Scale. *Journal of Advanced Nursing*, 29(2), 307–315.

Ware, J. E., Davies-Avery, A., & Stewart, A. I. (1978). The measurement and meaning of patient satisfaction. *Health & Medical Care Services Review*, 1(1), 1, 3–14.

Wolf, L. R., Giardino, E. R., Osborne, P. A., & Ambrose, M. S. (1994). Dimensions of nurse caring. *Image—The Journal of Nursing Scholarship*, 26(2), 107–111.

Client Satisfaction: Case Management   3015

Definition: Extent of positive perception of case management services

OUTCOME TARGET RATING: Maintain at_____   Increase to_____

		Not at all satisfied	Somewhat satisfied	Moderately satisfied	Very satisfied	Completely satisfied	
OUTCOME OVERALL RATING		1	2	3	4	5	
Indicators:							
301501	Availability of case manager	1	2	3	4	5	NA
301502	Availability of supplies needed for care	1	2	3	4	5	NA
301503	Availability of equipment needed for care	1	2	3	4	5	NA
301504	Assistance with contacting physician	1	2	3	4	5	NA
301505	Assistance with gaining access to health providers	1	2	3	4	5	NA
301506	Referrals made to appropriate health providers	1	2	3	4	5	NA
301507	Coordination of health care resources	1	2	3	4	5	NA
301508	Coordination of health providers	1	2	3	4	5	NA
301509	Coordination of care	1	2	3	4	5	NA
301510	Wait times for getting an appointment	1	2	3	4	5	NA
301511	Information provided about support groups	1	2	3	4	5	NA
301512	Consideration for feelings	1	2	3	4	5	NA
301513	Consideration of opinions	1	2	3	4	5	NA
301514	Concern shown for individual needs	1	2	3	4	5	NA
301515	Information provided about options for care	1	2	3	4	5	NA
301516	Information provided about cost of care	1	2	3	4	5	NA
301517	Consideration of cost of care	1	2	3	4	5	NA
301518	Avoidance of unnecessary treatments and procedures	1	2	3	4	5	NA
301519	Referral regarding costs and finances	1	2	3	4	5	NA
301520	Consistent information provided	1	2	3	4	5	NA
301521	Personal values considered	1	2	3	4	5	NA
301522	Personal preferences considered in care plan	1	2	3	4	5	NA
301523	Respect for cultural values	1	2	3	4	5	NA
301524	Respect for religious beliefs	1	2	3	4	5	NA
301525	Health providers work as a team	1	2	3	4	5	NA
301526	Safety issues are addressed	1	2	3	4	5	NA
301527	Family included in providing care	1	2	3	4	5	NA
301528	Confidentiality of client information maintained	1	2	3	4	5	NA
301529	Explanation provided in understand-able terms	1	2	3	4	5	NA
301530	Quality of instructional material provided	1	2	3	4	5	NA
301531	Included in decisions about care	1	2	3	4	5	NA
301532	Support for finding own solutions to problems	1	2	3	4	5	NA
301533	Information provided about legal rights	1	2	3	4	5	NA
301534	Information provided about course of illness	1	2	3	4	5	NA

Domain-Perceived Health (V)   *Class*-Satisfaction with Care (EE)   *4th edition 2008*

OUTCOME CONTENT REFERENCES:

Buck, P. W., & Alexander, L. B. (2005). Neglected voices: Consumers with serious mental illness speak about intensive case management. *Administration and Policy in Mental Health Services Research, 33*(4), 470–481.

Coffey, D. S. (2003). Connection and autonomy in the case management relationship. *Psychiatric Rehabilitation Journal, 26*(4), 404–412.

Finch, G. L., & Linderberg, J. (1999). Improving patient satisfaction through unit-based team case management. *Continuum (Chicago), 19*(2), 12–16.

Hadjistavropoulos, H. D., Sagan, M., Bierlein, C., & Lawson, K. (2003). Development of a case management quality questionnaire. *Case Management Journal, 4*(1), 8–17.

Huber, D. L. (Ed.). (2005). *Disease management: A guide for case managers.* St. Louis: Elsevier Saunders.

Kopelman, T., Huber, D. L., Kopelman, B. C., Sarrazin, M. V., & Hall, J. A. (2006). Client satisfaction with rural substance abuse case management services. *Care Management Journal, 7*(4), 179–190.

Mark, B. A., & Wan, T. T. H. (2005). Testing measurement equivalence in a patient satisfaction instrument. *Western Journal of Nursing Research, 27*(6), 772–787.

Rossi, P. (1999). *Case management in health care: A practical guide.* Philadelphia: Saunders.

Client Satisfaction: Communication 3002

Definition: Extent of positive perception of information exchanged between client and nursing staff

OUTCOME TARGET RATING: Maintain at_____ Increase to_____

OUTCOME OVERALL RATING	Not at all satisfied 1	Somewhat satisfied 2	Moderately satisfied 3	Very satisfied 4	Completely satisfied 5	
Indicators:						
300201 Staff introduce self	1	2	3	4	5	NA
300202 Use of client's preferred name	1	2	3	4	5	NA
300203 Staff speak clearly	1	2	3	4	5	NA
300204 Staff listen to client	1	2	3	4	5	NA
300205 Staff encourage questions	1	2	3	4	5	NA
300206 Staff repeat information as often as needed	1	2	3	4	5	NA
300207 Staff take time when communicating	1	2	3	4	5	NA
300208 Staff present information in understandable way	1	2	3	4	5	NA
300209 Staff make sure information is understood	1	2	3	4	5	NA
300210 Staff use non-judgmental communication	1	2	3	4	5	NA
300211 Questions answered clearly	1	2	3	4	5	NA
300212 Questions answered completely	1	2	3	4	5	NA
300213 Questions answered in a reasonable length of time	1	2	3	4	5	NA
300214 Consistent information given by nursing staff	1	2	3	4	5	NA
300215 Personal values considered in communication	1	2	3	4	5	NA
300216 Personal preferences considered	1	2	3	4	5	NA
300217 Discrepancies in information are resolved in a timely manner	1	2	3	4	5	NA
300218 Alternative communication methods used as needed	1	2	3	4	5	NA

Domain-Perceived Health (V) *Class-Satisfaction with Care (EE)* 3rd edition 2004

OUTCOME CONTENT REFERENCES:

Davis, J., Davis, M., & Riggs, H. (1999). Taking the measure of patient satisfaction. *Nursing Times, 95*(24), 52–53.

Deitrick, L., Bokovoy, J., Stern, G., & Panik, A. (2006). Dance of the call bells: Using ethnography to evaluate patient satisfaction with quality of care. *Journal of Nursing Care Quality, 21*(4), 316–324.

Hegedus, K. S. (1999). Providers' and consumers' perspective of nurses' caring behaviours. *Journal of Advanced Nursing, 30*(5), 1090–1096.

Hinshaw, A. S., & Atwood, J. R. (1982). A patient satisfaction instrument: Precision by replication. *Nursing Research, 31*(3), 170–175.

LaMonica, E. L., Oberst, M. T., Madea, A. R., & Wolf, R. M. (1986). Development of a patient satisfaction scale. *Research in Nursing & Health, 9*(1), 43–50.

Larrabee, J. H., Ostrow, C. L., Withrow, M. L., Janney, M. A., Hobbs, G. R., Jr., & Burant, C. (2004). Predictors of patient satisfaction with inpatient hospital nursing care. *Research in Nursing & Health, 27*(4), 254–268.

Laschinger, H. S., Hall, L. M., Pedersen, C., & Almost, J. (2004). A psychometric analysis of the patient satisfaction with nursing care quality questionnaire: An actionable approach to measuring patient satisfaction. *Journal of Nursing Care Quality, 20*(3), 220–230.

Lynn, M. R., & McMillen, B. J. (1999). Do nurses know what patients think is important in nursing care? *Journal of Nursing Care Quality, 13*(5), 65–74.

Mark, B. A., & Wan, T. T. H. (2005). Testing measurement equivalence in a patient satisfaction instrument. *Western Journal of Nursing Research, 27*(6), 772–787.

McCabe, C. (2004). Nurse-patient communication: An exploration of patients' experiences. *Issues in Clinical Nursing, 13*(1), 41–49.

McGilton, K., Boscart, V., Irwin-Robinson, H., & Spanjevic, L. (2006). Communication enhancement: Nurse and patient satisfaction outcomes in a complex continuing care facility. *Journal of Advanced Nursing, 54*(1), 35–44

Risser, N. L. (1975). Development of an instrument to measure patient satisfaction with nurses and nursing care in primary care settings. *Nursing Research, 24*(1), 45–52.

Walsh, M., & Walsh, A. (1999). Measuring patient satisfaction with nursing care: Experience of using the Newcastle Satisfaction with Nursing Scale. *Journal of Advanced Nursing, 29*(2), 307–315.

Ware, J. E., Davies-Avery, A., & Stewart, A. I. (1978). The measurement and meaning of patient satisfaction. *Health & Medical Care Services Review, 1*(1), 1, 3–14.

Wolf, L. R., Giardino, E. R., Osborne, P. A., & Ambrose, M. S. (1994). Dimensions of nurse caring. *Image—The Journal of Nursing Scholarship, 26*(2), 107–111.

Yellen, E. (2003). The influence of nurse-sensitive variables on patient satisfaction. *AORN Journal, 78*, 783–793.

Yellen, E., Davis, G. C., & Ricard, R. (2002). The measurement of patient satisfaction. *Journal of Nursing Care Quality, 16*(4), 23–29.

Client Satisfaction: Continuity of Care   3003

Definition: Extent of positive perception of coordination of care as the client moves from one care setting to another

OUTCOME TARGET RATING: Maintain at_____ Increase to_____

OUTCOME OVERALL RATING		Not at all satisfied	Somewhat satisfied	Moderately satisfied	Very satisfied	Completely satisfied	
		1	2	3	4	5	
Indicators:							
300301	Coordination of care	1	2	3	4	5	NA
300302	Personal preferences included in care plan	1	2	3	4	5	NA
300303	Client/family included in planning care	1	2	3	4	5	NA
300321	Client/family included in discharge planning	1	2	3	4	5	NA
300304	Client resources identified in discharge planning	1	2	3	4	5	NA
300305	Safety issues are addressed in care plan	1	2	3	4	5	NA
300306	Time to prepare for transfer	1	2	3	4	5	NA
300307	Information provided about what to expect when transferred	1	2	3	4	5	NA
300308	Opportunity provided to express concerns about managing self-care	1	2	3	4	5	NA
300309	Information provided to manage self-care	1	2	3	4	5	NA
300310	Opportunity to demonstrate care activities	1	2	3	4	5	NA
300311	Staff offer suggestions for solutions to concerns and questions	1	2	3	4	5	NA
300312	Discussion of strategies to meet care needs	1	2	3	4	5	NA
300313	Discussion of strategies to meet household needs	1	2	3	4	5	NA
300314	Personal preparation to deal with potential health problems	1	2	3	4	5	NA
300315	Discussion of guidelines for returning to sexual activities	1	2	3	4	5	NA
300316	Discussion of strategies for returning to work	1	2	3	4	5	NA
300317	Discussion of strategies for returning to homemaking activities	1	2	3	4	5	NA
300318	Discussion of strategies for returning to community activities	1	2	3	4	5	NA
300319	Assistance with managing relocation costs and finances	1	2	3	4	5	NA
300320	Health providers work as a team	1	2	3	4	5	NA

Domain-Perceived Health (V)   *Class*-Satisfaction with Care (EE)   3rd edition 2004; revised 2008

OUTCOME CONTENT REFERENCES:

Eriksen, L. (1988). Measuring patient satisfaction with nursing care: A magnitude estimation approach. In C. F. Waltz & O. W. Stickland (Eds.), *Measurement of nursing outcomes* (Vol. 1, pp. 523–527). New York: Springer.

Gesell, S. B., & Gregory, N. (2003). Identifying priority actions for improving patient satisfaction with outpatient cancer care. *Journal of Nursing Care Quality, 19*(3), 226–233.

Larrabee, J. H., Ostrow, C. L., Withrow, M. L., Janney, M. A., Hobbs, G. R., Jr., & Burant, C. (2004). Predictors of patient satisfaction with inpatient hospital nursing care. *Research in Nursing & Health, 27*(4), 254–268.

Laschinger, H. S., Hall, L. M., Pedersen, C., & Almost, J. (2004). A psychometric analysis of the patient satisfaction with nursing care quality questionnaire: An actionable approach to measuring patient satisfaction. *Journal of Nursing Care Quality, 20*(3), 220–230.

Mark, B. A., & Wan, T. T. H. (2005). Testing measurement equivalence in a patient satisfaction instrument. *Western Journal of Nursing Research, 27*(6), 772–787.

Ware, J. E., Davies-Avery, A., & Stewart, A. I. (1978). The measurement and meaning of patient satisfaction. *Health & Medical Care Services Review, 1*(1), 1, 3–14.

C

Client Satisfaction: Cultural Needs Fulfillment   3004

Definition: Extent of positive perception of integration of cultural beliefs, values and social structures into nursing care

OUTCOME TARGET RATING: Maintain at_____   Increase to_____

	Not at all satisfied	Somewhat satisfied	Moderately satisfied	Very satisfied	Completely satisfied	
OUTCOME OVERALL RATING	1	2	3	4	5	
Indicators:						
300401 Respect for cultural beliefs	1	2	3	4	5	NA
300402 Respect for cultural health behaviors	1	2	3	4	5	NA
300403 Respect for personal values	1	2	3	4	5	NA
300404 Respect for personal perspectives	1	2	3	4	5	NA
300405 Respect for traditions	1	2	3	4	5	NA
300406 Respect for religious beliefs	1	2	3	4	5	NA
300407 Respect for spiritual beliefs	1	2	3	4	5	NA
300408 Incorporation of cultural beliefs in health teaching	1	2	3	4	5	NA
300409 Care consistent with cultural beliefs	1	2	3	4	5	NA
300410 Use of creative methods to establish communication due to language differences	1	2	3	4	5	NA
300411 Consideration for cultural expectations	1	2	3	4	5	NA
300412 Respect for family members' participation in care	1	2	3	4	5	NA
300413 Respect for family members' participation in decisions	1	2	3	4	5	NA

Domain-Perceived Health (V)   *Class*-Satisfaction with Care (EE)   *3rd edition 2004*

OUTCOME CONTENT REFERENCES:

Ali, N. S., & Khalil, H. Z. (1993). A comparison of American and Egyptian cancer patients' attitudes and unmet needs. *Cancer Nursing, 16*(3), 193–203.

Arruda, E. N., Larson, P. J., & Meleis, A. I. (1992). Comfort: Immigrant Hispanic cancer patient's views. *Cancer Nursing, 15*(6), 387–394.

Austin, W., Gallop, R., McCay, E., Peternelj-Taylor, C., & Bayer, M. (1999). Culturally competent care for psychiatric clients who have a history of sexual abuse. *Clinical Nursing Research, 8*(1), 5–25.

Capers, C. F. (1994). Mental health issues and African-Americans. *Mental Health Nursing, 29*(1), 57–72.

Chmielarczyk, V. (1991). Transcultural nursing: Providing culturally congruent care to the Hausa of Northwest Africa. *Journal of Transcultural Nursing, 3*(1), 15–19.

Cravener, P. (1992). Establishing therapeutic alliance across cultural barriers. *Journal of Psychosocial Nursing, 30*(12), 10–14.

Denman-Vitale, S., & Murillo, E. K. (1999). Effective promotion of breastfeeding among Latin American women newly immigrated to the United States. *Holistic Nursing Practice, 13*(4), 51–60.

Granda-Cameron, C. (1999). The experience of having cancer in Latin America. *Cancer Nursing, 22*(1), 51–57.

Larrabee, J. H., Ostrow, C. L., Withrow, M. L., Janney, M. A., Hobbs, G. R., Jr., & Burant, C. (2004). Predictors of patient satisfaction with inpatient hospital nursing care. *Research in Nursing & Health, 27*(4), 254–268.

Laschinger, H. S., Hall, L. M., Pedersen, C., & Almost, J. (2004). A psychometric analysis of the patient satisfaction with nursing care quality questionnaire: An actionable approach to measuring patient satisfaction. *Journal of Nursing Care Quality, 20*(3), 220–230.

Mark, B. A., & Wan, T. T. (2005). Testing measurement equivalence in a patient satisfaction instrument. *Western Journal of Nursing Research, 27*(6), 772–787.

Sommer, B. (1995). How we do it: Special considerations for Orthodox Jewish patients in the emergency department. *Journal of Emergency Nursing, 21*(6), 569–570.

Tripp-Reimer, T., Choi, E., Skemp Kelley, L., & Enslein, J. C. (2001). Cultural barriers to care: Inverting the problem. *Diabetes Spectrum, 14*(1), 13–22.

Weaver, H. N. (1999). Transcultural nursing with Native Americans: Critical knowledge, skills, and attitudes. *Journal of Transcultural Nursing, 10*(3), 197–202.

Willis, W. O. (1999). Culturally competent nursing care during the perinatal period. *Journal of Perinatal and Neonatal Nursing, 13*(3), 45–59.

Wilson, A. H., Pittman, K., & Wold, J. L. (2000). Listening to the quiet voices of Hispanic migrant children about health. *Journal of Pediatric Nursing, 15*(3), 137–147.

Yellen, E. (2003). The influence of nurse-sensitive variables on patient satisfaction. *AORN Journal, 78*(5), 783–793.

Yellen, E., Davis, G. C., & Ricard, R. (2002). The measurement of patient satisfaction. *Journal of Nursing Care Quality, 16*(4), 23–29.

C

Client Satisfaction: Functional Assistance   3005

Definition: Extent of positive perception of nursing assistance to achieve mobility and self-care

OUTCOME TARGET RATING: Maintain at_____   Increase to_____

		Not at all satisfied	Somewhat satisfied	Moderately satisfied	Very satisfied	Completely satisfied	
OUTCOME OVERALL RATING		1	2	3	4	5	
Indicators:							
300501	Included in planning for optimal mobility and self-care	1	2	3	4	5	NA
300502	Included in planning time schedule for self-care	1	2	3	4	5	NA
300503	Encouraged to be as active as possible	1	2	3	4	5	NA
300504	Assistance with physical activity	1	2	3	4	5	NA
300505	Exercise routine provided to gain or maintain mobility	1	2	3	4	5	NA
300506	Exercise routine provided to gain or maintain flexibility	1	2	3	4	5	NA
300507	Equipment provided to enhance mobility	1	2	3	4	5	NA
300516	Information provided for correct use of other devices	1	2	3	4	5	NA
300509	Room space provided for equipment needed to support functional independence	1	2	3	4	5	NA
300510	Safety taught in all activities	1	2	3	4	5	NA
300511	Opportunity to do self-care unless assistance requested	1	2	3	4	5	NA
300512	Assistance with care	1	2	3	4	5	NA
300513	Allowed to choose own clothing	1	2	3	4	5	NA
300514	Allowed to choose food for meals	1	2	3	4	5	NA
300515	Information provided to manage medication	1	2	3	4	5	NA

Domain-Perceived Health (V)   *Class*-Satisfaction with Care (EE)   3rd edition 2004; revised 2008

OUTCOME CONTENT REFERENCES:

Hinshaw, A. S., & Atwood, J. R. (1982). A patient satisfaction instrument: Precision by replication. *Nursing Research, 31*(3), 170–175.

LaMonica, E. L., Oberst, M. T., Madea, A. R., & Wolf, R. M. (1986). Development of a patient satisfaction scale. *Research in Nursing & Health, 9*(1), 43–50.

Larrabee, J. H., Ostrow, C. L., Withrow, M. L., Janney, M. A., Hobbs, G. R., Jr., & Burant, C. (2004). Predictors of patient satisfaction with inpatient hospital nursing care. *Research in Nursing & Health, 27*(4), 254–268.

Laschinger, H. S., Hall, L. M., Pedersen, C., & Almost, J. (2004). A psychometric analysis of the patient satisfaction with nursing care quality questionnaire: An actionable approach to measuring patient satisfaction. *Journal of Nursing Care Quality, 20*(3), 220–230.

Mark, B. A., & Wan, T. T. H. (2005). Testing measurement equivalence in a patient satisfaction instrument. *Western Journal of Nursing Research, 27*(6), 772–787.

Risser, N. L. (1975). Development of an instrument to measure patient satisfaction with nurses and nursing care in primary care settings. *Nursing Research, 24*(1), 45–52.

Ware, J. E., Davies-Avery, A., & Stewart, A. I. (1978). The measurement and meaning of patient satisfaction. *Health & Medical Care Services Review, 1*(1), 1, 3–14.

Client Satisfaction: Pain Management 3016

Definition: Extent of positive perception of nursing care to relieve pain

OUTCOME TARGET RATING: Maintain at_____ Increase to_____

C

OUTCOME OVERALL RATING	Not at all satisfied 1	Somewhat satisfied 2	Moderately satisfied 3	Very satisfied 4	Completely satisfied 5	
Indicators:						
301601 Pain controlled	1	2	3	4	5	NA
301602 Pain level regularly monitored	1	2	3	4	5	NA
301603 Side effects of medication monitored	1	2	3	4	5	NA
301604 Actions taken to relieve pain	1	2	3	4	5	NA
301605 Actions taken to provide comfort	1	2	3	4	5	NA
301606 Information provided to manage medication use	1	2	3	4	5	NA
301607 Personal preferences considered	1	2	3	4	5	NA
301608 Information provided about options for pain management	1	2	3	4	5	NA
301609 Pain management consistent with cultural beliefs	1	2	3	4	5	NA
301610 Preventive approaches used for pain management	1	2	3	4	5	NA
301611 Information provided about activity restrictions	1	2	3	4	5	NA
301612 Information provided about pain relief	1	2	3	4	5	NA
301613 Information provided about options for pain management after discharge	1	2	3	4	5	NA
301614 Referrals made to support groups	1	2	3	4	5	NA
301615 Health providers work as a team to manage pain	1	2	3	4	5	NA
301616 Referral to pain-management health professionals as needed	1	2	3	4	5	NA
301617 Safety issues addressed with pain medication use	1	2	3	4	5	NA

Domain-Perceived Health (V)   *Class-Satisfaction with Care (EE)*   *4th edition 2008*

OUTCOME CONTENT REFERENCES:

Herr, K., & Kwekkeboom, K. (Eds.). (2003). Chronic pain management. *Nursing Clinics of North America, 38*(3), 403–560.

Hinshaw, A. S., & Atwood, J. R. (1982). A patient satisfaction instrument: Precision by replication. *Nursing Research, 31*(3), 170–175.

Hogan, S. L. (2005). Patient satisfaction with pain management in the emergency department. *Topics in Emergency Medicine, 27*(4), 284–294.

Innis, J., Bikaunieks, N., Petryshen, P., Zellermeyer, V., & Ciccarelli, L. (2004). Patient satisfaction and pain management: An educational approach. *Journal of Nursing Care Quality, 19*(4), 322–327.

LaMonica, E. L., Oberst, M. T., Madea, A. R., & Wolf, R. M. (1986). Development of a patient satisfaction scale. *Research in Nursing and Health, 9*(1), 43–50.

Larrabee, J. H., Ostrow, C. L., Withrow, M. L., Janney, M. A., Hobbs, G. R., Jr., & Burant, C. (2004). Predictors of patient satisfaction with inpatient hospital nursing care. *Research in Nursing & Health, 27*(4), 254–268.

Laschinger, H. S., Hall, L. M., Pedersen, C., & Almost, J. (2004). A psychometric analysis of the patient satisfaction with nursing care quality questionnaire: An actionable approach to measuring patient satisfaction. *Journal of Nursing Care Quality, 20*(3), 220–230.

Mark, B. A., & Wan, T. T. (2005). Testing measurement equivalence in a patient satisfaction instrument. *Western Journal of Nursing Research, 27*(6), 772–787.

Risser, N. L. (1975). Development of an instrument to measure patient satisfaction with nurses and nursing care in primary care settings. *Nursing Research, 24*(1), 45–52.

Sjoling, M., Nordahl, G., Olofsson, N., & Asplund, K. (2003). The impact of preoperative information on state anxiety, postoperative pain and satisfaction with pain management. *Patient Education and Counseling, 51*(2), 169–176.

Sterman, E., Gauker, S., & Krieger, J. (2003). A comprehensive approach to improving cancer pain management and patient satisfaction. *Oncology Nursing Forum, 30*(5), 857–864.

Ware, J. E., Davies-Avery, A., & Stewart, A. I. (1978). The measurement and meaning of patient satisfaction. *Health & Medical Care Services Review, 1*(1), 1, 3–14.

Client Satisfaction: Physical Care 3006

Definition: Extent of positive perception of nursing care to maintain body functions and cleanliness

OUTCOME TARGET RATING: Maintain at_____ Increase to_____

	Not at all satisfied	Somewhat satisfied	Moderately satisfied	Very satisfied	Completely satisfied	
OUTCOME OVERALL RATING	1	2	3	4	5	
Indicators:						
300601 Assistance with selecting food and fluid	1	2	3	4	5	NA
300602 Assistance with eating	1	2	3	4	5	NA
300603 Time for meals	1	2	3	4	5	NA
300604 Fluids available within restriction	1	2	3	4	5	NA
300605 Assistance with mouth care	1	2	3	4	5	NA
300606 Assistance with toileting	1	2	3	4	5	NA
300607 Normal bowel habits maintained	1	2	3	4	5	NA
300608 Normal bladder habits maintained	1	2	3	4	5	NA
300609 Assistance with bathing	1	2	3	4	5	NA
300610 Assistance with hair care	1	2	3	4	5	NA
300611 Assistance with nail care	1	2	3	4	5	NA
300612 Skin care routine maintained	1	2	3	4	5	NA
300613 Special skin care followed	1	2	3	4	5	NA
300614 Assistance with maintaining comfort	1	2	3	4	5	NA
300615 Time for rest	1	2	3	4	5	NA
300616 Sleep routine maintained	1	2	3	4	5	NA
300617 Assistance with ambulation	1	2	3	4	5	NA
300618 Opportunity for exercise	1	2	3	4	5	NA
300619 Special exercises provided	1	2	3	4	5	NA
300620 Assistance with repositioning	1	2	3	4	5	NA
300621 Assistance with transfer	1	2	3	4	5	NA

Domain-Perceived Health (V) *Class*-Satisfaction with Care (EE) *3rd edition 2004*

OUTCOME CONTENT REFERENCES:

Davis, B. A., & Bush, H. A. (1995). Developing effective measurement tools: A case study of the consumer emergency care satisfaction scale. *Journal of Nursing Care Quality, 9*(2), 26–35.

Hinshaw, A. S., & Atwood, J. R. (1982). A patient satisfaction instrument: Precision by replication. *Nursing Research, 31*(3), 170–175.

LaMonica, E. L., Oberst, M. T., Madea, A. R., & Wolf, R. M. (1986). Development of a patient satisfaction scale. *Research in Nursing & Health, 9*(1), 43–50.

Larrabee, J. H., Ostrow, C. L., Withrow, M. L., Janney, M. A., Hobbs, G. R., Jr., & Burant, C. (2004). Predictors of patient satisfaction with inpatient hospital nursing care. *Research in Nursing & Health, 27*(4), 254–268.

Laschinger, H. S., Hall, L. M., Pedersen, C., & Almost, J. (2004). A psychometric analysis of the patient satisfaction with nursing care quality questionnaire: An actionable approach to measuring patient satisfaction. *Journal of Nursing Care Quality, 20*(3), 220–230.

Lynn, M. R., & McMillen, B. J. (1999). Do nurses know what patients think is important in nursing care? *Journal of Nursing Care Quality, 13*(5), 65–74.

Mark, B. A., & Wan, T. T. (2005). Testing measurement equivalence in a patient satisfaction instrument. *Western Journal of Nursing Research, 27*(6), 772–787.

Ryden, M. B., Gross, C. R., Savik, K., Snyder, M., Oh, H. L., Jang, Y., Wang, J., & Krichbaum, K. E. (2000). Development of a measure of resident satisfaction with the nursing home. *Research in Nursing & Health, 23*(3), 237–245.

Ware, J. E., Davies-Avery, A., & Stewart, A. I. (1978). The measurement and meaning of patient satisfaction. *Health & Medical Care Services Review, 1*(1), 1, 3–14.

Wolf, L. R., Giardino, E. R., Osborne, P. A., & Ambrose, M. S. (1994). Dimensions of nurse caring. *Image—The Journal of Nursing Scholarship, 26*(2), 107–111.

Client Satisfaction: Physical Environment 3007

Definition: Extent of positive perception of living environment, treatment environment, equipment and supplies in acute or long-term care settings

OUTCOME TARGET RATING: Maintain at_____ Increase to_____

OUTCOMES OVERALL RATING	Not at all satisfied	Somewhat satisfied	Moderately satisfied	Very satisfied	Completely satisfied	
	1	2	3	4	5	
Indicators:						
300701 Cleanliness of room	1	2	3	4	5	NA
300702 Cleanliness of bathroom	1	2	3	4	5	NA
300703 Cleanliness of equipment	1	2	3	4	5	NA
300704 Control of room lighting	1	2	3	4	5	NA
300705 Comfort of room temperature	1	2	3	4	5	NA
300721 Control of odors	1	2	3	4	5	NA
300706 Comfort of bathroom temperature	1	2	3	4	5	NA
300707 Comfort of treatment room temperature	1	2	3	4	5	NA
300708 Comfort of room humidity	1	2	3	4	5	NA
300709 Control of noise	1	2	3	4	5	NA
300710 Control of number of people in room	1	2	3	4	5	NA
300711 Supplies and equipment within reach	1	2	3	4	5	NA
300712 Call light within reach	1	2	3	4	5	NA
300713 Access to telephone	1	2	3	4	5	NA
300714 Access to television	1	2	3	4	5	NA
300715 Access to radio	1	2	3	4	5	NA
300716 Attractiveness of room	1	2	3	4	5	NA
300717 Availability of chairs for family and visitors	1	2	3	4	5	NA
300718 Availability of space nearby for family and visitors	1	2	3	4	5	NA
300719 Orientation of family and visitors to facilities	1	2	3	4	5	NA
300720 Space in room for personal items	1	2	3	4	5	NA

Domain-Perceived Health (V) **Class**-Satisfaction with Care (EE) 3rd edition 2004; revised 2008

OUTCOME CONTENT REFERENCES:

Abdellah, F. G., & Levine, E. (1957). Developing a measure of patient and personnel satisfaction with nursing care. *Nursing Research, 5*(3), 100–108.

Eriksen, L. (1988). Measuring patient satisfaction with nursing care: A magnitude estimation approach. In C. F. Waltz & O. W. Stickland (Eds.), *Measurement of nursing outcomes* (Vol. 1, pp. 523–527). New York: Springer.

Gesell, S. B., & Gregory, N. (2003). Identifying priority actions for improving patient satisfaction with outpatient cancer care. *Journal of Nursing Care Quality, 19*(3), 226–233.

Larrabee, J. H., Ostrow, C. L., Withrow, M. L., Janney, M. A., Hobbs, G. R., Jr., & Burant, C. (2004). Predictors of patient satisfaction with inpatient hospital nursing care. *Research in Nursing & Health, 27*(4), 254–268.

Laschinger, H. S., Hall, L. M., Pedersen, C., & Almost, J. (2004). A psychometric analysis of the patient satisfaction with nursing care quality questionnaire: An actionable approach to measuring patient satisfaction. *Journal of Nursing Care Quality, 20*(3), 220–230.

Lynn, M. R., & McMillen, B. J. (1999). Do nurses know what patients think is important in nursing care? *Journal of Nursing Care Quality, 13*(5), 65–74.

Mark, B. A., & Wan, T. T. (2005). Testing measurement equivalence in a patient satisfaction instrument. *Western Journal of Nursing Research, 27*(6), 772–787.

Ryden, M. B., Gross, C. R., Savik, K., Snyder, M., Oh, H. L., Jang, Y., Wang, J., & Krichbaum, K. E. (2000). Development of a measure of resident satisfaction with the nursing home. *Research in Nursing & Health, 23*(3), 237–245.

Ware, J. E., Davies-Avery, A., & Stewart, A. I. (1978). The measurement and meaning of patient satisfaction. *Health & Medical Care Services Review, 1*(1), 1, 3–14.

C

Client Satisfaction: Protection of Rights 3008

Definition: Extent of positive perception of protection of a client's legal and moral rights provided by nursing staff

OUTCOME TARGET RATING: Maintain at_____ Increase to_____

OUTCOME OVERALL RATING	Not at all satisfied 1	Somewhat satisfied 2	Moderately satisfied 3	Very satisfied 4	Completely satisfied 5	
Indicators:						
300801 Maintenance of privacy	1	2	3	4	5	NA
300802 Care consistent with religious and spiritual needs	1	2	3	4	5	NA
300803 Confidentiality of client information maintained	1	2	3	4	5	NA
300804 Requests respected	1	2	3	4	5	NA
300805 Personal preferences for care considered	1	2	3	4	5	NA
300806 Use of client's preferred name	1	2	3	4	5	NA
300807 Introduced to staff	1	2	3	4	5	NA
300808 Introduced to roommate(s)	1	2	3	4	5	NA
300809 Information provided about available services of other disciplines	1	2	3	4	5	NA
300810 Information provided about support groups	1	2	3	4	5	NA
300811 Allowed to choose between care options	1	2	3	4	5	NA
300812 Included in decisions about care	1	2	3	4	5	NA
300813 Information provided about legal rights	1	2	3	4	5	NA
300814 Information provided about advance directives	1	2	3	4	5	NA
300815 Avoidance of repetitive questions by more than one provider	1	2	3	4	5	NA

Domain-Perceived Health (V)   *Class*-Satisfaction with Care (EE)   *3rd edition 2004*

OUTCOME CONTENT REFERENCES:

Eriksen, L. (1988). Measuring patient satisfaction with nursing care: A magnitude estimation approach. In C. F. Waltz & O. W. Stickland (Eds.), *Measurement of nursing outcomes* (Vol. 1, pp. 523–527). New York: Springer.

Hegedus, K. S. (1999). Providers' and consumers' perspective of nurses' caring behaviours. *Journal of Advanced Nursing*, 30(5), 1090–1096.

LaMonica, E. L., Oberst, M. T., Madea, A. R., & Wolf, R. M. (1986). Development of a patient satisfaction scale. *Research in Nursing & Health*, 9(1), 43–50.

Larrabee, J. H., Ostrow, C. L., Withrow, M. L., Janney, M. A., Hobbs, G. R., Jr., & Burant, C. (2004). Predictors of patient satisfaction with inpatient hospital nursing care. *Research in Nursing & Health*, 27(4), 254–268.

Laschinger, H. S., Hall, L. M., Pedersen, C., & Almost, J. (2004). A psychometric analysis of the patient satisfaction with nursing care quality questionnaire: An actionable approach to measuring patient satisfaction. *Journal of Nursing Care Quality*, 20(3), 220–230.

Mark, B. A., & Wan, T. T. (2005). Testing measurement equivalence in a patient satisfaction instrument. *Western Journal of Nursing Research*, 27(6), 772–787.

Ryden, M. B., Gross, C. R., Savik, K., Snyder, M., Oh, H. L., Jang, Y., Wang, J., & Krichbaum, K. E. (2000). Development of a measure of resident satisfaction with the nursing home. *Research in Nursing & Health*, 23(3), 237–245.

Ware, J. E., Davies-Avery, A., & Stewart, A. I. (1978). The measurement and meaning of patient satisfaction. *Health & Medical Care Services Review*, 1(1), 1, 3–14.

Wolf, L. R., Giardino, E. R., Osborne, P. A., & Ambrose, M. S. (1994). Dimensions of nurse caring. *Image—The Journal of Nursing Scholarship*, 26(2), 107–111.

Client Satisfaction: Psychological Care 3009

Definition: Extent of positive perception of nursing assistance to cope with emotional issues and perform mental activities

OUTCOME TARGET RATING: Maintain at_____ Increase to_____

OUTCOME OVERALL RATING	Not at all satisfied 1	Somewhat satisfied 2	Moderately satisfied 3	Very satisfied 4	Completely satisfied 5	
Indicators:						
300901 Information provided about course of illness	1	2	3	4	5	NA
300902 Information provided about expected improvement	1	2	3	4	5	NA
300917 Information provided about usual emotional responses to disease	1	2	3	4	5	NA
300918 Information provided about usual emotional responses to treatment regimen	1	2	3	4	5	NA
300904 Assistance with identifying community support groups for client	1	2	3	4	5	NA
300905 Assistance with identifying community support groups for family	1	2	3	4	5	NA
300906 Discussion of strategies to cope with mental impairments	1	2	3	4	5	NA
300907 Emotional support provided	1	2	3	4	5	NA
300908 Counseling provided to improve mental functioning	1	2	3	4	5	NA
300909 Counseling provided to improve emotional stability	1	2	3	4	5	NA
300910 Counseling provided to improve social interactions	1	2	3	4	5	NA
300919 Assistance with finding counseling services	1	2	3	4	5	NA
300912 Support for finding own solutions to problems	1	2	3	4	5	NA
300913 Support for expressing feelings	1	2	3	4	5	NA
300914 Support for working through feelings of loss	1	2	3	4	5	NA
300915 Support for identifying ways to cope with stress	1	2	3	4	5	NA
300916 Support for adjusting to functional changes	1	2	3	4	5	NA
300920 Assistance to address spiritual needs	1	2	3	4	5	NA

Domain-Perceived Health (V)   *Class*-Satisfaction with Care (EE)   *3rd edition 2004; revised 2008*

OUTCOME CONTENT REFERENCES:
Davis, B. A., & Bush, H. A. (1995). Developing effective measurement tools: A case study of the consumer emergency care satisfaction scale. *Journal of Nursing Care Quality, 9*(2), 26–35.
Gesell, S. B., & Gregory, N. (2003). Identifying priority actions for improving patient satisfaction with outpatient cancer care. *Journal of Nursing Care Quality, 19*(3), 226–233.
Larrabee, J. H., Ostrow, C. L., Withrow, M. L., Janney, M. A., Hobbs, G. R., Jr., & Burant, C. (2004). Predictors of patient satisfaction with inpatient hospital nursing care. *Research in Nursing & Health, 27*(4), 254–268.
Laschinger, H. S., Hall, L. M., Pedersen, C., & Almost, J. (2004). A psychometric analysis of the patient satisfaction with nursing care quality questionnaire: An actionable approach to measuring patient satisfaction. *Journal of Nursing Care Quality, 20*(3), 220–230.
Lynn, M. R., & McMillen, B. J. (1999). Do nurses know what patients think is important in nursing care? *Journal of Nursing Care Quality, 13*(5), 65–74.
Mark, B. A., & Wan, T. T. (2005). Testing measurement equivalence in a patient satisfaction instrument. *Western Journal of Nursing Research, 27*(6), 772–787.
Nussbaum, G. B. (2003). Spirituality in critical care: Patient comfort and satisfaction. *Critical Care Nursing Quarterly, 26*(3), 214–220.
Ryden, M. B., Gross, C. R., Savik, K., Snyder, M., Oh, H. L., Jang, Y., Wang, J., & Krichbaum, K. E. (2000). Development of a measure of resident satisfaction with the nursing home. *Research in Nursing & Health, 23*(3), 237–245.
Ware, J. E., Davies-Avery, A., & Stewart, A. I. (1978). The measurement and meaning of patient satisfaction. *Health & Medical Care Services Review, 1*(1), 1, 3–14.

C

Client Satisfaction: Safety   3010

Definition: Extent of positive perception of procedures, information and nursing care to prevent harm or injury

OUTCOME TARGET RATING: Maintain at_____   Increase to_____

		Not at all satisfied	Somewhat satisfied	Moderately satisfied	Very satisfied	Completely satisfied	
OUTCOME OVERALL RATING		1	2	3	4	5	
Indicators:							
301001	Explanation of safety rules and procedures	1	2	3	4	5	NA
301002	Prompt response to injury by staff	1	2	3	4	5	NA
301003	Client identified before receiving medication	1	2	3	4	5	NA
301014	Protective devices used to prevent harm	1	2	3	4	5	NA
301005	Assistance with transfer	1	2	3	4	5	NA
301006	Assistance with ambulation	1	2	3	4	5	NA
301007	Assistance with toileting	1	2	3	4	5	NA
301008	Assistance with bathing	1	2	3	4	5	NA
301009	Warning signs of high-risk environment clearly displayed	1	2	3	4	5	NA
301015	Fall prevention strategies	1	2	3	4	5	NA
301011	Information provided about treatment risks and complications	1	2	3	4	5	NA
301012	Maintenance of safe environment when cognitive function is impaired	1	2	3	4	5	NA
301013	Maintenance of protective environment when at risk for self-injury	1	2	3	4	5	NA

Domain-*Perceived Health (V)*   **Class**-*Satisfaction with Care (EE)*   *3rd edition 2004; revised 2008*

OUTCOME CONTENT REFERENCES:

Abdellah, F. G., & Levine, E. (1957). Developing a measure of patient and personnel satisfaction with nursing care. *Nursing Research*, 5(3), 100–108.

Eriksen, L. (1988). Measuring patient satisfaction with nursing care: A magnitude estimation approach. In C. F. Waltz & O. W. Stickland (Eds.), *Measurement of nursing outcomes* (Vol. 1, pp. 523–527). New York: Springer.

Larrabee, J. H., Ostrow, C. L., Withrow, M. L., Janney, M. A., Hobbs, G. R., Jr., & Burant, C. (2004). Predictors of patient satisfaction with inpatient hospital nursing care. *Research in Nursing & Health*, 27(4), 254–268.

Laschinger, H. S., Hall, L. M., Pedersen, C., & Almost, J. (2004). A psychometric analysis of the patient satisfaction with nursing care quality questionnaire: An actionable approach to measuring patient satisfaction. *Journal of Nursing Care Quality*, 20(3), 220–230.

Lynn, M. R., & McMillen, B. J. (1999). Do nurses know what patients think is important in nursing care? *Journal of Nursing Care Quality*, 13(5), 65–74.

Mark, B. A., & Wan, T. T. (2005). Testing measurement equivalence in a patient satisfaction instrument. *Western Journal of Nursing Research*, 27(6), 772–787.

Ryden, M. B., Gross, C. R., Savik, K., Snyder, M., Oh, H. L., Jang, Y., Wang, J., & Krichbaum, K. E. (2000). Development of a measure of resident satisfaction with the nursing home. *Research in Nursing & Health*, 23(3), 237–245.

Ware, J. E., Davies-Avery, A., & Stewart, A. I. (1978). The measurement and meaning of patient satisfaction. *Health & Medical Care Services Review*, 1(1), 1, 3–14.

Client Satisfaction: Symptom Control   3011

Definition: Extent of positive perception of nursing care to relieve symptoms of illness

OUTCOME TARGET RATING: Maintain at_____   Increase to_____

		Not at all satisfied	Somewhat satisfied	Moderately satisfied	Very satisfied	Completely satisfied	
OUTCOME OVERALL RATING		1	2	3	4	5	
Indicators:							
301101	Patterns of symptoms identified	1	2	3	4	5	NA
301102	Severity of symptoms identified	1	2	3	4	5	NA
301103	Duration of symptoms identified	1	2	3	4	5	NA
301104	Investigation of cause of symptoms	1	2	3	4	5	NA
301105	Actions taken to prevent symptoms	1	2	3	4	5	NA
301106	Symptoms responded to promptly	1	2	3	4	5	NA
301115	Care to control symptoms	1	2	3	4	5	NA
301116	Care to control pain	1	2	3	4	5	NA
301109	Actions taken to provide comfort	1	2	3	4	5	NA
301110	Symptoms regularly monitored	1	2	3	4	5	NA
301111	Monitored for unusual symptoms	1	2	3	4	5	NA
301112	Monitored for control of symptoms	1	2	3	4	5	NA
301113	Monitored for comfort	1	2	3	4	5	NA
301114	Referrals made to other health providers	1	2	3	4	5	NA

Domain-Perceived Health (V)   **Class**-Satisfaction with Care (EE)   *3rd edition 2004; revised 2008*

OUTCOME CONTENT REFERENCES:

Hogan, S. L. (2005). Patient satisfaction with pain management in the emergency department. *Topics in Emergency Medicine, 27*(4), 284–294.

Innis, J., Bikaunieks, N., Petryshen, P., Zellermeyer, V., & Ciccarelli, L. (2004). Patient satisfaction and pain management: An educational approach. *Journal of Nursing Care Quality, 19*(4), 322–327.

Larrabee, J. H., Ostrow, C. L., Withrow, M. L., Janney, M. A., Hobbs, G. R., Jr., & Burant, C. (2004). Predictors of patient satisfaction with inpatient hospital nursing care. *Research in Nursing & Health, 27*(4), 254–268.

Laschinger, H. S., Hall, L. M., Pedersen, C., & Almost, J. (2004). A psychometric analysis of the patient satisfaction with nursing care quality questionnaire: An actionable approach to measuring patient satisfaction. *Journal of Nursing Care Quality, 20*(3), 220–230.

Mark, B. A., & Wan, T. T. H. (2005). Testing measurement equivalence in a patient satisfaction instrument. *Western Journal of Nursing Research, 27*(6), 772–787.

Marsh, G. W. (1999). Measuring patient satisfaction outcomes across provider disciplines. *Journal of Nursing Measurement, 7*(1), 47–62.

Ryden, M. B., Gross, C. R., Savik, K., Snyder, M., Oh, H. L., Jang, Y., Wang, J., & Krichbaum, K. E. (2000). Development of a measure of resident satisfaction with the nursing home. *Research in Nursing & Health, 23*(3), 237–245.

Sterman, E., Gauker, S., & Krieger, J. (2003). A comprehensive approach to improving cancer pain management and patient satisfaction. *Oncology Nursing Forum, 30*(5), 857–864.

Ware, J. E., Davies-Avery, A., & Stewart, A. I. (1978). The measurement and meaning of patient satisfaction. *Health & Medical Care Services Review, 1*(1), 1, 3–14.

C

Client Satisfaction: Teaching 3012

Definition: Extent of positive perception of instruction provided by nursing staff to improve knowledge, understanding, and participation in care

OUTCOME TARGET RATING: Maintain at_____ Increase to_____

OUTCOME OVERALL RATING		Not at all satisfied 1	Somewhat satisfied 2	Moderately satisfied 3	Very satisfied 4	Completely satisfied 5	
Indicators:							
301210	Personal knowledge considered before teaching	1	2	3	4	5	NA
301219	Explanations provided in under standable terms	1	2	3	4	5	NA
301222	Explanation of medical diagnosis	1	2	3	4	5	NA
301223	Explanation of nursing care	1	2	3	4	5	NA
301203	Explanation of diagnostic tests and preparation	1	2	3	4	5	NA
301204	Explanation of results of diagnostic tests	1	2	3	4	5	NA
301205	Explanation of medication therapeutic effects	1	2	3	4	5	NA
301206	Explanation of medication side effects	1	2	3	4	5	NA
301207	Explanation of reasons for treatment	1	2	3	4	5	NA
301208	Explanation of self-care responsibilities for treatment	1	2	3	4	5	NA
301209	Explanation of self-care responsibilities for medication management	1	2	3	4	5	NA
301212	Explanation of activity restrictions	1	2	3	4	5	NA
301213	Discussion of strategies to improve physical strength	1	2	3	4	5	NA
301214	Discussion of strategies to improve physical endurance	1	2	3	4	5	NA
301215	Discussion of strategies to improve health	1	2	3	4	5	NA
301211	Information provided about signs of complications	1	2	3	4	5	NA
301216	Explanation of available health resources	1	2	3	4	5	NA
301217	Explanation of costs of care	1	2	3	4	5	NA
301218	Time for client learning	1	2	3	4	5	NA
301220	Quality of instructional material	1	2	3	4	5	NA
301221	Staff supportive of learning process	1	2	3	4	5	NA

Domain-Perceived Health (V) *Class*-Satisfaction with Care (EE) 3rd edition 2004; revised 2008

OUTCOME CONTENT REFERENCES:

Abramowitz, S., Cote, A. A., & Berry, E. (1987). *Quality Review Bulletin, 13*(4), 122–130.

Davis, B. A., & Bush, H. A. (1995). Developing effective measurement tools: A case study of the consumer emergency care satisfaction scale. *Journal of Nursing Care Quality, 9*(2), 26–35.

Gesell, S. B., & Gregory, N. (2003). Identifying priority actions for improving patient satisfaction with outpatient cancer care. *Journal of Nursing Care Quality, 19*(3), 226–233.

Hinshaw, A. S., & Atwood, J. R. (1982). A patient satisfaction instrument: Precision by replication. *Nursing Research, 31*(3), 170–175.

Larrabee, J. H., Ostrow, C. L., Withrow, M. L., Janney, M. A., Hobbs, G. R., Jr., & Burant, C. (2004). Predictors of patient satisfaction with inpatient hospital nursing care. *Research in Nursing & Health, 27*(4), 254–268.

Laschinger, H. S., Hall, L. M., Pedersen, C., & Almost, J. (2004). A psychometric analysis of the patient satisfaction with nursing care quality questionnaire: An actionable approach to measuring patient satisfaction. *Journal of Nursing Care Quality, 20*(3), 220–230.

Mark, B. A., & Wan, T. T. (2005). Testing measurement equivalence in a patient satisfaction instrument. *Western Journal of Nursing Research, 27*(6), 772–787.

Marsh, G. W. (1999). Measuring patient satisfaction outcomes across provider disciplines. *Journal of Nursing Measurement, 7*(1), 47–62.

Risser, N. L. (1975). Development of an instrument to measure patient satisfaction with nurses and nursing care in primary care settings. *Nursing Research, 24*(1), 45–52.

Ryden, M. B., Gross, C. R., Savik, K., Snyder, M., Oh, H. L., Jang, Y., Wang, J., & Krichbaum, K. E. (2000). Development of a measure of resident satisfaction with the nursing home. *Research in Nursing & Health, 23*(3), 237–245.

Ware, J. E., Davies-Avery, A., & Stewart, A. I. (1978). The measurement and meaning of patient satisfaction. *Health & Medical Care Services Review, 1*(1), 1, 3–14.

Client Satisfaction: Technical Aspects of Care 3013

Definition: Extent of positive perception of nursing staff's knowledge and expertise used in providing care

OUTCOME TARGET RATING: Maintain at_____ Increase to_____

OUTCOME OVERALL RATING	Not at all satisfied 1	Somewhat satisfied 2	Moderately satisfied 3	Very satisfied 4	Completely satisfied 5	
Indicators:						
301301	Correct care provided	1	2	3	4	5	NA
301302	Organization of care	1	2	3	4	5	NA
301303	Thoroughness of care	1	2	3	4	5	NA
301304	Capability of staff	1	2	3	4	5	NA
301305	Registered nurse knowledge of disease process	1	2	3	4	5	NA
301316	Registered nurse knowledge of procedures	1	2	3	4	5	NA
301307	Registered nurse knowledge of medication	1	2	3	4	5	NA
301308	Registered nurse knowledge of health history	1	2	3	4	5	NA
301309	Consistency in performance of care	1	2	3	4	5	NA
301310	Consistency of staff providing care	1	2	3	4	5	NA
301311	Comfort attended to during treatments	1	2	3	4	5	NA
301312	Gentleness of staff	1	2	3	4	5	NA
301317	Competence of staff	1	2	3	4	5	NA
301314	Responsiveness of staff to emergencies	1	2	3	4	5	NA
301315	Supplies and equipment not wasted	1	2	3	4	5	NA

Domain-Perceived Health (V)   *Class-Satisfaction with Care (EE)*   *3rd edition 2004; revised 2008*

OUTCOME CONTENT REFERENCES:

Abdellah, F. G., & Levine, E. (1957). Developing a measure of patient and personnel satisfaction with nursing care. *Nursing Research, 5*(3), 100–108.

Eriksen, L. (1988). Measuring patient satisfaction with nursing care: A magnitude estimation approach. In C. F. Waltz & O. W. Stickland (Eds.), *Measurement of nursing outcomes* (Vol. 1, pp. 523–527). New York: Springer.

Hinshaw, A. S., & Atwood, J. R. (1982). A patient satisfaction instrument: Precision by replication. *Nursing Research, 31*(3), 170–175.

LaMonica, E. L., Oberst, M. T., Madea, A. R., & Wolf, R. M. (1986). Development of a patient satisfaction scale. *Research in Nursing and Health, 9*(1), 43–50.

Larrabee, J. H., Ostrow, C. L., Withrow, M. L., Janney, M. A., Hobbs, G. R., Jr., & Burant, C. (2004). Predictors of patient satisfaction with inpatient hospital nursing care. *Research in Nursing & Health, 27*(4), 254–268.

Laschinger, H. S., Hall, L. M., Pedersen, C., & Almost, J. (2004). A psychometric analysis of the patient satisfaction with nursing care quality questionnaire: An actionable approach to measuring patient satisfaction. *Journal of Nursing Care Quality, 20*(3), 220–230.

Mark, B. A., & Wan, T. T. (2005). Testing measurement equivalence in a patient satisfaction instrument. *Western Journal of Nursing Research, 27*(6), 772–787.

Marsh, G. W. (1999). Measuring patient satisfaction outcomes across provider disciplines. *Journal of Nursing Measurement, 7*(1), 47–62.

Risser, N. L. (1975). Development of an instrument to measure patient satisfaction with nurses and nursing care in primary care settings. *Nursing Research, 24*(1), 45–52.

Ware, J. E., Davies-Avery, A., & Stewart, A. I. (1978). The measurement and meaning of patient satisfaction. *Health & Medical Care Services Review, 1*(1), 1, 3–14.

Wolf, L. R., Giardino, E. R., Osborne, P. A., & Ambrose, M. S. (1994). Dimensions of nurse caring. *Image—The Journal of Nursing Scholarship, 26*(2), 107–111.

Cognition 0900

Definition: Ability to execute complex mental processes

OUTCOME TARGET RATING: Maintain at_____ Increase to_____

		Severely compromised	Substantially compromised	Moderately compromised	Mildly compromised	Not compromised	
OUTCOME OVERALL RATING		1	2	3	4	5	
Indicators:							
090014	Communication clear for age	1	2	3	4	5	NA
090015	Communication appropriate for age	1	2	3	4	5	NA
090013	Comprehension of the meaning of situations	1	2	3	4	5	NA
090003	Attentiveness	1	2	3	4	5	NA
090004	Concentration	1	2	3	4	5	NA
090005	Cognitive orientation	1	2	3	4	5	NA
090006	Immediate memory	1	2	3	4	5	NA
090007	Recent memory	1	2	3	4	5	NA
090008	Remote memory	1	2	3	4	5	NA
090009	Information processing	1	2	3	4	5	NA
090010	Alternatives weighed when making decisions	1	2	3	4	5	NA
090011	Appropriate decision-making	1	2	3	4	5	NA
090016	Complex calculation skills	1	2	3	4	5	NA

Domain-Physiologic Health (II) **Class-**Neurocognitive (J) *1st edition 1997; revised 2004, 2008*

OUTCOME CONTENT REFERENCES:

Abraham, I., & Reel, S. (1993). Cognitive nursing interventions with long-term care residents: Effects on neurocognitive dimensions. *Archives of Psychiatric Nursing, 6*(6), 356–365.

Dellasega, C. (1992). Home health nurses' assessments of cognition. *Applied Nursing Research, 5*(3), 127–133.

Erlanger, D. M., Kaushik, T., Broshek, D., Freeman, J., Feldman, D., & Festa, J. (2002). Development and validation of a web-based screening tool for monitoring cognitive status. *Journal of Head Trauma Rehabilitation 17*(5), 458–476.

+Folstein, M. F., Folstein, S. E., & McHugh, P. R. (1975). "Mini-Mental State"—A practical method for grading the cognitive state of patients for the clinician. *Journal of Psychiatric Research, 12*(3), 189–198.

Foreman, M., Gilles, D., & Wagner, D. (1989). Impaired cognition in the critically ill elderly patient: Clinical implications. *Critical Care Nursing Quarterly, 12*(1), 61–73.

Gerdner, L. A., & Hall, G. R. (2001). Chronic confusion. In M. Maas, K. Buckwalter, M. Hardy, T. Tripp-Reimer, M. Titler, & J. Specht (Eds.), *Nursing care of older adults: Diagnoses, outcomes & interventions* (pp. 421–441). St. Louis: Mosby.

Inaba-Roland, K., & Maricle, R. (1992). Assessing delirium in the acute care setting. *Heart & Lung, 21*(1), 48–55.

Kupferer, S., Uebele, J., & Levin, D. (1988). Geriatric ambulatory surgery patients: Assessing cognitive functions. *AORN Journal, 47*(3), 752–766.

Mason, P. (1989). Cognitive assessment parameters and tools for the critically injured adult. *Critical Care Nursing Clinics of North America, 1*(1), 45–53.

Shih, R. A., Glass, T. A., Bandeen-Roche, K., Carlson, M. C., Bolla, K. I., Todd, A. C., & Schwartz, B. S. (2006). Environmental lead exposure and cognitive function in community-dwelling older adults. *Neurology, 67*(9), 1556–1562.

Souder, E., & O'Sullivan, P. S. (2000). Nursing documentation versus standardized assessment of cognitive status in hospitalized medical patients. *Applied Nursing Research, 13*(1), 29–36.

Strub, R. L., & Black, F. W. (2000). *The mental status examination in neurology* (4th ed.). Philadelphia: F. A. Davis.

Vellinga, A., Smit, J. H., van Leeuwen, E., van Tilburg, W., & Jonker, C. (2004). Instruments to assess decision-making capacity: An overview. *International Psychogeriatrics, 16*(4), 397–419.

Wakefield, B., Mentes, J., Mobily, P., Tripp-Reimer, T., Culp, K. R., Rapp, C. G., Gaspar, P., Kundrat, M., Wadle, K. R., & Akins, J. (2001). Acute confusion. In M. Maas, K. Buckwalter, M. Hardy, T. Tripp-Reimer, M. Titler, & J. Specht (Eds.), *Nursing care of older adults: Diagnoses, outcomes & interventions* (pp. 442–454). St. Louis: Mosby.

Cognitive Orientation 0901

Definition: Ability to identify person, place, and time accurately

OUTCOME TARGET RATING: Maintain at_____ Increase to_____

		Severely compromised	Substantially compromised	Moderately compromised	Mildly compromised	Not compromised	
OUTCOME OVERALL RATING		1	2	3	4	5	
Indicators:							
090101	Identifies self	1	2	3	4	5	NA
090102	Identifies significant other	1	2	3	4	5	NA
090103	Identifies current place	1	2	3	4	5	NA
090104	Identifies correct day	1	2	3	4	5	NA
090105	Identifies correct month	1	2	3	4	5	NA
090106	Identifies correct year	1	2	3	4	5	NA
090107	Identifies correct season	1	2	3	4	5	NA
090109	Identifies significant current events	1	2	3	4	5	NA

Domain-*Physiologic Health (II)* **Class**-*Neurocognitive (J)* *1st edition 1997; revised 2004*

OUTCOME CONTENT REFERENCES:

Abraham, I. L., & Reel, S. J. (1993). Cognitive nursing interventions and long-term care residents: Effects on neurocognitive dimensions. *Archives of Psychiatric Nursing, 6*(6), 356–365.

Agostinelli, B., Demers, K., Garrigan, D., & Waszynski, C. (1994). Targeted interventions: Use of the mini-mental state exam. *Journal of Gerontological Nursing, 20*(8), 15–23.

Aird, T., & McIntosh, M. (2004). Nursing assessment. Nursing tools and strategies to assess cognition and confusion. *British Journal of Nursing 13*(10), 621–626.

Crimlisk, J. T., & Grande, M. M. (2004). Neurologic assessment skills for the acute medical surgical nurse. *Orthopaedic Nursing, 23*(1), 3–11.

Critical Care Network. (2003). Check mental status or risk missing problems: Quick assessment checks for neurological deficit. *Hospital Case Management, 11*(5), 72–74.

Dellasega, C. (1992). Home health nurses' assessments of cognition. *Applied Nursing Research, 5*(3), 127–133.

Foreman, M., Gilles, D., & Wagner, D. (1989). Impaired cognition in the critically ill elderly patient: Clinical implications. *Critical Care Nursing Quarterly, 12*(1), 61–73.

Foreman, M., Theis, S., & Anderson, M. A. (1993). Adverse events in the hospitalized elderly. *Clinical Nursing Research, 2*(3) 360–370.

Gerdner, L. A., & Hall, G. R. (2001). Chronic confusion. In M. Maas, K. Buckwalter, M. Hardy, T. Tripp-Reimer, M. Titler, & J. Specht (Eds.), *Nursing care of older adults: Diagnoses, outcomes & interventions* (pp. 421–441). St. Louis: Mosby.

Hickey, J.V. (2003). *The clinical practice of neurological and neurosurgical nursing* (5th ed.). Philadelphia: Lippincott Williams & Wilkins.

Inaba-Roland, K., & Maricle, R. (1992). Assessing delirium in the acute care setting. *Heart & Lung, 21*(1), 48–55.

Mason, P. (1989). Cognitive assessment parameters and tools for the critically injured adult. *Critical Care Nursing Clinics of North America, 1*(1), 45–53.

Meyer, J., Xu, G., Thornby, J., Chowdhury, M., & Quach, M. (2002). Longitudinal analysis of abnormal domains comprising mild cognitive impairment (MCI) during aging. *Journal of Neurological Sciences, 201*(1–2), 19–25.

+Pfeiffer, E. (1975). A short portable mental status questionnaire for the assessment of organic brain deficit in elderly patients. *American Geriatrics Society, 23*(10), 433–441.

Souder, E., & O'Sullivan, P. S. (2000). Nursing documentation versus standardized assessment of cognitive status in hospitalized medical patients. *Applied Nursing Research, 13*(1), 29–36.

Strub, R. L., & Black, F. W. (2000). *The mental status examination in neurology* (4th ed.). Philadelphia: F. A. Davis.

Thibault, J. M., & Steiner, R. W. P. (2004). Efficient identification of adults with depression and dementia. *American Family Physician, 70*(6), 1101–1110.

C

Comfort Status   2008

Definition: Overall physical, psychospiritual, sociocultural, and environmental ease and safety of an individual

OUTCOME TARGET RATING: Maintain at_____ Increase to_____

		Severely compromised	Substantially compromised	Moderately compromised	Mildly compromised	Not compromised	
OUTCOME OVERALL RATING		1	2	3	4	5	
Indicators:							
200801	Physical well-being	1	2	3	4	5	NA
200802	Symptom control	1	2	3	4	5	NA
200803	Psychological well-being	1	2	3	4	5	NA
200804	Physical surroundings	1	2	3	4	5	NA
200805	Room temperature	1	2	3	4	5	NA
200806	Social support from family	1	2	3	4	5	NA
200807	Social support from friends	1	2	3	4	5	NA
200808	Social relationships	1	2	3	4	5	NA
200809	Spiritual life	1	2	3	4	5	NA
200810	Care consistent with cultural beliefs	1	2	3	4	5	NA
200811	Care consistent with needs	1	2	3	4	5	NA
200812	Ability to communicate needs	1	2	3	4	5	NA

Domain-Perceived Health (V) *Class*-Health & Life Quality (U) 4th edition 2008

OUTCOME CONTENT REFERENCES:
Gropper, E. (1992). Promoting health by promoting comfort. *Nursing Forum, 27*(2), 5–8.
Hamilton, J. (1989). Comfort and the hospitalized chronically ill. *Journal of Gerontological Nursing, 15*(4), 28–33.
Kennedy, G. (1991). *A nursing investigation of comfort and comforting care of the acutely ill patient.* Unpublished doctoral dissertation, The University of Texas, Austin.
Kolcaba, K. (2003). *Comfort theory and practice: A vision for holistic health care and research.* New York: Springer.
Kolcaba, K., & DiMarco, M. (2005). Comfort theory and its application to pediatric nursing. *Pediatric Nursing, 31*(3), 187–194.
Kolcaba, K., Panno, J., & Holder, C. (2000). Acute care for elders (ACE): A holistic model for geriatric orthopaedic nursing care. *Journal of Orthopaedic Nursing, 19*(6), 53–60.
Tipton, L. (2001). A qualitative study of hope and the environment of persons living with cancer. *Dissertation Abstracts International, 62*(03), 1326B. (UMI No. 3008460).

Comfort Status: Environment   2009

Definition: Environmental ease, comfort, and safety of surroundings

OUTCOME TARGET RATING: Maintain at_____ Increase to_____

		Severely compromised	Substantially compromised	Moderately compromised	Mildly compromised	Not compromised	
OUTCOME OVERALL RATING		1	2	3	4	5	
Indicators:							
200901	Needed supplies and equipment within reach	1	2	3	4	5	NA
200902	Room temperature	1	2	3	4	5	NA
200903	Environment conducive to sleep	1	2	3	4	5	NA
200904	Contentment with physical surroundings	1	2	3	4	5	NA
200905	Orderliness of environment	1	2	3	4	5	NA
200906	Cleanliness of environment	1	2	3	4	5	NA

Comfort Status: Environment—*cont'd*

	Severely compromised	Substantially compromised	Moderately compromised	Mildly compromised	Not compromised	
200907	Floor free of clutter	1	2	3	4	5	NA
200908	Safety devices used appropriately	1	2	3	4	5	NA
200909	Room lighting	1	2	3	4	5	NA
200910	Privacy	1	2	3	4	5	NA
200911	Availability of space for visitors	1	2	3	4	5	NA
200912	Comfortable bed	1	2	3	4	5	NA
200913	Comfortable furniture	1	2	3	4	5	NA
200914	Needed environmental adaptations	1	2	3	4	5	NA
200915	Peaceful environment	1	2	3	4	5	NA
200916	Control of noise	1	2	3	4	5	NA
200917	Control of odors	1	2	3	4	5	NA

Domain-Perceived Health (V)   *Class*-Health & Life Quality (U)   4th edition 2008

OUTCOME CONTENT REFERENCES:

Gropper, E. (1992). Promoting health by promoting comfort. *Nursing Forum, 27*(2), 5–8.

Hamilton, J. (1989). Comfort and the hospitalized chronically ill. *Journal of Gerontological Nursing, 15*(4), 28–33.

Kennedy, G. (1991). *A nursing investigation of comfort and comforting care of the acutely ill patient.* Unpublished doctoral dissertation, The University of Texas, Austin.

Kolcaba, K. (2003). *Comfort theory and practice: A vision for holistic health care and research.* New York: Springer.

Kolcaba, K., Panno, J., & Holder, C. (2000). Acute care for elders (ACE): A holistic model for geriatric orthopaedic nursing care. *Journal of Orthopaedic Nursing, 19*(6), 53–60.

Oliver, D., Daly, F., Martin, F. C., & McMurdo, M. E. (2004). Risk factors and risk assessment tools for falls in hospital in-patients: A systematic review. *Age and Ageing, 33*(2), 122–130.

Sherwood, G., Thomas, E., Bennett, D., & Lewis, P. (2002). A teamwork model to promote patient safety in critical care. *Critical Care Nursing Clinics of North America, 14*(4), 333–340.

Tipton, L. (2001). A qualitative study of hope and the environment of persons living with cancer. *Dissertation Abstracts International, 62*(03), 1326B. (UMI No. 3008460).

Comfort Status: Physical   **2010**

Definition: Physical ease related to bodily sensations and homeostatic mechanisms

OUTCOME TARGET RATING: Maintain at_____   Increase to_____

	Severely compromised	Substantially compromised	Moderately compromised	Mildly compromised	Not compromised	
OUTCOME OVERALL RATING	1	2	3	4	5	
Indicators:						
201001	Symptom control	1	2	3	4	5	NA
201002	Physical well-being	1	2	3	4	5	NA
201003	Muscular relaxation	1	2	3	4	5	NA
201004	Comfortable position	1	2	3	4	5	NA
201005	Comfortable clothing	1	2	3	4	5	NA
201006	Personal grooming and hygiene	1	2	3	4	5	NA
201007	Food intake	1	2	3	4	5	NA
201008	Fluid intake	1	2	3	4	5	NA
201009	Energy level	1	2	3	4	5	NA
201010	Body temperature	1	2	3	4	5	NA
201011	Airway patency	1	2	3	4	5	NA
201012	Oxygen saturation	1	2	3	4	5	NA

Continued

C

Comfort Status: Physical—cont'd

		Severe	Substantial	Moderate	Mild	None	
201013	Itching	1	2	3	4	5	NA
201014	Labored breathing	1	2	3	4	5	NA
201015	Air hunger	1	2	3	4	5	NA
201016	Restless legs syndrome	1	2	3	4	5	NA
201017	Muscle aches	1	2	3	4	5	NA
201018	Headache	1	2	3	4	5	NA
201019	Nausea	1	2	3	4	5	NA
201020	Vomiting	1	2	3	4	5	NA
201021	Urinary incontinence	1	2	3	4	5	NA
201022	Bowel incontinence	1	2	3	4	5	NA
201023	Diarrhea	1	2	3	4	5	NA
201024	Constipation	1	2	3	4	5	NA

Domain-Perceived Health (V)   **Class**-Health & Life Quality (U)   4th edition 2008

OUTCOME CONTENT REFERENCES:

Dowd, T., Kolcaba, K., & Steiner, R. (2000). Cognitive strategies to enhance comfort and decrease episodes of urinary incontinence. *Holistic Nursing Practice*, *14*(2), 91–102.

Gropper, E. (1992). Promoting health by promoting comfort. *Nursing Forum*, *27*(2), 5–8.

Hamilton, J. (1989). Comfort and the hospitalized chronically ill. *Journal of Gerontological Nursing*, *15*(4), 28–33.

Kennedy, G. (1991). *A nursing investigation of comfort and comforting care of the acutely ill patient.* Unpublished doctoral dissertation, The University of Texas, Austin.

Kolcaba, K. (2003). *Comfort theory and practice: A vision for holistic health care and research.* New York: Springer.

Tipton, L. (2001). A qualitative study of hope and the environment of persons living with cancer. *Dissertation Abstracts International*, *62*(03), 1326B. (UMI No. 3008460).

Comfort Status: Psychospiritual   2011

Definition: Psychospiritual ease related to self-concept, emotional well-being, source of inspiration, and meaning and purpose in one's life

OUTCOME TARGET RATING: Maintain at_____   Increase to_____

		Severely compromised	Substantially compromised	Moderately compromised	Mildly compromised	Not compromised	
OUTCOME OVERALL RATING		1	2	3	4	5	
Indicators:							
201101	Psychological well-being	1	2	3	4	5	NA
201102	Faith	1	2	3	4	5	NA
201103	Hope	1	2	3	4	5	NA
201104	Self-concept	1	2	3	4	5	NA
201105	Internal picture of self	1	2	3	4	5	NA
201106	Calm and tranquil affect	1	2	3	4	5	NA
201107	Expressions of optimism	1	2	3	4	5	NA
201108	Goal setting	1	2	3	4	5	NA
201109	Meaning and purpose in life	1	2	3	4	5	NA
201110	Spiritual contentment	1	2	3	4	5	NA
201111	Connectedness with inner self	1	2	3	4	5	NA

Comfort Status: Psychospiritual—cont'd

		Severe	Substantial	Moderate	Mild	None	
201112	Depression	1	2	3	4	5	NA
201113	Anxiety	1	2	3	4	5	NA
201114	Stress	1	2	3	4	5	NA
201115	Fear	1	2	3	4	5	NA
201116	Loss of faith	1	2	3	4	5	NA
201117	Sense of spiritual abandonment	1	2	3	4	5	NA
201118	Suicidal thoughts	1	2	3	4	5	NA

Domain-Perceived Health (V)   **Class**-Health & Life Quality (U)   *4th edition 2008*

OUTCOME CONTENT REFERENCES:
Gropper, E. (1992). Promoting health by promoting comfort. *Nursing Forum, 27*(2), 5–8.
Hamilton, J. (1989). Comfort and the hospitalized chronically ill. *Journal of Gerontological Nursing, 15*(4), 28–33.
Kennedy, G. (1991). *A nursing investigation of comfort and comforting care of the acutely ill patient*. Unpublished doctoral dissertation, The University of Texas, Austin.
Kolcaba, K. (2003). *Comfort theory and practice: A vision for holistic health care and research*. New York: Springer.
Kolcaba, K., & Fisher, E. (1996). A holistic perspective on comfort care as an advance directive. *Critical Care Nursing Quarterly, 18*(4), 66–76.
Puchalski, C., Kilpatrick, S., McCullough, M., & Larson, D. (2003). A systematic review of spiritual and religious variables in Palliative Medicine, American Journal of Hospice and Palliative Care, Hospice Journal, Journal of Palliative Care, and Journal of Pain and Symptom Management. *Palliative and Supportive Care, 1*, 7–13.
Tipton, L. (2001). A qualitative study of hope and the environment of persons living with cancer. *Dissertation Abstracts International, 62*(03), 1326B. (UMI No. 3008460).

Comfort Status: Sociocultural   2012

Definition: Social ease related to interpersonal, family, and societal relationships within a cultural context

OUTCOME TARGET RATING: Maintain at_____   Increase to_____

		Severely compromised	Substantially compromised	Moderately compromised	Mildly compromised	Not compromised	
OUTCOME OVERALL RATING		1	2	3	4	5	
Indicators:							
201201	Social support from family	1	2	3	4	5	NA
201202	Social support from friends	1	2	3	4	5	NA
201203	Relationships with family	1	2	3	4	5	NA
201204	Relationships with friends	1	2	3	4	5	NA
201205	Trust in relationships with family	1	2	3	4	5	NA
201206	Trust in relationships with friends	1	2	3	4	5	NA
201207	Social interactions with others	1	2	3	4	5	NA
201208	Care consistent with cultural beliefs	1	2	3	4	5	NA
201209	Availability of culture-specific foods	1	2	3	4	5	NA
201210	Incorporation of cultural beliefs into daily activities	1	2	3	4	5	NA
201211	Use of spoken language	1	2	3	4	5	NA
201212	Ability to communicate needs	1	2	3	4	5	NA
201213	Use of strategies to enhance communication	1	2	3	4	5	NA
201214	Willingness to call on others for help	1	2	3	4	5	NA
201215	Use of disclosure	1	2	3	4	5	NA

Domain-Perceived Health (V)   **Class**-Health & Life Quality (U)   *4th edition 2008*

OUTCOME CONTENT REFERENCES:

Gropper, E. (1992). Promoting health by promoting comfort. *Nursing Forum, 27*(2), 5–8.

Hamilton, J. (1989). Comfort and the hospitalized chronically ill. *Journal of Gerontological Nursing, 15*(4), 28–33.

Kennedy, G. (1991). *A nursing investigation of comfort and comforting care of the acutely ill patient*. Unpublished doctoral dissertation, The University of Texas, Austin.

Kolcaba, K. (2003). *Comfort theory and practice: A vision for holistic health care and research*. New York: Springer.

Leininger, M., & McFarland, M. (2002). *Transcultural nursing concepts, theories, research, & practices* (3rd ed.). New York: McGraw-Hill.

Tipton, L. (2001). A qualitative study of hope and the environment of persons living with cancer. *Dissertation Abstracts International, 62*(03), 1326B. (UMI No. 3008460).

C

Comfortable Death   2007

Definition: Physical, psychospiritual, sociocultural and environmental ease with the impending end of life

OUTCOME TARGET RATING: Maintain at_____   Increase to_____

OUTCOME OVERALL RATING	Severely compromised 1	Substantially compromised 2	Moderately compromised 3	Mildly compromised 4	Not compromised 5	
Indicators:						
200701 Calm affect	1	2	3	4	5	NA
200720 Physical environment	1	2	3	4	5	NA
200721 Room temperature	1	2	3	4	5	NA
200722 Psychological well-being	1	2	3	4	5	NA
200703 Airway patency	1	2	3	4	5	NA
200704 Body temperature	1	2	3	4	5	NA
200705 Comfortable position	1	2	3	4	5	NA
200723 Muscular relaxation	1	2	3	4	5	NA
200724 Support from family	1	2	3	4	5	NA
200725 Support from friends	1	2	3	4	5	NA
200726 Spiritual life	1	2	3	4	5	NA
200708 Personal hygiene	1	2	3	4	5	NA
200709 Oral hygiene	1	2	3	4	5	NA
200710 Food and fluid intake as desired	1	2	3	4	5	NA
200727 Expression of readiness for impending death	1	2	3	4	5	NA

	Severe	Substantial	Moderate	Mild	None	
200711 Moaning	1	2	3	4	5	NA
200712 Suffering	1	2	3	4	5	NA
200713 Thrashing	1	2	3	4	5	NA
200714 Pain	1	2	3	4	5	NA
200715 Itching	1	2	3	4	5	NA
200716 Retching or vomiting	1	2	3	4	5	NA
200717 Diarrhea	1	2	3	4	5	NA
200718 Labored breathing	1	2	3	4	5	NA
200719 Air hunger	1	2	3	4	5	NA
200728 Hyperactivity	1	2	3	4	5	NA
200729 Grimacing	1	2	3	4	5	NA
200730 Rebound tenderness	1	2	3	4	5	NA
200731 Jerking	1	2	3	4	5	NA
200732 Restlessness	1	2	3	4	5	NA

Domain-Perceived Health (V)   **Class**-Health & Life Quality (U)   *3rd edition 2004; revised 2008*

OUTCOME CONTENT REFERENCES:
Byock, I. (1997). *Dying well: The prospect for growth at the end of life*. New York: Riverhead Books.
Ferrell, B. R. (1999). Caring at the end of life. *Reflections, 25*(4), 31–37.
Gropper, E. (1992). Promoting health by promoting comfort. *Nursing Forum, 27*(2), 5–8.
Hamilton, J. (1989). Comfort and the hospitalized chronically ill. *Journal of Gerontological Nursing, 15*(4), 28–33.
Kennedy, G. (1991). *A nursing investigation of comfort and comforting care of the acutely ill patient*. Unpublished doctoral dissertation, The University of Texas, Austin.
Kolcaba, K. (2003). *Comfort theory and practice: A vision for holistic health care and research*. New York: Springer.
Kolcaba, K., & DiMarco, M. (2005). Comfort theory and its application to pediatric nursing. *Pediatric Nursing, 31*(3), 187–194.
Kolcaba, K., & Fisher, E. (1996). A holistic perspective on comfort care as an advance directive. *Critical Care Nursing Quarterly, 18*(4), 66–76.

Communication 0902

Definition: Reception, interpretation, and expression of spoken, written and non-verbal messages

OUTCOME TARGET RATING: Maintain at_____   Increase to_____

OUTCOME OVERALL RATING	Severely compromised 1	Substantially compromised 2	Moderately compromised 3	Mildly compromised 4	Not compromised 5	
Indicators:						
090201 Use of written language	1	2	3	4	5	NA
090202 Use of spoken language	1	2	3	4	5	NA
090203 Use of pictures and drawings	1	2	3	4	5	NA
090204 Use of sign language	1	2	3	4	5	NA
090205 Use of non-verbal language	1	2	3	4	5	NA
090206 Acknowledgment of messages received	1	2	3	4	5	NA
090210 Accurate interpretation of messages received	1	2	3	4	5	NA
090207 Directs messages to correct recipient	1	2	3	4	5	NA
090208 Exchanges messages accurately with others	1	2	3	4	5	NA

Domain-*Physiologic Health (II)*   **Class**-*Neurocognitive (J)*   *1st edition 1997; revised 2004*

OUTCOME CONTENT REFERENCES:
Arnold, E., & Boggs, K. (1999). *Interpersonal relationships: Professional communications skills for nurses* (3rd ed.). Philadelphia: W. B. Saunders.
Emick-Herring, B. (2001). Impaired communication. In M. Maas, K. Buckwalter, M. Hardy, T. Tripp-Reimer, M. Titler, & J. Specht (Eds.), *Nursing care of older adults: Diagnoses, outcomes & interventions* (pp. 664–678). St. Louis: Mosby.
+Harvey, R., & Jellinek, H. (1981). Functional performance assessment: A program approach. *Archives Physical Medicine & Rehabilitation, 62*(9), 456–460.
Potter, P. A., & Perry, A. G. (2001). *Fundamentals of nursing* (5th ed.). St. Louis: Mosby.
Strub, R. L., & Black, F. W. (2000). *The mental status examination in neurology* (4th ed.). Philadelphia: F. A. Davis.

C

Communication: Expressive 0903

Definition: Expression of meaningful verbal and/or non-verbal messages

OUTCOME TARGET RATING: Maintain at_____ Increase to_____

OUTCOME OVERALL RATING	Severely compromised 1	Substantially compromised 2	Moderately compromised 3	Mildly compromised 4	Not compromised 5	
Indicators:						
090301 Use of written language	1	2	3	4	5	NA
090302 Use of spoken language: vocal	1	2	3	4	5	NA
090303 Use of spoken language: esophageal	1	2	3	4	5	NA
090304 Clarity of speech	1	2	3	4	5	NA
090305 Use of pictures and drawings	1	2	3	4	5	NA
090306 Use of sign language	1	2	3	4	5	NA
090307 Use of non-verbal language	1	2	3	4	5	NA
090308 Directs messages to correct recipient	1	2	3	4	5	NA

Domain-*Physiologic Health (II)* **Class**-*Neurocognitive (J)* *1st edition 1997; revised 2004*

OUTCOME CONTENT REFERENCES:
Arnold, E., & Boggs, K. (1999). *Interpersonal relationships: Professional communications skills for nurses* (3rd ed.). Philadelphia: W. B. Saunders.
Emick-Herring, B. (2001). Impaired communication. In M. Maas, K. Buckwalter, M. Hardy, T. Tripp-Reimer, M. Titler, & J. Specht (Eds.), *Nursing care of older adults: Diagnoses, outcomes & interventions* (pp. 664–678). St. Louis: Mosby.
+Harvey, R., & Jellinek, H. (1981). Functional performance assessment: A program approach. *Archives of Physical Medicine & Rehabilitation, 62*(9), 456–460.
Potter, P. A., & Perry, A. G. (2001). *Fundamentals of nursing* (5th ed.). St. Louis: Mosby.
Strub, R. L., & Black, F. W. (2000). *The mental status examination in neurology* (4th ed.). Philadelphia: F. A. Davis.

Communication: Receptive 0904

Definition: Reception and interpretation of verbal and/or non-verbal messages

OUTCOME TARGET RATING: Maintain at_____ Increase to_____

OUTCOME OVERALL RATING	Severely compromised 1	Substantially compromised 2	Moderately compromised 3	Mildly compromised 4	Not compromised 5	
Indicators:						
090401 Interpretation of written language	1	2	3	4	5	NA
090402 Interpretation of spoken language	1	2	3	4	5	NA
090403 Interpretation of pictures and drawings	1	2	3	4	5	NA
090404 Interpretation of sign language	1	2	3	4	5	NA
090405 Interpretation of non-verbal language	1	2	3	4	5	NA
090406 Acknowledgment of messages received	1	2	3	4	5	NA

Domain-*Physiologic Health (II)* **Class**-*Neurocognitive (J)* *1st edition 1997; revised 2000, 2004*

OUTCOME CONTENT REFERENCES:
Arnold, E., & Boggs, K. (1999). *Interpersonal relationships: Professional communications skills for nurses* (3rd ed.). Philadelphia: W. B. Saunders.
Emick-Herring, B. (2001). Impaired communication. In M. Maas, K. Buckwalter, M. Hardy, T. Tripp-Reimer, M. Titler, & J. Specht (Eds.), *Nursing care of older adults: Diagnoses, outcomes & interventions* (pp. 664–678). St. Louis: Mosby.
+Harvey, R., & Jellinek, H. (1981). Functional performance assessment: A program approach. *Archives of Physical Medicine & Rehabilitation, 62*(9), 456–460.
Potter, P. A., & Perry, A. G. (2001). *Fundamentals of nursing* (5th ed.). St. Louis: Mosby.
Strub, R. L., & Black, F. W. (2000). *The mental status examination in neurology* (4th ed.). Philadelphia: F. A. Davis.

Community Competence 2700

Definition: Capacity of a community to collectively problem solve to achieve community goals

OUTCOME TARGET RATING: Maintain at_____ Increase to_____

OUTCOME OVERALL RATING	Poor 1	Fair 2	Good 3	Very good 4	Excellent 5	
Indicators:						
270001 Participation rates in community activities	1	2	3	4	5	NA
270003 Consideration of common and competing interests among groups when solving problems	1	2	3	4	5	NA
270004 Representation of all segments of the community in problem solving	1	2	3	4	5	NA
270005 Community issues articulated in media	1	2	3	4	5	NA
270006 Community issues articulated in community forums	1	2	3	4	5	NA
270007 Focus on community versus individual agendas	1	2	3	4	5	NA
270021 Collaboration among community groups to resolve problems	1	2	3	4	5	NA
270009 Consensus on goals and priorities	1	2	3	4	5	NA
270010 Consensus on actions to implement the goals	1	2	3	4	5	NA
270011 Communication among members and groups	1	2	3	4	5	NA
270012 Effective use of conflict management strategies	1	2	3	4	5	NA
270013 Procurement of resources	1	2	3	4	5	NA
270014 Use of external resources to meet goals	1	2	3	4	5	NA
270015 Flexibility of structures and processes that guide community decision-making	1	2	3	4	5	NA
270016 Participation rate in local government elections	1	2	3	4	5	NA
270017 Participation rate in school elections	1	2	3	4	5	NA
270018 Members attendance at community forums	1	2	3	4	5	NA
270019 Attainment of community goals	1	2	3	4	5	NA

Domain-Community Health (VII)   *Class*-Community Well-Being (BB)   *2nd edition 2000; revised 2004, 2008*

OUTCOME CONTENT REFERENCES:

Denham, A., Quinn, S., & Gamble, D. (1998). Community organizing for health promotion in the rural south: An exploration of community competence. *Family and Community Health, 21*(1), 1–21.

Eng, E., & Parker, E. (1994). Measuring community competence in the Mississippi Delta: The interface between program evaluation and empowerment. *Health Education Quarterly, 21*(2), 119–120.

Goeppinger, L., Lassiter, P., & Wilcox, B. (1982). Community health is community competence. *Nursing Outlook, 30*(8), 464–467.

Stanhope, M., & Lancaster, J. (2000). *Community health nursing* (5th ed.). St. Louis: Mosby.

Community Disaster Readiness 2804

Definition: Community preparedness to respond to a natural or man-made calamitous event

OUTCOME TARGET RATING: Maintain at_____ Increase to_____

		Not adequate	Slightly adequate	Moderately adequate	Substantially adequate	Totally adequate	
OUTCOME OVERALL RATING		1	2	3	4	5	
Indicators:							
280401	Identification of potential types of disasters	1	2	3	4	5	NA
280432	Plan to protect water	1	2	3	4	5	NA
280433	Plan to protect food supplies	1	2	3	4	5	NA
280404	Policy designating temporary administrative authority	1	2	3	4	5	NA
280405	Public health laboratory facilities	1	2	3	4	5	NA
280406	Public health disease surveillance system	1	2	3	4	5	NA
280434	Plan to access electronic health records	1	2	3	4	5	NA
280408	Mass immunization plan	1	2	3	4	5	NA
280409	Surge capacity of hospital resources	1	2	3	4	5	NA
280435	Written plan for mobilization of personnel	1	2	3	4	5	NA
280436	Written plan for evacuation	1	2	3	4	5	NA
280437	Written plan for triage	1	2	3	4	5	NA
280438	Current written plan for communication	1	2	3	4	5	NA
280439	Current written plan for resource appropriation	1	2	3	4	5	NA
280411	Essential agency involvement in planning	1	2	3	4	5	NA
280412	Assignment of agency responsibilities in the event of disaster	1	2	3	4	5	NA
280413	Ongoing training for disaster response personnel	1	2	3	4	5	NA
280414	Plan to protect health and safety of response personnel	1	2	3	4	5	NA
280415	Notification network to alert response personnel	1	2	3	4	5	NA
280416	Notification network to alert government and support agencies	1	2	3	4	5	NA
280417	Operational communication equipment	1	2	3	4	5	NA
280440	Plan for alternative communication among disaster personnel	1	2	3	4	5	NA
280441	Plan for alternative communication among agency networks	1	2	3	4	5	NA
280419	Functional warning mechanisms	1	2	3	4	5	NA
280420	Operational alternative utility resources	1	2	3	4	5	NA
280421	Emergency power backup	1	2	3	4	5	NA
280422	Equipment and supply availability	1	2	3	4	5	NA
280423	Equipment and supply maintenance	1	2	3	4	5	NA
280424	Designated, equipped shelters	1	2	3	4	5	NA
280425	Emergency shelter capacity	1	2	3	4	5	NA
280442	Plan to protect animals	1	2	3	4	5	NA
280426	Regular mass casualty drills with evaluation	1	2	3	4	5	NA
280427	Public education on disaster warning and response	1	2	3	4	5	NA
280428	Media plan for public information updates	1	2	3	4	5	NA
280443	Plan for coordination of victim health care	1	2	3	4	5	NA
280444	Plan for documentation of victim health care	1	2	3	4	5	NA
280430	Plan for availability of mental health care services	1	2	3	4	5	NA
280431	Written post disaster plan	1	2	3	4	5	NA

Domain-Community Health (VII) *Class-Community Health Protection (CC)* *3rd edition 2004; revised 2008*

OUTCOME CONTENT REFERENCES:
American Public Health Association. (2002). *One year after the terrorist attacks: Is public health prepared?* Washington, DC: Author.
Chaffee, M. W. (2005). Hospital response to acute-onset disasters: The state of the science in 2005. *Nursing Clinics of North America, 40*(3), 565–577.
Hassmiller, S. (2000). Disaster management. In M. Stanhope & J. Lancaster (Eds.), *Community and public health nursing* (5th ed.). St. Louis: Mosby.
Landesman, L. Y. (2001). *Public health management of disasters: The practice guide.* Washington, DC: American Public Health Association.
Millin, M. G., Jenkins, J. L., & Kirsch, T. (2006). A comparative analysis of two external health care disaster responses following Hurricane Katrina. *Prehospital Emergency Care, 10*(4), 451–456.
Rowney, R. (2005). The role of public health nursing in emergency preparedness and response. *Nursing Clinics of North America, 40*(3), 499–509.
Santamaria, B. (1995). Nursing in a disaster. In C. M. Smith & F. A. Maurer (Eds.), *Community health nursing: Theory and practice.* Philadelphia: W. B. Saunders.
Stratton, S. J., & Tyler, R. D. (2006). Characteristics of medical surge capacity demand for sudden-impact disasters. *Society for Academic Emergency Medicine, 13*(11), 1193–1197.

Community Disaster Response 2806

Definition: Community response following a natural or man-made calamitous event

OUTCOME TARGET RATING: Maintain at_____   Increase to_____

		Not adequate	Slightly adequate	Moderately adequate	Substantially adequate	Totally adequate	
OUTCOME OVERALL RATING		1	2	3	4	5	
Indicators:							
280609	Command authority identified	1	2	3	4	5	NA
280613	Operation of communication system	1	2	3	4	5	NA
280608	Mobilization of personnel	1	2	3	4	5	NA
280617	Information provided to public	1	2	3	4	5	NA
280611	Triage of injured individuals	1	2	3	4	5	NA
280612	Evacuation of injured individuals	1	2	3	4	5	NA
280610	Evacuation of population	1	2	3	4	5	NA
280601	Availability of safe water	1	2	3	4	5	NA
280602	Availability of safe food	1	2	3	4	5	NA
280603	Availability of medication	1	2	3	4	5	NA
280604	Availability of supplies	1	2	3	4	5	NA
280605	Availability of shelters	1	2	3	4	5	NA
280606	Availability of hospital resources	1	2	3	4	5	NA
280607	Availability of personnel	1	2	3	4	5	NA
280637	Availability of sanitation activities	1	2	3	4	5	NA
280623	Availability of functional equipment	1	2	3	4	5	NA
280614	Government agencies notified of needs	1	2	3	4	5	NA
280615	Support agencies notified of needs	1	2	3	4	5	NA
280618	Response of government agencies in carrying out responsibilities	1	2	3	4	5	NA
280619	Response of support agencies in carrying out responsibilities	1	2	3	4	5	NA
280620	Coordination efforts of local, state, federal, international, and non-governmental agencies	1	2	3	4	5	NA
280621	Performance of response personnel	1	2	3	4	5	NA
280622	Operation of emergency power	1	2	3	4	5	NA
280624	Availability of decontamination equipment	1	2	3	4	5	NA
280625	Access to electronic health records	1	2	3	4	5	NA
280626	Mental health care available for population	1	2	3	4	5	NA
280627	Mental health care available for response personnel	1	2	3	4	5	NA
280628	Response of public health laboratory facilities	1	2	3	4	5	NA
280629	Accurate disposition logs of patient and evacuees	1	2	3	4	5	NA
280630	Data collected on injury patterns	1	2	3	4	5	NA
280631	Data collected on disease incidence	1	2	3	4	5	NA

Continued

C

Community Disaster Response—cont'd

		Not adequate	Slightly adequate	Moderately adequate	Substantially adequate	Totally adequate	
280632	Mass immunization plan	1	2	3	4	5	NA
280633	Availability of morgue facilities	1	2	3	4	5	NA
280634	Provision of care for animals	1	2	3	4	5	NA
280635	Replacement of prescribed medication for individuals with chronic illness	1	2	3	4	5	NA
280636	Post disaster follow-up	1	2	3	4	5	NA

Domain-Community Health (VII)   *Class*-Community Health Protection (CC)   4th edition 2008; revised 2013

OUTCOME CONTENT REFERENCES:

Bass, M. L., Freidhoff, T., & Murphy, E. (2006). Providing consistent medical coverage at community events: North Carolina Rex Hospital's emergency response team. *Journal of Emergency Nursing, 32*(1), 75–77.

Chaffee, M. W. (2005). Hospital response to acute-onset disasters: The state of the science in 2005. *Nursing Clinics of North America, 40*(3), 565–577.

Millin, M. G., Jenkins, J. L., & Kirsch, T. (2006), A comparative analysis of two external health care disaster responses following Hurricane Katrina. *Prehospital Emergency Care, 10*(4), 451–456.

Milsten, A. (2000). Hospital responses to acute-onset disasters: A review. *Prehospital Disaster Medicine, 15*(1), 32–45.

Mitchell, A. M., Sakraida, T. J., & Zalice, K. K. (2005). Disaster care: Psychological considerations. *Nursing Clinics of North America, 40*(3), 535–550.

Tarantino, D. (2006). Asian tsunami relief: Department of defense public health response: Policy and strategic coordination considerations. *Military Medicine, 171*(10), 15–18.

Community Grief Response

2703

Definition: Community response to members' grief that involves loss of life or property

OUTCOME TARGET RATING: Maintain at_____ Increase to_____

		Not adequate	Slightly adequate	Moderately adequate	Substantially adequate	Totally adequate	
OUTCOME OVERALL RATING		1	2	3	4	5	

Indicators:

270301	Assessment of members' needs by leaders	1	2	3	4	5	NA
270302	Coordination of grief response efforts	1	2	3	4	5	NA
270303	Cooperation among members	1	2	3	4	5	NA
270304	Identification of mental health needs of members	1	2	3	4	5	NA
270305	Availability of mental health services	1	2	3	4	5	NA
270306	Opportunities of community recovery activities	1	2	3	4	5	NA
270307	Members' participation in recovery activities	1	2	3	4	5	NA
270308	Community post-trauma response program	1	2	3	4	5	NA
270309	Availability of humanitarian aid	1	2	3	4	5	NA
270310	Community information articulated in media	1	2	3	4	5	NA
270311	Community needs articulated in community forums	1	2	3	4	5	NA
270312	Recognition of members' problems	1	2	3	4	5	NA
270313	Resettlement options	1	2	3	4	5	NA
270314	Community psychosocial integration	1	2	3	4	5	NA
270315	Members' engagement in response to event	1	2	3	4	5	NA
270316	Psychosocial support systems utilization	1	2	3	4	5	NA
270317	Availability of group interventions	1	2	3	4	5	NA
270318	Availability of stabilizing processes	1	2	3	4	5	NA
270319	Availability of coping groups	1	2	3	4	5	NA

Community Grief Response—cont'd

		Not adequate	Slightly adequate	Moderately adequate	Substantially adequate	Totally adequate	
270320	Ability of community to adapt to traumatic losses	1	2	3	4	5	NA
270321	Creation of jobs	1	2	3	4	5	NA
270322	Preservation of jobs	1	2	3	4	5	NA
270323	Revitalization of neighborhoods	1	2	3	4	5	NA
270324	Distribution of economic resources	1	2	3	4	5	NA

Domain-*Community Health (VII)*   *Class*-*Community Well-Being (BB)*   *5th edition 2013*

OUTCOME CONTENT REFERENCES:

Adams, L. M., & Canclini, S. B. (2008). Disaster readiness: A community-university partnership. *Online Journal of Issues in Nursing, 13*(3).

Hilliker, L. (2008). The reporting of grief by one newspaper of record for the U.S.: The New York Times. *Omega: Journal of Death & Dying, 57*(3), 261–278.

Ingram, M., Sabo, S., Rothers, J., Wennerstrom, A., & de Zapien, J. G. (2008). Community health workers and community advocacy: Addressing health disparities. *Journal of Community Health, 33*(6), 417–424.

Jayasinghe, N., Glosan, C., Evans, S., Spielman, L., & Difede, J. (2008). Anger and posttraumatic stress disorder in disaster relief workers exposed to the September 11, 2001 World Trade Center disaster: One-year follow-up study. *Journal of Nervous & Mental Disease, 196*(11), 844–846.

Macy, R. D., Behar, L., Paulson, R., Delman, J., Schmid, L., & Smith, S. F. (2004). Community-based, acute posttraumatic stress management: A description and evaluation of a psychosocial-intervention continuum. *Harvard Review of Psychiatry, 12*(4), 217–228.

International Work Group on Death, Dying, and Bereavement. (2002). Assumptions and principles about psychosocial aspects of disasters. *Death Studies, 26*(6), 449–462.

van den Berg, B., Grievink, L., Gutschmidt, K., Lang, T., Palmer, S., Ruijten, M., Stumpel, R., & Yzermans, J. (2008). The public health dimension of disasters— health outcome assessment of disasters. *Prehospital & Disaster Medicine, 23*(4): s55–s59.

Walsh, F. (2007). Traumatic loss and major disasters: Strengthening family and community resilience. *Family Process, 46*(2), 207–227.

World Health Organization. (2005). *Psychosocial care of tsunami-affected populations: Manual for community level workers.* New Delhi, India: Author.

World Health Organization. (2005). *Psychosocial care of tsunami-affected populations: Physician's manual.* New Delhi, India: Author.

Community Health Screening Effectiveness   2807

Definition: Quality of community actions to screen members for potential health risks or presymptomatic conditions

OUTCOME TARGET RATING: Maintain at_____   Increase to_____

		Poor	Fair	Good	Very good	Excellent	
OUTCOME OVERALL RATING		1	2	3	4	5	

Indicators:

280701	Identification of high-risk conditions prevalent in the population	1	2	3	4	5	NA
280702	Identification of conditions that can benefit from early detection and treatment	1	2	3	4	5	NA
280703	Selection of screening focused on early detection	1	2	3	4	5	NA
280704	Identification of screening needs for infants	1	2	3	4	5	NA
280705	Identification of screening needs for toddlers and preschoolers	1	2	3	4	5	NA
280706	Identification of screening needs for school age children	1	2	3	4	5	NA
280707	Identification of screening needs for adults	1	2	3	4	5	NA
280708	Education of members of importance of screening	1	2	3	4	5	NA
280709	Identification of screening frequency requirements	1	2	3	4	5	NA
280710	Advertisement of screening opportunities	1	2	3	4	5	NA
280711	Identification of resources needed for screening	1	2	3	4	5	NA
280712	Coordination with health care organizations that provide screening	1	2	3	4	5	NA
280713	Outreach to target populations	1	2	3	4	5	NA
280714	Identification of cultural implications of screening	1	2	3	4	5	NA

Continued

Community Health Screening Effectiveness—cont'd

		Poor	Fair	Good	Very good	Excellent	
280715	Evaluation of cost-to-benefit ratio for specific screening	1	2	3	4	5	NA
280716	Provision of screening for prevalent conditions in the community	1	2	3	4	5	NA
280717	Provision of screening for infants	1	2	3	4	5	NA
280718	Provision of screening for toddlers and preschoolers	1	2	3	4	5	NA
280719	Provision of screening for school-age children	1	2	3	4	5	NA
280720	Provision of screening for adults	1	2	3	4	5	NA
280721	Provision of screening for elders	1	2	3	4	5	NA
280722	Mechanism for follow-up	1	2	3	4	5	NA
280723	Mechanism for referral	1	2	3	4	5	NA
280724	Support from influential community members	1	2	3	4	5	NA
280725	Target population participation rates in screening	1	2	3	4	5	NA

Domain-*Community Health (VII)* **Class**-*Community Health Protection (CC)* *5th edition 2013*

OUTCOME CONTENT REFERENCES:

Macha, K., & McDonough, J. P. (2012). *Epidemiology for advanced nursing practice*. Sudbury, MA: Jones & Bartlett.

Nguyen, T., Tanjasiri, S., Kagawa-Singer, M., Tran, J., & Foo, M. (2008). Community health navigators for breast- and cervical-cancer screening among Cambodian and Laotian women: Intervention strategies and relationship-building processes. *Health Promotion Practice, 9*(4), 356–357.

Nies, M. A., & McEwen, M. (2007). *Community/public health nursing: Promoting the health of populations* (4th ed.). Philadelphia: Elsevier Saunders.

Raz, A. E. (2009). Can population-based carrier screening be left to the community? *Journal of Genetic Counseling, 18*(2), 114–118.

Shannon, P., & Anderson, P. R. (2008). Developmental screening in community health care centers and pediatric practices: An evaluation of the baby steps program. *Intellectual and Developmental Disabilities, 46*(4), 281–289.

Community Health Status   2701

Definition: General state of well-being of a community or population

OUTCOME TARGET RATING: Maintain at_____   Increase to_____

		Poor	Fair	Good	Very good	Excellent	
OUTCOME OVERALL RATING		1	2	3	4	5	
Indicators:							
270111	Health status of infants	1	2	3	4	5	NA
270112	Health status of children	1	2	3	4	5	NA
270113	Health status of adolescents	1	2	3	4	5	NA
270114	Health status of adults	1	2	3	4	5	NA
270115	Health status of elders	1	2	3	4	5	NA
270132	Health status of minority populations	1	2	3	4	5	NA
270101	Participation rates in preventive health care services	1	2	3	4	5	NA
270102	Prevalence of health promotion programs	1	2	3	4	5	NA
270103	Prevalence of health protection programs	1	2	3	4	5	NA
270104	School enrollment rate	1	2	3	4	5	NA
270105	School attendance rate	1	2	3	4	5	NA
270106	Participation rates in worksite health programs	1	2	3	4	5	NA
270107	Participation rates in community health programs	1	2	3	4	5	NA

C

Community Health Status—cont'd

		Poor	Fair	Good	Very good	Excellent	
270108	Participation rates in school health programs	1	2	3	4	5	NA
270109	Evidence of health protection measures	1	2	3	4	5	NA
270110	Members with adequate health insurance coverage	1	2	3	4	5	NA
270116	Attendance at programs for healthy pregnancy	1	2	3	4	5	NA
270117	Compliance with environmental health standards	1	2	3	4	5	NA
270124	Mortality rates	1	2	3	4	5	NA
270133	Maternal mortality rates	1	2	3	4	5	NA
270119	Morbidity rates	1	2	3	4	5	NA
270120	Mental health illness rates	1	2	3	4	5	NA
270125	Chronic disease rates	1	2	3	4	5	NA
270134	Substance abuse rates for adults	1	2	3	4	5	NA
270135	Substance abuse rates for adolescents	1	2	3	4	5	NA
270136	Smoking rates	1	2	3	4	5	NA
270126	Sexually transmitted disease rates	1	2	3	4	5	NA
270137	Preterm birth rates	1	2	3	4	5	NA
270138	Low birth weight rates	1	2	3	4	5	NA
270121	Injury rates	1	2	3	4	5	NA
270122	Crime statistics	1	2	3	4	5	NA
270139	Homicide rates	1	2	3	4	5	NA
270127	Health surveillance data systems in place	1	2	3	4	5	NA
270128	Community health standards for health measurement and evaluation are defined	1	2	3	4	5	NA
270129	Monitoring of community health standards for health measurement and evaluation	1	2	3	4	5	NA
270130	Community demographics represented in health care planning and evaluation	1	2	3	4	5	NA

Domain-*Community Health (VII)* **Class**-*Community Well-Being (BB)* *2nd edition 2000; revised 2004, 2008*

OUTCOME CONTENT REFERENCES:
Deal, L. (1994). The effectiveness of community health nursing interventions: A literature review. *Public Health Nursing, 2*(5), 315–322.
Stanhope, M., & Lancaster, J. (2000). *Community health nursing* (5th ed.). St. Louis: Mosby.
Stoto, M. (1997). Sharing responsibility for the public's health: A new perspective from the Institute of Medicine. *Journal of Public Health Management and Practice, 3*(5), 22–34.
U.S. Department of Health and Human Services. (2000). *Healthy people 2010.* Washington, DC: Government Printing Office.
U.S. Department of Health and Human Services. (1991). *Healthy people 2000: National health promotion and disease prevention objectives.* (DHHS Pub No (PHS) 91-50012). Washington, DC: Government Printing Office.

C

Community Immune Status 2800

Definition: Resistance of community members to the invasion and spread of an infectious agent that could threaten public health

OUTCOME TARGET RATING: Maintain at_____ Increase to_____

		Poor	Fair	Good	Very good	Excellent	
OUTCOME OVERALL RATING		1	2	3	4	5	
Indicators:							
280001	Immunization rates equal to or greater than current national standards	1	2	3	4	5	NA
280002	Incidence of vaccine-preventable disease at or below recommended national rate	1	2	3	4	5	NA
280003	Prevalence of vaccine-preventable disease at or below recommended national rate	1	2	3	4	5	NA
280004	Surveillance of immunization status in schools	1	2	3	4	5	NA
280005	Surveillance of immunization status in group living facilities (e.g., jails, group homes)	1	2	3	4	5	NA
280006	Surveillance of communicable disease	1	2	3	4	5	NA
280007	Screening of at-risk populations for infections	1	2	3	4	5	NA
280008	Compliance with immunization recommendations	1	2	3	4	5	NA
280009	Culturally appropriate public education on the risks and benefits of immunization	1	2	3	4	5	NA
280010	Availability of low-cost immunizations	1	2	3	4	5	NA
280011	Enforcement of required immunizations prior to school attendance	1	2	3	4	5	NA

Domain-Community Health (VII)   *Class*-Community Well-Being (BB)   2nd edition 2000; revised 2004, 2013

OUTCOME CONTENT REFERENCES:
Centers for Disease Control and Prevention. (2011). Prevention and control of influenza with vaccines: Recommendations of the Advisory Committee on Immunization Practices (ACIP), 2011. *Morbidity and Mortality Weekly Report, 60*(33), 1128–1132.
Centers for Disease Control and Prevention. (2011). National and state vaccination coverage among adolescents aged 13 through 17 years—United States, 2010. *Morbidity and Mortality Weekly Report, 60*(33), 1117–1123
Johnson, H. (2011). Childhood immunization—Who gets what, when? *Practice Nurse, 41*(12), 14–18.
Stanhope, M., & Lancaster, J. (2000). *Community health nursing* (5th ed.). St. Louis: Mosby.
U.S. Department of Health and Human Services. (2000). *Healthy people 2010*. Washington, DC: Government Printing Office.
U.S. Preventive Services Task Force. (2010). *The guide to clinical preventive services 2010-2011* (AHRQ Publication No. 10-05145). Rockville, MD: Agency for Healthcare Research and Quality.

Community Program Effectiveness 2808

Definition: Quality of coordinated program activities that promote health and prevent, reduce, or eliminate health problems for an aggregate or population

OUTCOME TARGET RATING: Maintain at_____ Increase to_____

		Poor	Fair	Good	Very good	Excellent	
OUTCOME OVERALL RATING		1	2	3	4	5	
Indicators:							
280801	Program goals consistent with community assessment	1	2	3	4	5	NA
280802	Achievable program goals	1	2	3	4	5	NA
280803	Consistency of content with program goals	1	2	3	4	5	NA
280804	Consistency of methods with program goals	1	2	3	4	5	NA
280805	Quality of program methods	1	2	3	4	5	NA
280806	Timetable for program activities	1	2	3	4	5	NA
280807	Marketing plans for the program	1	2	3	4	5	NA
280808	Participation rate in program	1	2	3	4	5	NA
280809	Reduction in targeted health risks for participants	1	2	3	4	5	NA
280810	Improvement of health status of participants	1	2	3	4	5	NA
280811	Financial resources for program	1	2	3	4	5	NA
280812	Qualified program personnel	1	2	3	4	5	NA
280813	Program goals supported by data	1	2	3	4	5	NA
280814	Cost-benefit analyses support program	1	2	3	4	5	NA
280815	Measurement of program goals	1	2	3	4	5	NA
280816	Participants' satisfaction with program	1	2	3	4	5	NA
280817	Community members' satisfaction with program	1	2	3	4	5	NA
280818	Support from influential community representatives						
280819	Plans for sustaining successful program	1	2	3	4	5	NA

Domain-Community Health (VII)   *Class-Community Health Protection (CC)*   *5th edition 2013*

OUTCOME CONTENT REFERENCES:

Andrulis, D., & Brach, C. (2007). Integrating literacy, culture, and language to improve health care quality for diverse populations. *American Journal of Health Behavior, 31*(Suppl. 1), S122–S133.

Anema, M., Brown, B., & Stringfield, Y. (2003). Organizing and presenting: Program outcome data. *Nursing Education Perspectives, 24*(6), 306–310.

Brand, A., Walker, D., Hargreaves, M., & Rosenbach, M. (2010). Intermediate outcomes, strategies, and challenges of eight healthy start projects. *Maternal and Child Health Journal, 14*(5), 854–865.

Meade, C., Menard, J., Thervil, C., Rivera, M. (2009). Addressing cancer disparities through community engagement: Improving breast health among Haitian women. *Oncology Nursing Forum, 36*(6), 716–722.

Moodie, M., Carter, R., Swinburn, B., & Haby, M. (2010). The cost-effectiveness of Australia's active after-school communities program. *Obesity, 18*(8), 1585–1592.

Ovbiagele, B., Saver, J. L., Fredieu, A., Suzuki, S., McNair, N., Dandekar, A., Razinia, T., & Kidwell, C. S. (2004). PROTECT: A coordinated stroke treatment program to prevent recurrent thromboembolic events. *Neurology, 63*(7), 1217–1222.

Rome, S. (2002). Developing a fall-prevention program for patients. *American Journal of Nursing, 102*(6), 24A–24D.

Scriven, A., & Speller, V. (2007). Global issues and challenges beyond Ottawa: The way forward. *Promotion & Education, 14*(4), 269–273.

Smith, I., Koegel, R., Koegel, L., Openden, D., Fossum, K., & Bryson, S., (2010). Effectiveness of a novel community-based early intervention model for children with autistic spectrum disorder. *American Journal of Intellectual and Developmental Disabilities, 115*(6), 504–523.

Swallow, A. D., & Dykes, P. C. (2004). Tobacco cessation at Greenwich Hospital. *American Journal of Nursing, 104*(12), 61–62.

Woodward, D. (2005). Developing a pain management program through continuous improvement strategies. *Journal of Nursing Care Quality, 20*(3), 261–267.

Community Resiliency 2704

Definition: Community actions to collectively adapt and function in response to adverse socio-economic, geopolitical, and physical environmental challenges

OUTCOME TARGET RATING: Maintain at_____ Increase to_____

OUTCOME OVERALL RATING		Poor 1	Fair 2	Good 3	Very good 4	Excellent 5	
Indicators:							
270401	Community assessment plan	1	2	3	4	5	NA
270402	Community resources prepared to respond	1	2	3	4	5	NA
270403	Ongoing training for communication requirements	1	2	3	4	5	NA
270404	Currency of response plan	1	2	3	4	5	NA
270405	Community mobilization following adversity	1	2	3	4	5	NA
270406	Key leaders' monitoring of socio-economic environment	1	2	3	4	5	NA
270407	Key leaders' monitoring of geopolitical environment	1	2	3	4	5	NA
270408	Key leaders' monitoring of physical environment	1	2	3	4	5	NA
270409	Key leaders' coordination response	1	2	3	4	5	NA
270410	Key leaders' conflict-resolution strategies	1	2	3	4	5	NA
270411	Key leaders' encouragement of hope for the future	1	2	3	4	5	NA
270412	Continuation of routine community services	1	2	3	4	5	NA
270413	Availability of health care services	1	2	3	4	5	NA
270414	Availability of mental health care services	1	2	3	4	5	NA
270415	Availability of resources to maintain basic needs	1	2	3	4	5	NA
270416	Information provided in a timely manner	1	2	3	4	5	NA
270417	Use of communication networks	1	2	3	4	5	NA
270418	Inter-organizational collaboration within the community	1	2	3	4	5	NA
270419	Collaboration with state agencies	1	2	3	4	5	NA
270420	Collaboration with federal agencies	1	2	3	4	5	NA
270421	Support agencies notified of needs	1	2	3	4	5	NA
270422	Access to external resources	1	2	3	4	5	NA
270423	Policies that enable participation of grass-roots organizations	1	2	3	4	5	NA
270424	Support of members affected by change in environment	1	2	3	4	5	NA
270425	Community discussion of impact of changes in environment	1	2	3	4	5	NA
270426	Community expression of confidence in overcoming adversity	1	2	3	4	5	NA
270427	Community cooperation to meet challenges	1	2	3	4	5	NA
270428	Community support groups	1	2	3	4	5	NA
270429	Community adaptation to changes	1	2	3	4	5	NA
270430	Community preparation for future challenges	1	2	3	4	5	NA

Domain-Community Health (VII)　**Class**-Community Well-Being (BB)　5th edition 2013

OUTCOME CONTENT REFERENCES:

Nuwayhid, I., Huda, Z., Rouham, Y., & Cortas, C. (2011). Summer 2006 war on Lebanon: A lesson in community resilience. *Global Public Health*, *6*(5), 505–519.

Norris, F. H., & Stevens, S. P. (2007). Community resilience and the principles of mass trauma intervention. *Psychiatry: Interpersonal & Biological Processes*, *70*(4), 320–327.

Vaughan, E., & Tinker, T. (2009). Effective health risk communication about pandemic influenza for vulnerable populations. *American Journal of Public Health*, *99*(Suppl. 2), S324–S332.

Wyche, K., Pfefferbaum, R., Pfefferbaum, B., Norris, F., Wisnieski, D., & Younger, H. (2011). Exploring community resilience in workforce communities of first responders serving Katrina survivors. *American Journal of Orthopsychiatry*, *81*(1), 18–30.

Community Risk Control: Chronic Disease 2801

Definition: Community actions to eliminate or reduce the incidence of chronic diseases and related complications

OUTCOME TARGET RATING: Maintain at_____ Increase to_____

		Poor	Fair	Good	Very good	Excellent	
OUTCOME OVERALL RATING		1	2	3	4	5	
Indicators:							
280101	Provision of public education programs on chronic disease	1	2	3	4	5	NA
280102	Target population participation rates in risk-reduction programs	1	2	3	4	5	NA
280103	Availability of preventive screening programs	1	2	3	4	5	NA
280104	Target population participation rates in preventive screening programs	1	2	3	4 .	5	NA
280105	Availability of chronic disease self-management education programs	1	2	3	4	5	NA
280106	Proportion of target population participation rates in chronic disease self-management education programs	1	2	3	4	5	NA
280107	Availability of health care services to treat chronic disease	1	2	3	4	5	NA
280118	Provision of health care services to fit target population	1	2	3	4	5	NA
280119	Monitoring of incidence of chronic disease	1	2	3	4	5	NA
280120	Monitoring of prevalence of chronic disease	1	2	3	4	5	NA
280121	Monitoring of chronic disease morbidity	1	2	3	4	5	NA
280122	Monitoring of chronic disease mortality	1	2	3	4	5	NA
280123	Monitoring of chronic disease complications	1	2	3	4	5	NA
280111	Compliance with national standards for chronic disease prevention and management	1	2	3	4	5	NA
280112	Incidence of chronic disease at or below state or national rates	1	2	3	4	5	NA
280114	Prevalence of chronic disease at or below state or national rates	1	2	3	4	5	NA
280124	Public policies that promote health	1	2	3	4	5	NA
280125	Public policies that prevent disease	1	2	3	4	5	NA
280116	Procurement and allocation of funding for chronic disease prevention programs	1	2	3	4	5	NA
280126	Evidence of advocacy efforts for prevention of chronic illness	1	2	3	4	5	NA
280127	Evidence of advocacy efforts for management of chronic illness	1	2	3	4	5	NA

Domain-*Community Health (VII)*   **Class**-*Community Health Protection (CC)*   *2nd edition 2000; revised 2004, 2008, 2013*

OUTCOME CONTENT REFERENCES:
Clemen-Stone, S., McGuire, S. L., & Eigsti, D. G. (2002). *Comprehensive community health nursing: Family, aggregate, and community practice* (6th ed.). St. Louis: Mosby.
Robinson, K. L., Driedger, M. S., Elliot, S. J., & Eyles, J. (2006). Understanding facilitators of and barriers to health promotion practice. *Health Promotion Practice*, 7(4), 467–476.
Stanhope, M., & Lancaster, J. (2000). *Community health nursing* (5th ed.). St. Louis: Mosby.
U.S. Department of Health and Human Services. (2000). *Healthy people 2010*. Washington, DC: Government Printing Office.
U.S. Department of Health and Human Services. (2010). *The guide to clinical preventive services 2010–2011: Recommendations of the U.S. Preventive Services Task Force*. Rockville, MD: Agency for Healthcare Research and Quality.

Community Risk Control: Communicable Disease 2802

Definition: Community actions to eliminate or reduce the spread of infectious agents that threaten public health

OUTCOME TARGET RATING: Maintain at_____ Increase to_____

OUTCOME OVERALL RATING	Poor 1	Fair 2	Good 3	Very good 4	Excellent 5	
Indicators:						
280201 Screening of all targeted high-risk groups	1	2	3	4	5	NA
280202 Surveillance for infectious disease outbreaks including a system of data collection, reporting and follow-up	1	2	3	4	5	NA
280203 Investigation and notification of contacts concerning risk for infectious disease	1	2	3	4	5	NA
280204 Disease occurrences reported as mandated	1	2	3	4	5	NA
280205 Availability of treatment services for infected individuals	1	2	3	4	5	NA
280206 Provision of products to decrease disease spread	1	2	3	4	5	NA
280207 Established polices and surveillance for assuring safe food storage, handling, and preparation	1	2	3	4	5	NA
280208 Water testing consistent with local, state and federal regulations	1	2	3	4	5	NA
280209 Promotion of community wide immunization	1	2	3	4	5	NA
280220 Plan for mass immunization	1	2	3	4	5	NA
280210 Enforcement of infection-surveillance programs	1	2	3	4	5	NA
280221 Enforcement of infection-control programs	1	2	3	4	5	NA
280211 Availability of chemoprophylaxis for travelers	1	2	3	4	5	NA
280212 Evidence of environmental controls	1	2	3	4	5	NA
280213 Enforcement of environmental monitoring policies	1	2	3	4	5	NA
280214 Enforcement of domestic animal vaccination	1	2	3	4	5	NA
280215 Availability of health care services to treat communicable diseases	1	2	3	4	5	NA
280216 Access to health care services	1	2	3	4	5	NA
280217 Culturally appropriate public education about transmission of infectious disease	1	2	3	4	5	NA
280218 Policies supporting control of infectious disease	1	2	3	4	5	NA
280222 Monitoring of communicable disease morbidity	1	2	3	4	5	NA
280223 Monitoring of communicable disease mortality	1	2	3	4	5	NA
280224 Monitoring of communicable disease complications	1	2	3	4	5	NA

Domain-*Community Health (VII)* **Class**-*Community Health Protection (CC)* *2nd edition 2000; revised 2004, 2008*

OUTCOME CONTENT REFERENCES:
Stanhope, M., & Lancaster, J. (2000). *Community health nursing* (5th ed.). St. Louis: Mosby.
U.S. Department of Health and Human Services. (1991). *Healthy people 2000: National health promotion and disease prevention objectives* (DHHS Pub No (PHS) 91-50012). Washington, DC: Government Printing Office.
U.S. Department of Health and Human Services. (2000). *Healthy people 2010.* Washington, DC: Government Printing Office.
Veenema, T. G., & Toke, J. (2006). Early detection and surveillance for biopreparedness and emerging infectious diseases. *Online Journal of Issues in Nursing,* *11*(1), 47–59.

Community Risk Control: Lead Exposure   2803

Definition: Community actions to eliminate or reduce lead exposure and poisoning

OUTCOME TARGET RATING: Maintain at_____   Increase to_____

		Poor	Fair	Good	Very good	Excellent	
OUTCOME OVERALL RATING		1	2	3	4	5	
Indicators:							
280314	Problem assessment by community stakeholders and policy makers	1	2	3	4	5	NA
280315	Organization of lead screening programs that includes focus on preschools	1	2	3	4	5	NA
280316	Culturally appropriate marketing of screening programs to high-risk groups	1	2	3	4	5	NA
280301	Use of lead screening programs by targeted high-risk groups	1	2	3	4	5	NA
280317	Organization of referral and treatment services for exposed individuals	1	2	3	4	5	NA
280302	Referral of exposed individuals to treatment	1	2	3	4	5	NA
280318	Treatment of individuals with exposure to lead	1	2	3	4	5	NA
280303	Surveillance for sources of lead	1	2	3	4	5	NA
280304	Abatement of known lead sources in the community	1	2	3	4	5	NA
280305	Programs to identify nutritional deficiencies in targeted high-risk groups	1	2	3	4	5	NA
280306	Programs to correct nutritional deficiencies in targeted high-risk groups	1	2	3	4	5	NA
280307	Provision of culturally appropriate public education about lead poisoning prevention	1	2	3	4	5	NA
280319	Participation rates of high-risk groups in education programs	1	2	3	4	5	NA
280308	Policies that require the removal of lead-based paint from all buildings	1	2	3	4	5	NA
280321	Funds dedicated to screening of lead hazards	1	2	3	4	5	NA
280322	Funds dedicated to elimination of lead hazards	1	2	3	4	5	NA
280310	Incidence of elevated lead levels at or below recommended national standards	1	2	3	4	5	NA
280311	Enforcement of home-buyer notification	1	2	3	4	5	NA
280320	Advocacy on behalf of renters of pre-1950 homes	1	2	3	4	5	NA
280312	Enforcement of emission standards	1	2	3	4	5	NA

Domain-Community Health (VII)   *Class-Community Health Protection (CC)*   *2nd edition 2000; revised 2004, 2008, 2013*

OUTCOME CONTENT REFERENCES:

Kincl, L. D., Dietrich, K. N., & Bhattacharya, A. (2006). Injury trends for adolescents with early childhood lead exposure. *Journal of Adolescent Health, 39*(4), 604–606.

Morgan, L. (1996). Children and lead: A model of care for community health providers. *Family and Community Health, 19*(1), 42–48.

Needleman, H. (1998). Childhood lead poisoning: The promise and abandonment of primary prevention. *American Journal of Public Health, 88*(12), 1871–1876.

Needleman, H., Schell, A., Bellinger, D., Leviton, A., & Allred, E. (1990). The long-term effects of exposure to low doses of lead in childhood. *The New England Journal of Medicine, 22*(2), 83–90.

Rischitelli, G., Nygren, P., Biougatsos, C., Feeman, M., & Helfand, M. (2006). Screening for elevated lead levels in childhood and pregnancy: An update summary of evidence for the US Preventive Services Task Force. *Pediatrics, 118*(6), 1867–1895.

Schwartz, J. (1994). Societal benefits of reducing lead exposure. *Environmental Research, 66*(1), 105–124.

Shih, R. A., Glass, T. A., Bandeen-Roche, K., Carlson, M. C., Bolla, K. I., Todd, A. C., & Schwartz, B. S. (2006). Environmental lead exposure and cognitive function in community-dwelling older adults. *Neurology, 67*(9), 1556–1562.

C

Community Risk Control: Obesity 2809

Definition: Community actions to reduce obesity and related chronic diseases

OUTCOME TARGET RATING: Maintain at_____ Increase to_____

OUTCOME OVERALL RATING	Poor 1	Fair 2	Good 3	Very good 4	Excellent 5	

Indicators:

		Poor 1	Fair 2	Good 3	Very good 4	Excellent 5	
280901	Identification of cultural components of the obesity epidemic	1	2	3	4	5	NA
280902	Screening of high-risk members across the lifespan	1	2	3	4	5	NA
280903	Provision of community education programs on prevention of obesity	1	2	3	4	5	NA
280904	Participation rates of high-risk members in educational programs	1	2	3	4	5	NA
280905	Provision of children's programs to encourage physical activity	1	2	3	4	5	NA
280906	Participation rates in children's programs that encourage physical activity	1	2	3	4	5	NA
280907	Education of parents on importance of physical activity	1	2	3	4	5	NA
280908	Provision of healthy meals in lunch programs	1	2	3	4	5	NA
280909	Provision of family events that encourage active lifestyles	1	2	3	4	5	NA
280910	Provision of school-based obesity prevention programs	1	2	3	4	5	NA
280911	Provision of community programs to encourage activity	1	2	3	4	5	NA
280912	Provision of educational programs focused on healthy diet	1	2	3	4	5	NA
280913	Availability of community resources to support weight loss	1	2	3	4	5	NA
280914	Availability of affordable healthy food and beverages in public service venues	1	2	3	4	5	NA
280915	Limitation of unhealthy food and beverages advertisements	1	2	3	4	5	NA
280916	Incentives for food retailers to offer healthy food and beverage choices	1	2	3	4	5	NA
280917	Availability of fresh produce for purchase	1	2	3	4	5	NA
280918	Access to recreational facilities	1	2	3	4	5	NA
280919	Community facilities for physical activities	1	2	3	4	5	NA
280920	Availability of bicycle paths	1	2	3	4	5	NA
280921	Availability of walking paths	1	2	3	4	5	NA
280922	Availability of parks	1	2	3	4	5	NA
280923	Community coalitions to address obesity epidemic	1	2	3	4	5	NA
280924	Monitoring the incidence of obesity	1	2	3	4	5	NA
280925	Monitoring the incidence of diabetes	1	2	3	4	5	NA
280926	Monitoring the incidence of cardiovascular disease	1	2	3	4	5	NA
280927	Monitoring obesity complications	1	2	3	4	5	NA
280928	Public policies that promote healthy living	1	2	3	4	5	NA
280929	Procurement and allocation of funding for obesity prevention programs	1	2	3	4	5	NA

Domain-Community Health (VII)   *Class*-Community Health Protection (CC)   *5th edition 2013*

OUTCOME CONTENT REFERENCES:

Anderson, S., & Whitaker, R. (2010). Household routines and obesity in US preschool-aged children. *Pediatrics, 125*(3), 420–428.

Bauer, K., Neumark-Sztainer, D., Hannan, P., Fulkerson, J., & Story, M. (2011). Relationships between the family environment and school-based obesity prevention efforts: Can school programs help adolescents who are most in need? *Health Education Research, 26*(4), 675–688.

Cappellano, K. (2011). Let's move—Tools to fuel a healthier population. *Nutrition Today, 46*(3), 149–154.

Khan, L., Sobush, K., Keener, D., Goodman, K., Lowry, A., Kakierek, J., & Zaro, S. (2009). Recommended community strategies and measurements to prevent obesity in the United States. *Morbidity and Mortality Weekly Report, 58*(RR-7), 1–26.

Kwapiszewski, R., & Wallace, A. (2011). A pilot program to identify and reverse childhood obesity in a primary care clinic. *Clinical Pediatrics, 50*(7), 630–635.

Tucker, S., Foster, L., Murphy, J., Olsen, G., Orth, K., Voss, J., Aleman, M., & Lohse, C. (2011). A school based community partnership for promoting healthy habits for life. *Journal of Community Health, 36*(3), 414–422.

Uusitupa, M., Tuomilehto, J., & Puska, P. (2011). Are we really active in the prevention of obesity and type 2 diabetes at the community level? *Nutrition, Metabolism, & Cardiovascular Diseases, 21*(5), 380–389.

Community Risk Control: Unhealthy Cultural Traditions 2810

Definition: Community actions to promote customs, beliefs, values, and laws that support members' health and lifestyle modifications within the culture

OUTCOME TARGET RATING: Maintain at_____ Increase to_____

		Poor	Fair	Good	Very good	Excellent	
OUTCOME OVERALL RATING		1	2	3	4	5	

Indicators:

281001	Systematic assessment of cultural practices within the community	1	2	3	4	5	NA
281002	Representation of all segments of the community	1	2	3	4	5	NA
281003	Mobilization of community members to identify healthy cultural practices	1	2	3	4	5	NA
281004	Mobilization of community members to identify harmful cultural practices	1	2	3	4	5	NA
281005	Mobilization of community members to eliminate harmful cultural practices	1	2	3	4	5	NA
281006	Use of influential community representatives to foster recommended changes	1	2	3	4	5	NA
281007	Availability of financial resources	1	2	3	4	5	NA
281008	Educational programs for reinforcement of healthy cultural practices	1	2	3	4	5	NA
281009	Educational opportunities to discuss harmful cultural practices	1	2	3	4	5	NA
281010	Promotion of laws against harmful practices	1	2	3	4	5	NA
281011	Enforcement of existing legislation	1	2	3	4	5	NA
281012	Incentives for healthy behavior	1	2	3	4	5	NA
281013	Treatment of members with conditions related to harmful practice	1	2	3	4	5	NA
281014	Availability of referral systems for counseling	1	2	3	4	5	NA
281015	Availability of culturally relevant resources	1	2	3	4	5	NA
281016	Capacity of the community to monitor harmful practices	1	2	3	4	5	NA
281017	Modifications of harmful cultural practices to make them safe	1	2	3	4	5	NA
281018	Elimination of harmful cultural practices	1	2	3	4	5	NA
281019	Reinforcement of healthy cultural practices	1	2	3	4	5	NA

Domain-Community Health (VII)   **Class**-Community Health Protection (CC)   5th edition 2013

OUTCOME CONTENT REFERENCES:

Al-Qattan, M., & Al-Zahrani, K. (2009). A review of burns related to traditions, social habits, religious activities, festivals and traditional medical practices. *Burns, 35*(4), 476–481.

Bell, R., Hillers, V., & Thomas, T. (1999). Hispanic grandmothers preserve cultural traditions and reduce foodborne illness by conducting safe cheese workshops. *Journal of the American Dietetic Association, 99*(9), 1114–1116.

Natoli, L., Renzaho, A., & Rinaudo, T. (2008). Reducing harmful traditional practices in Adjibar, Ethiopia: Lessons learned from the Adjibar safe motherhood project. *Contemporary Nurse, 29*(1), 110–119.

Smeltzer, S., Bare, B., Hinkle, J., & Cheever, K. (2008). *Brunner and Suddarth's textbook of medical-surgical nursing* (11th ed., pp. 127–138). Philadelphia: Lippincott Williams Wilkins.

The United Nations Children's Fund. (2005). *Female genital mutilation/cutting: A statistical exploration 2005*. New York: Author.

World Health Organization. (2001). *Female genital mutilation: Integrating the prevention and the management of the health complications into the curricula of nursing and midwifery—a teacher's guide*. Geneva, Switzerland: Author.

Community Risk Control: Violence 2805

Definition: Community actions to eliminate or reduce intentional violent acts resulting in serious physical or psychological harm

OUTCOME TARGET RATING: Maintain at_____ Increase to_____

		Poor	Fair	Good	Very good	Excellent	
OUTCOME OVERALL RATING		1	2	3	4	5	
Indicators:							
280501	Systematic assessment of at-risk groups	1	2	3	4	5	NA
280502	Support programs for high-risk groups	1	2	3	4	5	NA
280503	Intervention programs for high-risk groups	1	2	3	4	5	NA
280504	Existence of weapon control policies	1	2	3	4	5	NA
280505	Enforcement of weapon control policies	1	2	3	4	5	NA
280506	Strategies to reduce violent content in the media	1	2	3	4	5	NA
280507	Control of violent content in the media	1	2	3	4	5	NA
280508	Educational programs on violence prevention	1	2	3	4	5	NA
280509	Competence in recognizing violence by community leaders	1	2	3	4	5	NA
280510	Competence in managing violence by community leaders	1	2	3	4	5	NA
280511	Acceptance of population diversity	1	2	3	4	5	NA
280512	Enforcement of laws against hate crimes by community leaders	1	2	3	4	5	NA
280513	Systematic monitoring of community violence levels	1	2	3	4	5	NA

Domain-*Community Health (VII)* **Class**-*Community Health Protection (CC)* *3rd edition 2004*

OUTCOME CONTENT REFERENCES:
Bell, C. C. (1997). Community violence: Causes, prevention, and intervention. *Journal of the National Medical Association, 89*(10), 657–662.
Campbell, J., & Landenburger, K. (2000). Violence and human abuse. In M. Stanhope & J. Lancaster (Eds.), *Community and public health nursing* (5th ed., pp. 747–778). St. Louis: Mosby.
Jones, F. C. (1997). Community violence, children and youth: Considerations for programs, policy and nursing roles. *Pediatric Nursing, 23*(2), 131–137.
Kroposki, M., & Alexander, J. (1998). Measuring community health nursing outcomes. *South Carolina Nurse, 5*(4), 17–18.

Community Violence Level 2702

Definition: Incidence of violent acts compared with local, state, or national values

OUTCOME TARGET RATING: Maintain at_____ Increase to_____

		Poor	Fair	Good	Very good	Excellent	
COMMUNITY VIOLENCE LEVEL OVERALL RATING		1	2	3	4	5	
Indicators:							
270201	Homicide rate	1	2	3	4	5	NA
270202	Suicide rate	1	2	3	4	5	NA
270203	Sexual assault rate	1	2	3	4	5	NA
270204	Physical assault rate	1	2	3	4	5	NA
270205	Child abuse rate	1	2	3	4	5	NA
270206	Elder abuse rate	1	2	3	4	5	NA
270207	Partner abuse rate	1	2	3	4	5	NA
270208	Hate crime rate	1	2	3	4	5	NA

Domain-*Community Health (VII)* **Class**-*Community Well-Being (BB)* *3rd edition 2004*

OUTCOME CONTENT REFERENCES:

Bell, C. C. (1997). Community violence: Causes, prevention, and intervention. *Journal of the National Medical Association, 89*(10), 657–662.

Campbell, J., & Landenburger, K. (2000). Violence and human abuse. In M. Stanhope & J. Lancaster (Eds.), *Community and public health nursing* (5th ed., pp. 747–778). St. Louis: Mosby.

Jones, F. C. (1997). Community violence, children and youth: Considerations for programs, policy and nursing roles. *Pediatric Nursing, 23*(2), 131–137.

Lutenbacher, M., Cooper, W. O., & Faccia, K. (2002). Planning youth violence prevention efforts: Decision-making across community sectors. *Journal of Adolescent Health, 30*(5), 346–354.

U.S. Department of Health and Human Services. (2000). *Healthy people 2010.* Washington, DC: Government Printing Office.

C

Compliance Behavior   1601

Definition: Personal actions to follow recommendations from a health professional for a specific health condition

OUTCOME TARGET RATING: Maintain at_____   Increase to_____

OUTCOME OVERALL RATING	Never demonstrated 1	Rarely demonstrated 2	Sometimes demonstrated 3	Often demonstrated 4	Consistently demonstrated 5	
Indicators:						
160104 Accepts diagnosis	1	2	3	4	5	NA
160114 Seeks reputable information about diagnosis	1	2	3	4	5	NA
160115 Seeks reputable information about treatment	1	2	3	4	5	NA
160102 Discusses prescribed treatment regimen with health professional	1	2	3	4	5	NA
160103 Performs treatment regimen as prescribed	1	2	3	4	5	NA
160105 Keeps appointments with health professional	1	2	3	4	5	NA
160111 Reports changes in symptoms to health professional	1	2	3	4	5	NA
160106 Modifies treatment regimen as directed by health professional	1	2	3	4	5	NA
160112 Monitors treatment response	1	2	3	4	5	NA
160113 Monitors medication therapeutic effects	1	2	3	4	5	NA
160107 Performs self-screening when directed	1	2	3	4	5	NA
160108 Performs activities of daily living as prescribed	1	2	3	4	5	NA
160109 Seeks external reinforcement for performance of health behaviors	1	2	3	4	5	NA

Domain-Health Knowledge & Behavior (IV)   *Class*-Health Behavior (Q)   *1st edition 1997; revised 2004, 2008, 2013*

OUTCOME CONTENT REFERENCES:

Barotsky, I., Sergenbaker, P., & Mills, M. (1979). Compliance and quality of life assessment. In J. Cohen (Ed.), *New directions in patient compliance* (pp. 59–74). Lexington, MA: D.C. Health.

Burkhart, P. V., Dunbar-Jacob, J. M., & Rohay, J. M. (2001). Accuracy of children's self-reported adherence to treatment. *Journal of Nursing Scholarship, 33*(1), 27–32.

+DiMatteo, M. R., Hays, R. D., & Sherbourne, C. D. (1992). Adherence to cancer regimens: Implications for treating the older patient. *Oncology, 6*(Suppl. 2), 50–57.

Epstein, L., & Cluss, P. A. (1982). A behavioral perspective on adherence to long-term medical regimens. *Journal of Consulting and Clinical Psychology, 50*(6), 950–971.

Folden, S. L. (1993). Definitions of health and health goals of participants in a community-based pulmonary rehabilitation program. *Public Health Nursing, 10*(1), 31–35.

Heiby, E., & Carlson, J. (1986). The health compliance model. *The Journal of Compliance in Health Care, 1*(2), 135–152.

Jensen, L., & Allen, M. (1993). Wellness: The dialect of illness. *Image—The Journal of Nursing Scholarship, 25*(3), 220–224.

King, I. M. (1988). Measuring health goal attainment in patients. In C. F. Waltz & O. L. Strickland (Eds.), *Measurement of nursing outcomes* (vol. I, pp. 108–127). New York: Springer.

Kravits, R., Hays, R. D., Sherbourne, C. D., DiMatteo, M. R., Rogers, W. H., Ordway, L., & Greenfield, S. (1993). Recall of recommendations and adherence to advice among patients with chronic medical conditions. *Archives of Internal Medicine, 153*(16), 1869–1878.

Oldridge, N. (1982). Compliance and exercise in primary and secondary prevention of coronary heart disease: A review. *Preventive Medicine, 11*(1), 56–70.

Compliance Behavior: Prescribed Activity 1632

Definition: Personal actions to follow daily physical activities recommended by a health professional for a specific health condition

OUTCOME TARGET RATING: Maintain at_____ Increase to_____

OUTCOME OVERALL RATING		Never demonstrated 1	Rarely demonstrated 2	Sometimes demonstrated 3	Often demonstrated 4	Consistently demonstrated 5	
Indicators:							
163201	Discusses activity recommendations with health professional	1	2	3	4	5	NA
163202	Identifies expected benefits of physical activity	1	2	3	4	5	NA
163203	Identifies barriers to implement prescribed physical activity	1	2	3	4	5	NA
163204	Sets achievable short-term activity goals with health professional	1	2	3	4	5	NA
163205	Sets achievable long-term activity goals with health professional	1	2	3	4	5	NA
163206	Follows target heart rate set by health professional	1	2	3	4	5	NA
163207	Uses strategies to promote safety	1	2	3	4	5	NA
163208	Uses strategies to allocate time for physical activity	1	2	3	4	5	NA
163209	Uses strategies to increase endurance	1	2	3	4	5	NA
163210	Participates in daily prescribed physical activity	1	2	3	4	5	NA
163211	Monitors heart rate	1	2	3	4	5	NA
163212	Monitors respiratory rate	1	2	3	4	5	NA
163213	Seeks external reinforcement for performance of health behaviors	1	2	3	4	5	NA

Compliance Behavior: Prescribed Activity—*cont'd*

	Never demonstrated	Rarely demonstrated	Sometimes demonstrated	Often demonstrated	Consistently demonstrated	
163214 Uses diary to monitor progress in prescribed physical activity	1	2	3	4	5	NA
163215 Modifies physical activity as directed by health professional	1	2	3	4	5	NA
163216 Identifies symptoms that need to be reported	1	2	3	4	5	NA
163217 Reports symptoms experienced during activity to health professional	1	2	3	4	5	NA

Domain-*Health Knowledge & Behavior (IV)*   **Class**-*Health Behavior (Q)*   *5th edition 2013*

OUTCOME CONTENT REFERENCES:

Barbour, K. A., & Miller, N. H. (2008). Adherence to exercise training in heart failure: A review. *Heart Failure Reviews, 13(1)*, 81–89.

Leijon, M., Bendtsen, P., Stahle, A., Ekberg, K., Festin, K., & Nilsen, P. (2010). Factors associated with patients self-reported adherence to prescribed physical activity in routine primary health care. *BMC Family Practice, 11,* 38.

Lippke, S., Ziegelmann, J., & Schwarzer, R. (2004). Behavioral intentions and action plans promote physical exercise: A longitudinal study with orthopedic rehabilitation patients. *Journal of Sport & Exercise Psychology, 26(3)*, 470–483.

Mayoux-Benhamou, A., Quintrec, J., Ravaud, P., Champion, K., Dernis, E., Zerkak, D., Roy, C., Kahan, A., Revel, M., & Dougados, M. (2008). Influence of patient education on exercise compliance in rheumatoid arthritis: A prospective 12-month randomized control trial. *The Journal of Rheumatology, 35(2)*, 216–223.

National Institute on Aging. (2009). *Exercise & physical activity: Your everyday guide from the National Institute on Aging.* Bethesda, MD: Author.

Pang, M. Y., Eng, J. J., Dawson, A. S., & Gylfadóttir, S. (2006). The use of aerobic exercise training in improving aerobic capacity in individuals with stroke: A meta-analysis. *Clinical Rehabilitation 20(2)*, 97–111.

Resnick, B., Orwig, D., Yu-Yahiro, J., Hawkes, W., Shardell, M., Hebel, J., Zimmerman, S., Golden, J., Werner, M., & Magaziner, J. (2007). Testing the effectiveness of the Exercise Plus Program in older women post-hip fracture. *Annals of Behavioral Medicine, 34(1)*, 67–76.

Compliance Behavior: Prescribed Diet   1622

Definition: Personal actions to follow food and fluid intake recommended by a health professional for a specific health condition

OUTCOME TARGET RATING: Maintain at_____   Increase to_____ .

	Never demonstrated	Rarely demonstrated	Sometimes demonstrated	Often demonstrated	Consistently demonstrated	
OUTCOME OVERALL RATING	1	2	3	4	5	

Indicators:

	Never demonstrated	Rarely demonstrated	Sometimes demonstrated	Often demonstrated	Consistently demonstrated	
162201 Participates in setting achievable dietary goals with health professional	1	2	3	4	5	NA
162202 Selects food and fluid consistent with prescribed diet	1	2	3	4	5	NA
162203 Uses nutritional information on labels to guide selections	1	2	3	4	5	NA
162204 Selects portions consistent with prescribed diet	1	2	3	4	5	NA
162205 Eats food consistent with prescribed diet	1	2	3	4	5	NA
162206 Drinks fluid consistent with prescribed diet	1	2	3	4	5	NA

Continued

Compliance Behavior: Prescribed Diet—cont'd

		Never demonstrated	Rarely demonstrated	Sometimes demonstrated	Often demonstrated	Consistently demonstrated	
162207	Avoids food and fluid not allowed on diet	1	2	3	4	5	NA
162208	Follows recommendations for between-meal food and fluid	1	2	3	4	5	NA
162209	Prepares food and fluid following dietary restrictions	1	2	3	4	5	NA
162210	Follows recommendations for number of meals per day	1	2	3	4	5	NA
162211	Plans meals consistent with prescribed diet	1	2	3	4	5	NA
162212	Plans strategies for situations that affect food and fluid intake	1	2	3	4	5	NA
162213	Alters diet within restrictions when activity level changes	1	2	3	4	5	NA
162214	Follows recommendations for diet staging	1	2	3	4	5	NA
162215	Uses a diary to monitor food and fluid intake over time	1	2	3	4	5	NA
162216	Aligns diet with cultural beliefs	1	2	3	4	5	NA
162217	Chooses foods consistent with cultural beliefs	1	2	3	4	5	NA
162218	Avoids food and fluid that interact with medications	1	2	3	4	5	NA
162219	Avoids food and fluid that interact with herbal remedies	1	2	3	4	5	NA
162220	Avoids food and fluid that trigger allergic reactions	1	2	3	4	5	NA

Domain-*Health Knowledge & Behavior (IV)*   **Class**-*Health Behavior (Q)*   *4th edition 2008*

OUTCOME CONTENT REFERENCES:

American Diabetes Association. (2004). Nutrition principles and recommendations in diabetes. *Diabetes Care, 27*(Suppl. 1), S36–S46.

Brownell, K., & Fairburn, C. (Eds.). (2002). *Eating disorders and obesity: A comprehensive handbook* (2nd ed.). New York: Guilford Press.

Dudek, S. G. (2007). *Nutrition essentials for nursing practice* (5th rev. ed.). Philadelphia: Lippincott Williams & Wilkins.

Frandsen, K. B., & Kristensen, J. S. (2002). Diet and lifestyle in type 2 diabetes: The patient's perspective. *Practical Diabetes International, 19*(3), 77–80.

Lee, A., & Newman, J. (2003). Celiac diet: Its impact on quality of life. *Journal of the American Dietetic Association, 103*(11), 1533–1535.

Rosenberg, I. (Ed.). (2002). The 5 lifestyle steps for lowering blood pressure. *Tufts University Health & Nutrition Letter, 21*(6), 7.

Compliance Behavior: Prescribed Medication   1623

Definition: Personal actions to administer medication safely to meet therapeutic effects for a specific condition as recommended by a health professional

OUTCOME TARGET RATING: Maintain at_____   Increase to_____

OUTCOME OVERALL RATING	Never demonstrated 1	Rarely demonstrated 2	Sometimes demonstrated 3	Often demonstrated 4	Consistently demonstrated 5	
Indicators:						
162301 Keeps a list of all medication with dose and frequency	1	2	3	4	5	NA
162302 Obtains required medication	1	2	3	4	5	NA
162303 Informs health professional of all medication being taken	1	2	3	4	5	NA
162304 Takes all medication at intervals prescribed	1	2	3	4	5	NA
162305 Takes correct dose	1	2	3	4	5	NA
162306 Modifies dose as instructed	1	2	3	4	5	NA
162307 Takes medication with or without food as prescribed	1	2	3	4	5	NA
162308 Avoids alcohol if contraindicated	1	2	3	4	5	NA
162309 Avoids food and fluids that are contraindicated	1	2	3	4	5	NA
162310 Administers topical medication correctly	1	2	3	4	5	NA
162311 Follows medication precautions	1	2	3	4	5	NA
162312 Monitors medication therapeutic effects	1	2	3	4	5	NA
162313 Monitors medication side effects	1	2	3	4	5	NA
162314 Monitors medication adverse effects	1	2	3	4	5	NA
162315 Uses strategies to minimize side effects	1	2	3	4	5	NA
162316 Reports therapeutic response to health professional	1	2	3	4	5	NA
162317 Reports adverse effects to health professional	1	2	3	4	5	NA
162318 Stores medication properly	1	2	3	4	5	NA
162319 Arranges for refills to ensure adequate supply	1	2	3	4	5	NA
162320 Monitors medication expiration date	1	2	3	4	5	NA
162321 Disposes of medication properly	1	2	3	4	5	NA
162322 Disposes of syringes and needles properly	1	2	3	4	5	NA
162323 Administers subcutaneous medication correctly	1	2	3	4	5	NA
162324 Administers intramuscular medication correctly	1	2	3	4	5	NA
162325 Administers intravenous medication correctly	1	2	3	4	5	NA
162326 Maintains asepsis with non-parenteral medication	1	2	3	4	5	NA
162327 Monitors injection insertion sites	1	2	3	4	5	NA
162328 Rotates injection sites	1	2	3	4	5	NA
162329 Maintains needed supplies	1	2	3	4	5	NA
162330 Stores supplies correctly	1	2	3	4	5	NA
162331 Disposes of sharps correctly	1	2	3	4	5	NA
162332 Obtains required laboratory tests	1	2	3	4	5	NA

Domain-Health Knowledge & Behavior (IV)   *Class*-Health Behavior (Q)   4th edition 2008; revised 2013

OUTCOME CONTENT REFERENCES:

Janssen, B., Gaebel, W., Haerter, M., Komaharadi, F., Lindel, B., & Weinmann, S. (2006). Evaluation of factors influencing medication compliance in inpatient treatment of psychotic disorders. *Psychopharmacology, 187*(2), 229–236.

Johnson, M. J. (2006). Development of the purposeful action medication-taking questionnaire. *Western Journal of Nursing Research, 28*(3), 335–351.

Roose, S. P. (2003). Compliance: The impact of adverse events and tolerability on the physician's treatment decisions. *European Neuropsychopharmacology, 13*(Suppl. 3), S85–S92.

Schmitz, J. M., Sayre, S. L., Stotts, A. L., Rothfleisch, J., & Mooney, M. E. (2005). Medication compliance during a smoking cessation clinical trial: A brief intervention using MEMS feedback. *Journal of Behavioral Medicine, 28*(2), 139–147.

C

Concentration 0905

Definition: Ability to focus on a specific stimulus

OUTCOME TARGET RATING: Maintain at_____   Increase to_____

		Severely compromised	Substantially compromised	Moderately compromised	Mildly compromised	Not compromised	
OUTCOME OVERALL RATING		1	2	3	4	5	
Indicators:							
090501	Maintains attention	1	2	3	4	5	NA
090502	Maintains focus	1	2	3	4	5	NA
090503	Responds to visual cues	1	2	3	4	5	NA
090504	Responds to auditory cues	1	2	3	4	5	NA
090505	Responds to tactile cues	1	2	3	4	5	NA
090506	Responds to olfactory cues	1	2	3	4	5	NA
090507	Responds to language cues	1	2	3	4	5	NA
090508	Spells 'world' backwards	1	2	3	4	5	NA
090515	Counts backward from 20 by 3s	1	2	3	4	5	NA
090516	Counts backward from 100 by 7s	1	2	3	4	5	NA
090510	Names the months of the year backward, starting with January	1	2	3	4	5	NA
090511	Draws a circle	1	2	3	4	5	NA
090514	Draws a triangle	1	2	3	4	5	NA
090512	Draws a pentagon	1	2	3	4	5	NA

Domain-*Physiologic Health (II)*   **Class**-*Neurocognitive (J)*   *1st edition 1997; revised 2004, 2008*

OUTCOME CONTENT REFERENCES:

Abraham, I., & Reel, S. (1993). Cognitive nursing interventions with long-term care residents: Effects on neurocognitive dimensions. *Archives of Psychiatric Nursing, 6*(6), 356–365.

Agostinelli, B., Demers, K., Garrigan, D., & Waszynski, C. (1994). Targeted interventions: Use of the Mini-Mental State Exam. *Journal of Gerontological Nursing, 20*(8), 15–23.

Dellasega, C. (1992). Home health nurses' assessments of cognition. *Applied Nursing Research, 5*(3), 127–133.

+Folstein, M. F., Folstein, S. E., & McHugh, P. R. (1975). "Mini-Mental State"—A practical method for grading the cognitive state of patients for the clinician. *Journal of Psychiatric Research, 12*(3), 189–198.

Foreman, M., Gilles, D., & Wagner, D. (1989). Impaired cognition in the critically ill elderly patient: Clinical implications. *Critical Care Nursing Quarterly, 12*(1), 61–73.

Kupferer, S., Uebele, J., & Levin, D. (1988). Geriatric ambulatory surgery patients: Assessing cognitive functions. *AORN Journal, 47*(3), 752–766.

Mason, P. (1989). Cognitive assessment parameters and tools for the critically injured adult. *Critical Care Nursing Clinics of North America, 1*(1), 45–53.

Norris, J. A., & Hoffman, P. R. (1996). Attaining, sustaining, and focusing attention: Intervention for children with ADHD. *Seminars in Speech & Language, 17*(1), 59–71.

O'Keeffe, S. T., & Gosney, M. A. (1997). Assessing attentiveness in older hospital patients: Global assessment versus tests of attention. *Journal of the American Geriatrics Society, 45*(4), 470–473.

Strub, R. L., & Black, F. W. (2000). *The mental status examination in neurology* (4th ed.). Philadelphia: F. A. Davis.

Coordinated Movement   0212

Definition: Ability of muscles to work together voluntarily for purposeful movement

OUTCOME TARGET RATING: Maintain at_____   Increase to_____

		Severely compromised	Substantially compromised	Moderately compromised	Mildly compromised	Not compromised	
OUTCOME OVERALL RATING		1	2	3	4	5	
Indicators:							
021201	Strength of muscle contraction	1	2	3	4	5	NA
021202	Muscle tone	1	2	3	4	5	NA
021203	Speed of movement	1	2	3	4	5	NA
021204	Smooth movement	1	2	3	4	5	NA
021205	Control of movement	1	2	3	4	5	NA
021206	Steadiness of movement	1	2	3	4	5	NA
021207	Balanced movement	1	2	3	4	5	NA
021208	Muscle tension	1	2	3	4	5	NA
021209	Movement in desired direction	1	2	3	4	5	NA
021210	Movement with desired timing	1	2	3	4	5	NA
021211	Movement at desired speed	1	2	3	4	5	NA
021212	Movement with desired precision	1	2	3	4	5	NA

Domain-*Functional Health (I)*   **Class**-*Mobility (C)*   *3rd edition 2004*

OUTCOME CONTENT REFERENCES:

Buchner, D. M. (1995). Clinical assessments of physical activity in older adults. In L. Z. Rubenstein, D. Wieland, & R. Bernabei (Eds.), *Geriatric assessment technology: The state of the art* (pp. 147–159). New York: Springer.

Crawford, S. G., Wilson, B. N., & Dewey, D. (2001). Identifying developmental coordination disorder: Consistency between tests. *Physical & Occupational Therapy in Pediatrics, 20*(2/3), 29–50.

DiFabio, R. P., Paul, S., Emasithi, A., & Greany, J. F. (2001). Evaluating eye-body coordination during unrestrained functional activity in older persons. *The Journals of Gerontology. Series A, Biological Sciences & Medical Sciences, 56*(9), M571–M574.

Guyton, A. C. (1992). *Human physiology and mechanisms of disease* (5th ed.). Philadelphia: W.B. Saunders.

Harris, T. (1997). Muscle mass and strength: Relation to function in population studies. *Journal of Nutrition, 127*(Suppl. 5), 1004S–1006S.

Junaid, K., Harris, S. R., Fulmer, K. A., & Carswell, A. (2000). Teachers' use of the MABC checklist to identify children with motor coordination difficulties. *Pediatric Physical Therapy, 12*(4), 158–163.

Matteson, M. A., McConnell, E. S., & Linton, A. D. (1997). *Gerontological nursing: Concepts and practice* (2nd ed.). Philadelphia: W. B. Saunders.

Novy, D. M., Simmonds, M. J., & Lee, C. E. (2002). Physical performance tasks: What are the underlying constructs? *Archives of Physical Medicine & Rehabilitation, 83*(1), 44–47.

Riggio, S., & Jagoda, A. (1999). The rapid neurologic examination, part 2: Movement, reflexes, sensation, balance: Know the signs that lead to the site of the pathologic response. *Journal of Critical Illness, 14*(7), 368–372.

Schmitz, T. J. (2001). Coordination assessment. In S. B. O'Sullivan & T. J. Schmitz (Eds.), *Physical rehabilitation: Assessment and treatment* (4th ed., pp. 157–175). Philadelphia: F. A. Davis.

Coping 1302

Definition: Personal actions to manage stressors that tax an individual's resources

OUTCOME TARGET RATING: Maintain at_____ Increase to_____

OUTCOME OVERALL RATING	Never demonstrated 1	Rarely demonstrated 2	Sometimes demonstrated 3	Often demonstrated 4	Consistently demonstrated 5	
Indicators:						
130201	Identifies effective coping patterns	1	2	3	4	5	NA
130202	Identifies ineffective coping patterns	1	2	3	4	5	NA
130203	Verbalizes sense of control	1	2	3	4	5	NA
130204	Reports decrease in stress	1	2	3	4	5	NA
130205	Verbalizes acceptance of situation	1	2	3	4	5	NA
130220	Seeks reputable information about diagnosis	1	2	3	4	5	NA
130221	Seeks reputable information about treatment	1	2	3	4	5	NA
130207	Modifies lifestyle to reduce stress	1	2	3	4	5	NA
130208	Adapts to life changes	1	2	3	4	5	NA
130222	Uses personal support system	1	2	3	4	5	NA
130210	Uses behaviors to reduce stress	1	2	3	4	5	NA
130211	Identifies multiple coping strategies	1	2	3	4	5	NA
130212	Uses effective coping strategies	1	2	3	4	5	NA
130213	Avoids unduly stressful situations	1	2	3	4	5	NA
130214	Verbalizes need for assistance	1	2	3	4	5	NA
130223	Obtains assistance from health professional	1	2	3	4	5	NA
130216	Reports decrease in physical symptoms of stress	1	2	3	4	5	NA
130217	Reports decrease in negative feelings	1	2	3	4	5	NA
130218	Reports increase in psychological comfort	1	2	3	4	5	NA

Domain-Psychosocial Health (III)   *Class*-Psychosocial Adaptation (N)   *1st edition 1997; revised 2004, 2008*

OUTCOME CONTENT REFERENCES:

Baldree, K., Murphy, S., & Powers, M. (1982). Stress identification and coping patterns in patients on hemodialysis. *Nursing Research*, *31*(2), 107–112.

+Carver, C. S. (1997). You want to measure coping but your protocol's too long: Consider the Brief COPE. *International Journal of Behavioral Medicine*, *4*(1), 92–100.

+Carver, C. S., Scheier, M. F., & Weintraub, J. K. (1989). Assessing coping strategies: A theoretically based approach. *Journal of Personality and Social Psychology*, *56*(2), 267–283.

Folkman, S., Lazarus, R., Gruen, R., & Delongis, A. (1986). Appraisal, coping, health status, and psychological symptoms. *Journal of Personality and Social Psychology*, *50*(3), 571–579.

McHaffie, H. (1992). The assessment of coping. *Clinical Nursing Research*, *1*(1), 67–79.

Panzarine, S. (1985). Coping: Conceptual and methodological issues. *Advances in Nursing Science*, *7*(4), 49–57.

Stolley, J. M. (2001). Ineffective individual coping. In M. Maas, K. Buckwalter, M. Hardy, T. Tripp-Reimer, M. Titler, & J. Specht (Eds.), *Nursing care of older adults: Diagnoses, outcomes & interventions* (pp. 766–777). St. Louis: Mosby.

Whiting, G., & Buckwalter, K. C. (2001). Grieving. In M. Maas, K. Buckwalter, M. Hardy, T. Tripp-Reimer, M. Titler, & J. Specht (Eds.), *Nursing care of older adults: Diagnoses, outcomes & interventions* (pp. 631–650). St. Louis: Mosby.

Cup Feeding Establishment: Infant 1018

Definition: Establishment of cup feeding for hydration and nourishment of an infant

OUTCOME TARGET RATING: Maintain at_____ Increase to_____

C

		Not adequate	Slightly adequate	Moderately adequate	Substantially adequate	Totally adequate	
OUTCOME OVERALL RATING		1	2	3	4	5	
Indicators:							
101801	Placement of tongue in cup	1	2	3	4	5	NA
101802	Laps or sips milk or formula	1	2	3	4	5	NA
101803	Production of noisy splashing sounds	1	2	3	4	5	NA
101804	Audible swallow	1	2	3	4	5	NA
101805	Periodic burping	1	2	3	4	5	NA
101806	Feeding tolerance	1	2	3	4	5	NA
101807	Feedings per day	1	2	3	4	5	NA
101808	Contentment after feeding	1	2	3	4	5	NA
101809	Urine output appropriate for age	1	2	3	4	5	NA
101810	Stools appropriate for age	1	2	3	4	5	NA
101811	Weight gain appropriate for age	1	2	3	4	5	NA

Domain-*Physiologic Health (II)*   **Class**-*Digestion & Nutrition (K)*   *5th edition 2013*

OUTCOME CONTENT REFERENCES:

American Dental Association. (2004). From baby bottle to cup: Choose training cups carefully, use them temporarily. *Journal of the American Dental Association, 135*(3), 387.

Brown, S. J., Alexander, J., & Thomas, P. (1999). Feeding outcome in breast-fed term babies supplemented by cup or bottle. *Midwifery, 15*(2), 92–96.

Cloherty, M., Alexander, J., Holloway, I., Galvin, K., & Inch, S. (2005). The cup-versus-bottle debate: A theme from an ethnographic study of the supplementation of breastfed infants in hospitals in the United Kingdom. *Journal of Human Lactation, 21*(2), 151–162.

Dowling, D. A., Meier, P. P., DiFiore, J. M., Blatz, M., & Martin, R. J. (2002). Cup feeding for preterm infants: Mechanics and safety. *Journal of Human Lactation, 18*(1), 13–20.

Kuehl, J. (1997). Cup feeding the newborn: What you should know. *Journal of Perinatal & Neonatal Nursing, 11*(2), 56–60.

Rocha, N. M., Martinez, F. E., & Jorge, S. M. (2002). Cup or bottle for preterm infants; effects on oxygen saturation, weight gain and breastfeeding. *Journal of Human Lactation, 18*(2), 132–138.

Samuel, P. (1998). Cup feeding: How and when to use it with term babies. *Practising Midwife, 1*(12), 33–35.

Thorley, V. (1997). Cup feeding: Problems created by incorrect use. *Journal of Human Lactation, 13*(1), 54–55.

Cup Feeding Performance

1019

Definition: Caregiver actions to provide fluids to an infant using a cup

OUTCOME TARGET RATING: Maintain at_____ Increase to_____

OUTCOME OVERALL RATING		Never demonstrated 1	Rarely demonstrated 2	Sometimes demonstrated 3	Often demonstrated 4	Consistently demonstrated 5	
Indicators:							
101901	Washes hands prior to feeding	1	2	3	4	5	NA
101902	Prepares formula according to directions	1	2	3	4	5	NA
101903	Uses a small clean cup without a spout	1	2	3	4	5	NA
101904	Uses formula before expiration date	1	2	3	4	5	NA
101905	Stores mixed formula correctly	1	2	3	4	5	NA
101906	Stores breast milk correctly	1	2	3	4	5	NA
101907	Tests temperature of fluid prior to feeding	1	2	3	4	5	NA
101908	Responds to infant hunger cues	1	2	3	4	5	NA
101909	Positions infant correctly while feeding	1	2	3	4	5	NA
101910	Positions cup correctly while feeding	1	2	3	4	5	NA
101911	Burps infant at frequent intervals	1	2	3	4	5	NA
101912	Allows infant to pace feeding	1	2	3	4	5	NA
101913	Responds to infant cues to stop feeding	1	2	3	4	5	NA
101914	Repositions infant in response to choking	1	2	3	4	5	NA

Domain-*Physiologic Health (II)*   **Class**-*Digestion & Nutrition (K)*   *5th edition 2013*

OUTCOME CONTENT REFERENCES:
American Dental Association (2004). From baby bottle to cup: Choose training cups carefully, use them temporarily. *Journal of the American Dental Association,* 135(3), 387.
Brown, S. J, Alexander, J., & Thomas, P. (1999). Feeding outcome in breast-fed term babies supplemented by cup or bottle. *Midwifery, 15*(2), 92–96.
Cloherty, M., Alexander, J., Holloway, I., Galvin, K., & Inch, S. (2005). The cup-versus-bottle debate: A theme from an ethnographic study of the supplementation of breastfed infants in hospitals in the United Kingdom. *Journal of Human Lactation, 21*(2), 151–162.
Dowling, D. A., Meier, P. P., DiFiore, J. M., Blatz, M., & Martin, R. J. (2002). Cup feeding for preterm infants: Mechanics and safety. *Journal of Human Lactation, 18*(1), 13–20.
Kuehl, J. (1997). Cup feeding the newborn: What you should know. *Journal of Perinatal & Neonatal Nursing, 11*(2), 56–60.
Rocha, N. M., Martinez, F. E., & Jorge, S. M. (2002). Cup or bottle for preterm infants; effects on oxygen saturation, weight gain and breastfeeding. *Journal of Human Lactation, 18*(2), 132–138.
Samuel, P. (1998). Cup feeding: How and when to use it with term babies. *Practising Midwife, 1*(12), 33–35.
Thorley, V. (1997). Cup feeding: Problems created by incorrect use. *Journal of Human Lactation, 13*(1), 54–55.

Decision-Making 0906

Definition: Ability to make judgments and choose between two or more alternatives

OUTCOME TARGET RATING: Maintain at_____   Increase to_____

OUTCOME OVERALL RATING	Severely compromised 1	Substantially compromised 2	Moderately compromised 3	Mildly compromised 4	Not compromised 5	
Indicators:						
090601 Identifies relevant information	1	2	3	4	5	NA
090602 Identifies alternatives	1	2	3	4	5	NA
090603 Identifies potential consequences of each alternative	1	2	3	4	5	NA
090604 Identifies needed resources to support each alternative	1	2	3	4	5	NA
090611 Identifies time frame necessary to support each alternative	1	2	3	4	5	NA
090612 Identifies sequence necessary to support each alternative	1	2	3	4	5	NA
090605 Recognizes contradiction with others' desires	1	2	3	4	5	NA
090606 Acknowledges social context of the situation	1	2	3	4	5	NA
090607 Acknowledges relevant legal implications	1	2	3	4	5	NA
090608 Weighs alternatives	1	2	3	4	5	NA
090609 Selects among alternatives	1	2	3	4	5	NA

Domain-*Physiologic Health (II)*   **Class**-*Neurocognitive (J)*   *1st edition 1997; revised 2004, 2008*

OUTCOME CONTENT REFERENCES:

Abraham, I., & Reel, S. (1993). Cognitive nursing interventions with long-term care residents: Effects on neurocognitive dimensions. *Archives of Psychiatric Nursing, 6*(6), 356–365.

Agostinelli, B., Demers, K., Garrigan, D., & Waszynski, C. (1994). Targeted interventions: Use of the Mini-Mental State Exam. *Journal of Gerontological Nursing, 20*(8), 15–23.

Dellasega, C. (1992). Home health nurses' assessments of cognition. *Applied Nursing Research, 5*(3), 127–133.

Foreman, M., Gilles, D., & Wagner, D. (1989). Impaired cognition in the critically ill elderly patient: Clinical implications. *Critical Care Nursing Quarterly, 12*(1), 61–73.

Jubeck, M. (1992). Are you sensitive to the cognitive needs of the elderly? *Home Healthcare Nurse, 10*(5), 20–25.

Kendall, E., Shum, D., Halson, D., Bunning, S., & Teb, M. (1997). The assessment of social problem-solving ability following traumatic brain injury. *Journal of Head Trauma Rehabilitation, 12*(3), 68–78.

Kupferer, S., Uebele, J., & Levin, D. (1988). Geriatric ambulatory surgery patients: Assessing cognitive functions. *AORN Journal, 47*(3), 752–766.

Mason, P. (1989). Cognitive assessment parameters and tools for the critically injured adult. *Critical Care Nursing Clinics of North America, 1*(1), 45–53.

Strub, R. L., & Black, F. W. (2000). *The mental status examination in neurology* (4th ed.). Philadelphia: F. A. Davis.

+Uniform Data System for Medical Rehabilitation. (1997). *Guide for the Uniform Data Set for Medical Rehabilitation* (including the FIM™ instrument) (version 5.1). Buffalo, NY: Author.

Vellinga, A., Smit, J. H., van Leeuwen, E., van Tilburg, W., & Jonker, C. (2004). Instruments to assess decision-making capacity: An overview. *International Psychogeriatrics, 16*(4), 397–419.

D

Delirium Level 0916

Definition: Severity of disturbance in consciousness and cognition that develops over a short period of time and is reversible

OUTCOME TARGET RATING: Maintain at_____ Increase to_____

OUTCOME OVERALL RATING		Severe 1	Substantial 2	Moderate 3	Mild 4	None 5	
Indicators:							
091601	Disorientation of time	1	2	3	4	5	NA
091602	Disorientation of place	1	2	3	4	5	NA
091603	Disorientation of person	1	2	3	4	5	NA
091604	Psychomotor activity	1	2	3	4	5	NA
091605	Impaired cognition	1	2	3	4	5	NA
091606	Impaired memory	1	2	3	4	5	NA
091607	Difficulty following complex commands	1	2	3	4	5	NA
091608	Difficulty interpreting environmental stimuli	1	2	3	4	5	NA
091609	Difficulty maintaining focus	1	2	3	4	5	NA
091610	Difficulty maintaining conversation	1	2	3	4	5	NA
091611	Misinterpretation of cues	1	2	3	4	5	NA
091612	Meaningless verbalizations	1	2	3	4	5	NA
091613	Altered level of consciousness	1	2	3	4	5	NA
091614	Reduction in abstract reasoning	1	2	3	4	5	NA
091615	Restlessness	1	2	3	4	5	NA
091616	Agitation	1	2	3	4	5	NA
091617	Disruption of sleep-wake pattern	1	2	3	4	5	NA
091618	Labile mood	1	2	3	4	5	NA
091619	Sundowning	1	2	3	4	5	NA
091620	Hallucinations	1	2	3	4	5	NA
091621	Delusions	1	2	3	4	5	NA

Domain-*Physiologic Health (II)*   **Class**-*Neurocognitive (J)*   *4th edition 2008; revised 2013*

OUTCOME CONTENT REFERENCES:

Foreman, M. D., Mion, L. C., Tryostad, L., & Fletcher, K. (1999). Standard of practice protocol: Acute confusion/delirium. *Geriatric Nursing, 20*(3), 147–152.

Johnson, M. (2001). Assessing confused patients. *Journal of Neurology, Neurosurgery and Psychiatry, 71*(Suppl. 1), i7–i12.

Miller, J., Neelon, V., Champagne, M., Bailey, D., Ng'andu, N., Belyea, M., Jarrell, E., Montoya, L., & Williams, A. (1997). The assessment of acute confusion as part of nursing care. *Applied Nursing Research, 10*(3), 143–151.

Rapp, C. G., Wakefield, B., Kundrat, M., Mentes, J., Tripp-Reimer, T., Culp, K., Mobily, P., Akins, J., & Onega, L. L. (2000). Acute confusion assessment instruments: Clinical versus research usability. *Applied Nursing Research, 13*(1), 37–45.

Trzepacz, P. T. (1999). The delirium rating scale: Its use in consultation-liaison research. *Psychosomatics, 40*(3), 193–204.

Wakefield, B., Mentes, J., Mobily, P., Tripp-Reimer, T., Culp, K. R., Rapp, C. G., Gaspar, P., Kundrat, M., Wadle, K. R., & Akins, J. (2001). Acute confusion. In M. Maas, K. Buckwalter, M. Hardy, T. Tripp-Reimer, M. Titler & J. Specht (Eds.), *Nursing care of older adults: Diagnoses, outcomes & interventions* (pp. 442–454). St. Louis: Mosby.

Dementia Level 0920

Definition: Severity of irreversible disturbances in consciousness and cognition that leads to mental, physical, and social functional losses over an extended period of time

OUTCOME TARGET RATING: Maintain at_____ Increase to_____

OUTCOME OVERALL RATING	Severe 1	Substantial 2	Moderate 3	Mild 4	None 5	
Indicators:						
092001 Difficulty remembering recent events	1	2	3	4	5	NA
092002 Difficulty remembering names	1	2	3	4	5	NA
092003 Difficulty recognizing family members	1	2	3	4	5	NA
092004 Difficulty remembering names of familiar objects	1	2	3	4	5	NA
092005 Difficulty finding way to familiar places	1	2	3	4	5	NA
092006 Difficulty maintaining conversation	1	2	3	4	5	NA
092007 Difficulty interpreting physiological cues	1	2	3	4	5	NA
092008 Difficulty processing information	1	2	3	4	5	NA
092009 Difficulty following complex commands	1	2	3	4	5	NA
092010 Difficulty problem solving	1	2	3	4	5	NA
092011 Difficulty expressing needs	1	2	3	4	5	NA
092012 Difficulty performing basic activities of daily living	1	2	3	4	5	NA
092013 Difficulty performing instrumental activities of daily living	1	2	3	4	5	NA
092014 Difficulty interpreting environmental stimuli	1	2	3	4	5	NA
092015 Unsafe wandering	1	2	3	4	5	NA
092016 Immobility	1	2	3	4	5	NA
092017 Disorientation of time	1	2	3	4	5	NA
092018 Disorientation of place	1	2	3	4	5	NA
092019 Disorientation of person	1	2	3	4	5	NA
092020 Bowel incontinence	1	2	3	4	5	NA
092021 Urinary incontinence	1	2	3	4	5	NA
092022 Disruption of sleep/wake pattern	1	2	3	4	5	NA
092023 Disruption of social activities	1	2	3	4	5	NA
092024 Depression	1	2	3	4	5	NA
092025 Agitation	1	2	3	4	5	NA
092026 Restlessness	1	2	3	4	5	NA
092027 Aggression	1	2	3	4	5	NA
092028 Suspiciousness	1	2	3	4	5	NA
092029 Social withdrawal	1	2	3	4	5	NA
092030 Change in personality	1	2	3	4	5	NA
092031 Altered level of consciousness	1	2	3	4	5	NA

Domain-*Physiologic Health (II)* **Class**-*Neurocognitive (J)* 5th edition 2013

OUTCOME CONTENT REFERENCES:

Dosa, D., Intrator, O., McNicoll, L., Cang, Y., & Teno, J. (2007). Preliminary derivation of a nursing home confusion assessment method based on data from the minimum data set. *Journal of the American Geriatrics Society, 55*(7), 1099–1105.

Gerdner, L. A., & Richards-Hall, G. (2001). Chronic confusion. In Maas, M., Buckwalter, K. C., Hardy, M. D., Tripp-Reimer, T., Titler, M., & Specht, J. P. (Eds.). *Nursing care of older adults: Diagnoses, outcomes, & interventions.* St. Louis: Mosby.

Kratz, K. (2008). Use of the acute confusion protocol: A research utilization project. *Journal of Nursing Care Quality, 23*(4), 331–337.

Moyle, W., Olorenshaw, R., Wallis, M., Borbasi, S. (2008). Best practice for the management of older people with dementia in the acute care setting: A review of the literature. *International Journal of Older People Nursing, 3*(2), 121–130.

Reisberg, B., Ferris, S. H., deLeon, M. J., & Crook, T. (1982). The global deterioration scale for assessment of primary degenerative dementia. *American Journal of Psychiatry, 139*(9), 1136–1139.

Shelby, M. (2006). Confusion in the elderly. *Practice Nurse, 32*(9), 45–48.

Depression Level 1208

Definition: Severity of melancholic mood and loss of interest in life events

OUTCOME TARGET RATING: Maintain at_____ Increase to_____

OUTCOME OVERALL RATING	Severe 1	Substantial 2	Moderate 3	Mild 4	None 5	
Indicators:						
120801 Depressed mood	1	2	3	4	5	NA
120802 Loss of interest in activities	1	2	3	4	5	NA
120827 Negative life events	1	2	3	4	5	NA
120803 Lack of pleasure in activities	1	2	3	4	5	NA
120804 Impaired concentration	1	2	3	4	5	NA
120805 Inappropriate guilt	1	2	3	4	5	NA
120828 Excessive guilt	1	2	3	4	5	NA
120806 Fatigue	1	2	3	4	5	NA
120807 Feelings of worthlessness	1	2	3	4	5	NA
120808 Psychomotor retardation	1	2	3	4	5	NA
120829 Psychomotor agitation	1	2	3	4	5	NA
120809 Insomnia	1	2	3	4	5	NA
120830 Hypersomnia	1	2	3	4	5	NA
120810 Weight gain	1	2	3	4	5	NA
120831 Weight loss	1	2	3	4	5	NA
120811 Increased appetite	1	2	3	4	5	NA
120832 Decreased appetite	1	2	3	4	5	NA
120835 Recurrent thoughts of death	1	2	3	4	5	NA
120836 Recurrent thoughts of suicide	1	2	3	4	5	NA
120813 Indecisiveness	1	2	3	4	5	NA
120814 Sadness	1	2	3	4	5	NA
120815 Crying spells	1	2	3	4	5	NA
120816 Anger	1	2	3	4	5	NA
120817 Hopelessness	1	2	3	4	5	NA
120818 Loneliness	1	2	3	4	5	NA
120819 Low self-esteem	1	2	3	4	5	NA
120820 Decreased libido	1	2	3	4	5	NA
120821 Decreased activity level	1	2	3	4	5	NA
120822 Lack of spontaneity	1	2	3	4	5	NA
120823 Irritability	1	2	3	4	5	NA
120833 Recreational drug use	1	2	3	4	5	NA
120834 Increased alcohol use	1	2	3	4	5	NA
120825 Poor personal hygiene	1	2	3	4	5	NA

Domain-Psychosocial Health (III) *Class-Psychological Well-Being (M)* 2nd edition 2000; revised 2004, 2008

OUTCOME CONTENT REFERENCES:

American Psychiatric Association. (2000). *Diagnostic and statistical manual of mental disorders* (4th ed. text revision). Washington, DC: Author.

Brink, T. L., Yesavage, J. A., Lum, O., Heersema, P. H., Adey, M., & Rose, T. L. (1982). Screening tests for geriatric depression. *Clinical Gerontologist, 1*(1), 37–43.

Kendler, K. S., Karkowski, L. M., & Prescott, C. A. (1999). Causal relationship between stressful life events and the onset of major depression. *American Journal of Psychiatry, 156*(6), 837–841.

Kraaij, V., Arensman, E., & Spinhoven, P. (2002). Negative life events and depression in elderly persons: A meta-analysis. *Journal of Gerontology Series B—Psychological Sciences, 57*(1), P87–P94.

Lloyd-Williams, M., Friedman, T., & Rudd, N. (2001). An analysis of the validity of the Hospital Anxiety and Depression Scale as a screening tool in patients with advanced metastatic cancer. *Journal of Pain & Symptom Management, 22*(6), 990–996.

Oakley, L. D., & Kane, J. (1999). Personal and social illness demands related to depression. *Archives of Psychiatric Nursing, 13*(6), 294–302.

Raue, P. J., Brown, E. L., & Bruce, M. L. (2002). Assessing behavior health using OASIS: Part 1: Depression and suicidality. *Home Healthcare Nurse, 20*(3), 154–162.

Depression Self-Control

1409

Definition: Personal actions to minimize melancholy and maintain interest in life events

OUTCOME TARGET RATING: Maintain at_____   Increase to_____

D

OUTCOME OVERALL RATING	Never demonstrated 1	Rarely demonstrated 2	Sometimes demonstrated 3	Often demonstrated 4	Consistently demonstrated 5	
Indicators:						
140901 Monitors ability to concentrate	1	2	3	4	5	NA
140902 Monitors intensity of depression	1	2	3	4	5	NA
140903 Identifies precursors of depression	1	2	3	4	5	NA
140904 Plans strategies to reduce effects of precursors	1	2	3	4	5	NA
140905 Monitors behavioral manifestations of depression	1	2	3	4	5	NA
140906 Reports adequate sleep	1	2	3	4	5	NA
140907 Reports improved libido	1	2	3	4	5	NA
140908 Monitors physical manifestations of depression	1	2	3	4	5	NA
140909 Reports improved mood	1	2	3	4	5	NA
140910 Maintains stable weight	1	2	3	4	5	NA
140911 Follows treatment regimen	1	2	3	4	5	NA
140923 Uses medication as prescribed	1	2	3	4	5	NA
140924 Sets realistic goals	1	2	3	4	5	NA
140925 Delays big decision until feeling better	1	2	3	4	5	NA
140926 Participates in enjoyable activities	1	2	3	4	5	NA
140913 Follows exercise plan	1	2	3	4	5	NA
140914 Adheres to therapy schedule	1	2	3	4	5	NA
140915 Reports changes in symptoms to a health provider	1	2	3	4	5	NA
140920 Avoids alcohol misuse	1	2	3	4	5	NA
140921 Avoids non-prescription drug misuse	1	2	3	4	5	NA
140922 Avoids recreational drug use	1	2	3	4	5	NA
140918 Maintains personal hygiene	1	2	3	4	5	NA

Domain-*Psychosocial Health (III)*   **Class**-*Self-Control (O)*   *2nd edition 2000; revised 2004, 2008*

OUTCOME CONTENT REFERENCES:

Adams, P. (2000). Insight: A mental health prevention intervention. *Nursing Clinics of North America, 35*(2), 329–338.

American Psychiatric Association. (2000). *Diagnostic and statistical manual of mental disorders* (4th ed. text revision). Washington, DC: Author.

Cronin, J., Nash, V., Ray-Mihm, R., & Tucker, S. (2001). Relationship between psychiatric clinical assessment scores and patients' daily activities. *Journal of the American Psychiatric Nurses Association, 7*(5), 145–154.

Jaret, P. (1999). Fitness. Move the body, heal the mind. *Health, 13*(1), 50–51.

Johnson, C. D. (1999). Therapeutic recreation treats depression in the elderly. *Home Health Care Services Quarterly, 18*(2), 79–90.

Lantz, M. S. (2001). The psychiatric consultant. Suicide in late life: Identifying and managing at-risk older patients. *Geriatrics, 56*(7), 47–48.

Laliberte, R. (1999). How to manage your moods. *New Choices: Living Even Better After 50, 39*(6), 44–47.

Peden, A. R., Hall, L. A., Rayens, M. K., & Beebe, L. L. (2000). Reducing negative thinking and depressive symptoms in college women. *Journal of Nursing Scholarship, 32*(2), 145–151.

Tucker, S., & Darley, J. (2001). How to detect and manage depression in older people. *Nursing Times, 97*(45), 36–37.

Development: Late Adulthood 0121

Definition: Cognitive, psychosocial, and moral progression from 65 years of age and older

OUTCOME TARGET RATING: Maintain at_____   Increase to_____

		Never demonstrated	Rarely demonstrated	Sometimes demonstrated	Often demonstrated	Consistently demonstrated	
OUTCOME OVERALL RATING		1	2	3	4	5	
Indicators:							
012101	Maintains cognitive function	1	2	3	4	5	NA
012102	Maintains language skills	1	2	3	4	5	NA
012103	Maintains problem solving skills	1	2	3	4	5	NA
012104	Maintains lifelong learning	1	2	3	4	5	NA
012105	Exhibits realistic outlook about abilities	1	2	3	4	5	NA
012106	Compensates if deterioration in memory occurs	1	2	3	4	5	NA
012107	Copes with personal loss	1	2	3	4	5	NA
012108	Copes with own mortality	1	2	3	4	5	NA
012109	Maintains life interests	1	2	3	4	5	NA
012110	Exhibits sense of pride	1	2	3	4	5	NA
012111	Exhibits sense of accomplishment	1	2	3	4	5	NA
012112	Maintains relationships with immediate family	1	2	3	4	5	NA
012113	Maintains relationships with extended family	1	2	3	4	5	NA
012114	Maintains close relationships with friends	1	2	3	4	5	NA
012115	Copes with adult children in the home	1	2	3	4	5	NA
012116	Performs positive role in lives of grandchildren	1	2	3	4	5	NA
012117	Adjusts to parenting role of grandchildren	1	2	3	4	5	NA
012118	Adjusts to retirement	1	2	3	4	5	NA
012119	Develops new interests	1	2	3	4	5	NA
012120	Adapts to changing needs for assistance	1	2	3	4	5	NA
012121	Accepts assistance from others	1	2	3	4	5	NA
012122	Adjusts to change in financial income	1	2	3	4	5	NA
012123	Adjusts to change in living arrangements	1	2	3	4	5	NA
012124	Adjusts to change in marital status	1	2	3	4	5	NA
012125	Adjusts to change in marital relationship	1	2	3	4	5	NA
012126	Adjusts to sexual function changes	1	2	3	4	5	NA
012127	Practices safe sex	1	2	3	4	5	NA
012128	Adapts to functional impairment	1	2	3	4	5	NA
012129	Avoids substance misuse	1	2	3	4	5	NA
012130	Challenges ageism stereotypes	1	2	3	4	5	NA
012131	Derives support from religious or spiritual beliefs	1	2	3	4	5	NA
012132	Seeks understanding to meaning of own life	1	2	3	4	5	NA

D

Development: Late Adulthood—cont'd

	Never demonstrated	Rarely demonstrated	Sometimes demonstrated	Often demonstrated	Consistently demonstrated	
012133	Adheres to laws that protect welfare of others	1	2	3	4	5	NA
012134	Acknowledges personal values	1	2	3	4	5	NA
012135	Acknowledges values of others	1	2	3	4	5	NA
012136	Acknowledges personal opinions	1	2	3	4	5	NA
012137	Acknowledges opinions of others	1	2	3	4	5	NA
012138	Refrains from violating the rights of others	1	2	3	4	5	NA
012139	Respects others	1	2	3	4	5	NA
012140	Respects the environment	1	2	3	4	5	NA
012141	Supports equality in treatment of others	1	2	3	4	5	NA
012142	Recognizes that mutual trust is necessary in healthy relationships	1	2	3	4	5	NA

	Consistently demonstrated	Often demonstrated	Sometimes demonstrated	Rarely demonstrated	Never demonstrated	
012143	Exhibits anger	1	2	3	4	5	NA
012144	Exhibits inappropriate trust in others	1	2	3	4	5	NA
012145	Exhibits loneliness	1	2	3	4	5	NA
012146	Exhibits depression	1	2	3	4	5	NA
012147	Exhibits anxiety	1	2	3	4	5	NA
012148	Dwells on past	1	2	3	4	5	NA

Domain-*Functional Health (I)*   **Class**-*Growth & Development (B)*   4th edition 2008

OUTCOME CONTENT REFERENCES:

Andreoletti, C., Weratti, B. W., & Lachan, M. E. (2006). Age differences in the relationship between anxiety and recall. *Aging & Mental Health, 10*(3), 265–271.

Eva, K. W. (2003). Stemming the tide: Cognitive aging theories and their implications for continuing education in the health professions. *Journal of Continuing Education in the Health Professions, 23*(3), 133–140.

Isaacowitz, D. M., Vaillant, G. E., & Seligman, M. E. P. (2003). Strengths and satisfaction across the adult lifespan. *International Journal of Aging & Human Development, 57*(2), 181–201.

Newman, R. S., & German, D. J. (2005). Life span effects of lexical factors on oral naming. *Language & Speech, 48*(Pt 2), 123–156.

Papalia, D. E., Olds, S. W., & Feldman, R. D. (2007). *Human development* (10th ed.). New York: McGraw Hill.

Skultety, K. M., & Whitbourne, S. K. (2004). Gender differences in identity processes and self-esteem in middle and later adulthood. *Journal of Women & Aging, 16*(1/2), 175–188.

Spira, M. (2006). Mapping your future—a proactive approach to aging. *Journal of Gerontological Social Work, 47*(1/2), 71–87.

Troyer, A. K., Hafliger, A., Cadieux, M. J., & Craik, F. I. M. (2006). Name and face learning in older adults effects of level of processing, self-generation, and intention to learn. *Journals of Gerontology Series B: Psychological Sciences & Social Sciences, 61B*(2), 67–74.

Valentijn, S. A., van Boxtel, M. P., van Hooren, S. A., Bosma, H., Beckers, H. J., Ponds, R. W., Jolles, J. (2005). Change in sensory functioning predicts change in cognitive functioning: Results from a 6-year follow-up in the Maastricht aging study. *Journal of the American Geriatrics Society, 53*(3), 374–380.

Development: Middle Adulthood

Definition: Cognitive, psychosocial, and moral progression from 40 through 64 years of age

OUTCOME TARGET RATING: Maintain at_____   Increase to_____

		Never demonstrated	Rarely demonstrated	Sometimes demonstrated	Often demonstrated	Consistently demonstrated	
OUTCOME OVERALL RATING		1	2	3	4	5	
Indicators:							
012201	Exhibits high-level cognitive function	1	2	3	4	5	NA
012202	Uses expanded language skills	1	2	3	4	5	NA
012203	Uses accumulated knowledge in decision-making	1	2	3	4	5	NA
012204	Exhibits high-level problem solving skills	1	2	3	4	5	NA
012205	Exhibits creativity	1	2	3	4	5	NA
012206	Maintains lifelong learning	1	2	3	4	5	NA
012207	Exhibits success in chosen occupation	1	2	3	4	5	NA
012208	Exhibits occupational flexibility	1	2	3	4	5	NA
012209	Copes with personal loss	1	2	3	4	5	NA
012210	Copes with career burnout	1	2	3	4	5	NA
012211	Expresses optimism about the present	1	2	3	4	5	NA
012212	Expresses optimism about the future	1	2	3	4	5	NA
012213	Adjusts to children leaving home	1	2	3	4	5	NA
012214	Copes with adult children in the home	1	2	3	4	5	NA
012215	Performs positive role in lives of grandchildren	1	2	3	4	5	NA
012216	Adjusts to parenting role of grandchildren	1	2	3	4	5	NA
012217	Exhibits strong sense of self	1	2	3	4	5	NA
012218	Maintains a healthy, intimate relationship with partner	1	2	3	4	5	NA
012219	Maintains relationships with immediate family	1	2	3	4	5	NA
012220	Maintains relationships with extended family	1	2	3	4	5	NA
012221	Develops close relationships with friends	1	2	3	4	5	NA
012222	Adjusts to sexual function changes	1	2	3	4	5	NA
012223	Practices safe sex	1	2	3	4	5	NA
012224	Adjusts to midlife changes	1	2	3	4	5	NA
012225	Avoids substance misuse	1	2	3	4	5	NA
012226	Adheres to laws that protect welfare of others	1	2	3	4	5	NA
012227	Acknowledges personal values	1	2	3	4	5	NA
012228	Acknowledges values of others	1	2	3	4	5	NA
012229	Acknowledges personal opinions	1	2	3	4	5	NA
012230	Acknowledges opinions of others	1	2	3	4	5	NA
012231	Refrains from violating rights of others	1	2	3	4	5	NA
012232	Respects others	1	2	3	4	5	NA

D

Development: Middle Adulthood—*cont'd*

		Never demonstrated	Rarely demonstrated	Sometimes demonstrated	Often demonstrated	Consistently demonstrated	
012233	Respects the environment	1	2	3	4	5	NA
012234	Supports equality in treatment of others	1	2	3	4	5	NA
012235	Recognizes that mutual trust is necessary in healthy relationships	1	2	3	4	5	NA

		Consistently demonstrated	Often demonstrated	Sometimes demonstrated	Rarely demonstrated	Never demonstrated	
012236	Dwells on past	1	2	3	4	5	NA
012237	Exhibits unresolved anger	1	2	3	4	5	NA
012238	Exhibits unresolved emotional issues	1	2	3	4	5	NA
012239	Exhibits incapacitating fear	1	2	3	4	5	NA
012240	Exhibits unsafe risk-taking behaviors	1	2	3	4	5	NA
012241	Exhibits impulsivity	1	2	3	4	5	NA

Domain-Functional Health (I)   **Class**-Growth & Development (B)   4th edition 2008

OUTCOME CONTENT REFERENCES:

Hartman-Stein, P. E., & Potkanowicz, E. S. (2003). Behavioral determinants of healthy aging: Good news for the baby boomer generation. *Online Journal of Issues in Nursing, 8*(2).

Isaacowitz, D. M., Vaillant, G. E., & Seligman, M. E. (2003). Strengths and satisfaction across the adult lifespan. *International Journal of Aging & Human Development, 57*(2), 181–201.

Newman, R. S., & German, D. J. (2005). Life span effects of lexical factors on oral naming. *Language & Speech, 48*(Pt 2), 123–156.

Papalia, D. E., Olds, S. W., & Feldman, R. D. (2007). *Human development* (10th ed.). New York: McGraw Hill.

Skultety, K. M., & Whitbourne, S. K. (2004). Gender differences in identity processes and self-esteem in middle and later adulthood. *Journal of Women & Aging, 16*(1/2), 175–188.

Development: Young Adulthood   **0123**

Definition: Cognitive, psychosocial, and moral progression from 18 through 39 years of age

OUTCOME TARGET RATING: Maintain at_____   Increase to_____

		Never demonstrated	Rarely demonstrated	Sometimes demonstrated	Often demonstrated	Consistently demonstrated	
OUTCOME OVERALL RATING		1	2	3	4	5	
Indicators:							
012301	Expresses complex thoughts	1	2	3	4	5	NA
012302	Expands language skills	1	2	3	4	5	NA
012303	Makes educational choices	1	2	3	4	5	NA
012304	Makes occupational choices	1	2	3	4	5	NA
012305	Establishes gainful employment	1	2	3	4	5	NA
012306	Establishes pattern of lifelong learning	1	2	3	4	5	NA
012307	Exhibits stable personality traits	1	2	3	4	5	NA
012308	Adjusts lifestyle according to life events	1	2	3	4	5	NA
012309	Embraces sexual identity	1	2	3	4	5	NA
012310	Practices safe sex	1	2	3	4	5	NA
012311	Maintains a healthy, intimate relationship with partner	1	2	3	4	5	NA

Continued

D

Development: Young Adulthood—cont'd

		Never demonstrated	Rarely demonstrated	Sometimes demonstrated	Often demonstrated	Consistently demonstrated	
012312	Maintains relationships with immediate family	1	2	3	4	5	NA
012313	Maintains relationships with extended family	1	2	3	4	5	NA
012314	Develops new friendships	1	2	3	4	5	NA
012315	Copes with personal loss	1	2	3	4	5	NA
012316	Adapts to parental role	1	2	3	4	5	NA
012336	Exhibits self-esteem	1	2	3	4	5	NA
012317	Exhibits autonomy	1	2	3	4	5	NA
012318	Exhibits self-control	1	2	3	4	5	NA
012319	Exhibits personal responsibility	1	2	3	4	5	NA
012320	Avoids substance misuse	1	2	3	4	5	NA
012321	Adheres to laws that protect the welfare of others	1	2	3	4	5	NA
012322	Acknowledges personal values	1	2	3	4	5	NA
012323	Acknowledges values of others	1	2	3	4	5	NA
012324	Acknowledges personal opinions	1	2	3	4	5	NA
012325	Acknowledges opinions of others	1	2	3	4	5	NA
012326	Refrains from violating the rights of others	1	2	3	4	5	NA
012327	Respects others	1	2	3	4	5	NA
012328	Respects the environment	1	2	3	4	5	NA

		Consistently demonstrated	Often demonstrated	Sometimes demonstrated	Rarely demonstrated	Never demonstrated	
012329	Dwells on past	1	2	3	4	5	NA
012330	Exhibits unresolved anger	1	2	3	4	5	NA
012331	Exhibits unresolved emotional issues	1	2	3	4	5	NA
012332	Exhibits incapacitating fear	1	2	3	4	5	NA
012333	Exhibits inappropriate mistrust in others	1	2	3	4	5	NA
012334	Exhibits unsafe risk-taking behaviors	1	2	3	4	5	NA
012335	Exhibits impulsivity	1	2	3	4	5	NA

Domain-*Functional Health (I)*   **Class**-*Growth & Development (B)*   *4th edition 2008; revised 2013*

OUTCOME CONTENT REFERENCES:
Andreoletti, C., Weratti, B. W., & Lachan, M. E. (2006). Age differences in the relationship between anxiety and recall. *Aging & Mental Health, 10*(3), 265–271.
Isaacowitz, D. M., Vaillant, G. E., & Seligman, M. E. P. (2003). Strengths and satisfaction across the adult lifespan. *International Journal of Aging & Human Development, 57*(2), 181–201.
McLaren, L., Kuh, D., Hardy, R., & Gauvin, L. (2004). Positive and negative body-related comments and their relationship with body dissatisfaction in middle-aged women. *Psychology & Health, 19*(2), 261–272.
Newman, R. S., & German, D. J. (2005). Life span effects of lexical factors on oral naming. *Language & Speech, 48*(Pt 2), 123–156.
Papalia, D. E., Olds, S. W., & Feldman, R. D. (2007). *Human development* (10th ed.). New York: McGraw Hill.

Dignified Life Closure   1307

Definition: Personal actions to maintain control when approaching end of life

OUTCOME TARGET RATING: Maintain at_____   Increase to_____

D

OUTCOME OVERALL RATING		Never demonstrated 1	Rarely demonstrated 2	Sometimes demonstrated 3	Often demonstrated 4	Consistently demonstrated 5	
Indicators:							
130701	Puts affairs in order	1	2	3	4	5	NA
130702	Expresses hopefulness	1	2	3	4	5	NA
130703	Participates in decisions related to care	1	2	3	4	5	NA
130704	Participates in decisions about hospitalization	1	2	3	4	5	NA
130705	Participates in decisions about resuscitation status	1	2	3	4	5	NA
130706	Controls decisions about organ donation	1	2	3	4	5	NA
130707	Participates in planning funeral	1	2	3	4	5	NA
130708	Maintains current will	1	2	3	4	5	NA
130709	Maintains advance directives	1	2	3	4	5	NA
130710	Resolves important issues	1	2	3	4	5	NA
130711	Shares feelings about dying	1	2	3	4	5	NA
130712	Reconciles relationships	1	2	3	4	5	NA
130713	Completes meaningful goals	1	2	3	4	5	NA
130714	Maintains sense of control of remaining time	1	2	3	4	5	NA
130715	Exchanges affection with others	1	2	3	4	5	NA
130716	Disengages gradually from significant others	1	2	3	4	5	NA
130717	Recalls lifetime memories	1	2	3	4	5	NA
130718	Reviews life's accomplishments	1	2	3	4	5	NA
130719	Discusses spiritual experiences	1	2	3	4	5	NA
130720	Discusses spiritual concerns	1	2	3	4	5	NA
130721	Maintains physical independence	1	2	3	4	5	NA
130722	Controls treatment choices	1	2	3	4	5	NA
130723	Controls food/drink intake	1	2	3	4	5	NA
130724	Controls personal possessions	1	2	3	4	5	NA
130725	Expresses readiness for death	1	2	3	4	5	NA

Domain-*Psychosocial Health (III)*   **Class**-*Psychosocial Adaptation (N)*   *3rd edition 2004; revised 2013*

OUTCOME CONTENT REFERENCES:

Callanan, M., & Kelley, P. (1992). *Final gifts*. New York: Poseidon Press.

Cicirelli, V. G. (1997). Elders' end-of-life decisions: Implications for hospice care. *Hospice Journal: Physical, Psychosocial, & Pastoral Care of the Dying, 12*(1), 57–72.

Ferrell, B. R. (1993). To know suffering. *Oncology Nursing Forum, 20*(10), 1471–1477.

McCanse, R. P. (1995). The McCanse Readiness for Death Instrument (MRDI): A reliable and valid measure for hospice care. *Hospice Journal, 10*(1), 15–26.

Potter, P. A., & Perry, A. G. (2001). *Fundamentals of nursing* (5th ed.). St. Louis: Mosby.

Quill, T. E. (1993). *Death and dignity: Making choices and taking charge*. New York: W. W. Norton.

Schmele, J. A. (1995). Perceptions of a dying patient of the quality of care and caring: An interview with Ivan Hanson. *Journal of Nursing Care Quality, 9*(4), 31–42.

Discharge Readiness: Independent Living 0311

Definition: Readiness of a patient to relocate from a health care institution to living independently

OUTCOME TARGET RATING: Maintain at_____ Increase to_____

		Never demonstrated	Rarely demonstrated	Sometimes demonstrated	Often demonstrated	Consistently demonstrated	
OUTCOME OVERALL RATING		1	2	3	4	5	
Indicators:							
031113	Obtains needed assistance	1	2	3	4	5	NA
031114	Uses personal support system	1	2	3	4	5	NA
031106	Describes signs & symptoms to health professional	1	2	3	4	5	NA
031107	Describes prescribed treatments	1	2	3	4	5	NA
031108	Describes risks for complications	1	2	3	4	5	NA
031115	Manages own non-parenteral medication	1	2	3	4	5	NA
031116	Manages own parenteral medication	1	2	3	4	5	NA
031110	Performs activities of daily living (ADLs) independently	1	2	3	4	5	NA
031111	Performs instrumental activities of daily living (IADLs) independently	1	2	3	4	5	NA
031112	Makes appropriate judgments	1	2	3	4	5	NA
031117	Participates in discharge planning	1	2	3	4	5	NA

		Consistently demonstrated	Often demonstrated	Sometimes demonstrated	Rarely demonstrated	Never demonstrated	
031101	Fever	1	2	3	4	5	NA
031102	Infection	1	2	3	4	5	NA
031103	Confusion	1	2	3	4	5	NA

Domain-Functional Health (I)   **Class**-Self-Care (D)   *3rd edition 2004; revised 2008*

OUTCOME CONTENT REFERENCES:

Barnes, S. (2000). Ambulatory surgery. Are you watching the clock? Let criteria define discharge readiness. *Journal of Perianesthesia Nursing, 15*(3), 174–176.

Bull, M. J., Hansen, H. E., & Gross, C. R. (2000). Differences in family caregiver outcomes by their level of involvement in discharge planning. *Applied Nursing Research, 13*(2), 76–82.

Costa, M. J. (2001). The lived perioperative experience of ambulatory surgery patients. *AORN Journal, 74*(6), 874–876, 878–881.

Harris, M. D. (1999). Medicare & the nurse. 10 DRGs that can affect home care referrals. *Home Healthcare Nurse, 17*(2), 127–129.

Higson, J., & Bolland, R. (2001). Paediatric discharge criteria lead to improved outcomes. *Times, 97*(35), 30–31.

Kuc, J. A., & Pietro, J. (1999). Safe discharge from the PACU and ambulatory care setting. *Journal of Nursing Law, 6*(2), 7–14.

Walker, C. R., Watters, N., Nadon, C., Graham, K., & Niday, P. (1999). Discharge of mothers and babies from hospital after birth of a healthy full-term infant: Developing criteria through a community-wide consensus process. *Canadian Journal of Public Health, 90*(5), 313–315.

Discharge Readiness: Supported Living 0312

Definition: Readiness of a patient to relocate from a health care institution to a lower level of supported living

OUTCOME TARGET RATING: Maintain at_____ Increase to_____

		Never demonstrated	Rarely demonstrated	Sometimes demonstrated	Often demonstrated	Consistently demonstrated	
OUTCOME OVERALL RATING		1	2	3	4	5	
Indicators:							
031201	Patient needs consistent with staff support	1	2	3	4	5	NA
031202	Patient needs consistent with family support	1	2	3	4	5	NA
031203	Oriented to care at new residence	1	2	3	4	5	NA
031204	Accepts transfer to new residence	1	2	3	4	5	NA
031205	Describes special needs	1	2	3	4	5	NA
031206	Describes short-term plan	1	2	3	4	5	NA
031207	Describes long-term plan	1	2	3	4	5	NA
031208	Describes plan for continuity of care	1	2	3	4	5	NA
031209	Participates in discharge planning	1	2	3	4	5	NA

Domain-*Functional Health (I)* **Class**-*Self-Care (D)* *3rd edition 2004; revised 2008*

OUTCOME CONTENT REFERENCES:

Bosek, M. S. D., Burton, L. A., & Savage, T. A. (1999). The patient who could not be discharged: How far should patient autonomy extend? *JONA's Healthcare Law, Ethics, & Regulation, 1*(4), 23–30.

Bull, M. J., Hansen, H. E., & Gross, C. R. (2000). Differences in family caregiver outcomes by their level of involvement in discharge planning. *Applied Nursing Research, 13*(2), 76–82.

Chan, L., & Ciol, M. (2000). Medicare's payment system: Its effect on discharges to skilled nursing facilities from rehabilitation hospitals. *Archives of Physical Medicine & Rehabilitation, 81*(6), 715–719.

Discomfort Level 2109

Definition: Severity of observed or reported mental or physical discomfort

OUTCOME TARGET RATING: Maintain at_____ Increase to_____

		Severe	Substantial	Moderate	Mild	None	
OUTCOME OVERALL RATING		1	2	3	4	5	
Indicators:							
210901	Pain	1	2	3	4	5	NA
210902	Anxiety	1	2	3	4	5	NA
210903	Moaning	1	2	3	4	5	NA
210904	Suffering	1	2	3	4	5	NA
210905	Thrashing	1	2	3	4	5	NA
210906	Stress	1	2	3	4	5	NA
210907	Fear	1	2	3	4	5	NA
210908	Depression	1	2	3	4	5	NA
210909	Hallucinations	1	2	3	4	5	NA
210910	Delusions	1	2	3	4	5	NA
210911	Paranoid thoughts	1	2	3	4	5	NA
210912	Obsessive-compulsive behaviors	1	2	3	4	5	NA
210913	Hyperactivity	1	2	3	4	5	NA
210914	Restlessness	1	2	3	4	5	NA

Continued

D

Discomfort Level—cont'd

	Severe	Substantial	Moderate	Mild	None	
210915	Restless legs syndrome	1	2	3	4	5	NA
210916	Itching	1	2	3	4	5	NA
210917	Muscle aches	1	2	3	4	5	NA
210918	Grimacing	1	2	3	4	5	NA
210919	Facial tension	1	2	3	4	5	NA
210920	Rebound tenderness	1	2	3	4	5	NA
210921	Jerking	1	2	3	4	5	NA
210922	Poor body positioning	1	2	3	4	5	NA
210923	Labored breathing	1	2	3	4	5	NA
210924	Air hunger	1	2	3	4	5	NA
210925	Loss of appetite	1	2	3	4	5	NA
210926	Chilling	1	2	3	4	5	NA
210927	Hypothermia	1	2	3	4	5	NA
210928	Nausea	1	2	3	4	5	NA
210929	Vomiting	1	2	3	4	5	NA
210930	Diarrhea	1	2	3	4	5	NA
210931	Bowel incontinence	1	2	3	4	5	NA
210932	Constipation	1	2	3	4	5	NA
210933	Urinary incontinence	1	2	3	4	5	NA
210934	Inability to communicate	1	2	3	4	5	NA
210935	Suicidal thoughts	1	2	3	4	5	NA
210936	Loss of faith	1	2	3	4	5	NA
210937	Sense of spiritual abandonment	1	2	3	4	5	NA

Domain-*Perceived Health (V)*   **Class**-*Symptom Status (V)*   *4th edition 2008*

OUTCOME CONTENT REFERENCES:
Gropper, E. I. (1992). Promoting health by promoting comfort. *Nursing Forum, 27*(2), 5–8.
Hamilton, J. (1989). Comfort and the hospitalized chronically ill. *Journal of Gerontological Nursing, 15*(4), 28–33.
Kennedy, G. T. (1991). *A nursing investigation of comfort and comforting care of the acutely ill patient.* Unpublished doctoral dissertation, The University of Texas, Austin.
Kolcaba, K. (2003). *Comfort theory and practice: A vision for holistic health care and research.* New York: Springer.
Kolcaba, K., & DiMarco, M. (2005). Comfort theory and its application to pediatric nursing. *Pediatric Nursing, 31*(3), 187–194.
Tipton, L. (2001). *A qualitative study of hope and the environment of persons living with cancer. Dissertation Abstracts International, 62*(03), 1326B. (UMI No. 3008460).

Distorted Thought Self-Control

1403

Definition: Self-restraint of disruptions in perception, thought processes, and thought content

OUTCOME TARGET RATING: Maintain at_____ Increase to_____

	Never demonstrated	Rarely demonstrated	Sometimes demonstrated	Often demonstrated	Consistently demonstrated	
OUTCOME OVERALL RATING	1	2	3	4	5	
Indicators:						
140301 Recognizes hallucinations or delusions are occurring	1	2	3	4	5	NA
140302 Refrains from attending to hallucinations or delusions	1	2	3	4	5	NA
140303 Refrains from responding to hallucinations or delusions	1	2	3	4	5	NA

Distorted Thought Self-Control—*cont'd*

		Never demonstrated	Rarely demonstrated	Sometimes demonstrated	Often demonstrated	Consistently demonstrated	
140304	Monitors frequency of hallucinations or delusions	1	2	3	4	5	NA
140305	Describes content of hallucinations or delusions	1	2	3	4	5	NA
140306	Reports decrease in hallucinations or delusions	1	2	3	4	5	NA
140307	Asks for validation of reality	1	2	3	4	5	NA
140308	Maintains affect consistent with mood	1	2	3	4	5	NA
140309	Interacts with others appropriately	1	2	3	4	5	NA
140310	Perceives environment accurately	1	2	3	4	5	NA
140311	Exhibits logical thought flow patterns	1	2	3	4	5	NA
140312	Exhibits reality-based thinking	1	2	3	4	5	NA
140313	Exhibits appropriate thought content	1	2	3	4	5	NA
140314	Exhibits ability to grasp ideas of others	1	2	3	4	5	NA

Domain-*Psychosocial Health (III)* **Class**-*Self-Control (O)* *1st edition 1997; revised 2000, 2004*

OUTCOME CONTENT REFERENCES:
Andreasen, N. C., & Black, D. (2001). *Introductory textbook of psychiatry* (3rd ed.). Washington, DC: American Psychiatric.
Buccheri, R., Trygstad, L., Kanas, N., & Dowling, G. (1997). Symptom management of auditory hallucinations in schizophrenia: Results of 1-year follow up. *Journal of Psychosocial Nursing & Mental Health Services, 35*(12), 20–28, 37–38.
Buccheri, R., Trygstad, L., Kanas, N., Waldron, B., & Dowling, G. (1996). Auditory hallucinations in schizophrenia: Group experience in examining symptom management and behavioral strategies. *Journal of Psychosocial Nursing & Mental Health Services, 34*(2), 12–26, 44–45.
+Cummings, J. L. (1997). The Neuropsychiatric Inventory: Assessing psychopathology in dementia patients. *Neurology, 48* (Suppl. 6), S10–S16.
Frederick, J., & Cotanch, P. (1995). Self-help techniques for auditory hallucinations in schizophrenia. *Issues in Mental Health Nursing, 16*(3), 213–224.
Grimaldi, D., & Cousins, A. (1985). Paranoia. *Journal of Emergency Nursing, 11*(4), 201–204.
MacRae, A. (1997). The model of functional deficits associated with hallucinations. *American Journal of Occupational Therapy, 51*(1), 57–63.
Rosenthal, T. T., & McGuinness, T. M. (1986). Dealing with delusional patients: Discovering the distorted truth. *Issues in Mental Health Nursing, 8*(2), 143–154.
Stuart, G. W., & Laraia, M. T. (2001). *Principles and practice of psychiatric nursing* (7th ed.). St. Louis: Mosby.

Drug Abuse Cessation Behavior 1630

Definition: Personal actions to eliminate drug use that poses a threat to health

OUTCOME TARGET RATING: Maintain at_____ Increase to_____

		Never demonstrated	Rarely demonstrated	Sometimes demonstrated	Often demonstrated	Consistently demonstrated	
OUTCOME OVERALL RATING		1	2	3	4	5	
Indicators:							
163001	Expresses willingness to stop drug use	1	2	3	4	5	NA
163002	Expresses belief in the ability to stop drug use	1	2	3	4	5	NA
163003	Identifies benefits of eliminating harmful drug use	1	2	3	4	5	NA
163004	Identifies negative consequences of drug use	1	2	3	4	5	NA

Continued

D

Drug Abuse Cessation Behavior—cont'd

		Never demonstrated	Rarely demonstrated	Sometimes demonstrated	Often demonstrated	Consistently demonstrated	
163005	Develops effective strategies to eliminate drug use	1	2	3	4	5	NA
163006	Identifies barriers to harmful drug use elimination	1	2	3	4	5	NA
163007	Adjusts drug use elimination strategies as needed	1	2	3	4	5	NA
163008	Commits to drug elimination strategies	1	2	3	4	5	NA
163009	Follows selected drug elimination strategies	1	2	3	4	5	NA
163010	Participates in screening for associated health problems	1	2	3	4	5	NA
163011	Uses strategies to cope with withdrawal symptoms	1	2	3	4	5	NA
163012	Uses behavior modification strategies	1	2	3	4	5	NA
163013	Uses effective coping strategies	1	2	3	4	5	NA
163014	Obtains assistance from health professional	1	2	3	4	5	NA
163015	Uses personal support system	1	2	3	4	5	NA
163016	Uses reputable sources of information	1	2	3	4	5	NA
163017	Uses drug replacement therapy	1	2	3	4	5	NA
163018	Uses alternative therapy	1	2	3	4	5	NA
163019	Identifies emotional states that affect drug use	1	2	3	4	5	NA
163020	Adjusts lifestyle to promote drug elimination	1	2	3	4	5	NA
163021	Participates in drug withdrawal program	1	2	3	4	5	NA
163022	Participates in counseling	1	2	3	4	5	NA
163023	Monitors for signs of depression	1	2	3	4	5	NA
163024	Uses prescribed medication as recommended	1	2	3	4	5	NA
163025	Uses non-prescription medication as recommended	1	2	3	4	5	NA
163026	Uses available support groups	1	2	3	4	5	NA
163027	Uses available community resources	1	2	3	4	5	NA
163028	Eliminates harmful drug use	1	2	3	4	5	NA

Domain-*Health Knowledge & Behavior (IV)*   **Class**-*Health Behavior (Q)*   *4th edition 2008*

OUTCOME CONTENT REFERENCES:

Giesbrecht, N., & Haydon, E. (2006). Community-based interventions and alcohol, tobacco and other drugs: Foci, outcomes and implications. *Drug and Alcohol Review, 25*(6), 633–646.

Gossop, M., Marsden, J., Stewart, D., Treacy, S. (2002). Change and stability of change after treatment of drug misuse: 2-year outcomes from the National Treatment Outcome Research Study (UK). *Addictive Behaviors, 27*(2), 155–166.

Kaminer, Y., Burleson, J. A., & Goldberger, R. (2002). Cognitive-behavioral coping skills and psychoeducation therapies for adolescent substance abuse. *Journal of Nervous and Mental Disease, 190*(11), 737–745.

Kenna, G. A., Nielsen, D. M., Mello, P., Schiesl, A., & Swift, R. M. (2007). Pharmacotherapy of dual substance abuse and dependence. *CNS Drugs, 21*(3), 213–237.

Litten, R. Z., & Allen, J. P. (1999). Medications for alcohol, illicit drug, and tobacco dependence: An update of research findings. *Journal of Substance Abuse Treatment, 16*(2), 105–112.

Simpson, D. D. (1997). Effectiveness of drug abuse treatment: A review of research from field settings. In J. A. Egertson, D. M. Fox, & A. I. Leshner (Eds.), *Treating drug abusers effectively*. Oxford: Blackwell.

Williams, R. J., Chang, S. Y., & Addiction Centre Adolescent Research Group. (2000). A comprehensive and comparative review of adolescent substance abuse treatment outcome. *Clinical Psychology: Science and Practice, 7*(2), 138–166.

Winters, K. C., Stinchfield, R., Latimer, W. W., & Lee, S. (2007). Long-term outcome of substance-dependent youth following 12-step treatment. *Journal of Substance Abuse Treatment, 33*(1), 61–69.

Dry Eye Severity

2110

Definition: Severity of signs and symptoms of insufficient tears

OUTCOME TARGET RATING: Maintain at_____   Increase to_____

		Severe	Substantial	Moderate	Mild	None	
OUTCOME OVERALL RATING		1	2	3	4	5	
Indicators:							
211001	Decreased tear production	1	2	3	4	5	NA
211002	Incomplete eyelid closure	1	2	3	4	5	NA
211003	Redness of conjunctiva	1	2	3	4	5	NA
211004	Burning eye sensation	1	2	3	4	5	NA
211005	Itchy eye sensation	1	2	3	4	5	NA
211006	Gritty sensation	1	2	3	4	5	NA
211007	Foreign body sensation	1	2	3	4	5	NA
211008	Eye pain	1	2	3	4	5	NA
211009	Excessive watering	1	2	3	4	5	NA
211010	Blurred vision	1	2	3	4	5	NA
211011	Excessive mucous secretions	1	2	3	4	5	NA
211012	Sensitivity to light	1	2	3	4	5	NA

Domain-*Perceived Health (V)*   **Class**-*Symptom Status (V)*   *5th edition 2013*

OUTCOME CONTENT REFERENCES:

Dawson, D. (2005). Development of a new eye care guideline for critically ill patients. *Intensive Critical Care Nursing, 21*(2), 119–122.

Tavares, F., Fernandes, R. S., Bernardes, T. F., Bonfioli, A. A., & Soares, E. J. (2010). Dry eye disease. *Seminars in Ophthalmology, 25*(3), 84–93.

Versura, P., Nanni, P., Bavelloni, A., Blalock, W. L., Piazzi, M., Roda, A., & Campos, E. C. (2010). Tear proteomics in evaporative dry eye disease. *Eye, 24*(8), 1396–1402.

Eating Disorder Self-Control 1411

E

Definition: Personal actions to eliminate maladaptive behaviors and to adopt and maintain healthy eating patterns and optimum body weight

OUTCOME TARGET RATING: Maintain at_____ Increase to_____

		Never demonstrated	Rarely demonstrated	Sometimes demonstrated	Often demonstrated	Consistently demonstrated	
OUTCOME OVERALL RATING		1	2	3	4	5	
Indicators:							
141101	Selects a healthy target weight	1	2	3	4	5	NA
141102	Participates in setting achievable dietary goals with health professional	1	2	3	4	5	NA
141103	Sets achievable weight gain goals	1	2	3	4	5	NA
141104	Sets achievable weight loss goals	1	2	3	4	5	
141105	Monitors body weight	1	2	3	4	5	NA
141106	Maintains progress toward target weight	1	2	3	4	5	NA
141107	Follows a healthy eating plan	1	2	3	4	5	NA
141108	Identifies emotional states that affect food and fluid intake	1	2	3	4	5	NA
141109	Identifies social situations that affect food and fluid intake	1	2	3	4	5	NA
141110	Plans strategies for situations that affect food and fluid intake	1	2	3	4	5	NA
141111	Identifies maladaptive eating behaviors	1	2	3	4	5	NA
141112	Verbalizes a desire to decrease maladaptive eating behaviors	1	2	3	4	5	NA
141113	Eliminates maladaptive eating behaviors	1	2	3	4	5	NA
141114	Follows treatment plan	1	2	3	4	5	NA
141115	Identifies daily food and fluid intake that meets nutritional needs	1	2	3	4	5	NA
141116	Consumes daily caloric intake appropriate for metabolic needs	1	2	3	4	5	NA
141117	Consumes daily nutrient intake appropriate for metabolic needs	1	2	3	4	5	NA
141118	Maintains body weight appropriate for height	1	2	3	4	5	NA
141119	Uses strategies to manage stress	1	2	3	4	5	NA
141120	Engages in recommended exercise routine	1	2	3	4	5	NA
141121	Identifies an accurate perception of body image	1	2	3	4	5	NA
141122	Expresses satisfaction with body image	1	2	3	4	5	NA
141123	Expresses positive esteem	1	2	3	4	5	NA
141124	Expresses satisfaction with personal self control	1	2	3	4	5	NA
141125	Identifies supportive family relationships	1	2	3	4	5	NA
141126	Uses medication as prescribed	1	2	3	4	5	NA
141127	Expresses determination to recover from eating disorder	1	2	3	4	5	NA

Eating Disorder Self-Control—cont'd

		Consistently demonstrated	Often demonstrated	Sometimes demonstrated	Rarely demonstrated	Never demonstrated	
141128	Nutritional deficits	1	2	3	4	5	NA
141129	Preoccupation with food	1	2	3	4	5	NA
141130	Preoccupation with weight	1	2	3	4	5	NA
141131	Purging	1	2	3	4	5	NA
141132	Bingeing	1	2	3	4	5	NA
141133	Overuse of diuretics	1	2	3	4	5	NA
141134	Overuse of laxatives	1	2	3	4	5	NA
141135	Depression	1	2	3	4	5	NA
141136	Substance abuse	1	2	3	4	5	NA
141137	Suicidal thoughts	1	2	3	4	5	NA
141138	Irregular menstrual cycles	1	2	3	4	5	NA
141139	Excessive exercise	1	2	3	4	5	NA

Domain-*Psychosocial Health (III)* **Class**-*Self-Control (O)* 5th edition 2013

OUTCOME CONTENT REFERENCES

Berkman, N., Bulik, C., Brownley, K., Lohr, K., Sedway, J., Rooks, A., & Gartlehner, G. (April). Management of eating disorders. Evidence report/technology assessment No. 135. (Prepared by the RTI International-University of North Carolina Evidence-Based Practice Center under Contract No. 290-02-0016.) Publication No. 06-E010. Rockville, MD: Agency for Healthcare Research and Quality.

Berkman, N., Lohr, K., & Bulik, C. (2007). Outcomes of eating disorder: A systematic review of the literature. *International Journal of Eating Disorders, 40*(4), 293–309.

Fichter, M., Quadflieg, N., & Hedlund, S. (2006). Twelve-year course and outcome predictors of anorexia nervosa. *International Journal of Eating Disorders, 39*(2), 87–100.

Kong, S. (2005). Day treatment programme for patients with eating disorders: Randomized controlled trial. *Journal of Advanced Nursing, 51*(1), 5–14.

Patching, J., & Lawler, J. (2009). Understanding women's experiences of developing an eating disorder and recovering: A life-history approach. *Nursing Inquiry, 16*(1), 10–21.

Sadock, B. J., & Sadock, V. A. (2007). *Kaplan & Sadock's synopsis of psychiatry: Behavioral sciences/clinical psychiatry* (10th ed.). Philadelphia: Lippincott, Williams, & Wilkins.

Stuart, G. W. (2009). *Principles and practice of psychiatric nursing* (9th ed.). St. Louis: Mosby Elsevier.

Electrolyte & Acid/Base Balance **0600**

Definition: Balance of electrolytes and non-electrolytes in the intracellular and extracellular compartments of the body

OUTCOME TARGET RATING: Maintain at_____ Increase to_____

		Severe deviation from normal range	Substantial deviation from normal range	Moderate deviation from normal range	Mild deviation from normal range	No deviation from normal range	
OUTCOME OVERALL RATING		1	2	3	4	5	
Indicators:							
060001	Apical heart rate	1	2	3	4	5	NA
060002	Apical heart rhythm	1	2	3	4	5	NA
060003	Respiratory rate	1	2	3	4	5	NA
060004	Respiratory rhythm	1	2	3	4	5	NA
060005	Serum sodium	1	2	3	4	5	NA
060006	Serum potassium	1	2	3	4	5	NA
060007	Serum chloride	1	2	3	4	5	NA
060008	Serum calcium	1	2	3	4	5	NA
060009	Serum magnesium	1	2	3	4	5	NA
060010	Serum pH	1	2	3	4	5	NA

Continued

E

Electrolyte & Acid/Base Balance—cont'd

		Severe deviation from normal range	Substantial deviation from normal range	Moderate deviation from normal range	Mild deviation from normal range	No deviation from normal range	
060011	Serum albumin	1	2	3	4	5	NA
060012	Serum creatinine	1	2	3	4	5	NA
060013	Serum bicarbonate	1	2	3	4	5	NA
060024	Serum carbon dioxide	1	2	3	4	5	NA
060025	Serum osmolarity	1	2	3	4	5	NA
060026	Serum glucose	1	2	3	4	5	NA
060027	Serum hematocrit	1	2	3	4	5	NA
060014	Blood urea nitrogen	1	2	3	4	5	NA
060028	Blood urea nitrogen to creatinine ratio	1	2	3	4	5	NA
060015	Urine pH	1	2	3	4	5	NA
060029	Urine sodium	1	2	3	4	5	NA
060030	Urine chloride	1	2	3	4	5	NA
060031	Urine creatinine	1	2	3	4	5	NA
060032	Urine osmolarity	1	2	3	4	5	NA
060022	Urine specific gravity	1	2	3	4	5	NA
060019	Neuromuscular non-irritability	1	2	3	4	5	NA
060023	Sensation in extremities	1	2	3	4	5	NA

		Severe	Substantial	Moderate	Mild	None	
060033	Impaired cognition	1	2	3	4	5	NA
060034	Fatigue	1	2	3	4	5	NA
060035	Muscle weakness	1	2	3	4	5	NA
060036	Muscle cramps	1	2	3	4	5	NA
060037	Abdominal cramps	1	2	3	4	5	NA
060038	Nausea	1	2	3	4	5	NA
060039	Dysrhythmia	1	2	3	4	5	NA
060040	Restlessness	1	2	3	4	5	NA
060041	Paresthesia	1	2	3	4	5	NA

Domain-Physiologic Health (II)   **Class**-Fluid & Electrolytes (G)   1st edition 1997; revised 2004, 2008

OUTCOME CONTENT REFERENCES:

Cherry, R. (1992). Furosemide facts. *Emergency Medical Services, 21*(9), 79.

Cullen, L. (1992). Interventions related to fluid and electrolytes. *Nursing Clinics of North America, 27*(2), 60, 62, 79.

Innerarity, S. A. (1997). *Fluids and electrolytes* (3rd ed.). Springhouse, PA: Springhouse.

McCance, K. L., & Huether, S. E. (2002). *Pathophysiology: The biologic basis for disease in adults and children* (4th ed.). St. Louis: Mosby.

Methany, N. (2000). *Fluid and electrolyte balance: Nursing considerations* (4th ed.). Philadelphia: Lippincott Williams & Wilkins.

Norris, C. (1982). *Concept clarification in nursing*. Rockville, MD: Aspen.

Schuller, D., Mitchell, J., Calendrino, F., & Schuster, D. (1991). Fluid balance during pulmonary edema: Is fluid gain a marker or a cause of post-operative outcome? *Chest, 100*(4), 1068–1075.

Vullo-Navich, K., Smith, S., Andrews, M., Levine, A. M., Tischer, J. F., & Veglia, J. M. (1998). Comfort and incidence of abnormal serum sodium, BUN, creatinine and osmolality in dehydration of terminal illness. *The American Journal of Hospice & Palliative Care, 15*(2), 77–84.

Electrolyte Balance 0606

Definition: Concentration of serum ions necessary to maintain equilibrium among electrolytes

OUTCOME TARGET RATING: Maintain at_____ Increase to_____

		Severe deviation from normal range	Substantial deviation from normal range	Moderate deviation from normal range	Mild deviation from normal range	No deviation from normal range	
OUTCOME OVERALL RATING		1	2	3	4	5	
Indicators:							
060601	Decreased serum sodium	1	2	3	4	5	NA
060602	Increased serum sodium	1	2	3	4	5	NA
060603	Decreased serum potassium	1	2	3	4	5	NA
060604	Increased serum potassium	1	2	3	4	5	NA
060605	Decreased serum chloride	1	2	3	4	5	NA
060606	Increased serum chloride	1	2	3	4	5	NA
060607	Decreased serum calcium	1	2	3	4	5	NA
060608	Increased serum calcium	1	2	3	4	5	NA
060609	Decreased serum magnesium	1	2	3	4	5	NA
060610	Increased serum magnesium	1	2	3	4	5	NA
060611	Decreased serum phosphorus	1	2	3	4	5	NA
060612	Increased serum phosphorus	1	2	3	4	5	NA

Domain-*Physiologic Health (II)* **Class**-*Fluid & Electrolytes (G)* *5th edition 2013*

OUTCOME CONTENT REFERENCES:
Appel, S. J., & Downs, C. A. (2007). Steady a disturbed equilibrium. Accurately interpret the acid-base balance of acutely ill patients. *Nursing Critical Care, 2*(4), 45–53.
LeMone, P., Burke, K., & Bauldoff, G. (2011). *Medical-surgical nursing: Critical thinking in patient care, Vol. 1* (5th ed.). Upper Saddle River, NJ: Pearson Education.
Roberts, K. (2005). Pediatric fluid and electrolyte balance: Critical care case studies. *Critical Care Nursing Clinics of North America, 17*(4), 361–373.
Smeltzer, S., Bare, B., Hinkle, J., & Cheever, K. (2008). *Brunner & Suddarth's textbook of medical-surgical nursing* (11th ed.). Philadelphia: Lippincott Williams & Wilkins.

Elopement Occurrence 1919

Definition: Number of times that an individual with a cognitive impairment escapes a secure area

OUTCOME TARGET RATING: Maintain at_____ Increase to_____

		10 and over	7-9	4-6	1-3	None	
OUTCOME OVERALL RATING		1	2	3	4	5	
Indicators:							
191901	Leaves place of residence unattended	1	2	3	4	5	NA
191902	Leaves secure area unattended	1	2	3	4	5	NA
191903	Opens exterior door	1	2	3	4	5	NA
191904	Slips away from group activities	1	2	3	4	5	NA
191905	Leaves with visitors	1	2	3	4	5	NA
191906	Leaves with others	1	2	3	4	5	NA
191907	Climbs out window	1	2	3	4	5	NA

Specify period of time: 24 hours /1 week /1 month

Domain-*Health Knowledge & Behavior (IV)* **Class**-*Risk Control & Safety (T)* *4th edition 2008*

OUTCOME CONTENT REFERENCES:

Algase, D. L., Son, G., Beattie, E., Song, J., Leitsch, S., & Yao, L. (2004). The interrelatedness of wandering and wayfinding in a community sample of persons with dementia. *Dementia and Geriatric Cognitive Disorders, 17*(3), 231–239.

Aud, M. A. (2004). Dangerous wandering: Elopements of older adults with dementia from long-term care facilities. *American Journal of Alzheimer's Disorders and Other Dementias, 19*(6), 361–368.

Dewing, J. (2006). Wandering into the future: Reconceptualizing wandering 'a natural and good thing.' *International Journal of Older People Nursing, 1*(4), 239–249.

Lai, C. K. Y., & Arthur, D. G. (2003). Wandering behavior in persons with dementia. *Journal of Advanced Nursing, 44*(2), 173–182.

E

Elopement Propensity Risk 1920

Definition: The propensity of an individual with cognitive impairment to escape a secure area

OUTCOME TARGET RATING: Maintain at_____ Increase to_____

	Consistently demonstrated	Often demonstrated	Sometimes demonstrated	Rarely demonstrated	Never demonstrated	
OUTCOME OVERALL RATING	1	2	3	4	5	
Indicators:						
192001 Wanders	1	2	3	4	5	NA
192002 Appears agitated	1	2	3	4	5	NA
192003 Refuses to remove coat	1	2	3	4	5	NA
192004 Packs bag to leave	1	2	3	4	5	NA
192005 Attempts to leave secure area	1	2	3	4	5	NA
192006 Leaves secure area unobserved	1	2	3	4	5	NA
192007 Leaves yard when outside	1	2	3	4	5	NA
192008 Appears sad	1	2	3	4	5	NA
192009 Weeps	1	2	3	4	5	NA
192010 Appears frightened	1	2	3	4	5	NA
192011 Asks others for assistance to leave	1	2	3	4	5	NA
192012 Attempts to leave with visitors	1	2	3	4	5	NA
192013 States wants to go home	1	2	3	4	5	NA
192014 Threatens to leave	1	2	3	4	5	NA
192015 Attempts to disengage alarm	1	2	3	4	5	NA

Domain-Health Knowledge & Behavior (IV) *Class*-Risk Control & Safety (T) 4th edition 2008

OUTCOME CONTENT REFERENCES:

Algase, D. L., Son, G., Beattie, E., Song, J., Leitsch, S., & Yao, L. (2004). The interrelatedness of wandering and wayfinding in a community sample of persons with dementia. *Dementia and Geriatric Cognitive Disorders, 17*(3), 231–239.

Aud, M. A. (2004). Dangerous wandering: Elopements of older adults with dementia from long-term care facilities. *American Journal of Alzheimer's Disorders and Other Dementias, 19*(6), 361–368.

Dewing, J. (2006). Wandering into the future: Reconceptualizing wandering 'a natural and good thing.' *International Journal of Older People Nursing, 1*(4), 239–249.

Greenberg, H., Blank, H. R., & Argrett, S. (1968). The anatomy of elopement from an acute adolescent service: Escape from engagement. *Psychiatric Quarterly, 42*(1), 28–47.

Lai, C. K. Y., & Arthur, D. G. (2003). Wandering behavior in persons with dementia. *Journal of Advanced Nursing, 44*(2), 173–182.

Endurance 0001

Definition: Capacity to sustain activity

OUTCOME TARGET RATING: Maintain at_____   Increase to_____

		Severely compromised	Substantially compromised	Moderately compromised	Mildly compromised	Not compromised	
OUTCOME OVERALL RATING		1	2	3	4	5	
Indicators:							
000101	Performance of usual routine	1	2	3	4	5	NA
000102	Physical activity	1	2	3	4	5	NA
000104	Concentration	1	2	3	4	5	NA
000106	Muscle endurance	1	2	3	4	5	NA
000108	Libido	1	2	3	4	5	NA
000109	Energy restored after rest	1	2	3	4	5	NA
000112	Blood oxygen level with activity	1	2	3	4	5	NA
000113	Hemoglobin	1	2	3	4	5	NA
000114	Hematocrit	1	2	3	4	5	NA
000115	Blood glucose	1	2	3	4	5	NA
000116	Serum electrolytes	1	2	3	4	5	NA
		Severe	**Substantial**	**Moderate**	**Mild**	**None**	
000110	Exhaustion	1	2	3	4	5	NA
000111	Lethargy	1	2	3	4	5	NA
000118	Fatigue	1	2	3	4	5	NA

Domain-*Functional Health (I)*   **Class**-*Energy Maintenance (A)*   *1st edition 1997; revised 2004, 2008, 2013*

OUTCOME CONTENT REFERENCES:

Ades, P. A., Ballor, D. L., Ashikaga, T., Utton, J. L., & Streekumaran Nair, K. (1996). Weight training improves walking endurance in healthy elderly persons, *Annals of Internal Medicine, 124*(6), 568–572.

+Dartmouth Primary Care Cooperative Information Project. (1987). *COOP Charts.* Hanover, NH: Department of Community and Family Medicine, Dartmouth Medical School.

Ellis, J. R., & Nowlis, E. A. (1994). *Providing nursing care within the nursing process* (5th ed.). Philadelphia: J. B. Lippincott.

Johns, M. E. (1991). Activity and exercise. In S. Wingate (Ed.), *Cardiac nursing: A clinical management and patient care resource* (pp. 141–145). Gaithersburg, MD: Aspen.

Lubkin, I. M. (2002). *Chronic illness: Impact and interventions* (5th ed.). Sudbury, MA: Jones and Bartlett.

Potter, P. A., & Perry, A. G. (2001). *Fundamentals of nursing* (5th ed.). St. Louis: Mosby.

Pugh, L. C., & Milligan, R. (1993). A framework for the study of childbearing fatigue. *Advances in Nursing Science, 15*(4), 60–70.

Tiesinga, L. J., Dassen, T. W. N., & Halfens, R.J.G. (1996). Fatigue: A summary of the definitions, dimensions, and indicators. *Nursing Diagnosis, 7*(2), 51–62.

Titler, M. G. (2001). Activity intolerance. In M. Maas, K. Buckwalter, M. Hardy, T. Tripp-Reimer, M. Titler, & J. Specht (Eds.), *Nursing care of older adults: Diagnoses, outcomes & interventions* (pp. 324–336). St. Louis: Mosby.

Topf, M. (1992). Effects of personal control over hospital noise on sleep. *Research in Nursing & Health, 15*(1), 19–28.

Energy Conservation 0002

Definition: Personal actions to manage energy for initiating and sustaining activity

OUTCOME TARGET RATING: Maintain at_____   Increase to_____

		Never demonstrated	Rarely demonstrated	Sometimes demonstrated	Often demonstrated	Consistently demonstrated	
OUTCOME OVERALL RATING		1	2	3	4	5	
Indicators:							
000201	Balances activity and rest	1	2	3	4	5	NA
000202	Uses naps to restore energy	1	2	3	4	5	NA
000203	Recognizes energy limitations	1	2	3	4	5	NA
000204	Uses energy conservation techniques	1	2	3	4	5	NA
000209	Organizes activities to conserve energy	1	2	3	4	5	NA
000205	Adapts lifestyle to energy level	1	2	3	4	5	NA
000206	Maintains adequate nutrition	1	2	3	4	5	NA
000207	Reports adequate endurance for activity	1	2	3	4	5	NA

Domain-Functional Health (I)   **Class**-Energy Maintenance (A)   1st edition 1997; revised 2004

OUTCOME CONTENT REFERENCES:
Dixon, J. K., Dixon, J. P., & Hickey, M. (1993). Energy as a central factor in the self assessment of health. *Advances in Nursing Science, 15*(4), 1–12.
+Lee, K. A., Hicks, G., & Nino-Murcia, G. (1991). Validity and reliability of a scale to assess fatigue. *Psychiatry Research, 36*(3), 291–298.
Lubkin, I. M. (2002). *Chronic illness: Impact and interventions* (5th ed.). Sudbury, MA: Jones and Bartlett.
McCance, K. L., & Huether, S. E. (2002). *Pathophysiology: The biologic basis for disease in adults and children* (4th ed.). St. Louis: Mosby.
Potter, P. A., & Perry, A. G. (2001). *Fundamentals of nursing* (5th ed.). St. Louis: Mosby.

Exercise Participation 1633

Definition: Personal actions to perform a self-planned, structured, and repetitive regimen to maintain or advance the level of fitness and health

OUTCOME TARGET RATING: Maintain at_____   Increase to_____

		Never demonstrated	Rarely demonstrated	Sometimes demonstrated	Often demonstrated	Consistently demonstrated	
OUTCOME OVERALL RATING		1	2	3	4	5	
Indicators:							
163301	Plans appropriate exercise with health provider before starting exercise	1	2	3	4	5	NA
163302	Identifies barriers to exercise program	1	2	3	4	5	NA
163303	Sets realistic short-term goals	1	2	3	4	5	NA
163304	Sets realistic long-term goals	1	2	3	4	5	NA
163305	Sets target heart rate based on health status	1	2	3	4	5	NA
163306	Achieves target heart rate during exercise	1	2	3	4	5	NA
163307	Balances life routine to include exercise	1	2	3	4	5	NA
163308	Participates in regular exercise	1	2	3	4	5	NA
163309	Performs exercise correctly	1	2	3	4	5	NA

Exercise Participation—*cont'd*

		Never demonstrated	Rarely demonstrated	Sometimes demonstrated	Often demonstrated	Consistently demonstrated	
163310	Wears appropriate clothing for exercise	1	2	3	4	5	NA
163311	Uses strategies to overcome exercise barriers	1	2	3	4	5	NA
163312	Performs exercise in safe environment	1	2	3	4	5	NA
163313	Uses strategies to prevent physical injury	1	2	3	4	5	NA
163314	Uses equipment correctly	1	2	3	4	5	NA
163315	Uses protective devices	1	2	3	4	5	NA
163316	Uses proper warm-up techniques	1	2	3	4	5	NA
163317	Uses proper cool down techniques	1	2	3	4	5	NA
163318	Monitors heart rate	1	2	3	4	5	NA
163319	Monitors respiratory rate	1	2	3	4	5	NA
163320	Monitors progress	1	2	3	4	5	NA
163321	Engages in moderate-intensity aerobic exercise to increase endurance	1	2	3	4	5	NA
163322	Engages in exercises to increase strength	1	2	3	4	5	NA
163323	Engages in exercises to maintain flexibility	1	2	3	4	5	NA
163324	Engages in exercises to maintain balance	1	2	3	4	5	NA
163325	Plans for disruption in exercise program	1	2	3	4	5	NA
163326	Varies exercise	1	2	3	4	5	NA
163327	Adheres to exercise program	1	2	3	4	5	NA
163328	Optimizes opportunities to exercise	1	2	3	4	5	NA
163329	Uses strategies to make exercise interesting	1	2	3	4	5	NA
163330	Maintains fluid balance	1	2	3	4	5	NA
163331	Maintains caloric requirements based on exercise	1	2	3	4	5	NA
163332	Uses personal support system	1	2	3	4	5	NA
163333	Uses community resources	1	2	3	4	5	NA
163334	Contacts a health provider as needed	1	2	3	4	5	NA

Domain-*Health Knowledge & Behavior (IV)* **Class**-*Health Behavior (Q)* *5th edition 2013*

OUTCOME CONTENT REFERENCES:

Haskell, W., Lee, I-M., Pate, R., Powell, K., Blair, S., Franklin, B., Macera, C., Heath, G., Thompson, P., & Bauman, A. (2007). Physical activity and public health: Updated recommendation for adults from the American College of Sports Medicine and the American Heart Association. *Circulation, 116*(9), 1081–1093.

Jung, M. E., & Brawley, L. R. (2010). Concurrent management of exercise with other valued life goals: Comparison of frequent and less frequent exercisers. *Psychology of Sport and Exercise, 11*(5), 372–377.

National Institute on Aging. (2009). *Exercise & physical activity: Your everyday guide from the National Institute on Aging.* Bethesda, MD: Author.

Resnick, B., & D'Adamo, C. (2011) Factors associated with exercise among older adults in a continuing care retirement community. *Rehabilitation Nursing, 36*(2), 47–53, 82.

Shields, C. A., & Brawley, L. R. (2006). Preferring proxy-agency: Impact on self-efficacy for exercise. *Journal of Health Psychology, 11*(6), 904–914.

Fall Prevention Behavior | 1909

Definition: Personal or family caregiver actions to minimize risk factors that might precipitate falls in the personal environment

OUTCOME TARGET RATING: Maintain at_____ Increase to_____

		Never demonstrated	Rarely demonstrated	Sometimes demonstrated	Often demonstrated	Consistently demonstrated	
OUTCOME OVERALL RATING		1	2	3	4	5	
Indicators:							
190923	Asks for assistance	1	2	3	4	5	NA
190903	Places barriers to prevent falls	1	2	3	4	5	NA
190905	Uses handrails as needed	1	2	3	4	5	NA
190915	Uses grab bars as needed	1	2	3	4	5	NA
190914	Uses rubber mats in tub/shower	1	2	3	4	5	NA
190910	Uses well-fitting tied shoes	1	2	3	4	5	NA
190901	Uses assistive devices correctly	1	2	3	4	5	NA
190918	Uses vision-correcting devices	1	2	3	4	5	NA
190902	Provides assistance with mobility	1	2	3	4	5	NA
190919	Uses safe transfer procedure	1	2	3	4	5	NA
190922	Provides adequate lighting	1	2	3	4	5	NA
190909	Uses stools and ladders safely	1	2	3	4	5	NA
190906	Eliminates clutter, spills, glare from floors	1	2	3	4	5	NA
190907	Removes rugs	1	2	3	4	5	NA
190908	Arranges for removal of snow and ice from walking surfaces	1	2	3	4	5	NA
190911	Adjusts toilet height as needed	1	2	3	4	5	NA
190912	Adjusts chair height as needed	1	2	3	4	5	NA
190913	Adjusts bed height as needed	1	2	3	4	5	NA
190916	Controls restlessness	1	2	3	4	5	NA
190917	Uses precautions when taking medication that increase risk for falls	1	2	3	4	5	NA

Domain-*Health Knowledge & Behavior (IV)*   **Class**-*Risk Control & Safety (T)*   *1st edition 1997; revised 2004, 2013*

OUTCOME CONTENT REFERENCES:

Abreu, N., Hutchins, J., Matson, J., Polizzi, N., & Seymour, C. J. (1998). Effect of group versus home visit safety education and prevention strategies for falling in community-dwelling elderly persons. *Home Health Care Management & Practice, 10*(4), 57–65.

Johnson, M., Cusick, A., & Chang, S. (2001). Home-screen: A short scale to measure fall risk in the home. *Public Health Nursing, 18*(3), 169–177.

Kilpack, V., Boehm, J., Smith, N., & Mudge, B. (1991). Using research-based interventions to decrease patient falls. *Applied Nursing Research, 4*(2), 50–56.

Meller, J. L., & Shermeta, D. W. (1987). Falls in urban children. *American Journal of Diseases of Children, 14*(12), 1271–1275.

Moss, A. B. (1992). Are the elderly safe at home? *Journal of Community Health Nursing, 9*(1), 13–19.

O'Connor, M. S., Boyle, W. E., O'Connor, G. T., & Letellier, R. (1992). Self-reported safety practices in child care facilities. *American Journal of Preventative Medicine, 8*(1), 14–18.

Scott, V. J., Votova, K., & Gallagher, E. (2006). Falls prevention training for community health workers: Strategies and actions for independent living (SAIL). *Journal of Gerontological Nursing, 32*(10), 48–56.

Urton, M. M. (1991). A community home inspection approach to preventing falls among the elderly. *Public Health Reports, 106*(2), 192–196.

Falls Occurrence 1912

Definition: Number of times an individual falls

OUTCOME TARGET RATING: Maintain at_____ Increase to_____

	10 and over	7-9	4-6	1-3	None	
OUTCOME OVERALL RATING	1	2	3	4	5	
Indicators:						
191201 Falls while standing still	1	2	3	4	5	NA
191202 Falls while walking	1	2	3	4	5	NA
191203 Falls while sitting	1	2	3	4	5	NA
191204 Falls from bed	1	2	3	4	5	NA
191205 Falls while transferring	1	2	3	4	5	NA
191206 Falls climbing steps	1	2	3	4	5	NA
191207 Falls descending steps	1	2	3	4	5	NA
191209 Falls going to bathroom	1	2	3	4	5	NA
191210 Falls while bending over	1	2	3	4	5	NA

Specify period of time: 24 hours /1 week /1 month

Domain-*Health Knowledge & Behavior (IV)* **Class**-*Risk Control & Safety (T)* *1st edition 1997; revised 2004, 2008*

OUTCOME CONTENT REFERENCES:
Baker, L. (1992). Developing a safety plan that works for patients and nurses. *Rehabilitation Nursing, 17*(5), 264–266.
Nelson, R. C., & Amin, M. A. (1990). Falls in the elderly. *Emergency Care of the Elderly, 8*(2), 309–323.
Schoenfelder, D. P., & Van Why, K. (1997). A fall prevention educational program for community dwelling seniors. *Public Health Nursing, 14*(6), 383–390.
Schroeder, P. (1995). Benchmarking patient falls. *Nursing Quality Connection, 4*(5), 5.
Sorock, G. S. (1988). Falls among the elderly: Epidemiology and prevention. *American Journal of Preventive Medicine, 4*(5), 282–288.

Family Coping 2600

Definition: Capacity of the family to manage stressors that tax family resources

OUTCOME TARGET RATING: Maintain at_____ Increase to_____

	Never demonstrated	Rarely demonstrated	Sometimes demonstrated	Often demonstrated	Consistently demonstrated	
OUTCOME OVERALL RATING	1	2	3	4	5	
Indicators:						
260020 Establishes role flexibility	1	2	3	4	5	NA
260002 Enables member role flexibility	1	2	3	4	5	NA
260003 Confronts family problems	1	2	3	4	5	NA
260005 Manages family problems	1	2	3	4	5	NA
260006 Involves family members in decision-making	1	2	3	4	5	NA
260007 Expresses feelings and emotions openly among members	1	2	3	4	5	NA
260021 Uses strategies to manage family conflict	1	2	3	4	5	NA
260009 Uses family-centered stress reduction strategies	1	2	3	4	5	NA
260010 Cares for needs of all family members	1	2	3	4	5	NA
260011 Establishes family priorities	1	2	3	4	5	NA

Continued

F

Family Coping—*cont'd*

		Never demonstrated	Rarely demonstrated	Sometimes demonstrated	Often demonstrated	Consistently demonstrated	
260012	Establishes schedule for family routines and activities	1	2	3	4	5	NA
260019	Shares responsibility for family tasks	1	2	3	4	5	NA
260013	Arranges for respite care	1	2	3	4	5	NA
260014	Plans for emergencies	1	2	3	4	5	NA
260015	Maintains financial stability	1	2	3	4	5	NA
260022	Reports need for family assistance	1	2	3	4	5	NA
260023	Obtains family assistance	1	2	3	4	5	NA
260024	Uses available family support system	1	2	3	4	5	NA
260025	Uses available community resources	1	2	3	4	5	NA

Domain-Family Health (VI)   **Class**-Family Well-Being (X)   2nd edition 2000; revised 2004, 2008, 2013

OUTCOME CONTENT REFERENCES:
Friedman, M. (1991). An instrument to evaluate effectiveness in family functioning. *Western Journal of Nursing Research, 13*(2), 220–241.
Hymovich, D. P. (1983). The Chronicity Impact and Coping Instrument: Parent Questionnaire. *Nursing Research, 32*(5), 275–281.
Lohan, J. A., & Murphy, S. A. (2002). Family functioning and family typology after an adolescent or young adult's sudden violent death. *Journal of Family Nursing, 8*(1), 32–49.
McCubbin, H. I. (1987). Family coping inventory. In H. I. McCubbin, & A. I. Thomas (Eds.), *Family assessment: Research and practice*. Madison, WI: University of Wisconsin-Madison.
Ryan-Wenger, N. M. (1990). Development and psychometric properties of the Schoolagers' Coping Strategies Inventory. *Nursing Research, 39*(6), 344–349.

Family Functioning   2602

Definition: Capacity of a family to meet the needs of its members during developmental transitions

OUTCOME TARGET RATING: Maintain at_____   Increase to_____

		Never demonstrated	Rarely demonstrated	Sometimes demonstrated	Often demonstrated	Consistently demonstrated	
OUTCOME OVERALL RATING		1	2	3	4	5	
Indicators:							
260201	Socializes new family members	1	2	3	4	5	NA
260202	Cares for dependent members	1	2	3	4	5	NA
260203	Regulates behavior of members	1	2	3	4	5	NA
260204	Allocates responsibilities among members	1	2	3	4	5	NA
260206	Maintains stable core of traditions	1	2	3	4	5	NA
260208	Adapts to developmental transitions	1	2	3	4	5	NA
260209	Adapts to unexpected crises	1	2	3	4	5	NA
260210	Obtains adequate resources to meet needs of members	1	2	3	4	5	NA
260211	Creates environment where members can openly express feelings	1	2	3	4	5	NA
260212	Accepts diversity among members	1	2	3	4	5	NA
260213	Involves members in problem solving	1	2	3	4	5	NA
260214	Involves members in conflict resolution	1	2	3	4	5	NA

F

Family Functioning—*cont'd*

		Never demonstrated	Rarely demonstrated	Sometimes demonstrated	Often demonstrated	Consistently demonstrated	
260221	Members receptive to new ideas	1	2	3	4	5	NA
260205	Members perform expected roles	1	2	3	4	5	NA
260222	Members support one another	1	2	3	4	5	NA
260223	Members assist one another	1	2	3	4	5	NA
260216	Members spend time with one another	1	2	3	4	5	NA
260217	Members express commitment to family	1	2	3	4	5	NA
260218	Members express loyalty to family	1	2	3	4	5	NA
260219	Members participate in community activities	1	2	3	4	5	NA

Domain-*Family Health (VI)* **Class**-*Family Well-Being (X)* *2nd edition 2000; revised 2004, 2008, 2013*

OUTCOME CONTENT REFERENCES:

Friedman, M. M., Bowden, V., & Jones, E. (2003). *Family nursing: Research theory & practice* (5th ed.). New Jersey: Prentice Hall.

Friedman, M. (1991). An instrument to evaluate effectiveness in family functioning. *Western Journal of Nursing Research, 13*(2), 220–241.

Nishka, K. J. (2001). Mexican American family survival, continuity, and growth: The parental perspective. *Nursing Science Quarterly, 14*(4), 322–329.

Quayhagen, M. P., & Roth, P. A. (1989). From models to measures in assessment of mature families. *Journal of Professional Nursing, 5*(3), 144–151.

Roberts, C. S., & Feetham, S. A. (1982). Assessing family functioning across three areas of relationships. *Nursing Research, 31*(4), 231–235.

Swain, K. J., & Harrigan, M. P. (1995). *Measures of family functioning for research and practice.* New York: Springer.

Tamplin, A., & Goodyer, I. M. (2001). Family functioning in adolescents at high and low risk for major depressive disorder. *European Child & Adolescent Psychiatry, 10*(3), 170–190.

Family Health Status   2606

Definition: Overall health and social competence of a family

OUTCOME TARGET RATING: Maintain at_____ Increase to_____

		Severely compromised	Substantially compromised	Moderately compromised	Mildly compromised	Not compromised	
OUTCOME OVERALL RATING		1	2	3	4	5	
Indicators:							
260605	Physical health of members	1	2	3	4	5	NA
260606	Physical activity of members	1	2	3	4	5	NA
260618	Mental health of members	1	2	3	4	5	NA
260601	Immunization of members	1	2	3	4	5	NA
260628	Screening for infections of members	1	2	3	4	5	NA
260612	Physical development of members	1	2	3	4	5	NA
260613	Psychosocial development of members	1	2	3	4	5	NA
260617	Adjustment to disabilities	1	2	3	4	5	NA
260602	Appropriate child care provisions	1	2	3	4	5	NA
260603	Appropriate dependent adult care provisions	1	2	3	4	5	NA
260604	Access to health care	1	2	3	4	5	NA
260629	Age-appropriate health screening of members	1	2	3	4	5	NA

Continued

Family Health Status—cont'd

		Severely compromised	Substantially compromised	Moderately compromised	Mildly compromised	Not compromised	
260607	School attendance of members	1	2	3	4	5	NA
260608	School achievement of members	1	2	3	4	5	NA
260609	Parental employment	1	2	3	4	5	NA
260610	Appropriate housing	1	2	3	4	5	NA
260611	Nutritious food supply	1	2	3	4	5	NA
260630	Financial resources	1	2	3	4	5	NA
260615	Appropriate health care resources	1	2	3	4	5	NA
260616	Appropriate social services resources	1	2	3	4	5	NA
		Severe	Substantial	Moderate	Mild	None	
260620	Domestic violence	1	2	3	4	5	NA
260621	Physical abuse of members	1	2	3	4	5	NA
260624	Psychological abuse of members	1	2	3	4	5	NA
260625	Alcohol abuse	1	2	3	4	5	NA
260626	Tobacco use	1	2	3	4	5	NA
260627	Recreational drug use	1	2	3	4	5	NA
260631	Gambling addiction	1	2	3	4	5	NA

Domain-Family Health (VI)   **Class**-Family Well-Being (X)   2nd edition 2000; revised 2004, 2008, 2013

OUTCOME CONTENT REFERENCES:
Children's Defense Fund. (1997). *The state of America's children: Leave no child behind—Yearbook 1997*. Washington, DC: Author.
Cody, W. K. (1999). The view of family within the human becoming theory. In R. R. Parse (Ed.), *Illuminations: The human becoming theory in practice and research*. Sudbury, MA: Jones and Bartlett.
DeVoe, E. R., & Kantor, G. K. (2002). Measurement issues in child maltreatment and family violence prevention programs. *Trauma, Violence & Abuse, 3*(1), 15–39.
Donnelly, E. (1993). Family health assessment. *Home Healthcare Nurse, 11*(2), 30–37.
Ford-Gilboe, M. (2002). Developing knowledge about family health promotion by testing the development model of health and nursing. *Journal of Family Nursing, 8*(2), 140–156.
Friedman, M. (1991). An instrument to evaluate effectiveness in family functioning. *Western Journal of Nursing Research, 13*(2), 220–241.
Garwick, A. W., Patterson, J. M., Meschke, L. L., Bennett, F. C., & Blum, R. W. (2002). The uncertainty of preadolescents' chronic health conditions and family distress. *Journal of Family Nursing, 8*(1), 11–31.
Graham, K. Y. (1995). Childbearing family health: A wake up call. *Public Health Nursing, 12*(3), 141.
Nishka, K. J. (2001). Mexican American family survival, continuity, and growth: The parental perspective. *Nursing Science Quarterly, 14*(4), 322–329.
Quayhagen, M. P., & Roth, P. A. (1989). From models to measures in assessment of mature families. *Journal of Professional Nursing, 5*(3), 144–151.
Reutter, L. (1984). Family health assessment—An integrated approach. *Journal of Advanced Nursing, 9*(4), 391–399.

Family Integrity 2603

Definition: Capacity of family members to maintain cohesion and emotional bonding

OUTCOME TARGET RATING: Maintain at_____ Increase to_____

		Never demonstrated	Rarely demonstrated	Sometimes demonstrated	Often demonstrated	Consistently demonstrated	
OUTCOME OVERALL RATING		1	2	3	4	5	
Indicators:							
260305	Interacts frequently with extended family	1	2	3	4	5	NA
260308	Involves members in conflict resolution	1	2	3	4	5	NA
260309	Involves members in problem solving	1	2	3	4	5	NA
260310	Encourages individual autonomy and independence	1	2	3	4	5	NA
260311	Prepares and eats meals together	1	2	3	4	5	NA
260312	Participates in leisure-time activities together	1	2	3	4	5	NA
260313	Participates in family rituals	1	2	3	4	5	NA
260314	Participates in family traditions	1	2	3	4	5	NA
260315	Members provide support during times of crisis	1	2	3	4	5	NA
260301	Members express loyalty	1	2	3	4	5	NA
260302	Members express strong ties to family	1	2	3	4	5	NA
260303	Members express affection to one another	1	2	3	4	5	NA
260304	Members assist one another in performing roles and daily tasks	1	2	3	4	5	NA
260306	Members share thoughts, feelings, interests, concerns	1	2	3	4	5	NA
260307	Members communicate openly and honestly with one another	1	2	3	4	5	NA

Domain-*Family Health (VI)*   **Class**-*Family Well-Being (X)*   *2nd edition 2000; revised 2004, 2013*

OUTCOME CONTENT REFERENCES:
Friedman, M. M., Bowden, V., & Jones, E. (2003). *Family nursing: Research theory & practice* (5th ed.). New Jersey: Prentice Hall.
Swain, K. J., & Harrigan, M. P. (1995). *Measures of family functioning for research and practice.* New York: Springer.
Thomasgard, M., & Metz, W. P. (1999). Parent-child relationship disorders: What do the child vulnerability scale and the parent protection scale measure? *Clinical Pediatrics, 38*(6), 347–356.

Family Normalization 2604

Definition: Capacity of a family to develop strategies for optimal functioning when a member has a chronic illness or disability

OUTCOME TARGET RATING: Maintain at_____ Increase to_____

OUTCOME OVERALL RATING	Never demonstrated 1	Rarely demonstrated 2	Sometimes demonstrated 3	Often demonstrated 4	Consistently demonstrated 5	
Indicators:						
260417 Acknowledges potential of impairment to alter family routines	1	2	3	4	5	NA
260403 Maintains usual family routines	1	2	3	4	5	NA
260405 Adapts family routines to accommodate needs of affected member	1	2	3	4	5	NA
260406 Meets physical needs of family members	1	2	3	4	5	NA
260407 Meets psychosocial needs of family members	1	2	3	4	5	NA
260408 Meets developmental needs of family members	1	2	3	4	5	NA
260418 Reports family life returned to precrisis state	1	2	3	4	5	NA
260419 Maintains activities and routines as appropriate	1	2	3	4	5	NA
260420 Maintains usual expectations for member	1	2	3	4	5	NA
260412 Provides activities appropriate to age and ability for affected member	1	2	3	4	5	NA
260413 Structures activities to avoid embarrassment of affected member	1	2	3	4	5	NA
260414 Structures environment to avoid embarrassment of affected member	1	2	3	4	5	NA
260415 Uses community support groups	1	2	3	4	5	NA

Domain-Family Health (VI) *Class*-Family Well-Being (X) *2nd edition 2000; revised 2004, 2008, 2013*

OUTCOME CONTENT REFERENCES:
Bossert, E., Holaday, B., Harkins, A., & Turner-Henson, A. (1990). Strategies of normalization used by parents of chronically ill school age children. *Journal of Child Psychiatric Nursing, 3*(2), 57–61.

Knafl, K., Brietmayer, B., Gallo, A., & Zoeller, L. (1996). Family response to childhood chronic illness: Description of management styles. *Journal of Pediatric Nursing, 11*(5), 315–316.

Knafl, K. A., & Deatrick, J. A. (1986). How families manage chronic conditions: An analysis of the concept of normalization. *Research in Nursing and Health, 9*(3), 215–222.

Knafl, K. A., & Gilliss, C. L. (2002). Families and chronic illness: A synthesis of current research. *Journal of Family Nursing, 8*(3), 178–198.

Wade, S. L., Taylor, H. G., Drotar, D., Stancin, T., Yeates, K. O., & Minich, N. M. (2002). A prospective study of long-term caregiver and family adaptation following brain injury in children. *Journal of Health Trauma Rehabilitation, 17*(2), 96–111.

Family Participation in Professional Care 2605

Definition: Capacity of a family to be involved in decision-making, care delivery, and evaluation of care provided by health care personnel

OUTCOME TARGET RATING: Maintain at_____ Increase to_____

OUTCOME OVERALL RATING	Never demonstrated 1	Rarely demonstrated 2	Sometimes demonstrated 3	Often demonstrated 4	Consistently demonstrated 5	
Indicators:						
260501 Participates in planning care	1	2	3	4	5	NA
260502 Participates in providing care	1	2	3	4	5	NA
260503 Provides relevant information	1	2	3	4	5	NA
260504 Obtains required information	1	2	3	4	5	NA
260505 Identifies factors that affect care	1	2	3	4	5	NA
260506 Collaborates in determining treatment	1	2	3	4	5	NA
260507 Defines needs and problems relevant to care	1	2	3	4	5	NA
260508 Makes decisions when patient is unable to do so	1	2	3	4	5	NA
260509 Participates in decisions with patient	1	2	3	4	5	NA
260510 Participates in mutual goal setting for care	1	2	3	4	5	NA
260511 Evaluates effectiveness of care	1	2	3	4	5	NA
260513 Participates in discharge planning	1	2	3	4	5	NA

Domain-*Family Health (VI)* **Class**-*Family Well-Being (X)* *2nd edition 2000; revised 2008, 2013*

OUTCOME CONTENT REFERENCES:

Biley, F. C. (1992). Some determinants that effect patient participation in decision-making about nursing care. *Journal of Advanced Nursing, 17*(4), 414–421.

Brownlea, A. (1987). Participation: Myths, realities and prognosis. *Social Science and Medicine, 25*(6), 605–614.

Ende, J., Kazis, L., Ash, A., & Moskowitz, M. A. (1989). Measuring patients' desire for autonomy: Decision making and information-seeking preferences among medical patients. *Journal of General Internal Medicine, 4*(1), 23–30.

Janis, I. L., & Rodin, J. (1979). Attribution, control and decision making: Social psychology and health care. In G. D. Stone, F. Cohen & N. E. Adler (Eds.), *Health psychology*. San Francisco: Jossey-Bass.

McEwen, J. (1985). Primary health care: The challenge of participation. In U. Laaser, R. Senault, & H. Viefhues (Eds.), *Primary health care in the making*. Heidelberg: Springer-Verlag.

Richardson, A., & Bray, C. (1987). *Promoting health through participation*. London: Policy Studies Institute.

Stanhope, M., & Lancaster, J. (2000). *Community health nursing* (5th ed.). St Louis: Mosby.

Family Resiliency 2608

Definition: Capacity of a family to positively adapt and function following a significant adversity or crisis

OUTCOME TARGET RATING: Maintain at_____ Increase to_____

OUTCOME OVERALL RATING	Never demonstrated 1	Rarely demonstrated 2	Sometimes demonstrated 3	Often demonstrated 4	Consistently demonstrated 5	
Indicators:						
260801 Mobilizes quickly following adversity	1	2	3	4	5	NA
260802 Proposes practical, constructive solutions for disputes	1	2	3	4	5	NA
260803 Adapts to adversities as challenges	1	2	3	4	5	NA
260804 Tolerates separations when required	1	2	3	4	5	NA
260805 Discusses meaning of crisis	1	2	3	4	5	NA
260806 Expresses confidence in overcoming adversities	1	2	3	4	5	NA
260807 Maintains values, goals, and dreams	1	2	3	4	5	NA
260809 Supports members	1	2	3	4	5	NA
260810 Cooperates to meet challenges	1	2	3	4	5	NA
260811 Nurtures members	1	2	3	4	5	NA
260812 Protects members	1	2	3	4	5	NA
260813 Communicates clearly among members	1	2	3	4	5	NA
260814 Clarifies ambiguous communication	1	2	3	4	5	NA
260815 Uses conflict resolution strategies	1	2	3	4	5	NA
260816 Shares humor	1	2	3	4	5	NA
260817 Reports learning and growth	1	2	3	4	5	NA
260818 Maintains usual family routines	1	2	3	4	5	NA
260819 Prepares for future challenges	1	2	3	4	5	NA
260820 Supports individuality and independence among members	1	2	3	4	5	NA
260821 Accepts respite from extended family	1	2	3	4	5	NA
260822 Accepts respite from friends	1	2	3	4	5	NA
260823 Accepts assistance with direct care from extended family	1	2	3	4	5	NA
260824 Accepts assistance with direct care from friends	1	2	3	4	5	NA
260825 Accepts assistance with instrumental activities of daily living from extended family	1	2	3	4	5	NA
260826 Accepts assistance with instrumental activities of daily living from friends	1	2	3	4	5	NA
260827 Seeks emotional support from extended family	1	2	3	4	5	NA
260828 Seeks emotional support from friends	1	2	3	4	5	NA
260829 Uses community resources for assistance	1	2	3	4	5	NA

F

Family Resiliency—cont'd

		Never demonstrated	Rarely demonstrated	Sometimes demonstrated	Often demonstrated	Consistently demonstrated	
260830	Uses community groups for emotional support	1	2	3	4	5	NA
260831	Adjusts schedules to support and assist members	1	2	3	4	5	NA
260832	Uses health care team for information and assistance	1	2	3	4	5	NA

Domain-Family Health (VI) *Class*-Family Well-Being (X) *3rd edition 2004; revised 2008, 2013*

F

OUTCOME CONTENT REFERENCES:

Armstrong, M. I., Birnie-Lefcovitch, S., & Ungar, M. (2005). Pathways between social support, family well being, quality of parenting, and child resilience: What we know. *Journal of Child & Family Studies, 14*(2), 269–281.

Black, C., & Ford-Gilboe, M. (2004). Adolescent mothers: Resilience, family health work and health-promoting practices. *Journal of Advanced Nursing, 48*(4), 351–360.

McCubbin, M., Balling, K., Possin, P., Frierdich, S., & Bryne, B. (2002). Family resiliency in childhood cancer. *Family Relations, 51*(2), 103–111.

Patterson, J. M. (2002). Integrating family resilience and family stress theory. *Journal of Marriage and Family, 64*(2), 349–360.

Walsh, F. (2002). A family resilience framework: Innovative practice applications. *Family Relations, 51*(2), 130–137.

Family Risk Control: Obesity **2610**

Definition: Capacity of a family to understand, prevent, or eliminate obesity among members

OUTCOME TARGET RATING: Maintain at_____   Increase to_____

		Never demonstrated	Rarely demonstrated	Sometimes demonstrated	Often demonstrated	Consistently demonstrated	
OUTCOME OVERALL RATING		1	2	3	4	5	
Indicators:							
261001	Acknowledges risk factors	1	2	3	4	5	NA
261002	Acknowledges consequences of obesity	1	2	3	4	5	NA
261003	Seeks reputable information about obesity prevention	1	2	3	4	5	NA
261004	Obtains reputable information about weight loss strategies	1	2	3	4	5	NA
261005	Identifies target weight for members	1	2	3	4	5	NA
261006	Members commit to healthy eating plan	1	2	3	4	5	NA
261007	Monitors environmental factors that encourage overeating	1	2	3	4	5	NA
261008	Monitors family eating patterns	1	2	3	4	5	NA
261009	Monitors food portion sizes to maintain healthy weight	1	2	3	4	5	NA
261010	Prepares healthy meals together	1	2	3	4	5	NA
261011	Eats meals together	1	2	3	4	5	NA
261012	Understands importance of eating breakfast	1	2	3	4	5	NA

Continued

Family Risk Control: Obesity—cont'd

		Never demonstrated	Rarely demonstrated	Sometimes demonstrated	Often demonstrated	Consistently demonstrated	
261013	Provides healthy breakfast choices	1	2	3	4	5	NA
261014	Provides healthy snacks	1	2	3	4	5	NA
261015	Drinks water for adequate hydration	1	2	3	4	5	NA
261016	Adjusts recipes to decrease calories	1	2	3	4	5	NA
261017	Reads food labels for nutritional content	1	2	3	4	5	NA
261018	Introduces healthy new items into family's diet	1	2	3	4	5	NA
261019	Makes healthy choices when eating out	1	2	3	4	5	NA
261020	Limits availability of high caloric food	1	2	3	4	5	NA
261021	Limits availability of high caloric fluid	1	2	3	4	5	NA
261022	Limits saturated fat intake	1	2	3	4	5	NA
261023	Limits consumption of sweetened beverages	1	2	3	4	5	NA
261024	Eliminates using food as reward	1	2	3	4	5	NA
261025	Limits electronic screen time	1	2	3	4	5	NA
261026	Encourages involvement in regular exercise	1	2	3	4	5	NA
261027	Promotes active family activities	1	2	3	4	5	NA
261028	Encourages involvement in sports	1	2	3	4	5	NA
261029	Modifies family routine to increase activity level of members	1	2	3	4	5	NA
261030	Maintains healthy sleep routines of members	1	2	3	4	5	NA
261031	Uses available community resources to increase activity level	1	2	3	4	5	NA

Domain-*Family Health (VI)*   **Class**-*Family Well-Being (X)*   *5th edition 2013*

OUTCOME CONTENT REFERENCES:

Anderson, S., & Whitaker, R. (2010). Household routines and obesity in US preschool-aged children. *Pediatrics, 125*(3), 420–428.

Cappellano, K. (2011). Let's move—Tools to fuel a healthier population. *Nutrition Today, 46*(3), 149–154.

Cowart, L., Biro, D., Wasserman, T., Stein, R., Reider, L., & Brown, B. (2010). Designing and pilot-testing a church-based community program to reduce obesity among African Americans. *The ABNF Journal, 21*(1), 4–10.

Henkemans, O., van der Boog, P., Lindenberg, J., van der Mast, C., Neerinex, M., & Zwetsloot-Schonk, B. (2009). An online lifestyle diary with a persuasive computer assistant providing feedback on self-management. *Technology and Health Care, 17*(3), 253–267.

Jordan-Welch, M., & Harbaugh, B. (2008). End the epidemic of childhood obesity one family at a time. *American Nurse Today, 3*(6), 26–31.

Kitzman-Ulrich, H., Wilson, D., St. George, S., Lawman, H., Segal, M., & Fairchild, A. (2010). The integration of a family systems approach for understanding youth obesity, physical activity, and dietary programs. *Clinical Child & Family Psychology Review, 13*(3), 231–253.

Wen, L., Simpson, J., Baur, L., Rissel, C., & Flood, V. (2011). Family functioning and obesity risk behaviors: Implications for early obesity intervention. *Obesity, 19*(6), 1252–1258.

Family Social Climate   **2601**

Definition: Capacity of a family to provide a supportive milieu as characterized by family member relationships and goals

OUTCOME TARGET RATING: Maintain at_____   Increase to_____

		Never demonstrated	Rarely demonstrated	Sometimes demonstrated	Often demonstrated	Consistently demonstrated	
OUTCOME OVERALL RATING		1	2	3	4	5	
Indicators:							
260101	Participates in activities together	1	2	3	4	5	NA
260102	Participates in family traditions	1	2	3	4	5	NA
260103	Attends religious services together	1	2	3	4	5	NA
260121	Maintains relationships with extended family members	1	2	3	4	5	NA
260122	Maintains relationships with friends	1	2	3	4	5	NA
260105	Participates in leisure activities	1	2	3	4	5	NA
260119	Participates in community events	1	2	3	4	5	NA
260106	Establishes family rules	1	2	3	4	5	NA
260123	Establishes family routine	1	2	3	4	5	NA
260124	Maintains family routine	1	2	3	4	5	NA
260108	Maintains clean home	1	2	3	4	5	NA
260109	Supports one another	1	2	3	4	5	NA
260110	Provides privacy for members	1	2	3	4	5	NA
260111	Supports individuality and independence among members	1	2	3	4	5	NA
260125	Encourages maturity enhancing activities	1	2	3	4	5	NA
260126	Encourages life-long learning	1	2	3	4	5	NA
260112	Shares the decision-making process	1	2	3	4	5	NA
260113	Works cooperatively to meet family goals	1	2	3	4	5	NA
260114	Shares feelings with one another	1	2	3	4	5	NA
260120	Shares problems with one another	1	2	3	4	5	NA
260115	Discusses issues relevant to family	1	2	3	4	5	NA
260116	Solves problems together	1	2	3	4	5	NA
260117	Promotes cohesion	1	2	3	4	5	NA

Domain-Family Health (VI)   *Class*-Family Well-Being (X)   2nd edition 2000; revised 2004, 2008, 2013

OUTCOME CONTENT REFERENCES:

Burston, A., Puckering, C., & Kearney, E. (2005). At HOME in Scotland: Validation of the home observation for measurement of the environment inventory. *Child: Care, Health & Development, 31*(5), 533–538.

Folden, S. L. (2001). The politics of the family. In P. L. Munhall (Ed.), *The emergence of family into the 21st century*. Sudbury, MA: Jones and Bartlett.

Moos, R. H. (1974). *Family Environment Scale—Form R*. Palo Alto, CA: Consulting Psychologists Press.

Soubhi, H., Potvin, L., & Paradis, G. (2004). Family process and parent's leisure time physical activity. *American Journal of Health Behavior, 28*(3), 218–230.

Swain, K. J., & Harrigan, M. P. (1995). *Measures of family functioning for research and practice*. New York: Springer.

F

Family Support During Treatment 2609

Definition: Capacity of a family to be present and to provide emotional support for an individual undergoing treatment

OUTCOME TARGET RATING: Maintain at_____   Increase to_____

OUTCOME OVERALL RATING	Never demonstrated 1	Rarely demonstrated 2	Sometimes demonstrated 3	Often demonstrated 4	Consistently demonstrated 5	

Indicators:

260901	Members express desire to support ill member	1	2	3	4	5	NA
260902	Members express feelings and emotions of concern for ill member	1	2	3	4	5	NA
260903	Members ask how they may assist	1	2	3	4	5	NA
260904	Requests information about procedure	1	2	3	4	5	NA
260905	Requests information about patient condition	1	2	3	4	5	NA
260906	Members maintain communication with ill member	1	2	3	4	5	NA
260907	Members encourage ill member	1	2	3	4	5	NA
260908	Members provide comforting touch to ill member	1	2	3	4	5	NA
260915	Seeks social support for ill member	1	2	3	4	5	NA
260916	Seeks spiritual support for ill member	1	2	3	4	5	NA
260910	Collaborates with ill member in determining care	1	2	3	4	5	NA
260911	Collaborates with health providers in determining care	1	2	3	4	5	NA
260912	Members verbalize meaning of health crisis	1	2	3	4	5	NA
260913	Contacts other members as desired by ill member	1	2	3	4	5	NA
260914	Provides accurate information to other members	1	2	3	4	5	NA
260917	Participates in discharge planning	1	2	3	4	5	NA

Domain-Family Health (VI)   **Class**-Family Well-Being (X)   3rd edition 2004; revised 2008, 2013

OUTCOME CONTENT REFERENCES:

American Heart Association. (2000). Guidelines 2000 for cardiopulmonary resuscitation and emergency cardiovascular care, part 2: Ethical aspects of CPR and ECC. *Circulation, 102*(Suppl. 8), I12–I21.

Breen, M., Coombes, L, & Bradbourne, C. (2009). Supportive care for children and young people during cancer treatment. *Community Practitioner, 82*(9), 28–31.

Bull, M. J., Hansen, H. E., & Gross, C. R. (2000). Differences in family caregiver outcomes by their level of involvement in discharge planning. *Applied Nursing Research, 13*(2), 76–82.

Eichhorn, D. J., Meyers, T. A., Guzzetta, C. E., Clark, A. P., Klein, J. D., & Calvin, A. O. (2001). During invasive procedures and resuscitation: Hearing the voice of the patient. *American Journal of Nursing, 101*(5), 48–55.

Emergency Nurses Association. (1998). Emergency Nurses Association position statement: Family presence at the bedside during invasive procedures and/or resuscitation. *Journal of Emergency Nursing, 21*(2), 26A.

Emergency Nurses Association. (2000). *Presenting the option for family presence* (2nd ed.). Des Plaines, IL: Author.

Meyers, T. A., Eichhorn, D. J., & Guzzetta, C. E. (1998). Do families want to be present during CPR? A retrospective survey. *Journal of Emergency Nursing, 24*(5), 400–405.

Meyers, T. A., Eichhorn, D. J., Guzzetta, C. E., Clark, A. P., Klein, J. D., Taliaferro, E., & Calvin, A. (2000). Family presence during invasive procedures and resuscitation. *American Journal of Nursing, 100*(2), 32–42.

Rhee, H., Belyea, M., & Brasch, J. (2010). Family support and asthma outcomes in adolescents: Barriers to adherence as a mediator. *Journal of Adolescent Health, 47*(5), 472–478.

Fatigue: Disruptive Effects   0008

Definition: Severity of observed or reported disruptive effects of chronic fatigue on daily functioning

OUTCOME TARGET RATING: Maintain at_____ Increase to_____

		Severe	Substantial	Moderate	Mild	None	
OUTCOME OVERALL RATING		1	2	3	4	5	
Indicators:							
000801	Malaise	1	2	3	4	5	NA
000802	Lethargy	1	2	3	4	5	NA
000803	Decreased energy	1	2	3	4	5	NA
000804	Interference with activities of daily living	1	2	3	4	5	NA
000805	Impaired home maintenance	1	2	3	4	5	NA
000806	Disruption of routine	1	2	3	4	5	NA
000807	Interference with treatment regimen	1	2	3	4	5	NA
000808	Decreased appetite	1	2	3	4	5	NA
000809	Altered nutritional status	1	2	3	4	5	NA
000810	Impaired physical activity	1	2	3	4	5	NA
000811	Impaired role performance	1	2	3	4	5	NA
000812	Impaired work performance	1	2	3	4	5	NA
000813	Impaired school performance	1	2	3	4	5	NA
000814	Absenteeism from work	1	2	3	4	5	NA
000815	Absenteeism from school	1	2	3	4	5	NA
000816	Disruption of interpersonal relationships	1	2	3	4	5	NA
000817	Interference with leisure activities	1	2	3	4	5	NA
000818	Pessimistic about current health status	1	2	3	4	5	NA
000819	Pessimistic about future health status	1	2	3	4	5	NA
000820	Impaired recall	1	2	3	4	5	NA
000821	Impaired mood	1	2	3	4	5	NA
000822	Impaired life enjoyment	1	2	3	4	5	NA
000823	Psychological co-morbidity	1	2	3	4	5	NA

Domain-*Functional Health (I)*   **Class**-*Energy Maintenance (A)*   5th edition 2013

OUTCOME CONTENT REFERENCES:

Knoop, H., Stulemeijer, M., de Jong, L., Fiselier, T., & Bleijenberg, G. (2008). Efficacy of cognitive behavioral therapy for adolescents with chronic fatigue syndrome: Long-term follow-up of a randomized, controlled trial. *Pediatrics, 121*(3), e619–e625.

Lowry, T. J., & Pakenham, K. I. (2008). Health-related quality of life in chronic fatigue syndrome: Predictors of physical functioning and psychological distress. *Psychology, Health & Medicine, 13*(2), 222–238.

Sohl, S. J., & Friedberg, F. (2008). Memory for fatigue in chronic fatigue syndrome. *Behavioral Medicine, 34*(1), 29–35.

Taylor, R. R., & Kielhofner, G. W. (2005). Work-related impairment and employment-focused rehabilitation options for individuals with chronic fatigue syndrome: A review. *Journal of Mental Health, 14*(3), 253–267.

Fatigue Level   **0007**

Definition: Severity of observed or reported prolonged generalized fatigue

OUTCOME TARGET RATING: Maintain at_____ Increase to_____

OUTCOME OVERALL RATING	Severe 1	Substantial 2	Moderate 3	Mild 4	None 5	
Indicators:						
000701 Exhaustion	1	2	3	4	5	NA
000702 Lassitude	1	2	3	4	5	NA
000703 Depressed mood	1	2	3	4	5	NA
000704 Loss of appetite	1	2	3	4	5	NA
000705 Decreased libido	1	2	3	4	5	NA
000706 Impaired concentration	1	2	3	4	5	NA
000707 Decreased motivation	1	2	3	4	5	NA
000708 Headaches	1	2	3	4	5	NA
000709 Sore throat	1	2	3	4	5	NA
000710 Tender lymph nodes	1	2	3	4	5	NA
000711 Muscle pain	1	2	3	4	5	NA
000712 Joint pain	1	2	3	4	5	NA
000713 Post exertional malaise	1	2	3	4	5	NA
000714 Stress level	1	2	3	4	5	NA

	Severely compromised	Substantially compromised	Moderately compromised	Mildly compromised	Not compromised	
000715 Activities of daily living	1	2	3	4	5	NA
000716 Instrumental activities of daily living	1	2	3	4	5	NA
000717 Work performance	1	2	3	4	5	NA
000718 Lifestyle performance	1	2	3	4	5	NA
000719 Rest quality	1	2	3	4	5	NA
000720 Sleep quality	1	2	3	4	5	NA
000721 Balance of activity and rest	1	2	3	4	5	NA
000722 Alertness	1	2	3	4	5	NA
000723 Hematocrit	1	2	3	4	5	NA
000724 Oxygen saturation	1	2	3	4	5	NA
000725 Thyroid function	1	2	3	4	5	NA
000726 Immune function	1	2	3	4	5	NA
000727 Neurological function	1	2	3	4	5	NA
000728 Metabolism	1	2	3	4	5	NA

Domain-*Functional Health (I)*   **Class**-*Energy Maintenance (A)*   *4th edition 2008*

OUTCOME CONTENT REFERENCES:

Aaronson, L. S., Teel, C., Cassmeyer, V., Neuberger, G. B., Pallikkathayil, L., Pierce, J., Press, A. N., Williams, P. D., & Wingate, A. (1999). Defining and measuring fatigue. *Image—Journal of Nursing Scholarship, 31*(1), 45–51.

Chalder, T., Berelowitz, K., Pawlikowska, T., Watts, L., Wessely, S., Wright, D., & Wallace, E. P. (1993). Development of a fatigue scale. *Journal of Psychosomatic Research, 37*(2), 147–153.

Hampton, T. (2006). Chronic fatigue syndrome answers sought. *JAMA: Journal of the American Medical Association, 296*(24), 2915.

Jason, L. A., Corradi, K., Gress, S., Williams, S., & Torres-Harding, S. (2006). Causes of death among patients with chronic fatigue syndrome. *Health Care for Women International, 27*(7), 615–626.

Krupp, L. B., LaRocca, N. G., Muir Nash, J., & Steinberg, A. D. (1989). The fatigue severity scale: Application to patients with multiple sclerosis and systemic lupus erythematosus. *Archives of Neurology, 46*(10), 1121–1123.

Michielsen, H. J., De Vries, J., Van Heck, G., Van de Vijven, F. J., Sijtsma, K. (2004). Examination of the dimensionality of fatigue: The construction of the Fatigue Assessment Scale (FAS). *European Journal of Psychological Assessment 20*(1), 39–48.

Piper, B. F., Dibble, S. L., Dodd, M. J., Weiss, M. C., Slaughter, R. E., & Paul, S. M. (1998). The revised Piper fatigue scale: Psychometric evaluation in women with breast cancer. *Oncology Nursing Forum, 25*(4), 67–84.

Smets, E. M., Garssen, B., Bonke, B., & De Haes, J. C. (1995). The Multidimensional Fatigue Inventory (MFI) psychometric qualities of an instrument to assess fatigue. *Journal of Psychosomatic Research, 39*(3), 315–325.

Tiesinga, L., Dassen, T., Halfens, R., & van Den Heuvel, W. (2001). Sensitivity, specificity, and usefulness of the Dutch Fatigue Scale. *Nursing Diagnosis, 12*(3), 93–106.

Fear Level 1210

Definition: Severity of manifested apprehension, tension, or uneasiness arising from an identifiable source

OUTCOME TARGET RATING: Maintain at_____ Increase to_____

OUTCOME OVERALL RATING	Severe 1	Substantial 2	Moderate 3	Mild 4	None 5	
Indicators:						
121001 Distress	1	2	3	4	5	NA
121002 Tendency to blame others	1	2	3	4	5	NA
121003 Self-absorption	1	2	3	4	5	NA
121004 Lack of self-confidence	1	2	3	4	5	NA
121005 Restlessness	1	2	3	4	5	NA
121006 Irritability	1	2	3	4	5	NA
121007 Outbursts of anger	1	2	3	4	5	NA
121008 Difficulty concentrating	1	2	3	4	5	NA
121009 Difficulty learning	1	2	3	4	5	NA
121010 Difficulty problem solving	1	2	3	4	5	NA
121011 Decreased perceptual field	1	2	3	4	5	NA
121012 Perceived inadequacy in interpersonal relationships	1	2	3	4	5	NA
121013 Exaggerated concern about life events	1	2	3	4	5	NA
121014 Preoccupation with life events	1	2	3	4	5	NA
121015 Preoccupation with source of fear	1	2	3	4	5	NA
121016 Increased blood pressure	1	2	3	4	5	NA
121017 Increased radial pulse rate	1	2	3	4	5	NA
121018 Increased respiratory rate	1	2	3	4	5	NA
121019 Dilated pupils	1	2	3	4	5	NA
121020 Sweating	1	2	3	4	5	NA
121021 Feeling faint	1	2	3	4	5	NA
121022 Muscle tension	1	2	3	4	5	NA
121023 Facial tension	1	2	3	4	5	NA
121024 Frequent urination	1	2	3	4	5	NA
121025 Diarrhea	1	2	3	4	5	NA
121026 Inability to sleep	1	2	3	4	5	NA
121027 Skin pallor	1	2	3	4	5	NA
121028 Fatigue	1	2	3	4	5	NA
121029 Withdrawal	1	2	3	4	5	NA
121030 Avoidance behavior	1	2	3	4	5	NA
121031 Verbalized fear	1	2	3	4	5	NA
121032 Crying	1	2	3	4	5	NA
121033 Dread	1	2	3	4	5	NA
121034 Panic	1	2	3	4	5	NA
121035 Terror	1	2	3	4	5	NA

Domain-Psychosocial Health (III)   **Class**-Psychological Well-Being (M)   *3rd edition 2004; revised 2008*

OUTCOME CONTENT REFERENCES:

American Psychiatric Association. (2000). *Diagnostic and statistical manual of mental disorders* (4th ed. text revision). Washington, DC: Author.

Charron, H. S. (1998). Anxiety disorders. In E. M. Varcarolis (Ed.), *Foundations of psychiatric mental health nursing* (3rd ed., pp. 443–477). Philadelphia: W. B. Saunders.

Kim, M., Sertella, R., Gulanick, M., Moyer, K., Parsons, E., Scherbel, J., Stafford, M., Suhayada, R., & Yocum, C. (1984). Clinical validation of cardiovascular nursing diagnoses. In M. Kim, G. McFarland, & A. McLane (Eds.), *Classification of nursing diagnoses: Proceedings of the fifth national conference* (pp. 128–137). St. Louis: Mosby.

Taylor-Loughran, A. E., O'Brien, M. E., Lachapelle, R., & Rangel, S. (1989). Defining characteristics of the nursing diagnoses fear and anxiety: A validation study. *Applied Nursing Research, 2*(4), 178–186.

Whitley, G. G., & Tousman, S. A. (1996). A multivariate approach for validation of anxiety and fear. *Nursing Diagnoses, 7*(3), 116–124.

Fear Level: Child   1213

Definition: Severity of manifested apprehension, tension, or uneasiness arising from an identifiable source in a child from 1 year through 17 years of age

OUTCOME TARGET RATING: Maintain at_____ Increase to_____

OUTCOME OVERALL RATING	Severe 1	Substantial 2	Moderate 3	Mild 4	None 5	
Indicators:						
121302 Increased heart rate	1	2	3	4	5	NA
121303 Headaches	1	2	3	4	5	NA
121304 Stomachaches	1	2	3	4	5	NA
121305 Frequent urination	1	2	3	4	5	NA
121306 Frequent diarrhea	1	2	3	4	5	NA
121307 Fatigue	1	2	3	4	5	NA
121308 Weight loss	1	2	3	4	5	NA
121310 Sweating	1	2	3	4	5	NA
121311 Crying	1	2	3	4	5	NA
121312 Emotional lability	1	2	3	4	5	NA
121313 Stammering	1	2	3	4	5	NA
121314 Irritability	1	2	3	4	5	NA
121315 Excessive giggling	1	2	3	4	5	NA
121316 Avoidance behavior	1	2	3	4	5	NA
121317 Withdrawal	1	2	3	4	5	NA
121318 Increased school absence	1	2	3	4	5	NA
121319 Cheating	1	2	3	4	5	NA
121320 Difficulty staying on task	1	2	3	4	5	NA
121321 Difficulty concentrating	1	2	3	4	5	NA
121322 Tics	1	2	3	4	5	NA
121323 Nail biting	1	2	3	4	5	NA
121324 Finger sucking	1	2	3	4	5	NA
121325 Hair chewing	1	2	3	4	5	NA
121326 Chewing clothing	1	2	3	4	5	NA
121327 Fidgeting	1	2	3	4	5	NA
121328 Rocking motion	1	2	3	4	5	NA
121329 Shaking	1	2	3	4	5	NA
121330 Violent behavior	1	2	3	4	5	NA
121331 Violence displayed in drawings	1	2	3	4	5	NA
121332 Destructive behavior	1	2	3	4	5	NA
121333 Stealing	1	2	3	4	5	NA
121334 Regressive behavior	1	2	3	4	5	NA
121335 Excessive approval-seeking behavior	1	2	3	4	5	NA
121336 Demanding behavior	1	2	3	4	5	NA
121337 Fabrication of stories	1	2	3	4	5	NA
121338 Continuous questioning	1	2	3	4	5	NA
121339 Clinging behavior	1	2	3	4	5	NA
121340 Injury-faking behavior	1	2	3	4	5	NA
121341 Self-destructive behavior	1	2	3	4	5	NA
121342 Recreational drug use	1	2	3	4	5	NA
121343 Alcohol use	1	2	3	4	5	NA
121344 Excessive self-denigration	1	2	3	4	5	NA
121345 Dread	1	2	3	4	5	NA
121346 Panic	1	2	3	4	5	NA
121347 Terror	1	2	3	4	5	NA

Domain-Psychosocial Health (III)   *Class*-Psychological Well-Being (M)   *3rd edition 2004; revised 2008*

OUTCOME CONTENT REFERENCES:

Berliner, L., & Saunders, B. E. (1996). Treating fear and anxiety in sexually abused children. *Child Maltreatment, 1*(4), 294–310.

Byrne, B. (2000). Relationships between anxiety, fear, self-esteem and coping strategies in adolescence. *Adolescence, 35*(137), 201–216.

Carlson, K. L., Broome, M., & Vessey, J. A. (2000). Using distraction to reduce reported pain, fear and behavioral distress in children and adolescents: A multi-site study. *Journal of the Society of Pediatric Nursing, 5*(2), 75–85.

Carr, T. D., Lemanek, K. L., & Armstrong, F. D. (1998). Pain and fear ratings: Clinical implications of age and gender differences. *Journal of Pain and Symptom Management, 15*(5), 305–313.

Carroll, M. K., & Ryan-Wenger, N. A. (1999). School-age children's fears, anxiety and human figure drawings. *Journal of Pediatric Health Care, 13*(1), 24–31.

Nicastro, E. A., & Whetsell, M. V. (1999). Children's fears. *Journal of Pediatric Nursing, 14*(6), 392–402.

Potter, P. A., & Perry, A. G. (2001). *Fundamentals of nursing* (5th ed.). St. Louis: Mosby.

Wilson, A. H., & Yorker, B. (1996). Fears of medical events among school-age children with emotional disorders, parents, and health care providers. *Issues in Mental Health Nursing, 18*(1), 57–71.

Wong, D. L., Hockenberry-Eaton, M., Wilson, D., Winkelstein, M. L., Ahmann, E., & DiVito-Thomas, P. A. (1999). *Whaley & Wong's nursing care of infants and children* (6th ed.). St. Louis: Mosby.

F

Fear Self-Control   **1404**

Definition: Personal actions to eliminate or reduce disabling feelings of apprehension, tension, or uneasiness from an identifiable source

OUTCOME TARGET RATING: Maintain at_____   Increase to_____

		Never demonstrated	Rarely demonstrated	Sometimes demonstrated	Often demonstrated	Consistently demonstrated	
OUTCOME OVERALL RATING		1	2	3	4	5	
Indicators:							
140401	Monitors intensity of fear	1	2	3	4	5	NA
140402	Eliminates precursors of fear	1	2	3	4	5	NA
140403	Seeks information to reduce fear	1	2	3	4	5	NA
140404	Avoids source of fear when possible	1	2	3	4	5	NA
140405	Plans coping strategies for fearful situations	1	2	3	4	5	NA
140406	Uses effective coping strategies	1	2	3	4	5	NA
140407	Uses relaxation techniques to reduce fear	1	2	3	4	5	NA
140408	Monitors duration of episodes	1	2	3	4	5	NA
140409	Monitors length of time between episodes	1	2	3	4	5	NA
140410	Maintains role performance	1	2	3	4	5	NA
140411	Maintains social relationships	1	2	3	4	5	NA
140412	Maintains concentration	1	2	3	4	5	NA
140413	Maintains control over life	1	2	3	4	5	NA
140414	Maintains physical functioning	1	2	3	4	5	NA
140415	Maintains a sense of purpose despite fear	1	2	3	4	5	NA
140416	Remains productive	1	2	3	4	5	NA
140417	Controls fear response	1	2	3	4	5	NA

Domain-Psychosocial Health (III)   *Class-Self Control (O)*   *1st edition 1997; revised 2000, 2004*

OUTCOME CONTENT REFERENCES:
+Marks, I. M., & Mathews, A. M. (1979). Brief standard self-rating for phobic patients. *Behavior Research and Therapy, 17*(3), 263–267.

McAuley, E., Mihalko, S. L., & Rosengren, K. (1997). Self-efficacy and balance correlates of fear of falling in the elderly. *Journal of Aging and Physical Activity, 5(4)*, 329–340.

McFarland, G. K., & McFarlane, E. A. (1997). *Nursing diagnosis & intervention: Planning for patient care* (3rd ed.). St. Louis: Mosby.

Moorhead, S. A., & Brighton, V. A. (2001). Anxiety and fear. In M. Maas, K. Buckwalter, M. Hardy, T. Tripp-Reimer, M. Titler, & J. Specht (Eds.), *Nursing care of older adults: Diagnoses, outcomes & interventions* (pp. 571–592). St. Louis: Mosby.

Stuart, G. W., & Laraia, M. T. (2001). *Principles and practice of psychiatric nursing* (7th ed.). St. Louis: Mosby.

Whitley, G. G., & Tousman, S. A. (1996). A multivariate approach for validation of anxiety and fear. *Nursing Diagnosis, 7*(3), 116–124.

Wilson, A. H., & Yorker, B. (1997). Fears of medical events among school-age children with emotional disorders, parents, and health care providers. *Issues in Mental Health Nursing, 18*(1), 57–71.

F

Fetal Status: Antepartum 0111

Definition: Extent to which fetal signs are within normal limits from conception to the onset of labor

OUTCOME TARGET RATING: Maintain at_____   Increase to_____

		Severe deviation from normal range	Substantial deviation from normal range	Moderate deviation from normal range	Mild deviation from normal range	No deviation from normal range	
OUTCOME OVERALL RATING		1	2	3	4	5	
Indicators:							
011101	Fetal heart rate (120-160)	1	2	3	4	5	NA
011102	Deceleration patterns in electronic fetal monitor findings	1	2	3	4	5	NA
011103	Fetal heart rate variability	1	2	3	4	5	NA
011104	Fetal ultrasound findings	1	2	3	4	5	NA
011105	Fetal movement frequency	1	2	3	4	5	NA
011106	Fetal movement pattern	1	2	3	4	5	NA
011107	Nonstress test	1	2	3	4	5	NA
011108	Contraction stress test	1	2	3	4	5	NA
011109	Auscultated acceleration test	1	2	3	4	5	NA
011110	Biophysical profile score	1	2	3	4	5	NA
011111	Amniotic fluid sample findings	1	2	3	4	5	NA
011112	Umbilical artery blood flow velocity	1	2	3	4	5	NA
011114	Doppler umbilical flow study	1	2	3	4	5	NA
011115	Surfactant levels/ratio	1	2	3	4	5	NA
011116	Chorionic villi sampling	1	2	3	4	5	NA
011117	Quadruple screen	1	2	3	4	5	NA
011118	Echocardiography	1	2	3	4	5	NA
011119	Nuchal translucency testing (NTT)	1	2	3	4	5	NA
011120	Acoustic stimulation test	1	2	3	4	5	NA
011121	First trimester combined screening	1	2	3	4	5	NA

Domain-Functional Health (I)   *Class*-Growth & Development (B)   *2nd edition 2000; revised 2004, 2013*

OUTCOME CONTENT REFERENCES:
Alus, M., Okumus, H., Mete, S., & Guclu, S. (2007). The effects of different maternal positions on non-stress test: An experimental study. *Journal of Clinical Nursing, 16*(3), 562–568.
Armour, K. (2004). Using surveillance to improve maternal and fetal outcomes: Antepartum maternal-fetal assessment. *AWHONN Lifelines, 8*(3), 232–240.
Hale, R. (2009). Non-invasive techniques for fetal monitoring in pregnancy and labour. *British Journal of Midwifery, 17*(10), 661–776.
Ladewig, P., London, M., & Davidson, M. (2010). *Contemporary maternal-newborn nursing care* (7th ed.). New York: Pearson.

Fetal Status: Intrapartum   0112

F

Definition: Extent to which fetal signs are within normal limits from onset of labor to delivery

OUTCOME TARGET RATING: Maintain at_____   Increase to_____

		Severe deviation from normal range	Substantial deviation from normal range	Moderate deviation from normal range	Mild deviation from normal range	No deviation from normal range	
OUTCOME OVERALL RATING		1	2	3	4	5	
Indicators:							
011201	Baseline fetal heart rate (120-160)	1	2	3	4	5	NA
011213	Periodic fetal heart rate deceleration	1	2	3	4	5	NA
011214	Fetal heart rate variability	1	2	3	4	5	NA
011204	Amniotic fluid color	1	2	3	4	5	NA
011205	Amniotic fluid amount	1	2	3	4	5	NA
011206	Fetal position	1	2	3	4	5	NA
011207	Fetal presenting part	1	2	3	4	5	NA
011209	Fetal scalp blood pH	1	2	3	4	5	NA
011210	Fetal scalp stimulation response	1	2	3	4	5	NA
011212	Fetal pulse oximetry	1	2	3	4	5	NA
011215	Episodic fetal heart rate patterns	1	2	3	4	5	NA
011216	Fetal heart rate accelerations with movement	1	2	3	4	5	NA
011217	Fetal heart rate accelerations with stimulation	1	2	3	4	5	NA

Domain-Functional Health (I)   *Class-Growth & Development (B)*   *2nd edition 2000; revised 2004, 2008, 2013*

OUTCOME CONTENT REFERENCES:
Kelly, M., Johnson, E., Lee, V., Massey, L., Purser, D., Ring, K., Sanderson, S., Styles, J., & Wood, D. (2010). Delayed versus immediate pushing in second stage of labor. *MCN: The American Journal of Maternal Child Nursing, 35*(2), 81–88.
Ladewig, P., London, M., & Davidson, M. (2010). *Contemporary maternal-newborn nursing care* (7th ed.). New York: Pearson.
Maccones, G., Hankins, G., Spong, C., Hauth, J., & Moore, T. (2008). The 2008 National Institute of Child Health and Human Development workshop report on electronic fetal monitoring: Update on definitions, interpretation, and research guidelines. *Journal of Obstetric, Gynecologic & Neonatal Nursing, 37*(5), 1–6.

Fluid Balance 0601

Definition: Water balance in the intracellular and extracellular compartments of the body

OUTCOME TARGET RATING: Maintain at_____   Increase to_____

OUTCOME OVERALL RATING		Severely compromised 1	Substantially compromised 2	Moderately compromised 3	Mildly compromised 4	Not compromised 5	
Indicators:							
060101	Blood pressure	1	2	3	4	5	NA
060122	Radial pulse rate	1	2	3	4	5	NA
060102	Mean arterial pressure	1	2	3	4	5	NA
060103	Central venous pressure	1	2	3	4	5	NA
060104	Pulmonary wedge pressure	1	2	3	4	5	NA
060105	Peripheral pulses	1	2	3	4	5	NA
060107	24-hour intake and output balance	1	2	3	4	5	NA
060109	Stable body weight	1	2	3	4	5	NA
060116	Skin turgor	1	2	3	4	5	NA
060117	Moist mucous membranes	1	2	3	4	5	NA
060118	Serum electrolytes	1	2	3	4	5	NA
060119	Hematocrit	1	2	3	4	5	NA
060120	Urine specific gravity	1	2	3	4	5	NA

		Severe	Substantial	Moderate	Mild	None	
060106	Orthostatic hypotension	1	2	3	4	5	NA
060108	Adventitious breath sounds	1	2	3	4	5	NA
060110	Ascites	1	2	3	4	5	NA
060111	Neck vein distention	1	2	3	4	5	NA
060112	Peripheral edema	1	2	3	4	5	NA
060113	Soft, sunken eyeballs	1	2	3	4	5	NA
060114	Confusion	1	2	3	4	5	NA
060115	Thirst	1	2	3	4	5	NA
060123	Muscle cramps	1	2	3	4	5	NA
060124	Dizziness	1	2	3	4	5	NA

Domain-*Physiologic Health (II)*   **Class**-*Fluid & Electrolytes (G)*   *1st edition 1997; revised 2004*

OUTCOME CONTENT REFERENCES:
Bosquet, G. L. (1990). Congestive heart failure: A review of nonpharmacologic therapies. *Journal of Cardiovascular Nursing, 4*(3), 35–46.
Chowdhury, A., & Lobo, D. (2011). Fluids and gastrointestinal function. *Current Opinion in Clinical Nutrition & Metabolic Care, 14*(5), 469–476.
Coats, A. J. S., Adamopoulos, S., Meyer, T. E., Conway, J., & Sleight, P. (1990). Effects of physical training in chronic heart failure. *The Lancet, 335*(8681), 63–66.
Coyle, E. F. (2004). Fluid and fuel intake during exercise. *Journal of Sports Sciences, 22*(1), 39–55.
Fukada, N. (1990). Outcome standards for the client with congestive heart failure. *Journal of Cardiovascular Nursing, 4*(3), 59–70.
Kraft, P. A. (2000). The osmotic shift. *Journal of Intravenous Nursing, 23*(4), 220–224.
Medina, J. (2000). *Standards for acute and critical care nursing practice* (3rd ed.). Irvine, CA: American Association of Critical-Care Nurses.
Reese, J. L. (2001). Fluid volume deficit—dehydration: Isotonic, hypotonic, and hypertonic. In M. Maas, K. Buckwalter, M. Hardy, T. Tripp-Reimer, M. Titler, & J. Specht (Eds.), *Nursing care of older adults: Diagnoses, outcomes & interventions* (pp. 183–200). St. Louis: Mosby.
Toto, K. H. (1998). Fluid balance assessment: The total perspective. *Critical Care Clinics of North America, 10*(4), 383–400.
Vullo-Navich, K., Smith, S., Andrews, M., Levine, A. M., Tischer, J. F., & Veglia, J. M. (1998). Comfort and incidence of abnormal serum sodium, BUN, creatinine and osmolality in dehydration of terminal illness. *The American Journal of Hospice & Palliative Care, 15*(2), 77–84.

F

Fluid Overload Severity   **0603**

Definition: Severity of signs and symptoms of excess intracellular and extracellular fluids

OUTCOME TARGET RATING: Maintain at_____   Increase to_____

	Severe	Substantially	Moderately	Mild	None	
OUTCOME OVERALL RATING	1	2	3	4	5	
Indicators:						
060301 Periorbital edema	1	2	3	4	5	NA
060302 Hand edema	1	2	3	4	5	NA
060303 Sacral edema	1	2	3	4	5	NA
060304 Ankle edema	1	2	3	4	5	NA
060305 Leg edema	1	2	3	4	5	NA
060306 Ascites	1	2	3	4	5	NA
060307 Increased abdominal girth	1	2	3	4	5	NA
060308 Generalized edema	1	2	3	4	5	NA
060309 Venous congestion	1	2	3	4	5	NA
060310 Rales	1	2	3	4	5	NA
060311 Malaise	1	2	3	4	5	NA
060312 Lethargy	1	2	3	4	5	NA
060313 Headache	1	2	3	4	5	NA
060314 Confusion	1	2	3	4	5	NA
060315 Seizures	1	2	3	4	5	NA
060316 Coma	1	2	3	4	5	NA
060317 Increased blood pressure	1	2	3	4	5	NA
060318 Weight gain	1	2	3	4	5	NA
060319 Decreased urine output	1	2	3	4	5	NA
060320 Decreased specific urine gravity	1	2	3	4	5	NA
060321 Decreased urine color	1	2	3	4	5	NA
060322 Decreased serum sodium	1	2	3	4	5	NA
060323 Increased serum sodium	1	2	3	4	5	NA

Domain-*Physiologic Health (II)*   **Class**-*Fluid & Electrolytes (G)*   *3rd edition 2004; revised 2013*

OUTCOME CONTENT REFERENCES:

Edwards, S. L. (2000). Fluid overload and monitoring indices. *Professional Nurse, 15*(9), 568–572.

Kelly, A. L. (1999). Left ventricular systolic heart failure resulting in acute pulmonary edema: Pathophysiology and nursing management in the emergency department. *Australian Emergency Nursing Journal, 2*(1), 5–9.

Smeltzer, S. C., & Bare, B. G. (Eds.). (2003). *Brunner and Suddarth's textbook of medical-surgical nursing* (10th ed.). Philadelphia: Lippincott Williams & Wilkins.

F

Gait

0222

Definition: Ability to walk with correct body alignment, with smooth gait cycle, and at a steady pace

OUTCOME TARGET RATING: Maintain at_____ Increase to_____

		Severely compromised	Substantially compromised	Moderately compromised	Mildly compromised	Not compromised	
OUTCOME OVERALL RATING		1	2	3	4	5	
Indicators:							
022201	Steadiness of gait	1	2	3	4	5	NA
022202	Balance while walking	1	2	3	4	5	NA
022203	Walking posture	1	2	3	4	5	NA
022204	Walks in straight line	1	2	3	4	5	NA
022205	Length of stride	1	2	3	4	5	NA
022206	Step symmetry	1	2	3	4	5	NA
022207	Speed appropriate for activity	1	2	3	4	5	NA
022208	Base of support	1	2	3	4	5	NA
022209	Arm swing	1	2	3	4	5	NA
022210	Range of right knee flexion	1	2	3	4	5	NA
022211	Range of left knee flexion	1	2	3	4	5	NA
022212	Range of right hip flexion	1	2	3	4	5	NA
022213	Range of left hip flexion	1	2	3	4	5	NA

		Severe	Substantial	Moderate	Mild	None	
022214	Hesitancy	1	2	3	4	5	NA
022215	Limping	1	2	3	4	5	NA
022216	Shuffling gait	1	2	3	4	5	NA
022217	Weaving	1	2	3	4	5	NA
022218	Stumbling	1	2	3	4	5	NA
022219	Hopping	1	2	3	4	5	NA
022220	Leaning from side to side	1	2	3	4	5	NA
022221	Twisting hips	1	2	3	4	5	NA
022222	Lifting of knees as in marching	1	2	3	4	5	NA
022223	Stiff-legged walk	1	2	3	4	5	NA
022224	Forward stooped posture	1	2	3	4	5	NA

Domain-Functional Health (I)   **Class**-Mobility (C)   5th edition 2013

OUTCOME CONTENT REFERENCES:

Harris, M. H., Holden, M. K., Cahalin, L. P., Fitzpatrick, D., Lowe, S., & Canavan, P. K. (2008). Gait in older adults: A review of the literature with an emphasis toward achieving favorable clinical outcomes, Part I. *Clinical Geriatrics, 16*(7), 32–44.

Harris, M. H., Holden, M. K., Cahalin, L. P., Fitzpatrick, D., Lowe, S., & Canavan, P. K. (2008). Gait in older adults: A review of the literature with an emphasis toward achieving favorable clinical outcomes, Part II. *Clinical Geriatrics, 16*(8), 37–45.

Otsuki, T., Nawata, K., & Okuno, M. (1999). Quantitative evaluation of gait pattern in patients with osteoarthrosis of the knee before and after total knee arthroplasty. Gait analysis using a pressure measuring system. *Journal of Orthopaedic Science, 4*(2), 99–105.

Romei, M., Galli, M., Motta, F., Schwartz, M., & Crivellni, M. (2004). Use of the normalcy index for the evaluation of gait pathology. *Gait &Posture, 19*(1), 85–90.

Salzman, B. (2010). Gait and balance disorders in older adults. *American Family Physician, 82*(1), 61–68.

Tinetti, M. E. (1986). Performance-oriented assessment of mobility problems in elderly patients. *Journal of the American Geriatric Society, 34*(2), 119–126.

Gastrointestinal Function 1015

Definition: Ability of the gastrointestinal tract to ingest and digest food products, absorb nutrients, and eliminate waste

OUTCOME TARGET RATING: Maintain at_____ Increase to_____

OUTCOME OVERALL RATING		Severely compromised 1	Substantially compromised 2	Moderately compromised 3	Mildly compromised 4	Not compromised 5	
Indicators:							
101501	Food tolerance	1	2	3	4	5	NA
101524	Appetite	1	2	3	4	5	NA
101525	Gastric emptying time	1	2	3	4	5	NA
101503	Frequency of stools	1	2	3	4	5	NA
101504	Color of stool	1	2	3	4	5	NA
101505	Consistency of stool	1	2	3	4	5	NA
101506	Amount of stool	1	2	3	4	5	NA
101508	Bowel sounds	1	2	3	4	5	NA
101509	Color of gastric aspirates	1	2	3	4	5	NA
101510	Amount of residuals in gastric aspirates	1	2	3	4	5	NA
101526	pH of gastric aspirates	1	2	3	4	5	NA
101527	Serum albumin	1	2	3	4	5	NA
101528	Hematocrit	1	2	3	4	5	NA
101529	Blood glucose	1	2	3	4	5	NA

		Severe	Substantial	Moderate	Mild	None	
101513	Abdominal pain	1	2	3	4	5	NA
101514	Abdominal distention	1	2	3	4	5	NA
101515	Abdominal tenderness	1	2	3	4	5	NA
101516	Regurgitation	1	2	3	4	5	NA
101530	Gastric reflux	1	2	3	4	5	NA
101517	Increase in visible peristalsis	1	2	3	4	5	NA
101520	Blood in stool	1	2	3	4	5	NA
101521	White blood count elevation	1	2	3	4	5	NA
101522	White blood count depression	1	2	3	4	5	NA
101523	White blood count differential	1	2	3	4	5	NA
101531	Indigestion	1	2	3	4	5	NA
101532	Nausea	1	2	3	4	5	NA
101533	Vomiting	1	2	3	4	5	NA
101534	Hematemesis	1	2	3	4	5	NA
101535	Diarrhea	1	2	3	4	5	NA
101536	Constipation	1	2	3	4	5	NA
101537	Weight loss	1	2	3	4	5	NA
101538	Gastrointestinal bleeding	1	2	3	4	5	NA

Domain-Physiologic Health (II) *Class*-Digestion & Nutrition (K) 4th edition 2008, 2013

OUTCOME CONTENT REFERENCES:

Chowdhury, A., & Lobo, D. (2011). Fluids and gastrointestinal function. *Current Opinion in Clinical Nutrition & Metabolic Care, 14*(5), 469–476.

Hockenberry, M., & Wilson, D. (2011). *Wong's nursing care of infants and children* (9th ed.). St. Louis: Mosby.

LeMone, P., Burke, K., & Bauldoff, G. (2011). *Medical-surgical nursing: Critical thinking in patient care* (5th ed., pp. 560–587). Upper Saddle River, NJ: Pearson Education.

Smeltzer, S., Bare, B., Hinkle, J., & Cheever, K. (2010). Assessment of digestive and gastrointestinal function. In *Textbook of medical-surgical nursing* (12th ed., pp. 978–996). Philadelphia: Lippincott Williams & Wilkins.

Viteri, F. (2010). INCAP studies of hematologic and gastrointestinal function in healthy individuals and those with protein-energy malnutrition and infection. *Food and Nutrition Bulletin, 31*(1), 130–140.

G

Grief Resolution 1304

Definition: Personal actions to adjust thoughts, feelings, and behaviors to actual or impending loss

OUTCOME TARGET RATING: Maintain at_____ Increase to_____

		Never demonstrated	Rarely demonstrated	Sometimes demonstrated	Often demonstrated	Consistently demonstrated	
OUTCOME OVERALL RATING		1	2	3	4	5	
Indicators:							
130401	Resolves feelings about loss	1	2	3	4	5	NA
130402	Expresses spiritual beliefs about death	1	2	3	4	5	NA
130403	Verbalizes reality of loss	1	2	3	4	5	NA
130404	Verbalizes acceptance of loss	1	2	3	4	5	NA
130405	Describes meaning of the loss	1	2	3	4	5	NA
130406	Participates in planning service	1	2	3	4	5	NA
130409	Discusses unresolved conflict(s)	1	2	3	4	5	NA
130410	Reports absence of somatic distress	1	2	3	4	5	NA
130411	Reports decreased preoccupation with loss	1	2	3	4	5	NA
130412	Maintains living environment	1	2	3	4	5	NA
130413	Maintains personal grooming and hygiene	1	2	3	4	5	NA
130414	Reports adequate sleep	1	2	3	4	5	NA
130415	Reports adequate nutrition intake	1	2	3	4	5	NA
130416	Reports normal sexual desire	1	2	3	4	5	NA
130417	Seeks social support	1	2	3	4	5	NA
130418	Shares loss with significant others	1	2	3	4	5	NA
130419	Reports increased involvement in social activities	1	2	3	4	5	NA
130420	Progresses through stages of grief	1	2	3	4	5	NA
130421	Expresses positive expectations about the future	1	2	3	4	5	NA

Domain-*Psychosocial Health (III)*   **Class**-*Psychosocial Adaptation (N)*   *1st edition 1997; revised 2004, 2013*

OUTCOME CONTENT REFERENCES:

Batemen, A., Broderick, D., Gleason, L., Kardon, R., Flaherty, C., & Anderson, S. (1992). Dysfunctional grieving. *Journal of Psychosocial Nursing, 30*(12), 5–9.

Cooley, M. E. (1992). Bereavement care: A role for nurses. *Cancer Nursing, 15*(2), 125–129.

Freitag-Koontz, M. J. (1988). Parents' grief reaction to the diagnosis of their infants' severe neurologic impairment and static encephalopathy. *Journal of Perinatal and Neonatal Nursing, 2*(2), 45–57.

Gibbons, M. B. (1992). A child dies, a child survives: The impact of sibling loss. *Journal of Pediatric Health Care, 6*(2), 45–57.

Harrigan, R., Naber, M., Jensen, K., Tse, A., & Perez, D. (1993). Perinatal grief: Response to the loss of an infant. *Neonatal Network, 12*(5), 25–31.

Kallenberg, K., & Soderfeldt, B. (1992). Three years later: Grief, view of life, and personal crisis after the death of a family member. *Journal of Palliative Care, 8*(4), 13–19.

Kirschling, J. M., & McBride, A. B. (1989). Effects of age and sex on the experience of widowhood. *Western Journal of Nursing Research, 11*(2), 207–218.

Kuntz, B. (1991). Exploring the grief of adolescents after the death of a parent. *Journal of Child and Adolescent Psychiatric and Mental Health Nursing, 4*(3), 105–109.

+Prigerson, H. G., Maciejewski, P. K., Reynolds, C. F., Bierhals, A., Newsom, J. T., Fasiczka, A., Frank, E., Doman, J., & Miller, M. (1995). Inventory of complicated grief: A scale to measure maladaptive symptoms of loss. *Psychiatry Research, 59*(1–2), 65–79.

Whiting, G., & Buckwalter, K. C. (2001). Grieving. In M. Maas, K. Buckwalter, M. Hardy, T. Tripp-Reimer, M. Titler, & J. Specht (Eds.), *Nursing care of older adults: Diagnoses, outcomes & interventions* (pp. 631–650). St. Louis: Mosby.

Growth 0110

Definition: Normal increase in bone size and body weight during growth years

OUTCOME TARGET RATING: Maintain at_____ Increase to_____

	Severe deviation from normal range	Substantial deviation from normal range	Moderate deviation from normal range	Mild deviation from normal range	No deviation from normal range	
OUTCOME OVERALL RATING	1	2	3	4	5	
Indicators:						
011001 Weight percentile for sex	1	2	3	4	5	NA
011002 Weight percentile for age	1	2	3	4	5	NA
011003 Weight percentile for height	1	2	3	4	5	NA
011004 Rate of weight gain	1	2	3	4	5	NA
011005 Rate of height gain	1	2	3	4	5	NA
011006 Length/height percentile for age	1	2	3	4	5	NA
011007 Length/height percentile for sex	1	2	3	4	5	NA
011008 Head circumference percentile for age	1	2	3	4	5	NA
011009 Bone mass index	1	2	3	4	5	NA
011010 Mean body mass	1	2	3	4	5	NA

Domain-*Functional Health (I)* **Class**-*Growth & Development (B)* *1st edition 1997; revised 2004*

OUTCOME CONTENT REFERENCES:

Allen, K. D., Warzak, W. J., Greger, N. G., Bernotas, T. D., & Huseman, C. A. (1993). Psychosocial adjustment of children with isolated growth hormone deficiency. *Children's Health Care, 22*(1), 61–72.

Blinkin, N. J., Yip, R., Fleshood, L., & Trowbridge, F. L. (1988). Birth weight and childhood growth. *Pediatrics, 82*(6), 828–834.

Georgieff, M. K., Hoffman, J. S., Pereira, G. R., Bernbaum, J., & Hoffman-Williamson, M. (1985). Effect of neonatal caloric deprivation on head growth and 1-year developmental status in preterm infants. *Journal of Pediatrics, 107*(4), 581–587.

Hockenberry, M. J., Wilson, D., Winkelstein, M. L., & Kline, N. E. (2003). *Wong's nursing care of infants and children* (7th ed.). St. Louis: Mosby.

Jung, E., & Czajka-Narins, D. M. (1985). Birth weight doubling and tripling times: An updated look at the effects of birth weight, sex, race and type of feeding. *The American Journal of Clinical Nutrition, 42*(8), 182–189.

Sapala, S. (1994). Pediatric management problems. *Pediatric Nursing, 20*(1), 54–55.

Tanner, J. M., & Davies, P. S. W. (1985). Clinical longitudinal standards for height and height velocity for North American children. *The Journal of Pediatrics, 107*(3), 317–329.

Guilt Resolution 1310

Definition: Personal actions to adjust intense and frequent thoughts, feelings, and behaviors due to actual or perceived self-blame

OUTCOME TARGET RATING: Maintain at_____ Increase to_____

	Never demonstrated	Rarely demonstrated	Sometimes demonstrated	Often demonstrated	Consistently demonstrated	
OVERALL OUTCOME RATING	1	2	3	4	5	
Indicators:						
131001 Expresses the causes of guilt	1	2	3	4	5	NA
131002 Identifies feelings of guilt	1	2	3	4	5	NA
131003 Monitors intensity of feelings	1	2	3	4	5	NA

Continued

Guilt Resolution—*cont'd*

		Never demonstrated	Rarely demonstrated	Sometimes demonstrated	Often demonstrated	Consistently demonstrated	
131004	Monitors frequency of feelings	1	2	3	4	5	NA
131005	Expresses the personal meaning of guilt	1	2	3	4	5	NA
131006	Identifies a realistic perception of the cause of guilt	1	2	3	4	5	NA
131007	Identifies guilt as a common reaction	1	2	3	4	5	NA
131008	Identifies exaggerated negative feelings	1	2	3	4	5	NA
131009	Identifies irrational thoughts	1	2	3	4	5	NA
131010	Shares feelings of guilt with significant others	1	2	3	4	5	NA
131011	Shares feelings of guilt with health providers	1	2	3	4	5	NA
131012	Uses strategies to decrease guilt	1	2	3	4	5	NA
131013	Reports absence of somatic distress	1	2	3	4	5	NA
131014	Follows recommended treatment	1	2	3	4	5	NA
131015	Uses effective coping strategies	1	2	3	4	5	NA
131016	Uses support services	1	2	3	4	5	NA
131017	Reports improved mood	1	2	3	4	5	NA
131018	Reports increased involvement in social activities	1	2	3	4	5	NA
131019	Expresses positive expectations about the future	1	2	3	4	5	NA
131020	Reports decreased preoccupation with guilt	1	2	3	4	5	NA
131021	Resolves feelings of guilt	1	2	3	4	5	NA
131022	Verbalizes acceptance of guilt	1	2	3	4	5	NA
131023	Adapts to life changes	1	2	3	4	5	NA

Domain-*Psychosocial Health (III)*   **Class**-*Psychosocial Adaptation (N)*   5th edition 2013

OUTCOME CONTENT REFERENCES:

Abrams, R. D., & Finesinger, J. E. (1953). Guilt reactions in patients with cancer. *Cancer, 6*(3), 474–482.

Antai-Otong, D. (2008). Crisis intervention and management: The role of adaptation. In D. Antai-Otang (2nd ed.), *Psychiatric nursing: biological & behavioral concepts* (pp. 961–983.). Clifton Park, NY: Thomson Delmar Learning.

Arnold, E. C., & Boggs, K. U. (2011). Communicating with clients in crisis. In E. C. Arnold and K. U. Boggs (Eds.), *Interpersonal relationships: Professional communication skills for nurses* (6th ed., pp. 415–435). St. Louis: Elsevier Saunders.

Fortinash, K. M. (2008). Grief and loss. In K. M. Fortinash and P. A. Holoday-Worret (Eds.), *Psychiatric mental health nursing* (4th ed., pp. 593). St. Louis: Mosby Elsevier.

Nishith, P., Nixon, R. D. V., & Resick, P. A. (2005). Resolution of trauma-related guilt following treatment of PTSD in female rape victims: A result of cognitive processing therapy targeting comorbid depression? *Journal of affective disorders, 86*(2–3), 259–265.

Health Beliefs 1700

Definition: Personal convictions that influence health behaviors

OUTCOME TARGET RATING: Maintain at_____ Increase to_____

		Very weak	Weak	Moderate	Strong	Very strong	
OUTCOME OVERALL RATING		1	2	3	4	5	
Indicators:							
170001	Perceived importance of taking action	1	2	3	4	5	NA
170002	Perceived threat from inaction	1	2	3	4	5	NA
170003	Perceived benefits of action	1	2	3	4	5	NA
170004	Perceived internal control of action	1	2	3	4	5	NA
170005	Perceived control of health outcome	1	2	3	4	5	NA
170006	Perceived reduction of threat from action	1	2	3	4	5	NA
170007	Perceived improvement in lifestyle from action	1	2	3	4	5	NA
170008	Perceived ability to perform action	1	2	3	4	5	NA
170009	Perceived resources to perform action	1	2	3	4	5	NA
170010	Perceived absence of barriers to action	1	2	3	4	5	NA

Domain-Health Knowledge & Behavior (IV)   **Class**-Health Beliefs (R)   1st edition 1997

OUTCOME CONTENT REFERENCES:
+Champion, V. L. (1993). Instrument refinement for breast cancer screening behaviors. *Nursing Research, 42*(3), 139–143.
Clarke, V. A., Lovegrove, H., Williams, A., & Machperson, M. (2000). Unrealistic optimism and the Health Belief Model. *Journal of Behavioral Medicine, 23*(4), 367–376.
Gillis, A. J. (1993). Determinants of health promoting lifestyle: An integrative review. *Journal of Advanced Nursing, 18*(3), 345–353.
Glick, O. J., & Ressler, C. (2001). Altered health maintenance. In M. Maas, K. Buckwalter, M. Hardy, T. Tripp-Reimer, M. Titler, & J. Specht (Eds.), *Nursing care of older adults: Diagnoses, outcomes & interventions* (pp. 6–22). St. Louis: Mosby.
Hayes, D., & Ross, C. (1987). Concern with appearance, health beliefs, and eating habits. *Journal of Health and Social Behavior, 28*(6), 120–130.
+Kim, K. K., Horan, M. L., Gendler, P., & Patel, M. K. (1991). Development and evaluation of the osteoporosis health belief scale. *Research in Nursing & Health, 14*(2), 155–163.
Robertson, D., & Keller, C. (1992). Relationships among health beliefs, self-efficacy, and exercise adherence in patients with coronary artery disease. *Heart & Lung, 21*(1), 56–63.
Thompson, J., McFarland, G. K., & Hirsch, J. E. (2002). *Mosby's clinical nursing* (5th ed.). St. Louis: Mosby.

Health Beliefs: Perceived Ability to Perform 1701

Definition: Personal conviction that one can carry out a given health behavior

OUTCOME TARGET RATING: Maintain at_____ Increase to_____

		Very weak	Weak	Moderate	Strong	Very strong	
OUTCOME OVERALL RATING		1	2	3	4	5	
Indicators:							
170101	Perception that health behavior is not too complex	1	2	3	4	5	NA
170102	Perception that health behavior requires reasonable effort	1	2	3	4	5	NA
170103	Perception that the frequency of health behavior is not excessive	1	2	3	4	5	NA
170104	Perception of likelihood of performing health behavior over time	1	2	3	4	5	NA
170105	Confidence related to past experience with health behavior	1	2	3	4	5	NA
170106	Confidence related to past experience with similar health behaviors	1	2	3	4	5	NA

Continued

H

Health Beliefs: Perceived Ability to Perform—cont'd

		Very weak	Weak	Moderate	Strong	Very strong	
170107	Confidence related to observation of successful experiences of others	1	2	3	4	5	NA
170108	Confidence in ability to perform health behavior	1	2	3	4	5	NA

Domain-Health Knowledge & Behavior (IV) *Class*-Health Beliefs (R) 1st edition 1997; revised 2004

OUTCOME CONTENT REFERENCES:
Bauer, M. S., Williford, W. O., McBride, L., McBride, K., & Shea, N. M. (2005). Perceived barriers to health care access in a treated population. *International Journal of Psychiatry in Medicine, 35*(1), 13–26.
Calfee, C. S., Katz, P. P., Yelin, E. H., Iribarren, C., & Eisner, M. D. (2007). The influence of perceived control of asthma on health outcomes. *Chest, 130*(5), 1312–1318.
+Champion, V. L. (1993). Instrument refinement for breast cancer screening behaviors. *Nursing Research, 42*(3), 139–143.
Clarke, V. A., Lovegrove, H., Williams, A., & Machperson, M. (2000). Unrealistic optimism and the Health Belief Model. *Journal of Behavioral Medicine, 23*(4), 367–376.
de Weerdt, I., Visser, A., & van der Veen, E. (1989). Attitude behaviour theories and diabetes education programmes. *Patient Education and Counseling, 14*(1), 3–19.
Hayes, D., & Ross, C. (1987). Concern with appearance, health beliefs, and eating habits. *Journal of Health and Social Behavior, 28*(6), 120–130.
Jemmot, L., & Jemmot, J. (1992). Increasing condom-use intentions among sexually active black adolescent women. *Nursing Research, 41*(5), 273–278.
Jensen, K., Banwart, L., Venhaus, R., Popkess-Vawter, S., & Perkins, S. B. (1993). Advanced rehabilitation nursing care of coronary angioplasty patients using self-efficacy theory. *Journal of Advanced Nursing, 18*(6), 926–931.
Kim, K. K., Horan, M. L., Gendler, P., & Patel, M. K. (1991). Development and evaluation of the Osteoporosis Health Belief Scale. *Research in Nursing & Health, 14*(2), 155–163.
Lowe, N. K. (1993). Maternal confidence for labor: Development of the Childbirth Self-Efficacy Inventory. *Research in Nursing & Health, 16*(2), 141–149.
Robertson, D., & Keller, C. (1992). Relationships among health beliefs, self-efficacy, and exercise adherence in patients with coronary artery disease. *Heart & Lung, 21*(1), 56–63.
+Smith, M. S., Wallston, K. A., & Smith, C. A. (1995). The development and validation of the Perceived Health Competence Scale. *Health Education Research, 10*(1), 51–64.

Health Beliefs: Perceived Control 1702

Definition: Personal conviction that one can influence a health outcome

OUTCOME TARGET RATING: Maintain at_____ Increase to_____

		Very weak	Weak	Moderate	Strong	Very strong	
OUTCOME OVERALL RATING		1	2	3	4	5	
Indicators:							
170201	Perceived responsibility for health decisions	1	2	3	4	5	NA
170202	Requested involvement in health decisions	1	2	3	4	5	NA
170203	Efforts at gathering information	1	2	3	4	5	NA
170204	Belief that own decisions control health outcomes	1	2	3	4	5	NA
170205	Belief that own actions control health outcomes	1	2	3	4	5	NA
170206	Willingness to designate surrogate decision-maker	1	2	3	4	5	NA
170207	Willingness to have current living will	1	2	3	4	5	NA

Domain-Health Knowledge & Behavior (IV) *Class*-Health Beliefs (R) 1st edition 1997

OUTCOME CONTENT REFERENCES:
Calnan, M., & Moss, S. (1984). The Health Belief Model and compliance with education given at a class in breast self-examination. *Journal of Health and Social Behavior, 25*(2), 198–210.
+Champion, V. L. (1993). Instrument refinement for breast cancer screening behaviors. *Nursing Research, 42*(3), 139–143.
Clarke, V. A., Lovegrove, H., Williams, A., & Machperson, M. (2000). Unrealistic optimism and the Health Belief Model. *Journal of Behavioral Medicine, 23*(4), 367–376.
Gillis, A. J. (1993). Determinants of health promoting lifestyle: An integrative review. *Journal of Advanced Nursing, 18*(3), 345–353.
Hayes, D., & Ross, C. (1987). Concern with appearance, health beliefs, and eating habits. *Journal of Health and Social Behavior, 28*(6), 120–130.
+Wallston, K. A., & Wallston, B. S. (1981). Health Locus of Control Scales. In H. Lefcourt (Ed.), *Research with the locus of control construct* (Vol. 1, pp.189–243). New York: Academic Press.
+Wallston, K. A., Wallston, B. S., & DeVellis, R. (1978). Development of the Multidimensional Health Locus of Control (MHLC) Scales. *Health Education Monographs, 6*(2), 160–170.

Health Beliefs: Perceived Resources 1703

Definition: Personal conviction that one has adequate means to carry out a health behavior

OUTCOME TARGET RATING: Maintain at_____ Increase to_____

	Very weak	Weak	Moderate	Strong	Very strong	
OUTCOME OVERALL RATING	1	2	3	4	5	
Indicators:						
170301 Perceived support of significant others	1	2	3	4	5	NA
170302 Perceived support of friends	1	2	3	4	5	NA
170303 Perceived support of neighbors	1	2	3	4	5	NA
170304 Perceived support of health provider	1	2	3	4	5	NA
170305 Perceived support of self-help groups	1	2	3	4	5	NA
170306 Perceived functional ability	1	2	3	4	5	NA
170307 Perceived energy to act	1	2	3	4	5	NA
170309 Perceived adequacy of time	1	2	3	4	5	NA
170310 Perceived adequacy of personal finances	1	2	3	4	5	NA
170311 Perceived adequacy of health insurance	1	2	3	4	5	NA
170318 Perceived access to medication	1	2	3	4	5	NA
170312 Perceived access to equipment	1	2	3	4	5	NA
170313 Perceived access to supplies	1	2	3	4	5	NA
170314 Perceived access to health care services	1	2	3	4	5	NA
170315 Perceived access to transportation	1	2	3	4	5	NA
170316 Perceived access to physical assistance	1	2	3	4	5	NA

Domain-*Health Knowledge & Behavior (IV)* **Class**-*Health Beliefs (R)* *1st edition 1997; revised 2004*

OUTCOME CONTENT REFERENCES:
+Becker, H., Stuifbergen, A. K., & Sands, D. (1991). Development of a scale to measure barriers to health promotion activities among persons with disabilities. *American Journal of Health Promotion, 5*(6), 449–454.
+Champion, V. L. (1993). Instrument refinement for breast cancer screening behaviors. *Nursing Research, 42*(3), 139–143.
Clarke, V. A., Lovegrove, H., Williams, A., & Machperson, M. (2000). Unrealistic optimism and the Health Belief Model. *Journal of Behavioral Medicine, 23*(4), 367–376.
Gillis, A. J. (1993). Determinants of health promoting lifestyle: An integrative review. *Journal of Advanced Nursing, 18*(3), 345–353.
Kim, K. K., Horan, M. L., Gendler, P., & Patel, M. K. (1991). Development and evaluation of the osteoporosis health belief scale. *Research in Nursing & Health, 14*(2), 155–163.
Robertson, D., & Keller, C. (1992). Relationships among health beliefs, self-efficacy, and exercise adherence in patients with coronary artery disease. *Heart & Lung, 21*(1), 56–63.

Health Beliefs: Perceived Threat 1704

Definition: Personal conviction that a threatening health problem is serious and has potential negative consequences for lifestyle

OUTCOME TARGET RATING: Maintain at_____ Increase to_____

	Very weak	Weak	Moderate	Strong	Very strong	
OUTCOME OVERALL RATING	1	2	3	4	5	
Indicators:						
170401 Perceived threat to health	1	2	3	4	5	NA
170403 Perceived vulnerability to progressive health problems	1	2	3	4	5	NA
170404 Concern regarding illness or injury	1	2	3	4	5	NA
170405 Concern regarding potential complications	1	2	3	4	5	NA
170406 Perceived severity of illness or injury	1	2	3	4	5	NA

Continued

H

Health Beliefs: Perceived Threat—cont'd

		Very weak	Weak	Moderate	Strong	Very strong	
170407	Perceived severity of complications	1	2	3	4	5	NA
170408	Perceived threat of discomfort from illness or injury	1	2	3	4	5	NA
170409	Perception that condition may be of long duration	1	2	3	4	5	NA
170410	Perceived impact on current lifestyle	1	2	3	4	5	NA
170411	Perceived impact on future lifestyle	1	2	3	4	5	NA
170412	Perceived impact on functional status	1	2	3	4	5	NA
170414	Perceived threat of death	1	2	3	4	5	NA

Domain-Health Knowledge & Behavior (IV)   *Class*-Health Beliefs (R)   *1st edition 1997; revised 2004*

OUTCOME CONTENT REFERENCES:

Calnan, M., & Moss, S. (1984). The health belief model and compliance with education given at a class in breast self-examination. *Journal of Health and Social Behavior, 25*(2), 198–210.

+Champion, V. L. (1993). Instrument refinement for breast cancer screening behaviors. *Nursing Research, 42*(3), 139–143.

Clarke, V. A., Lovegrove, H., Williams, A., & Machperson, M. (2000). Unrealistic optimism and the Health Belief Model. *Journal of Behavioral Medicine, 23*(4), 367–376.

de Weerdt, I., Visser, A., & van der Veen, E. (1989). Attitude behaviour theories and diabetes education programmes. *Patient Education and Counseling, 14*(1), 3–19.

Dunn, S., Beeney, L., Hoskins, P., & Turtle, J. (1990). Knowledge and attitude change as predictors of metabolic improvement in diabetes education. *Social Science and Medicine, 31*(10), 1135–1141.

+Kim, K. K., Horan, M. L., Gendler, P., & Patel, M. K. (1991). Development and evaluation of the osteoporosis health belief scale. *Research in Nursing & Health, 14*(2), 155–163.

Robertson, D., & Keller, C. (1992). Relationships among health beliefs, self-efficacy, and exercise adherence in patients with coronary artery disease. *Heart & Lung, 21*(1), 56–63.

Thompson, J., McFarland, G., & Hirsch, J. (2002). *Mosby's clinical nursing* (5th ed.). St. Louis: Mosby.

Health Orientation
1705

Definition: Personal commitment to health behaviors as lifestyle priorities

OUTCOME TARGET RATING: Maintain at_____   Increase to_____

		Very weak	Weak	Moderate	Strong	Very strong	
OUTCOME OVERALL RATING		1	2	3	4	5	
Indicators:							
170501	Focus on wellness	1	2	3	4	5	NA
170514	Focus on maintaining health behaviors	1	2	3	4	5	NA
170502	Focus on disease prevention	1	2	3	4	5	NA
170503	Focus on maintaining role performance	1	2	3	4	5	NA
170504	Focus on maintaining functional abilities	1	2	3	4	5	NA
170505	Focus on adjustment to life situations	1	2	3	4	5	NA
170506	Focus on overall well-being	1	2	3	4	5	NA
170507	Expectation that individual is responsible for health-related choices	1	2	3	4	5	NA
170508	Perception that health behavior is relevant to one's health	1	2	3	4	5	NA
170515	Perceived importance of incorporating health behaviors with cultural beliefs	1	2	3	4	5	NA
170512	Perception that health is a high priority in making lifestyle choices	1	2	3	4	5	NA

Domain-Health Knowledge & Behavior (IV)   *Class*-Health Beliefs (R)   *1st edition 1997; revised 2004*

OUTCOME CONTENT REFERENCES:

Gillis, A. J. (1993). Determinants of health promoting lifestyle: An integrative review. *Journal of Advanced Nursing, 18*(3), 345–353.

Glick, O. J., & Ressler, C. (2001). Altered health maintenance. In M. Maas, K. Buckwalter, M. Hardy, T. Tripp-Reimer, M. Titler, & J. Specht (Eds.), *Nursing care of older adults: Diagnoses, outcomes & interventions* (pp. 6–22). St. Louis: Mosby.

Kulbok, P., & Baldwin, J. (1992). From preventive health behavior to health promotion: Advancing a positive construct of health. *Advances in Nursing Science, 14*(4), 50–64.

Palank, C. (1991). Determinants of health promoting behavior. *Nursing Clinics of North America, 26*(4), 815–832.

Pender, N. J. (1990). Expressing health through lifestyle patterns. *Nursing Science Quarterly, 3*(3), 115–122.

+Walker, S. N., Sechrist, K. R., & Pender, N. J. (1987). The Health-Promoting Lifestyle Profile: Development and psychometric characteristics. *Nursing Research, 36*(2), 76–81.

+Walker, S. N., Sechrist, K. R., & Pender, N. J. (1995). *The Health-Promoting Lifestyle Profile II.* Omaha, NE: University of Nebraska at Omaha.

Ziebland, S., Evans, J., McPherson, A. (2006). The choice is yours? How women with ovarian cancer make sense of treatment choices. *Patient Education and Counseling, 62*(3), 361–367.

Health Promoting Behavior   1602

Definition: Personal actions to sustain or increase wellness

OUTCOME TARGET RATING: Maintain at_____   Increase to_____

OUTCOME OVERALL RATING	Never demonstrated 1	Rarely demonstrated 2	Sometimes demonstrated 3	Often demonstrated 4	Consistently demonstrated 5	
Indicators:						
160201 Uses risk avoidance behaviors	1	2	3	4	5	NA
160202 Monitors environment for risks	1	2	3	4	5	NA
160203 Monitors personal behavior for risks	1	2	3	4	5	NA
160221 Balances activity and rest	1	2	3	4	5	NA
160222 Maintains adequate sleep	1	2	3	4	5	NA
160205 Uses effective stress reduction techniques	1	2	3	4	5	NA
160206 Maintains social relationships	1	2	3	4	5	NA
160207 Performs healthy behaviors routinely	1	2	3	4	5	NA
160208 Supports healthful public policy	1	2	3	4	5	NA
160209 Uses financial resources to promote health	1	2	3	4	5	NA
160210 Uses social support to promote health	1	2	3	4	5	NA
160212 Obtains recommended immunizations	1	2	3	4	5	NA
160213 Obtains recommended health screenings	1	2	3	4	5	NA
160214 Follows healthy diet	1	2	3	4	5	NA
160223 Drinks eight glasses of water daily	1	2	3	4	5	NA
160224 Obtains regular check-ups	1	2	3	4	5	NA
160215 Uses effective weight control strategies	1	2	3	4	5	NA
160216 Uses effective exercise routine	1	2	3	4	5	NA
160217 Avoids exposure to infectious disease	1	2	3	4	5	NA
160225 Avoids exposure to secondhand smoke	1	2	3	4	5	NA
160218 Avoids alcohol misuse	1	2	3	4	5	NA
160219 Avoids tobacco use	1	2	3	4	5	NA
160220 Avoids recreational drug use	1	2	3	4	5	NA

Domain-Health Knowledge & Behavior (IV)   **Class**-Health Behavior (Q)   *1st edition 1997; revised 2004, 2008*

OUTCOME CONTENT REFERENCES:

Green, L., & Raeburn, J. (1990). Contemporary development in health promotion. In N. Bracht (Ed.), *Health promotion at the community level* (pp. 29–44). Thousand Oaks, CA: Sage.

Johnson, P. H., & Kittleson, M. J. (2003). A qualitative exploration of health behaviors and the associated factor among university students from different cultures. *The International Journal of Health Education, 6*, 14–25.

Kulbok, P., & Baldwin, J. (1992). From preventive health behavior to health promotion: Advancing a positive construct of health. *Advances in Nursing Science, 14*(4), 50–64.

Leenerts, M. H., Teel, C. S., & Pendleton, M. K. (2002). Building a model of self-care for health promotion in aging. *Journal of Nursing Scholarship, 34*(4), 355–361.

Mechanic, D., & Cleary, P. (1980). Factors associated with maintenance of positive behavior. *Preventive Medicine, 9*(6), 805–814.

Resnick, B. (2000). Health promotion practices of the older adult. *Public Health Nursing, 17*(3), 160–168.

Seeman, T. E. (2000). Health promoting effects of friends and family on health outcomes in older adults. *American Journal of Health Promotion, 14*(6), 362–370.

Simons-Morton, D. G., Mullen, P. D., Mains, D. A., Tabak, E. R., & Green, L. W. (1992). Characteristics of controlled studies of patient education and counseling for preventive health behavior. *Patient Education and Counseling, 19*(2), 175–204.

Stevenson, J. S. (2001). Health seeking behaviors. In M. Maas, K. Buckwalter, M. Hardy, T. Tripp-Reimer, M. Titler, & J. Specht (Eds.), *Nursing care of older adults: Diagnoses, outcomes & interventions* (pp. 75–85). St. Louis: Mosby.

+Walker, S. N., Sechrist, K. R., & Pender, N. J. (1987). The Health-Promoting Lifestyle Profile: Development and psychometric characteristics. *Nursing Research, 36*(2), 76–81.

+Walker, S. N., Sechrist, K. R., & Pender, N. J. (1995). *The Health-Promoting Lifestyle Profile II.* Omaha, NE: University of Nebraska at Omaha.

H

Health Seeking Behavior 1603

Definition: Personal actions to promote optimal wellness, recovery, and rehabilitation

OUTCOME TARGET RATING: Maintain at_____   Increase to_____

	Never demonstrated	Rarely demonstrated	Sometimes demonstrated	Often demonstrated	Consistently demonstrated	
OUTCOME OVERALL RATING	1	2	3	4	5	
Indicators:						
160301 Asks health-related questions	1	2	3	4	5	NA
160302 Completes health-related tasks	1	2	3	4	5	NA
160303 Performs self-screening	1	2	3	4	5	NA
160313 Obtains assistance from health professional	1	2	3	4	5	NA
160305 Performs activities of daily living consistent with tolerance	1	2	3	4	5	NA
160306 Describes strategies to eliminate unhealthy behavior	1	2	3	4	5	NA
160314 Performs self-initiated health behavior	1	2	3	4	5	NA
160308 Performs prescribed health behavior	1	2	3	4	5	NA
160315 Uses reputable health information	1	2	3	4	5	NA
160310 Describes strategies to optimize health	1	2	3	4	5	NA
160316 Seeks assistance when needed	1	2	3	4	5	NA

Domain-*Health Knowledge & Behavior (IV)*   **Class**-*Health Behavior (Q)*   *1st edition 1997; revised 2004, 2008, 2013*

OUTCOME CONTENT REFERENCES:

Folden, S. L. (1993). Definitions of health and health goals of participants in a community-based pulmonary rehabilitation program. *Public Health Nursing, 10*(1), 31–35.

Frich, J. C., Ose, L., Malterud, K., & Fugelli, P. (2006). Perceived vulnerability to heart disease in patients with familial hypercholesterolemia: A qualitative interview study. *Annals of Family Medicine, 4*(3), 198–204.

Jensen, L., & Allen, M. (1993). Wellness: The dialect of illness. *Image—The Journal of Nursing Scholarship, 25*(3), 220–224.

Kaplan, M., Kiernan, N. E., & James, L. (2006). Intergenerational family conversations and decision making about eating healthfully. *Journal of Nutrition Education & Behavior, 38*(5), 298–306.

Macnee, C. L., Edwards, J., Kaplan, A., Reed, S., Bradford, S., Walls, J., & Schaller-Ayers, J. M. (2006). Evaluation of NOC standardized outcome of "health seeking behavior" in nurse-managed clinics. *Journal of Nursing Care Quality, 21*(3), 242–247.

Mansfield, A. K., Addis, M. E., Mahalik, J. R. (2003). "Why won't he go to the doctor?": The psychology of men's help seeking. *International Journal of Men's Health, 2*(2), 93–109.

Nicoteri, J. A., & Arnold, E. C. (2005). The development of health care-seeking behaviors in traditional-age undergraduate college students. *Journal of the American Academy of Nurse Practitioners, 17*(10), 411–415.

Pender, N. J. (1990). Expressing health through lifestyle patterns. *Nursing Science Quarterly, 3*(3), 115–122.

Pender, N. J., & Pender, A. R. (1986). Attitudes, subjective norms, and intentions to engage in health behaviors. *Nursing Research, 35*(1), 15–18.

Stevenson, J. S. (2001). Health seeking behaviors. In M. Maas, K. Buckwalter, M. Hardy, T. Tripp-Reimer, M. Titler, & J. Specht (Eds.), *Nursing care of older adults: Diagnoses, outcomes & interventions* (pp. 75–85). St. Louis: Mosby.

+Walker, S. N., Sechrist, K. R., & Pender, N. J. (1987). The Health-Promoting Lifestyle Profile: Development and psychometric characteristics. *Nursing Research, 36*(2), 76–81.

+Walker, S. N., Sechrist, K. R., & Pender, N. J. (1995). *The Health-Promoting Lifestyle Profile II.* Omaha, NE: University of Nebraska at Omaha.

Woods, N. (1989). Conceptualizations of self-care: Toward health-oriented models. *Advances in Nursing Science, 12*(1), 1–13.

Hearing Compensation Behavior   1610

Definition: Personal actions to identify, monitor, and compensate for hearing loss

OUTCOME TARGET RATING: Maintain at_____ Increase to_____

		Never demonstrated	Rarely demonstrated	Sometimes demonstrated	Often demonstrated	Consistently demonstrated	
OUTCOME OVERALL RATING		1	2	3	4	5	
Indicators:							
161001	Monitors symptoms of hearing deterioration	1	2	3	4	5	NA
161002	Positions self to advantage hearing	1	2	3	4	5	NA
161003	Reminds others to use techniques that advantage hearing	1	2	3	4	5	NA
161004	Eliminates background noise	1	2	3	4	5	NA
161005	Uses sign language	1	2	3	4	5	NA
161006	Uses lip reading	1	2	3	4	5	NA
161007	Uses closed captioning for television viewing	1	2	3	4	5	NA
161009	Uses hearing supportive devices	1	2	3	4	5	NA
161012	Uses hearing aids correctly	1	2	3	4	5	NA
161010	Cares for internal hearing assistive devices correctly	1	2	3	4	5	NA
161011	Cares for external hearing assistive devices correctly	1	2	3	4	5	NA
161013	Uses support services for hearing impaired	1	2	3	4	5	NA

Domain-*Health Knowledge & Behavior (IV)*   **Class**-*Health Behavior (Q)*   *2nd edition 2000; revised 2004, 2008*

OUTCOME CONTENT REFERENCES:
Burrell, L. O. (Ed.). (1992). *Adult nursing in hospital and community settings.* Norwalk, CT: Appleton & Lange.
Phipps, W. J., Monahan, F. D., Sands, J. K., Marek, J., & Neighbors, M. (Eds.). (2003). *Medical-surgical nursing: Concepts and clinical practice* (7th ed.). St. Louis: Mosby.
Smeltzer, S. C., & Bare, B. G. (Eds.). (2003). *Brunner and Suddarth's textbook of medical-surgical nursing* (10th ed.). Philadelphia: Lippincott Williams & Wilkins.

H

Heedfulness of Affected Side 0918

Definition: Personal actions to acknowledge, protect, and cognitively integrate affected body part(s) into self

OUTCOME TARGET RATING: Maintain at_____   Increase to_____

	Never demonstrated	Rarely demonstrated	Sometimes demonstrated	Often demonstrated	Consistently demonstrated	
OUTCOME OVERALL RATING	1	2	3	4	5	
Indicators:						
091801 Acknowledges affected side as being integral to self	1	2	3	4	5	NA
091802 Protects affected side when ambulating	1	2	3	4	5	NA
091803 Protects affected side when positioning	1	2	3	4	5	NA
091804 Protects affected side when transferring	1	2	3	4	5	NA
091805 Protects affected side during rest or sleep	1	2	3	4	5	NA
091806 Performs daily care to affected side	1	2	3	4	5	NA
091807 Arranges environment to compensate for physical or sensory deficits	1	2	3	4	5	NA
091808 Changes body orientation to enable unaffected side to compensate for physical or sensory deficits	1	2	3	4	5	NA
091809 Uses visual scanning as a compensatory strategy	1	2	3	4	5	NA
091810 Promotes strength and dexterity of affected limb	1	2	3	4	5	NA
091811 Prevents underuse of affected limb	1	2	3	4	5	NA
091812 Maintains postural control	1	2	3	4	5	NA

Domain-*Physiologic Health (II)*   **Class**-*Neurocognitive (J)*   *4th edition 2008; revised 2013*

OUTCOME CONTENT REFERENCES:

Duncan, P. W., Zorowitz, R., Bates, B., Choi, J. Y., Glasberg, J. J., Graham, G. D., Katz, R. C., Lamberty, K., & Reker, D. (2005). Management of adult stroke rehabilitation care: A clinical practice guideline. *Stroke, 36*(9), e100–143.

Intercollegiate Stroke Working Party. (2004). *National clinical guidelines for stroke* (2nd ed.). London: Clinical Effectiveness and Evaluation Unit of the Royal College of Physicians.

Perennou, D. A., Leblond, C., Amblard, B., Micallef, J. P., Herisson, C., & Pelissier, Y. (2001). Transcutaneous electric nerve stimulation reduces neglect-related postural instability after stroke. *Archives of Physical Medicine and Rehabilitation, 82*(4), 440–448.

Punt, T. D., & Riddoch, M. J. (2006). Motor neglect: Implications for movement and rehabilitation following stroke. *Disability and Rehabilitation, 28*(13–14), 857–864.

Ringman, J. M., Saver, J. L., Woolson, R. F., Clarke, W. R., & Adams, H. P. (2004). Frequency, risk factors, anatomy, and course of unilateral neglect in an acute stroke cohort. *Neurology, 63*(3), 468–474.

Slater, D. I., Curtin, S., Johns, J. S., Schmidt, C., Tipton, J. L., & Newbury, R. E. (2006). *Middle cerebral artery stroke.* Retrieved January 22, 2007 from http://www.emedicine.com/pmr/topic77.htm

Weitzel, E. A. (2001). Unilateral neglect. In M. Maas, K. Buckwalter, M. Hardy, T. Tripp-Reimer, M. Titler, & J. Specht (Eds.), *Nursing care of older adults: Diagnoses, outcomes, and interventions* (pp. 492–502). St. Louis: Mosby.

Hemodialysis Access   1105

Definition: Functionality of a dialysis access site and health of surrounding tissues

OUTCOME TARGET RATING: Maintain at_____   Increase to_____

	Severely compromised	Substantially compromised	Moderately compromised	Mildly compromised	Not compromised	
OUTCOME OVERALL RATING	1	2	3	4	5	
Indicators:						
110501 Blood volume flow through fistula/shunt	1	2	3	4	5	NA
110502 Site skin color	1	2	3	4	5	NA
110517 Access site skin temperature	1	2	3	4	5	NA
110505 Bruit	1	2	3	4	5	NA
110506 Thrill	1	2	3	4	5	NA
110509 Distal peripheral pulses	1	2	3	4	5	NA
110510 Distal peripheral skin temperature	1	2	3	4	5	NA
110511 Distal peripheral skin color	1	2	3	4	5	NA
110514 Clotting time	1	2	3	4	5	NA
	Severe	**Substantial**	**Moderate**	**Mild**	**None**	
110503 Drainage at site	1	2	3	4	5	NA
110507 Hematoma at site	1	2	3	4	5	NA
110508 Bleeding at site	1	2	3	4	5	NA
110512 Distal peripheral edema	1	2	3	4	5	NA
110515 Tenderness at site	1	2	3	4	5	NA
110513 Cannula displacement	1	2	3	4	5	NA

Domain-*Physiologic Health (II)*   **Class**-*Tissue Integrity (L)   2nd edition 2000; revised 2004, 2013*

OUTCOME CONTENT REFERENCES

Broscious, S. K., & Castagnola, J. (2006). Chronic kidney disease: Acute manifestations and role of critical care nurses. *Critical Care Nurse, 26*(4), 17–28.

Eisenbud, M. D. (1996). *The handbook of dialysis access.* Columbus, OH: Anadem.

Lancaster, L. E. (Ed.). (1995). *ANNA's core curriculum for nephrology nurses* (section X, 3rd ed.). Pitman, NJ: Anthony J. Janetti.

Levine, D. Z. (1997). *Caring for the renal patient* (3rd ed.). Philadelphia: W. B. Saunders.

Gutch, C. F., Stoner, M. H., & Corea, A. L. (1999). *Review of hemodialysis for nurses and dialysis personnel* (6th ed.). St. Louis: Mosby.

Rabani, A., & Jafarian, A. (2005). Function and complications of arteriovenous fistula in chronic hemodialysis patients (a report from two referral centers). *Journal of Medical Council of Islamic Republic of Iran, 22*(4), 369.

Hope 1201

Definition: Optimism that is personally satisfying and life-supporting

OUTCOME TARGET RATING: Maintain at_____ Increase to_____

		Never demonstrated	Rarely demonstrated	Sometimes demonstrated	Often demonstrated	Consistently demonstrated	
OUTCOME OVERALL RATING		1	2	3	4	5	
Indicators:							
120101	Expresses expectation of a positive future	1	2	3	4	5	NA
120102	Expresses faith	1	2	3	4	5	NA
120103	Expresses will to live	1	2	3	4	5	NA
120104	Expresses reasons to live	1	2	3	4	5	NA
120105	Expresses meaning in life	1	2	3	4	5	NA
120106	Expresses optimism	1	2	3	4	5	NA
120107	Expresses belief in self	1	2	3	4	5	NA
120108	Expresses belief in others	1	2	3	4	5	NA
120109	Expresses inner peace	1	2	3	4	5	NA
120110	Expresses sense of self-control	1	2	3	4	5	NA
120111	Exhibits a zest for life	1	2	3	4	5	NA
120112	Sets goals	1	2	3	4	5	NA

Domain-*Psychosocial Health (III)* **Class**-*Psychological Well-Being (M)* *1st edition 1997; revised 2004*

OUTCOME CONTENT REFERENCES:

+Beckman, E. E., Leber, W. R., Watkins, J. T., Boyer, J. L., & Cook, J. B. (1986). Development of an instrument to measure Beck's cognitive triad: The Cognitive Triad Inventory. *Journal of Consulting and Clinical Psychology, 54*(4), 566–567.

Farran, C. J. (2001). Hopelessness. In M. Maas, K. Buckwalter, M. Hardy, T. Tripp-Reimer, M. Titler, & J. Specht (Eds.), *Nursing care of older adults: Diagnoses, outcomes & interventions* (pp. 601–612). St. Louis: Mosby.

Hall, B. (1990). The struggle of the diagnosed terminally ill person to maintain hope. *Nursing Science Quarterly, 3*(4), 177–184.

Herth, K. (1993). Hope in the family caregiver of terminally ill people. *Journal of Advanced Nursing, 18*(4), 538–548.

Hunt-Raleigh, E. (1992). Sources of hope in chronic illness. *Oncology Nursing Forum, 3*(19), 443–448.

Owen, D. (1989). Nurses' perspectives on the meaning of hope in patients with cancer: A qualitative study. *Oncology Nursing Forum, 1*(16), 75–79.

Sowers, W. (2005). Transforming systems of care: The American Association of Community Psychiatrists guidelines for recovery oriented services. *Community Mental Health Journal, 41*(6), 757–774.

Stephenson, C. (1991). The concept of hope revisited for nursing. *Journal of Advanced Nursing, 16*(12), 1456–1461.

Hydration 0602

Definition: Adequate water in the intracellular and extracellular compartments of the body

OUTCOME TARGET RATING: Maintain at_____   Increase to_____

		Severely compromised	Substantially compromised	Moderately compromised	Mildly compromised	Not compromised	
OUTCOME OVERALL RATING		1	2	3	4	5	
Indicators:							
060201	Skin turgor	1	2	3	4	5	NA
060202	Moist mucous membranes	1	2	3	4	5	NA
060215	Fluid intake	1	2	3	4	5	NA
060211	Urine output	1	2	3	4	5	NA
060216	Serum sodium	1	2	3	4	5	NA
060217	Tissue perfusion	1	2	3	4	5	NA
060218	Cognitive function	1	2	3	4	5	NA
		Severe	Substantial	Moderate	Mild	None	
060205	Thirst	1	2	3	4	5	NA
060219	Dark urine	1	2	3	4	5	NA
060208	Soft, sunken eyeballs	1	2	3	4	5	NA
060220	Sunken fontanel	1	2	3	4	5	NA
060212	Decreased blood pressure	1	2	3	4	5	NA
060221	Rapid, thready pulse	1	2	3	4	5	NA
060213	Increased hematocrit	1	2	3	4	5	NA
060222	Increased blood urea nitrogen	1	2	3	4	5	NA
060223	Weight loss	1	2	3	4	5	NA
060224	Muscle cramps	1	2	3	4	5	NA
060225	Muscle twitching	1	2	3	4	5	NA
060226	Diarrhea	1	2	3	4	5	NA
060227	Body temperature elevation	1	2	3	4	5	NA

Domain-*Physiologic Health (II)*   **Class**-*Fluid & Electrolytes (G)*   *1st edition 1997; revised 2004, 2013*

OUTCOME CONTENT REFERENCES:

Arieff, A. (1986). Hyponatremia, convulsions, respiratory arrest, and permanent brain damage after elective surgery in healthy women. *The New England Journal of Medicine, 314*(24), 1529–1534.

Carcillo, J. A., Davis, A. L., & Zaritsky, A. (1991). Role of early fluid resuscitation in pediatric septic shock. *Journal of the American Medical Association, 266*(9), 1242–1245.

Gilski, D. (1993). Controversies in patient management after cardiac surgery. *Journal of Cardiovascular Nursing, 7*(4), 1–13.

Hill, P., & Aldag, J. (1991). Potential indicators of insufficient milk supply syndrome. *Research in Nursing & Health, 14*(1), 11–19.

Innerarity, S. A. (1997). *Fluids and electrolytes* (3rd ed.). Springhouse, PA: Springhouse.

The Joanna Briggs Institute for Evidence Based Nursing and Midwifery. (2000). Identification and nursing management of dysphagia in adults with neurological impairment. *Best Practice, 4*(2), Blackwell Science-Asia, Australia.

Mentes, J., Culp, K., Wakefield, B., Gaspar, P., Rapp, C., Mobily, P., & Tripp-Reimer, T. (1998). Dehydration as a precipitating factor in the development of acute confusion in the frail elderly. In B. Vellas, J. Albarde, & P. Garry (Eds.), *Facts, research, and intervention in geriatrics: Hydration and aging* (pp. 83–100). Paris: Serdi.

Reese, J. L. (2001). Fluid volume deficit—dehydration: Isotonic, hypotonic, and hypertonic. In M. Maas, K. Buckwalter, M. Hardy, T. Tripp-Reimer, M. Titler, & J. Specht (Eds.), *Nursing care of older adults: Diagnoses, outcomes & interventions* (pp. 183–200). St. Louis: Mosby.

Wakefield, B., Mentes, J., Digglemann, L., & Culp, K. (2002). Monitoring hydration status in elderly veterans. *Western Journal of Nursing Research, 24*(2), 132–142.

Hyperactivity Level 0915

Definition: Severity of patterns of inattention or impulsivity in a child from 1 year through 17 years of age

OUTCOME TARGET RATING: Maintain at_____ Increase to_____

		Severe	Substantial	Moderate	Mild	None	
OUTCOME OVERALL RATING		1	2	3	4	5	
Indicators:							
091501	Inattention	1	2	3	4	5	NA
091524	Difficulty listening	1	2	3	4	5	NA
091503	Difficulty organizing tasks	1	2	3	4	5	NA
091504	Inability to stay on task	1	2	3	4	5	NA
091525	Difficulty completing tasks	1	2	3	4	5	NA
091506	Difficulty with tasks that require sustained cognitive effort	1	2	3	4	5	NA
091507	Careless mistakes	1	2	3	4	5	NA
091508	Frequency of losing things	1	2	3	4	5	NA
091509	Excessive distractibility	1	2	3	4	5	NA
091510	Excessive forgetfulness	1	2	3	4	5	NA
091511	Impulsivity	1	2	3	4	5	NA
091512	Excessive fidgeting	1	2	3	4	5	NA
091513	Inability to remain seated	1	2	3	4	5	NA
091526	Excessive running	1	2	3	4	5	NA
091527	Excessive climbing	1	2	3	4	5	NA
091515	Excessive motor behavior	1	2	3	4	5	NA
091516	Difficulty playing quietly	1	2	3	4	5	NA
091517	Excessive talking	1	2	3	4	5	NA
091518	Blurts out answers before the question is completed	1	2	3	4	5	NA
091519	Difficulty waiting turn	1	2	3	4	5	NA
091520	Excessive interrupting of others	1	2	3	4	5	NA
091521	Intrusive, abrasive, loud, interpersonal interactions	1	2	3	4	5	NA
091522	Inappropriate aggressive behavior	1	2	3	4	5	NA
091523	Difficulty keeping hands to self	1	2	3	4	5	NA

Domain-*Physiologic Health (II)* **Class**-*Neurocognitive (J)* *3rd edition 2004; revised 2008*

OUTCOME CONTENT REFERENCES:

American Psychiatric Association. (2000). *Diagnostic and statistical manual of mental disorders* (4th ed. text revision). Washington, DC: Author.

Caldwell, C. L., Wasson, D., Anderson, M. A., Brighton, V., & Dixon, L. (2005). Development of the nursing outcome (NOC) label: Hyperactivity level. *Journal of Child and Adolescent Psychiatric Nursing, 18*(3), 95–102.

Caldwell, C. L., Wasson, D., Brighton, V., Dixon, L., & Anderson, M. A. (2003). Personal autonomy: Development of a NOC label. *International Journal of Nursing Terminologies & Classifications, 14*(4), 12–13.

Hechtman, L. (2000). Assessment and diagnosis of attention deficit/hyperactive disorder. *Child and Adolescent Psychiatric Clinics of North America, 9*(3), 481–498.

Novak, L. L. (1999). Attention deficit hyperactivity disorder. In M. R. Dambro (Ed.), *Griffith's 5-minute clinical consult*. Philadelphia: Lippincott Williams & Wilkins.

Sharma, V., Newcorn, J. H., Matier-Sharma, K., & Halperin, J. M. (1997). Attention-deficit and disruptive behavior disorders. In A. Tasman (Ed.), *Psychiatry*. Philadelphia: W. B. Saunders.

Hypercalcemia Severity

0607

Definition: Severity of signs and symptoms of increased serum calcium

OUTCOME TARGET RATING: Maintain at_____   Increase to_____

		Severe	Substantial	Moderate	Mild	None	
OUTCOME OVERALL RATING		1	2	3	4	5	
Indicators:							
060701	Increase in serum calcium	1	2	3	4	5	NA
060702	Electrocardiogram changes	1	2	3	4	5	NA
060703	Decreased heart rate	1	2	3	4	5	NA
060704	Increased blood pressure	1	2	3	4	5	NA
060705	Muscle weakness	1	2	3	4	5	NA
060706	Muscle pain	1	2	3	4	5	NA
060707	Decreased coordination	1	2	3	4	5	NA
060708	Constipation	1	2	3	4	5	NA
060709	Anorexia	1	2	3	4	5	NA
060710	Nausea	1	2	3	4	5	NA
060711	Vomiting	1	2	3	4	5	NA
060712	Abdominal pain	1	2	3	4	5	NA
060713	Bone pain	1	2	3	4	5	NA
060714	Increased urine output	1	2	3	4	5	NA
060715	Thirst	1	2	3	4	5	NA
060716	Dehydration	1	2	3	4	5	NA
060717	Hypoactive deep tendon reflexes	1	2	3	4	5	NA
060718	Pathological fractures	1	2	3	4	5	NA
060719	Urinary tract stones	1	2	3	4	5	NA
060720	Impaired memory	1	2	3	4	5	NA
060721	Confusion	1	2	3	4	5	NA
060722	Headaches	1	2	3	4	5	NA
060723	Depression	1	2	3	4	5	NA
060724	Lethargy	1	2	3	4	5	NA
060725	Acute psychosis	1	2	3	4	5	NA
060726	Coma	1	2	3	4	5	NA

Domain-*Physiologic Health (II)*   **Class**-*Fluid & Electrolyte (G)*   *5th edition 2013*

OUTCOME CONTENT REFERENCES:

Koltin, D., Rachmiel, M., Wong, B., Cole, D., Harvey, E., & Sochett, E. (2011). Mild infantile hypercalcemia: Diagnostic tests and outcomes. *The Journal of Pediatrics, 159*(2), 215–221.

LeMone, P., Burke, K., & Bauldoff, G. (2011). *Medical-surgical nursing: Critical thinking in patient care* (5th ed., pp. 543–544). Upper Saddle River, NJ: Pearson Education.

Mosby Elsevier. (2009). *Mosby's dictionary of medicine, nursing, and health professions* (8th ed., p. 906). St. Louis: Author.

Smeltzer, S., Bare, B., Hinkle, J., & Cheever, K. (2008). *Brunner & Suddarth's textbook of medical-surgical nursing* (11th ed., pp. 327–328). Philadelphia: Lippincott Williams & Wilkins.

Vroman, R. (2011). Electrolyte imbalances—Part 4: Calcium balance disorders. *EMS World, 40*(5), 60–61.

H

Hyperchloremia Severity

0608

Definition: Severity of signs and symptoms of increased serum chloride

OUTCOME TARGET RATING: Maintain at_____   Increase to_____

		Severe	Substantial	Moderate	Mild	None	
OUTCOME OVERALL RATING		1	2	3	4	5	
Indicators:							
060801	Increase in serum chloride	1	2	3	4	5	NA
060802	Increase in serum sodium	1	2	3	4	5	NA
060803	Decrease in serum pH	1	2	3	4	5	NA
060804	Decrease in serum bicarbonate	1	2	3	4	5	NA
060805	Increase in urine chloride	1	2	3	4	5	NA
060806	Increased respiratory rate	1	2	3	4	5	NA
060807	Increased depth of respirations	1	2	3	4	5	NA
060808	Hypertension	1	2	3	4	5	NA
060809	Dyspnea	1	2	3	4	5	NA
060810	Lethargy	1	2	3	4	5	NA
060811	Weakness	1	2	3	4	5	NA
060812	Impaired cognition	1	2	3	4	5	NA
060813	Increased heart rate	1	2	3	4	5	NA
060814	Arrhythmias	1	2	3	4	5	NA
060815	Pitting edema	1	2	3	4	5	NA
060816	Coma	1	2	3	4	5	NA

Domain-Physiologic Health (II)   **Class**-Fluid & Electrolyte (G)   5th edition 2013

OUTCOME CONTENT REFERENCES:
LePane, C., Peleman, R., & Kinzie, J. (2012). Chronic diarrhea with hyperchloremic acidosis and hypokalemia. *Gastroenterology, 142*(1), e22-e23.
Smeltzer, S., Bare, B., Hinkle, J., & Cheever, K. (2008). *Brunner & Suddarth's textbook of medical-surgical nursing* (11th ed., p. 334). Philadelphia: Lippincott Williams & Wilkins.

Hyperglycemia Severity

2111

Definition: Severity of signs and symptoms of elevated blood glucose levels

OUTCOME TARGET RATING: Maintain at_____   Increase to_____

		Severe	Substantial	Moderate	Mild	None	
OUTCOME OVERALL RATING		1	2	3	4	5	
Indicators:							
211101	Increased urine output	1	2	3	4	5	NA
211102	Increased thirst	1	2	3	4	5	NA
211103	Excessive hunger	1	2	3	4	5	NA
211104	Malaise	1	2	3	4	5	NA
211105	Fatigue	1	2	3	4	5	NA
211106	Headaches	1	2	3	4	5	NA
211107	Blurred vision	1	2	3	4	5	NA
211108	Unexplained weight loss	1	2	3	4	5	NA
211109	Loss of appetite	1	2	3	4	5	NA
211110	Nausea	1	2	3	4	5	NA
211111	Dry mouth	1	2	3	4	5	NA
211112	Fruity breath	1	2	3	4	5	NA
211113	Yeast infections	1	2	3	4	5	NA

Hyperglycemia Severity—cont'd

	Severe	Substantial	Moderate	Mild	None	
211114 Electrolyte disturbances	1	2	3	4	5	NA
211115 Impaired concentration	1	2	3	4	5	NA
211116 Mental status changes	1	2	3	4	5	NA
211117 Elevated blood glucose	1	2	3	4	5	NA
211118 Elevated A1C (glycated hemoglobin)	1	2	3	4	5	NA

Domain-Perceived Health (V)   *Class*-Symptom Status (V)   5th edition 2013

OUTCOME CONTENT REFERENCES:
Hartwig, M. S. (2010). A prevention framework for managing type 2 diabetes. *Arkansas Nursing News, 5*(2), 11–19.
Kaufman, F. R. (2009). Hyperglycemia management in students with diabetes. *NASN School Nursing, 24*(3), 108–110.
LeMone, P., Burke, K., & Bauldoff, G. (2011). *Medical-surgical nursing: Critical thinking in patient care* (5th ed., pp. 539–541). Upper Saddle River, NJ: Pearson Education.
Weiss, S., Alexander, J., & Agus, M. (2010). Extreme stress hyperglycemia during acute illness in a pediatric emergency department. *Pediatric Emergency Care, 26*(9), 626–632.

Hyperkalemia Severity   0609

Definition: Severity of signs and symptoms of increased serum potassium

OUTCOME TARGET RATING: Maintain at_____   Increase to_____

	Severe	Substantial	Moderate	Mild	None	
OUTCOME OVERALL RATING	1	2	3	4	5	
Indicators:						
060901 Increase in serum potassium	1	2	3	4	5	NA
060902 Electrocardiogram changes	1	2	3	4	5	NA
060903 Increased heart rate	1	2	3	4	5	NA
060904 Decreased blood pressure	1	2	3	4	5	NA
060905 Arrhythmias	1	2	3	4	5	NA
060906 Anxiety	1	2	3	4	5	NA
060907 Muscle weakness	1	2	3	4	5	NA
060908 Flaccid paralysis	1	2	3	4	5	NA
060909 Paresthesias	1	2	3	4	5	NA
060910 Nausea	1	2	3	4	5	NA
060911 Intestinal colic	1	2	3	4	5	NA
060912 Abdominal cramps	1	2	3	4	5	NA
060913 Diarrhea	1	2	3	4	5	NA
060914 Neuromuscular irritability	1	2	3	4	5	NA
060915 Restlessness	1	2	3	4	5	NA
060916 Headache	1	2	3	4	5	NA
060917 Seizures	1	2	3	4	5	NA
060918 Coma	1	2	3	4	5	NA

Domain-Physiologic Health (II)   *Class*-Fluid & Electrolyte (G)   5th edition 2013

OUTCOME CONTENT REFERENCES:
Crawford, A., & Harris, H. (2011). Balancing act: Na^+ sodium K^+ potassium. *Nursing, 41*(7), 44–50.
Lehnhardt, A., & Kemper, M. (2011). Pathogenesis, diagnosis, and management of hyperkalemia. *Pediatric Nephrology, 26*(3), 377–384.
Mosby Elsevier. (2009). *Mosby's dictionary of medicine, nursing, and health professions* (8th ed., p. 908). St. Louis: Author.
Palmer, B. (2010). A physiologic-based approach to the evaluation of a patient with hyperkalemia. *American Journal of Kidney Diseases, 56*(2), 387–393.
Smeltzer, S., Bare, B., Hinkle, J., & Cheever, K. (2008). *Brunner & Suddarth's textbook of medical-surgical nursing* (11th ed., pp. 323–324). Philadelphia: Lippincott Williams & Wilkins.
Vraets, A., Lin, Y., & Callum, J. (2011). Transfusion-associated hyperkalemia. *Transfusion Medicine Reviews, 25*(3), 184–196.

H

Hypermagnesemia Severity 0610

Definition: Severity of signs and symptoms of increased serum magnesium

OUTCOME TARGET RATING: Maintain at_____ Increase to_____

	Severe	Substantial	Moderate	Mild	None	
OUTCOME OVERALL RATING	1	2	3	4	5	
Indicators:						
061001 Increase in serum magnesium	1	2	3	4	5	NA
061002 Decreased blood pressure	1	2	3	4	5	NA
061003 Electrocardiogram changes	1	2	3	4	5	NA
061004 Decreased heart rate	1	2	3	4	5	NA
061005 Decreased respiratory rate	1	2	3	4	5	NA
061006 Hypoactive deep tendon reflexes	1	2	3	4	5	NA
061007 Soft tissue calcifications	1	2	3	4	5	NA
061008 Clumping of platelets	1	2	3	4	5	NA
061009 Delayed thrombin formation	1	2	3	4	5	NA
061010 Nausea	1	2	3	4	5	NA
061011 Vomiting	1	2	3	4	5	NA
061012 Weakness	1	2	3	4	5	NA
061013 Flushing	1	2	3	4	5	NA
061014 Diaphoresis	1	2	3	4	5	NA
061015 Drowsiness	1	2	3	4	5	NA
061016 Cardiac arrest	1	2	3	4	5	NA
061017 Coma	1	2	3	4	5	NA

Domain-*Physiologic Health (II)*   **Class**-*Fluid & Electrolyte (G)*   *5th edition 2013*

OUTCOME CONTENT REFERENCES:
Crawford, A., & Harris, H. (2011). Balancing act: Hypomagnesemia & hypermagnesemia. *Nursing, 41*(10), 52–55.
LeMone, P., Burke, K., & Bauldoff, G. (2011). *Medical-surgical nursing: Critical thinking in patient care* (5th ed., p. 219). Upper Saddle River, NJ: Pearson Education.
Mosby Elsevier. (2009). *Mosby's dictionary of medicine, nursing, and health professions* (8th ed., p. 909). St. Louis: Author.
Smeltzer, S., Bare, B., Hinkle, J., & Cheever, K. (2008). *Brunner & Suddarth's textbook of medical-surgical nursing* (11th ed., pp. 330–331). Philadelphia: Lippincott Williams & Wilkins.
Vroman, R. (2011). Electrolyte imbalances—Part 3: Magnesium balance disorders. *EMS World, 40*(4), 52–54.

Hypernatremia Severity 0611

Definition: Severity of signs and symptoms of increased serum sodium

OUTCOME TARGET RATING: Maintain at_____ Increase to_____

	Severe	Substantial	Moderate	Mild	None	
OUTCOME OVERALL RATING	1	2	3	4	5	
Indicators:						
061101 Increase in serum sodium	1	2	3	4	5	NA
061102 Increased urine output	1	2	3	4	5	NA
061103 Decrease in urine sodium	1	2	3	4	5	NA
061104 Increase in urine specific gravity	1	2	3	4	5	NA
061105 Increased blood pressure	1	2	3	4	5	NA
061106 Increased heart rate	1	2	3	4	5	NA
061107 Dry skin and mucous membranes	1	2	3	4	5	NA
061108 Thirst	1	2	3	4	5	NA
061109 Anorexia	1	2	3	4	5	NA
061110 Nausea	1	2	3	4	5	NA

Hypernatremia Severity—cont'd

	Severe	Substantial	Moderate	Mild	None	
061111 Vomiting	1	2	3	4	5	NA
061112 Headache	1	2	3	4	5	NA
061113 Restlessness	1	2	3	4	5	NA
061114 Dizziness	1	2	3	4	5	NA
061115 Confusion	1	2	3	4	5	NA
061116 Muscle twitching	1	2	3	4	5	NA
061117 Seizures	1	2	3	4	5	NA
061118 Pulmonary edema	1	2	3	4	5	NA
061119 Weight gain	1	2	3	4	5	NA
061120 Papilledema	1	2	3	4	5	NA
061121 Coma	1	2	3	4	5	NA

Domain-Physiologic Health (II)   **Class**-Fluid & Electrolyte (G)   5th edition 2013

H

OUTCOME CONTENT REFERENCES:

Crawford, A., & Harris, H. (2011). Balancing act: Na$^+$ sodium K$^+$ potassium. *Nursing, 41*(7), 44–50.

Mosby Elsevier. (2009). *Mosby's dictionary of medicine, nursing, and health professions* (8th ed., p. 910). St. Louis: Author.

Smeltzer, S., Bare, B., Hinkle, J., & Cheever, K. (2008). *Brunner & Suddarth's textbook of medical-surgical nursing* (11th ed., pp. 319–320). Philadelphia: Lippincott Williams & Wilkins.

Yee, A., & Rabinstein, A. (2010). Neurologic presentations of acid-base imbalance, electrolyte abnormalities, and endocrine emergencies. *Neurologic Clinics, 28*(1), 1–16.

Hyperphosphatemia Severity   0612

Definition: Severity of signs and symptoms of increased serum phosphorus

OUTCOME TARGET RATING: Maintain at_____   Increase to_____

	Severe	Substantial	Moderate	Mild	None	
OUTCOME OVERALL RATING	1	2	3	4	5	
Indicators:						
061201 Increase in serum phosphorus	1	2	3	4	5	NA
061202 Decreased blood pressure	1	2	3	4	5	NA
061203 Arrhythmias	1	2	3	4	5	NA
061204 Increased heart rate	1	2	3	4	5	NA
061205 Numbness	1	2	3	4	5	NA
061206 Tingling of fingers and hands	1	2	3	4	5	NA
061207 Tingling around mouth	1	2	3	4	5	NA
061208 Muscle cramps	1	2	3	4	5	NA
061209 Muscle spasms	1	2	3	4	5	NA
061210 Muscle weakness	1	2	3	4	5	NA
061211 Hyperactive deep tendon reflexes	1	2	3	4	5	NA
061212 Anorexia	1	2	3	4	5	NA
061213 Nausea	1	2	3	4	5	NA
061214 Vomiting	1	2	3	4	5	NA
061215 Tetany	1	2	3	4	5	NA
061216 Seizures	1	2	3	4	5	NA
061217 Vascular calcifications	1	2	3	4	5	NA
061218 Soft tissue calcifications	1	2	3	4	5	NA

Domain-Physiologic Health (II)   **Class**-Fluid & Electrolyte (G)   5th edition 2013

OUTCOME CONTENT REFERENCES:

Hruska, K., Mathew, S., Lund, R., Qiu, P., & Pratt, R. (2008). Hyperphosphatemia of chronic kidney disease. *Kidney International, 74*(2), 148–157.

LeMone, P., Burke, K., & Bauldoff, G. (2011). *Medical-surgical nursing: Critical thinking in patient care* (5th ed., p. 221). Upper Saddle River, NJ: Pearson Education.

Smeltzer, S., Bare, B., Hinkle, J., & Cheever, K. (2008). *Brunner & Suddarth's textbook of medical-surgical nursing* (11th ed., p. 332). Philadelphia: Lippincott Williams & Wilkins.

Hypertension Severity   2112

Definition: Severity of signs and symptoms of chronic elevated blood pressure

OUTCOME TARGET RATING: Maintain at_____   Increase to_____

		Severe	Substantial	Moderate	Mild	None	
OUTCOME OVERALL RATING		1	2	3	4	5	
Indicators:							
211201	Fatigue	1	2	3	4	5	NA
211202	Nosebleeds	1	2	3	4	5	NA
211203	Irregular heartbeat	1	2	3	4	5	NA
211204	Blurred vision	1	2	3	4	5	NA
211205	Temporary paralysis	1	2	3	4	5	NA
211206	Alterations in speech	1	2	3	4	5	NA
211207	Headaches	1	2	3	4	5	NA
211208	Dizziness	1	2	3	4	5	NA
211209	Breathlessness	1	2	3	4	5	NA
211210	Excessive sweating	1	2	3	4	5	NA
211211	Nocturia	1	2	3	4	5	NA
211212	Tinnitus	1	2	3	4	5	NA
211213	Confusion	1	2	3	4	5	NA
211214	Convulsions	1	2	3	4	5	NA
211215	Nausea	1	2	3	4	5	NA
211216	Elevation of systolic blood pressure	1	2	3	4	5	NA
211217	Elevation of diastolic blood pressure	1	2	3	4	5	NA

Domain-Perceived Health (V)   *Class*-Symptom Status (V)   5th edition 2013

OUTCOME CONTENT REFERENCES:

Chummun, H. (2009). Hypertension—A contemporary approach to nursing care. *British Journal of Nursing, 18*(13), 784–789.

DeSimone, M. E., & Crowe, A. (2009). Nonpharmacological approaches in the management of hypertension. *Journal of the American Academy of Nurse Practitioners, 21*, 189–196.

Good, L. B. (2010). Hypertension highlights: Blood pressure targets, global risk factors, and diabetes: the latest data are not encouraging. *Medscape Cardiology.* Retrieved from www.medscape.com/viewarticle/715584

Guidelines and Protocols Advisory Committee. (2008). Hypertension—Detection diagnosis and management. Retrieved from http://www.bcguidelines.ca/gpac/guideline_hypertension.html

National Heart, Lung, and Blood Institute (NHLBI). (2003). *JNC 7 express: The seventh report of the Joint National Committee on Prevention, Detection, Evaluation, and Treatment of High Blood Pressure.* Bethesda, MD: Author.

Hypocalcemia Severity 0613

Definition: Severity of signs and symptoms of decreased serum calcium

OUTCOME TARGET RATING: Maintain at_____ Increase to_____

OUTCOME OVERALL RATING	Severe 1	Substantial 2	Moderate 3	Mild 4	None 5	
Indicators:						
061301 Decrease in serum calcium	1	2	3	4	5	NA
061302 Decreased clotting time	1	2	3	4	5	NA
061303 Decreased heart rate	1	2	3	4	5	NA
061304 Electrocardiogram changes	1	2	3	4	5	NA
061305 Hypotension	1	2	3	4	5	NA
061306 Anxiety	1	2	3	4	5	NA
061307 Pain	1	2	3	4	5	NA
061308 Numbness of extremities	1	2	3	4	5	NA
061309 Tingling of fingers and toes	1	2	3	4	5	NA
061310 Tingling around mouth	1	2	3	4	5	NA
061311 Hyperactive deep tendon reflexes	1	2	3	4	5	NA
061312 Pain	1	2	3	4	5	NA
061313 Bone pain	1	2	3	4	5	NA
061314 Bone fracture	1	2	3	4	5	NA
061315 Positive Trousseau's sign	1	2	3	4	5	NA
061316 Positive Chvostek's sign	1	2	3	4	5	NA
061317 Muscle cramps	1	2	3	4	5	NA
061318 Carpopedal spasms	1	2	3	4	5	NA
061319 Laryngeal spasms	1	2	3	4	5	NA
061320 Bronchospasm	1	2	3	4	5	NA
061321 Neuromuscular irritability	1	2	3	4	5	NA
061322 Depression	1	2	3	4	5	NA
061323 Confusion	1	2	3	4	5	NA
061324 Impaired memory	1	2	3	4	5	NA
061325 Delirium	1	2	3	4	5	NA
061326 Hallucinations	1	2	3	4	5	NA
061327 Tetany	1	2	3	4	5	NA
061328 Seizures	1	2	3	4	5	NA
061329 Increased urine output	1	2	3	4	5	NA

Domain-*Physiologic Health (II)* **Class**-*Fluid & Electrolyte (G)* *5th edition 2013*

OUTCOME CONTENT REFERENCES:
LeMone, P., Burke, K., & Bauldoff, G. (2011). *Medical-surgical nursing: Critical thinking in patient care* (5th ed., pp. 213–216). Upper Saddle River, NJ: Pearson Education.
Mosby Elsevier. (2009). *Mosby's dictionary of medicine, nursing, and health professions* (8th ed., p. 917). St. Louis: Author.
Smeltzer, S., Bare, B., Hinkle, J., & Cheever, K. (2008). *Brunner & Suddarth's textbook of medical-surgical nursing* (11th ed., pp. 325–327). Philadelphia: Lippincott Williams & Wilkins.
Vroman, R. (2011). Electrolyte imbalances—Part 4: Calcium balance disorders. *EMS World, 40*(5), 60–61.
Zhou, P., & Markowitz, M. (2009). Hypocalcemia in infants and children. *Pediatrics in Review, 30*(5), 190–192.

H

Hypochloremia Severity

0614

Definition: Severity of signs and symptoms of decreased serum chloride

OUTCOME TARGET RATING: Maintain at_____   Increase to_____

		Severe	Substantial	Moderate	Mild	None	
OUTCOME OVERALL RATING		1	2	3	4	5	
Indicators:							
061401	Decrease in serum chloride	1	2	3	4	5	NA
061402	Decrease in serum sodium	1	2	3	4	5	NA
061403	Increase in serum pH	1	2	3	4	5	NA
061404	Increase in serum bicarbonate	1	2	3	4	5	NA
061405	Increase in serum carbon dioxide content	1	2	3	4	5	NA
061406	Decrease in urine chloride	1	2	3	4	5	NA
061407	Agitation	1	2	3	4	5	NA
061408	Neuromuscular irritability	1	2	3	4	5	NA
061409	Tremors	1	2	3	4	5	NA
061410	Muscle cramps	1	2	3	4	5	NA
061411	Hyperactive deep tendon reflexes	1	2	3	4	5	NA
061412	Tetany	1	2	3	4	5	NA
061413	Decreased respiratory rate	1	2	3	4	5	NA
061414	Shallow respirations	1	2	3	4	5	NA
061415	Arrhythmias	1	2	3	4	5	NA
061416	Seizures	1	2	3	4	5	NA
061417	Coma	1	2	3	4	5	NA

Domain-*Physiologic Health (II)*   **Class**-*Fluid & Electrolyte (G)*   *5th edition 2013*

OUTCOME CONTENT REFERENCES:

O'Dell, E., Tibby, S., Durward, A., & Murdoch, I. (2007). Hyperchloremia is the dominant cause of metabolic acidosis in the postresuscitation phase of pediatric meningococcal sepsis. *Pediatric Critical Care, 35*(10), 2390–2394.

Smeltzer, S., Bare, B., Hinkle, J., & Cheever, K. (2008). *Brunner & Suddarth's textbook of medical-surgical nursing* (11th ed., pp. 333–334). Philadelphia: Lippincott Williams & Wilkins.

Yee, A., & Rabinstein, A. (2010). Neurologic presentations of acid-base imbalance, electrolyte abnormalities, and endocrine emergencies. *Neurologic Clinics, 28*(1), 1–16.

Hypoglycemia Severity

2113

Definition: Severity of signs and symptoms of decreased blood glucose levels

OUTCOME TARGET RATING: Maintain at_____   Increase to_____

		Severe	Substantial	Moderate	Mild	None	
OUTCOME OVERALL RATING		1	2	3	4	5	
Indicators:							
211301	Shakiness	1	2	3	4	5	NA
211302	Sweating	1	2	3	4	5	NA
211303	Nervousness	1	2	3	4	5	NA
211304	Heart palpitations	1	2	3	4	5	NA
211305	Lightheadedness	1	2	3	4	5	NA
211306	Hunger	1	2	3	4	5	NA
211307	Weakness	1	2	3	4	5	NA
211308	Dizziness	1	2	3	4	5	NA
211309	Sleepiness	1	2	3	4	5	NA
211310	Impaired vision	1	2	3	4	5	NA

Hypoglycemia Severity—cont'd

		Severe	Substantial	Moderate	Mild	None	
211311	Nightmares	1	2	3	4	5	NA
211312	Irritability	1	2	3	4	5	NA
211313	Fatigue	1	2	3	4	5	NA
211314	Headaches	1	2	3	4	5	NA
211315	Paresthesia	1	2	3	4	5	NA
211316	Slurred speech	1	2	3	4	5	NA
211317	Impaired concentration	1	2	3	4	5	NA
211318	Abnormal behavior	1	2	3	4	5	NA
211319	Confusion	1	2	3	4	5	NA
211320	Seizure	1	2	3	4	5	NA
211321	Coma	1	2	3	4	5	NA
211322	Decreased blood glucose levels	1	2	3	4	5	NA

Domain-Perceived Health (V)   **Class**-Symptom Status (V)   5th edition 2013

H

OUTCOME CONTENT REFERENCES:

American Diabetes Association Workgroup on Hypoglycemia. (2005). Defining and reporting hypoglycemia in diabetes. *Diabetes Care, 28*(5), 1245–1249.
Clarke, W., Jones, T., Rewers, A., Dunger, D., Klingensmith, G. (2009). Assessment and management of hypoglycemia in children and adolescents with diabetes. *Pediatric Diabetes, 10*(Suppl. 12), 134–145.
Cryer, P. E. (2010). Hypoglycemia in type 1 diabetes mellitus. *Endocrinology and Metabolism Clinics of North America, 39*(3), 641–654.
Goldstein, P. C. (2009). Assessment and treatment of hypoglycemia in elders: Cautions and recommendations. *Medsurg Nursing, 18*(4), 215–241.
Hartwig, M. (2009). A prevention framework for managing type 2 diabetes. *Arkansas Nursing News, 5*(2), 11–19.
LeMone, P., Burke, K., & Bauldoff, G. (2011). *Medical-surgical nursing: Critical thinking in patient care* (5th ed., pp. 543–544). Upper Saddle River, NJ: Pearson Education.

Hypokalemia Severity   0615

Definition: Severity of signs and symptoms of decreased serum potassium

OUTCOME TARGET RATING: Maintain at_____   Increase to_____

		Severe	Substantial	Moderate	Mild	None	
OUTCOME OVERALL RATING		1	2	3	4	5	
Indicators:							
061501	Decrease in serum potassium	1	2	3	4	5	NA
061502	Orthostatic hypotension	1	2	3	4	5	NA
061503	Decreased blood pressure	1	2	3	4	5	NA
061504	Arrhythmias	1	2	3	4	5	NA
061505	Changes in electrocardiogram	1	2	3	4	5	NA
061506	Fatigue	1	2	3	4	5	NA
061507	Lethargy	1	2	3	4	5	NA
061508	Apathy	1	2	3	4	5	NA
061509	Mental depression	1	2	3	4	5	NA
061510	Confusion	1	2	3	4	5	NA
061511	Anorexia	1	2	3	4	5	NA
061512	Nausea	1	2	3	4	5	NA
061513	Vomiting	1	2	3	4	5	NA
061514	Decreased bowel motility	1	2	3	4	5	NA
061515	Constipation	1	2	3	4	5	NA
061516	Polyuria	1	2	3	4	5	NA
061517	Abdominal distention	1	2	3	4	5	NA
061518	Muscle weakness	1	2	3	4	5	NA

Continued

Hypokalemia Severity—cont'd

		Severe	Substantial	Moderate	Mild	None	
061519	Decreased muscle tone	1	2	3	4	5	NA
061520	Flaccid paralysis	1	2	3	4	5	NA
061521	Paresthesias	1	2	3	4	5	NA
061522	Leg cramps	1	2	3	4	5	NA
061523	Hypoactive deep tendon reflexes	1	2	3	4	5	NA
061524	Coma	1	2	3	4	5	NA

Domain-Physiologic Health (II)　*Class*-Fluid & Electrolyte (G)　5th edition 2013

OUTCOME CONTENT REFERENCES:

Burger, C. (2004). Hypokalemia: Averting crisis with early recognition and intervention. *American Journal of Nursing, 104*(11), 61–65.

Crawford, A., & Harris, H. (2011). Balancing act: Na$^+$ sodium K$^+$ potassium. *Nursing, 41*(7), 44–50.

LeMone, P., Burke, K., & Bauldoff, G. (2011). *Medical-surgical nursing: Critical thinking in patient care* (5th ed., pp. 205–206). Upper Saddle River, NJ: Pearson Education.

Lin, S., Yang, S., & Chau, T. (2010). A practical approach to genetic hypokalemia. *Electrolyte & Blood Pressure, 8*(1), 38–50.

Mosby Elsevier. (2009). *Mosby's dictionary of medicine, nursing, and health professions* (8th ed., p. 920). St. Louis: Author.

Smeltzer, S., Bare, B., Hinkle, J., & Cheever, K. (2008). *Brunner & Suddarth's textbook of medical-surgical nursing* (11th ed., pp. 321–333). Philadelphia: Lippincott Williams & Wilkins.

Hypomagnesemia Severity　　　　0616

Definition: Severity of signs and symptoms of decreased serum magnesium

OUTCOME TARGET RATING: Maintain at＿＿＿＿　　Increase to＿＿＿＿＿

		Severe	Substantial	Moderate	Mild	None	
OUTCOME OVERALL RATING		1	2	3	4	5	
Indicators:							
061601	Decrease in serum magnesium	1	2	3	4	5	NA
061602	Increased blood pressure	1	2	3	4	5	NA
061603	Electrocardiogram changes	1	2	3	4	5	NA
061604	Neuromuscular irritability	1	2	3	4	5	NA
061605	Positive Babinski	1	2	3	4	5	NA
061606	Positive Trousseau's sign	1	2	3	4	5	NA
061607	Positive Chvostek's sign	1	2	3	4	5	NA
061608	Hyperactive deep tendon reflexes	1	2	3	4	5	NA
061609	Leg cramps	1	2	3	4	5	NA
061610	Nausea	1	2	3	4	5	NA
061611	Vomiting	1	2	3	4	5	NA
061612	Mood changes	1	2	3	4	5	NA
061613	Vertigo	1	2	3	4	5	NA
061614	Depression	1	2	3	4	5	NA
061615	Agitation	1	2	3	4	5	NA
061616	Apprehension	1	2	3	4	5	NA
061617	Delirium	1	2	3	4	5	NA
061618	Confusion	1	2	3	4	5	NA
061619	Psychosis	1	2	3	4	5	NA
061620	Insomnia	1	2	3	4	5	NA
061621	Combativeness	1	2	3	4	5	NA

Domain-Physiologic Health (II)　*Class*-Fluid & Electrolyte (G)　5th edition 2013

OUTCOME CONTENT REFERENCES:
LeMone, P., Burke, K., & Bauldoff, G. (2011). *Medical-surgical nursing: Critical thinking in patient care* (5th ed., pp. 218–219). Upper Saddle River, NJ: Pearson Education.
Mosby Elsevier. (2009). *Mosby's dictionary of medicine, nursing, and health professions* (8th ed., p. 920). St. Louis: Author.
Smeltzer, S., Bare, B., Hinkle, J., & Cheever, K. (2008). *Brunner & Suddarth's textbook of medical-surgical nursing* (11th ed., pp. 329–330). Philadelphia: Lippincott Williams & Wilkins.

Hyponatremia Severity   0617

Definition: Severity of signs and symptoms of decreased serum sodium

OUTCOME TARGET RATING: Maintain at_____ Increase to_____

OUTCOME OVERALL RATING	Severe 1	Substantial 2	Moderate 3	Mild 4	None 5	
Indicators:						
061701 Decrease in serum sodium	1	2	3	4	5	NA
061702 Decrease in urine sodium	1	2	3	4	5	NA
061703 Decrease in urine specific gravity	1	2	3	4	5	NA
061704 Orthostatic hypertension	1	2	3	4	5	NA
061705 Decreased blood pressure	1	2	3	4	5	NA
061706 Increased heart rate	1	2	3	4	5	NA
061707 Dry skin and mucous membranes	1	2	3	4	5	NA
061708 Anorexia	1	2	3	4	5	NA
061709 Nausea	1	2	3	4	5	NA
061710 Vomiting	1	2	3	4	5	NA
061711 Headache	1	2	3	4	5	NA
061712 Apathy	1	2	3	4	5	NA
061713 Impaired concentration	1	2	3	4	5	NA
061714 Lethargy	1	2	3	4	5	NA
061715 Fatigue	1	2	3	4	5	NA
061716 Dizziness	1	2	3	4	5	NA
061717 Confusion	1	2	3	4	5	NA
061718 Muscle cramps	1	2	3	4	5	NA
061719 Muscle weakness	1	2	3	4	5	NA
061720 Muscle twitching	1	2	3	4	5	NA
061721 Seizures	1	2	3	4	5	NA
061722 Edema	1	2	3	4	5	NA
061723 Weight gain	1	2	3	4	5	NA

Domain-*Physiologic Health (II)*   **Class**-*Fluid & Electrolyte (G)*   *5th edition 2013*

OUTCOME CONTENT REFERENCES:
Crawford, A., & Harris, H. (2011). Balancing act: Na^+ sodium K^+ potassium. *Nursing, 41*(7), 44–50.
Mosby Elsevier. (2009). *Mosby's dictionary of medicine, nursing, and health professions* (8th ed., p. 921). St. Louis: Author.
Shapiro, D., Sonnenblick, M., Galperin, I., Melkonyan, L., & Munter, G. (2010). Severe hyponatraemia in elderly hospitalized patients: Prevalence, aetiology and outcome. *Internal Medicine Journal, 40*(8), 574–580.
Smeltzer, S., Bare, B., Hinkle, J., & Cheever, K. (2008). *Brunner & Suddarth's textbook of medical-surgical nursing* (11th ed., pp. 316, 318–319). Philadelphia: Lippincott Williams & Wilkins.
Verbalis, J., Goldsmith, S., Greenberg, A., Schrier, R., & Sterns, R. (2007). Hyponatremia treatment guidelines 2007: Expert panel recommendations. *American Journal of Medicine, 120*(11A), S1–S21.
Vroman, R. (2011). Electrolyte imbalances—Part 3: Sodium balance disorders. *EMS World, 40*(2), 37–43.

Hypophosphatemia Severity 0618

Definition: Severity of signs and symptoms of decreased serum phosphorus

OUTCOME TARGET RATING: Maintain at_____   Increase to_____

		Severe	Substantial	Moderate	Mild	None	
OUTCOME OVERALL RATING		1	2	3	4	5	
Indicators:							
061801	Decrease in serum phosphorus	1	2	3	4	5	NA
061802	Paresthesias	1	2	3	4	5	NA
061803	Muscle weakness	1	2	3	4	5	NA
061804	Impaired swallowing	1	2	3	4	5	NA
061805	Bone pain	1	2	3	4	5	NA
061806	Chest pain	1	2	3	4	5	NA
061807	Cardiomyopathy	1	2	3	4	5	NA
061808	Confusion	1	2	3	4	5	NA
061809	Irritability	1	2	3	4	5	NA
061810	Fatigue	1	2	3	4	5	NA
061811	Seizures	1	2	3	4	5	NA
061812	Respiratory failure	1	2	3	4	5	NA
061813	Tissue hypoxia	1	2	3	4	5	NA
061814	Susceptibility to infections	1	2	3	4	5	NA
061815	Double vision	1	2	3	4	5	NA
061816	Joint stiffness	1	2	3	4	5	NA
061817	Bleeding disorders	1	2	3	4	5	NA
061818	Impaired white blood cell function	1	2	3	4	5	NA

Domain-Physiologic Health (II)   *Class-Fluid & Electrolyte (G)*   5th edition 2013

OUTCOME CONTENT REFERENCES:
LeMone, P., Burke, K., & Bauldoff, G. (2011). *Medical-surgical nursing: Critical thinking in patient care* (5th ed., p. 220). Upper Saddle River, NJ: Pearson Education.
Smeltzer, S., Bare, B., Hinkle, J., & Cheever, K. (2008). *Brunner & Suddarth's textbook of medical-surgical nursing* (11th ed., p. 331). Philadelphia: Lippincott Williams & Wilkins.

Hypotension Severity 2114

Definition: Severity of signs and symptoms of episodic low blood pressure

OUTCOME TARGET RATING: Maintain at_____   Increase to_____

		Severe	Substantial	Moderate	Mild	None	
OUTCOME OVERALL RATING		1	2	3	4	5	
Indicators:							
211401	Pallor	1	2	3	4	5	NA
211402	Clammy skin	1	2	3	4	5	NA
211403	Chronic cold extremities	1	2	3	4	5	NA
211404	Rapid respirations	1	2	3	4	5	NA
211405	Shallow respirations	1	2	3	4	5	NA
211406	Thready pulse	1	2	3	4	5	NA
211407	Irregular heart rate	1	2	3	4	5	NA
211408	Syncope	1	2	3	4	5	NA
211409	Blurred vision	1	2	3	4	5	NA
211410	Seizure activity	1	2	3	4	5	NA
211411	Anxiety	1	2	3	4	5	NA

Hypotension Severity—cont'd

		Severe	Substantial	Moderate	Mild	None	
211412	Dizziness	1	2	3	4	5	NA
211413	Lightheadedness on standing abruptly	1	2	3	4	5	NA
211414	Orthostatic hypotension	1	2	3	4	5	NA
211415	Obstructive sleep apnea	1	2	3	4	5	NA
211416	Mouth breathing	1	2	3	4	5	NA
211417	Nocturnal asthma	1	2	3	4	5	NA
211418	Snoring	1	2	3	4	5	NA
211419	Fatigue	1	2	3	4	5	NA
211420	Delirium	1	2	3	4	5	NA
211421	Low systolic blood pressure	1	2	3	4	5	NA
211422	Low diastolic blood pressure	1	2	3	4	5	NA

Domain-Perceived Health (V)   **Class-**Symptom Status (V)   5th edition 2013

OUTCOME CONTENT REFERENCES:

Arbogast, S., Alshekhlee, A., Hussain, Z., McNeeley, K., & Chelimksy, T. (2009). Hypotension unawareness in profound orthostatic hypotension. *The American Journal of Medicine, 122*(6), 574–580.

Dabrowski, G. P., Steinberg, S. M., Ferrara, J. J., & Flint, L. M. (2000). A critical assessment of endpoints of shock resuscitation. *Surgical Clinics of North America, 80*(3), 825–844.

Guilleminault, C., Faul, J., & Stoohs, R. (2001). Sleep-disordered breathing and hypotension. *American Journal of Respiratory and Critical Care Medicine, 164*(7), 1242–1247.

Guilleminault, C., Khramsov, A., Stoohs, R. A., Kushida, C., Pelayo, R., Kreutzer, M. L., & Chowdhuri, S. (2004). Abnormal blood pressure in prepubertal children with sleep-disordered breathing. *Pediatric Research, 55*(1), 76–84.

Lipsky, A. M., Gausche-Hill, M., Henneman, P. L., Loffredo, A. J., Eckhardt, P. B., Cryer, H. G., deVirgilio, C., Klein, S. L., Bongard, F. S., & Lewis, R. J. (2006). Prehospital hypotension is a predictor of the need for an emergent, therapeutic operation in trauma patients with normal systolic blood pressure in the emergency department. *Journal of Trauma, Injury, Infection and Critical Care, 61*(5), 1228–1233.

Mathew, T. P., Menown, I. B., McCarty, D., Gracey, H., Hill, L., Adgey, A. A. (2003). Impact of pre-hospital care in patients with acute myocardial infarction compared with those first managed in-hospital. *European Heart Journal, 24*(2), 161–171.

Shapiro, N. I., Kociszewski, C., Harrison, T., Chang, Y., Wedel, S. K., Thomas, S. H. (2003). Isolated prehospital hypotension after traumatic injuries: A predictor of mortality? *Journal of Emergency Medicine, 25*(2), 175–179.

Stell, A., Sinnott, R., Jiang, J., Donald, R., Chambers, I., Citerio, G., Enblad, P., Gregson, B., Howells, T., Kiening, K., Nilsson, P., Ragauskas, A., Sahuquillo, J., & Piper, I. (2009). Federating distributed clinical data for the prediction of adverse hypotensive events. *Philosophical Transactions. Series A, Mathematical, Physical, and Engineering Sciences, 367*(1898), 2679–2690.

Weiss, A., Chagnac, A., Beloosesky, Y., Weinstein, T., Grinblat, J., & Grossman, E. (2004). Orthostatic hypotension in the elderly: Are the diagnostic criteria adequate? *Journal of Human Hypertension, 18*(5), 301–305.

H

Identity

1202

Definition: Distinguishes between self and non-self and characterizes one's essence

OUTCOME TARGET RATING: Maintain at_____   Increase to_____

OUTCOME OVERALL RATING	Never demonstrated 1	Rarely demonstrated 2	Sometimes demonstrated 3	Often demonstrated 4	Consistently demonstrated 5	
Indicators:						
120201 Verbalizes affirmations of personal identity	1	2	3	4	5	NA
120202 Exhibits congruent verbal and non-verbal behavior about self	1	2	3	4	5	NA
120203 Verbalizes clear sense of personal identity	1	2	3	4	5	NA
120204 Differentiates self from environment	1	2	3	4	5	NA
120205 Differentiates self from other human beings	1	2	3	4	5	NA
120206 Perceives environment accurately	1	2	3	4	5	NA
120207 Performs social roles	1	2	3	4	5	NA
120208 Verbalizes own value system	1	2	3	4	5	NA
120209 Challenges faulty beliefs about self	1	2	3	4	5	NA
120210 Challenges negative images of self	1	2	3	4	5	NA
120211 Recognizes interpersonal versus intrapersonal conflict	1	2	3	4	5	NA
120212 Establishes personal boundaries	1	2	3	4	5	NA
120213 Verbalizes trust in self	1	2	3	4	5	NA

Domain-Psychosocial Health (III)   *Class*-Psychological Well-Being (M)   *1st edition 1997; revised 2004*

OUTCOME CONTENT REFERENCES:

Barnard, D. (1990). Healing the damaged self: Identity, intimacy, and meaning in the lives of the chronically ill. *Perspectives in Biology & Medicine, 33*(4), 535–546.

Erickson, E. (1968). *Identity, youth and crisis.* New York: W. W. Norton & Company.

Gara, M. A., Rosenberg, S., & Cohen, B. (1987). Personal identity and the schizophrenic process: An integration. *Psychiatry, 50*(3), 267–278.

Grotevant, H. D., & Adams, G. R. (1984). Development of an objective measure to assess ego identity in adolescence: Validation and replication. *Journal of Youth and Adolescence, 13*(5), 419–437.

Hernandez, J. T., & Diclemente, R. J. (1992). Self-control and ego identity development as predictors of unprotected sex in late adolescent males. *Journal of Adolescence, 15*(4), 437–447.

Marcia, J. E. (1966). Development and validations of ego identity status. *Journal of Personality and Social Psychology, 3*(5), 551–558.

Marcia, J. E. (1967). Ego identity status: Relationships to change in self-esteem, general adjustment, and authoritarianism. *Journal of Personality, 35*(1), 118–133.

Oldaker, S. (1985). Identity confusion: Nursing diagnoses for adolescents. *Nursing Clinics of North America, 20*(4), 763–773.

Streitmatter, J. (1993). Gender differences in identity development: An examination of longitudinal data. *Adolescence, 28*(109), 55–66.

Streitmatter, J. (1993). Identity status and identity style: A replication study. *Journal of Adolescence, 16*(2), 211–215.

Stuart, G. W., & Laraia, M. T. (2001). *Principles and practice of psychiatric nursing* (7th ed.). St. Louis: Mosby.

+Tan, A. L., Kendis, R. J., Fine, J. T., & Porac, J. (1977). A short measure of Eriksonian ego identity. *Journal of Personality Assessment, 41*(3), 279–284.

Immobility Consequences: Physiological   0204

Definition: Severity of compromise in physiological functioning due to impaired physical mobility

OUTCOME TARGET RATING: Maintain at_____   Increase to_____

	Severe	Substantial	Moderate	Mild	None	
OUTCOME OVERALL RATING	1	2	3	4	5	
Indicators:						
020401 Pressure sore(s)	1	2	3	4	5	NA
020402 Constipation	1	2	3	4	5	NA
020403 Stool impaction	1	2	3	4	5	NA
020405 Hypoactive bowel	1	2	3	4	5	NA
020406 Paralytic ileus	1	2	3	4	5	NA
020407 Urinary calculi	1	2	3	4	5	NA
020408 Urinary retention	1	2	3	4	5	NA
020409 Fever	1	2	3	4	5	NA
020410 Urinary tract infection	1	2	3	4	5	NA
020413 Bone fracture	1	2	3	4	5	NA
020415 Contracted joints	1	2	3	4	5	NA
020416 Ankylosed joints	1	2	3	4	5	NA
020417 Orthostatic hypotension	1	2	3	4	5	NA
020418 Venous thrombosis	1	2	3	4	5	NA
020419 Lung congestion	1	2	3	4	5	NA
020422 Pneumonia	1	2	3	4	5	NA
020424 Venous stasis	1	2	3	4	5	NA

	Severely compromised	Substantially compromised	Moderately compromised	Mildly compromised	Not compromised	
020404 Nutritional status	1	2	3	4	5	NA
020411 Muscle strength	1	2	3	4	5	NA
020412 Muscle tone	1	2	3	4	5	NA
020414 Joint movement	1	2	3	4	5	NA
020420 Cough effectiveness	1	2	3	4	5	NA
020421 Vital capacity	1	2	3	4	5	NA

Domain-Functional Health (I)   *Class*-Mobility (C)   *1st edition 1997; revised 2000, 2004, 2013*

OUTCOME CONTENT REFERENCES:

Bloomfield, S. A. (1997). Changes in musculoskeletal structure and function with prolonged bed rest. *Medicine & Science in Sports & Exercise, 29*(2), 197–206.

Greenleaf, J. E. (1997). Intensive exercise training during bed rest attenuates deconditioning. *Medicine & Science in Sports & Exercise, 29*(2), 207–215.

Irvin, D. J., & White, M. (2004). The importance of accurately assessing orthostatic hypotension. *Geriatric Nursing, 25*(2), 99–101.

Kottke, F. J., & Lehmann, J. F. (1990). *Krusen's handbook of physical medicine and rehabilitation* (4th ed.). Philadelphia: W. B. Saunders.

Maas, M., & Specht, J. P. (2001). Impaired physical mobility. In M. Maas, K. Buckwalter, M. Hardy, T. Tripp-Reimer, M. Titler, & J. Specht (Eds.), *Nursing care of older adults: Diagnoses, outcomes & interventions* (pp. 337–365). St. Louis: Mosby.

Milde, F. K. (1981). Physiological immobilization. In L. Hart, J. Reese, & M. Fearing (Eds.), *Concepts common to acute illness: Identification and management* (pp. 67–109). St. Louis: Mosby.

Olson, E. V., Johnson, B. J., Thompson, L. F., McCarthy, J. S., Edmonds, R. E., Schroeder, L. M., & Wade, M. (1967). The hazards of immobility. *American Journal of Nursing, 67*(4), 780–797.

Potter, P. A., & Perry, A. G. (1997). Mobility and immobility. In P. A. Potter & A. G. Perry (Eds.), *Fundamentals of nursing: Concepts, process, and practice* (4th ed., pp. 1460–1520). St. Louis: Mosby.

Rubin, M. (1988). The physiology of bedrest. *American Journal of Nursing, 88*(1), 50–55.

Immobility Consequences: Psycho-Cognitive   0205

Definition: Severity of compromise in psycho-cognitive functioning due to impaired physical mobility

OUTCOME TARGET RATING: Maintain at_____ Increase to_____

		Severe	Substantial	Moderate	Mild	None	
OUTCOME OVERALL RATING		1	2	3	4	5	
Indicators:							
020504	Perceptual distortions	1	2	3	4	5	NA
020507	Exaggerated emotions	1	2	3	4	5	NA
020508	Sleep disturbance	1	2	3	4	5	NA
020510	Negative body image	1	2	3	4	5	NA
020513	Depression	1	2	3	4	5	NA
020514	Apathy	1	2	3	4	5	NA

		Severely compromised	Substantially compromised	Moderately compromised	Mildly compromised	Not compromised	
020501	Alertness	1	2	3	4	5	NA
020502	Cognitive status	1	2	3	4	5	NA
020503	Attentiveness	1	2	3	4	5	NA
020505	Kinesthetic sense	1	2	3	4	5	NA
020509	Self-esteem	1	2	3	4	5	NA
020511	Ability to act	1	2	3	4	5	NA

Domain-Functional Health (I)   **Class**-Mobility (C)   *1st edition 1997; revised 2004*

OUTCOME CONTENT REFERENCES:

Friedrich, R. M., & Lively, S. I. (1981). Psychological immobilization. In L. Hart, J. Reese, & M. Fearing (Eds.), *Concepts common to acute illness: Identification and management* (pp. 51–66). St. Louis: Mosby.

Greenleaf, J. E. (1997). Intensive exercise training during bed rest attenuates deconditioning. *Medicine & Science in Sports & Exercise, 29*(2), 207–215.

Maas, M., & Specht, J. P. (2001). Impaired physical mobility. In M. Maas, K. Buckwalter, M. Hardy, T. Tripp-Reimer, M. Titler, & J. Specht (Eds.), *Nursing care of older adults: Diagnoses, outcomes & interventions* (pp. 337–365). St. Louis: Mosby.

Rubin, M. (1988). How bedrest changes perception. *American Journal of Nursing, 88*(1), 55–56.

Immune Hypersensitivity Response   0707

Definition: Severity of inappropriate immune responses

OUTCOME TARGET RATING: Maintain at_____ Increase to_____

		Severe	Substantial	Moderate	Mild	None	
OUTCOME OVERALL RATING		1	2	3	4	5	
Indicators:							
070701	Alterations in skin	1	2	3	4	5	NA
070702	Alterations in mucosa	1	2	3	4	5	NA
070703	Allergic reactions	1	2	3	4	5	NA
070704	Localized inflammatory responses	1	2	3	4	5	NA
070705	Autoimmune events	1	2	3	4	5	NA
070706	Vasculitis	1	2	3	4	5	NA
070707	Transplant rejection	1	2	3	4	5	NA
070708	Graft versus host response	1	2	3	4	5	NA
070709	Itching	1	2	3	4	5	NA
070710	Jaundice	1	2	3	4	5	NA

Immune Hypersensitivity Response—cont'd

	Severe	Substantial	Moderate	Mild	None	
070711	Level of auto-antibodies or auto-antigens	1	2	3	4	5	NA
070712	Increased bilirubin	1	2	3	4	5	NA
070713	Alterations in complete blood count	1	2	3	4	5	NA
070714	Alterations in differential white blood count	1	2	3	4	5	NA
070715	Alterations in complement levels	1	2	3	4	5	NA
070716	Alterations in T4-cell level	1	2	3	4	5	NA
070717	Alterations in T8-cell level	1	2	3	4	5	NA

	Severely compromised	Substantially compromised	Moderately compromised	Mildly compromised	Not compromised	
070718	Respiratory function	1	2	3	4	5	NA
070719	Cardiac function	1	2	3	4	5	NA
070720	Gastrointestinal function	1	2	3	4	5	NA
070721	Renal function	1	2	3	4	5	NA
070722	Neurological function	1	2	3	4	5	NA
070723	Joint mobility	1	2	3	4	5	NA

Domain-*Physiologic Health (II)*   **Class**-*Immune Response (H)*   *3rd edition 2004*

OUTCOME CONTENT REFERENCES:
Birney, M. H. (1991). Psychoneuroimmunology: A holistic framework for the study of stress and illness. *Holistic Nursing Practice, 5*(4), 32–38.
Brandt, B. (1990). Nursing protocol for the patient with neutropenia. *Oncology Nursing Forum, 17*(Suppl. 1), 9–15.
McCance, K. L., & Huether, S. E. (2002). *Pathophysiology: The biologic basis for disease in adults and children* (4th ed.). St. Louis: Mosby.
Phillips, M. C., & Olson, L. R. (1993). The immunologic role of the gastrointestinal tract. *Critical Care Nursing Clinics of North America, 5*(1), 107–118.
Van Wynsberghe, D., Noback, C. R., & Carola, R. (1995). *Human anatomy and physiology* (3rd ed.). New York: McGraw-Hill.
Workman, M. L. (1993). The immune system: Your defensive partner and offensive foe. *AACN, 4*(3), 453–470.

Immune Status   **0702**

Definition: Natural and acquired appropriately targeted resistance to internal and external antigens

OUTCOME TARGET RATING: Maintain at_____   Increase to_____

	Severely compromised	Substantially compromised	Moderately compromised	Mildly compromised	Not compromised	
OUTCOME OVERALL RATING	1	2	3	4	5	
Indicators:						
070203	Gastrointestinal function	1	2	3	4	5	NA
070204	Respiratory function	1	2	3	4	5	NA
070205	Genitourinary function	1	2	3	4	5	NA
070207	Body temperature	1	2	3	4	5	NA
070208	Skin integrity	1	2	3	4	5	NA
070209	Mucosa integrity	1	2	3	4	5	NA
070211	Immunizations current	1	2	3	4	5	NA
070221	Screenings for infections current	1	2	3	4	5	NA
070212	Antibody titers	1	2	3	4	5	NA
070213	Skin test reaction with exposure	1	2	3	4	5	NA
070214	Absolute white blood count	1	2	3	4	5	NA
070215	Differential white blood count	1	2	3	4	5	NA

Continued

Immune Status—cont'd

		Severely compromised	Substantially compromised	Moderately compromised	Mildly compromised	Not compromised	
070216	T4-cell level	1	2	3	4	5	NA
070217	T8-cell level	1	2	3	4	5	NA
070218	Complement levels	1	2	3	4	5	NA
070219	Thymus x-ray findings	1	2	3	4	5	NA
		Severe	Substantial	Moderate	Mild	None	
070201	Recurrent infections	1	2	3	4	5	NA
070202	Tumors	1	2	3	4	5	NA
070206	Weight loss	1	2	3	4	5	NA
070210	Chronic fatigue	1	2	3	4	5	NA

Domain-*Physiologic Health (II)*   **Class**-*Immune Response (H)*   *1st edition 1997; revised 2004, 2008*

I

OUTCOME CONTENT REFERENCES:

Birney, M. H. (1991). Psychoneuroimmunology: A holistic framework for the study of stress and illness. *Holistic Nursing Practice, 5*(4), 32–38.

Brandt, B. (1990). Nursing protocol for the patient with neutropenia. *Oncology Nursing Forum, 17*(Suppl. 1), 9–15.

Hymes, D. J. (1985). Primary immunodeficiency disorders in the neonate. *Neonatal Network: The Journal of Neonatal Nursing, 3*(4), 40–48.

Lentz, A. K., & Feezor, R. J. (2003). Principles of immunology. *Nutritional Clinical Practice, 18*(6), 451–460.

Mayer, L. (2003). Mucosal immunity. *Pediatrics, 111*(6), 1595–1600.

McCance, K. L., & Huether, S. E. (2002). *Pathophysiology: The biologic basis for disease in adults and children* (4th ed.). St. Louis: Mosby.

Phillips, M. C., & Olson, L. R. (1993). The immunologic role of the gastrointestinal tract. *Critical Care Nursing Clinics of North America, 5*(1), 107–118.

Ungvarski, P. J., & Flaskerud, J. H. (1999). *HIV/AIDS: A guide to primary care management* (4th ed.). Philadelphia: W. B. Saunders.

Urakawa, K., & Yokoyama, K. (2004). Can relaxation programs with music enhance human immune function? *Journal of Alternative and Complementary Medicine, 10*(4), 605

Van Wynsberghe, D., Noback, C. R., & Carola, R. (1995). *Human anatomy and physiology* (3rd ed.). New York: McGraw-Hill.

Weber, R. (2003). Our innate immune system: Barking at the doorbell. *Dermatological Nursing, 15*(5), 471.

Workman, M. L. (1993). The immune system: Your defensive partner and offensive foe. *AACN, 4*(3), 453–470.

Immunization Behavior   **1900**

Definition: Personal actions to obtain immunization to prevent a communicable disease

OUTCOME TARGET RATING: Maintain at_____   Increase to_____

		Never demonstrated	Rarely demonstrated	Sometimes demonstrated	Often demonstrated	Consistently demonstrated	
OUTCOME OVERALL RATING		1	2	3	4	5	
Indicators:							
190001	Acknowledges disease risk without immunization	1	2	3	4	5	NA
190002	Describes risks associated with specific immunization	1	2	3	4	5	NA
190003	Describes contraindications to specific immunization	1	2	3	4	5	NA
190004	Brings updated vaccination card to each visit	1	2	3	4	5	NA
190005	Obtains immunizations recommended for age by the American Academy of Pediatrics or United States Public Health Service	1	2	3	4	5	NA

Immunization Behavior—*cont'd*

	Never demonstrated	Rarely demonstrated	Sometimes demonstrated	Often demonstrated	Consistently demonstrated	
190006 Describes relief measures for vaccine side effects	1	2	3	4	5	NA
190007 Reports any adverse reactions	1	2	3	4	5	NA
190009 Confirms date of next immunization	1	2	3	4	5	NA
190010 Obtains immunizations recommended with chronic illness by the American Academy of Pediatrics or United States Public Health Service	1	2	3	4	5	NA
190011 Obtains immunizations recommended for occupational risk by the American Academy of Pediatrics or United States Public Health Service	1	2	3	4	5	NA
190012 Obtains immunizations recommended for travel by the American Academy of Pediatrics or United States Public Health Service	1	2	3	4	5	NA
190013 Identifies community resources for immunization	1	2	3	4	5	NA

Domain-*Health Knowledge & Behavior (IV)* **Class**-*Risk Control & Safety (T)*   *1st edition 1997; revised 2000, 2004*

OUTCOME CONTENT REFERENCES:

Forshner, L., & Garza, A. (1999). Childhood vaccines: An update. *RN, 62*(4), 32–37.

Notice to readers: Recommended childhood immunization schedule—United States, 2002. (2002). *Morbidity and Mortality Weekly Report, 51*(2), 31–33.

Paulson, P. R., & Hammer, A. L. (2002). Updates & kidbits. Pediatric immunization update 2002. *Pediatric Nursing, 28*(2), 173–181.

Preboth, M. (2000). Practice guidelines. ACIP recommendations for the prevention of hepatitis A through immunization. *American Family Physician, 61*(7), 2246–2248.

Selekman, J. (1994). The guidelines for immunizations have changed again! *Pediatric Nursing, 20*(4), 376–378.

Sharts-Hopko, N. C. (1994). Current immunization guidelines. *MCN: American Journal of Maternal Child Nursing, 19*(2), 82–84.

Smith, C., & Maurer, F. (1995). *Community health nursing: Theory and practice.* Philadelphia: W. B. Saunders.

Zimmerman, R. K., & Ball, J. A. (2001). Adult vaccinations. *Primary Care: Clinics in Office Practice, 28*(4), 763–790.

I

Impulse Self-Control 1405

Definition: Self-restraint of compulsive or impulsive behaviors

OUTCOME TARGET RATING: Maintain at_____ Increase to_____

		Never demonstrated	Rarely demonstrated	Sometimes demonstrated	Often demonstrated	Consistently demonstrated	
OUTCOME OVERALL RATING		1	2	3	4	5	
Indicators:							
140501	Identifies harmful impulsive behaviors	1	2	3	4	5	NA
140502	Identifies feelings that lead to impulsive actions	1	2	3	4	5	NA
140503	Identifies behaviors that lead to impulsive actions	1	2	3	4	5	NA
140504	Identifies consequences of impulsive actions	1	2	3	4	5	NA
140505	Recognizes risks in environment	1	2	3	4	5	NA
140514	Avoids high-risk environments	1	2	3	4	5	NA
140515	Avoids high-risk situations	1	2	3	4	5	NA
140507	Controls impulses	1	2	3	4	5	NA
140516	Obtains assistance when experiencing impulses	1	2	3	4	5	NA
140509	Uses available social support	1	2	3	4	5	NA
140517	Keeps referral appointments	1	2	3	4	5	NA
140511	Upholds contract to control behavior	1	2	3	4	5	NA
140512	Maintains self-control without supervision	1	2	3	4	5	NA

Domain-Psychosocial Health (III)   **Class**-Self-Control (O)   1st edition 1997; revised 2000, 2004, 2008

OUTCOME CONTENT REFERENCES:

American Psychiatric Association Practice Guidelines. (1993). Practice guidelines for eating disorders. *American Journal of Psychiatry, 150*(2), 207–228.

Dyckoff, D., Goldstein, L., & Levine-Schacht, L. (1996). The investigation of behavioral contracting in patients with borderline personality disorder. *Journal of the American Psychiatric Nurses Association, 2*(3), 71–76.

Gallop, R. (1992). Self-destructive and impulsive behavior in the patient with borderline personality disorder: Rethinking hospital treatment and management. *Archives of Psychiatric Nursing, 6*(6), 366–373.

Gallop, R., McCay, E., & Esplen, M. T. (1992). The conceptualization of impulsivity for psychiatric nursing practice. *Archives of Psychiatric Nursing, 6*(6), 366–373.

Ingram, T. N. (2001). Risk for violence: Self-directed or directed at others. In M. Maas, K. Buckwalter, M. Hardy, T. Tripp-Reimer, M. Titler, & J. Specht (Eds.), *Nursing care of older adults: Diagnoses, outcomes & interventions* (pp. 696–705). St. Louis: Mosby.

+Lazzaro, T. A., Beggs, D. L., & McNeil, K. A. (1969). The development and validation of the Self-Report Test of Impulse Control. *Journal of Clinical Psychology, 25*(4), 434–438.

Miller, L. J. (1990). The formal treatment contract in the inpatient management of borderline personality disorder. *Hospital and Community Psychiatry, 41*(9) 985–987.

Staples, N. R., & Schwartz, M. (1990). Anorexia nervosa support group: Providing transitional support. *Journal of Psychosocial Nursing and Mental Health Services, 28*(2), 6–10.

Stuart, G. W., & Laraia, M. T. (2001). *Principles and practice of psychiatric nursing* (7th ed.). St. Louis: Mosby.

Infant Nutritional Status

1020

Definition: Amount of nutrients ingested and absorbed to meet metabolic needs and foster growth of an infant

OUTCOME TARGET RATING: Maintain at_____ Increase to_____

		Not adequate	Slightly adequate	Moderately adequate	Substantially adequate	Totally adequate	
OUTCOME OVERALL RATING		1	2	3	4	5	
Indicators:							
102001	Nutrient intake	1	2	3	4	5	NA
102002	Oral food intake	1	2	3	4	5	NA
102003	Oral fluid intake	1	2	3	4	5	NA
102004	Food tolerance	1	2	3	4	5	NA
102005	Weight/height ratio	1	2	3	4	5	NA
102006	Hydration	1	2	3	4	5	NA
102007	Growth	1	2	3	4	5	NA
102008	Blood glucose	1	2	3	4	5	NA
102009	Hemoglobin	1	2	3	4	5	NA
102010	Total iron binding capacity	1	2	3	4	5	NA
102011	Serum albumin	1	2	3	4	5	NA
102012	Caloric intake	1	2	3	4	5	NA
102013	Protein intake	1	2	3	4	5	NA
102014	Fat intake	1	2	3	4	5	NA
102015	Carbohydrate intake	1	2	3	4	5	NA
102016	Vitamin intake	1	2	3	4	5	NA
102017	Mineral intake	1	2	3	4	5	NA
102018	Iron intake	1	2	3	4	5	NA
102019	Calcium intake	1	2	3	4	5	NA
102020	Sodium intake	1	2	3	4	5	NA
102021	Tube feeding intake	1	2	3	4	5	NA
102022	Intravenous fluid intake	1	2	3	4	5	NA
102023	Parenteral fluid intake	1	2	3	4	5	NA

Domain-*Physiologic Health (II)* **Class**-*Digestion & Nutrition (K)* *5th edition 2013*

OUTCOME CONTENT REFERENCES:

Abrams, S. A. (2006). Building bones in babies: Can and should we exceed the human milk-fed infant's rate of bone calcium accretion? *Nutrition Reviews, 64*(11), 487–494.

Calamaro, C. J., & Selekman, J. (2000). Infant nutrition in the first year of life: Tradition or science? *Pediatric Nursing, 26*(2), 211–216.

D'Anci, K. E., Constant, F., & Rosenberg, I. H. (2006). Hydration and cognitive function in children. *Nutrition Reviews, 64*(10, Part 1), 457–464.

Hodges, E., Houck, G., & Kindermann, T. (2007). Reliability of the nursing child assessment feeding scale during toddlerhood. *Issues in Comprehensive Pediatric Nursing, 30*(3), 109–130.

Mentro, A., Steward, D., & Garvin, B. (2002). Infant feeding responsiveness: A conceptual analysis. *Journal of Advanced Nursing, 37*(2), 208–216.

Wheeler, B., & Wilson, D. (2007). Health promotion of the newborn and family. In M. J. Hockenberry & D. Wilson (Eds.), *Wong's nursing care of infants and children* (8th ed., pp. 525–531). St. Louis: Mosby Elsevier.

Wilson, D. (2007). Health promotion of the infant and family. In M. J. Hockenberry & D. Wilson (Eds.), *Wong's nursing care of infants and children* (8th ed., pp. 289–298). St. Louis: Mosby Elsevier.

I

Infection Severity 0703

Definition: Severity of signs and symptoms of infection

OUTCOME TARGET RATING: Maintain at_____ Increase to_____

OUTCOME OVERALL RATING	Severe 1	Substantial 2	Moderate 3	Mild 4	None 5	
Indicators:						
070301 Rash	1	2	3	4	5	NA
070302 Uncrusted vesicles	1	2	3	4	5	NA
070303 Foul-smelling discharge	1	2	3	4	5	NA
070304 Purulent sputum	1	2	3	4	5	NA
070305 Purulent drainage	1	2	3	4	5	NA
070306 Pyuria	1	2	3	4	5	NA
070307 Fever	1	2	3	4	5	NA
070329 Hypothermia	1	2	3	4	5	NA
070330 Temperature instability	1	2	3	4	5	NA
070333 Pain	1	2	3	4	5	NA
070334 Tenderness	1	2	3	4	5	NA
070309 Gastrointestinal symptoms	1	2	3	4	5	NA
070310 Lymphadenopathy	1	2	3	4	5	NA
070311 Malaise	1	2	3	4	5	NA
070312 Chilling	1	2	3	4	5	NA
070313 Unexplained cognitive impairment	1	2	3	4	5	NA
070331 Lethargy	1	2	3	4	5	NA
070332 Loss of appetite	1	2	3	4	5	NA
070319 Chest x-ray infiltration	1	2	3	4	5	NA
070320 Blood culture colonization	1	2	3	4	5	NA
070335 Vascular access device colonization	1	2	3	4	5	NA
070321 Sputum culture colonization	1	2	3	4	5	NA
070322 Cerebrospinal fluid culture colonization	1	2	3	4	5	NA
070323 Wound site culture colonization	1	2	3	4	5	NA
070324 Urine culture colonization	1	2	3	4	5	NA
070325 Stool culture colonization	1	2	3	4	5	NA
070326 White blood count elevation	1	2	3	4	5	NA
070327 White blood count depression	1	2	3	4	5	NA

Site of infection: _____

Domain-Physiologic Health (II)   **Class**-Immune Response (H)   *1st edition 1997; revised 2004, 2008, 2013*

OUTCOME CONTENT REFERENCES:
Albrutyn, E., & Talbot, G. H. (1987). Surveillance strategies: A primer. *Infection Control, 8*(11), 459–464.
Birnbaum, D. (1987). Nosocomial infection surveillance programs. *Infection Control, 8*(11), 474–479.
Burns, M. V. (1998). *Pathophysiology: A self-instructional program* (pp. 151–207). Stamford, CT: Appleton & Lange.
Carter, C., & Pottinger, J. M. (2001). Risk for infection. In M. Maas, K. Buckwalter, M. Hardy, T. Tripp-Reimer, M. Titler, & J. Specht (Eds.), *Nursing care of older adults: Diagnoses, outcomes & interventions* (pp. 47–62). St. Louis: Mosby.
Haley, R. W., Aber, R. C., & Bennett, J. V. (1986). Surveillance of nosocomial infections. In J. V. Bennett & D. S. Brachman (Eds.), *Hospital infections* (2nd ed., pp. 51–71). Boston: Little, Brown & Company.
Levy, C. R., Eilertsen, T., Kramer, A. M., & Hutt, E. (2006). Which clinical indicators and resident characteristics are associated with health care practitioner nursing home visits or hospital transfer for urinary tract infections? *Journal of the American Medical Directors Association, 7*(8), 493–498.
Yamashita, H., Tsukayama, H., Hori, N., Kimura, T., & Tanno, Y. (2000). Incidence of adverse reactions associated with acupuncture. *Journal of Alternative & Complementary Medicine, 6*(4), 345–350.

Infection Severity: Newborn 0708

Definition: Severity of signs and symptoms of infection during the first 28 days of life

OUTCOME TARGET RATING: Maintain at_____ Increase to_____

		Severe	Substantial	Moderate	Mild	None	
OUTCOME OVERALL RATING		1	2	3	4	5	
Indicators:							
070801	Temperature instability	1	2	3	4	5	NA
070802	Hypothermia	1	2	3	4	5	NA
070803	Tachypnea	1	2	3	4	5	NA
070804	Tachycardia	1	2	3	4	5	NA
070805	Bradycardia	1	2	3	4	5	NA
070806	Arrhythmias	1	2	3	4	5	NA
070807	Hypotension	1	2	3	4	5	NA
070808	Hypertension	1	2	3	4	5	NA
070809	Pale	1	2	3	4	5	NA
070810	Mottled skin	1	2	3	4	5	NA
070811	Cyanosis	1	2	3	4	5	NA
070812	Cold, clammy skin	1	2	3	4	5	NA
070813	Vomiting	1	2	3	4	5	NA
070814	Diarrhea	1	2	3	4	5	NA
070815	Abdominal distension	1	2	3	4	5	NA
070816	Feeding intolerance	1	2	3	4	5	NA
070817	Lethargy	1	2	3	4	5	NA
070818	Irritability	1	2	3	4	5	NA
070819	Seizures	1	2	3	4	5	NA
070820	Jitteriness	1	2	3	4	5	NA
070821	High-pitched cry	1	2	3	4	5	NA
070822	Rash	1	2	3	4	5	NA
070823	Uncrusted vesicles	1	2	3	4	5	NA
070824	Foul-smelling discharge	1	2	3	4	5	NA
070825	Purulent drainage	1	2	3	4	5	NA
070826	Conjunctivitis	1	2	3	4	5	NA
070827	Infected umbilicus	1	2	3	4	5	NA
070828	Blood culture colonization	1	2	3	4	5	NA
070829	Wound site culture colonization	1	2	3	4	5	NA
070830	Urine culture colonization	1	2	3	4	5	NA
070831	Stool culture colonization	1	2	3	4	5	NA
070832	Chest x-ray infiltration	1	2	3	4	5	NA
070833	Cerebrospinal fluid culture colonization	1	2	3	4	5	NA
070834	White blood count elevation	1	2	3	4	5	NA
070835	White blood count depression	1	2	3	4	5	NA

Site of infection: _____

Domain-*Physiologic Health (II)* **Class**-*Immune Response (H)* *3rd edition 2004; revised 2013*

OUTCOME CONTENT REFERENCES:
Albrutyn, E., & Talbot, G. H. (1987). Surveillance strategies: A primer. *Infection Control, 8*(11), 459–464.
Antonow, J. A., Smout, R. J., Gassaway, J., Horn, S. D., & Wilson, D. F. (2001). Variation among 10 pediatric hospitals: Sepsis evaluations for infants with bronchiolitis. *Journal of Nursing Care Quality, 15*(3), 39–49.
Deacon, J., & O'Neill, P. (Eds.). (1999). *Core curriculum for neonatal intensive care nursing* (2nd ed.). Philadelphia: W. B. Saunders.
Griffin, M. P., & Moorman, J. R. (2001). Toward the early diagnosis of neonatal sepsis and sepsis-like illness using novel heart rate analysis. *Pediatrics, 107*(1), 97–104.
Mattson, S., & Smith, J. E. (Eds.). (2000). *Core curriculum for maternal-newborn nursing* (2nd ed.). Philadelphia: W. B. Saunders.
Mullany, L. C., Darmstadt, G. L., Katz, J., Khatry, S. K., LeClerq, S. C., Adhikari, R. K., & Tielsch, J. M. (2006). *Archives of Disease in Childhood—Fetal & Neonatal Edition, 91*(2), F99–F104.

Information Processing

Definition: Ability to acquire, organize, and use information

OUTCOME TARGET RATING: Maintain at_____ Increase to_____

		Severely compromised	Substantially compromised	Moderately compromised	Mildly compromised	Not compromised	
OUTCOME OVERALL RATING		1	2	3	4	5	
Indicators:							
090701	Identifies common objects	1	2	3	4	5	NA
090709	Comprehends a sentence	1	2	3	4	5	NA
090710	Comprehends a paragraph	1	2	3	4	5	NA
090711	Comprehends a story	1	2	3	4	5	NA
090716	Comprehends universal symbols	1	2	3	4	5	NA
090703	Verbalizes a coherent message	1	2	3	4	5	NA
090704	Exhibits organized thought processes	1	2	3	4	5	NA
090705	Exhibits logical thought processes	1	2	3	4	5	NA
090712	Explains similarity between two items	1	2	3	4	5	NA
090713	Explains dissimilarity between two items	1	2	3	4	5	NA
090714	Adds several numbers	1	2	3	4	5	NA
090715	Subtracts several numbers	1	2	3	4	5	NA

Domain-*Physiologic Health (II)* **Class**-*Neurocognitive (J)* *1st edition 1997; revised 2004, 2008*

OUTCOME CONTENT REFERENCES:

Abraham, I., & Reel, S. (1993). Cognitive nursing interventions with long-term care residents: Effects on neurocognitive dimensions. *Archives of Psychiatric Nursing, 6*(6), 356–365.

Agostinelli, B., Demers, K., Garrigan, D., & Waszynski, C. (1994). Targeted interventions: Use of the mini-mental state exam. *Journal of Gerontological Nursing, 20*(8), 15–23.

Dellasega, C. (1992). Home health nurses' assessments of cognition. *Applied Nursing Research, 5*(3), 127–133.

+Folstein, M. F., Folstein, S. E., & McHugh, P. R. (1975). "Mini-Mental State"—A practical method for grading the cognitive state of patients for the clinician. *Journal of Psychiatric Research, 12*(3), 189–198.

Foreman, M., Theis, S., & Anderson, M. A. (1993). Adverse events in the hospitalized elderly. *Clinical Nursing Research, 2*(3) 360–370.

Gerdner, L. A., & Hall, G. R. (2001). Chronic confusion. In M. Maas, K. Buckwalter, M. Hardy, T. Tripp-Reimer, M. Titler, & J. Specht (Eds.), *Nursing care of older adults: Diagnoses, outcomes & interventions* (pp. 421–441). St. Louis: Mosby.

Inaba-Roland, K., & Maricle, R. (1992). Assessing delirium in the acute care setting. *Heart & Lung, 21*(1), 48–55.

Mason, P. (1989). Cognitive assessment parameters and tools for the critically injured adult. *Critical Care Nursing Clinics of North America, 1*(1), 45–53.

Prins, N., van Dijk, E., den Heijer, T., Vermeer, S., Jolles, J., Koudstaal, P., Hofman, A., & Breteler, M. (2005). Cerebral small-vessel disease and decline in information processing speed, executive function and memory. *Brain: A Journal of Neurology, 128*(Part 9), 2034–2041.

Strub, R. L., & Black, F. W. (2000). *The mental status examination in neurology* (4th ed.). Philadelphia: F. A. Davis.

Joint Movement

0206

Definition: Active range of motion of all joints with self-initiated movement

OUTCOME TARGET RATING: Maintain at_____ Increase to_____

		Severe deviation from normal range	Substantial deviation from normal range	Moderate deviation from normal range	Mild deviation from normal range	No deviation from normal range	
OUTCOME OVERALL RATING		1	2	3	4	5	
Indicators:							
020601	Jaw	1	2	3	4	5	NA
020602	Neck	1	2	3	4	5	NA
020620	Spine	1	2	3	4	5	NA
020603	Fingers (right)	1	2	3	4	5	NA
020604	Fingers (left)	1	2	3	4	5	NA
020605	Thumb (right)	1	2	3	4	5	NA
020606	Thumb (left)	1	2	3	4	5	NA
020607	Wrist (right)	1	2	3	4	5	NA
020608	Wrist (left)	1	2	3	4	5	NA
020609	Elbow (right)	1	2	3	4	5	NA
020610	Elbow (left)	1	2	3	4	5	NA
020611	Shoulder (right)	1	2	3	4	5	NA
020612	Shoulder (left)	1	2	3	4	5	NA
020613	Ankle (right)	1	2	3	4	5	NA
020614	Ankle (left)	1	2	3	4	5	NA
020615	Knee (right)	1	2	3	4	5	NA
020616	Knee (left	1	2	3	4	5	NA
020617	Hip (right)	1	2	3	4	5	NA
020618	Hip (left)	1	2	3	4	5	NA

Domain-*Functional Health (I)*   **Class**-*Mobility (C)*   *1st edition 1997; revised 2008*

OUTCOME CONTENT REFERENCES:
Bickley, L. (2002). *Bates' guide to physical examination and history taking* (8th ed.). Philadelphia: Lippincott Williams & Wilkins.
Hoeman, S. (2002). *Rehabilitation nursing: Process, application, and outcomes* (3rd ed.). St. Louis: Mosby.
Seidel, H. M., Ball, J. W., Dains, J. E., & Benedict, G. W. (2003). *Mosby's guide to physical examination* (5th ed.). St. Louis: Mosby.

Joint Movement: Ankle

0213

Definition: Active range of motion of the ankle with self-initiated movement

OUTCOME TARGET RATING: Maintain at_____ Increase to_____

		Severe deviation from normal range	Substantial deviation from normal range	Moderate deviation from normal range	Mild deviation from normal range	No deviation from normal range	
OUTCOME OVERALL RATING		1	2	3	4	5	
Indicators:							
021301	Dorsal flexion 20 degrees (R)	1	2	3	4	5	NA
021302	Plantar flexion 45 degrees (R)	1	2	3	4	5	NA
021303	Inversion 30 degrees (R)	1	2	3	4	5	NA
021304	Eversion 20 degrees (R)	1	2	3	4	5	NA

Continued

Joint Movement: Ankle—cont'd

		Severe deviation from normal range	Substantial deviation from normal range	Moderate deviation from normal range	Mild deviation from normal range	No deviation from normal range	
021305	Rotation (R)	1	2	3	4	5	NA
021306	Dorsal flexion 20 degrees (L)	1	2	3	4	5	NA
021307	Plantar flexion 45 degrees (L)	1	2	3	4	5	NA
021308	Inversion 30 degrees (L)	1	2	3	4	5	NA
021309	Eversion 20 degrees (L)	1	2	3	4	5	NA
021310	Rotation (L)	1	2	3	4	5	NA

Specify: Right (R)_____ Left (L)_____ Both_____

Domain-*Functional Health (I)* **Class**-*Mobility (C)* *3rd edition 2004*

OUTCOME CONTENT REFERENCES:
Bickley, L. (2002). *Bates' guide to physical examination and history taking* (8th ed.). Philadelphia: Lippincott Williams & Wilkins.
Hoeman, S. (2002). *Rehabilitation nursing: Process, application, and outcomes* (3rd ed.). St. Louis: Mosby.
Seidel, H. M., Ball, J. W., Dains, J. E., & Benedict, G. W. (2003). *Mosby's guide to physical examination* (5th ed.). St. Louis: Mosby.

Joint Movement: Elbow   0214

Definition: Active range of motion of the elbow with self-initiated movement

OUTCOME TARGET RATING: Maintain at_____ Increase to_____

		Severe deviation from normal range	Substantial deviation from normal range	Moderate deviation from normal range	Mild deviation from normal range	No deviation from normal range	
OUTCOME OVERALL RATING		1	2	3	4	5	
Indicators:							
021401	Extension 0 degrees (R)	1	2	3	4	5	NA
021402	Flexion 160 degrees (R)	1	2	3	4	5	NA
021403	Supination 90 degrees (R)	1	2	3	4	5	NA
021404	Pronation 90 degrees (R)	1	2	3	4	5	NA
021405	Extension 0 degrees (L)	1	2	3	4	5	NA
021406	Flexion 160 degrees (L)	1	2	3	4	5	NA
021407	Supination 90 degrees (L)	1	2	3	4	5	NA
021408	Pronation 90 degrees (L)	1	2	3	4	5	NA

Specify: Right (R)_____ Left (L)_____ Both_____

Domain-*Functional Health (I)* **Class**-*Mobility (C)* *3rd edition 2004*

OUTCOME CONTENT REFERENCES:
Bickley, L. (2002). *Bates' guide to physical examination and history taking* (8th ed.). Philadelphia: Lippincott Williams & Wilkins.
Hoeman, S. (2002). *Rehabilitation nursing: Process, application, and outcomes* (3rd ed.). St. Louis: Mosby.
Seidel, H. M., Ball, J. W., Dains, J. E., & Benedict, G. W. (2003). *Mosby's guide to physical examination* (5th ed.). St. Louis: Mosby.

Joint Movement: Fingers   0215

Definition: Active range of motion of the fingers with self-initiated movement

OUTCOME TARGET RATING: Maintain at_____   Increase to_____

		Severe deviation from normal range	Substantial deviation from normal range	Moderate deviation from normal range	Mild deviation from normal range	No deviation from normal range	
OUTCOME OVERALL RATING		1	2	3	4	5	
Indicators:							
021501	Metacarpophalangeal extension 0 degrees (R)	1	2	3	4	5	NA
021502	Metacarpophalangeal flexion 90 degrees (R)	1	2	3	4	5	NA
021503	Metacarpophalangeal hyperflexion 30 degrees (R)	1	2	3	4	5	NA
021504	Proximal interphalangeal extension 0 degrees (R)	1	2	3	4	5	NA
021505	Proximal interphalangeal flexion 100-120 degrees (R)	1	2	3	4	5	NA
021506	Distal interphalangeal extension 0 degrees (R)	1	2	3	4	5	NA
021507	Distal interphalangeal flexion 45-80 degrees (R)	1	2	3	4	5	NA
021508	Metacarpophalangeal extension 0 degrees (L)	1	2	3	4	5	NA
021509	Metacarpophalangeal flexion 90 degrees (L)	1	2	3	4	5	NA
021510	Metacarpophalangeal hyperflexion 30 degrees (L)	1	2	3	4	5	NA
021511	Proximal interphalangeal extension 0 degrees (L)	1	2	3	4	5	NA
021512	Proximal interphalangeal flexion 100-120 degrees (L)	1	2	3	4	5	NA
021513	Distal interphalangeal extension 0 degrees (L)	1	2	3	4	5	NA
021514	Distal interphalangeal flexion 45-80 degrees (L)	1	2	3	4	5	NA

Specify: Right hand (R)_____   Left hand (L)_____   Both_____

Domain-Functional Health (I)   *Class*-Mobility (C)   *3rd edition 2004*

OUTCOME CONTENT REFERENCES:
Bickley, L. (2002). *Bates' guide to physical examination and history taking* (8th ed.). Philadelphia: Lippincott Williams & Wilkins.
Hoeman, S. (2002). *Rehabilitation nursing: Process, application, and outcomes* (3rd ed.). St. Louis: Mosby.
Seidel, H. M., Ball, J. W., Dains, J. E., & Benedict, G. W. (2003). *Mosby's guide to physical examination* (5th ed.). St. Louis: Mosby.

Joint Movement: Hip   0216

Definition: Active range of motion of the hip with self-initiated movement

OUTCOME TARGET RATING: Maintain at_____   Increase to_____

		Severe deviation from normal range	Substantial deviation from normal range	Moderate deviation from normal range	Mild deviation from normal range	No deviation from normal range	
OUTCOME OVERALL RATING		1	2	3	4	5	
Indicators:							
021601	Flexion knee straight 90 degrees (R)	1	2	3	4	5	NA
021602	Extension knee straight 0 degrees (R)	1	2	3	4	5	NA
021603	Hyperextension knee straight 15 degrees (R)	1	2	3	4	5	NA
021604	Flexion knee bent 120 degrees (R)	1	2	3	4	5	NA
021605	Abduction 45 degrees (R)	1	2	3	4	5	NA
021606	Adduction 30 degrees (R)	1	2	3	4	5	NA
021607	Internal rotation 40 degrees (R)	1	2	3	4	5	NA
021608	External rotation 45 degrees (R)	1	2	3	4	5	NA
021609	Flexion knee straight 90 degrees (L)	1	2	3	4	5	NA
021610	Extension knee straight 0 degrees (L)	1	2	3	4	5	NA
021611	Hyperextension knee straight 15 degrees (L)	1	2	3	4	5	NA
021612	Flexion knee bent 120 degrees (L)	1	2	3	4	5	NA
021613	Abduction 45 degrees (L)	1	2	3	4	5	NA
021614	Adduction 30 degrees (L)	1	2	3	4	5	NA
021615	Internal rotation 40 degrees (L)	1	2	3	4	5	NA
021616	External rotation 45 degrees (L)	1	2	3	4	5	NA

Specify: Right (R)_____   Left (L)_____   Both_____

Domain-Functional Health (I)   **Class**-Mobility (C)   3rd edition 2004

OUTCOME CONTENT REFERENCES:
Bickley, L. (2002). *Bates' guide to physical examination and history taking* (8th ed.). Philadelphia: Lippincott Williams & Wilkins.
Hoeman, S. (2002). *Rehabilitation nursing: Process, application, and outcomes* (3rd ed.). St. Louis: Mosby.
Seidel, H. M., Ball, J. W., Dains, J. E., & Benedict, G. W. (2003). *Mosby's guide to physical examination* (5th ed.). St. Louis: Mosby.

Joint Movement: Knee   0217

Definition: Active range of motion of the knee with self-initiated movement

OUTCOME TARGET RATING: Maintain at_____   Increase to_____

		Severe deviation from normal range	Substantial deviation from normal range	Moderate deviation from normal range	Mild deviation from normal range	No deviation from normal range	
OUTCOME OVERALL RATING		1	2	3	4	5	
Indicators:							
021701	Extension 0 degrees (R)	1	2	3	4	5	NA
021702	Flexion 130 degrees (R)	1	2	3	4	5	NA
021703	Hyperextension 15 degrees (R)	1	2	3	4	5	NA
021704	Extension 0 degrees (L)	1	2	3	4	5	NA
021705	Flexion 130 degrees (L)	1	2	3	4	5	NA
021706	Hyperextension 15 degrees (L)	1	2	3	4	5	NA

Specify: Right (R)_____   Left (L)_____   Both_____

Domain-Functional Health (I)   **Class**-Mobility (C)   *3rd edition 2004*

OUTCOME CONTENT REFERENCES:
Bickley, L. (2002). *Bates' guide to physical examination and history taking* (8th ed.). Philadelphia: Lippincott Williams & Wilkins.
Hoeman, S. (2002). *Rehabilitation nursing: Process, application, and outcomes* (3rd ed.). St. Louis: Mosby.
Seidel, H. M., Ball, J. W., Dains, J. E., & Benedict, G. W. (2003). *Mosby's guide to physical examination* (5th ed.). St. Louis: Mosby.

J

Joint Movement: Neck   0218

Definition: Active range of motion of the neck with self-initiated movement

OUTCOME TARGET RATING: Maintain at_____   Increase to_____

		Severe deviation from normal range	Substantial deviation from normal range	Moderate deviation from normal range	Mild deviation from normal range	No deviation from normal range	
OUTCOME OVERALL RATING		1	2	3	4	5	
Indicators:							
021801	Flexion 45 degrees	1	2	3	4	5	NA
021802	Extension 55 degrees	1	2	3	4	5	NA
021803	Lateral bending 40 degrees (R)	1	2	3	4	5	NA
021804	Lateral bending 40 degrees (L)	1	2	3	4	5	NA
021805	Rotation	1	2	3	4	5	NA

Domain-Functional Health (I)   **Class**-Mobility (C)   *3rd edition 2004*

OUTCOME CONTENT REFERENCES:
Bickley, L. (2002). *Bates' guide to physical examination and history taking* (8th ed.). Philadelphia: Lippincott Williams & Wilkins.
Hoeman, S. (2002). *Rehabilitation nursing: Process, application, and outcomes* (3rd ed.). St. Louis: Mosby.
Seidel, H. M., Ball, J. W., Dains, J. E., & Benedict, G. W. (2003). *Mosby's guide to physical examination* (5th ed.). St. Louis: Mosby.

Joint Movement: Passive

0207

Definition: Joint movement with assistance

OUTCOME TARGET RATING: Maintain at_____   Increase to_____

		Severe deviation from normal range	Substantial deviation from normal range	Moderate deviation from normal range	Mild deviation from normal range	No deviation from normal range	
OUTCOME OVERALL RATING		1	2	3	4	5	
Indicators:							
020702	Neck	1	2	3	4	5	NA
020703	Fingers (right)	1	2	3	4	5	NA
020705	Thumb (right)	1	2	3	4	5	NA
020707	Wrist (right)	1	2	3	4	5	NA
020709	Elbow (right)	1	2	3	4	5	NA
020711	Shoulder (right)	1	2	3	4	5	NA
020713	Ankle (right)	1	2	3	4	5	NA
020715	Knee (right)	1	2	3	4	5	NA
020717	Hip (right)	1	2	3	4	5	NA
020704	Fingers (left)	1	2	3	4	5	NA
020706	Thumb (left)	1	2	3	4	5	NA
020708	Wrist (left)	1	2	3	4	5	NA
020710	Elbow (left)	1	2	3	4	5	NA
020712	Shoulder (left)	1	2	3	4	5	NA
020714	Ankle (left)	1	2	3	4	5	NA
020716	Knee (left)	1	2	3	4	5	NA
020718	Hip (left)	1	2	3	4	5	NA

Domain-*Functional Health (I)*   **Class**-*Mobility (C)*   *1st edition 1997; revised 2004*

OUTCOME CONTENT REFERENCES:
Bickley, L. (2002). *Bates' guide to physical examination and history taking* (8th ed.). Philadelphia: Lippincott Williams & Wilkins.
Hoeman, S. (2002). *Rehabilitation nursing: Process, application, and outcomes* (3rd ed.). St. Louis: Mosby.
Seidel, H. M., Ball, J. W., Dains, J. E., & Benedict, G. W. (2003). *Mosby's guide to physical examination* (5th ed.). St. Louis: Mosby.

Joint Movement: Shoulder

0219

Definition: Active range of motion of the shoulder with self-initiated movement

OUTCOME TARGET RATING: Maintain at_____   Increase to_____

		Severe deviation from normal range	Substantial deviation from normal range	Moderate deviation from normal range	Mild deviation from normal range	No deviation from normal range	
OUTCOME OVERALL RATING		1	2	3	4	5	
Indicators:							
021901	Forward flexion 180 degrees (R)	1	2	3	4	5	NA
021902	Extension 50 degrees (R)	1	2	3	4	5	NA
021903	External rotation 90 degrees (R)	1	2	3	4	5	NA
021904	Internal rotation 90 degrees (R)	1	2	3	4	5	NA
021905	Abduction 180 degrees (R)	1	2	3	4	5	NA
021906	Adduction 50 degrees (R)	1	2	3	4	5	NA
021907	Forward flexion 180 degrees (L)	1	2	3	4	5	NA

Joint Movement: Shoulder—*cont'd*

	Severe deviation from normal range	Substantial deviation from normal range	Moderate deviation from normal range	Mild deviation from normal range	No deviation from normal range	
021908 Extension 50 degrees (L)	1	2	3	4	5	NA
021909 External rotation 90 degrees (L)	1	2	3	4	5	NA
021910 Internal rotation 90 degrees (L)	1	2	3	4	5	NA
021911 Abduction 180 degrees (L)	1	2	3	4	5	NA
021912 Adduction 50 degrees (L)	1	2	3	4	5	NA

Specify: Right (R)_____   Left (L)_____   Both_____

Domain-Functional Health (I)   *Class*-Mobility (C)   *3rd edition 2004*

OUTCOME CONTENT REFERENCES:
Bickley, L. (2002). *Bates' guide to physical examination and history taking* (8th ed.). Philadelphia: Lippincott Williams & Wilkins.
Hoeman, S. (2002). *Rehabilitation nursing: Process, application, and outcomes* (3rd ed.). St. Louis: Mosby.
Seidel, H. M., Ball, J. W., Dains, J. E., & Benedict, G. W. (2003). Mosby's *guide to physical examination* (5th ed.). St. Louis: Mosby.

J

Joint Movement: Spine   0220

Definition: Active range of motion of the spine with self-initiated movement

OUTCOME TARGET RATING: Maintain at_____   Increase to_____

	Severe deviation from normal range	Substantial deviation from normal range	Moderate deviation from normal range	Mild deviation from normal range	No deviation from normal range	
OUTCOME OVERALL RATING	1	2	3	4	5	
Indicators:						
022001 Extension 30 degrees	1	2	3	4	5	NA
022002 Flexion 90 degrees	1	2	3	4	5	NA
022003 Lateral bending 35 degrees (R)	1	2	3	4	5	NA
022004 Rotation (R)	1	2	3	4	5	NA
022005 Lateral bending 35 degrees (L)	1	2	3	4	5	NA
022006 Rotation (L)	1	2	3	4	5	NA

Domain-Functional Health (I)   *Class*-Mobility (C)   *3rd edition 2004*

OUTCOME CONTENT REFERENCES:
Bickley, L. (2002). *Bates' guide to physical examination and history taking* (8th ed.). Philadelphia: Lippincott Williams & Wilkins.
Hoeman, S. (2002). *Rehabilitation nursing: Process, application, and outcomes* (3rd ed.). St. Louis: Mosby.
Seidel, H. M., Ball, J. W., Dains, J. E., & Benedict, G. W. (2003). *Mosby's guide to physical examination* (5th ed.). St. Louis: Mosby.

Joint Movement: Wrist   0221

Definition: Active range of motion of the wrist with self-initiated movement

OUTCOME TARGET RATING: Maintain at_____ Increase to_____

	Severe deviation from normal range	Substantial deviation from normal range	Moderate deviation from normal range	Mild deviation from normal range	No deviation from normal range	
OUTCOME OVERALL RATING	1	2	3	4	5	
Indicators:						
022101 Radial deviation 20 degrees (R)	1	2	3	4	5	NA
022102 Ulnar deviation 55 degrees (R)	1	2	3	4	5	NA
022103 Flexion 90 degrees (R)	1	2	3	4	5	NA
022104 Extension 70 degrees (R)	1	2	3	4	5	NA
022105 Radial deviation 20 degrees (L)	1	2	3	4	5	NA
022106 Ulnar deviation 55 degrees (L)	1	2	3	4	5	NA
022107 Flexion 90 degrees (L)	1	2	3	4	5	NA
022108 Extension 70 degrees (L)	1	2	3	4	5	NA

Specify: Right (R)_____ Left (L)_____ Both_____

Domain-*Functional Health (I)*   **Class**-*Mobility (C)*   *3rd edition 2004*

OUTCOME CONTENT REFERENCES:

Bickley, L. *(2002). Bates' guide to physical examination and history taking (8th ed.).* Philadelphia: Lippincott Williams & Wilkins.

Hoeman, S. (2002). *Rehabilitation nursing: Process, application, and outcomes* (3rd ed.). St. Louis: Mosby.

Seidel, H. M., Ball, J. W., Dains, J. E., & Benedict, G. W. (2003). *Mosby's guide to physical examination* (5th ed.). St. Louis: Mosby.

Kidney Function   0504

Definition: Ability of the kidneys to regulate body fluids, filter blood and eliminate waste products through the formation of urine

OUTCOME TARGET RATING: Maintain at_____ Increase to_____

		Severely compromised	Substantially compromised	Moderately compromised	Mildly compromised	Not compromised	
OUTCOME OVERALL RATING		1	2	3	4	5	
Indicators:							
050424	8-hour urine output	1	2	3	4	5	NA
050402	24-hour intake and output balance	1	2	3	4	5	NA
050425	Skin turgor	1	2	3	4	5	NA
050405	Urine specific gravity	1	2	3	4	5	NA
050406	Urine color	1	2	3	4	5	NA
050408	Urine pH	1	2	3	4	5	NA
050409	Urine electrolytes	1	2	3	4	5	NA
050410	Arterial bicarbonate (HCO_3)	1	2	3	4	5	NA
050411	Arterial pH	1	2	3	4	5	NA

		Severe	Substantial	Moderate	Mild	None	
050426	Increased blood urea nitrogen	1	2	3	4	5	NA
050427	Increased serum creatinine	1	2	3	4	5	NA
050428	Increased serum potassium	1	2	3	4	5	NA
050429	Increased urine glucose	1	2	3	4	5	NA
050430	Increased urine protein	1	2	3	4	5	NA
050431	Increased white blood cells	1	2	3	4	5	NA
050414	Hematuria	1	2	3	4	5	NA
050415	Urine ketones	1	2	3	4	5	NA
050416	Urine abnormal microscopic findings	1	2	3	4	5	NA
050417	Kidney stone formation	1	2	3	4	5	NA
050418	Weight gain	1	2	3	4	5	NA
050419	Hypertension	1	2	3	4	5	NA
050420	Nausea	1	2	3	4	5	NA
050421	Fatigue	1	2	3	4	5	NA
050422	Malaise	1	2	3	4	5	NA
050423	Anemia	1	2	3	4	5	NA
050432	Edema	1	2	3	4	5	NA

K

Domain-Physiologic Health (II) *Class-Elimination (F)* *3rd edition 2004; revised 2013*

OUTCOME CONTENT REFERENCES:
Broscious, S. K., & Castagnola, J. (2006). Chronic kidney disease: Acute manifestations and role of critical care nurses. *Critical Care Nurse, 26*(4), 17–28.
Guyton, A. C., Hall, J. E., & Schmitt, W. (1997). *Human physiology and mechanisms of disease* (6th ed.). Philadelphia: W. B. Saunders.
LeMone, P., Burke, K., & Bauldoff, G. (2011). *Medical-surgical nursing: Critical thinking in patient care* (5th ed., pp. 768–782). Upper Saddle River, NJ: Pearson Education.
Potter, P., Perry, A., Stockert, P., & Hall, A. (2013). *Fundamentals of nursing* (8th ed.). St. Louis: Elsevier Mosby.
Roth, C., & Culp, K. (2001). Renal osteodystrophy in elderly patients with end-stage renal disease. *Journal of Gerontological Nursing, 27*(7), 46–51.
Smeltzer, S., Bare, B., Hinkle, J., & Cheever, K. (2008). *Brunner & Suddarth's textbook of medical-surgical nursing* (11th ed., pp. 1492–1513). Philadelphia: Lippincott Williams & Wilkins.

Knowledge: Acute Illness Management 1844

Definition: Extent of understanding conveyed about a reversible illness, its treatment, and the prevention of complications

OUTCOME TARGET RATING: Maintain at_____ Increase to_____

OUTCOME OVERALL RATING		No knowledge 1	Limited knowledge 2	Moderate knowledge 3	Substantial knowledge 4	Extensive knowledge 5	
Indicators:							
184401	Cause and contributing factors	1	2	3	4	5	NA
184402	Usual course of illness	1	2	3	4	5	NA
184403	Benefits of illness management	1	2	3	4	5	NA
184404	Signs and symptoms of illness	1	2	3	4	5	NA
184405	Signs and symptoms of complications	1	2	3	4	5	NA
184406	Strategies to prevent complications	1	2	3	4	5	NA
184407	Strategies to prevent exposing others to illness	1	2	3	4	5	NA
184408	Strategies to manage comfort	1	2	3	4	5	NA
184409	Available treatment options	1	2	3	4	5	NA
184410	Correct use of non-prescription medications	1	2	3	4	5	NA
184411	Correct use of prescribed medication	1	2	3	4	5	NA
184412	Medication therapeutic effects	1	2	3	4	5	NA
184413	Medication side effects	1	2	3	4	5	NA
184414	Medication adverse effects	1	2	3	4	5	NA
184415	Potential medication interactions	1	2	3	4	5	NA
184416	Treatment regimen	1	2	3	4	5	NA
184417	Personal responsibilities for treatment regimen	1	2	3	4	5	NA
184418	Importance of compliance to treatment regimen	1	2	3	4	5	NA
184419	Cultural influences on compliance with treatment regimen	1	2	3	4	5	NA
184420	Importance of adequate rest	1	2	3	4	5	NA
184421	Diet modifications	1	2	3	4	5	NA
184422	Strategies to cope with adverse effects of illness	1	2	3	4	5	NA
184423	Reputable sources of acute illness information related to illness	1	2	3	4	5	NA
184424	When to obtain assistance from a health professional	1	2	3	4	5	NA

Domain-Health Knowledge & Behavior (IV)   **Class**-Health Knowledge (S)   5th edition 2013

OUTCOME CONTENT REFERENCES:
Jones, R., White, P., Armstrong, D., Ashworth, M., & Peters, M. (2010). *Managing acute illness*. London: The King's Fund.
LeMone, P., Burke, K., & Bauldoff, G. (2011). *Medical-surgical nursing: Critical thinking in patient care* (5th ed.). Upper Saddle River, NJ: Pearson Education.
Potter, P., Perry, A., Stockert, P., & Hall, A. (2013). *Fundamentals of nursing* (8th ed.). St. Louis: Elsevier Mosby.

Knowledge: Anticoagulation Therapy Management 1845

Definition: Extent of understanding conveyed about the therapeutic purposes, actions, and risks of chemical agents that lengthen blood clotting time

OUTCOME TARGET RATING: Maintain at_____ Increase to_____

		No knowledge	Limited knowledge	Moderate knowledge	Substantial knowledge	Extensive knowledge	
OUTCOME OVERALL RATING		1	2	3	4	5	
Indicators:							
184501	Specific thromboembolic disorder	1	2	3	4	5	NA
184502	Benefits of anticoagulation therapy	1	2	3	4	5	NA
184503	Correct use of prescribed medication	1	2	3	4	5	NA
184504	Adverse health effects of skipping medication	1	2	3	4	5	NA
184505	Importance of maintaining medication regimen	1	2	3	4	5	NA
184506	Medication therapeutic effects	1	2	3	4	5	NA
184507	Medication adverse effects	1	2	3	4	5	NA
184508	Medication side effects	1	2	3	4	5	NA
184509	Potential prescribed medication interactions with other agents	1	2	3	4	5	NA
184510	Potential non-prescription medication interactions with other agents	1	2	3	4	5	NA
184511	Herbal interactions	1	2	3	4	5	NA
184512	Prescribed diet	1	2	3	4	5	NA
184513	Food interactions	1	2	3	4	5	NA
184514	Importance of vitamin K restrictions	1	2	3	4	5	NA
184515	Therapeutic range of blood clotting time	1	2	3	4	5	NA
184516	Importance of required laboratory tests	1	2	3	4	5	NA
184517	Importance of regular blood clotting tests	1	2	3	4	5	NA
184518	Risk of bleeding	1	2	3	4	5	NA
184519	Risk of clotting	1	2	3	4	5	NA
184520	Importance of coordinated management with health professional	1	2	3	4	5	NA
184521	Importance of informing health professional of anticoagulation therapy	1	2	3	4	5	NA
184522	Strategies to reduce venous stasis	1	2	3	4	5	NA
184523	Strategies to reduce internal bleeding	1	2	3	4	5	NA
184524	Strategies to prevent physical injury	1	2	3	4	5	NA
184525	Signs and symptoms of internal bleeding	1	2	3	4	5	NA
184526	Signs of external bleeding	1	2	3	4	5	NA
184527	Signs and symptoms of embolism	1	2	3	4	5	NA
184528	Signs and symptoms of atrial fibrillation	1	2	3	4	5	NA
184529	Signs and symptoms of stroke	1	2	3	4	5	NA
184530	Signs and symptoms of transient ischemic attack	1	2	3	4	5	NA
184531	Importance of monitoring vital signs	1	2	3	4	5	NA
184532	Benefits of activity restrictions	1	2	3	4	5	NA
184533	High-risk activities	1	2	3	4	5	NA
184534	Importance of alcohol abstinence	1	2	3	4	5	NA
184535	Importance of tobacco abstinence	1	2	3	4	5	NA
184536	When to obtain assistance from a health professional	1	2	3	4	5	NA
184537	Caregiver's role in treatment plan	1	2	3	4	5	NA

K

Continued

Knowledge: Anticoagulation Therapy Management—cont'd

	No knowledge	Limited knowledge	Moderate knowledge	Substantial knowledge	Extensive knowledge	
184538	Reputable sources of anticoagulation therapy information	1	2	3	4	5	NA
184539	Plan for obtaining immediate treatment if adverse signs and symptoms occur	1	2	3	4	5	NA

Domain-Health Knowledge & Behavior (IV)   **Class**-Health Knowledge (S)   5th edition 2013

OUTCOME CONTENT REFERENCES:

Findlay, J., Keogh, M., & Cooper, L. (2010). Venous thromboembolism prophylaxis: The role of the nurse. *British Journal of Nursing, 19*(16), 1028–1032.

Fitzgerald, J. (2010). Venous thromboembolism: Have we made headway? *Orthopaedic Nursing, 29*(4), 226–234.

Headley, C. M., & Melander, S. (2011). When it may be a pulmonary embolism. *Nephrology Nursing Journal, 38*(2), 127–152.

Houman Fekrazad, M., Lopes, R. D., Stashenko, G. J., Alexander, J. H., & Garcia, D. (2009). Treatment of venous thromboembolism: Guidelines translated for the clinician. *Journal of Thrombosis and Thrombolysis, 28*(3), 270–275.

Lancaster, S. L., Owens, A., Bryant, A. S., Ramey, L. S., Nicholson, J., Gossett, K., Forni, J. T., & Padgett, T. M. (2010). Emergency: Upper-extremity deep vein thrombosis. *AJN: American Journal of Nursing, 110*(5), 48–52.

Shaughnessy, K. (2007). Massive pulmonary embolism. *Critical Care Nurse, 27*(1), 39–40, 42–51.

Van Damme, S., Van Deyk, K., Budts, W., Verhamme, P., & Moons, P. (2011). Patient knowledge of and adherence to oral anticoagulation therapy after mechanical heart-valve replacement for congenital or acquired valve defects. *Heart and Lung, 40*(2), 139–146.

Yee, C. A. (2010). Conquering pulmonary embolism. *OR Nurse, 4*(5), 18–24.

K

Knowledge: Arthritis Management   1831

Definition: Extent of understanding conveyed about arthritis, its treatment, and the prevention of disease progression and complications

OUTCOME TARGET RATING: Maintain at_____   Increase to_____

	No knowledge	Limited knowledge	Moderate knowledge	Substantial knowledge	Extensive knowledge	
OUTCOME OVERALL RATING	1	2	3	4	5	
Indicators:						
183101	Cause and contributing factors	1	2	3	4	5	NA
183102	Usual course of disease	1	2	3	4	5	NA
183103	Signs and symptoms of early disease	1	2	3	4	5	NA
183104	Signs and symptoms of worsening disease	1	2	3	4	5	NA
183105	Potential body changes due to disease	1	2	3	4	5	NA
183106	Benefits of disease management	1	2	3	4	5	NA
183107	Strategies to balance activity and rest	1	2	3	4	5	NA
183108	Energy conservation techniques	1	2	3	4	5	NA
183109	Benefits of regular exercise	1	2	3	4	5	NA
183110	Modification of daily activities	1	2	3	4	5	NA
183111	Factors that decrease the ability to perform physical activity	1	2	3	4	5	NA
183112	Effective exercise routine	1	2	3	4	5	NA
183113	Strategies to protect joints	1	2	3	4	5	NA
183114	Strategies to manage pain	1	2	3	4	5	NA

Knowledge: Arthritis Management—cont'd

		No knowledge	Limited knowledge	Moderate knowledge	Substantial knowledge	Extensive knowledge	
183115	Surgical treatment options	1	2	3	4	5	NA
183116	Medical treatment options	1	2	3	4	5	NA
183117	Medication therapeutic effects	1	2	3	4	5	NA
183118	Medication side effects	1	2	3	4	5	NA
183119	Medication adverse effects	1	2	3	4	5	NA
183120	When to obtain assistance from a health professional	1	2	3	4	5	NA
183121	Health beliefs that affect adherence to treatment	1	2	3	4	5	NA
183122	Adverse health effects of being overweight	1	2	3	4	5	NA
183123	Diet modifications	1	2	3	4	5	NA
183124	Correct use of assistive devices	1	2	3	4	5	NA
183125	Home safety measures	1	2	3	4	5	NA
183126	Fall prevention strategies	1	2	3	4	5	NA
183127	Available support groups	1	2	3	4	5	NA
183128	Reputable sources of arthritis information	1	2	3	4	5	NA

Domain-*Health Knowledge & Behavior (IV)*   **Class**-*Health Knowledge (S)*   *4th edition 2008; revised 2013*

K

OUTCOME CONTENT REFERENCES:

Bellamy, N., Buchanan, W. W., Goldsmith, C. H., Campbell, J., & Stitt, L. W. (1988). Validation study of WOMAC: A health status instrument for measuring clinically important patient relevant outcomes to antirheumatic drug therapy in patients with osteoarthritis of the hip or knee. *Journal of Rheumatology, 15*(12), 1796–1840.

Branch, V. K., Lipsky, K., Nieman, T., & Lipsky, P. E. (1999). Positive impact of an intervention by arthritis patient educators on knowledge and satisfaction of patients in a rheumatology practice. *Arthritis Care and Research, 12*(6), 370–375.

Davies, G. M., Watson, D. J., & Bellamy, N. (1999). Comparison of the responsiveness and relative effect size of the Western Ontario and McMaster Universities Osteoarthritis Index and the Short-Form Medical Outcomes Study Survey in a randomized, clinical trial of osteoarthritis patients. *Arthritis Care Research, 12*(3), 172–179.

Edworthy, S. M., Devins, G. M., Watson, M. M. (1995). The arthritis knowledge questionnaire. *Arthritis and Rheumatism, 38*(5), 590–600.

Figaro, M. K, Williams-Russo, P., Allegrante, J. P. (2005). Expectation and outlook: The impact of patient preference on arthritis care among African Americans. *Journal of Ambulatory Care Management, 28*(1), 41–48.

Hammond, A., & Lincoln, N. (1999). The Joint Protection Knowledge Assessment (JPKA): Reliability and validity. *British Journal of Occupational Therapy, 62*(3), 117–122.

Hill, J., & Bird, H. (2007). Patient knowledge and misconceptions of osteoarthritis assessed by a validated self-completed knowledge questionnaire (PKQ-OA). *Rheumatology, 46*(5), 796–800.

Memel, D. S., & Kirwan, J. R. (1999). General practitioners' knowledge of functional and social factors in patients with rheumatoid arthritis. *Health and Social Care in the Community, 7*(6), 387–393.

Neame, R., & Hammond, A. (2005). Beliefs about medications: a questionnaire survey of people with rheumatoid arthritis. *Rheumatology, 44*(6), 762–767.

Neame, R., Hammond, A., & Deighton, C. (2005). Need for information and for involvement in decision making among patients with rheumatoid arthritis: A questionnaire survey. *Arthritis Care & Research, 53*(2), 249–255.

Knowledge: Asthma Management 1832

Definition: Extent of understanding conveyed about asthma, its treatment, and the prevention of complications

OUTCOME TARGET RATING: Maintain at_____ Increase to_____

		No knowledge	Limited knowledge	Moderate knowledge	Substantial knowledge	Extensive knowledge	
OUTCOME OVERALL RATING		1	2	3	4	5	
Indicators:							
183201	Signs and symptoms of asthma	1	2	3	4	5	NA
183202	Benefits of disease management	1	2	3	4	5	NA
183203	Cause and contributing factors	1	2	3	4	5	NA
183204	Usual course of disease	1	2	3	4	5	NA
183205	Potential complications of asthma	1	2	3	4	5	NA
183206	Strategies to manage asthma	1	2	3	4	5	NA
183207	Asthma management goals	1	2	3	4	5	NA
183208	Importance of continual access to inhaler	1	2	3	4	5	NA
183209	Effects on lifestyle	1	2	3	4	5	NA
183210	Relationship of physical and emotional stress to condition	1	2	3	4	5	NA
183211	Importance of compliance with treatment regimen	1	2	3	4	5	NA
183212	Importance of compliance with medication regimen	1	2	3	4	5	NA
183213	Actions to take in an emergency	1	2	3	4	5	NA
183214	Options for assistance with medical emergencies	1	2	3	4	5	NA
183215	Proper technique to measure peak expiratory flow	1	2	3	4	5	NA
183216	When to use peak flow meter	1	2	3	4	5	NA
183217	Conditions that trigger asthma	1	2	3	4	5	NA
183218	Strategies to manage controllable environmental risk factors	1	2	3	4	5	NA
183219	Benefits of ongoing self-monitoring	1	2	3	4	5	NA
183220	Effective breathing techniques	1	2	3	4	5	NA
183221	Recommended physical activity	1	2	3	4	5	NA
183222	Activity restrictions	1	2	3	4	5	NA
183223	Leisure activity recommendations	1	2	3	4	5	NA
183224	Medication used for asthma	1	2	3	4	5	NA
183225	Strategies to balance activity and rest	1	2	3	4	5	NA
183226	Medication therapeutic effects	1	2	3	4	5	NA
183227	Medication side effects	1	2	3	4	5	NA
183228	Medication adverse effects	1	2	3	4	5	NA
183229	When to obtain assistance from a health professional	1	2	3	4	5	NA
183230	When to obtain emergency treatment	1	2	3	4	5	NA
183231	Available support groups	1	2	3	4	5	NA
183232	Available community resources	1	2	3	4	5	NA
183233	Reputable sources of asthma information	1	2	3	4	5	NA

Domain-Health Knowledge & Behavior (IV) **Class**-Health Knowledge (S) *4th edition 2008; revised 2013*

OUTCOME CONTENT REFERENCES:
American Academy of Allergy, Asthma, and Immunology (AAAAI). (1999). Pediatric asthma: Promoting best practice guide for managing asthma. Milwaukee, WI: Author.
Baker, V., Friedman, J., & Schmitt, R. (2002a). Asthma management, part I: An overview of the problem and current trends. *Journal of School Nursing, 18*(3), 128–137.
Baker, V., Friedman, J., & Schmitt, R. (2002b). Asthma management, part II: Pharmacologic management. *Journal of School Nursing, 18*(5), 257–269.
Lung, C. L., & Lung, M. L. (2003). General principles of asthma management: Symptom monitoring. *Nursing Clinics of North America, 38*(4), 585–596.
National Heart, Lung, and Blood Institute and National Asthma Education and Prevention Program (NAEPP). (2007). *Expert panel report 3: Guidelines for the diagnosis and management of asthma* (Publication No. 07-4051). Bethesda, MD: U.S. Department of Health and Human Services.
Yawn, B. P. (2005). Asthma. In D. L. Huber (Ed.), *Disease management: A guide for case managers* (pp. 100–131). St. Louis: Elsevier Saunders.
Yoos, H. L., Philipson, E., McMullen, A. (2003). Asthma management across the life span: The child with asthma. *Nursing Clinics of North America, 38*(4), 635–652.

Knowledge: Body Mechanics 1827

Definition: Extent of understanding conveyed about proper body alignment, balance and coordinated movement

OUTCOME TARGET RATING: Maintain at_____   Increase to_____

		No knowledge	Limited knowledge	Moderate knowledge	Substantial knowledge	Extensive knowledge	
OUTCOME OVERALL RATING		1	2	3	4	5	
Indicators:							
182701	Natural spinal curves	1	2	3	4	5	NA
182702	Proper standing posture	1	2	3	4	5	NA
182703	Proper sitting posture	1	2	3	4	5	NA
182704	Proper lying posture	1	2	3	4	5	NA
182705	Proper lifting techniques	1	2	3	4	5	NA
182706	Exercises to improve posture	1	2	3	4	5	NA
182707	Exercises to improve muscle flexibility	1	2	3	4	5	NA
182708	Exercises to improve joint mobility	1	2	3	4	5	NA
182709	Exercises to improve muscle strength	1	2	3	4	5	NA
182710	Exercises to strengthen lower abdominal muscles	1	2	3	4	5	NA
182711	Positional causes of muscle or joint pain from sitting	1	2	3	4	5	NA
182712	Positional causes of muscle or joint pain from lying	1	2	3	4	5	NA
182713	Positional causes of muscle or joint pain from lifting	1	2	3	4	5	NA
182714	Common symptoms of back injury	1	2	3	4	5	NA
182715	Personal risk activities	1	2	3	4	5	NA

Domain-Health Knowledge & Behavior (IV)   **Class**-Health Knowledge (S)   *3rd edition 2004; revised 2008*

OUTCOME CONTENT REFERENCES:
American Physical Therapy Association. (1996). *Taking care of your back: A physical therapist's perspective*. Washington, DC: Author.
American Physical Therapy Association. (2000). *The secret of good posture: A physical therapist's perspective*. Washington, DC: Author.
Lieber, S. J., Rudy, T. E., & Boston, R. (1999). Effects of body mechanics training on performance of repetitive lifting. *The American Journal of Occupational Therapy, 54*(2), 166–175.
McConnell, E. A. (2002). Clinical do's & don'ts. Using proper body mechanics. *Nursing 2002, 32*(15), 17.
Neal, C. (1997). The assessment of knowledge and application of proper body mechanics in the workplace. *Orthopaedic Nursing, 16*(1), 66–69.
Perry, A. G., & Potter, P. A. (1998). *Clinical nursing skills and techniques*. (4th ed., pp. 877–884). St. Louis: Mosby.
Porteau-Cassard, L., Zabraniecki, L., Dromer, C., & Fournie, B. (1999). A back school program at the Toulouse-Purpan teaching hospital. Evaluation of 144 patients. *Revue Du Rhumatisme, English Edition, 66*(10), 477–483.
Richardson, C. A., Snijders, C. J., Hides, J. A., Damen, L., Pas, M. S., & Storm, J. (2002). The relation between the transversus abdominis muscles, sacroiliac joint mechanics, and low back pain. *Spine, 27*(4), 399–405.
Sorrentino, S. A. (2000). *Mosby's textbook for nursing assistants*. (5th ed., pp. 242–247). St. Louis: Mosby.

K

Knowledge: Bottle Feeding

1846

Definition: Extent of understanding conveyed about providing fluids to an infant using a bottle

OUTCOME TARGET RATING: Maintain at_____ Increase to_____

		No knowledge	Limited knowledge	Moderate knowledge	Substantial knowledge	Extensive knowledge	
OUTCOME OVERALL RATING		1	2	3	4	5	
Indicators:							
184601	Infant hunger cues	1	2	3	4	5	NA
184602	Safety of different types of bottles	1	2	3	4	5	NA
184603	Proper nipple type and hole size	1	2	3	4	5	NA
184604	Importance of hand sanitation	1	2	3	4	5	NA
184605	Preparation of infant formula	1	2	3	4	5	NA
184606	Methods to clean bottles and nipples	1	2	3	4	5	NA
184607	Proper storage of milk	1	2	3	4	5	NA
184608	Proper storage of mixed formula	1	2	3	4	5	NA
184609	Importance of checking expiration date	1	2	3	4	5	NA
184610	Proper methods to warm bottle	1	2	3	4	5	NA
184611	Importance of testing temperature of fluid prior to feeding infant	1	2	3	4	5	NA
184612	Proper infant positioning while feeding	1	2	3	4	5	NA
184613	Proper bottle position while feeding	1	2	3	4	5	NA
184614	Methods to burp infant	1	2	3	4	5	NA
184615	Importance of burping at periodic intervals	1	2	3	4	5	NA
184616	Infant cues to stop feeding	1	2	3	4	5	NA
184617	Reasons for avoidance of water for newborn	1	2	3	4	5	NA
184618	Proper technique to respond to choking	1	2	3	4	5	NA

Domain-Health Knowledge & Behavior (IV)   **Class**-Health Knowledge (S)   5th edition 2013

OUTCOME CONTENT REFERENCES:
Borghese-Lang, T., Morrison, L., Ogle, A., & Wright, A. (2003). Successful bottle feeding of the young infant. _Journal of Pediatric Health Care, 17_(2), 94–101.
Lowdermilk, D., & Perry, S. (2007). _Maternity & women's health care_ (9th ed.). Philadelphia: Elsevier.
Hockenberry, J. J., Wilson, D., & Winkelstein, M. L. (2005). _Wong's essentials of pediatric nursing._ (7th ed.). St. Louis: Mosby.
Thomas, J. (2007). A parent's guide to bottle feeding your premature baby. _Advances in Neonatal Care, 7_(6), 319–320.

Knowledge: Breastfeeding 1800

Definition: Extent of understanding conveyed about lactation and nourishment of an infant through breastfeeding

OUTCOME TARGET RATING: Maintain at_____ Increase to_____

OUTCOME OVERALL RATING	No knowledge 1	Limited knowledge 2	Moderate knowledge 3	Substantial knowledge 4	Extensive knowledge 5	
Indicators:						
180001 Benefits of breastfeeding	1	2	3	4	5	NA
180002 Physiology of lactation	1	2	3	4	5	NA
180020 Fluid intake requirements for mother	1	2	3	4	5	NA
180003 Breastmilk composition, letdown process, foremilk versus hindmilk	1	2	3	4	5	NA
180004 Infant hunger cues	1	2	3	4	5	NA
180005 Proper technique for attaching infant to the breast	1	2	3	4	5	NA
180006 Proper infant positioning while nursing	1	2	3	4	5	NA
180007 Nutritive versus non-nutritive sucking	1	2	3	4	5	NA
180008 Evaluation of infant swallowing	1	2	3	4	5	NA
180009 Proper technique to break infant suction	1	2	3	4	5	NA
180024 Methods to burp infant	1	2	3	4	5	NA
180010 Signs of adequate milk supply	1	2	3	4	5	NA
180011 Signs of well-nourished infant	1	2	3	4	5	NA
180012 Nipple evaluation	1	2	3	4	5	NA
180013 Signs of mastitis, blocked ducts, nipple trauma	1	2	3	4	5	NA
180014 Reasons for early avoidance of artificial nipples	1	2	3	4	5	NA
180021 Reasons for avoidance of water and supplements for infant	1	2	3	4	5	NA
180015 Proper breastmilk expression and storage techniques	1	2	3	4	5	NA
180016 Substances that transfer from mother to infant through breastmilk	1	2	3	4	5	NA
180022 Relationship between breastfeeding and infant immunity	1	2	3	4	5	NA
180017 Signs of weaning readiness	1	2	3	4	5	NA
180018 Strategies to access health care services	1	2	3	4	5	NA
180023 Available support groups	1	2	3	4	5	NA

Domain-Health Knowledge & Behavior (IV)   **Class**-Health Knowledge (S)   *1st edition 1997; revised 2004, 2008, 2013*

OUTCOME CONTENT REFERENCES:
Biancizzo, M. (2003). *Breastfeeding the newborn* (2nd ed.). St. Louis: Mosby.
Dowling, D., & Thanattherakul, W. (2001). Nipple confusion, alternative feeding methods, and breast-feeding supplementation: State of the science. *Newborn and Infant Nursing Reviews. 1*(4), 217–223.
Giglia, R., & Binns, C. (2006). Alcohol and lactation: A systematic review. *Nutrition & Dietetics, 63*(2), 103–116.
Lawrence, R. A., & Lawrence, R. M. (1999). *Breastfeeding: A guide for the medical profession* (5th ed.). St. Louis: Mosby.
Li, R., Rock, V. J., & Grummer-Strawn, L. (2007). Changes in public attitudes toward breastfeeding in the United States, 1999–2003. *Journal of the American Dietetic Association, 107*(1), 122–127.
Lovelady, C. A., Fuller, C. J., Geigerman, C. M., Hunter, C. P., & Kinsella, T. A. (2004). Immune status of physically active women during lactation. *Medicine & Science in Sports & Exercise, 36*(6), 1001–1007.
McCarter-Spaulding, D. E. (2005). Medications in pregnancy and lactation. *MCN: American Journal of Maternal Child Nursing. 30*(1), 24–29.
Shrago, L., & Bocar, D. (1990). The infant's contribution to breastfeeding. *Journal of Obstetric, Gynecologic, and Neonatal Nursing, 19*(3), 209–213.
Spangler, A. (1992). *Amy Spangler's breastfeeding: A parent's guide*. Atlanta: A. Spangler.
Walker, M. (1989). Functional assessment of infant breastfeeding patterns. *Birth: Issues in Perinatal Care and Education, 16*(3), 140–147.

K

Knowledge: Cancer Management   1833

Definition: Extent of understanding conveyed about cancer, its treatment and the prevention of disease progression and complications

OUTCOME TARGET RATING: Maintain at_____   Increase to_____

		No knowledge	Limited knowledge	Moderate knowledge	Substantial knowledge	Extensive knowledge	
OUTCOME OVERALL RATING		1	2	3	4	5	
Indicators:							
183301	Abnormal screening results	1	2	3	4	5	NA
183302	Signs and symptoms of cancer	1	2	3	4	5	NA
183303	Specific cancer diagnosis	1	2	3	4	5	NA
183304	Cause and contributing factors	1	2	3	4	5	NA
183305	Usual course of disease	1	2	3	4	5	NA
183306	Stages of cancer	1	2	3	4	5	NA
183307	Signs and symptoms of recurrence	1	2	3	4	5	NA
183308	Available treatment options	1	2	3	4	5	NA
183309	Alternative treatments	1	2	3	4	5	NA
183310	Purpose of different treatment options	1	2	3	4	5	NA
183311	Benefits of different treatment options	1	2	3	4	5	NA
183312	Tests and procedures involved in treatment regimen	1	2	3	4	5	NA
183313	Steps in treatment regimen	1	2	3	4	5	NA
183314	Medication therapeutic effects	1	2	3	4	5	NA
183315	Medication adverse effects	1	2	3	4	5	NA
183316	Medication side effects	1	2	3	4	5	NA
183317	Potential complications of treatment	1	2	3	4	5	NA
183318	Signs and symptoms of complications	1	2	3	4	5	NA
183319	Precautions to prevent complications of treatment	1	2	3	4	5	NA
183320	Self-care responsibilities for ongoing treatment	1	2	3	4	5	NA
183321	Physical effects of cancer treatment	1	2	3	4	5	NA
183322	Effects on lifestyle	1	2	3	4	5	NA
183323	Effects on employment	1	2	3	4	5	NA
183324	Effects on sexuality	1	2	3	4	5	NA
183325	Strategies to cope with adverse effects of disease	1	2	3	4	5	NA
183326	Survival rate	1	2	3	4	5	NA
183327	Self-care issues during recovery	1	2	3	4	5	NA
183328	Importance of positive attitude for coping with cancer	1	2	3	4	5	NA
183335	Importance of informing genetic risk to family members	1	2	3	4	5	NA
183329	Reputable sources of cancer information	1	2	3	4	5	NA
183330	Available community resources	1	2	3	4	5	NA
183331	Available support groups	1	2	3	4	5	NA
183332	Financial resources for assistance	1	2	3	4	5	NA
183333	Health beliefs that affect adherence to treatment	1	2	3	4	5	NA
183334	Benefits of disease management	1	2	3	4	5	NA

Specify cancer: _____

Domain-Health Knowledge & Behavior (IV)   *Class*-Health Knowledge (S)   *4th edition 2008; revised 2013*

OUTCOME CONTENT REFERENCES:

Carlson, R. (2006, August 10). HPV vaccine, now FDA-approved, shown to protect against vaginal, vulvar intraepithelial neoplasias. *Oncology Times Meeting Reporter*, pp. 2–3.

Dein, S. (2004). Explanatory models of and attitudes towards cancer in different cultures. *The Lancet Oncology, 5*(2), 119–124.

Rutten, L. J., Arora, N. K., Bakos, A. D., Aziz, N., & Rowland, J. (2005). Information needs and sources of information among cancer patients: A systematic review of research (1980–2003). *Patient Education and Counseling, 57*(3), 250–261.

Shokar, N. K., Veron, S. W., & Weller, S. C. (2005). Cancer and colorectal cancer: Knowledge, beliefs, and screening preferences of a diverse patient population. *Family Medicine, 37*(5), 341–347.

Sterman, E., Gauker, S., & Krieger, J. (2003). A comprehensive approach to improving cancer pain management and patient satisfaction. *Oncology Nursing Forum, 30*(5), 857–864.

Waller, J., McCaffery, K., & Wardle, J. (2004). Measuring cancer knowledge: Comparing prompted and unprompted recall. *British Journal of Psychology, 95*(Pt 2), 219–234.

Knowledge: Cancer Threat Reduction 1834

Definition: Extent of understanding conveyed about causes, prevention and early detection of cancer

OUTCOME TARGET RATING: Maintain at_____   Increase to_____

		No knowledge	Limited knowledge	Moderate knowledge	Substantial knowledge	Extensive knowledge	
OUTCOME OVERALL RATING		1	2	3	4	5	
Indicators:							
183401	Warning signs of cancer	1	2	3	4	5	NA
183402	Cause and contributing factors	1	2	3	4	5	NA
183421	Genetic risk factors	1	2	3	4	5	NA
183403	Genetic testing	1	2	3	4	5	NA
183404	Recommended cancer screenings	1	2	3	4	5	NA
183405	Cancer screening procedures	1	2	3	4	5	NA
183406	Recommended self-screenings for cancer detection	1	2	3	4	5	NA
183407	Benefits of adequate sleep	1	2	3	4	5	NA
183408	Benefits of regular exercise	1	2	3	4	5	NA
183409	Importance of oral screening	1	2	3	4	5	NA
183410	Diet recommendations for reducing risk	1	2	3	4	5	NA
183411	Correct use of nutritional supplements	1	2	3	4	5	NA
183412	Correct use of prescribed medication	1	2	3	4	5	NA
183413	Strategies to avoid exposure to carcinogens	1	2	3	4	5	NA
183414	Strategies to protect skin from sun exposure	1	2	3	4	5	NA
183415	Strategies to prevent cervical cancer	1	2	3	4	5	NA
183416	Strategies to manage controllable environmental risk factors	1	2	3	4	5	NA
183417	Adverse health effects of tobacco use	1	2	3	4	5	NA
183418	Safe sexual practices	1	2	3	4	5	NA
183419	When to obtain assistance from a health professional	1	2	3	4	5	NA
183420	Reputable sources of cancer prevention information	1	2	3	4	5	NA

Domain-*Health Knowledge & Behavior (IV)*   **Class**-*Health Knowledge (S)*   *4th edition 2008; revised 2013*

OUTCOME CONTENT REFERENCES:

Carlson, R. (2006, August 10). HPV vaccine, now FDA-approved, shown to protect against vaginal, vulvar intraepithelial neoplasias. *Oncology Times Meeting Reporter*, pp. 2–3.

Patterson, R. E., Kristal, A. R., & White, E. (1996). Do beliefs, knowledge, and perceived norms about diet and cancer predict dietary change? *American Journal of Public Health, 86*(10), 1394–1400.

Rutten, L. J. F., Arora, N. K., Bakos, A. D., Aziz, N., & Rowland, J. (2005). Information needs and sources of information among cancer patients: A systematic review of research (1980–2003). *Patient Education and Counseling, 57*(3), 250–261.

Waller, J., McCaffery, K., & Wardle, J. (2004). Measuring cancer knowledge: Comparing prompted and unprompted recall. *British Journal of Psychology, 95*(Pt 2), 219–234.

Knowledge: Cardiac Disease Management 　1830

Definition: Extent of understanding conveyed about heart disease, its treatment, and the prevention of disease progression and complications

OUTCOME TARGET RATING: Maintain at_____ 　Increase to_____

OUTCOME OVERALL RATING	No knowledge	Limited knowledge	Moderate knowledge	Substantial knowledge	Extensive knowledge	
	1	2	3	4	5	
Indicators:						
183001 Usual course of disease	1	2	3	4	5	NA
183002 Signs and symptoms of early disease	1	2	3	4	5	NA
183003 Signs and symptoms of worsening disease	1	2	3	4	5	NA
183004 Benefits of disease management	1	2	3	4	5	NA
183005 Strategies to reduce risk factors	1	2	3	4	5	NA
183028 Strategies to decrease treatment side effects	1	2	3	4	5	NA
183006 Importance of completing cardiac rehabilitation	1	2	3	4	5	NA
183007 Family's role in treatment plan	1	2	3	4	5	NA
183008 Methods to measure blood pressure	1	2	3	4	5	NA
183029 Methods to monitor heart rate	1	2	3	4	5	NA
183009 Strategies to limit sodium intake	1	2	3	4	5	NA
183010 Benefits of following a low-fat, low-cholesterol diet	1	2	3	4	5	NA
183011 Strategies to increase diet compliance	1	2	3	4	5	NA
183012 Strategies to limit fluid intake	1	2	3	4	5	NA
183013 Importance of monitoring weight	1	2	3	4	5	NA
183014 Importance of alcohol restrictions	1	2	3	4	5	NA
183015 Importance of tobacco abstinence	1	2	3	4	5	NA
183030 Recommended work activity	1	2	3	4	5	NA
183031 Recommended physical activity	1	2	3	4	5	NA
183032 Recommended leisure activity	1	2	3	4	5	NA
183017 Benefits of regular exercise	1	2	3	4	5	NA
183018 Energy conservation techniques	1	2	3	4	5	NA
183019 Guidelines for sexual activity	1	2	3	4	5	NA
183020 Potential sexual difficulties	1	2	3	4	5	NA
183021 Medication therapeutic effects	1	2	3	4	5	NA
183033 Medication side effects	1	2	3	4	5	NA
183034 Medication adverse effects						
183022 Strategies to manage stress	1	2	3	4	5	NA
183038 Importance of obtaining influenza seasonal vaccine	1	2	3	4	5	NA
183039 Importance of obtaining pneumonia vaccine	1	2	3	4	5	NA
183035 When to obtain assistance from a health professional	1	2	3	4	5	NA
183025 Care options for assistance with medical emergencies	1	2	3	4	5	NA
183026 Importance of family learning cardiopulmonary resuscitation	1	2	3	4	5	NA
183027 Cultural influences on compliance to treatment regimen	1	2	3	4	5	NA
183036 Available support groups	1	2	3	4	5	NA
183037 Reputable sources of cardiac disease information	1	2	3	4	5	NA

Domain-Health Knowledge & Behavior (IV) 　*Class*-Health Knowledge (S) 　*3rd edition 2004; revised 2008, 2013*

OUTCOME CONTENT REFERENCES:

Alm-Roijer, C., Stagmo, M., Uden, G., & Erhardt, L. (2004). Better knowledge improves adherence to lifestyle changes and medication in patients with coronary heart disease. *European Journal of Cardiovascular Nursing, 3*(4), 321–330.

Cannon, C., Battler, A., Brindis, R., Cox, J., Ellis, S., Every, N., Flaherty, J., Harrington, R., Krumholz, H., Simoons, M., Van De Werf, F., & Weintraub, W. S. (2001). ACC key data elements and definitions for measuring the clinical management and outcomes of patients with acute coronary syndromes: A report of the American College of Cardiology task force on clinical data standards. *Journal of the American College of Cardiology, 38*(7), 2114–2130.

Dunbar, S. B., Jacobson, L. H., & Deaton, C. (1998). Heart failure: Strategies to enhance patient self-management. *AACN Clinical Issues: Advanced Practice in Acute & Critical Care, 9*(2), 244–256.

Dusseldorp, E., Van Elderan, T., Maes, S., Meulman, J., & Kraaij, V. (1999). A meta-analysis of psychoeducational programs for coronary heart disease patients. *Health Psychology, 18*(5), 506–519.

Johnson, J., & Pearson, V. (2000). The effects of a structured education course on stroke survivors living in the community. *Rehabilitation Nursing, 25*(2), 59–65.

Kimble, L. P., & Kunik, C. L. (2000). Knowledge and use of sublingual nitroglycerin and cardiac-related quality of life in patients with chronic stable angina. *Journal of Pain & Symptom Management, 19*(2), 109–117.

Silcox, P. D. (2005). Congestive heart failure. In D. L. Huber (Ed.), *Disease management: A guide for case managers* (pp. 71–80). St. Louis: Elsevier Saunders.

Knowledge: Child Physical Safety   1801

Definition: Extent of understanding conveyed about safely caring for a child from 1 year through 17 years of age

OUTCOME TARGET RATING: Maintain at_____　　Increase to_____

OUTCOME OVERALL RATING		No knowledge	Limited knowledge	Moderate knowledge	Substantial knowledge	Extensive knowledge	
		1	2	3	4	5	
Indicators:							
180101	Appropriate activities for child's developmental level	1	2	3	4	5	NA
180119	Diving hazards	1	2	3	4	5	NA
180103	Strategies to prevent drowning	1	2	3	4	5	NA
180104	Strategies to prevent electrical shock	1	2	3	4	5	NA
180105	Benefits of protective helmet	1	2	3	4	5	NA
180120	First-aid techniques	1	2	3	4	5	NA
180108	Correct use of safety seats and seat belts	1	2	3	4	5	NA
180121	Age-appropriate cardiopulmonary resuscitation techniques	1	2	3	4	5	NA
180122	Heimlich maneuver	1	2	3	4	5	NA
180106	Strategies to prevent choking	1	2	3	4	5	NA
180111	Strategies to prevent farm accidents	1	2	3	4	5	NA
180123	Strategies to prevent motor vehicle accidents	1	2	3	4	5	NA
180124	Strategies to prevent cycle accidents	1	2	3	4	5	NA
180112	Strategies to prevent falls	1	2	3	4	5	NA
180113	Strategies to prevent playground accidents	1	2	3	4	5	NA
180114	Strategies to prevent burns	1	2	3	4	5	NA
180115	Correct use of smoke detectors	1	2	3	4	5	NA
180116	Proper surveillance of outdoor play	1	2	3	4	5	NA
180117	Importance of teaching stranger awareness	1	2	3	4	5	NA
180125	Strategies to prevent tobacco use	1	2	3	4	5	NA
180126	Strategies to prevent alcohol use	1	2	3	4	5	NA
180127	Strategies to prevent recreational drug use	1	2	3	4	5	NA
180128	Strategies to prevent firearm injuries	1	2	3	4	5	NA
180129	Strategies to prevent participation in violence	1	2	3	4	5	NA
180130	Strategies to prevent medication misuse	1	2	3	4	5	NA
180131	Strategies to prevent exposure to toxic chemicals	1	2	3	4	5	NA

Domain-*Health Knowledge & Behavior (IV)*　　**Class**-*Health Knowledge (S)*　　*1st edition 1997; revised 2004, 2008*

OUTCOME CONTENT REFERENCES:

Eichelberger, M. R., Gotschall, C. S., Feely, H. B., Harstad, P., & Bowman, L. M. (1990). Parental attitudes and knowledge of child safety. *American Journal of Diseases of Children, 144*(6), 714–720.

Gilk, D., Kronenfeld, J., & Jackson, K. (1993). Safety behaviors among parents of preschoolers. *Health Values, 17*(1), 18–25.

Grossman, D. C., & Rivera, F. P. (1992). Injury control in childhood. *Pediatric Clinics of North America, 39*(3), 471–484.

Rivera, F. P., & Howard, D. (1982). Parental knowledge of child development and injury risks. *Developmental and Behavioral Pediatrics, 3*(2), 103–105.

Wortel, E., Geus, G. H., Kok, G., & van Woerkum, C. (1994). Injury control in pre-school children: A review of parental safety measures and the behavioral determinants. *Health Education Research, 9*(2), 201–213.

Knowledge: Chronic Disease Management   1847

Definition: Extent of understanding conveyed about a specific chronic disease, its treatment, and the prevention of disease progression and complications

OUTCOME TARGET RATING: Maintain at_____   Increase to_____

OUTCOME OVERALL RATING	No knowledge 1	Limited knowledge 2	Moderate knowledge 3	Substantial knowledge 4	Extensive knowledge 5	
Indicators:						
184701 Cause and contributing factors	1	2	3	4	5	NA
184702 Usual course of disease	1	2	3	4	5	NA
184703 Benefits of disease management	1	2	3	4	5	NA
184704 Signs and symptoms of chronic disease	1	2	3	4	5	NA
184705 Signs and symptoms of disease progression	1	2	3	4	5	NA
184706 Signs and symptoms of complications	1	2	3	4	5	NA
184707 Strategies to prevent complications	1	2	3	4	5	NA
184708 Strategies to balance activity and rest	1	2	3	4	5	NA
184709 Strategies to manage pain	1	2	3	4	5	NA
184710 Available treatment options	1	2	3	4	5	NA
184711 Correct use of prescribed medication	1	2	3	4	5	NA
184712 Medication therapeutic effects	1	2	3	4	5	NA
184713 Medication side effects	1	2	3	4	5	NA
184714 Medication adverse effects	1	2	3	4	5	NA
184715 Potential medication interactions	1	2	3	4	5	NA
184716 Required laboratory tests	1	2	3	4	5	NA
184717 Procedures involved in treatment regimen	1	2	3	4	5	NA
184718 Personal responsibilities for treatment regimen	1	2	3	4	5	NA
184719 Importance of compliance with treatment regimen	1	2	3	4	5	NA
184720 Recommended immunizations	1	2	3	4	5	NA
184721 Cultural influences on compliance to treatment regimen	1	2	3	4	5	NA
184722 Prescribed diet	1	2	3	4	5	NA
184723 Strategies for tobacco cessation	1	2	3	4	5	NA
184724 Strategies to cope with adverse effects of disease	1	2	3	4	5	NA
184725 Financial resources for assistance	1	2	3	4	5	NA
184726 Available support groups	1	2	3	4	5	NA
184727 Available community resources	1	2	3	4	5	NA
184728 Reputable sources of chronic disease information related to disease	1	2	3	4	5	NA
184729 When to obtain assistance from a health professional	1	2	3	4	5	NA
184730 Actions to take in an emergency	1	2	3	4	5	NA

Domain-Health Knowledge & Behavior (IV)   ***Class**-Health Knowledge (S)*   *5th edition 2013*

OUTCOME CONTENT REFERENCES:
Bourbeau, J. (2008). Clinical decision processes and patient engagement in self-management. *Disease Manage Health Outcome 16*(6), 327–333.
Chen, K. H., Chen, M. L., Lee, S., Cho, H. Y., & Weng, L. C. (2008). Self-management behaviours for patients with chronic obstructive pulmonary disease: A qualitative study. *Journal of Advanced Nursing 64*(6), 595–604.
Gallagher, R., Donoghue, J., Chenoweth, L., & Stein-Parbury, J. (2008). Self-management in older patients with chronic illness. *International Journal of Nursing Practice, 14*(5), 373–382.
Hibbard, J. H., Greene, J., & Tusler, M. (2009). Improving the outcomes of disease management by tailoring care to the patient's level of activation. *The American Journal of Managed Care, 15*(6), 353–360.
Rosser, B. A., & Eccleaton, C. E. (2009). Promoting self-management through technology: SMART solutions for long-term health conditions. *Journal of Integrated Care, 17*(6), 10–19.

Knowledge: Chronic Obstructive Pulmonary Disease Management   1848

Definition: Extent of understanding conveyed about chronic obstructive pulmonary disease, its treatment, and the prevention of disease progression and complications

OUTCOME TARGET RATING: Maintain at_____   Increase to_____

		No knowledge	Limited knowledge	Moderate knowledge	Substantial knowledge	Extensive knowledge	
OUTCOME OVERALL RATING		1	2	3	4	5	
Indicators:							
184801	Cause and contributing factors	1	2	3	4	5	NA
184802	Specific disease process	1	2	3	4	5	NA
184803	Risk factors for disease progression	1	2	3	4	5	NA
184804	Signs and symptoms of chronic obstructive pulmonary disease	1	2	3	4	5	NA
184805	Signs and symptoms of disease relapse	1	2	3	4	5	NA
184806	Benefits of disease management	1	2	3	4	5	NA
184807	Signs and symptoms of complications	1	2	3	4	5	NA
184808	Strategies to prevent complications	1	2	3	4	5	NA
184809	Strategies to adapt lifestyle to energy level	1	2	3	4	5	NA
184810	Strategies to balance activity and rest	1	2	3	4	5	NA
184811	Energy conservation techniques	1	2	3	4	5	NA
184812	Medication therapeutic effects	1	2	3	4	5	NA
184813	Medication side effects	1	2	3	4	5	NA
184814	Medication adverse effects	1	2	3	4	5	NA
184815	Correct use of prescribed medication	1	2	3	4	5	NA
184816	Importance of completing prescribed antibiotics	1	2	3	4	5	NA
184817	Correct use of inhaler	1	2	3	4	5	NA
184818	Safety issues related to oxygen use	1	2	3	4	5	NA
184819	Actions to take in an emergency	1	2	3	4	5	NA
184820	Importance of compliance with treatment regimen	1	2	3	4	5	NA
184821	Importance of compliance with medication regimen	1	2	3	4	5	NA
184822	Prescribed procedures	1	2	3	4	5	NA
184823	Adequate fluid intake	1	2	3	4	5	NA
184824	Strategies to manage chronic obstructive pulmonary disease	1	2	3	4	5	NA
184825	Strategies for smoking cessation	1	2	3	4	5	NA
184826	Strategies to prevent disease progression	1	2	3	4	5	NA
184827	Strategies to manage controllable environmental risk factors	1	2	3	4	5	NA
184828	Effective breathing techniques	1	2	3	4	5	NA
184829	Effects on lifestyle	1	2	3	4	5	NA
184830	When to obtain assistance from a health professional	1	2	3	4	5	NA
184831	When to obtain emergency treatment	1	2	3	4	5	NA
184832	Importance of obtaining pneumonia vaccine	1	2	3	4	5	NA
184833	Importance of obtaining influenza seasonal vaccine	1	2	3	4	5	NA
184834	Importance of follow-up care	1	2	3	4	5	NA
184835	Benefits of pulmonary rehabilitation program	1	2	3	4	5	NA
184836	Available support groups	1	2	3	4	5	NA
184837	Available community resources	1	2	3	4	5	NA

K

***Domain**-Health Knowledge & Behavior (IV)*   ***Class**-Health Knowledge (S)*   *5th edition 2013*

OUTCOME CONTENT REFERENCES:

Horsley, L. (2008). ACP guideline recommends diagnosis and management strategies for COPD. *American Family Physician, 78*(3), 401–402.

Kuebler, K. K., Buchsel, P. C., Balkstra, C. R. (2008). Differentiating chronic obstructive pulmonary disease from asthma. *Journal of the American Academy of Nurse Practitioners, 20*(9), 445–454.

Kuzma, A. M., Meli, Y., Meldrum, C., Jellen, P., Butler-Lebair, M., Koczen-Doyle, D., Rising, P., Stavrolakes, K., & Brogan, F. (2008). Multidisciplinary care of the patient with chronic obstructive pulmonary disease. *Proceedings of the American Thoracic Society, 5*(4), 567–571.

Kyung, K. A., Chin, P. A., (2007). The effect of a pulmonary rehabilitation programme on older patients with chronic pulmonary disease. *Journal of Clinical Nursing, 17*(1), 118–125.

Lewis, S. L., Heitkemper, M. M., Dirksen, S. R., O'Brien, P. G., & Bucher, L. (2007). *Medical-surgical nursing: Assessment and management of clinical problems* Philadelphia: Mosby.

Ries, A. L. (2008). Pulmonary rehabilitation: Summary of an evidence-based guideline. *Respiratory Care, 53*(9), 1203–1207.

Knowledge: Conception Prevention — 1821

Definition: Extent of understanding conveyed about prevention of unintended pregnancy

OUTCOME TARGET RATING: Maintain at_____   Increase to_____

		No knowledge	Limited knowledge	Moderate knowledge	Substantial knowledge	Extensive knowledge	
OUTCOME OVERALL RATING		1	2	3	4	5	
Indicators:							
182105	How conception occurs	1	2	3	4	5	NA
182116	Advantages of having a child	1	2	3	4	5	NA
182117	Disadvantages of having a child	1	2	3	4	5	NA
182107	Influence of personal values on chosen contraceptive method	1	2	3	4	5	NA
182108	Periodic rhythm method	1	2	3	4	5	NA
182109	Chemical barrier methods	1	2	3	4	5	NA
182110	Hormonal therapy methods	1	2	3	4	5	NA
182111	Mechanical barrier methods	1	2	3	4	5	NA
182112	Surgical treatment options	1	2	3	4	5	NA
182101	How chosen contraceptive method works	1	2	3	4	5	NA
182102	Correct use of chosen contraceptive method	1	2	3	4	5	NA
182103	Effectiveness of chosen contraceptive method	1	2	3	4	5	NA
182104	Effects of chosen contraceptive on sexually transmitted disease transmission	1	2	3	4	5	NA

Domain-Health Knowledge & Behavior (IV)   **Class**-Health Knowledge (S)   2nd edition 2000; revised 2004, 2008, 2013

OUTCOME CONTENT REFERENCES:

Hatcher, R. A., Trussell, J., Stewart, F., Cates, W., Jr., Stewart, G. K., Guest, F., & Kowal, D. (1998). *Contraceptive technology* (17th ed.). New York: Irvington.

Howard, M. (1991). *How to help your teenager postpone sexual involvement.* Lexington, NY: Continuum.

Miller, B., Card, J., Paikoff, R. J., & Peterson, J. (1992). *Preventing adolescent pregnancy.* Newbury Park, CA: Sage.

K

Knowledge: Coronary Artery Disease Management 1849

Definition: Extent of understanding conveyed about coronary heart disease, its treatment, and the prevention of disease progression and complications

OUTCOME TARGET RATING: Maintain at_____ Increase to_____

		No knowledge	Limited knowledge	Moderate knowledge	Substantial knowledge	Extensive knowledge	
OUTCOME OVERALL RATING		1	2	3	4	5	
Indicators:							
184901	Usual course of disease	1	2	3	4	5	NA
184902	Cause and contributing factors	1	2	3	4	5	NA
184903	Signs and symptoms of early disease	1	2	3	4	5	NA
184904	Signs and symptoms of worsening disease	1	2	3	4	5	NA
184905	Types of pain associated with disease	1	2	3	4	5	NA
184906	Strategies to reduce risk factors	1	2	3	4	5	NA
184907	Importance of completing cardiac rehabilitation	1	2	3	4	5	NA
184908	Methods to monitor blood pressure	1	2	3	4	5	NA
184909	Methods to monitor heart rate	1	2	3	4	5	NA
184910	Methods to monitor heart rhythm	1	2	3	4	5	NA
184911	Benefits of disease management	1	2	3	4	5	NA
184912	Medication schedule	1	2	3	4	5	NA
184913	Medication therapeutic effects	1	2	3	4	5	NA
184914	Medication side effects	1	2	3	4	5	NA
184915	Medication adverse effects						
184916	Importance of limiting sodium intake	1	2	3	4	5	NA
184917	Benefits of following a low-fat, low-cholesterol diet	1	2	3	4	5	NA
184918	Strategies to increase diet compliance	1	2	3	4	5	NA
184919	Strategies to maintain optimal weight	1	2	3	4	5	NA
184920	Benefits of maintaining optimal weight	1	2	3	4	5	NA
184921	Importance of alcohol restrictions	1	2	3	4	5	NA
184922	Importance of tobacco abstinence	1	2	3	4	5	NA
184923	Rationale for regular exercise	1	2	3	4	5	NA
184924	Guidelines for activity level	1	2	3	4	5	NA
184925	Guidelines for sexual activity	1	2	3	4	5	NA
184926	Strategies to prevent blood clots	1	2	3	4	5	NA
184927	Adverse health effects of stress on coronary artery disease	1	2	3	4	5	NA
184928	Adverse health effects of anger on coronary artery disease	1	2	3	4	5	NA
184929	Strategies to manage stress	1	2	3	4	5	NA
184930	Strategies to manage anger	1	2	3	4	5	NA
184931	Importance of obtaining influenza seasonal vaccine	1	2	3	4	5	NA
184932	Importance of obtaining pneumonia vaccine	1	2	3	4	5	NA
184933	Importance of periodic screening of cholesterol level	1	2	3	4	5	NA
184934	Importance of periodic screening of blood glucose level	1	2	3	4	5	NA
184935	Rationale for controlling blood glucose level	1	2	3	4	5	NA
184936	When to obtain assistance from a health professional	1	2	3	4	5	NA
184937	Care options for assistance with medical emergencies	1	2	3	4	5	NA
184938	Family's role in treatment plan	1	2	3	4	5	NA

K

Continued

Knowledge: Coronary Artery Disease Management—*cont'd*

		No knowledge	Limited knowledge	Moderate knowledge	Substantial knowledge	Extensive knowledge	
184939	Importance of family learning cardiopulmonary resuscitation	1	2	3	4	5	NA
184940	Cultural influences on compliance to treatment regimen	1	2	3	4	5	NA
184941	Available support groups	1	2	3	4	5	NA
184942	Reputable sources of cardiac disease information	1	2	3	4	5	NA

Domain-*Health Knowledge & Behavior (IV)* **Class**-*Health Knowledge (S)* *5th edition 2013*

OUTCOME CONTENT REFERENCES:

Arnetz, J., Winblad, U., Hoglund, A., Lindahl, B., Spangberg, K., Wallentin, L., Wang, Y., Ager, J., & Arnetz, B. (2010). Is patient involvement during hospitalization for acute myocardial infarction associated with post-discharge treatment outcome? *Health Expectations, 13*(3), 298–311.

Cannon, C. P., Battler, A., Brindis, R. G., Cox, J. L., Ellis, S. G., Every, N. R., Flaherty, J. T., Harrington, R. A., Krumholz, H. M., Simoons, M. L., Van De Werf, F. J. J., & Weintraub, W. S. (2001). ACC key data elements and definitions for measuring the clinical management and outcomes of patients with acute coronary syndromes: A report of the American College of Cardiology task force on clinical data standards (acute coronary syndrome writing committee). *Journal of the American College of Cardiology, 38,* 2114–2130.

Kimble, L. P., & Kunik, C. L. (2000). Knowledge and use of sublingual nitroglycerin and cardiac-related quality of life in patients with chronic stable angina. *Journal of Pain & Symptom Management, 19*(2), 109–117.

National Heart, Lung, and Blood Institute. (2011). Coronary artery disease. Retrieved from http://www.nhlbi.nih.gov/health/dci/Diseases/Cad/CAD_WhatIs.html

Smeltzer, S., Bare, B., Hinkle, J., & Cheever, K. (2008). *Brunner and Suddarth's textbook of medical-surgical nursing* (11th ed., pp. 859–912). Philadelphia: Lippincott Williams & Wilkins.

Knowledge: Cup Feeding   1850

Definition: Extent of understanding conveyed about providing fluids to an infant using a small cup

OUTCOME TARGET RATING: Maintain at_____   Increase to_____

		No knowledge	Limited knowledge	Moderate knowledge	Substantial knowledge	Extensive knowledge	
OUTCOME OVERALL RATING		1	2	3	4	5	
Indicators:							
185001	Infant hunger cues	1	2	3	4	5	NA
185002	Proper infant positioning while feeding	1	2	3	4	5	NA
185003	Importance of cup sanitation	1	2	3	4	5	NA
185004	Proper storage of milk	1	2	3	4	5	NA
185005	Proper placement of cup brim	1	2	3	4	5	NA
185006	Proper placement of tongue	1	2	3	4	5	NA
185007	Regulation of milk flow	1	2	3	4	5	NA
185008	Time required for feeding	1	2	3	4	5	NA
185009	Methods to monitor infant swallowing	1	2	3	4	5	NA
185010	Proper technique to respond to choking	1	2	3	4	5	NA
185011	Methods to allow infant to pace feeding	1	2	3	4	5	NA
185012	Importance of burping at periodic intervals	1	2	3	4	5	NA
185013	Methods to burp infant	1	2	3	4	5	NA
185014	Infant cues to stop feeding	1	2	3	4	5	NA
185015	Reasons for avoidance of water for newborn	1	2	3	4	5	NA
185016	Signs of well-nourished infant	1	2	3	4	5	NA

Domain-*Health Knowledge & Behavior (IV)* **Class**-*Health Knowledge (S)* *5th edition 2013*

OUTCOME CONTENT REFERENCES:

American Dental Association. (2004). From baby bottle to cup: Choose training cups carefully, use them temporarily. *Journal of the American Dental Association, 135*(3), 387.

Brown, S. J., Alexander, J., & Thomas, P. (1999). Feeding outcome in breast-fed term babies supplemented by cup or bottle. *Midwifery, 15*(2), 92–96.

Cloherty, M., Alexander, J., Holloway, I., Galvin, K., & Inch, S. (2005). The cup-versus-bottle debate: A theme from an ethnographic study of the supplementation of breastfed infants in hospitals in the United Kingdom. *Journal of Human Lactation, 21*(2), 151–162.

Dowling, D. A., Meier, P. P., DiFiore, J. M., Blatz, M., & Martin, R. J. (2002). Cup feeding for preterm infants: Mechanics and safety. *Journal of Human Lactation, 18*(1), 13–20.

Kuehl, J. (1997). Cup feeding the newborn: What you should know. *Journal of Perinatal & Neonatal Nursing, 11*(2), 56–60.

Rocha, N. M., Martinez, F. E., & Jorge, S. M. (2002). Cup or bottle for preterm infants: Effects on oxygen saturation, weight gain and breastfeeding. *Journal of Human Lactation, 18*(2), 132–138.

Samuel, P. (1998). Cup feeding: How and when to use it with term babies. *Practising Midwife, 1*(12), 33–35.

Thorley, V. (1997). Cup feeding: Problems created by incorrect use. *Journal of Human Lactation, 13*(1), 54–55.

Knowledge: Dementia Management 1851

Definition: Extent of understanding conveyed about progressive dementia, its course over an extended period of time, and plan for supportive care as the disease progresses

OUTCOME TARGET RATING: Maintain at_____ Increase to_____

		No knowledge 1	Limited knowledge 2	Moderate knowledge 3	Substantial knowledge 4	Extensive knowledge 5	
OUTCOME OVERALL RATING		1	2	3	4	5	
Indicators:							
185101	Signs and symptoms of onset	1	2	3	4	5	NA
185102	Type of dementia	1	2	3	4	5	NA
185103	Stages of dementia	1	2	3	4	5	NA
185104	Usual course of neurological losses	1	2	3	4	5	NA
185105	Signs and symptoms of neurological losses	1	2	3	4	5	NA
185106	Usual progression of functional losses	1	2	3	4	5	NA
185107	Signs and symptoms of functional losses	1	2	3	4	5	NA
185108	Importance of sharing feelings about losses	1	2	3	4	5	NA
185109	Importance of stimulating remaining mental functions	1	2	3	4	5	NA
185110	Compensatory strategies for memory losses	1	2	3	4	5	NA
185111	Compensatory strategies for losses in judgment	1	2	3	4	5	NA
185112	Compensatory strategies to remember names	1	2	3	4	5	NA
185113	Compensatory strategies to remember instructions	1	2	3	4	5	NA
185114	Compensatory strategies to remember locations	1	2	3	4	5	NA
185115	Compensatory strategies to maintain personal safety	1	2	3	4	5	NA
185116	Strategies to maintain safety of others	1	2	3	4	5	NA
185117	Plan for care in later stages of dementia	1	2	3	4	5	NA
185118	Plan for end of life care	1	2	3	4	5	NA

K

Domain-Health Knowledge & Behavior (IV)   *Class*-Health Knowledge (S)   5th edition 2013

OUTCOME CONTENT REFERENCES:

Gerdner, L. A., & Richards-Hall, G. (2001). Chronic confusion. In M. Maas, K. C. Buckwalter, M. D. Hardy, T. Tripp-Reimer, M. Titler, & J. P. Specht (Eds.), *Nursing care of older adults: Diagnoses, outcomes & interventions.* St. Louis: Mosby.

Reisberg, B., Ferris, S. H., deLeon, M. J., & Crook, T. (1982). The global deterioration scale for assessment of primary degenerative dementia. *American Journal of Psychiatry, 139*(9), 1136–1139.

Taylor, R. (2007). *Alzheimer's from the inside out.* Baltimore: Health Professions Press.

Knowledge: Depression Management   1836

Definition: Extent of understanding conveyed about depression and interrelationships among causes, effects and treatments

OUTCOME TARGET RATING: Maintain at_____   Increase to_____

		No knowledge	Limited knowledge	Moderate knowledge	Substantial knowledge	Extensive knowledge	
OUTCOME OVERALL RATING		1	2	3	4	5	
Indicators:							
183601	Physical signs and symptoms of depression	1	2	3	4	5	NA
183602	Emotional signs and symptoms of depression	1	2	3	4	5	NA
183603	Chronic conditions that increase risk for depression	1	2	3	4	5	NA
183604	Benefits of disease management	1	2	3	4	5	NA
183605	Available treatment options	1	2	3	4	5	NA
183606	Personal treatment regimen	1	2	3	4	5	NA
183607	Relationship of treatment regimen to goals	1	2	3	4	5	NA
183608	Importance of completing treatment regimen	1	2	3	4	5	NA
183609	Personal treatment therapeutic effects	1	2	3	4	5	NA
183610	Importance of compliance with treatment regimen	1	2	3	4	5	NA
183611	Importance of compliance with medication regimen	1	2	3	4	5	NA
183612	Factors contributing to depression	1	2	3	4	5	NA
183613	Factors that alleviate depression	1	2	3	4	5	NA
183614	Strategies to reduce precursors of depression	1	2	3	4	5	NA
183615	Strategies to facilitate recovery	1	2	3	4	5	NA
183616	Adverse health effects of depression on daily functioning	1	2	3	4	5	NA
183617	Interrelationship of self-esteem and body image to depression	1	2	3	4	5	NA
183618	Relationship of substance use to depression	1	2	3	4	5	NA
183619	Medication therapeutic effects	1	2	3	4	5	NA
183620	Medication side effects	1	2	3	4	5	NA
183621	Medication adverse effects	1	2	3	4	5	NA
183622	Potential medication interactions	1	2	3	4	5	NA
183623	Available support groups	1	2	3	4	5	NA
183624	Available community resources	1	2	3	4	5	NA
183625	When to obtain assistance from a health professional	1	2	3	4	5	NA

Domain-Health Knowledge & Behavior (IV)   *Class*-Health Knowledge (S)   *4th edition 2008; revised 2013*

OUTCOME CONTENT REFERENCES:

Blazer, D. (2002). *Depression in late life* (3rd ed.). New York: Springer.

Crowe, M., Ward, N., Dunnachie, B., & Roberts, M. (2006). Characteristics of adolescent depression. *International Journal of Mental Health Nursing, 15*(1), 10–18.

Eller, L. S., Corless, I., Bunch, E. H., Kemppainen, J., Holzemer, W., Nokes, K., Portillo, C., & Nicholas, P. (2005). Self-care strategies for depressive symptoms in people with HIV disease. *Journal of Advanced Nursing, 51*(2), 119–130.

Patel, V., Branch, T., Mottur-Pilson, C., & Pinard, G. (2004). Public awareness about depression: The effectiveness of a patient guideline. *International Journal of Psychiatry in Medicine, 34*(1), 1–20.

Roes, N. A. (2006). Depression 101 for addiction counselors. *Addiction Professional, 4*(1), 36–37.

Knowledge: Diabetes Management   1820

Definition: Extent of understanding conveyed about diabetes, its treatment, and the prevention of complications

OUTCOME TARGET RATING: Maintain at_____   Increase to_____

		No knowledge	Limited knowledge	Moderate knowledge	Substantial knowledge	Extensive knowledge	
OUTCOME OVERALL RATING		1	2	3	4	5	
Indicators:							
182030	Cause and contributing factors	1	2	3	4	5	NA
182031	Signs and symptoms of early disease	1	2	3	4	5	NA
182002	Role of diet in blood glucose control	1	2	3	4	5	NA
182003	Prescribed meal plan	1	2	3	4	5	NA
182004	Strategies to increase diet compliance	1	2	3	4	5	NA
182005	Role of exercise in blood glucose control	1	2	3	4	5	NA
182032	Role of sleep in blood glucose control	1	2	3	4	5	NA
182006	Hyperglycemia and related symptoms	1	2	3	4	5	NA
182007	Hyperglycemia prevention	1	2	3	4	5	NA
182008	Procedures to be followed in treating hyperglycemia	1	2	3	4	5	NA
182009	Hypoglycemia and related symptoms	1	2	3	4	5	NA
182010	Hypoglycemia prevention	1	2	3	4	5	NA
182011	Procedures to be followed in treating hypoglycemia	1	2	3	4	5	NA
182012	Importance of maintaining blood glucose level within target range	1	2	3	4	5	NA
182013	Impact of acute illness on blood glucose level	1	2	3	4	5	NA
182033	How to use a monitoring device	1	2	3	4	5	NA
182015	Actions to take in response to blood glucose levels	1	2	3	4	5	NA
182016	Prescribed insulin regimen	1	2	3	4	5	NA
182034	Correct use of insulin	1	2	3	4	5	NA
182027	Proper technique to draw up and administer insulin	1	2	3	4	5	NA
182018	Plan for rotation of injection sites	1	2	3	4	5	NA
182019	Onset, peak and duration of prescribed insulin	1	2	3	4	5	NA
182035	Proper disposal of syringes and needles	1	2	3	4	5	NA
182020	Prescribed oral medication regimen	1	2	3	4	5	NA
182036	Correct use of prescribed medication	1	2	3	4	5	NA
182037	Correct use of non-prescription medication	1	2	3	4	5	NA
182038	Proper medication storage	1	2	3	4	5	NA
182039	Medication therapeutic effects	1	2	3	4	5	NA
182040	Medication side effects	1	2	3	4	5	NA
182041	Medication adverse effects	1	2	3	4	5	NA
182042	When to obtain assistance from a health professional	1	2	3	4	5	NA
182028	Correct procedure for urine ketone testing	1	2	3	4	5	NA
182029	Importance of dilated eye exam and vision testing by an ophthalmologist	1	2	3	4	5	NA
182023	Preventive foot care practices	1	2	3	4	5	NA
182043	Reputable sources of diabetes information	1	2	3	4	5	NA
182024	Benefits of disease management	1	2	3	4	5	NA

K

Domain-Health Knowledge & Behavior (IV)   *Class*-Health Knowledge (S)   *2nd edition 2000; revised 2004, 2008, 2013*

OUTCOME CONTENT REFERENCES:
Anderson, S. (1994). 7 care tips for managing patients with diabetes. *American Journal of Nursing, 94*(9), 36–38.
Boucher, J. L., Swift, C. S., Franz, M. J., Kulkami, K., Schafer, R. G., Pritchett, E., & Clark, N. G. (2007). Inpatient management of diabetes and hyperglycemia: Implications for nutrition practice and the food and nutrition professional. *Journal of the American Dietetic Association, 107*(1), 105–111.

Brody, G. (1992). Diabetic ketoacidosis and hyperosmolar hyperglycemic nonketotic coma. *Topics of Emergency Medicine, 14*(1), 12–22.

Cameron, B. L. (2002). Making diabetes management routine: How often do you and your patients screen for complications? *American Journal of Nursing, 102*(2), 26–33.

Carlson, M. (1994). Diabetic emergencies: A clinical review. *Journal of the American Academy of Physician Assistants, 7*(2), 79–86.

Clark, A. (1994). Complications and management of diabetes. *Critical Care Nursing of North America, 6*(4), 723–733.

Dalewitz, J., Khan, N., & Hershey, C. O. (2000). Barriers to control blood glucose in diabetes mellitus. *American Journal of Medical Quality, 15*(1), 16–25.

Franz, M. J. (Ed.). (2000). *A core curriculum for diabetes education* (4th ed.). Chicago: American Association of Diabetes Educators.

Ibrahem, I. A. (2006). Diabetes mellitus. In D. L. Huber (Ed.), *Disease management: A guide for case managers* (pp. 81–99). St. Louis: Elsevier Saunders.

Jones, T. (1994). From diabetic ketoacidosis to hyperglycemic hyperosmolar nonketotic syndrome. *Critical Care Nursing Clinics of North America, 6*(4), 703–721.

Loewen, S., & Haas, L. (1991). Complications of diabetes: Acute and chronic. *Nurse Practitioner Forum, 2*(3), 181–187.

Miller, D. K., & Fain, J. A. (2006). Diabetes self-management education. *Nursing Clinics of North America, 41*(4), 655–666.

Norton, R. (1995). The right mix of diet and exercise. *RN, 58*(4), 20–24.

Peragallo-Dittko, V. (1995). Diabetes 2000: Acute complications. *RN, 58*(8), 36–41.

Reising, D. L. (1995). Acute hypoglycemia: Keeping the bottom from falling out. *Nursing 25*(2), 41–48.

Knowledge: Disease Process 1803

Definition: Extent of understanding conveyed about a specific disease process and potential complications

OUTCOME TARGET RATING: Maintain at_____   Increase to_____

OUTCOME OVERALL RATING	No knowledge 1	Limited knowledge 2	Moderate knowledge 3	Substantial knowledge 4	Extensive knowledge 5	
Indicators:						
180302 Characteristics of specific disease	1	2	3	4	5	NA
180303 Cause and contributing factors	1	2	3	4	5	NA
180304 Risk factors	1	2	3	4	5	NA
180305 Physiological effects of disease	1	2	3	4	5	NA
180306 Signs and symptoms of disease	1	2	3	4	5	NA
180307 Usual course of disease process	1	2	3	4	5	NA
180308 Strategies to minimize disease progression	1	2	3	4	5	NA
180309 Potential complications of disease	1	2	3	4	5	NA
180310 Signs and symptoms of disease complications	1	2	3	4	5	NA
180313 Psychosocial effects of disease on self	1	2	3	4	5	NA
180314 Psychosocial effects of disease on family	1	2	3	4	5	NA
180315 Benefits of disease management	1	2	3	4	5	NA
180316 Available support groups	1	2	3	4	5	NA
180317 Reputable sources of disease-specific information	1	2	3	4	5	NA

Specify disease: _____

Domain-Health Knowledge & Behavior (IV)   **Class**-Health Knowledge (S)   *1st edition 1997; revised 2004, 2008, 2013*

OUTCOME CONTENT REFERENCES:

Bushnell, F. (1992). Self-care teaching for congestive heart failure patients. *Journal of Gerontological Nursing, 18*(10), 27–32.

Conn, V. S., Armer, J. M., & Hayes, K. S. (2001). Knowledge deficit. In M. Maas, K. Buckwalter, M. Hardy, T. Tripp-Reimer, M. Titler, & J. Specht (Eds.), *Nursing care of older adults: Diagnoses, outcomes & interventions* (pp. 503–515). St. Louis: Mosby.

Devins, G. M., Binik, Y. M., Mandin, H., Litourneau, P. K., Hollomby, D. J., Barre, P. E., & Prichard, S. (1990). The kidney disease questionnaire: A test for measuring patient knowledge about end-stage renal disease. *Journal of Clinical Epidemiology, 43*(3), 297–307.

Garrard, J., Joynes, J. O., Mullen, L., McNeil, L., Mensing, C., Feste, C., & Etzwiler, D. D. (1987). Psychometric study of patient knowledge test. *Diabetes Care, 10*(4), 500–509.

Gilden, J. L., Hendryx, M., Casia, C., & Singh, S. P. (1989). The effectiveness of diabetes education programs for older patients and their spouses. *Journal of American Geriatrics Society, 37*(11), 1023–1030.

Mazzuca, S. A., Moorman, N. H., Wheeler, M. L., Norton, J. A., Fineberg, N. S., Vinicor, F., Cohen, S. J., & Clark, C. M. (1986). The diabetes education study: A controlled trial of the effects of diabetes patient education. *Diabetes Care, 9*(1), 1–10.

Redman, B. (1993). Knowledge deficit (specify). In J. M. Thompson, G. K. McFarland, J. E. Hirsch, & S. M. Tucker (Eds.), *Mosby's clinical nursing* (3rd ed., pp. 1548–1552). St. Louis: Mosby.

Scherer, Y. K., Janelli, L. M., & Schmieder, L. E. (1992). A time-series perspective of effectiveness of a health teaching program on chronic obstructive pulmonary disease. *Journal of Healthcare Education and Training, 6*(3), 7–13.

Smith, M. M., Hicks, V. L., & Heyward, V. H. (1991). Coronary disease knowledge test: Developing a valid and reliable tool. *Nurse Practitioner, 16*(4), 28, 31, 35–38.

Wright, L. K. (2001). Sexual dysfunction. In M. Maas, K. Buckwalter, M. Hardy, T. Tripp-Reimer, M. Titler, & J. Specht (Eds.), *Nursing care of older adults: Diagnoses, outcomes & interventions* (pp. 733–749). St. Louis: Mosby.

Knowledge: Dysrhythmia Management 1852

Definition: Extent of understanding conveyed about cardiac conduction irregularity, its treatment, and the prevention of disease progression and complications

OUTCOME TARGET RATING: Maintain at_____ Increase to_____

		No knowledge	Limited knowledge	Moderate knowledge	Substantial knowledge	Extensive knowledge	
OUTCOME OVERALL RATING		1	2	3	4	5	
Indicators:							
185201	Type of dysrhythmia	1	2	3	4	5	NA
185202	Methods to monitor blood pressure	1	2	3	4	5	NA
185203	Methods to monitor heart rate	1	2	3	4	5	NA
185204	Methods to monitor heart rhythm	1	2	3	4	5	NA
185205	Signs and symptoms of dysrhythmia	1	2	3	4	5	NA
185206	Relationship of lightheadedness to dysrhythmia	1	2	3	4	5	NA
185207	Relationship of dizziness to dysrhythmia	1	2	3	4	5	NA
185208	Effects of exercise on heart rhythm	1	2	3	4	5	NA
185209	Effects of fever on heart rhythm	1	2	3	4	5	NA
185210	Effects of anxiety on heart rhythm	1	2	3	4	5	NA
185211	Effects of caffeine on heart rhythm	1	2	3	4	5	NA
185212	Effects of other stimulants on heart rhythm	1	2	3	4	5	NA
185213	Signs and symptoms of overexertion	1	2	3	4	5	NA
185214	Strategies to control anxiety	1	2	3	4	5	NA
185215	Factors that precede dysrhythmia onset	1	2	3	4	5	NA
185216	Strategies to eliminate causative factors	1	2	3	4	5	NA
185217	Effects on lifestyle	1	2	3	4	5	NA
185218	Strategies to cope with lifestyle changes	1	2	3	4	5	NA
185219	Adaptations for role performance	1	2	3	4	5	NA
185220	Guidelines for sexual activity	1	2	3	4	5	NA
185221	Benefits of prescribed medication	1	2	3	4	5	NA
185222	Importance of compliance with prescribed medication schedule	1	2	3	4	5	NA
185223	Medication schedule	1	2	3	4	5	NA
185224	Importance of maintaining medication blood levels	1	2	3	4	5	NA
185225	Medication therapeutic effects	1	2	3	4	5	NA
185226	Medication side effects	1	2	3	4	5	NA
185227	Medication adverse effects	1	2	3	4	5	NA
185228	Actions to take in an emergency	1	2	3	4	5	NA
185229	Importance of family learning cardiopulmonary resuscitation	1	2	3	4	5	NA
185230	Cultural influences on compliance to treatment regimen	1	2	3	4	5	NA
185231	Available support groups	1	2	3	4	5	NA
185232	Reputable sources of cardiac disease information	1	2	3	4	5	NA
185233	When to obtain assistance from a health professional	1	2	3	4	5	NA

Domain-*Health Knowledge & Behavior (IV)*   ***Class**-Health Knowledge (S)*   *5th edition 2013*

OUTCOME CONTENT REFERENCES:

National Heart, Lung, and Blood Institute. (2009). *Implantable cardioverter defibrillator.* Retrieved from http://www.nhlbi.nih.gov/health/dci/Diseases/icd/icd_whatis.html

National Heart, Lung, and Blood Institute. (2011). *Arrhythmia.* Retrieved from http://www.nhlbi.nih.gov/health/dci/Diseases/arr/arr_whatis.html

Xu, W., Sun, G., Lin, Z., Chen, M., Yang, B., Chen, H., & Cao, K. (2010). Knowledge, attitude, and behavior in patients with atrial fibrillation undergoing radiofrequency catheter ablation. *Journal of Interventional Cardiac Electrophysiology, 28*(3), 199–207.

K

Knowledge: Eating Disorder Management 1853

Definition: Extent of understanding conveyed about an eating disorder, its treatment, and the prevention of disease progression and complications

OUTCOME TARGET RATING: Maintain at_____   Increase to_____

OUTCOME OVERALL RATING		No knowledge 1	Limited knowledge 2	Moderate knowledge 3	Substantial knowledge 4	Extensive knowledge 5	
Indicators:							
185301	Healthy target weight	1	2	3	4	5	NA
185302	Healthy nutritional practices	1	2	3	4	5	NA
185303	Relationship among diet, exercise and weight	1	2	3	4	5	NA
185304	Achievable weight gain goals	1	2	3	4	5	NA
185305	Achievable weight loss goals	1	2	3	4	5	NA
185306	Adverse health effects of emotional states on food and fluid intake	1	2	3	4	5	NA
185307	Effects of social situations on food and fluid intake	1	2	3	4	5	NA
185308	Strategies for situations that affect food and fluid intake	1	2	3	4	5	NA
185309	Maladaptive eating responses	1	2	3	4	5	NA
185310	Daily fluid intake that meets body needs	1	2	3	4	5	NA
185311	Caloric intake appropriate for metabolic needs	1	2	3	4	5	NA
185312	Nutrient intake appropriate for individual needs	1	2	3	4	5	NA
185313	Signs and symptoms of nutritional deficits	1	2	3	4	5	NA
185314	Strategies to create a healthy attitude about food	1	2	3	4	5	NA
185315	Realistic exercise routine	1	2	3	4	5	NA
185316	Strategies to manage stress	1	2	3	4	5	NA
185317	Strategies to gain sense of personal control	1	2	3	4	5	NA
185318	Strategies to decrease preoccupation with food	1	2	3	4	5	NA
185319	Strategies to avoid purging behaviors	1	2	3	4	5	NA
185320	Strategies to avoid binging behaviors	1	2	3	4	5	NA
185321	Strategies to promote an accurate perception of body image	1	2	3	4	5	NA
185322	Strategies to promote satisfaction with body image	1	2	3	4	5	NA
185323	Strategies to promote self-esteem	1	2	3	4	5	NA
185324	Factors that trigger relapse	1	2	3	4	5	NA
185325	Strategies to prevent relapses	1	2	3	4	5	NA
185326	Signs and symptoms of depression	1	2	3	4	5	NA
185327	Strategies to reduce depression	1	2	3	4	5	NA
185328	Characteristics of supportive relationships	1	2	3	4	5	NA
185329	Prescribed medication regimen	1	2	3	4	5	NA
185330	Potential dangers of non-prescription medication	1	2	3	4	5	NA
185331	Available support groups	1	2	3	4	5	NA
185332	Available community resources	1	2	3	4	5	NA
185333	When to obtain assistance from a health professional	1	2	3	4	5	NA

Domain-Health Knowledge & Behavior (IV)   **Class**-Health Knowledge (S)   5th edition 2013

OUTCOME CONTENT REFERENCES:
Berkman, N., Bulik, C., Brownley, K., Lohr, K., Sedway, J., Rooks, A., & Gartlehner, G. (2006). Management of eating disorders. Evidence report/technology assessment No. 135. (Prepared by the RTI International-University of North Carolina Evidence-Based Practice Center under Contract No. 290-02-0016.) Publication No. 06-E010. Rockville, MD: Agency for Healthcare Research and Quality.
Berkman, N., Lohr, K., & Bulik, C. (2007). Outcomes of eating disorder: A systematic review of the literature. *International Journal of Eating Disorders, 40*(4), 293–309.
Fichter, M., Quadflieg, N., & Hedlund, S. (2006). Twelve-year course and outcome predictors of anorexia nervosa. *International Journal of Eating Disorders, 39*(2), 87–100.
Kong, S. (2005). Day treatment programme for patients with eating disorders: Randomized controlled trial. *Journal of Advanced Nursing, 51*(1), 5–14.
Patching, J., & Lawler, J. (2009). Understanding women's experiences of developing an eating disorder and recovering: A life-history approach. *Nursing Inquiry, 16*(1), 10–21.
Sadock, B. J., & Sadock, V. A. (2007). *Kaplan & Sadock's synopsis of psychiatry: Behavioral sciences/clinical psychiatry* (10th ed.). Philadelphia: Lippincott, Williams, & Wilkins.
Stuart, G. W. (2009). *Principles and practice of psychiatric nursing* (9th ed.). St. Louis: Mosby Elsevier.

Knowledge: Energy Conservation — 1804

Definition: Extent of understanding conveyed about energy conservation techniques

OUTCOME TARGET RATING: Maintain at_____ Increase to_____

OUTCOME OVERALL RATING	No knowledge 1	Limited knowledge 2	Moderate knowledge 3	Substantial knowledge 4	Extensive knowledge 5	
Indicators:						
180401 Recommended physical activity	1	2	3	4	5	NA
180402 Activity restrictions	1	2	3	4	5	NA
180403 Appropriate activities	1	2	3	4	5	NA
180404 Factors that increase energy expenditure	1	2	3	4	5	NA
180405 Factors that decrease energy expenditure	1	2	3	4	5	NA
180406 Energy limitations	1	2	3	4	5	NA
180407 Strategies to balance activity and rest	1	2	3	4	5	NA
180416 Energy conservation techniques	1	2	3	4	5	NA
180422 Methods to monitor heart rate	1	2	3	4	5	NA
180423 Effective breathing techniques	1	2	3	4	5	NA
180419 Proper body mechanics	1	2	3	4	5	NA
180420 Work simplification techniques	1	2	3	4	5	NA
180421 Correct use of assistive devices	1	2	3	4	5	NA

Domain-Health Knowledge & Behavior (IV)   **Class**-Health Knowledge (S)   1st edition 1997; revised 2004, 2008, 2013

OUTCOME CONTENT REFERENCES:
Conn, V. S., Armer, J. M., & Hayes, K. S. (2001). Knowledge deficit. In M. Maas, K. Buckwalter, M. Hardy, T. Tripp-Reimer, M. Titler, & J. Specht (Eds.), *Nursing care of older adults: Diagnoses, outcomes & interventions* (pp. 503–515). St. Louis: Mosby.
Hart, L. K., & Freel, M. I. (1982). Fatigue. In C. M. Norris (Ed.), *Concept clarification in nursing* (pp. 251–261). Rockville, MD: Aspen.
Lubkin, I. M. (2002). *Chronic illness: Impact and interventions* (5th ed.). Boston: Jones & Bartlett.
McFarlane, E. A. (1993). Activity intolerance. In J. M. Thompson, G. K. McFarland, J. E. Hirsch, & S. M. Tucker (Eds.), *Clinical nursing* (3rd ed., pp. 1498–1500). St. Louis: Mosby.
McFarlane, E. A. (1993). High risk for activity intolerance. In J. M. Thompson, G. K. McFarland, J. E. Hirsch, & S. M. Tucker (Eds.), *Clinical nursing* (3rd ed., pp. 1497–1498). St. Louis: Mosby.
Mock, V. L. (1993). Fatigue. In J. M. Thompson, G. K. McFarland, J. E. Hirsch, & S. M. Tucker (Eds.), *Clinical nursing* (3rd ed., pp. 1504–1506). St. Louis: Mosby.
Morris, M. L. (1982). Tiredness and fatigue. In C. M. Norris (Ed.), *Concept clarification in nursing* (pp. 263–275). Rockville, MD: Aspen.

K

Knowledge: Fall Prevention 1828

Definition: Extent of understanding conveyed about prevention of falls

OUTCOME TARGET RATING: Maintain at_____ Increase to_____

OUTCOME OVERALL RATING	No knowledge 1	Limited knowledge 2	Moderate knowledge 3	Substantial knowledge 4	Extensive knowledge 5	
Indicators:						
182801 Correct use of assistive devices	1	2	3	4	5	NA
182802 Correct use of safety devices	1	2	3	4	5	NA
182803 Appropriate footwear	1	2	3	4	5	NA
182804 Correct use of grab bars	1	2	3	4	5	NA
182805 Correct use of safety gates	1	2	3	4	5	NA
182806 Correct use of window guards	1	2	3	4	5	NA
182807 Correct use of environmental lighting	1	2	3	4	5	NA
182808 When to ask for personal assistance	1	2	3	4	5	NA
182809 Use of safe transfer procedure	1	2	3	4	5	NA
182810 Reasons for restraints	1	2	3	4	5	NA
182811 Exercises to reduce risk for falls	1	2	3	4	5	NA
182812 Prescribed medications that increase risk for falls	1	2	3	4	5	NA
182813 Chronic conditions that increase risk for falls	1	2	3	4	5	NA
182814 Acute illnesses that increase risk for falls	1	2	3	4	5	NA
182815 Blood pressure changes that increase risk for falls	1	2	3	4	5	NA
182816 Non-prescription medications that increase risk for falls	1	2	3	4	5	NA
182817 Strategies to safely ambulate	1	2	3	4	5	NA
182818 Importance of maintaining clear walkway	1	2	3	4	5	NA
182819 Safe use of stools and ladders	1	2	3	4	5	NA
182820 Use of rubber mats	1	2	3	4	5	NA
182821 Strategies to keep floor surfaces safe	1	2	3	4	5	NA

Domain-Health Knowledge & Behavior (IV)   *Class*-Health Knowledge (S)   *3rd edition 2004; revised 2008*

OUTCOME CONTENT REFERENCES:

Bexon, J., Echevarria, K. H., & Smith, G. B. (1999). Nursing outcome indicator: Preventing falls for elderly people. *Outcomes Management for Nursing Practice, 3*(3), 112–116.

Edwards, B. J., & Lee, S. (1998). Gait disorders and falls in a retirement home: A pilot study. *Annals of Long-Term Care, 6*(4), 140–143.

Fleck, M. M., & Forrester, D. A. (2001). The efficacy of an educational program to improve direct caregiver knowledge regarding fall prevention. *Journal for Nurses in Staff Development, 17*(1), 27–33.

Hendrich, A. L. (1996). *Falls, immobility, and restraints: A resource manual.* St. Louis: Mosby.

Malmivaara, A., Heliovaara, M., Knekt, P., Reunanen, A., & Aromaa, A. (1993). Risk factors for injurious falls leading to hospitalization or death in a cohort of 19,500 adults. *American Journal of Epidemiology, 138*(6), 384–394.

Patient information. Decreasing your risks of falls. *American Family Physician, 56*(7), 1823.

Schoenfelder, D. P., Crowell, C. M., & The Nursing Diagnosis Extension and Classification Research Team (1999). From risk for trauma to unintentional injury risk: Falls—a concept analysis. *Nursing Diagnoses, 10*(4), 149–157.

Stevens, J. A., & Olson, S. (2000). Reducing falls and resulting hip fractures among older women. *Morbidity & Mortality Weekly Report, 49* (RR-2), 1–12.

Wortel, E., & de Geus, G. H. (1993). Prevention of home related injuries of pre-school children: Safety measures taken by mothers. *Health Education Research, 8*(2), 217–231.

Knowledge: Fertility Promotion 1816

Definition: Extent of understanding conveyed about fertility testing and the conditions that affect conception

OUTCOME TARGET RATING: Maintain at_____ Increase to_____

OUTCOME OVERALL RATING	No knowledge 1	Limited knowledge 2	Moderate knowledge 3	Substantial knowledge 4	Extensive knowledge 5	
Indicators:						
181601 Effect of age	1	2	3	4	5	NA
181602 Effect of coital frequency	1	2	3	4	5	NA
181603 Effect of nutrition	1	2	3	4	5	NA
181604 Adverse health effects	1	2	3	4	5	NA
181606 Effect of heat on sperm count	1	2	3	4	5	NA
181607 Effect of tight clothes on sperm count	1	2	3	4	5	NA
181608 Effect of physical anomalies	1	2	3	4	5	NA
181609 Effect of pelvic surgery	1	2	3	4	5	NA
181610 Effect of pelvic infections	1	2	3	4	5	NA
181611 Influence of vaginal/uterine environment	1	2	3	4	5	NA
181612 Effect of hormone levels	1	2	3	4	5	NA
181613 Effect of thyroid function	1	2	3	4	5	NA
181614 Use of basal body temperature to predict ovulation	1	2	3	4	5	NA
181615 Symptothermal method	1	2	3	4	5	NA
181616 Ultrasonography	1	2	3	4	5	NA
181617 Influence of semen characteristics	1	2	3	4	5	NA
181618 Influence of sperm count	1	2	3	4	5	NA
181619 Postcoital test	1	2	3	4	5	NA
181620 Fertility monitoring devices	1	2	3	4	5	NA
181621 Options to reverse sterilization	1	2	3	4	5	NA
181622 Methods for semen collection	1	2	3	4	5	NA

Domain-Health Knowledge & Behavior (IV) *Class*-Health Knowledge (S) *2nd edition 2000; revised 2004, 2008, 2013*

K

OUTCOME CONTENT REFERENCES:

Fehring, R. J. (1991). New technology in natural family planning. *Journal of Obstetric, Gynecologic, and Neonatal Nursing, 20*(3), 199–205.

Grodstein, F., Goldman, M. B., & Cramer, D. W. (1994). Infertility in women and moderate alcohol use. *American Journal of Public Health, 84*(9), 1429–1432.

Halman, L. J., Abbey, A., & Andrews, F. M. (1992). Attitudes about infertility interventions among fertile and infertile couples. *American Journal of Public Health, 82*(2), 191–194.

Rudy, E. B., & Estok, P. (1992). Professional and lay interrater reliability of urinary luteinizing hormone surges measured by OvuQuick test. *Journal of Obstetric, Gynecologic, and Neonatal Nursing, 21*(5), 407–410.

Shane, J. M. (1993). Evaluation and treatment of infertility. *Clinical Symposia, 45*(2), 2–32.

Toner, J. P., & Flood, J. T. (1993). Fertility after the age of 40. *Obstetrics and Gynecology Clinics of North America, 20*(2), 261–272.

Knowledge: Health Behavior 1805

Definition: Extent of understanding conveyed about the promotion and protection of health

OUTCOME TARGET RATING: Maintain at_____ Increase to_____

OUTCOME OVERALL RATING		No knowledge 1	Limited knowledge 2	Moderate knowledge 3	Substantial knowledge 4	Extensive knowledge 5	
Indicators:							
180501	Healthy nutritional practices	1	2	3	4	5	NA
180502	Benefits of regular exercise	1	2	3	4	5	NA
180503	Strategies to manage stress	1	2	3	4	5	NA
180504	Normal sleep-wake patterns	1	2	3	4	5	NA
180505	Methods of family planning	1	2	3	4	5	NA
180506	Adverse health effects of tobacco use	1	2	3	4	5	NA
180507	Adverse health effects of alcohol use	1	2	3	4	5	NA
180508	Adverse health effects of recreational drug use	1	2	3	4	5	NA
180509	Safe use of prescribed medication	1	2	3	4	5	NA
180510	Safe use of non-prescription medication	1	2	3	4	5	NA
180511	Effects of caffeine use	1	2	3	4	5	NA
180512	Strategies to reduce the risk of accidental injury	1	2	3	4	5	NA
180513	Strategies to avoid exposure to environmental hazards	1	2	3	4	5	NA
180514	Strategies to prevent transmission of infectious disease	1	2	3	4	5	NA
180518	Health promotion services	1	2	3	4	5	NA
180519	Health protection services	1	2	3	4	5	NA
180516	Self-screening techniques	1	2	3	4	5	NA

Domain-Health Knowledge & Behavior (IV)   **Class**-Health Knowledge (S)   *1st edition 1997; revised 2004, 2008, 2013*

OUTCOME CONTENT REFERENCES:

Conn, V. S., Armer, J. M., & Hayes, K. S. (2001). Knowledge deficit. In M. Maas, K. Buckwalter, M. Hardy, T. Tripp-Reimer, M. Titler, & J. Specht (Eds.), *Nursing care of older adults: Diagnoses, outcomes & interventions* (pp. 503–515). St. Louis: Mosby.

Simons-Morton, D. G., Mullen, P. D., Mains, D. A., Tabak, E. R., & Green, L. W. (1992). Characteristics of controlled studies of patient education and counseling for preventive health behaviors. *Patient Education and Counseling, 19*(2), 174–204.

Spellbring, A. M. (1991). Nursing's role in health promotion. *Nursing Clinics of North America, 16*(4), 805–814.

Tanner, E. K. (1991). Assessment of a health-promotive lifestyle. *Nursing Clinics of North America, 26*(4), 845–854.

U.S. Department of Health and Human Services. (1990). *Healthy people 2000. National health promotion and disease prevention objectives*. Washington, DC: U.S. Government Printing Office.

Knowledge: Health Promotion 1823

Definition: Extent of understanding conveyed about information needed to obtain and maintain optimal health

OUTCOME TARGET RATING: Maintain at_____ Increase to_____

OUTCOME OVERALL RATING	No knowledge 1	Limited knowledge 2	Moderate knowledge 3	Substantial knowledge 4	Extensive knowledge 5	
Indicators:						
182308 Behaviors that promote health	1	2	3	4	5	NA
182309 Strategies to manage stress	1	2	3	4	5	NA
182310 Recommended health screenings	1	2	3	4	5	NA
182311 Recommended immunizations	1	2	3	4	5	NA
182321 Recommended self-screenings for cancer detection	1	2	3	4	5	NA
182312 Reputable health care resources	1	2	3	4	5	NA
182313 Prevention and control of infection	1	2	3	4	5	NA
182314 Behaviors to prevent unintentional injuries	1	2	3	4	5	NA
182315 Behaviors to protect skin from sun exposure	1	2	3	4	5	NA
182316 Safe management of medication	1	2	3	4	5	NA
182322 Adverse health effects of alcohol use	1	2	3	4	5	NA
182323 Adverse health effects of tobacco use	1	2	3	4	5	NA
182324 Adverse health effects of drug use	1	2	3	4	5	NA
182318 Healthy nutritional practices	1	2	3	4	5	NA
182319 Strategies for weight management	1	2	3	4	5	NA
182320 Effective exercise routine	1	2	3	4	5	NA
182325 Relationship among diet, exercise, and weight	1	2	3	4	5	NA
182326 Strategies to avoid exposure to environmental hazards	1	2	3	4	5	NA
182327 Risk for hereditary disease	1	2	3	4	5	NA
182328 Reputable sources of health promotion information	1	2	3	4	5	NA

Domain-*Health Knowledge & Behavior (IV)*   **Class**-*Health Knowledge (S)*   *2nd edition 2000; revised 2004, 2008, 2013*

OUTCOME CONTENT REFERENCES:
This is a general outcome that combines the following: Knowledge: Health Behavior, Knowledge: Health Resources, Knowledge: Personal Safety, Knowledge: Substance Use Control, and Knowledge: Diet.

K

Knowledge: Health Resources 1806

Definition: Extent of understanding conveyed about relevant health care resources

OUTCOME TARGET RATING: Maintain at_____ Increase to_____

	No knowledge	Limited knowledge	Moderate knowledge	Substantial knowledge	Extensive knowledge	
OUTCOME OVERALL RATING	1	2	3	4	5	
Indicators:						
180601 Reputable health care resources	1	2	3	4	5	NA
180602 When to obtain assistance from a health professional	1	2	3	4	5	NA
180603 Emergency measures	1	2	3	4	5	NA
180604 Emergency care resources	1	2	3	4	5	NA
180605 Importance of follow-up care	1	2	3	4	5	NA
180606 Plan for follow-up care	1	2	3	4	5	NA
180607 Available community resources	1	2	3	4	5	NA
180608 Strategies to access health care services	1	2	3	4	5	NA

Domain-Health Knowledge & Behavior (IV)   **Class**-Health Knowledge (S)   *1st edition 1997; revised 2004, 2008*

K

OUTCOME CONTENT REFERENCES:
Bull, M. J. (1994). Patients' and professionals' perceptions of quality in discharge planning. *Journal of Nursing Care Quality, 8*(2), 47–61.
Conn, V. S., Armer, J. M., & Hayes, K. S. (2001). Knowledge deficit. In M. Maas, K. Buckwalter, M. Hardy, T. Tripp-Reimer, M. Titler, & J. Specht (Eds.), *Nursing care of older adults: Diagnoses, outcomes & interventions* (pp. 503–515). St. Louis: Mosby.
Redman, B. (1993). Knowledge deficit (specify). In J. M. Thompson, G. K. McFarland, J. E. Hirsch, & S. M. Tucker (Eds.), *Mosby's clinical nursing* (3rd ed., pp. 1548–1552). St. Louis: Mosby.
Wyness, M. A. (1990). Evaluation of an educational program for patients taking warfarin. *Journal of Advanced Nursing, 15*(9), 1052–1063.

Knowledge: Healthy Diet 1854

Definition: Extent of understanding conveyed about a balanced nutritious diet

OUTCOME TARGET RATING: Maintain at_____ Increase to_____

	No knowledge	Limited knowledge	Moderate knowledge	Substantial knowledge	Extensive knowledge	
OUTCOME OVERALL RATING	1	2	3	4	5	
Indicators:						
185401 Achievable dietary goals	1	2	3	4	5	NA
185402 Optimal personal weight range	1	2	3	4	5	NA
185403 Relationship among diet, exercise and weight	1	2	3	4	5	NA
185404 Fluid intake appropriate for metabolic needs	1	2	3	4	5	NA
185405 Caloric intake appropriate for metabolic needs	1	2	3	4	5	NA
185406 Nutrient intake appropriate for individual needs	1	2	3	4	5	NA
185407 Recommended nutritional guidelines	1	2	3	4	5	NA
185408 Foods consistent with nutritional guidelines	1	2	3	4	5	NA
185409 Recommended daily amount of vitamins	1	2	3	4	5	NA
185410 Recommended daily amount of minerals	1	2	3	4	5	NA
185411 Dietary recommendations for healthy fats, proteins, and carbohydrates	1	2	3	4	5	NA
185412 Dietary recommendations for sodium	1	2	3	4	5	NA
185413 Guidelines for food portions	1	2	3	4	5	NA
185414 Interpretation of nutritional information on food labels	1	2	3	4	5	NA

Knowledge: Healthy Diet—cont'd

	No knowledge	Limited knowledge	Moderate knowledge	Substantial knowledge	Extensive knowledge	
185415 Nutritional value of whole-grain versus refined-grain products	1	2	3	4	5	NA
185416 Recommended daily protein servings	1	2	3	4	5	NA
185417 Recommended daily fruit servings	1	2	3	4	5	NA
185418 Recommended daily vegetable servings	1	2	3	4	5	NA
185419 Recommended daily dairy servings	1	2	3	4	5	NA
185420 Importance of eating breakfast	1	2	3	4	5	NA
185421 Importance of distributing food intake throughout the day	1	2	3	4	5	NA
185422 Strategies to increase diet compliance	1	2	3	4	5	NA
185423 Strategies to avoid saturated fats	1	2	3	4	5	NA
185424 Strategies to avoid foods with high caloric value and little nutritional value	1	2	3	4	5	NA
185425 Safety recommendations for food storage	1	2	3	4	5	NA
185426 Safety recommendations for food preparation	1	2	3	4	5	NA
185427 Guidelines for nutritional supplements	1	2	3	4	5	NA
185428 Potential food and medication interactions	1	2	3	4	5	NA
185429 Potential food and herbal supplement interactions	1	2	3	4	5	NA

Domain-*Health Knowledge & Behavior (IV)*   **Class**-*Health Knowledge (S)*   *5th edition 2013*

OUTCOME CONTENT REFERENCES:

Dickson-Spillman, M., & Siegrist, M. (2010). Consumers' knowledge of healthy diets and its correlation with dietary behavior. *Journal of Human Nutrition and Dietetics, 24*(1), 54–60.

Gassin, A. (2001). Helping to promote healthy diets and lifestyles: The role of the food industry. *Public Health Nutrition, 4*(6A), 1445–1450.

Guidelines to good health: What do the latest dietary guidelines mean to you and your food choices? (2011). *Tufts University Health & Nutrition Letter, 29*(3), 1–4.

Hockenberry, M. J., & Wilson, D. (2011). *Wong's nursing care of infants and children* (9th ed.). St. Louis: Elsevier.

Nazarki, L. (2009). Nutrition part 1: Maintaining a healthy diet. *British Journal of Healthcare Assistants, 3*(1), 25–28.

Richards, S. (2009). The building blocks of a healthy diet. *Practice Nurse, 38*(3), 12–17.

Richards, S. (2009). The building blocks of a healthy diet. Part 2. *Practice Nurse, 38*(4), 29–33.

U.S. Department of Agriculture and U.S. Dept of Health and Human Services. (2010). *Dietary guidelines for Americans 2010* (7th ed.). Washington, DC: U.S. Government Printing Office.

K

Knowledge: Healthy Lifestyle   **1855**

Definition: Extent of understanding conveyed about a healthy, balanced lifestyle consistent with one's values, strengths, and interests

OUTCOME TARGET RATING: Maintain at_____   Increase to_____

	No knowledge	Limited knowledge	Moderate knowledge	Substantial knowledge	Extensive knowledge	
OUTCOME OVERALL RATING	1	2	3	4	5	NA
Indicators:						
185501 Optimal personal weight range	1	2	3	4	5	NA
185502 Optimal body mass index range	1	2	3	4	5	NA
185503 Optimal body fat percentage	1	2	3	4	5	NA
185504 Strategies to maintain healthy diet	1	2	3	4	5	NA
185505 Importance of water for adequate hydration	1	2	3	4	5	NA
185506 Recommended daily fruit servings	1	2	3	4	5	NA
185507 Recommended daily vegetable servings	1	2	3	4	5	NA

Continued

Knowledge: Healthy Lifestyle—cont'd

		No knowledge	Limited knowledge	Moderate knowledge	Substantial knowledge	Extensive knowledge	
185508	Strategies to limit saturated fat and cholesterol intake	1	2	3	4	5	NA
185509	Strategies to limit sodium intake	1	2	3	4	5	NA
185510	Importance of food portions	1	2	3	4	5	NA
185511	Recommended vitamin supplements	1	2	3	4	5	NA
185512	Recommended mineral supplements	1	2	3	4	5	NA
185513	Strategies to avoid secondhand smoke	1	2	3	4	5	NA
185514	Strategies for tobacco cessation	1	2	3	4	5	NA
185515	Importance of alcohol use in moderation	1	2	3	4	5	NA
185516	Benefits of regular exercise	1	2	3	4	5	NA
185517	Importance of being physically active	1	2	3	4	5	NA
185518	Strategies to limit use of electronic devices	1	2	3	4	5	NA
185519	Personal factors affecting health behaviors	1	2	3	4	5	NA
185520	Environmental factors affecting health behaviors	1	2	3	4	5	NA
185521	Barriers to maintain healthy behaviors	1	2	3	4	5	NA
185522	Strategies to prevent disease	1	2	3	4	5	NA
185523	Strategies to prevent infection	1	2	3	4	5	NA
185524	Strategies to prevent accidents	1	2	3	4	5	NA
185525	Benefits of social support	1	2	3	4	5	NA
185526	Importance of constructively communicating thoughts, feelings, and emotions	1	2	3	4	5	NA
185527	Importance of preventive screenings	1	2	3	4	5	NA
185528	Importance of oral health care	1	2	3	4	5	NA
185529	Importance of protection against ultraviolet radiation	1	2	3	4	5	NA
185530	Adverse health effects of being overweight	1	2	3	4	5	NA
185531	Strategies to enhance self-esteem	1	2	3	4	5	NA
185532	Strategies to reduce stress	1	2	3	4	5	NA
185533	Importance of maintaining optimism	1	2	3	4	5	NA
185534	Importance of mental stimulation	1	2	3	4	5	NA
185535	Strategies to promote life balance	1	2	3	4	5	NA
185536	When to obtain assistance from a health professional	1	2	3	4	5	NA

Domain-Health Knowledge & Behavior (IV) **Class**-Health Knowledge (S) 5th edition 2013

OUTCOME CONTENT REFERENCES:

Downes, L. (2008). Motivators and barriers of a healthy lifestyle scale: Development and psychometric characteristics. *Journal of Nursing Measurement, 16*(1), 3–15.

Downes, L. (2010). Further validation of the motivators and barriers of a healthy lifestyle scale. *Southern Online Journal of Nursing Research, 10*(4).

Gellert, K., Aubert, R., & Mikami, J. (2010). Ke 'Ano Ola: Moloka'i's community-based healthy lifestyle modification program. *American Journal of Public Health, 100*(5), 779–783.

Golley, R., Perry, R., Magarey, A., & Daniels, L. (2007). Family-focused weight management program for five- to nine-year-olds incorporating parenting skills training with healthy lifestyle information to support behaviour modification. *Nutrition & Dietetics, 64*(3), 144–150.

Harrington, J., Perry, I., Lutomski, J., Fitzgerald, A., Shiely, F., McGee, H., Barry, M., Lente, E., Morgan, K., & Shelley, E. (2009). Living longer and feeling better: Healthy lifestyle, self-rated health, obesity and depression in Ireland. *European Journal of Public Health, 20*(1), 91–95.

Meinyk, B. (2009). Improving the mental health, healthy lifestyle choices, and physical health of Hispanic adolescents: A randomized controlled pilot study. *Journal of School Health, 79*(12), 575–584.

Ochieng, B. (2006). Factors affecting choice of a healthy lifestyle: Implications for nurses. *British Journal of Community Nursing, 17*(2), 78–81.

Olvera, N., Schere, R., McLeod, M., Graham, M., Knox, B., Hall, K., Butte, N., Bush, J., Smith, D., & Bloom, J. (2010). Bounce: An exploratory healthy lifestyle summer intervention for girls. *American Journal of Health Behavior, 34*(2), 144–155.

Stanner, S., Thompson, R., & Buttriss, J. (Eds.). (2009). *Healthy ageing: The role of nutrition and lifestyle.* London: Wiley-Blackwell.

Knowledge: Heart Failure Management   1835

Definition: Extent of understanding conveyed about heart failure, its treatment, and the prevention of disease progression and complications

OUTCOME TARGET RATING: Maintain at_____   Increase to_____

		No knowledge	Limited knowledge	Moderate knowledge	Substantial knowledge	Extensive knowledge	
OUTCOME OVERALL RATING		1	2	3	4	5	NA
Indicators:							
183501	Cause and contributing factors	1	2	3	4	5	NA
183502	Signs and symptoms of early disease	1	2	3	4	5	NA
183503	Benefits of disease management	1	2	3	4	5	NA
183530	Role of diagnostic tests for disease management	1	2	3	4	5	NA
183504	Basic actions of the heart	1	2	3	4	5	NA
183505	Signs and symptoms of progressive heart failure	1	2	3	4	5	NA
183538	Signs and symptoms of complications	1	2	3	4	5	NA
183507	Signs and symptoms of anemia	1	2	3	4	5	NA
183539	Barriers to self-care	1	2	3	4	5	NA
183540	Strategies to manage dyspnea	1	2	3	4	5	NA
183541	Strategies to manage tachycardia	1	2	3	4	5	NA
183542	Strategies to manage edema	1	2	3	4	5	NA
183512	Relationship of physical and emotional stress to condition	1	2	3	4	5	NA
183513	Psychosocial effects of heart failure	1	2	3	4	5	NA
183515	Strategies to control anxiety	1	2	3	4	5	NA
183543	Signs and symptoms of depression	1	2	3	4	5	NA
183544	Counseling available for depression	1	2	3	4	5	NA
183516	Treatments to improve cardiac performance	1	2	3	4	5	NA
183545	Health behaviors to promote physiologic stability	1	2	3	4	5	NA
183517	Strategies to promote peripheral circulation	1	2	3	4	5	NA
183546	Benefits of adequate rest	1	2	3	4	5	NA
183547	Benefits of regular exercise	1	2	3	4	5	NA
183548	Recommended physical activity	1	2	3	4	5	NA
183511	Signs and symptoms of overexertion	1	2	3	4	5	NA
183549	Strategies to prevent overexertion	1	2	3	4	5	NA
183519	Strategies to balance activity and rest	1	2	3	4	5	NA
183521	Strategies to increase resistance to infection	1	2	3	4	5	NA
183550	Recommended immunizations	1	2	3	4	5	NA
183523	Strategies to manage edema	1	2	3	4	5	NA
183524	Factors contributing to weight changes	1	2	3	4	5	NA
183525	Strategies to manage weight	1	2	3	4	5	NA
183551	Prescribed diet	1	2	3	4	5	NA
183526	Strategies to increase diet compliance	1	2	3	4	5	NA
183552	Recommended fluid intake	1	2	3	4	5	NA
183553	Importance of tobacco abstinence	1	2	3	4	5	NA
183554	Strategies for smoking cessation	1	2	3	4	5	NA
183555	Importance of alcohol restrictions	1	2	3	4	5	NA
183527	Medication therapeutic effects	1	2	3	4	5	NA
183528	Medication side effects	1	2	3	4	5	NA
183529	Medication adverse effects	1	2	3	4	5	NA
183531	Self-monitoring techniques	1	2	3	4	5	NA
183556	How to use a pulse oximetry	1	2	3	4	5	NA
183557	Correct use of oxygen	1	2	3	4	5	NA

K

Continued

Knowledge: Heart Failure Management—cont'd

	No knowledge	Limited knowledge	Moderate knowledge	Substantial knowledge	Extensive knowledge	
183532	Effects on lifestyle	1	2	3	4	5	NA
183533	Adaptations for role performance	1	2	3	4	5	NA
183558	Risks associated with travel	1	2	3	4	5	NA
183559	Adaptations for travel	1	2	3	4	5	NA
183534	Effects on sexuality	1	2	3	4	5	NA
183535	Adaptations for sexual performance	1	2	3	4	5	NA
183536	Available support groups	1	2	3	4	5	NA
183537	When to obtain assistance from a health professional	1	2	3	4	5	NA

Domain-Health Knowledge & Behavior (IV)   *Class*-Health Knowledge (S)   *4th edition 2008; revised 2013*

OUTCOME CONTENT REFERENCES:
Bonow, R. O., Bennett, S., Casey, D. E., Ganiats, T. G., Hlatky, M. A., et al. (2005). ACC/AHA clinical performance measures for adults with chronic heart failure: A report of the American College of Cardiology/American Heart Association Task Force on Performance Measures. *Circulation, 112,* 1853–1887.
Chen, A., Yehle, K., Plake, K., Murawski, M., & Mason, H. (2011). Health literacy and self-care of patients with heart failure. *Journal of Cardiovascular Nursing, 26*(6), 446–451.
House-Fancher, M. A., & Foell, H. Y. (2004). Nursing management: Heart failure and cardiomyopathy. In S. M. Lewis, M. M. Heitkemper, & S. R. Dirksen (Eds.), *Medical-surgical nursing* (6th ed., pp. 838–860). St. Louis: Mosby.
Lainscak, M., Blue, L., Clark, A. L., Dahlström, U., Dickstein, K., Ekman, I., McDonagh, T., McMurray, J. J., Ryder, M., Stewart, S., Strömberg, A., & Jaarsma, T. (2011). Self-care management of heart failure: Practical recommendations from the Patient Care Committee of the Heart Failure Association of the European Society of Cardiology. *European Journal of Heart Failure, 13*(2), 115–126.
Pina, I. L., Apstein, C. S., Balady, G. J., Belardinelli, R., Chaitman, B. R., Duscha, B. D., Fletcher, B. J., Fleg, J. L., Myers, J. N., & Sullivan, M. J. (2003). Exercise and heart failure: A statement from the American Heart Association Committee on Exercise, Rehabilitation, and Prevention. *Circulation, 107,* 1210–1225.
Silcox, P. D. (2005). Congestive heart failure. In D. L. Huber (Ed.), *Disease management: A guide for case managers* (pp. 71–80). St. Louis: Elsevier Saunders.

K

Knowledge: Hypertension Management   1837

Definition: Extent of understanding conveyed about high blood pressure, its treatment, and the prevention of complications

OUTCOME TARGET RATING: Maintain at_____   Increase to_____

	No knowledge	Limited knowledge	Moderate knowledge	Substantial knowledge	Extensive knowledge	
OUTCOME OVERALL RATING	1	2	3	4	5	
Indicators:						
183701 Normal range for systolic blood pressure	1	2	3	4	5	NA
183702 Normal range for diastolic blood pressure	1	2	3	4	5	NA
183703 Target blood pressure	1	2	3	4	5	NA
183704 Methods to measure blood pressure	1	2	3	4	5	NA
183705 Potential complications of hypertension	1	2	3	4	5	NA
183706 Available treatment options	1	2	3	4	5	NA
183707 Benefits of long-term treatment	1	2	3	4	5	NA
183708 Signs and symptoms of exacerbation of hypertension	1	2	3	4	5	NA
183709 Correct use of prescribed medication	1	2	3	4	5	NA
183710 Medication therapeutic effects	1	2	3	4	5	NA
183711 Medication side effects	1	2	3	4	5	NA
183712 Medication adverse effects	1	2	3	4	5	NA
183713 Importance of adherence to treatment	1	2	3	4	5	NA
183714 Importance of informing health professional of all current medication	1	2	3	4	5	NA

Knowledge: Hypertension Management—*cont'd*

	No knowledge	Limited knowledge	Moderate knowledge	Substantial knowledge	Extensive knowledge	
183715	Importance of keeping follow-up appointments	1	2	3	4	5	NA
183716	Benefits of ongoing self-monitoring	1	2	3	4	5	NA
183717	Recommended schedule for monitoring blood pressure	1	2	3	4	5	NA
183718	Benefits of weight loss	1	2	3	4	5	NA
183719	Benefits of lifestyle modifications	1	2	3	4	5	NA
183720	Strategies to manage stress	1	2	3	4	5	NA
183721	Prescribed diet	1	2	3	4	5	NA
183722	Strategies to change dietary habits	1	2	3	4	5	NA
183723	Strategies to limit sodium intake	1	2	3	4	5	NA
183724	Strategies to increase diet compliance	1	2	3	4	5	NA
183725	Adverse health effects of alcohol use	1	2	3	4	5	NA
183726	Importance of tobacco abstinence	1	2	3	4	5	NA
183727	Benefits of regular exercise	1	2	3	4	5	NA
183728	Reputable sources of hypertension information	1	2	3	4	5	NA
183729	Available support groups	1	2	3	4	5	NA
183730	When to obtain assistance from a health professional	1	2	3	4	5	NA
183731	Benefits of disease management	1	2	3	4	5	NA

Domain-*Health Knowledge & Behavior (IV)*   **Class**-*Health Knowledge (S)*   *4th edition 2008; revised 2013*

K

OUTCOME CONTENT REFERENCES:

Baster, T., & Baster-Brooks, C. (2005). Exercise and hypertension. *Australian Family Physician, 34*(6), 419–424.

Boulware, L. E., Daumit, G. L., Frick, K. D., Minkovitz, C. S., Lawrence, R. S., & Powe, N. R. (2001). An evidence-based review of patient-centered behavioral interventions for hypertension. *American Journal of Preventive Medicine, 21*(3), 221–232.

Egan, B., Zhao, Y., & Axon, R. (2010). US trends in prevalence, awareness, treatment, and control of hypertension, 1988-2008. *JAMA, 303*(20), 2043–2050.

Kaplan, N. M. (2004). Lifestyle modifications for prevention and treatment of hypertension. *The Journal of Clinical Hypertension, 6*(12), 716–719.

Knight, E. L., Bohn, R. L., Wang, P. S., Glynn, R. J., Mogun, H., & Avorn, J. (2001). Predictors of uncontrolled hypertension in ambulatory patients. *Hypertension, 38*(4), 809–814.

Morisky, D. E., Bowler, M. H., & Finlay, J. S. (1982). An educational and behavioral approach toward increasing patient activation in hypertension management. *Journal of Community Health, 7*(3), 171–182.

The National Collaborating Centre for Chronic Conditions. (2006). *Hypertension. Management of hypertension in adults in primary care: Partial update.* London: Royal College of Physicians.

Padwal, R., Campbell, N., Touyz, R. M. (2005). Applying the 2005 Canadian hypertension education program recommendations: 3. Lifestyle modifications to prevent and treat hypertension. *CMAJ: Canadian Medical Association Journal, 173*(7), 749–751.

Svetkey, L. P., Erlinger, T. P., Vollmer, W. M., Feldstein, A., Cooper, L. S., Appel, L. J., Ard, J. D., Elmer, P. J., Harsha, D., & Stevens, V. J. (2005). Effect of lifestyle modifications on blood pressure by race, sex, hypertension status, and age. *Journal of Human Hypertension, 19*(1), 21–31.

U.S. Department of Health and Human Services. (2003). *Your guide to lowering blood pressure.* Bethesda, MD: Author.

Zernike, W., & Henderson, A. (1998). Evaluating the effectiveness of two teaching strategies for patients diagnosed with hypertension. *Journal of Clinical Nursing, 7*(1), 37–44.

Knowledge: Infant Care 1819

Definition: Extent of understanding conveyed about caring for a baby from birth to first birthday

OUTCOME TARGET RATING: Maintain at_____   Increase to_____

		No knowledge	Limited knowledge	Moderate knowledge	Substantial knowledge	Extensive knowledge	
OUTCOME OVERALL RATING		1	2	3	4	5	
Indicators:							
181901	Normal infant characteristics	1	2	3	4	5	NA
181902	Normal growth and development	1	2	3	4	5	NA
181903	Proper holding of infant	1	2	3	4	5	NA
181904	Proper infant positioning	1	2	3	4	5	NA
181905	Infant safety practices	1	2	3	4	5	NA
181906	Swaddling	1	2	3	4	5	NA
181928	Age-appropriate cardiopulmonary resuscitation techniques	1	2	3	4	5	NA
181908	Nutritive versus non-nutritive sucking	1	2	3	4	5	NA
181909	Pros and cons of infant feeding choices	1	2	3	4	5	NA
181910	Infant feeding techniques	1	2	3	4	5	NA
181911	Signs and symptoms of dehydration	1	2	3	4	5	NA
181912	Signs and symptoms of jaundice	1	2	3	4	5	NA
181913	Infant bathing	1	2	3	4	5	NA
181914	Umbilical cord care	1	2	3	4	5	NA
181915	Infant diapering	1	2	3	4	5	NA
181916	Appropriate clothing for environment	1	2	3	4	5	NA
181917	Methods to measure body temperature	1	2	3	4	5	NA
181918	Infant sleep-wake patterns	1	2	3	4	5	NA
181919	Infant communication cues	1	2	3	4	5	NA
181920	Infant stimulation methods	1	2	3	4	5	NA
181921	Infant relaxation techniques	1	2	3	4	5	NA
181922	Strategies to adjust to addition of infant	1	2	3	4	5	NA
181923	Special care needs	1	2	3	4	5	NA
181924	Considerations when choosing a childcare provider	1	2	3	4	5	NA
181926	Precautions when pets are in the household	1	2	3	4	5	NA
181925	Available community resources	1	2	3	4	5	NA
181929	Available support groups	1	2	3	4	5	NA

Domain-Health Knowledge & Behavior (IV)   **Class**-Health Knowledge (S)   *2nd edition 2000; revised 2004, 2008, 2013*

OUTCOME CONTENT REFERENCES:
Association of Women's Health, Obstetricians and Neonatal Nurses. (1998). *Standards & guidelines for the professional nursing practice in the care of women and newborns* (5th ed.). Washington, DC: Author
Nichols, F., & Humenick, S. (2000). *Childbirth education: Practice, research and theory* (2nd ed.). Philadelphia: W. B. Saunders.
Reeder, S. J., Martin, L. L., & Koniak-Griffin, D. (1997). *Maternity nursing: Family, newborn, and women's health care* (18th ed.). Philadelphia: Lippincott.

Knowledge: Infection Management 1842

Definition: Extent of understanding conveyed about infection, its treatment, and the prevention of disease progression and complications

OUTCOME TARGET RATING: Maintain at_____ Increase to_____

OUTCOME OVERALL RATING	No knowledge 1	Limited knowledge 2	Moderate knowledge 3	Substantial knowledge 4	Extensive knowledge 5	
Indicators:						
184201 Mode of transmission	1	2	3	4	5	NA
184202 Factors contributing to infection transmission	1	2	3	4	5	NA
184203 Practices that reduce transmission	1	2	3	4	5	NA
184204 Signs and symptoms of infection	1	2	3	4	5	NA
184206 Monitoring procedures for infection	1	2	3	4	5	NA
184207 Importance of hand sanitation	1	2	3	4	5	NA
184208 Actions to increase resistance to infection	1	2	3	4	5	NA
184209 Treatment for diagnosed infection	1	2	3	4	5	NA
184210 Follow-up for diagnosed infection	1	2	3	4	5	NA
184211 Signs and symptoms of exacerbation of infection	1	2	3	4	5	NA
184212 Correct name of medication	1	2	3	4	5	NA
184213 Medication side effects	1	2	3	4	5	NA
184214 Medication therapeutic effects	1	2	3	4	5	NA
184215 Medication adverse effects	1	2	3	4	5	NA
184216 Potential medication interactions	1	2	3	4	5	NA
184217 Importance of adherence to treatment	1	2	3	4	5	NA
184218 Use of probiotics in the treatment of infection	1	2	3	4	5	NA
184219 Risk of drug resistance	1	2	3	4	5	NA
184220 Importance of completing medication regimen	1	2	3	4	5	NA
184221 Influences of nutrition on infection	1	2	3	4	5	NA
184222 Strategies to manage stress	1	2	3	4	5	NA
184223 Factors that affect immune response	1	2	3	4	5	NA
184224 Available support groups	1	2	3	4	5	NA
184225 Available community resources	1	2	3	4	5	NA
184226 When to obtain assistance from a health professional	1	2	3	4	5	NA

Domain-Health Knowledge & Behavior (IV)   **Class**-Health Knowledge (S)   4th edition 2008; revised 2013

OUTCOME CONTENT REFERENCES:

Centers for Disease Control and Prevention, National Center for HIV, STD, and TB Prevention & Division of Tuberculosis Elimination. (2000). *Core curriculum on tuberculosis* (4th ed.). Atlanta: U.S. Department of Health and Human Services.

Conn, V. S., Armer, J. M., & Hayes, K. S. (2001). Knowledge deficit. In M. Maas, K. Buckwalter, M. Hardy, T. Tripp-Reimer, M. Titler, & J. Specht (Eds.), *Nursing care of older adults: Diagnoses, outcomes & interventions* (pp. 503–515). St. Louis: Mosby.

Joseph, A. (2006). *The impact of the environment on infections in healthcare facilities.* Princeton, NJ: Robert Wood Johnson Foundation.

National Center for Nursing Research. (1990). *HIV infection: Prevention and care.* Bethesda, MD: U.S. Department of Health and Human Services.

Rotheram-Borus, M. J., Reid, M. A., & Rosario, M. (1994). Factors mediating changes in sexual HIV risk behaviors among gay and bisexual male adolescents. *American Journal of Public Health, 84*(12), 1938–1946.

Simons-Morton, D. G., Mullen, P. D., Mains, D. A., Tabak, E. R., & Green, L. W. (1992). Characteristics of controlled studies of patient education and counseling for preventive health behaviors. *Patient Education and Counseling, 19*(2), 174–204.

Statton, P., & Alexander, N. J. (1993). Prevention of sexually transmitted infections: Physical and chemical barrier methods. *Infectious Disease Clinics of North America, 7*(4), 841–859.

Ungvarski, P. J., & Flaskerud, J. H. (1999). *HIV/AIDS: A guide to primary care management* (4th ed.). Philadelphia: W. B. Saunders.

K

Knowledge: Inflammatory Bowel Disease Management 1856

Definition: Extent of understanding conveyed about the inflammatory bowel disease process, its treatment and the prevention of relapses or complications

OUTCOME TARGET RATING: Maintain at_____   Increase to_____

	No knowledge	Limited knowledge	Moderate knowledge	Substantial knowledge	Extensive knowledge	
OUTCOME OVERALL RATING	1	2	3	4	5	
Indicators:						
185601 Cause and contributing factors	1	2	3	4	5	NA
185602 Risk factors for disease progression	1	2	3	4	5	NA
185603 Usual course of disease	1	2	3	4	5	NA
185604 Signs and symptoms of inflammatory bowel disease	1	2	3	4	5	NA
185605 Area of bowel affected by disease	1	2	3	4	5	NA
185606 Signs and symptoms of disease relapse	1	2	3	4	5	NA
185607 Benefits of disease management	1	2	3	4	5	NA
185608 Strategies to balance activity and rest	1	2	3	4	5	NA
185609 Energy conservation techniques	1	2	3	4	5	NA
185610 Medication therapeutic effects	1	2	3	4	5	NA
185611 Medication side effects	1	2	3	4	5	NA
185612 Medication adverse effects	1	2	3	4	5	NA
185613 Medical treatment options	1	2	3	4	5	NA
185614 Surgical treatment options	1	2	3	4	5	NA
185615 Psychosocial effects of disease	1	2	3	4	5	NA
185616 Relationship of physical and emotional stress to condition	1	2	3	4	5	NA
185617 Role of diagnostic tests for disease management	1	2	3	4	5	NA
185618 Potential complications of disease	1	2	3	4	5	NA
185619 Strategies to minimize disease progression	1	2	3	4	5	NA
185620 Prescribed diet	1	2	3	4	5	NA
185621 Trigger foods	1	2	3	4	5	NA
185622 Strategies to modify nutritional requirements	1	2	3	4	5	NA
185623 Strategies to enhance bowel function	1	2	3	4	5	NA
185624 Factors that trigger relapse	1	2	3	4	5	NA
185625 Strategies to manage pain	1	2	3	4	5	NA
185626 Effects on lifestyle	1	2	3	4	5	NA
185627 Strategies to adapt lifestyle to energy level	1	2	3	4	5	NA
185628 Effects on sexuality	1	2	3	4	5	NA
185629 Potential effects of pregnancy	1	2	3	4	5	NA
185630 Activity restrictions during a relapse	1	2	3	4	5	NA
185631 Importance of tobacco abstinence	1	2	3	4	5	NA
185632 Impact of disease on growth and development	1	2	3	4	5	NA
185633 Available support groups	1	2	3	4	5	NA
185634 When to obtain assistance from a health professional	1	2	3	4	5	NA

Domain-Health Knowledge & Behavior (IV) **Class**-Health Knowledge (S)   5th edition 2013

OUTCOME CONTENT REFERENCES:

Bruno, M. (2004). Irritable bowel syndrome and inflammatory bowel disease in pregnancy. *Journal of Perinatal and Neonatal Nursing, 18*(4), 341–350.

Fletcher, P. C., & Schneider, M. A. (2006). Is there any food I can eat? Living with inflammatory bowel disease and/or irritable bowel syndrome. *Clinical Nurse Specialist, 20*(5), 241–247.

Fow, J., & Grossman, S. (2006). A comprehensive guide to patient-focused management strategies for Crohn disease. *Gastroenterology Nursing, 30*(2), 93–99.

MacDonald, A. (2006). Omega-3 fatty acids as adjunctive therapy in Crohns disease. *Gastroenterology Nursing, 29*(4), 295–304.

Razack, R., & Seidner, D. L. (2007). Nutrition in inflammatory bowel disease. *Current Opinion in Gastroenterology, 23*(4), 400–405.

Rufo, P. A., & Bousvaros, A. (2007). Challenges and progress in pediatric inflammatory bowel disease. *Current Opinion in Gastroenterology, 23*(4), 406–412.

Ruthruff, B. (2007). Clinical review of Crohn's disease. *Journal of the American Academy of Nurse Practitioners, 1*(9), 392–397.

Vizcarra, C. (2003). New perspectives and emerging therapies for immune-mediated inflammatory disorders. *Journal of Infusion Nursing, 26*(5), 319–325.

Zaidel, O., & Abreu, M. T. (2003). Crohn's disease: An evidence-based approach to medical management. *Journal of Clinical Outcomes Management, 10*(5), 279–290.

Knowledge: Kidney Disease Management 1857

Definition: Extent of understanding conveyed about kidney disease, its treatment, and the prevention of disease progression and complications

OUTCOME TARGET RATING: Maintain at_____   Increase to_____

OUTCOME OVERALL RATING	No knowledge 1	Limited knowledge 2	Moderate knowledge 3	Substantial knowledge 4	Extensive knowledge 5	
Indicators:						
185701 Specific kidney disease	1	2	3	4	5	NA
185702 Signs and symptoms of kidney disease	1	2	3	4	5	NA
185703 Usual course of disease	1	2	3	4	5	NA
185704 Cause and contributing factors	1	2	3	4	5	NA
185705 Risk factors for complications	1	2	3	4	5	NA
185706 Signs and symptoms of complications	1	2	3	4	5	NA
185707 Strategies to prevent complications	1	2	3	4	5	NA
185708 Strategies to minimize disease progression	1	2	3	4	5	NA
185709 Relationship of kidney disease to hypertension	1	2	3	4	5	NA
185710 Signs and symptoms of fluid volume excess	1	2	3	4	5	NA
185711 Strategies to reduce risk of bleeding	1	2	3	4	5	NA
185712 Activity precautions	1	2	3	4	5	NA
185713 Strategies to increase resistance to infection	1	2	3	4	5	NA
185714 Strategies to maintain adequate nutrition	1	2	3	4	5	NA
185715 Dietary restrictions	1	2	3	4	5	NA
185716 Fluid restrictions	1	2	3	4	5	NA
185717 Relationship of fluid intake and weight	1	2	3	4	5	NA
185718 Importance of monitoring intake and output	1	2	3	4	5	NA
185719 Required laboratory tests	1	2	3	4	5	NA
185720 Role of laboratory tests for disease management	1	2	3	4	5	NA
185721 Recommended schedule for monitoring blood pressure	1	2	3	4	5	NA
185722 Importance of maintaining blood glucose level within target range	1	2	3	4	5	NA
185723 Medication used for kidney disease	1	2	3	4	5	NA
185724 Medication therapeutic effects	1	2	3	4	5	NA
185725 Medication side effects	1	2	3	4	5	NA
185726 Medication adverse effects	1	2	3	4	5	NA
185727 Potential dangers of taking non-prescription medication	1	2	3	4	5	NA
185728 Importance of compliance with treatment regimen	1	2	3	4	5	NA
185729 Importance of adequate sleep	1	2	3	4	5	NA
185730 Strategies to cope with adverse effects of disease	1	2	3	4	5	NA
185731 Strategies to cope with changes in body image	1	2	3	4	5	NA
185732 Strategies to maintain intact oral mucosa	1	2	3	4	5	NA
185733 Strategies to decrease nausea	1	2	3	4	5	NA
185734 When to obtain assistance from a health professional	1	2	3	4	5	NA
185735 Available support groups	1	2	3	4	5	NA
185736 Available community resources	1	2	3	4	5	NA
185737 Benefits of disease management	1	2	3	4	5	NA

K

Domain-Health Knowledge & Behavior (IV)   **Class-**Health Knowledge (S)   5th edition 2013

OUTCOME CONTENT REFERENCES:
Agrawai, V., Barnes, M., Ghosh, A., & McCullough, P. (2009). Questionnaire instrument to assess knowledge of chronic kidney disease clinical practice guidelines among internal medicine residents. *Journal of Evaluation in Clinical Practice, 15*(4), 733–738.

Ali, B., & Gray-Vickrey, P. (2011). Limiting the damage from acute kidney injury. *Nursing 2011, 41*(3), 22–31.

Avery-Lynch, M. (2006). Intradialytic parenteral nutrition in hemodialysis patients: Acute and chronic intervention. *Canadian Association of Nephrology Nurses and Technologists, 16*(2), 30–33.

Bernstein, A. M., Treyzon, L., & Li, Z. (2007). Are high-protein, vegetable-based diets safe for kidney function? A review of the literature. *Journal of the American Dietetic Association, 107*(4), 644–655.

Combe, C., McCullough, K. P., Asano, Y., Ginsberg, N., Maroni, B. J., Pifer, T. B. K. (2004). Kidney Disease Outcomes Quality Initiative (K/DOQI) and the Dialysis Outcomes and Practice Pattern Study (DOPPS): Nutrition guidelines, indicators, and practices. *American Journal of Kidney Diseases,* 44(5, Suppl. 2), 539–546.

Davison, S. N., & Simpson, C. (2006). Hope and advance care planning in patients with end stage renal disease: Qualitative interview study. *British Medical Journal, 333*(7574), 886–890.

Guo, H., Kaira, P. A., Gilbertson, D. T., Liu, J, Chen, S. C., Collins, A. J., & Foley, R. N. (2007). Atherosclerotic renovascular disease in older US patients starting dialysis, 1996–2001. *Circulation, 115*(1), 50–58.

LeMone, P., Burke, K., & Bauldoff, G. (Eds.). (2011). *Medical-surgical nursing: Critical thinking in client care* (Vol. 1, 4th ed.). Upper Saddle River, NJ: Pearson Education.

McLennan, G. (2007). Vein preservation: An algorithmic approach to vascular access placement in patients with compromised renal function. *Journal of the Association for Vascular Access, 12*(2), 89–91.

Olivares, R. (2007). Important considerations in iron management and nutritional status in select hemodialysis populations. *Nephrology Nursing Journal, 34*(4), 425–434.

Rabindranath, K. S., Adams, J., Ali, T. Z., MacLeod, A. M., Vale, L., Cody, J., Wallace, S. A., & Daly, C. (2007). Continuous ambulatory peritoneal dialysis versus automated peritoneal dialysis for end-stage renal disease. *The Cochrane Database of Systematic Reviews,* Issue 2: CD006515.

Rabindranath, K. S., Dally, C., Butier, J. A., Roderick, P. H., Wallace, S., & MacLeod, A. M. (2005). Psychosocial interventions for depression in dialysis. *The Cochrane Database of Systematic Reviews,* Issue 3: CD004542.

Richard. C. J. (2006). Self-care management in adults undergoing hemodialysis. *Nephrology Nursing Journal, 33*(4), 387–394.

Shankar, A., Klein, R., & Klein, B. E. K. (2006). The association among smoking, heavy drinking, and chronic kidney disease. *American Journal of Epidemiology, 164*(3), 263–271.

K

Knowledge: Labor & Delivery   1817

Definition: Extent of understanding conveyed about labor and vaginal delivery

OUTCOME TARGET RATING: Maintain at_____   Increase to_____

OUTCOME OVERALL RATING	No knowledge	Limited knowledge	Moderate knowledge	Substantial knowledge	Extensive knowledge	
	1	2	3	4	5	
Indicators:						
181701 Birthing options	1	2	3	4	5	NA
181702 Role of the labor coach	1	2	3	4	5	NA
181703 Signs and symptoms of labor	1	2	3	4	5	NA
181704 Stages of labor and delivery	1	2	3	4	5	NA
181705 Strategies to control pain	1	2	3	4	5	NA
181706 Effective breathing techniques	1	2	3	4	5	NA
181707 Effective relaxation techniques	1	2	3	4	5	NA
181708 Effective positioning techniques	1	2	3	4	5	NA
181709 Potential medical procedures	1	2	3	4	5	NA
181710 Potential complications of birthing	1	2	3	4	5	NA
181711 Effective pushing techniques	1	2	3	4	5	NA
181714 Delivery of infant	1	2	3	4	5	NA
181712 Delivery of placenta	1	2	3	4	5	NA

Domain-*Health Knowledge & Behavior (IV)*   **Class**-*Health Knowledge (S)*   *2nd edition 2000; revised 2004, 2008*

OUTCOME CONTENT REFERENCES:

Association of Women's Health, Obstetric, and Neonatal Nurses. (2004). *Core curriculum for maternal-newborn nursing.* Washington, DC: Author.

Nichols, F., & Humenick, S. (2000). *Childbirth education: Practice, research and theory* (2nd ed.). Philadelphia: W. B. Saunders.

Reeder, S. J., Martin, L. L., & Koniak-Griffin, D. (1997). *Maternity nursing: Family, newborn, and women's health care* (18th ed.). Philadelphia: Lippincott.

Knowledge: Lipid Disorder Management 1858

Definition: Extent of understanding conveyed about hyperlipidemia, its treatment, and the prevention of complications

OUTCOME TARGET RATING: Maintain at_____ Increase to_____

		No knowledge	Limited knowledge	Moderate knowledge	Substantial knowledge	Extensive knowledge	
OUTCOME OVERALL RATING		1	2	3	4	5	
Indicators:							
185801	Cause and contributing factors	1	2	3	4	5	NA
185802	Signs and symptoms of complications	1	2	3	4	5	NA
185803	Required laboratory tests for monitoring lipid levels	1	2	3	4	5	NA
185804	Target lipid levels	1	2	3	4	5	NA
185805	Benefits of lifestyle modifications	1	2	3	4	5	NA
185806	Benefits of weight loss	1	2	3	4	5	NA
185807	Benefits of aerobic exercise	1	2	3	4	5	NA
185808	Prescribed diet	1	2	3	4	5	NA
185809	Strategies to change dietary habits	1	2	3	4	5	NA
185810	Correct use of prescribed medication	1	2	3	4	5	NA
185811	Potential medication interactions with food	1	2	3	4	5	NA
185812	Medication therapeutic effects	1	2	3	4	5	NA
185813	Medication side effects	1	2	3	4	5	NA
185814	Medication adverse effects	1	2	3	4	5	NA
185815	Importance of adherence to treatment	1	2	3	4	5	NA
185816	Recommendations for alcohol use	1	2	3	4	5	NA
185817	Importance of tobacco abstinence	1	2	3	4	5	NA
185818	Reputable sources of hyperlipidemia information	1	2	3	4	5	NA
185819	Available support groups	1	2	3	4	5	NA
185820	When to obtain assistance from a health professional	1	2	3	4	5	NA
185821	Benefits of hyperlipidemia management	1	2	3	4	5	NA

Domain-*Health Knowledge & Behavior (IV)* **Class**-*Health Knowledge (S)* *5th edition 2013*

OUTCOME CONTENT REFERENCES:
Bertolotti, M. (2009). High protein intake reduces intrahepatocellular lipid deposition in humans. *The American Journal of Clinical Nutrition*, 90(4), 1002–1009.
Elpers, M. (2008). Common obstacles in lipid management. *Critical Care Nursing Clinics of North America, 20*(3), 287–295.
Gatti, A., Maranghi, M., Bacci, S., Carallo, C., Gnasso, A., Mandosi, E., Fallarino, M., Morano, S., Trischitta, V., & Filetti, S. (2009). Poor glycemic control is an independent risk factor for low HDL cholesterol in patients with type 2 diabetes. *Diabetes Care, 32*(8), 1550–1552.
Iughetti, L., Bruzzi, P., & Predieri, B. (2010). Evaluation and management of hyperlipidemia in children and adolescents. *Current Opinion in Pediatrics, 22*(4), 485–493.
Lowenstein, C. J., & Cameron, S. J. (2010). High-density lipoprotein metabolism and endothelial function. *Current Opinion in Endocrinology, Diabetes & Obesity, 17*(2), 166–170.

K

Knowledge: Medication   1808

Definition: Extent of understanding conveyed about the safe use of medication

OUTCOME TARGET RATING: Maintain at_____   Increase to_____

	No knowledge	Limited knowledge	Moderate knowledge	Substantial knowledge	Extensive knowledge	
OUTCOME OVERALL RATING	1	2	3	4	5	

Indicators:

180801	Importance of informing health professional of all current medication	1	2	3	4	5	NA
180802	Correct name of medication	1	2	3	4	5	NA
180803	Appearance of medication	1	2	3	4	5	NA
180819	Medication therapeutic effects	1	2	3	4	5	NA
180805	Medication side effects	1	2	3	4	5	NA
180820	Medication adverse effects	1	2	3	4	5	NA
180807	Use of memory aids	1	2	3	4	5	NA
180808	Potential medication interactions	1	2	3	4	5	NA
180809	Potential medication interactions with other agents	1	2	3	4	5	NA
180810	Correct use of prescribed medication	1	2	3	4	5	NA
180821	Correct use of non-prescription medication	1	2	3	4	5	NA
180822	Proper technique for self-injection	1	2	3	4	5	NA
180811	Self-monitoring techniques	1	2	3	4	5	NA
180812	Proper medication storage	1	2	3	4	5	NA
180815	Proper disposal of medication	1	2	3	4	5	NA
180813	Proper care of administration devices	1	2	3	4	5	NA
180823	Proper disposal of syringes and needles	1	2	3	4	5	NA
180824	Strategies to obtain required medication	1	2	3	4	5	NA
180825	Strategies to obtain required supplies	1	2	3	4	5	NA
180826	Available financial support	1	2	3	4	5	NA
180816	Required laboratory tests for monitoring medication	1	2	3	4	5	NA
180817	Importance of using medical alert identification	1	2	3	4	5	NA

Specify medication(s): _____

Domain-Health Knowledge & Behavior (IV)   **Class**-Health Knowledge (S)   1st edition 1997; revised 2004, 2008, 2013

OUTCOME CONTENT REFERENCES:

Barry, K. (1993). Patient self-medication: An innovative approach to medication teaching. *Journal of Nursing Care Quality, 8*(1), 75–82.

Colley, C. A., & Lucas, L. M. (1993). Polypharmacy: The cure becomes the disease. *Journal of General Internal Medicine, 8*(5), 278–283.

Conn, V. S., Armer, J. M., & Hayes, K. S. (2001). Knowledge deficit. In M. Maas, K. Buckwalter, M. Hardy, T. Tripp-Reimer, M. Titler, & J. Specht (Eds.), *Nursing care of older adults: Diagnoses, outcomes & interventions* (pp. 503–515). St. Louis: Mosby.

Everitt, D. E., & Avorn, J. (1986). Drug prescribing for the elderly. *Archives of Internal Medicine, 146*(12), 2393–2396.

Kleoppel, J. W., & Henry, D. W. (1987). Teaching patients, families, and communities about their medications. In C.E. Smith (Ed.), *Patient education: Nurses in partnership with other health professionals* (pp. 271–296). Philadelphia: W. B. Saunders.

Proos, M., Reiley, P., Eagan, J., Stengrevics, S., Castile, J., & Arian, D. (1992). A study of the effects of self-medication on patients' knowledge of and compliance with their medication regimen. *Journal of Nursing Care Quality*, Special Report, 18–26.

Simons-Morton, D. G., Mullen, P. D., Mains, D. A., Tabak, E. R., & Green, L. W. (1992). Characteristics of controlled studies of patient education and counseling for preventive health behaviors. *Patient Education and Counseling, 19*(2), 174–204.

Togger, D. A., & Brenner, P. S. (2001). Metered dose inhalers. *American Journal of Nursing, 101*(10), 26–32, 38–39.

U.S. Department of Health and Human Services. (1990). *Healthy people 2000: National health promotion and disease prevention objectives.* Washington, DC: U.S. Government Printing Office.

Waddell, D. L., Hummel, M. E., & Sumners, A. D. (2001). Three herbs you should get to know. *American Journal of Nursing, 101*(4), 48–54.

Weitzel, E. A. (2001). Risk for poisoning: Drug toxicity. In M. Maas, K. Buckwalter, M. Hardy, T. Tripp-Reimer, M. Titler, & J. Specht (Eds.), *Nursing care of older adults: Diagnoses, outcomes & interventions* (pp. 34–46). St. Louis: Mosby.

Knowledge: Multiple Sclerosis Management 1838

Definition: Extent of understanding conveyed about multiple sclerosis, its treatment and the prevention of relapses or complications

OUTCOME TARGET RATING: Maintain at_____ Increase to_____

		No knowledge	Limited knowledge	Moderate knowledge	Substantial knowledge	Extensive knowledge	
OUTCOME OVERALL RATING		1	2	3	4	5	NA
Indicators:							
183801	Signs and symptoms of multiple sclerosis	1	2	3	4	5	NA
183802	Usual course of disease	1	2	3	4	5	NA
183803	Therapeutic effects of personal treatment regimen	1	2	3	4	5	NA
183804	Benefits of adequate rest	1	2	3	4	5	NA
183805	Relationship of fatigue to disease	1	2	3	4	5	NA
183806	Strategies to control fatigue	1	2	3	4	5	NA
183807	Factors that decrease energy expenditure	1	2	3	4	5	NA
183808	Energy conservation techniques	1	2	3	4	5	NA
183809	Strategies to manage stress	1	2	3	4	5	NA
183810	Factors that trigger relapse	1	2	3	4	5	NA
183811	Factors that trigger exacerbation	1	2	3	4	5	NA
183812	Strategies to control symptoms	1	2	3	4	5	NA
183813	Benefits of disease management	1	2	3	4	5	NA
183814	When to obtain assistance from a health professional	1	2	3	4	5	NA
183815	Medication therapeutic effects	1	2	3	4	5	NA
183816	Medication side effects	1	2	3	4	5	NA
183817	Medication adverse effects	1	2	3	4	5	NA
183818	Strategies to decrease treatment regimen side effects	1	2	3	4	5	NA
183819	Proper technique for self-injection	1	2	3	4	5	NA
183820	Potential prescribed medication interactions with other medication	1	2	3	4	5	NA
183821	Alternative treatments	1	2	3	4	5	NA
183822	Strategies to cope with limitations	1	2	3	4	5	NA
183823	Adverse health effects of extreme temperature on disease	1	2	3	4	5	NA
183824	Strategies to increase diet compliance	1	2	3	4	5	NA
183825	Strategies to increase resistance to infection	1	2	3	4	5	NA
183826	Strategies to balance activity and rest	1	2	3	4	5	NA
183827	Strategies to cope with unpredictability of disease	1	2	3	4	5	NA
183834	Strategies to enhance bladder function	1	2	3	4	5	NA
183835	Strategies to enhance bowel function	1	2	3	4	5	NA
183829	Surgical treatment options	1	2	3	4	5	NA
183830	Available support groups	1	2	3	4	5	NA
183831	Available community resources	1	2	3	4	5	NA
183832	Adaptations for role performance	1	2	3	4	5	NA
183833	Reputable sources of multiple sclerosis information	1	2	3	4	5	NA

K

Domain-*Health Knowledge & Behavior (IV)*   ***Class-****Health Knowledge (S)*   *4th edition 2008; revised 2013*

OUTCOME CONTENT REFERENCES:

Denis, L., Namey, M., Costello, K., Frenette, J., Gagnon, N., Harris, C., Lowden, D., McEwan, L., Morrison, W., & Poirier, J. (2004). Long-term treatment optimization in individuals with multiple sclerosis using disease-modifying therapies: A nursing approach. *Journal of Neuroscience Nursing. 36*(1):10–22.

Embrey, N., Lowndes, C., & Warner, R. (2003). Benchmarking best practice in relapse management of multiple sclerosis. *Nursing Standard. 17*(22):38–42.

Jarrett, L. (2003). Attitudes to long-term care in multiple sclerosis. *Nursing Standard. 17*(17), 39–43.

National Multiple Sclerosis Society. Retrieved from http://www.nmss.org

Ozuna, J. M. (2004). Nursing management: Chronic neurologic problems. In S. M. Lewis, M. M. Heitkemper, & S. R. Dirksen (Eds.), *Medical-surgical nursing: Assessment and management of clinical problems* (6th ed., pp. 1549–1580). St. Louis: Mosby.

Ward, N., & Winters, S. (2003). Results of a fatigue management programme in multiple sclerosis. *British Journal of Nursing. 12*(18), 1075–1080.

Knowledge: Osteoporosis Management 1859

Definition: Extent of understanding conveyed about osteoporosis, its treatment, and the prevention of disease progression and complications

OUTCOME TARGET RATING: Maintain at_____   Increase to_____

	No knowledge	Limited knowledge	Moderate knowledge	Substantial knowledge	Extensive knowledge	
OUTCOME OVERALL RATING	1	2	3	4	5	

Indicators:

185901	Cause and contributing factors	1	2	3	4	5	NA
185902	Signs and symptoms of osteoporosis	1	2	3	4	5	NA
185903	Relationship of bone metabolism and osteoporosis	1	2	3	4	5	NA
185904	Relationship of testosterone and estrogen levels and osteoporosis	1	2	3	4	5	NA
185905	Risk of fracture	1	2	3	4	5	NA
185906	Recommended daily calcium supplements	1	2	3	4	5	NA
185907	Recommended daily vitamin D supplements	1	2	3	4	5	NA
185908	Benefits of sunlight exposure for source of vitamin D	1	2	3	4	5	NA
185909	Prescribed diet	1	2	3	4	5	NA
185910	Strategies to change dietary habits	1	2	3	4	5	NA
185911	Benefits of weight-bearing exercises	1	2	3	4	5	NA
185912	Benefits of muscle-strengthening exercise	1	2	3	4	5	NA
185913	Benefits of lifestyle modifications	1	2	3	4	5	NA
185914	Medications that reduce bone density	1	2	3	4	5	NA
185915	Prescribed medication						
185916	Strategies to take prescribed medication as scheduled	1	2	3	4	5	NA
185917	Medication therapeutic effects	1	2	3	4	5	NA
185918	Medication side effects	1	2	3	4	5	NA
185919	Medication adverse effects	1	2	3	4	5	NA
185920	Course of treatment						
185921	Importance of adherence to treatment	1	2	3	4	5	NA
185922	Recommended bone mineral density testing	1	2	3	4	5	NA
185923	Importance of alcohol restrictions	1	2	3	4	5	NA
185924	Importance of tobacco abstinence	1	2	3	4	5	NA
185925	Strategies to prevent falls	1	2	3	4	5	NA
185926	Available social support	1	2	3	4	5	NA
185927	Available community resources	1	2	3	4	5	NA

Domain-Health Knowledge & Behavior (IV)   **Class**-Health Knowledge (S)   5th edition 2013

OUTCOME CONTENT REFERENCES:

Alexander, L., LaRosa, J. H., Bader, H., Garfield, S., & Alexander, W. J. (2010). *New dimensions in women's health* (5th ed.). Boston: Jones & Bartlett.

Costa-Paiva, L., Gomes, D., Morais, S., Pedro, A., & Pinto-Neto, A. (2011). Knowledge about osteoporosis in postmenopausal women undergoing antiresorptive treatment. *Maturitas, 69*(1), 81–85.

Daly, R., Ahlborg, H., Ringsberg, K., Gardsell, P., Sembo, I., Karlsson, M. (2008). Association between changes in habitual physical activity and changes in bone density, muscle strength, and functional performance in elderly men and women. *Journal of the American Geriatrics Society, 56*(12), 2252–2260.

Gaines, J., & Marx, K. (2011). Older men's knowledge about osteoporosis and educational interventions to increase osteoporosis knowledge in older men: A systematic review. *Maturitas, 68*(1), 5–12.

International Society for Clinical Densitometry (ISCD). (2004). *Pocket guide to bone mineral density testing.* Retrieved from http://www.iscd.org/visitors/pdfs/ISCD-CANADIANPanelOfficialPositions-BMDcard.pdf

Matheson, E., Mainous, A., & Carnemolla, M. (2009). The association between onion consumption and bone density in perimenopausal and postmenopausal non-Hispanic white women 50 years and older. *Menopause, 16*(4), 756–759.

National Institute of Arthritis and Musculoskeletal and Skin Diseases. (2009). *Bone mass measurement: What the numbers mean.* Retrieved from http://www.niams.nih.gov/Health_Info/Bone/Bone_Health/bone_mass_measure.asp

Nielsen, D., Ryg, J., Nielsen, W., Knold, B., Nissen, N., & Brixen, K. (2010). Patient education in groups increases knowledge of osteoporosis and adherence to treatment: A two-year randomized controlled trial. *Patient Education and Counseling, 81*(2), 155–160.

Papaloannou, A., Morin, S., Cheung, A., Atkinson, S., Brown, J., Feldman, S., et al. (2010). 2010 clinical practice guidelines for the diagnosis and management of osteoporosis in Canada: A summary. *Canadian Medical Association Journal, 182*(17), 1864–1873.

K

Knowledge: Ostomy Care   1829

Definition: Extent of understanding conveyed about maintenance of an ostomy for elimination

OUTCOME TARGET RATING: Maintain at_____   Increase to_____

		No knowledge	Limited knowledge	Moderate knowledge	Substantial knowledge	Extensive knowledge	
OUTCOME OVERALL RATING		1	2	3	4	5	
Indicators:							
182902	Purpose of ostomy	1	2	3	4	5	NA
182901	Function of ostomy	1	2	3	4	5	NA
182909	Supplies required to care for ostomy	1	2	3	4	5	NA
182915	Procedure to change ostomy bag	1	2	3	4	5	NA
182908	Schedule for changing ostomy bag	1	2	3	4	5	NA
182905	How to measure stoma	1	2	3	4	5	NA
182907	Complications related to stoma	1	2	3	4	5	NA
182916	Procedure to empty ostomy bag	1	2	3	4	5	NA
182903	Skin care needs around ostomy	1	2	3	4	5	NA
182904	Irrigation techniques	1	2	3	4	5	NA
182910	Flatus-producing foods	1	2	3	4	5	NA
182911	Diet modifications	1	2	3	4	5	NA
182912	Fluid intake requirements	1	2	3	4	5	NA
182913	Odor control mechanisms	1	2	3	4	5	NA
182914	Modification of daily activities	1	2	3	4	5	NA
182917	Available support groups	1	2	3	4	5	NA

Domain-Health Knowledge & Behavior (IV)   **Class**-Health Knowledge (S)   *3rd edition 2004; revised 2008, 2013*

OUTCOME CONTENT REFERENCES:
Bryant, D., & Fleischer, I. (2000). Changing an ostomy appliance. *Nursing, 30*(11), 51–53.
O'Shea, H. S. (2001). Teaching the adult ostomy patient. *Journal of Wound, Ostomy, and Continence Nursing, 28*(1), 47–54.
Thompson, J. (2000). A practical ostomy guide. *RN, 63*(11), 61–68.

K

Knowledge: Pain Management   1843

Definition: Extent of understanding conveyed about causes, symptoms, and treatment of pain

OUTCOME TARGET RATING: Maintain at_____   Increase to_____

		No knowledge	Limited knowledge	Moderate knowledge	Substantial knowledge	Extensive knowledge	
OUTCOME OVERALL RATING		1	2	3	4	5	
Indicators:							
184301	Cause and contributing factors	1	2	3	4	5	NA
184302	Signs and symptoms of pain	1	2	3	4	5	NA
184303	Strategies to control pain	1	2	3	4	5	NA
184304	Strategies to manage chronic pain	1	2	3	4	5	NA
184305	Prescribed medication regimen	1	2	3	4	5	NA
184306	Correct use of prescribed medication	1	2	3	4	5	NA
184307	Correct use of non-prescription medication	1	2	3	4	5	NA
184308	Safe use of prescribed medication	1	2	3	4	5	NA
184309	Safe use of non-prescription medication	1	2	3	4	5	NA
184310	Medication therapeutic effects	1	2	3	4	5	NA
184311	Medication side effects	1	2	3	4	5	NA
184312	Medication adverse effects	1	2	3	4	5	NA

Continued

Knowledge: Pain Management—cont'd

		No knowledge	Limited knowledge	Moderate knowledge	Substantial knowledge	Extensive knowledge	
184313	Potential medication interactions	1	2	3	4	5	NA
184314	Potential medication interactions with other agents	1	2	3	4	5	NA
184315	Safety issues related to medication	1	2	3	4	5	NA
184316	Proper medication storage	1	2	3	4	5	NA
184317	Proper disposal of medication	1	2	3	4	5	NA
184318	Importance of compliance with medication regimen	1	2	3	4	5	NA
184319	Importance of informing health professional of all current medication	1	2	3	4	5	NA
184320	Activity restrictions	1	2	3	4	5	NA
184321	Activity precautions	1	2	3	4	5	NA
184322	Effective positioning techniques	1	2	3	4	5	NA
184323	Effective relaxation techniques	1	2	3	4	5	NA
184324	Effective guided imagery	1	2	3	4	5	NA
184325	Effective distraction	1	2	3	4	5	NA
184326	Effective heat/cold application	1	2	3	4	5	NA
184327	Effective electrical stimulation	1	2	3	4	5	NA
184328	Effective meditation techniques	1	2	3	4	5	NA
184329	Benefits of transcutaneous electrical nerve stimulation	1	2	3	4	5	NA
184330	Benefits of hypnosis	1	2	3	4	5	NA
184331	Benefits of acupuncture	1	2	3	4	5	NA
184332	Benefits of biofeedback	1	2	3	4	5	NA
184333	Benefits of massage	1	2	3	4	5	NA
184334	Benefits of ongoing self-monitoring	1	2	3	4	5	NA
184335	Benefits of lifestyle modifications	1	2	3	4	5	NA
184336	Benefits of weight loss	1	2	3	4	5	NA
184337	Strategies for pain prevention	1	2	3	4	5	NA
184338	When to obtain assistance from a health professional	1	2	3	4	5	NA
184339	Available support groups	1	2	3	4	5	NA
184340	Available community resources	1	2	3	4	5	NA
184341	Reputable sources of pain control information	1	2	3	4	5	NA

Domain-Health Knowledge & Behavior (IV)   **Class**-Health Knowledge (S)   4th edition 2008; revised 2013

OUTCOME CONTENT REFERENCES:

Barnes, S. (2001). Pain management: What do patients need to know and when do they need to know it? *Journal of PeriAnesthesia Nursing, 16*(2), 107–108.

Henrotin, Y. E., Cedraschi, C., Duplan, B., Bazin, T., & Duquesnoy, B. (2006). Information and low back pain management: A systematic review. *Spine, 31*(11), E326–E334.

Herr, K., & Kwekkeboom, K. (Eds.). (2003). Chronic pain management. *Nursing Clinics of North America, 38*(3), 403–560.

Sjoling, M., Nordahl, G., Olofsson, N., & Asplund, K. (2003). The impact of preoperative information on state anxiety, postoperative pain and satisfaction with pain management. *Patient Education and Counseling, 51*(2), 169–176.

Knowledge: Parenting 1826

Definition: Extent of understanding conveyed about provision of a nurturing and constructive environment for a child from 1 year through 17 years of age

OUTCOME TARGET RATING: Maintain at_____   Increase to_____

OUTCOME OVERALL RATING		No knowledge 1	Limited knowledge 2	Moderate knowledge 3	Substantial knowledge 4	Extensive knowledge 5	
Indicators:							
182601	Normal growth and development	1	2	3	4	5	NA
182602	Normal child behavior	1	2	3	4	5	NA
182603	Safety needs	1	2	3	4	5	NA
182604	Injury prevention	1	2	3	4	5	NA
182605	Nutritional needs	1	2	3	4	5	NA
182606	Physical care needs	1	2	3	4	5	NA
182607	Psychological needs	1	2	3	4	5	NA
182608	Emotional needs	1	2	3	4	5	NA
182609	Stimulation needs	1	2	3	4	5	NA
182610	Socialization needs	1	2	3	4	5	NA
182611	Spiritual needs	1	2	3	4	5	NA
182612	Moral guidance needs	1	2	3	4	5	NA
182613	Health supervision needs	1	2	3	4	5	NA
182614	Illness prevention	1	2	3	4	5	NA
182615	Management of common health problems	1	2	3	4	5	NA
182616	Age-appropriate expectations	1	2	3	4	5	NA
182620	Methods of discipline appropriate for developmental age	1	2	3	4	5	NA
182621	Methods of discipline appropriate for unacceptable behavior	1	2	3	4	5	NA
182618	Basic care needs	1	2	3	4	5	NA
182619	Effective communication strategies	1	2	3	4	5	NA
182622	Motor vehicle safety measures	1	2	3	4	5	NA
182623	Strategies to manage controllable environmental risk factors	1	2	3	4	5	NA
182624	Strategies to prevent tobacco use	1	2	3	4	5	NA
182625	Strategies to prevent alcohol use	1	2	3	4	5	NA
182626	Strategies to prevent recreational drug use	1	2	3	4	5	NA
182627	Strategies to prevent exposure to toxic chemicals	1	2	3	4	5	NA
182628	Available support groups	1	2	3	4	5	NA

Domain-Health Knowledge & Behavior (IV)   **Class**-Health Knowledge (S)   *3rd edition 2004; revised 2008, 2013*

OUTCOME CONTENT REFERENCES:

Craft-Rosenberg, M., & Denehy, J. (Eds.). (2001). *Nursing interventions for infants, children, and families.* Thousand Oaks, CA: Sage.

Friedman, M. (1998). *Family nursing: Research, theory and practice* (4th ed.). Stamford, CT: Appleton & Lange.

Green, M., Palfrey, J. S. (Eds.). (2002). *Bright futures: Guidelines for health supervision of infants, children, and adolescents.* Arlington, VA: National Center for Education in Maternal and Child Health.

Murray, R., & Zenter, J. (1997). *Health assessment & promotion strategies through the life span* (6th ed.). Stamford, CT: Appleton & Lange.

Knowledge: Peripheral Artery Disease Management 1860

Definition: Extent of understanding conveyed about peripheral artery disease, its treatment and the prevention of disease progression and complications

OUTCOME TARGET RATING: Maintain at_____   Increase to_____

		No knowledge	Limited knowledge	Moderate knowledge	Substantial knowledge	Extensive knowledge	
OUTCOME OVERALL RATING		1	2	3	4	5	
Indicators:							
186001	Cause and contributing factors	1	2	3	4	5	NA
186002	Signs and symptoms of peripheral artery disease	1	2	3	4	5	NA
186003	Benefits of disease management	1	2	3	4	5	NA
186004	Relationship of claudication to peripheral artery disease	1	2	3	4	5	NA
186005	Signs and symptoms of intermittent claudication	1	2	3	4	5	NA
186006	Signs and symptoms of worsening disease	1	2	3	4	5	NA
186007	Stages of peripheral artery disease	1	2	3	4	5	NA
186008	Signs and symptoms of heart disease	1	2	3	4	5	NA
186009	Signs and symptoms of stroke	1	2	3	4	5	NA
186010	Adverse health effects of ischemia if untreated	1	2	3	4	5	NA
186011	Role of blood cholesterol in atherosclerosis	1	2	3	4	5	NA
186012	Importance of controlling blood cholesterol level	1	2	3	4	5	NA
186013	Medication that reduce risk of heart attack and stroke	1	2	3	4	5	NA
186014	Importance of tobacco abstinence	1	2	3	4	5	NA
186015	Importance of monitoring lower extremities skin color	1	2	3	4	5	NA
186016	Importance of monitoring lower extremities temperature	1	2	3	4	5	NA
186017	Importance of monitoring lower extremities sensation	1	2	3	4	5	NA
186018	Importance of monitoring lower extremities muscle strength	1	2	3	4	5	NA
186019	Benefits of prescribed exercise	1	2	3	4	5	NA
186020	Strategies to relieve discomfort	1	2	3	4	5	NA
186021	Strategies to comply with exercise program	1	2	3	4	5	NA
186022	Strategies to increase walking tolerance	1	2	3	4	5	NA
186023	Importance of monitoring blood pressure	1	2	3	4	5	NA
186024	Benefits of healthy diet	1	2	3	4	5	NA
186025	Importance of weight control	1	2	3	4	5	NA
186026	Importance of controlling blood glucose level	1	2	3	4	5	NA
186027	Surgical treatment options	1	2	3	4	5	NA

Specify extremity: _____

Domain-Health Knowledge & Behavior (IV)   **Class**-Health Knowledge (S)   5th edition 2013

OUTCOME CONTENT REFERENCES:

Brunelle, C., & Mulgrew, J. (2011). Exercise for intermittent claudication. *Physical Therapy, 91*(7), 991–1001.

Hirsch, A., Haskal, Z., Hertzer, N., Bakal, C., Creager, M., Halperin, J., et.al. (2006). ACC/AHA 2005 practice guidelines for the management of patients with peripheral artery disease (lower extremity, renal, mesenteric, and abdominal aortic). *Circulation, 113*(11), 463–654.

Peripheral Arterial Disease Coalition. (2007). Gaps in public knowledge of peripheral artery disease: The first national PAD public awareness survey. *Circulation, 116*(18), 2086–2094.

Lewis, S., Dirksen, S., Heitkemper, M., Bucher, L., & Camera, I. (2011). *Medical-surgical nursing: Assessment and management of clinical problems* (8th ed., pp. 874–880). St. Louis: Elsevier.

Selvin, E., Wattanakit, K., Steffes, M., Coresh, J., & Sharrett, A. (2006). HbA1c and peripheral arterial disease in diabetes: The atherosclerosis risk in communities study. *Diabetes Care, 29*(4), 877–882.

Knowledge: Personal Safety   1809

Definition: Extent of understanding conveyed about risk reduction and prevention of unintentional injuries to self

OUTCOME TARGET RATING: Maintain at_____   Increase to_____

OUTCOME OVERALL RATING	No knowledge 1	Limited knowledge 2	Moderate knowledge 3	Substantial knowledge 4	Extensive knowledge 5	
Indicators:						
180917 Age-specific safety risks	1	2	3	4	5	NA
180918 Personal high-risk behaviors	1	2	3	4	5	NA
180922 Personal behaviors that increase risk for injury	1	2	3	4	5	NA
180923 Health conditions that increase risk	1	2	3	4	5	NA
180919 Work safety risks	1	2	3	4	5	NA
180920 Community safety risks	1	2	3	4	5	NA
180901 Suffocation prevention	1	2	3	4	5	NA
180924 Aspiration precautions	1	2	3	4	5	NA
180925 Safe food preparation	1	2	3	4	5	NA
180926 Safe food storage	1	2	3	4	5	NA
180902 Fall prevention strategies	1	2	3	4	5	NA
180903 Risk reduction strategies	1	2	3	4	5	NA
180904 Home safety measures	1	2	3	4	5	NA
180905 Water safety	1	2	3	4	5	NA
180906 Fire safety	1	2	3	4	5	NA
180907 Burn prevention	1	2	3	4	5	NA
180908 Electrocution prevention	1	2	3	4	5	NA
180927 Strategies to avoid known allergens	1	2	3	4	5	NA
180928 Strategies to avoid environmental contaminants	1	2	3	4	5	NA
180909 Poison prevention	1	2	3	4	5	NA
180910 Bicycle safety guidelines	1	2	3	4	5	NA
180911 Pedestrian safety measures	1	2	3	4	5	NA
180912 Benefits of protective helmet	1	2	3	4	5	NA
180913 Firearm safety	1	2	3	4	5	NA
180915 Motor vehicle safety measures	1	2	3	4	5	NA
180916 Emergency procedures	1	2	3	4	5	NA
180929 Safe use of prescribed medication	1	2	3	4	5	NA
180930 Correct use of assistive devices	1	2	3	4	5	NA
180931 Safe sexual practices	1	2	3	4	5	NA
180932 Appropriate clothing for activity	1	2	3	4	5	NA
180933 Safety devices appropriate for activity	1	2	3	4	5	NA

K

Domain-Health Knowledge & Behavior (IV)   *Class*-Health Knowledge (S)   *1st edition 1997; revised 2004, 2008, 2013*

OUTCOME CONTENT REFERENCES:

Conn, V. S., Armer, J. M., & Hayes, K. S. (2001). Knowledge deficit. In M. Maas, K. Buckwalter, M. Hardy, T. Tripp-Reimer, M. Titler, & J. Specht (Eds.), *Nursing care of older adults: Diagnoses, outcomes & interventions* (pp. 503–515). St. Louis: Mosby.

Simons-Morton, D. G., Mullen, P. D., Mains, D. A., Tabak, E. R., & Green, L. W. (1992). Characteristics of controlled studies of patient education and counseling for preventive health behaviors. *Patient Education and Counseling, 19*(2), 174–204.

U.S. Department of Health and Human Services. (1990). *Healthy people 2000. National health promotion and disease prevention objectives.* Washington, DC: U.S. Government Printing Office.

Knowledge: Pneumonia Management 1861

Definition: Extent of understanding conveyed about pneumonia, its treatment, and the prevention of complications

OUTCOME TARGET RATING: Maintain at_____ Increase to_____

		No knowledge	Limited knowledge	Moderate knowledge	Substantial knowledge	Extensive knowledge	
OUTCOME OVERALL RATING		1	2	3	4	5	
Indicators:							
186101	Cause and contributing factors	1	2	3	4	5	NA
186102	Specific disease process	1	2	3	4	5	NA
186103	Risk factors for reoccurrence	1	2	3	4	5	NA
186104	Signs and symptoms of disease progression	1	2	3	4	5	NA
186105	Signs and symptoms of disease relapse	1	2	3	4	5	NA
186106	Benefits of disease management	1	2	3	4	5	NA
186107	Signs and symptoms of complications	1	2	3	4	5	NA
186108	Strategies to prevent complications	1	2	3	4	5	NA
186109	Strategies to balance activity and rest	1	2	3	4	5	NA
186110	Energy conservation techniques	1	2	3	4	5	NA
186111	Medication therapeutic effects	1	2	3	4	5	NA
186112	Medication side effects	1	2	3	4	5	NA
186113	Medication adverse effects	1	2	3	4	5	NA
186114	Potential medication interactions with other agents	1	2	3	4	5	NA
186115	Potential prescribed medication interactions with other medication	1	2	3	4	5	NA
186116	Safety issues related to medication	1	2	3	4	5	NA
186117	Correct use of prescribed medication	1	2	3	4	5	NA
186118	Importance of completing prescribed antibiotics	1	2	3	4	5	NA
186119	Diagnostic tests	1	2	3	4	5	NA
186120	Expected effects of treatment	1	2	3	4	5	NA
186121	Prescribed procedures	1	2	3	4	5	NA
186122	Correct use of bulb syringe to clear nasal airway	1	2	3	4	5	NA
186123	Correct procedure to administer nebulizer treatments at home	1	2	3	4	5	NA
186124	Correct method for performing chest percussion	1	2	3	4	5	NA
186125	Correct method for performing postural drainage	1	2	3	4	5	NA
186126	Adequate fluid intake	1	2	3	4	5	NA
186127	Strategies for smoking cessation	1	2	3	4	5	NA
186128	Strategies to avoid exposure to smoke	1	2	3	4	5	NA
186129	Importance of obtaining pneumonia vaccine	1	2	3	4	5	NA
186130	Importance of obtaining influenza seasonal vaccine	1	2	3	4	5	NA
186131	Follow-up care	1	2	3	4	5	NA
186132	Potential effects of other disease conditions	1	2	3	4	5	NA
186133	Potential effects of age on treatment	1	2	3	4	5	NA

Domain-Health Knowledge & Behavior (IV)   **Class**-Health Knowledge (S)   5th edition 2013

OUTCOME CONTENT REFERENCES:

Barakzai, M. D., & Fraser, D. (2008). Assessment of infection in older adults: Signs and symptoms in four body systems. *Journal of Gerontological Nursing, 34*(1), 7–12.

Burman, M. E., & Wright, W. L. (2007). Diagnosis and management of community-acquired pneumonia: Evidence-based practice. *The Journal for Nurse Practitioners, 3*(9), 633–640.

Donowitz, G. R., & Cox, H. L. (2007). Bacterial community-acquired pneumonia in older patients. *Clinics in Geriatric Medicine, 23*(3), 515–534.

Hockenberry, M., & Wilson, D. (2007) *Wong's nursing care of infants and children* (8th ed.). St. Louis: Elsevier Mosby.

Lewis, S. L., Heitkemper, M. M., Dirksen, S. R., O'Brien, P. G., & Bucher, L. (2007). *Medical-surgical nursing: Assessment and management of clinical problems.* St. Louis: Mosby.

Pines, J. M. (2007). Within the inflamed lung: Signs, symptoms, & treatment of pneumonia in adults & children. *JEMS: Journal of Emergency Medical Services, 32*(10), 64–76.

Vines-Douglas, G. (2008). Diagnosing and treating CAP in immunocompetent adults. *Journal of the American Academy of Physician Assistants, 21*(1), 26–30.

Knowledge: Postpartum Maternal Health 1818

Definition: Extent of understanding conveyed about maternal health in the period following birth of infant

OUTCOME TARGET RATING: Maintain at_____   Increase to_____

OUTCOME OVERALL RATING		No knowledge 1	Limited knowledge 2	Moderate knowledge 3	Substantial knowledge 4	Extensive knowledge 5	
Indicators:							
181801	Normal physical sensations following delivery	1	2	3	4	5	NA
181802	Routine monitoring	1	2	3	4	5	NA
181803	Normal vaginal discharge	1	2	3	4	5	NA
181804	Breast changes	1	2	3	4	5	NA
181805	Uterine involution patterns	1	2	3	4	5	NA
181806	Fundal massage	1	2	3	4	5	NA
181807	Perineal care	1	2	3	4	5	NA
181808	Episiotomy care	1	2	3	4	5	NA
181809	Cesarean section care	1	2	3	4	5	NA
181810	Coughing techniques following surgery	1	2	3	4	5	NA
181820	Recommended nutrient intake	1	2	3	4	5	NA
181821	Recommended fluid intake	1	2	3	4	5	NA
181822	Energy level changes	1	2	3	4	5	NA
181812	Strategies to balance activity and rest	1	2	3	4	5	NA
181813	Appropriate exercise	1	2	3	4	5	NA
181814	Time frame for resumption of sexual activity	1	2	3	4	5	NA
181815	Contraceptive options	1	2	3	4	5	NA
181816	Psychological changes	1	2	3	4	5	NA
181823	Postpartum body changes	1	2	3	4	5	NA
181824	Maternal role performance	1	2	3	4	5	NA
181825	Strategies to manage postpartum depression	1	2	3	4	5	NA
181826	Strategies to manage stress	1	2	3	4	5	NA
181827	Strategies to bond with infant	1	2	3	4	5	NA
181818	Available social support	1	2	3	4	5	NA
181828	When to obtain assistance from a health professional	1	2	3	4	5	NA

Domain-*Health Knowledge & Behavior (IV)*   **Class**-*Health Knowledge (S)*   *2nd edition 2000; revised 2004, 2008*

OUTCOME CONTENT REFERENCES:

Association of Women's Health, Obstetricians and Neonatal Nurses. (1998). *Standards & guidelines for the professional nursing practice in the care of women and newborns* (5th ed.). Washington, DC: Author

Crowell, D. T. (1995). Weight change in the postpartum period. A review of the literature. *Journal of Nurse Midwifery, 40*(5), 418–423.

Nichols, F., & Humenick, S. (2000). *Childbirth education: Practice, research and theory* (2nd ed.). Philadelphia: W. B. Saunders.

Reeder, S. J., Martin, L. L., & Koniak-Griffin, D. (1997). *Maternity nursing: Family, newborn, and women's health care* (18th ed.). Philadelphia: Lippincott.

K

K

Knowledge: Preconception Maternal Health 1822

Definition: Extent of understanding conveyed about maternal health prior to conception to ensure a healthy pregnancy

OUTCOME TARGET RATING: Maintain at_____ Increase to_____

		No knowledge	Limited knowledge	Moderate knowledge	Substantial knowledge	Extensive knowledge	
OUTCOME OVERALL RATING		1	2	3	4	5	
Indicators:							
182201	Factors to consider when deciding to become a parent	1	2	3	4	5	NA
182213	Usual course of pregnancy	1	2	3	4	5	NA
182203	Recommended diet	1	2	3	4	5	NA
182204	Strategies to balance activity and rest	1	2	3	4	5	NA
182214	Adverse health effects of alcohol use	1	2	3	4	5	NA
182215	Adverse health effects of tobacco use	1	2	3	4	5	NA
182216	Adverse health effects of drug use	1	2	3	4	5	NA
182206	Maternal risk factors	1	2	3	4	5	NA
182207	Environmental hazards at home that affect fetal development	1	2	3	4	5	NA
182211	Environmental hazards at work that affect fetal development	1	2	3	4	5	NA
182208	Risk for hereditary disease	1	2	3	4	5	NA
182217	Anatomic and physiologic changes of pregnancy	1	2	3	4	5	NA
182212	Strategies to adjust to addition of infant	1	2	3	4	5	NA

Domain-Health Knowledge & Behavior (IV)   **Class**-Health Knowledge (S)   2nd edition 2000; revised 2004, 2008, 2013

OUTCOME CONTENT REFERENCES:

Aneshensel, C. S., Becerra, R. M., Fielder, E. P., & Schuler, R. H. (1990). Onset of fertility-related events during adolescence: A prospective comparison of Mexican American and non-Hispanic white females. *American Journal of Public Health, 80*(8), 959–963.

Fehring, R. J. (1991). New technology in natural family planning. *Journal of Obstetric, Gynecologic, & Neonatal Nursing, 20*(3), 199–205.

Grodstein, F., Goldman, M. B., & Cramer, D. W. (1994). Infertility in women and moderate alcohol use. *American Journal of Public Health, 84*(9), 1429–1432.

Halman, L. J., Abbey, A., & Andrews, F. M. (1992). Attitudes about infertility interventions among fertile and infertile couples. *American Journal of Public Health, 82*(2), 191–194.

Rudy, E. B., & Estok, P. (1992). Professional and lay interrater reliability of urinary luteinizing hormone surges measured by OvuQuik test. *Journal of Obstetric, Gynecologic, & Neonatal Nursing, 21*(5), 407–411.

Shane, J. M. (1993). Evaluation and treatment of infertility. *Clinical Symposia, 45*(2), 2–32.

Summers, L. (1993). Preconception care: An opportunity to maximize health in pregnancy. *Journal of Nurse Midwifery, 38*(4), 188–198.

Toner, J. P., & Flood, J. T. (1993). Fertility after the age of 40. *Obstetrics & Gynecology Clinics of North America, 20*(2), 261–272.

Knowledge: Pregnancy 1810

Definition: Extent of understanding conveyed about promotion of a healthy pregnancy and prevention of complications

OUTCOME TARGET RATING: Maintain at_____ Increase to_____

		No knowledge	Limited knowledge	Moderate knowledge	Substantial knowledge	Extensive knowledge	
OUTCOME OVERALL RATING		1	2	3	4	5	
Indicators:							
181026	Importance of frequent prenatal care	1	2	3	4	5	NA
181027	Importance of prenatal education	1	2	3	4	5	NA
181003	Warning signs of pregnancy complications	1	2	3	4	5	NA

Knowledge: Pregnancy—*cont'd*

		No knowledge	Limited knowledge	Moderate knowledge	Substantial knowledge	Extensive knowledge	
181004	Major fetal developmental milestones	1	2	3	4	5	NA
181029	Fetal movement pattern	1	2	3	4	5	NA
181005	Anatomic and physiologic changes of pregnancy	1	2	3	4	5	NA
181006	Psychological changes associated with pregnancy	1	2	3	4	5	NA
181030	Emotional changes associated with pregnancy	1	2	3	4	5	NA
181007	Strategies to balance activity and rest	1	2	3	4	5	NA
181008	Proper body mechanics	1	2	3	4	5	NA
181009	Benefits of regular exercise	1	2	3	4	5	NA
181010	Healthy nutritional practices	1	2	3	4	5	NA
181011	Healthy weight gain pattern	1	2	3	4	5	NA
181031	Correct use of nutritional supplements	1	2	3	4	5	NA
181032	Correct use of medication	1	2	3	4	5	NA
181033	Correct use of non-prescription medication	1	2	3	4	5	NA
181013	Importance of dental care	1	2	3	4	5	NA
181014	Appropriate self-care for discomforts of pregnancy	1	2	3	4	5	NA
181015	Safe sexual practices	1	2	3	4	5	NA
181016	Correct use of motor vehicle safety devices	1	2	3	4	5	NA
181034	Birthing options	1	2	3	4	5	NA
181018	Signs and symptoms of labor	1	2	3	4	5	NA
181019	Effective labor techniques	1	2	3	4	5	NA
181020	Strategies to prevent infection	1	2	3	4	5	NA
181035	Signs of potential domestic abuse	1	2	3	4	5	NA
181021	Strategies to escape domestic abuse	1	2	3	4	5	NA
181022	Strategies to adjust to addition of infant	1	2	3	4	5	NA
181023	Environmental hazards	1	2	3	4	5	NA
181024	Teratogenic agents	1	2	3	4	5	NA
181036	Adverse health effects of tobacco use	1	2	3	4	5	NA
181037	Adverse health effects of alcohol use on fetus	1	2	3	4	5	NA
181038	Adverse health effects of illicit drug use on fetus	1	2	3	4	5	NA

Domain-*Health Knowledge & Behavior (IV)*   **Class**-*Health Knowledge (S)*   *2nd edition 2000; revised 2004, 2008, 2013*

OUTCOME CONTENT REFERENCES:

Association of Women's Health, Obstetric, and Neonatal Nurses. (2004). *Core curriculum for maternal-newborn nursing.* Washington, DC: Author

Bell, R., & O'Neill, M. (1994). Exercise and pregnancy: A review. *Birth, 21*(2), 85–95.

Freda, M. C., Andersen, H. F., Damus, K., & Merkatz, I. R. (1993). What pregnant women want to know: A comparison of client and provider perceptions. *Journal of Obstetric, Gynecologic, and Neonatal Nursing, 22*(3), 237.

Kearney, M. H., Murphy, S., Irwin, K., & Rosenbaum, M. (1995). Salvaging self: A grounded theory of pregnancy on crack cocaine. *Nursing Research, 44*(4), 208–213.

Lowdermilk, D. L., & Perry, S. E. (2004). *Maternity & women's health care* (8th ed.). St. Louis: Mosby.

McFarlane, J., Parker, B., & Soeken, K. (1996). Abuse during pregnancy: Associations with maternal health and infant birth weight. *Nursing Research, 45*(1), 37–42.

Olds, S. B., London, M. L., & Ladewig, P. W. (1996). *Maternal-newborn nursing: A family-centered approach* (5th ed.). Menlo Park, CA: Addison-Wesley.

K

Knowledge: Pregnancy & Postpartum Sexual Functioning 1839

Definition: Extent of understanding conveyed about sexual function during pregnancy and postpartum

OUTCOME TARGET RATING: Maintain at_____ Increase to_____

		No knowledge	Limited knowledge	Moderate knowledge	Substantial knowledge	Extensive knowledge	
OUTCOME OVERALL RATING		1	2	3	4	5	
Indicators:							
183901	Non-pregnant anatomy	1	2	3	4	5	NA
183902	Normal changes in body image	1	2	3	4	5	NA
183903	Physiology of female sexual functioning	1	2	3	4	5	NA
183904	Anatomic and physiologic changes of pregnancy	1	2	3	4	5	NA
183905	Psychological changes associated with pregnancy	1	2	3	4	5	NA
183906	Emotional changes associated with pregnancy	1	2	3	4	5	NA
183907	Anatomic and physiologic changes of postpartum	1	2	3	4	5	NA
183908	Psychological changes associated with postpartum	1	2	3	4	5	NA
183909	Emotional changes associated with postpartum	1	2	3	4	5	NA
183910	Potential changes in sexual desire and response	1	2	3	4	5	NA
183911	Intercourse restrictions during pregnancy	1	2	3	4	5	NA
183912	Intercourse restrictions during postpartum	1	2	3	4	5	NA
183913	Modification of coital position to prevent injury	1	2	3	4	5	NA
183914	Modification of coital position to prevent discomfort	1	2	3	4	5	NA
183915	Modification of sexual activity for mutual satisfaction	1	2	3	4	5	NA
183916	Use of vaginal water-based lubricant	1	2	3	4	5	NA
183917	Safe sexual practices	1	2	3	4	5	NA
183918	Strategies to prevent sexually transmitted diseases	1	2	3	4	5	NA
183919	Importance of contraception during early postpartum	1	2	3	4	5	NA
183920	Societal influences on personal sexual behavior	1	2	3	4	5	NA
183921	Cultural influences on personal sexual behavior	1	2	3	4	5	NA

Domain-*Health Knowledge & Behavior (IV)* **Class**-*Health Knowledge (S)* *4th edition 2008; revised 2013*

OUTCOME CONTENT REFERENCES:

Lowdermilk, D. L., & Perry, S. E. (2004). *Maternity & women's health care* (8th ed.). St. Louis: Mosby.

Matthey, S., Morgan, M., Healey, L., Barnett, B., Kavanagh, D. J., & Howie, P. (2002). Postpartum issues for expectant mothers and fathers. *JOGNN: Journal of Obstetric, Gynecologic, & Neonatal Nursing, 31*(4), 428–435.

Olds, S. B., London, M. L., Ladewig, P. W., & Davidson, M. R. (2004). *Maternal-newborn nursing & women's health care* (7th ed.). Upper Saddle River, NJ: Prentice Hall.

Knowledge: Prescribed Activity   1811

Definition: Extent of understanding conveyed about physical activity recommended by a health professional for a specific condition

OUTCOME TARGET RATING: Maintain at_____   Increase to_____

		No knowledge	Limited knowledge	Moderate knowledge	Substantial knowledge	Extensive knowledge	
OUTCOME OVERALL RATING		1	2	3	4	5	
Indicators:							
181101	Prescribed activity	1	2	3	4	5	NA
181102	Purpose of prescribed activity	1	2	3	4	5	NA
181103	Expected effects of prescribed activity	1	2	3	4	5	NA
181104	Prescribed activity restrictions	1	2	3	4	5	NA
181105	Prescribed activity precautions	1	2	3	4	5	NA
181121	Realistic goals about prescribed activity	1	2	3	4	5	NA
181116	Strategies to safely ambulate	1	2	3	4	5	NA
181122	Strategies to avoid injury	1	2	3	4	5	NA
181117	Appropriate footwear	1	2	3	4	5	NA
181106	Factors that decrease the ability to perform prescribed activity	1	2	3	4	5	NA
181107	Strategies to gradually increase prescribed activity	1	2	3	4	5	NA
181123	Strategies to incorporate physical activity into life routine	1	2	3	4	5	NA
181124	Strategies to monitor progress in prescribed physical activity	1	2	3	4	5	NA
181118	Methods to monitor heart rate	1	2	3	4	5	NA
181119	Methods to monitor respiratory rate	1	2	3	4	5	NA
181111	Realistic prescribed activity routine	1	2	3	4	5	NA
181110	Barriers to implementing prescribed activity routine	1	2	3	4	5	NA
181112	Proper performance of prescribed activity	1	2	3	4	5	NA
181120	Benefits of prescribed activity	1	2	3	4	5	NA

K

Domain-Health Knowledge & Behavior (IV)   *Class*-Health Knowledge (S)   *1st edition 1997; revised 2004, 2008, 2013*

OUTCOME CONTENT REFERENCES:

Bushnell, F. (1992). Self-care teaching for congestive heart failure patients. *Journal of Gerontological Nursing, 18*(10), 27–32.

Conn, V. S., Armer, J. M., & Hayes, K. S. (2001). Knowledge deficit. In M. Maas, K. Buckwalter, M. Hardy, T. Tripp-Reimer, M. Titler, & J. Specht (Eds.), *Nursing care of older adults: Diagnoses, outcomes & interventions* (pp. 503–515). St. Louis: Mosby.

Devins, G. M., Binik, Y. M., Mandin, H., Litourneau, P. K., Hollomby, D. J., Barre, P. E., & Prichard, S. (1990). The kidney disease questionnaire: A test for measuring patient knowledge about end-stage renal disease. *Journal of Clinical Epidemiology, 43*(3), 297–307.

Garrard, J., Joynes, J. O., Mullen, L., McNeil, L., Mensing, C., Feste, C., & Etzwiler, D. D. (1987). Psychometric study of patient knowledge test. *Diabetes Care, 10*(4), 500–509.

Gilden, J. L., Hendryx, M., Casia, C., & Singh, S. P. (1989). The effectiveness of diabetes education programs for older patients and their spouses. *Journal of American Geriatrics Society, 37*(11), 1023–1030.

Mazzuca, S. A., Moorman, N. H., Wheeler, M. L., Norton, J. A., Fineberg, N. S., Vinicor, F., Cohen, S. J., & Clark, C. M. (1986). The diabetes education study: A controlled trial of the effects of diabetes patient education. *Diabetes Care, 9*(1), 1–10.

Redman, B. (1993). Knowledge deficit (specify). In J. M. Thompson, G. K. McFarland, J. E. Hirsch, & S. M. Tucker (Eds.), *Mosby's clinical nursing* (3rd ed., pp. 1548–1552). St. Louis: Mosby.

Scherer, Y. K., Janelli, L. M., & Schmieder, L. E. (1992). A time-series perspective of effectiveness of a health teaching program on chronic obstructive pulmonary disease. *Journal of Healthcare Education and Training, 6*(3), 7–13.

Smith, M. M., Hicks, V. L., & Heyward, V. H. (1991). Coronary disease knowledge test: Developing a valid and reliable tool. *Nurse Practitioner, 16*(4), 28, 31, 35–38.

Knowledge: Prescribed Diet

1802

Definition: Extent of understanding conveyed about a diet recommended by a health professional for a specific health condition

OUTCOME TARGET RATING: Maintain at_____ Increase to_____

	No knowledge	Limited knowledge	Moderate knowledge	Substantial knowledge	Extensive knowledge	
OUTCOME OVERALL RATING	1	2	3	4	5	
Indicators:						
180201 Prescribed diet	1	2	3	4	5	NA
180202 Benefits of diet	1	2	3	4	5	NA
180203 Benefits of prescribed diet	1	2	3	4	5	NA
180204 Dietary goals	1	2	3	4	5	NA
180205 Relationship among diet, exercise, and weight	1	2	3	4	5	NA
180206 Food allowed in diet	1	2	3	4	5	NA
180218 Fluid allowed in diet	1	2	3	4	5	NA
180207 Food to avoid in diet	1	2	3	4	5	NA
180219 Fluid to avoid in diet	1	2	3	4	5	NA
180221 Food consistent with cultural beliefs	1	2	3	4	5	NA
180222 Recommended food intake distribution throughout the day	1	2	3	4	5	NA
180223 Recommended food portions	1	2	3	4	5	NA
180208 Interpretation of nutritional information on food labels	1	2	3	4	5	NA
180209 Guidelines for food preparation	1	2	3	4	5	NA
180211 Menu planning based on prescribed diet	1	2	3	4	5	NA
180212 Strategies to change dietary habits	1	2	3	4	5	NA
180213 Diet plans for social situations	1	2	3	4	5	NA
180224 Strategies for situations that affect food and fluid intake	1	2	3	4	5	NA
180217 Self-monitoring techniques	1	2	3	4	5	NA
180215 Potential food and medication interactions	1	2	3	4	5	NA
180225 Potential food and herbal supplement interactions	1	2	3	4	5	NA
180226 Strategies to increase diet compliance	1	2	3	4	5	NA

Specify diet: _____

Domain-*Health Knowledge & Behavior (IV)* **Class**-*Health Knowledge (S)* *1st edition 1997; revised 2004, 2008, 2013*

OUTCOME CONTENT REFERENCES:
Bloomgarden, Z. T., Karmally, W., Metzger, J., Brothers, M., Nechemias, C., Bookman, J., Faierman, D., Ginsberg-Fellner, F., Rayfield, E., & Brown, W. V. (1987). Randomized controlled trial of diabetic patient education: Improved knowledge without improved metabolic status. *Diabetes Care, 10*(3), 263–272.
Bushnell, F. (1992). Self-care teaching for congestive heart failure patients. *Journal of Gerontological Nursing, 18*(10), 27–32.
Conn, V. S., Armer, J. M., & Hayes, K. S. (2001). Knowledge deficit. In M. Maas, K. Buckwalter, M. Hardy, T. Tripp-Reimer, M. Titler, & J. Specht (Eds.), *Nursing care of older adults: Diagnoses, outcomes & interventions* (pp. 503–515). St. Louis: Mosby.
Devins, G. M., Binik, Y. M., Mandin, H., Litourneau, P. K., Hollomby, D. J., Barre, P. E., & Prichard, S. (1990). The Kidney Disease Questionnaire: A test for measuring patient knowledge about end-stage renal disease. *Journal of Clinical Epidemiology, 43*(3), 297–307.
Garrard, J., Joynes, J. O., Mullen, L., McNeil, L., Mensing, C., Feste, C., & Etzwiler, D. D. (1987). Psychometric study of patient knowledge test. *Diabetes Care, 10*(4), 500–509.
Gilden, J. L., Hendryx, M., Casia, C., & Singh, S. P. (1989). The effectiveness of diabetes education programs for older patients and their spouses. *Journal of American Geriatrics Society, 37*(11), 1023–1030.
Mazzuca, S. A., Moorman, N. H., Wheeler, M. L., Norton, J. A., Fineberg, N. S., Vinicor, F., Cohen, S. J., & Clark, C. M. (1986). The diabetes education study: A controlled trial of the effects of diabetes patient education. *Diabetes Care, 9*(1), 1–10.
Redman, B. (1993). Knowledge deficit (specify). In J. M. Thompson, G. K. McFarland, J. E. Hirsch, & S. M. Tucker (Eds.), *Mosby's clinical nursing* (3rd ed., pp. 1548–1552). St. Louis: Mosby.
Scherer, Y. K., Janelli, L. M., & Schmieder, L. E. (1992). A time-series perspective of effectiveness of a health teaching program on chronic obstructive pulmonary disease. *Journal of Healthcare Education and Training, 6*(3), 7–13.
Smith, M. M., Hicks, V. L., & Heyward, V. H. (1991). Coronary disease knowledge test: Developing a valid and reliable tool. *Nurse Practitioner, 16*(4), 28, 31, 35–38.

Knowledge: Preterm Infant Care 1840

Definition: Extent of understanding conveyed about the care of a premature infant born 24 to 37 weeks (term) gestation

OUTCOME TARGET RATING: Maintain at_____   Increase to_____

OUTCOME OVERALL RATING		No knowledge 1	Limited knowledge 2	Moderate knowledge 3	Substantial knowledge 4	Extensive knowledge 5	
Indicators:							NA
184001	Cause and contributing factors for prematurity	1	2	3	4	5	NA
184002	Premature infant characteristics	1	2	3	4	5	NA
184003	Major developmental milestones	1	2	3	4	5	NA
184004	Proper infant positioning	1	2	3	4	5	NA
184005	Infant sleep-wake pattern	1	2	3	4	5	NA
184006	Respiratory needs	1	2	3	4	5	NA
184007	Thermoregulation needs	1	2	3	4	5	NA
184008	Skin care needs	1	2	3	4	5	NA
184009	Physiologic monitoring needs	1	2	3	4	5	NA
184010	Hydration monitoring needs	1	2	3	4	5	NA
184011	Glucose monitoring needs	1	2	3	4	5	NA
184012	Pain management strategies	1	2	3	4	5	NA
184013	Prescribed medication	1	2	3	4	5	NA
184014	Diagnostic imaging tests	1	2	3	4	5	NA
184015	Laboratory tests	1	2	3	4	5	NA
184016	Nutritional needs	1	2	3	4	5	NA
184017	Importance of environmental control	1	2	3	4	5	NA
184018	Benefits of kangaroo care	1	2	3	4	5	NA
184019	Neonatal intensive care routine	1	2	3	4	5	NA
184020	Parenting strategies in the hospital	1	2	3	4	5	NA
184021	Strategies to enhance bonding with infant	1	2	3	4	5	NA
184022	Strategies to adjust to addition of infant	1	2	3	4	5	NA
184023	Strategies to enhance sibling support	1	2	3	4	5	NA
184024	Available support groups	1	2	3	4	5	NA
184025	Reputable sources of preterm infant care information	1	2	3	4	5	NA
184026	Financial resources for assistance	1	2	3	4	5	NA
184027	Discharge planning	1	2	3	4	5	NA

Domain-Health Knowledge & Behavior (IV)   **Class**-Health Knowledge (S)   *4th edition 2008; revised 2013*

OUTCOME CONTENT REFERENCES:
Merenstein, G. B. (2002). *Handbook of neonatal intensive care* (5th ed.). Mosby: St. Louis.
Zaichkin, J. (Ed.). (1996). *Newborn intensive care: What every parent needs to know*. Petaluma, CA: NICU.

Knowledge: Sexual Functioning

1815

Definition: Extent of understanding conveyed about sexual development and responsible sexual practices

OUTCOME TARGET RATING: Maintain at_____ Increase to_____

		No knowledge	Limited knowledge	Moderate knowledge	Substantial knowledge	Extensive knowledge	
OUTCOME OVERALL RATING		1	2	3	4	5	
Indicators:							
181501	Sexual anatomy	1	2	3	4	5	NA
181502	Function of sexual anatomy	1	2	3	4	5	NA
181503	Physical changes with puberty	1	2	3	4	5	NA
181504	Emotional changes with puberty	1	2	3	4	5	NA
181505	Reproduction	1	2	3	4	5	NA
181506	Physical changes with aging	1	2	3	4	5	NA
181507	Emotional changes with aging	1	2	3	4	5	NA
181508	Societal influences on personal sexual behavior	1	2	3	4	5	NA
181509	Safe sexual practices	1	2	3	4	5	NA
181513	Strategies for safe sex	1	2	3	4	5	NA
181510	Effective contraception	1	2	3	4	5	NA
181511	Strategies to prevent sexually transmitted diseases	1	2	3	4	5	NA
181514	Risk of multiple partners	1	2	3	4	5	NA
181515	Potential consequences of sexual activity	1	2	3	4	5	NA
181516	Benefits of delaying sexual activity	1	2	3	4	5	NA

Domain-*Health Knowledge & Behavior (IV)*   **Class**-*Health Knowledge (S)*   *2nd edition 2000; revised 2004, 2008, 2013*

OUTCOME CONTENT REFERENCES:
Howard, M. (1991). *How to help your teenager postpone sexual involvement*. Lexington, NY: Continuum.
Nass, G., Libby, R., & Fischer, M. P. (1989). *Sexual choices: An introduction to human sexuality* (2nd ed.). Monterey, CA: Wadsworth Health Sciences.
Neinstein, L. S. (2002). *Adolescent health care: A practical guide*. Philadelphia: Lippincott Williams & Wilkins.
Tuttle, B. (1984). Adult sexual response. In L.P. Higgins & J.W. Hawkins (Eds.), *Human sexuality across the life span: Implications for nursing practice* (pp. 39–76). Monterey, CA: Wadsworth Health Sciences Division.
Wright, L. K. (2001). Altered sexuality patterns. In M. Maas, K. Buckwalter, M. Hardy, T. Tripp-Reimer, M. Titler, & J. Specht (Eds.), *Nursing care of older adults: Diagnoses, outcomes & interventions* (pp. 750–761). St. Louis: Mosby.

Knowledge: Stress Management

1862

Definition: Extent of understanding conveyed about the stress process and strategies to reduce or cope with stress

OUTCOME TARGET RATING: Maintain at_____ Increase to_____

		No knowledge	Limited knowledge	Moderate knowledge	Substantial knowledge	Extensive knowledge	
OUTCOME OVERALL RATING		1	2	3	4	5	
Indicators:							
186201	Factors that cause stress	1	2	3	4	5	NA
186202	Factors that increase stress	1	2	3	4	5	NA
186203	Physical stress response	1	2	3	4	5	NA
186204	Cognitive stress response	1	2	3	4	5	NA
186205	Affective stress response	1	2	3	4	5	NA

K

Knowledge: Stress Management—cont'd

		No knowledge	Limited knowledge	Moderate knowledge	Substantial knowledge	Extensive knowledge	
186206	Behavioral stress response	1	2	3	4	5	NA
186207	Spiritual stress response	1	2	3	4	5	NA
186208	Role of stress in illness	1	2	3	4	5	NA
186209	Benefits of stress management	1	2	3	4	5	NA
186210	Cognitive therapy techniques	1	2	3	4	5	NA
186211	Stress inoculation techniques	1	2	3	4	5	NA
186212	Problem-solving approaches	1	2	3	4	5	NA
186213	Effective meditation techniques	1	2	3	4	5	NA
186214	Effective relaxation techniques	1	2	3	4	5	NA
186215	Effective stress reduction techniques	1	2	3	4	5	NA
186216	Effective communication techniques	1	2	3	4	5	NA
186217	Benefits of adequate sleep	1	2	3	4	5	NA
186218	Benefits of healthy diet	1	2	3	4	5	NA
186219	Benefits of regular exercise	1	2	3	4	5	NA
186220	Benefits of massage	1	2	3	4	5	NA
186221	Benefits of prayer	1	2	3	4	5	NA
186222	Benefits of hypnosis	1	2	3	4	5	NA
186223	Benefits of music	1	2	3	4	5	NA
186224	Effects on lifestyle	1	2	3	4	5	NA
186225	Benefits of lifestyle modifications	1	2	3	4	5	NA
186226	Alternative thoughts to replace negative and irrational thoughts	1	2	3	4	5	NA
186227	Available support groups	1	2	3	4	5	NA
186228	Strategies to increase social support	1	2	3	4	5	NA

Domain-Health Knowledge & Behavior (IV)   **Class**-Health Knowledge (S)   5th edition 2013

OUTCOME CONTENT REFERENCES:

Dusek, J. A., Hibberd, P. L., Buczynski, B., Chang, B., Dusek, K. C., Johnston, J. M., Wohlhueter, A. L., Benson, H., Zusman, R. M. (2008). Stress management versus lifestyle modification on systolic hypertension and medication elimination: A randomized trial. *Journal of Alternative & Complementary Medicine*, 14(2), 129–138.

Koertge, J., Janszky, I., Sundin, Ö., Blom, M., Georgiades, A., László, K. D., Alinaghizadeh, H., Ahnve, S. (2008). Effects of a stress management program on vital exhaustion and depression in women with coronary heart disease: A randomized controlled intervention study. *Journal of Internal Medicine*, 263(3), 281–293.

Lehrer, P. (2007). Principles and practice of stress management: Advances in the field. *Biofeedback*, 35(3), 82-84.

McCance, K., & Huether, S. (2009). *Pathophysiology: The biological basis for disease in adults and children* (6th ed.). St. Louis: Mosby.

Overholser, J. C., & Fisher, L. B. (2009). Contemporary perspectives on stress management: Medication, meditation or mitigation. *Journal of Contemporary Psychotherapy*, 39(3), 147–155.

Knowledge: Stroke Management   1863

Definition: Extent of understanding conveyed about stroke, its treatment, and the prevention of disease progression and complications

OUTCOME TARGET RATING: Maintain at_____   Increase to_____

		No knowledge	Limited knowledge	Moderate knowledge	Substantial knowledge	Extensive knowledge	
OUTCOME OVERALL RATING		1	2	3	4	5	
Indicators:							
186301	Specific type of stroke	1	2	3	4	5	NA
186302	Cause and contributing factors	1	2	3	4	5	NA
186303	Usual course of ischemic disease	1	2	3	4	5	NA

Continued

K

Knowledge: Stroke Management—cont'd

		No knowledge	Limited knowledge	Moderate knowledge	Substantial knowledge	Extensive knowledge	
186304	Signs and symptoms of ischemic disease	1	2	3	4	5	NA
186305	Usual course of hemorrhagic disease	1	2	3	4	5	NA
186306	Signs and symptoms of hemorrhagic disease	1	2	3	4	5	NA
186307	Psychosocial effects of disease	1	2	3	4	5	NA
186308	Relationship of physical and emotional stress to condition	1	2	3	4	5	NA
186309	Surgical treatment options	1	2	3	4	5	NA
186310	Available treatment options	1	2	3	4	5	NA
186311	Alternative treatment options	1	2	3	4	5	NA
186312	Medication therapeutic effects	1	2	3	4	5	NA
186313	Medication side effects	1	2	3	4	5	NA
186314	Medication adverse effects	1	2	3	4	5	NA
186315	When to obtain emergency treatment	1	2	3	4	5	NA
186316	Complications of stroke	1	2	3	4	5	NA
186317	Effects on lifestyle	1	2	3	4	5	NA
186318	Guidelines for sexual activity	1	2	3	4	5	NA
186319	Energy conservation techniques	1	2	3	4	5	NA
186320	Strategies to minimize disease progression	1	2	3	4	5	NA
186321	Strategies for smoking cessation	1	2	3	4	5	NA
186322	Strategies to manage hypertension	1	2	3	4	5	NA
186323	Strategies to adapt to sensory losses	1	2	3	4	5	NA
186324	Strategies to maintain skin integrity	1	2	3	4	5	NA
186325	Strategies to adapt to cognitive changes	1	2	3	4	5	NA
186326	Strategies to prevent aspiration	1	2	3	4	5	NA
186327	Importance of completing rehabilitation	1	2	3	4	5	NA
186328	Available support groups	1	2	3	4	5	NA
186329	Risk factors for complications	1	2	3	4	5	NA
186330	Reputable sources of stroke prevention information	1	2	3	4	5	NA

Domain-Health Knowledge & Behavior (IV) **Class**-Health Knowledge (S) 5th edition 2013

OUTCOME CONTENT REFERENCES:

Boss, B. (2005). Alterations of neurologic function. In K. L. McCance, & S. E. Huether, *Pathophysiology: The biological basis for disease in adults & children*. St. Louis: Mosby.

Carty, R., Mooraby, R., & Paterson, J. (2006). Stroke management. Evolution of a model for the thrombolysis of acute stroke patients. *British Journal of Nursing, 15*(8), 453–457.

Christian, A. H., Rosamond, W., White, A. R., & Mosca, L. (2007). Nine-year trends and racial and ethnic disparities in women's awareness of heart disease and stroke: An American Heart Association national study. *Journal of Women's Health, 16*(1), 68–81.

Draper, P., & Brocklehurst, H. (2007). The impact of stroke on the well-being of the patient's spouse: An exploratory study. *Journal of Clinical Nursing, 16*(2), 264–271.

Hutton, C. (2005). *After a stroke: 300 tips for making life easier*. New York: New York Demos Medical.

Johnson, M., Moorhead, S., Bulechek, G., Butcher, H., Maas, M., Swanson, E. (2012). Stroke. In *NOC and NIC linkages to NANDA-I and clinical conditions: Supporting critical reasoning and quality care* (3rd ed., pp. 352–355). St. Louis: Elsevier Mosby.

National Stroke Association. (2008). *Stroke facts*. Centennial, CO: Author.

National Stroke Association. (2008). *Stroke prevention guidelines*. Centennial, CO: Author.

World Health Organization. (2005). *Avoiding heart attacks and strokes: Don't be a victim—Protect yourself*. Geneva: Author.

Knowledge: Stroke Prevention 1864

Definition: Extent of understanding conveyed about the causes and the prevention of stroke

OUTCOME TARGET RATING: Maintain at_____   Increase to_____

		No knowledge	Limited knowledge	Moderate knowledge	Substantial knowledge	Extensive knowledge	
OUTCOME OVERALL RATING		1	2	3	4	5	
Indicators:							
186401	Signs and symptoms of stroke	1	2	3	4	5	NA
186402	Types of stroke and related syndromes	1	2	3	4	5	NA
186403	Cause and contributing factors	1	2	3	4	5	NA
186404	Therapies that increase risk	1	2	3	4	5	NA
186405	Lifestyle risk factors	1	2	3	4	5	NA
186406	Genetic risk factors	1	2	3	4	5	NA
186407	Tests to assess risk factors	1	2	3	4	5	NA
186408	Benefits of reducing risk factors	1	2	3	4	5	NA
186409	Stroke prevention guidelines	1	2	3	4	5	NA
186410	Strategies for smoking cessation	1	2	3	4	5	NA
186411	Strategies to manage hypertension	1	2	3	4	5	NA
186412	Importance of alcohol restrictions	1	2	3	4	5	NA
186413	Strategies to manage weight	1	2	3	4	5	NA
186414	Strategies to manage diabetes	1	2	3	4	5	NA
186415	Strategies to manage carotid artery disease	1	2	3	4	5	NA
186416	Strategies to manage atrial fibrillation	1	2	3	4	5	NA
186417	Strategies to manage high cholesterol	1	2	3	4	5	NA
186418	Strategies to promote exercise	1	2	3	4	5	NA
186419	Strategies to manage previous stroke events	1	2	3	4	5	NA
186420	Strategies to manage chronic bacterial infections	1	2	3	4	5	NA
186421	Prescribed diet	1	2	3	4	5	NA
186422	Strategies to maintain hydration	1	2	3	4	5	NA
186423	Anticoagulant preventive therapy	1	2	3	4	5	NA
186424	Alternative preventive therapies	1	2	3	4	5	NA
186425	When to obtain assistance from a health professional	1	2	3	4	5	NA
186426	Plan for obtaining immediate treatment if adverse signs and symptoms occur	1	2	3	4	5	NA

Domain-Health Knowledge & Behavior (IV)   **Class**-Health Knowledge (S)   5th edition 2013

OUTCOME CONTENT REFERENCES:

Boss, B. (2005). Alterations of neurologic function. In K. L. McCance, & S. E. Huether, *Pathophysiology: The biological basis for disease in adults & children*. St. Louis: Mosby.

Christian, A. H., Rosamond, W., White, A. R., & Mosca, L. (2007). Nine-year trends and racial and ethnic disparities in women's awareness of heart disease and stroke: An American Heart Association national study. *Journal of Women's Health, 16*(1), 68–81.

Johnson, M., Moorhead, S., Bulechek, G., Butcher, H., Maas, M., Swanson, E. (2012). Stroke. In *NOC and NIC linkages to NANDA-I and clinical conditions: Supporting critical reasoning and quality care* (3rd ed., pp. 352–355). St. Louis: Elsevier Mosby.

National Stroke Association. (2008). *Stroke facts*. Centennial, CO: Author.

National Stroke Association. (2008). *Stroke prevention guidelines*. Centennial, CO: Author.

World Health Organization. (2005). *Avoiding heart attacks and strokes: Don't be a victim—Protect yourself*. Geneva: Author.

K

Knowledge: Substance Use Control   1812

Definition: Extent of understanding conveyed about controlling the use of addictive drugs, toxic chemicals, tobacco, or alcohol

OUTCOME TARGET RATING: Maintain at_____   Increase to_____

		No knowledge	Limited knowledge	Moderate knowledge	Substantial knowledge	Extensive knowledge	
OUTCOME OVERALL RATING		1	2	3	4	5	
Indicators:							
181201	Personal risk for substance misuse	1	2	3	4	5	NA
181202	Adverse health effects of substance use	1	2	3	4	5	NA
181203	Benefits of eliminating substance use	1	2	3	4	5	NA
181205	Social consequences of substance use	1	2	3	4	5	NA
181206	Personal responsibility to manage substance misuse	1	2	3	4	5	NA
181207	Threats to substance use control	1	2	3	4	5	NA
181208	Support for substance use control	1	2	3	4	5	NA
181209	Strategies to prevent substance use	1	2	3	4	5	NA
181210	Strategies to manage substance use	1	2	3	4	5	NA
181211	Benefits of ongoing self-monitoring	1	2	3	4	5	NA
181212	Potential for relapse in efforts to control substance use	1	2	3	4	5	NA
181213	Strategies to prevent relapses in substance use	1	2	3	4	5	NA
181214	Signs of dependence during substance withdrawal	1	2	3	4	5	NA
181216	Signs and symptoms of substance withdrawal	1	2	3	4	5	NA
181217	Available support groups	1	2	3	4	5	NA

Specify substance: _____

K

Domain-*Health Knowledge & Behavior (IV)*   **Class**-*Health Knowledge (S)*   *1st edition 1997; revised 2004, 2008*

OUTCOME CONTENT REFERENCES:

Eells, M. A. (1991). Strategies for promotion of avoiding harmful substances. *Nursing Clinics of North America, 26*(40), 915–927.

Hall, J. A., & Williams, J. K. (2005). Substance abuse. In D. L. Huber (Ed.), *Disease management: A guide for case managers* (pp. 187–202). St. Louis: Elsevier Saunders.

Simons-Morton, D. G., Mullen, P. D., Mains, D. A., Tabak, E. R., & Green, L. W. (1992). Characteristics of controlled studies of patient education and counseling for preventive health behaviors. *Patient Education and Counseling, 19*(2), 174–204.

Tanner, E. K. (1991). Assessment of a health-promotive lifestyle. *Nursing Clinics of North America, 26*(4), 845–854.

U.S. Department of Health and Human Services. (1990). *Healthy people 2000, National health promotion and disease prevention objectives*. Washington, DC: U.S. Government Printing Office.

Knowledge: Thrombus Prevention

1865

Definition: Extent of understanding conveyed about causes, prevention, and early detection of blood clots within the circulatory system

OUTCOME TARGET RATING: Maintain at_____ Increase to_____

		No knowledge 1	Limited knowledge 2	Moderate knowledge 3	Substantial knowledge 4	Extensive knowledge 5	
OUTCOME OVERALL RATING		1	2	3	4	5	
Indicators:							
186501	Risk factors for venous stasis	1	2	3	4	5	NA
186502	Risk factors for intimal injury	1	2	3	4	5	NA
186503	Risk factors for hypercoagulation	1	2	3	4	5	NA
186504	Importance of lifelong vigilance for risk factors	1	2	3	4	5	NA
186505	Strategies to reduce venous stasis	1	2	3	4	5	NA
186506	Strategies to reduce intimal injury	1	2	3	4	5	NA
186507	Strategies to reduce hypercoagulation	1	2	3	4	5	NA
186508	Signs and symptoms of thrombi	1	2	3	4	5	NA
186509	Benefits of maintaining optimal weight	1	2	3	4	5	NA
186510	Importance of monitoring blood pressure	1	2	3	4	5	NA
186511	Benefits of activity restrictions	1	2	3	4	5	NA
186512	High-risk activities	1	2	3	4	5	NA
186513	Importance of alcohol restrictions	1	2	3	4	5	NA
186514	Importance of tobacco abstinence	1	2	3	4	5	NA
186515	Benefits of regular exercise	1	2	3	4	5	NA
186516	Medication therapeutic effects	1	2	3	4	5	NA
186517	Medication side effects	1	2	3	4	5	NA
186518	Medication adverse effects	1	2	3	4	5	NA
186519	Potential non-prescription medication interactions	1	2	3	4	5	NA
186520	Herbal interactions	1	2	3	4	5	NA
186521	Importance of maintaining medication regimen	1	2	3	4	5	NA
186522	When to obtain assistance from a health professional	1	2	3	4	5	NA
186523	Caregiver's role in treatment plan	1	2	3	4	5	NA
186524	Available support groups	1	2	3	4	5	NA
186525	Reputable sources of thrombus prevention information	1	2	3	4	5	NA
186526	Plan for obtaining immediate treatment if adverse signs and symptoms occur	1	2	3	4	5	NA

Domain-Health Knowledge & Behavior (IV)   *Class*-Health Knowledge (S)   5th edition 2013

OUTCOME CONTENT REFERENCES:

Agnelli, G., & Becattini, C. (2008). Treatment of DVT: How long is enough and how do you predict recurrence. *Journal of Thrombosis and Thrombolysis, 25*(1), 37–44.

Findlay, J., Keogh, M., & Cooper, L. (2010). Venous thromboembolism prophylaxis: The role of the nurse. *British Journal of Nursing (BJN), 19*(16), 1028–1032.

Fitzgerald, J. (2010). Venous thromboembolism: Have we made headway? *Orthopaedic Nursing, 29*(4), 226–234.

Headley, C. M., & Melander, S. (2011). When it may be a pulmonary embolism. *Nephrology Nursing Journal, 38*(2), 127–152.

Houman Fekrazad, M., Lopes, R. D., Stashenko, G. J., Alexander, J. H., & Garcia, D. (2009). Treatment of venous thromboembolism: Guidelines translated for the clinician. *Journal of Thrombosis and Thrombolysis, 28*(3), 270–275.

Kearon, C., Kahn, S., Agnelli, G., Goldhaber, S., Raskob, G., Comerota, A., American College of Chest Physicians. (2008). Antithrombotic therapy for venous thromboembolic disease: American College of Chest Physicians evidence-based clinical practice guidelines (8th ed.). *Chest, 133*(6 Suppl.), 454S–545S.

Lancaster, S. L., Owens, A., Bryant, A. S., Ramey, L. S., Nicholson, J., Gossett, K., Forni, J. T., & Padgett, T. M. (2010). Emergency: Upper-extremity deep vein thrombosis. *AJN: American Journal of Nursing, 110*(5), 48–52.

Lankshear, A., Harden, J., & Simms, J. (2010). Safe practice for patients receiving anticoagulant therapy. *Nursing Standard, 24*(20), 47–56.

Meetoo, D. (2010). In too deep: Understanding, detecting and managing DVT. *British Journal of Nursing (BJN), 19*(16), 1021–1022, 1024–1027.

Shaughnessy, K. (2007). Massive pulmonary embolism. *Critical Care Nurse, 27*(1), 39–40, 42–51.

Yee, C. A. (2010). Conquering pulmonary embolism. *OR Nurse, 4*(5), 18–24.

K

Knowledge: Time Management 1866

Definition: Extent of understanding conveyed about strategies to complete commitments within an expected timeframe with minimum stress

OUTCOME TARGET RATING: Maintain at_____ Increase to_____

		No knowledge	Limited knowledge	Moderate knowledge	Substantial knowledge	Extensive knowledge	
OUTCOME OVERALL RATING		1	2	3	4	5	
Indicators:							
186601	Importance of prioritizing commitments	1	2	3	4	5	NA
186602	Importance of setting short-term goals	1	2	3	4	5	NA
186603	Importance of setting long-term goals	1	2	3	4	5	NA
186604	Strategies to prioritize commitments	1	2	3	4	5	NA
186605	Realistic timeframe for each activity	1	2	3	4	5	NA
186606	Personal limitations that affect time management	1	2	3	4	5	NA
186607	Strategies to organize personal space	1	2	3	4	5	NA
186608	Strategies to structure commitments	1	2	3	4	5	NA
186609	Strategies to manage commitments within timeframe	1	2	3	4	5	NA
186610	Strategies to balance competing demands	1	2	3	4	5	NA
186611	Strategies to track progress toward completion of commitments	1	2	3	4	5	NA
186612	Strategies for delegating activities	1	2	3	4	5	NA
186613	Strategies to minimize interruptions	1	2	3	4	5	NA
186614	Strategies to reassess commitment priorities	1	2	3	4	5	NA
186615	Strategies to prevent feeling overwhelmed	1	2	3	4	5	NA
186616	Benefits of time management	1	2	3	4	5	NA

Domain-Health Knowledge & Behavior (IV) **Class**-Health Knowledge (S) 5th edition 2013

OUTCOME CONTENT REFERENCES:
Allen, D. (2001). *Getting things done: The art of stress-free productivity*. London: Penguin Books
Cohen, S., & Williamson, G. M. (1988). Perceived stress in a probability sample of the United States. In S. Spacapan & S. Oskamp (Eds.), *The social psychology of health*. Newbury Park, CA: Sage.
Johnson, S. (2004, September). Organizing your work and time. *Academic Physician & Scientist*, pp. 2–3

Knowledge: Treatment Procedure 1814

Definition: Extent of understanding conveyed about a procedure required as part of a treatment regimen

OUTCOME TARGET RATING: Maintain at_____ Increase to_____

		No knowledge	Limited knowledge	Moderate knowledge	Substantial knowledge	Extensive knowledge	
OUTCOME OVERALL RATING		1	2	3	4	5	
Indicators:							
181401	Treatment procedure	1	2	3	4	5	NA
181402	Purpose of procedure	1	2	3	4	5	NA
181403	Steps in procedure	1	2	3	4	5	NA
181405	Precautions related to procedure	1	2	3	4	5	NA
181406	Restrictions related to procedure	1	2	3	4	5	NA
181404	Correct use of equipment	1	2	3	4	5	NA
181407	Proper care of equipment	1	2	3	4	5	NA
181409	Appropriate action for complications	1	2	3	4	5	NA

K

Knowledge: Treatment Procedure—cont'd

		No knowledge	Limited knowledge	Moderate knowledge	Substantial knowledge	Extensive knowledge	
181410	Treatment side effects	1	2	3	4	5	NA
181412	Contraindications for procedure	1	2	3	4	5	NA

Specify procedure: _____

Domain-*Health Knowledge & Behavior (IV)*   **Class**-*Health Knowledge (S)*   *1st edition 1997; revised 2004, 2008*

OUTCOME CONTENT REFERENCES:
Conn, V. S., Armer, J. M., & Hayes, K. S. (2001). Knowledge deficit. In M. Maas, K. Buckwalter, M. Hardy, T. Tripp-Reimer, M. Titler, & J. Specht (Eds.), *Nursing care of older adults: Diagnoses, outcomes & interventions* (pp. 503–515). St. Louis: Mosby.
Redman, B. K. (2001). *The practice of patient education.* (9th ed.). St. Louis: Mosby.
Roe, B. H. (1990). Study of the effects of education on the management of urine drainage systems by patients and carers. *Journal of Advanced Nursing, 15*(5), 517–524.
Sarisley, C. (1987). Designing a teaching program for outpatient antibiotic therapy. *Journal of Nursing Staff Development, 3*(3), 128–135.
Smith, C. E. (1987). *Patient education: Nurses in partnership with other health professionals.* Orlando, FL: Gruen & Stratton.
Togger, D. A., & Brenner, P. S. (2001). Metered dose inhalers. *American Journal of Nursing, 101*(10), 26–32, 38–39.

Knowledge: Treatment Regimen

1813   **K**

Definition: Extent of understanding conveyed about a specific treatment regimen

OUTCOME TARGET RATING: Maintain at_____   Increase to_____

		No knowledge	Limited knowledge	Moderate knowledge	Substantial knowledge	Extensive knowledge	
OUTCOME OVERALL RATING		1	2	3	4	5	
Indicators:							
181310	Specific disease process	1	2	3	4	5	NA
181301	Benefits of treatment	1	2	3	4	5	NA
181302	Self-care responsibilities for ongoing treatment	1	2	3	4	5	NA
181303	Self-care responsibilities for emergency situations	1	2	3	4	5	NA
181315	Self-monitoring techniques	1	2	3	4	5	NA
181304	Expected effects of treatment	1	2	3	4	5	NA
181305	Prescribed diet	1	2	3	4	5	NA
181306	Prescribed medication regimen	1	2	3	4	5	NA
181307	Prescribed physical activity	1	2	3	4	5	NA
181308	Prescribed exercise	1	2	3	4	5	NA
181309	Prescribed procedure	1	2	3	4	5	NA
181316	Benefits of disease management	1	2	3	4	5	NA

Domain-*Health Knowledge & Behavior (IV)*   **Class**-*Health Knowledge (S)*   *1st edition 1997; revised 2004, 2008, 2013*

OUTCOME CONTENT REFERENCES:
Bushnell, F. (1992). Self-care teaching for congestive heart failure patients. *Journal of Gerontological Nursing, 18*(10), 27–32.
Conn, V. S., Armer, J. M., & Hayes, K. S. (2001). Knowledge deficit. In M. Maas, K. Buckwalter, M. Hardy, T. Tripp-Reimer, M. Titler, & J. Specht (Eds.), *Nursing care of older adults: Diagnoses, outcomes & interventions* (pp. 503–515). St. Louis: Mosby.
Devins, G. M., Binik, Y. M., Mandin, H., Litourneau, P. K., Hollomby, D. J., Barre, P. E., & Prichard, S. (1990). The kidney disease questionnaire: A test for measuring patient knowledge about end-stage renal disease. *Journal of Clinical Epidemiology, 43*(3), 297–307.
Garrard, J., Joynes, J. O., Mullen, L., McNeil, L., Mensing, C., Feste, C., & Etzwiler, D. D. (1987). Psychometric study of patient knowledge test. *Diabetes Care, 10*(4), 500–509.
Gilden, J. L., Hendryx, M., Casia, C., & Singh, S. P. (1989). The effectiveness of diabetes education programs for older patients and their spouses. *Journal of American Geriatrics Society, 37*(11), 1023–1030.
Mazzuca, S. A., Moorman, N. H., Wheeler, M. L., Norton, J. A., Fineberg, N. S., Vinicor, F., Cohen, S. J., & Clark, C. M. (1986). The diabetes education study: A controlled trial of the effects of diabetes patient education. *Diabetes Care, 9*(1), 1–10.
Redman, B. (1993). Knowledge deficit (specify). In J. M. Thompson, G. K. McFarland, J. E. Hirsch, & S. M. Tucker (Eds.), *Mosby's clinical nursing* (3rd ed., pp. 1548–1552). St. Louis: Mosby.

Scherer, Y. K., Janelli, L. M., & Schmieder, L. E. (1992). A time-series perspective of effectiveness of a health teaching program on chronic obstructive pulmonary disease. *Journal of Healthcare Education & Training, 6*(3), 7–13.

Smith, M. M., Hicks, V. L., & Heyward, V. H. (1991). Coronary disease knowledge test: Developing a valid and reliable tool. *Nurse Practitioner, 16*(4), 28, 31, 35–38.

Zwygart-Stauffacher, M. (2001). Ineffective management of therapeutic regimen. In M. Maas, K. Buckwalter, M. Hardy, T. Tripp-Reimer, M. Titler, & J. Specht (Eds.), *Nursing care of older adults: Diagnoses, outcomes & interventions* (pp. 86–92). St. Louis: Mosby.

Knowledge: Weight Management 1841

Definition: Extent of understanding conveyed about the promotion and maintenance of optimal body weight and fat percentage congruent with height, frame, gender and age

OUTCOME TARGET RATING: Maintain at_____   Increase to_____

		No knowledge	Limited knowledge	Moderate knowledge	Substantial knowledge	Extensive knowledge	
OUTCOME OVERALL RATING		1	2	3	4	5	
Indicators:							
184101	Optimal personal weight range	1	2	3	4	5	NA
184102	Optimal body mass index	1	2	3	4	5	NA
184103	Strategies to reach optimal weight	1	2	3	4	5	NA
184104	Strategies to maintain optimal weight	1	2	3	4	5	NA
184105	Relationship among diet, exercise and weight	1	2	3	4	5	NA
184106	Health risks related to overweight	1	2	3	4	5	NA
184107	Health risks related to underweight	1	2	3	4	5	NA
184108	Appetite versus hunger	1	2	3	4	5	NA
184109	Healthy nutritional practices	1	2	3	4	5	NA
184110	Adequate fluid intake	1	2	3	4	5	NA
184111	Strategies to modify food intake	1	2	3	4	5	NA
184112	Food cravings that trigger unhealthy eating	1	2	3	4	5	NA
184113	Emotional states that trigger unhealthy eating	1	2	3	4	5	NA
184114	Benefits of regular exercise	1	2	3	4	5	NA
184115	Exercises to maintain optimal weight	1	2	3	4	5	NA
184116	Barriers to implementing exercise routine	1	2	3	4	5	NA
184117	Strategies to modify behavior	1	2	3	4	5	NA
184118	Lifestyle changes to promote optimal weight	1	2	3	4	5	NA
184119	Benefits of prescribed weight loss medication	1	2	3	4	5	NA
184120	Potential dangers of non-prescription medication	1	2	3	4	5	NA
184121	Surgical treatment options for weight loss	1	2	3	4	5	NA
184122	Benefits of hypnosis	1	2	3	4	5	NA
184123	Benefits of alternative therapies	1	2	3	4	5	NA
184124	Benefits of social support	1	2	3	4	5	NA
184125	Risks associated with treatment options	1	2	3	4	5	NA
184126	Available support groups	1	2	3	4	5	NA
184127	Available community resources	1	2	3	4	5	NA
184128	Reputable sources of weight management information	1	2	3	4	5	NA
184129	Self-monitoring techniques	1	2	3	4	5	NA
184130	When to obtain assistance from a health professional	1	2	3	4	5	NA

Domain-Health Knowledge & Behavior (IV)   *Class-Health Knowledge (S)*   *4th edition 2008; revised 2013*

OUTCOME CONTENT REFERENCES:

Dennis, K. E. (2004). Weight management in women. *Nursing Clinics of North America, 39*(1), 231–241.

Huether, S., & McCance, K. (Eds.). (2002). *Pathophysiology: The biologic basis for disease in adults and children* (4th ed.). St. Louis: Mosby.

Lewis, S., Heitkemper, M., & Dirksen, S. (Eds.). (2004). *Medical-surgical nursing: Assessment and management of clinical problems* (6th ed., pp. 991–1000). St. Louis: Mosby.

National Heart, Lung, and Blood Institute. (2005). *Aim for a healthy weight* (NIH Publication No. 05-5213). Bethesda, MD: U.S. Department of Health and Human Services.

National Heart, Lung, and Blood Institute and the North American Association for the Study of Obesity. (2000). *The practical guide to the identification, evaluation, and treatment of overweight and obesity in adults* (NIH Publication No. 00-4084). Bethesda, MD: U.S. Department of Health and Human Services.

Leisure Participation 1604

Definition: Use of relaxing, interesting, and enjoyable activities to promote well-being

OUTCOME TARGET RATING: Maintain at_____ Increase to_____

OUTCOME OVERALL RATING	Never demonstrated 1	Rarely demonstrated 2	Sometimes demonstrated 3	Often demonstrated 4	Consistently demonstrated 5	
Indicators:						
160401 Participates in activities other than regular work	1	2	3	4	5	NA
160410 Participates in high physical demand leisure activities	1	2	3	4	5	NA
160411 Participates in low physical demand leisure activities	1	2	3	4	5	NA
160412 Selects leisure activities of interest	1	2	3	4	5	NA
160402 Expresses satisfaction with leisure activities	1	2	3	4	5	NA
160403 Uses appropriate social interaction skills	1	2	3	4	5	NA
160404 Feels relaxed from leisure activities	1	2	3	4	5	NA
160413 Enjoys leisure activities	1	2	3	4	5	NA
160405 Exhibits creativity through leisure activities	1	2	3	4	5	NA
160407 Identifies recreational options	1	2	3	4	5	NA

Domain-*Health Knowledge & Behavior (IV)*   **Class**-*Health Behavior (Q)*   *1st edition 1997; revised 2004, 2008*

OUTCOME CONTENT REFERENCES:

Ansello, E. F. (1985). *The activity coordinator as environmental press.* New York: The Haworth Press.

+Drummond, A. E. R., & Walker, M. F. (1994). The Nottingham Leisure Questionnaire for stroke patients. *British Journal of Occupational Therapy, 57*(11), 414–418.

Everard, K. M., Lach, H. W., Fisher, E. B., & Baum, M. C. (2000). Relationship of activity and social support to the functional health of older adults. *Journal of Gerontology. Series B, Psychological Sciences and Social Sciences, 55*(4), P208–P212.

Godin, G., Jobin, J., & Bouillon, J. (1986). Assessment of leisure time exercise behavior by self-report: A concurrent validity study. *Canadian Journal of Public Health, 77*(5), 359–362.

Gordon, M. D. (1987). Pediatric recreational therapy after thermal injury. *Journal of Burn Rehabilitation, 8*(4), 336–340.

Johnson, S. W., McSweeney, M., & Webster, R. E. (1989). Leisure: How to promote inpatient motivation after discharge. *Journal of Psychosocial Nursing, 27*(9), 29–31.

Jongbloed, L., & Morgan, D. (1991). An investigation of involvement in leisure activities after a stroke. *The American Journal of Occupational Therapy, 45*(5), 420–427.

Klein, M. M. (1985). The therapeutics of recreation. *Physical Occupational Therapy Pediatrics, 4*(3), 9–11.

Peterson, C. A., & Stumbo, N. J. (1999). *Therapeutic recreation program design: Principles and procedures* (3rd ed.). San Francisco: Benjamin Cummings.

Rantz, M. J., & Popejoy, L. (2001). Diversional activity deficit. In M. Maas, K. Buckwalter, M. Hardy, T. Tripp-Reimer, M. Titler, & J. Specht (Eds.), *Nursing care of older adults: Diagnoses, outcomes & interventions* (pp. 385–396). St. Louis: Mosby.

L

Lifestyle Balance 2013

Definition: Personal actions to live a healthy, balanced lifestyle consistent with one's values, strengths, and interests through conscious adherence to daily health habits and efforts to reduce or minimize stress

OUTCOME TARGET RATING: Maintain at_____ Increase to_____

OUTCOME OVERALL RATING		Never demonstrated 1	Rarely demonstrated 2	Sometimes demonstrated 3	Often demonstrated 4	Consistently demonstrated 5	
Indicators:							
201301	Recognizes need for balancing life activities	1	2	3	4	5	NA
201302	Seeks information about strategies to balance life activities	1	2	3	4	5	NA
201303	Considers personal needs and values when choosing life activities	1	2	3	4	5	NA
201304	Identifies personal strengths	1	2	3	4	5	NA
201305	Identifies major sources of stress	1	2	3	4	5	NA
201306	Uses strategies to reduce stress	1	2	3	4	5	NA
201307	Evaluates areas of perceived imbalance in lifestyle	1	2	3	4	5	NA
201308	Limits activities that contribute to a sense of feeling burdened	1	2	3	4	5	NA
201309	Uses strategies to balance work activities and family roles	1	2	3	4	5	NA
201310	Uses time management in daily routine	1	2	3	4	5	NA
201311	Organizes time and energy to meet personal goals	1	2	3	4	5	NA
201312	Modifies role responsibilities within the family as needed	1	2	3	4	5	NA
201313	Uses strategies to adapt to multiple role responsibilities	1	2	3	4	5	NA
201314	Engages in activities that meet psychological needs	1	2	3	4	5	NA
201315	Synchronizes daily activities with biological rhythms	1	2	3	4	5	NA
201316	Engages in activities that promote personal growth	1	2	3	4	5	NA
201317	Engages in activities consistent with personal values	1	2	3	4	5	NA

Domain-Perceived Health (V)   *Class*-Health & Life Quality (U)   5th edition 2013

OUTCOME CONTENT REFERENCES:

Christiansen, C. H., & Matuska, K. M. (2006). Lifestyle balance: A review of concepts and research. *Journal of Occupational Science, 13*(1), 49–61.

Grant, N., Wardle, J., & Steptoe, A. (2009). The relationship between life satisfaction and health behavior: A cross-cultural analysis of young adults. *International Journal of Behavioral Medicine, 16*(3), 259–268.

Hwang, J. E. (2010). Promoting healthy lifestyles with aging: Development and validation of the health enhancement lifestyle profile (HELP) using the Rasch measurement model. *American Journal of Occupational Therapy, 64*(5), 786–795.

Kennedy, C., & Miller, M. (2005). The future of fitness: Is "lifestyle enhancement" the wellness balance we should help clients seek in the coming years? *IDEA Fitness Journal, 2*(7), 104–108.

Lawrence, W., & Sherrod, D. (2009). Are you successfully balancing your work and home life? *Nursing Management, 40*(5), 51, 53.

Matuska, K. M., & Christiansen, C. H. (2008). A proposed model of lifestyle balance. *Journal of Occupational Science, 15*(1), 9–19.

Teta, J., & Teta, K. (December 2005). The impact of lifestyle choices and hormonal balance on coping with stress. *Townsend Letter for Doctors & Patients*, pp. 89–91.

Liver Function 0803

Definition: Ability of the liver to manufacture, store, alter, and secrete substances essential for metabolism and other body functions

OUTCOME TARGET RATING: Maintain at_____   Increase to_____

OUTCOME OVERALL RATING	Severely compromised	Substantially compromised	Moderately compromised	Mildly compromised	Not compromised	
	1	2	3	4	5	
Indicators:						
080301 Appetite	1	2	3	4	5	NA
080302 Color of stool	1	2	3	4	5	NA
080303 Sleep	1	2	3	4	5	NA
080304 Stamina	1	2	3	4	5	NA
080305 Albumin/globulin ratio	1	2	3	4	5	NA
080306 Skin turgor	1	2	3	4	5	NA
080307 Consciousness	1	2	3	4	5	NA

	Severe	Substantial	Moderate	Mild	None	
080308 Increased total serum bilirubin	1	2	3	4	5	NA
080309 Increased direct serum bilirubin	1	2	3	4	5	NA
080310 Prolonged prothrombin time	1	2	3	4	5	NA
080311 Serum ammonia level	1	2	3	4	5	NA
080312 Increased alanine transaminase (ALT) (SGPT)	1	2	3	4	5	NA
080313 Increased aspartate aminotransferase (AST) (SGOT)	1	2	3	4	5	NA
080314 Increased gamma-glutamyl transferase (GGT)	1	2	3	4	5	NA
080315 Jaundice	1	2	3	4	5	NA
080316 Pruritus	1	2	3	4	5	NA
080317 Spider angiomas	1	2	3	4	5	NA
080318 Petechiae	1	2	3	4	5	NA
080319 Palmar erythema	1	2	3	4	5	NA
080320 Tremor	1	2	3	4	5	NA
080321 Muscle atrophy	1	2	3	4	5	NA
080322 Ascites	1	2	3	4	5	NA
080323 Weight gain	1	2	3	4	5	NA
080324 Dilated abdominal wall veins	1	2	3	4	5	NA
080325 Increased abdominal girth	1	2	3	4	5	NA
080326 Abdominal pain	1	2	3	4	5	NA
080327 Liver tenderness	1	2	3	4	5	NA
080328 Bruising	1	2	3	4	5	NA
080329 Hematemesis	1	2	3	4	5	NA
080330 Blood in stools	1	2	3	4	5	NA
080331 Anorexia	1	2	3	4	5	NA
080332 Fatigue	1	2	3	4	5	NA
080333 Agitation	1	2	3	4	5	NA

Domain-*Physiologic Health (II)*   **Class**-*Metabolic Regulation (I)*   *5th edition 2013*

OUTCOME CONTENT REFERENCES:

Kortgen, A., Recknagel, P., & Bauer, M. (2010). How to assess liver function? *Current Opinion in Critical Care, 16*(2), 136–141.

LeMone, P., Burke, K., & Bauldoff, G. (2011). *Medical-surgical nursing: Critical thinking in patient care, vol. 1* (5th ed., pp. 727–748). Upper Saddle River, NJ: Pearson Education.

Smeltzer, S., Bare, B., Hinkle, J., & Cheever, K. (2008). *Brunner & Suddarth's textbook of medical-surgical nursing* (11th ed., pp. 1285–1340). Philadelphia: Lippincott Williams & Wilkins.

Loneliness Severity 1203

Definition: Severity of emotional, social, or existential signs and symptoms of isolation

OUTCOME TARGET RATING: Maintain at_____ Increase to_____

OUTCOME OVERALL RATING	Severe 1	Substantial 2	Moderate 3	Mild 4	None 5	
Indicators:						
120301 Sense of unfounded dread	1	2	3	4	5	NA
120302 Sense of desperation	1	2	3	4	5	NA
120303 Sense of extreme restlessness	1	2	3	4	5	NA
120304 Sense of hopelessness	1	2	3	4	5	NA
120305 Sense of not belonging	1	2	3	4	5	NA
120306 Sense of loss due to separation from another	1	2	3	4	5	NA
120307 Sense of social isolation	1	2	3	4	5	NA
120308 Sense of not being understood	1	2	3	4	5	NA
120309 Sense of being excluded	1	2	3	4	5	NA
120310 Sense that time seems endless	1	2	3	4	5	NA
120311 Difficulty in planning	1	2	3	4	5	NA
120312 Difficulty in establishing contact with others	1	2	3	4	5	NA
120313 Difficulty overcoming separateness	1	2	3	4	5	NA
120314 Difficulty in effecting a mutual relationship	1	2	3	4	5	NA
120315 Mood fluctuations	1	2	3	4	5	NA
120316 Impaired concentration	1	2	3	4	5	NA
120317 Non-assertiveness	1	2	3	4	5	NA
120318 Difficulty making decisions	1	2	3	4	5	NA
120328 Unhealthy eating pattern	1	2	3	4	5	NA
120320 Sleep disturbance	1	2	3	4	5	NA
120321 Headaches	1	2	3	4	5	NA
120322 Nausea	1	2	3	4	5	NA
120323 Decreased activity level	1	2	3	4	5	NA
120324 Pain	1	2	3	4	5	NA
120325 Spiritual discomfort	1	2	3	4	5	NA
120327 Depression	1	2	3	4	5	NA

Domain-*Psychosocial Health (III)*   **Class**-*Psychological Well-Being (M)*   *1st edition 1997; revised 2004, 2008, 2013*

OUTCOME CONTENT REFERENCES:
Copel, L. C. (1988). Loneliness: A conceptual model. *Journal of Psychosocial Nursing, 26*(1), 14–19.
Ellison, C. W. (1978). Loneliness: A social-developmental analysis. *Journal of Psychology and Theology, 6*(1), 3–17.
Peplau, H. E. (1955). Loneliness. *American Journal of Nursing, 55*(12), 1476–1481.
Peplau, L. A., & Pearlman, D. (Eds.). (1982). *Loneliness: A sourcebook of current theory, research, and therapy.* New York: John Wiley.
+Russell, D., Peplau, L. A., & Cutrona, C. E. (1980). The revised UCLA Loneliness Scale: Concurrent and discriminant validity evidence. *Journal of Personality and Social Psychology, 39*(3), 472–480.
+Russell, D., Peplau, L. A., & Ferguson, M. (1978). Developing a measure of loneliness. *Journal of Personality Assessment, 42*(3), 290–294.
Weiss, R. S. (Ed.). (1973). *Loneliness: The experience of emotional and social isolation.* Cambridge, MA: The MIT Press.
West, D. A., Kellner, R., & Moore-West, M. (1986). The effects of loneliness: A review of the literature. *Comparative Psychiatry, 27*(4), 351–363.

Maternal Status: Antepartum   2509

Definition: Extent to which maternal well-being is within normal limits from conception to the onset of labor

OUTCOME TARGET RATING: Maintain at_____   Increase to_____

		Severe deviation from normal range	Substantial deviation from normal range	Moderate deviation from normal range	Mild deviation from normal range	No deviation from normal range	
OUTCOME OVERALL RATING		1	2	3	4	5	
Indicators:							
250901	Emotional attachment to fetus	1	2	3	4	5	NA
250902	Coping with discomforts of pregnancy	1	2	3	4	5	NA
250903	Mood lability	1	2	3	4	5	NA
250904	Weight change	1	2	3	4	5	NA
250907	Cognitive status	1	2	3	4	5	NA
250908	Visual acuity	1	2	3	4	5	NA
250910	Neurological reflexes	1	2	3	4	5	NA
250916	Blood pressure	1	2	3	4	5	NA
250917	Radial pulse rate	1	2	3	4	5	NA
250926	Apical heart rate	1	2	3	4	5	NA
250929	Respiratory rate	1	2	3	4	5	NA
250918	Body temperature	1	2	3	4	5	NA
250919	Urine protein	1	2	3	4	5	NA
250920	Urine glucose	1	2	3	4	5	NA
250921	Blood glucose	1	2	3	4	5	NA
250922	Hemoglobin	1	2	3	4	5	NA
250923	Liver enzymes	1	2	3	4	5	NA
250924	Blood count	1	2	3	4	5	NA

		Severe	Substantial	Moderate	Mild	None	
250905	Edema	1	2	3	4	5	NA
250906	Headache	1	2	3	4	5	NA
250909	Seizure activity	1	2	3	4	5	NA
250911	Nausea	1	2	3	4	5	NA
250928	Vomiting	1	2	3	4	5	NA
250912	Abdominal pain	1	2	3	4	5	NA
250913	Epigastric pain	1	2	3	4	5	NA
250914	Vaginal bleeding	1	2	3	4	5	NA
250915	Vaginal discharge	1	2	3	4	5	NA
250927	Heartburn	1	2	3	4	5	NA
250930	Constipation	1	2	3	4	5	NA

M

Domain-Family Health (VI)   *Class*-Family Member Health Status (Z)   *2nd edition 2000; revised 2004, 2008, 2013*

OUTCOME CONTENT REFERENCES:

Armour, K. (2004). Using surveillance to improve maternal and fetal outcomes: Antepartum maternal-fetal assessment. *AWHONN Lifelines, 8*(3), 232–240.

Association of Women's Health, Obstetric and Neonatal Nurses. (1998). *Clinical competencies and educational guide: Limited ultrasound examinations in obstetric and gynecologic/infertility settings.* Washington, DC: Author.

Association of Women's Health, Obstetric and Neonatal Nurses. (1998). *Standards & guidelines for the professional nursing practice in the care of women and newborns* (5th ed.). Washington, DC: Author.

Chez, B. F., Skurnick, J. H., Chez, R. A., Verklan, M. T., Biggs, S., & Hage, M. L. (1990). Interpretations of nonstress tests by obstetric nurses. *Journal of Obstetric, Gynecologic, and Neonatal Nursing, 19*(3), 227–232.

Givens, S. R., & Moore, M. L. (1995). Status report on maternal and child health indicators. *Journal of Perinatal and Neonatal Nursing, 9*(1), 8–18.

Lowdermilk, D. L., & Perry, S. E. (2003). *Maternity nursing* (6th ed.). St. Louis: Mosby.

Nichols, F., & Humenick, S. (2000). *Childbirth education: Practice, research and theory* (2nd ed.). Philadelphia: W. B. Saunders.

Nurses Association of the American College of Obstetricians and Gynecologists. (1991). *NAACOBG standards for the nursing care of women and newborns* (4th ed.). Washington, DC: Author.

Reeder, S. J., Martin, L. L., & Koniak-Griffin, D. (1997). *Maternity nursing: Family, newborn, and women's health care* (18th ed.). Philadelphia: J. B. Lippincott.

Maternal Status: Intrapartum 2510

Definition: Extent to which maternal well-being is within normal limits from onset of labor to delivery

OUTCOME TARGET RATING: Maintain at_____ Increase to_____

OUTCOME OVERALL RATING		Severe deviation from normal range	Substantial deviation from normal range	Moderate deviation from normal range	Mild deviation from normal range	No deviation from normal range	
		1	2	3	4	5	
Indicators:							
251001	Coping with discomforts of labor	1	2	3	4	5	NA
251003	Use of techniques to facilitate labor	1	2	3	4	5	NA
251004	Uterine contraction frequency	1	2	3	4	5	NA
251005	Uterine contraction duration	1	2	3	4	5	NA
251006	Uterine contraction intensity	1	2	3	4	5	NA
251007	Progression of cervical dilation	1	2	3	4	5	NA
251009	Blood pressure	1	2	3	4	5	NA
251010	Radial pulse rate	1	2	3	4	5	NA
251021	Apical heart rate	1	2	3	4	5	NA
251011	Blood glucose	1	2	3	4	5	NA
251012	Body temperature	1	2	3	4	5	NA
251013	Urine output	1	2	3	4	5	NA
251014	Visual acuity	1	2	3	4	5	NA
251015	Cognitive status	1	2	3	4	5	NA
251016	Neurological reflexes	1	2	3	4	5	NA

		Severe	Substantial	Moderate	Mild	None	
251008	Vaginal bleeding	1	2	3	4	5	NA
251017	Seizure activity	1	2	3	4	5	NA
251018	Headache	1	2	3	4	5	NA
251019	Epigastric pain	1	2	3	4	5	NA
251022	Pain with contractions	1	2	3	4	5	NA
251023	Back pain	1	2	3	4	5	NA
251024	Nausea	1	2	3	4	5	NA
251025	Vomiting	1	2	3	4	5	NA

Domain-Family Health (VI)   **Class**-Family Member Health Status (Z)   *2nd edition 2000; revised 2004*

OUTCOME CONTENT REFERENCES:
Dickason, E. J., Schultz, M. O., & Silverman, B. L. (1994). *Maternal-infant nursing care* (3rd ed.). St. Louis: Mosby.
Hodnett, E. (1996). Nursing support of the laboring woman. *Journal of Obstetric and Neonatal Nursing, 25*(3), 257–263.
Lowe, N. K. (1996). The pain and discomfort of labor and birth. *Journal of Obstetric and Neonatal Nursing, 25*(1), 82–92.
Mattson, S. (Ed.). (2000). *Core curriculum for maternal-newborn nursing* (2nd ed.). Philadelphia: W. B. Saunders.

Maternal Status: Postpartum 2511

Definition: Extent to which maternal well-being is within normal limits from delivery of placenta to completion of involution

OUTCOME TARGET RATING: Maintain at_____ Increase to_____

		Severe deviation from normal range	Substantial deviation from normal range	Moderate deviation from normal range	Mild deviation from normal range	No deviation from normal range	
OUTCOME OVERALL RATING		1	2	3	4	5	
Indicators:							
251101	Mood equilibrium	1	2	3	4	5	NA
251102	Comfort	1	2	3	4	5	NA
251103	Blood pressure	1	2	3	4	5	NA
251104	Apical heart rate	1	2	3	4	5	NA
251123	Radial pulse rate	1	2	3	4	5	NA
251105	Peripheral circulation	1	2	3	4	5	NA
251106	Uterine fundal height	1	2	3	4	5	NA
251107	Lochia amount	1	2	3	4	5	NA
251124	Lochia color	1	2	3	4	5	NA
251108	Breast fullness	1	2	3	4	5	NA
251109	Breast comfort	1	2	3	4	5	NA
251110	Perineal healing	1	2	3	4	5	NA
251111	Incisional healing	1	2	3	4	5	NA
251112	Body temperature	1	2	3	4	5	NA
251114	Urinary elimination	1	2	3	4	5	NA
251115	Bowel elimination	1	2	3	4	5	NA
251116	Food and fluid intake	1	2	3	4	5	NA
251117	Physical activity	1	2	3	4	5	NA
251118	Endurance	1	2	3	4	5	NA
251119	Liver enzymes	1	2	3	4	5	NA
251120	Hemoglobin	1	2	3	4	5	NA
251121	White blood count	1	2	3	4	5	NA
251129	Blood glucose	1	2	3	4	5	NA

		Severe	Substantial	Moderate	Mild	None	
251113	Infection	1	2	3	4	5	NA
251125	Incisional pain	1	2	3	4	5	NA
251126	Fatigue	1	2	3	4	5	NA
251127	Vaginal bleeding	1	2	3	4	5	NA
251128	Depression	1	2	3	4	5	NA
251130	Lacerations	1	2	3	4	5	NA

Domain-*Family Health (VI)*   **Class**-*Family Member Health Status (Z)*   *2nd edition 2000; revised 2004, 2013*

OUTCOME CONTENT REFERENCES:
Association of Women's Health, Obstetricians and Neonatal Nurses. (1998). *Standards & guidelines for the professional nursing practice in the care of women and newborns* (5th ed.). Washington, DC: Author.
Beck, C. T. (1992). The lived experience of postpartum depression: A phenomenological study. *Nursing Research, 41*(3), 166–170.
Bond, L. (1993). Physiological changes. In S. Mattson & J. E. Smith (Eds.), *AWHONN: Core Curriculum for maternal newborn nursing.* Philadelphia: W. B. Saunders.
Nichols, F., & Humenick, S. (2000). *Childbirth education: Practice, research and theory* (2nd ed.). Philadelphia: W. B. Saunders.
Reeder, S. J., Martin, L. L., & Koniak-Griffin, D. (1997). *Maternity nursing: Family, newborn, and women's health care* (18th ed.). Philadelphia: J. B. Lippincott.

M

Mechanical Ventilation Response: Adult 0411

Definition: Alveolar exchange and tissue perfusion are effectively supported by mechanical ventilation

OUTCOME TARGET RATING: Maintain at_____ Increase to_____

OUTCOME OVERALL RATING		Severe deviation from normal range	Substantial deviation from normal range	Moderate deviation from normal range	Mild deviation from normal range	No deviation from normal range	
		1	2	3	4	5	
Indicators:							
041102	Respiratory rate	1	2	3	4	5	NA
041103	Respiratory rhythm	1	2	3	4	5	NA
041104	Depth of inspiration	1	2	3	4	5	NA
041126	Inspiratory capacity	1	2	3	4	5	NA
041106	Tidal volume	1	2	3	4	5	NA
041107	Vital capacity	1	2	3	4	5	NA
041108	FiO_2 (fraction of inspired oxygen) meets oxygen demand	1	2	3	4	5	NA
041109	PaO_2 (partial pressure of oxygen in arterial blood)	1	2	3	4	5	NA
041110	$PaCO_2$ (partial pressure of carbon dioxide in arterial blood)	1	2	3	4	5	NA
041111	Arterial pH	1	2	3	4	5	NA
041112	Oxygen saturation	1	2	3	4	5	NA
041113	Peripheral tissue perfusion	1	2	3	4	5	NA
041114	End tidal carbon dioxide	1	2	3	4	5	NA
041115	Pulmonary function tests	1	2	3	4	5	NA
041116	Chest x-ray findings	1	2	3	4	5	NA
041117	Ventilation perfusion balance	1	2	3	4	5	NA

		Severe	Substantial	Moderate	Mild	None	
041122	Asymmetrical chest wall movement	1	2	3	4	5	NA
041123	Asymmetrical chest wall expansion	1	2	3	4	5	NA
041124	Difficulty breathing with ventilator	1	2	3	4	5	NA
041127	Adventitious breath sounds	1	2	3	4	5	NA
041134	Atelectasis	1	2	3	4	5	NA
041125	Anxiety	1	2	3	4	5	NA
041128	Restlessness	1	2	3	4	5	NA
041129	Impaired skin integrity at tracheostomy site	1	2	3	4	5	NA
041130	Hypoxia	1	2	3	4	5	NA
041131	Pulmonary infection	1	2	3	4	5	NA
041132	Respiratory secretions	1	2	3	4	5	NA
041133	Difficulty communicating needs	1	2	3	4	5	NA

Type and mode of ventilation: _____

Domain-*Physiologic Health (II)*   **Class**-*Cardiopulmonary (E)*   *3rd edition 2004; revised 2008*

OUTCOME CONTENT REFERENCES:
Bickley, L. S., & Hoekelman, R. A. (1998). *Bates' guide to physical examination and history taking* (7th ed.). Philadelphia: Lippincott Williams & Wilkins.
Chlan, L. (2000). Music therapy as a nursing intervention for patients supported by mechanical ventilation. *AACN Clinical Issues, 11*(1), 128–138.
Coates, L. (2000). Care of the ventilated patient. *Nursing Standard, 14*(28), 60.
Hanneman, S. (1999). Protocols for practice: Applying research at the bedside. *Critical Care Nurse, 9*(5), 86–89.
Henderson, N. (1999). Mechanical ventilation. *Nursing Standard, 13*(44), 49–54.
Kelly-Heidenthal, P., & O'Connor, M. (1994). Nursing assessment of portable AP chest x-rays. *Dimensions of Critical Care Nursing, 13*(3), 127–132.
Smeltzer, S. C., & Bare, B. G. (2004). *Brunner & Suddarth's textbook of medical surgical nursing* (10th ed.). Philadelphia: Lippincott Williams & Wilkins.

Mechanical Ventilation Weaning Response: Adult   0412

Definition: Respiratory and psychological adjustment to progressive removal of mechanical ventilation

OUTCOME TARGET RATING: Maintain at_____   Increase to_____

		Severe deviation from normal range	Substantial deviation from normal range	Moderate deviation from normal range	Mild deviation from normal range	No deviation from normal range	
OUTCOME OVERALL RATING		1	2	3	4	5	
Indicators:							
041202	Spontaneous respiratory rate	1	2	3	4	5	NA
041203	Spontaneous respiratory rhythm	1	2	3	4	5	NA
041204	Spontaneous respiratory depth	1	2	3	4	5	NA
041205	Apical heart rate	1	2	3	4	5	NA
041208	PaO_2 (partial pressure of oxygen in arterial blood)	1	2	3	4	5	NA
041209	$PaCO_2$ (partial pressure of carbon dioxide in arterial blood)	1	2	3	4	5	NA
041210	Arterial pH	1	2	3	4	5	NA
041211	Oxygen saturation	1	2	3	4	5	NA
041212	Vital capacity	1	2	3	4	5	NA
041213	Tidal volume	1	2	3	4	5	NA
041214	Minute ventilation <10 L/minute	1	2	3	4	5	NA
041215	Positive end expiratory pressure	1	2	3	4	5	NA
041219	Chest x-ray findings	1	2	3	4	5	NA
041220	Ventilation perfusion balance	1	2	3	4	5	NA
		Severe	Substantial	Moderate	Mild	None	
041223	Difficulty breathing on own	1	2	3	4	5	NA
041224	Respiratory secretions	1	2	3	4	5	NA
041225	Anxiety	1	2	3	4	5	NA
041226	Fear	1	2	3	4	5	NA
041227	Impaired gag reflex	1	2	3	4	5	NA

M

Continued

Mechanical Ventilation Weaning Response: Adult—*cont'd*

		Severe	Substantial	Moderate	Mild	None	
041228	Impaired cough reflex	1	2	3	4	5	NA
041229	Impaired drive to breath	1	2	3	4	5	NA
041230	Adventitious breath sounds	1	2	3	4	5	NA
041231	Asymmetrical chest wall movement	1	2	3	4	5	NA
041232	Asymmetrical chest wall expansion	1	2	3	4	5	NA
041233	Atelectasis	1	2	3	4	5	NA
041234	Restlessness	1	2	3	4	5	NA
041235	Discomfort	1	2	3	4	5	NA
041236	Difficulty communicating needs	1	2	3	4	5	NA

Domain-*Physiologic Health (II)*   *Class*-*Cardiopulmonary (E)*   *3rd edition 2004; revised 2008*

OUTCOME CONTENT REFERENCES:

Burns, S. M., Fahey, S. A., Barton, D. M., & Clack, D. (1991). Weaning from mechanical ventilation: A method for assessment and intervention. *AACN Clinical Issues for Critical Care Nurses, 2*(3), 372–387.

Chlan, L. (2000). Music therapy as a nursing intervention for patients supported by mechanical ventilation. *AACN Clinical Issues, 11*(1), 128–138.

Coates, L. (2000). Care of the ventilated patient. *Nursing Standard, 14*(28), 60.

Hanneman, S. (1999). Protocols for practice: Applying research at the bedside. *Critical Care Nurse, 9*(5), 86–89.

Henderson, N. (1999). Mechanical ventilation. *Nursing Standard, 13*(44), 49–54.

Kelly-Heidenthal, P., & O'Connor, M. (1994). Nursing assessment of portable AP chest x-rays. *Dimensions of Critical Care Nursing, 13*(3), 127–132.

Morganroth, M. L., Morganroth, J. L., Nett, L. M., & Petty, T. L. (1984). Criteria for weaning from prolonged mechanical ventilation. *Archives of Internal Medicine, 144*(5), 1012–1016.

Smeltzer, S. C., & Bare, B. G. (2004). *Brunner & Suddarth's textbook of medical surgical nursing* (10th ed.). Philadelphia: Lippincott Williams & Wilkins.

Urban, N., Greenlee, K., Krumberger, J., & Winkelman, C. (1995). *Guidelines for critical care nursing.* St. Louis: Mosby.

Yang, K. L., & Tobin, M. J. (1991). A prospective study of indexes predicting the outcome trials of weaning a patient from mechanical ventilation. *New England Journal of Medicine, 324*(21), 1445–1450.

M

Medication Response 2301

Definition: Therapeutic and adverse effects of prescribed medication

OUTCOME TARGET RATING: Maintain at_____ Increase to_____

	Severely compromised	Substantially compromised	Moderately compromised	Mildly compromised	Not compromised	
OUTCOME OVERALL RATING	1	2	3	4	5	
Indicators:						
230101 Expected therapeutic effects	1	2	3	4	5	NA
230102 Expected change in blood chemistries	1	2	3	4	5	NA
230103 Expected change in symptoms	1	2	3	4	5	NA
230111 Maintenance of expected blood levels	1	2	3	4	5	NA
230112 Expected behavioral response	1	2	3	4	5	NA

	Severe	Substantial	Moderate	Mild	None	
230105 Allergic reaction	1	2	3	4	5	NA
230106 Adverse effects	1	2	3	4	5	NA
230107 Medication interactions	1	2	3	4	5	NA
230108 Medication intolerance	1	2	3	4	5	NA
230113 Adverse behavioral effects	1	2	3	4	5	NA

Specify medication: _____

Domain-*Physiologic Health (II)* **Class**-*Therapeutic Response (AA)* *2nd edition 2000; revised 2004, 2008*

M

OUTCOME CONTENT REFERENCES:

Arnold, G. J. (1998). Clinical recognition of adverse drug reactions: Obstacles and opportunities for the nursing profession. *Journal of Nursing Care Quality,* *13*(2), 45–55.

Hodgson, B. B., & Kizior, R. J. (2003). *Saunders nursing drug book 2003* (3rd ed.). Philadelphia: W. B. Saunders.

Katzung, B. G. (Ed.). (2000). *Basic and clinical pharmacology* (8th ed.). Norwalk, CT: Appleton & Lange.

Shannon, M. T., Wilson, B. A., & Stang, C. L. (1995). *Drugs and nursing implications* (8th ed.). Norwalk, CT: Appleton & Lange.

Springhouse. (1998). *Nurse practitioner's drug handbook* (2nd ed.). Springhouse, PA: Author.

Memory 0908

Definition: Ability to cognitively retrieve and report previously stored information

OUTCOME TARGET RATING: Maintain at_____ Increase to_____

		Severely compromised	Substantially compromised	Moderately compromised	Mildly compromised	Not compromised	
OUTCOME OVERALL RATING		1	2	3	4	5	
Indicators:							
090801	Recalls immediate information accurately	1	2	3	4	5	NA
090802	Recalls recent information accurately	1	2	3	4	5	NA
090803	Recalls remote information accurately	1	2	3	4	5	NA

Domain-Physiologic Health (II) *Class*-Neurocognitive (J) *1st edition 1997; revised 2004*

OUTCOME CONTENT REFERENCES:

Abraham, I., & Reel, S. (1993). Cognitive nursing interventions with long-term residents: Effects on neurocognitive dimensions. *Archives of Psychiatric Nursing,* 6(6), 356–365.

Agostinelli, B., Demers, K., Garrigan, D., & Waszynski, C. (1994). Targeted interventions: Use of the Mini-Mental State Exam. *Journal of Gerontological Nursing,* 20(8), 15–23.

Dellasega, C. (1992). Home health nurses' assessments of cognition. *Applied Nursing Research, 5*(3), 127–133.

Foreman, M., Theis, S., & Anderson, M. A. (1993). Adverse events in the hospitalized elderly. *Clinical Nursing Research, 2*(3), 360–370.

Gerdner, L. A., & Hall, G. R. (2001). Chronic confusion. In M. Maas, K. Buckwalter, M. Hardy, T. Tripp-Reimer, M. Titler, & J. Specht (Eds.), *Nursing care of older adults: Diagnoses, outcomes & interventions* (pp. 421–441). St. Louis: Mosby.

Mason, P. (1989). Cognitive assessment parameters and tools for the critically injured adult. *Critical Care Nursing Clinics of North America, 1*(1), 45–53.

+Pfeiffer, E. (1975). A short portable mental status questionnaire for the assessment of organic brain deficit in elderly patients. *American Geriatrics Society, 23*(10), 433–441.

Strub, R. L., & Black, F. W. (2000). *The mental status examination in neurology* (4th ed.). Philadelphia: F. A. Davis.

Metabolic Acidosis Severity 0619

Definition: Severity of signs and symptoms of decreased blood pH due to decreased bicarbonate and increased hydrogen ions

OUTCOME TARGET RATING: Maintain at_____ Increase to_____

		Severe	Substantial	Moderate	Mild	None	
OUTCOME OVERALL RATING		1	2	3	4	5	
Indicators:							
061901	Decreased blood plasma pH	1	2	3	4	5	NA
061902	Increased serum hydrogen ions	1	2	3	4	5	NA
061903	Decreased serum bicarbonate	1	2	3	4	5	NA
061904	Elevated anion gap	1	2	3	4	5	NA
061905	Increased serum potassium	1	2	3	4	5	NA
061906	Increased respiratory rate	1	2	3	4	5	NA
061907	Increased respiratory depth	1	2	3	4	5	NA
061908	Hypoxia	1	2	3	4	5	NA
061909	Kussmaul-Kien respiration	1	2	3	4	5	NA
061910	Arrhythmias	1	2	3	4	5	NA
061911	Peripheral vasodilation	1	2	3	4	5	NA
061912	Hypotension	1	2	3	4	5	NA

M

Metabolic Acidosis Severity—cont'd

		Severe	Substantial	Moderate	Mild	None	
061913	Cold, clammy skin	1	2	3	4	5	NA
061914	Headache	1	2	3	4	5	NA
061915	Drowsiness	1	2	3	4	5	NA
061916	Confusion	1	2	3	4	5	NA
061917	Abdominal pain	1	2	3	4	5	NA
061918	Anorexia	1	2	3	4	5	NA
061919	Nausea	1	2	3	4	5	NA
061920	Vomiting	1	2	3	4	5	NA
061921	Seizures	1	2	3	4	5	NA
061922	Decreased level of consciousness	1	2	3	4	5	NA

Domain-*Physiologic Health (II)* **Class**-*Fluid & Electrolytes (G)* *5th edition 2013*

OUTCOME CONTENT REFERENCES:

Appel, S. J., & Downs, C. A. (2007). Steady a disturbed equilibrium. Accurately interpret the acid-base balance of acutely ill patients. *Nursing Critical Care 2*(4), 45–53.

Aschner, J. L., & Poland, R. L. (2008). Sodium bicarbonate: Basically useless therapy. *Pediatrics, 122*(4), 831–835.

Clancy, J., & McVicar, A. (2007). Intermediate and long-term regulation of acid-base homeostasis. *British Journal of Nursing, 16*(17), 1076–1079.

Isenhour, J. L., & Slovis, C. M. (2008). Arterial blood gas analysis: A 3-step approach to acid-base disorders. *The Journal of Respiratory Diseases, 29*(2), 74–82.

Jones, M. B. (2010). Pediatric care: Basic interpretation of metabolic acidosis. *Critical Care Nurse, 30*(5), 63–70.

Kovacic, V., Roguljic, L., & Kovacic, V. (2003). Metabolic acidosis of chronically hemodialyzed patients. *American Journal of Nephrology, 23*(3), 158–164.

Lian, J. X. (2010). Interpreting and using the arterial blood gas analysis. *Nursing Critical Care, 5*(3), 26–36.

Porth, C. M. (2007). *Essentials of pathophysiology* (2nd ed.). Philadelphia: Lippincott Williams & Wilkins.

Powers, F. (1999). The role of chloride in acid-base balance. *Journal of Intravenous Nursing, 22*(5), 286–290.

Reddy, P., & Mooradian, A. (2009). Clinical utility of anion gap in deciphering acid-base disorders. *International Journal of Clinical Practice, 63*(10), 1516–1525.

Smeltzer, S. C., & Bare, B. G. (2004). *Brunner & Suddarth's textbook of medical surgical nursing* (Vol. 1, 10th ed.). Philadelphia: Lippincott Williams & Wilkins.

M

Metabolic Alkalosis Severity   0620

Definition: Severity of signs and symptoms of increased blood pH and bicarbonate due to conditions that cause excessive acid loss or increased bicarbonate retention

OUTCOME TARGET RATING: Maintain at_____   Increase to_____

		Severe	Substantial	Moderate	Mild	None	
OUTCOME OVERALL RATING							
Indicators:							
062001	Increased blood plasma pH	1	2	3	4	5	NA
062002	Decreased serum hydrogen ions	1	2	3	4	5	NA
062003	Increased serum bicarbonate	1	2	3	4	5	NA
062004	Decreased serum potassium	1	2	3	4	5	NA
062005	Decreased ionized serum calcium	1	2	3	4	5	NA
062006	Decreased respiratory rate	1	2	3	4	5	NA

Continued

Metabolic Alkalosis Severity—cont'd

	Severe	Substantial	Moderate	Mild	None	
062007 Decreased respiratory rhythm	1	2	3	4	5	NA
062008 Atrial tachycardia	1	2	3	4	5	NA
062009 Premature ventricular contractions	1	2	3	4	5	NA
062010 Dizziness	1	2	3	4	5	NA
062011 Seizures	1	2	3	4	5	NA
062012 Confusion	1	2	3	4	5	NA
062013 Tingling of extremities	1	2	3	4	5	NA
062014 Hyperactive reflexes	1	2	3	4	5	NA
062015 Hypertonic muscles	1	2	3	4	5	NA

Domain-*Physiologic Health (II)*   **Class**-*Fluid & Electrolytes (G)*   *5th edition 2013*

OUTCOME CONTENT REFERENCES:

Appel, S. J., & Downs, C. A. (2007). Steady a disturbed equilibrium: Accurately interpret the acid-base balance of acutely ill patients. *Nursing Critical Care 2*(4), 45–53.

Clancy, J., & McVicar, A. (2007). Intermediate and long-term regulation of acid-base homeostasis. *British Journal of Nursing, 16*(17), 1076–1079.

Huang, L. H., & Priestley, M. A. (2008). Alkalosis, metabolic. In Emedicine. Retrieved March 9, 2009, from http://emedicine.medscape.com/article/906819-overview

Isenhour, J. L., & Slovis, C. M. (2008). Arterial blood gas analysis: A 3-step approach to acid-base disorders. *The Journal of Respiratory Diseases, 29*(2), 74–82.

Khanna, A., & Kurtzman, N. A. (2001). Metabolic alkalosis. *Respiratory Care, 46*(4), 354–365.

Kraut, J. A., & Madeas, N. E. (2001). Approach to patients with acid-base disorders. *Respiratory Care, 46*(4), 392–402.

Lian, J. X. (2010). Interpreting and using the arterial blood gas analysis. *Nursing Critical Care, 5*(3), 26–36.

Lynch, F. (2009). Arterial blood gas analysis: Implications for nursing. *Paediatric Nursing, 21*(1), 41–44.

Porth, C. M. (2007). *Essentials of pathophysiology* (2nd ed.). Philadelphia: Lippincott Williams & Wilkins.

Ruholl, L. (2006). Arterial blood gases: Analysis and nursing responses. *MEDSURG Nursing, 15*(6), 343–351.

Smeltzer, S. C., & Bare, B. G. (2004). *Brunner & Suddarth's textbook of medical surgical nursing* (Vol. 1, 10th ed.). Philadelphia: Lippincott Williams & Wilkins.

M

Mobility   0208

Definition: Ability to move purposefully in own environment independently with or without assistive device

OUTCOME TARGET RATING: Maintain at_____   Increase to_____

	Severely compromised	Substantially compromised	Moderately compromised	Mildly compromised	Not compromised	
OUTCOME OVERALL RATING	1	2	3	4	5	
Indicators:						
020801 Balance	1	2	3	4	5	NA
020809 Coordination	1	2	3	4	5	NA
020810 Gait	1	2	3	4	5	NA
020803 Muscle movement	1	2	3	4	5	NA
020804 Joint movement	1	2	3	4	5	NA
020802 Body positioning performance	1	2	3	4	5	NA
020805 Transfer performance	1	2	3	4	5	NA
020811 Running	1	2	3	4	5	NA
020812 Jumping	1	2	3	4	5	NA

Mobility—*cont'd*

		Severely compromised	Substantially compromised	Moderately compromised	Mildly compromised	Not compromised	
020813	Crawling	1	2	3	4	5	NA
020806	Walking	1	2	3	4	5	NA
020814	Moves with ease	1	2	3	4	5	NA

***Domain*-**Functional Health (I)   ***Class*-**Mobility (C)   *1st edition 1997; revised 2004*

OUTCOME CONTENT REFERENCES:

Maas, M. L., & Specht, J. P. (2001). Impaired physical mobility. In M. Maas, K. Buckwalter, M. Hardy, T. Tripp-Reimer, M. Titler, & J. Specht (Eds.), *Nursing care of older adults: Diagnoses, outcomes & interventions* (pp. 337–365). St. Louis: Mosby.

+Podsiadlo, D., & Richardson, S. (1991). The timed "Up & Go": A test of basic functional mobility for frail elderly persons. *Journal of American Geriatrics Society, 39*(2), 142–148.

Rukenstein, L. Z., Wieland, D., & Bernakei, R. (Eds.). (1995). *Geriatric assessment technology: The state of the art.* New York: Springer.

Mood Equilibrium   1204

Definition: Appropriate adjustment of prevailing emotional tone in response to circumstances

OUTCOME TARGET RATING: Maintain at_____   Increase to_____

		Never demonstrated	Rarely demonstrated	Sometimes demonstrated	Often demonstrated	Consistently demonstrated	
OUTCOME OVERALL RATING		1	2	3	4	5	
Indicators:							
120401	Exhibits affect that fits situation	1	2	3	4	5	NA
120402	Exhibits non-labile mood	1	2	3	4	5	NA
120403	Exhibits impulse control	1	2	3	4	5	NA
120404	Reports adequate sleep	1	2	3	4	5	NA
120405	Exhibits concentration	1	2	3	4	5	NA
120406	Speaks at moderate pace	1	2	3	4	5	NA
120423	Maintains personal grooming and hygiene	1	2	3	4	5	NA
120411	Wears appropriate clothing for situation	1	2	3	4	5	NA
120412	Maintains stable weight	1	2	3	4	5	NA
120413	Exhibits normal appetite	1	2	3	4	5	NA
120424	Reports compliance with medication regimen	1	2	3	4	5	NA
120425	Reports compliance with treatment regimen	1	2	3	4	5	NA
120415	Shows interest in surroundings	1	2	3	4	5	NA

Continued

M

Mood Equilibrium—cont'd

	Never demonstrated	Rarely demonstrated	Sometimes demonstrated	Often demonstrated	Consistently demonstrated	
120417 Exhibits stable energy level	1	2	3	4	5	NA
120418 Accomplishes daily tasks	1	2	3	4	5	NA

	Consistently demonstrated	Often demonstrated	Sometimes demonstrated	Rarely demonstrated	Never demonstrated	
120407 Flight of ideas	1	2	3	4	5	NA
120408 Grandiosity	1	2	3	4	5	NA
120409 Euphoria	1	2	3	4	5	NA
120416 Suicide ideation	1	2	3	4	5	NA
120420 Depression	1	2	3	4	5	NA
120421 Lethargy	1	2	3	4	5	NA
120422 Hyperactivity	1	2	3	4	5	NA

Domain-*Psychosocial Health (III)*   **Class**-*Psychological Well-Being (M)*   *1st edition 1997; revised 2004, 2008*

OUTCOME CONTENT REFERENCES:

George, L. K., Blazer, D. B., Hughes, D. C., & Fowler, N. (1989). Social support and the outcome of major depression. *British Journal of Psychiatry, 154*(4), 478–485.

Keitner, G. I., & Miller, I. W. (1990). Family functioning and major depression: An overview. *American Journal of Psychiatry, 147*(9), 1128–1137.

Maynard, C. (1993). Psychoeducational approach to depression in women. *Journal of Psychosocial Nursing and Mental Health Services, 31*(12), 9–14.

Maynard, C. K. (1993). Comparison of effectiveness of group interventions for depression in women. *Archives of Psychiatric Nursing, 7*(5), 277–283.

Piven, M. L., & Buckwalter, K. C. (2001). Depression. In M. Maas, K. Buckwalter, M. Hardy, T. Tripp-Reimer, M. Titler, & J. Specht (Eds.), *Nursing care of older adults: Diagnoses, outcomes & interventions* (pp. 521–542). St. Louis: Mosby.

Porth, C. M. (2002). *Pathophysiology: Concepts of altered health states* (6th ed.). Philadelphia: Lippincott Williams & Wilkins.

Stuart, G. W., & Laraia, M. T. (2001). *Principles and practice of psychiatric nursing* (7th ed.). St. Louis: Mosby.

+Underwood, B., & Froming, W. J. (1980). The Mood Survey: A personality measure of happy and sad moods. *Journal of Personality Assessment, 44*(4), 404–413.

Motivation   1209

Definition: Inner urge that moves or prompts an individual to positive action(s)

OUTCOME TARGET RATING: Maintain at_____   Increase to_____

	Never demonstrated	Rarely demonstrated	Sometimes demonstrated	Often demonstrated	Consistently demonstrated	
OUTCOME OVERALL RATING	1	2	3	4	5	
Indicators:						
120901 Plans for the future	1	2	3	4	5	NA
120902 Develops an action plan	1	2	3	4	5	NA
120903 Obtains resources as needed	1	2	3	4	5	NA
120904 Obtains support as needed	1	2	3	4	5	NA
120905 Self-initiates goal-directed behavior	1	2	3	4	5	NA
120906 Seeks new experiences	1	2	3	4	5	NA
120907 Maintains positive self-esteem	1	2	3	4	5	NA
120908 Welcomes opportunity to make contributions	1	2	3	4	5	NA
120916 Maintains flexibility	1	2	3	4	5	NA

Motivation—cont'd

		Never demonstrated	Rarely demonstrated	Sometimes demonstrated	Often demonstrated	Consistently demonstrated	
120910	Expresses belief in ability to perform action	1	2	3	4	5	NA
120911	Expresses that performance will lead to desired outcome	1	2	3	4	5	NA
120912	Completes tasks	1	2	3	4	5	NA
120913	Accepts responsibility for actions	1	2	3	4	5	NA
120917	Anticipates intrinsic reward	1	2	3	4	5	NA
120918	Anticipates extrinsic reward	1	2	3	4	5	NA
120915	Expresses intent to act	1	2	3	4	5	NA

Domain-*Psychosocial Health (III)*   **Class**-*Psychological Well-Being (M)*   *3rd edition 2004; revised 2008*

OUTCOME CONTENT REFERENCES:
Ellis, J. R., & Hartley, C. L. (1999). *Managing and coordinating nursing care* (3rd ed.). Philadelphia: Lippincott Williams & Wilkins.
Glickstein, J. (1990). Motivation in geriatric rehabilitation. *Focus on Geriatric Care and Rehabilitation, 3*(8), 1–3.
Mali, P. (1978). *Improving total productivity: MBO strategies for business, government, and not-for-profit organizations*. New York: Wiley.
Marriner-Tomey, A. (1996). *Guide to nursing management and leadership* (5th ed.). St. Louis: Mosby.
Resnick, B. (1998). Motivating older adults to perform functional activities. *Journal of Gerontological Nursing, 24*(11), 23–20.
Resnick, B., Zimmerman, S. I., Magaziner, J., & Adelman, A. (1998). Use of the apathy evaluation scale as a measure of motivation in elderly people. *Rehabilitation Nursing, 23*(3), 141–147.
Vroom, V. (1964). *Work and motivation*. New York: Wiley.

M

Mutilation Self-Restraint **1406**

Definition: Personal actions to refrain from intentional self-inflicted injury (non-lethal)

OUTCOME TARGET RATING: Maintain at_____   Increase to_____

		Never demonstrated	Rarely demonstrated	Sometimes demonstrated	Often demonstrated	Consistently demonstrated	
OUTCOME OVERALL RATING		1	2	3	4	5	
Indicators:							
140601	Refrains from gathering means for self-injury	1	2	3	4	5	NA
140608	Obtains assistance as needed	1	2	3	4	5	NA
140604	Upholds contract to not harm self	1	2	3	4	5	NA
140605	Maintains self-control without supervision	1	2	3	4	5	NA
140606	Refrains from injuring self	1	2	3	4	5	NA
140609	Uses available support groups	1	2	3	4	5	NA
140610	Uses medication as prescribed	1	2	3	4	5	NA
140611	Participates in mental health promotion activities	1	2	3	4	5	NA
140612	Follows treatment regimen	1	2	3	4	5	NA
140613	Uses effective coping strategies	1	2	3	4	5	NA

Domain-*Psychosocial Health (III)*   **Class**-*Self-Control (O)*   *1st edition 1997; revised 2004, 2008, 2013*

Continued

OUTCOME CONTENT REFERENCES:

Burrow, S. (1994). Nursing management of self-mutilation. *British Journal of Nursing, 3*(8), 382–386.

Coler, M. S., & Vincent, K. G. (1995). Psychiatric mental health nursing. In K. V. Gettrust (Series Ed.), *Plans of care for specialty practice.* Albany, NY: Delmar.

Faye, P. (1995). Addictive characteristics of the behavior of self-mutilation. *Journal of Psychosocial Nursing and Mental Health Services, 33*(2), 19–22.

+Rojahn, J., Polster, L. M., Mulick, J. A., & Wisniewski, J. J. (1989). Reliability of the Behavior Problems Inventory. *Journal of the Multihandicapped Person, 2*(4), 283–293.

Stuart, G. W., & Laraia, M. T. (2001). *Principles and practice of psychiatric nursing* (7th ed.). St. Louis: Mosby.

Valente, S. M. (1991). Deliberate self-injury management in a psychiatric setting. *Journal of Psychosocial Nursing and Mental Health Services, 29*(12), 19–25.

Winchel, R. M. (1991). Self-injurious behavior. A review of the behavior and biology of self-mutilation. *American Journal of Psychiatry, 148*(3), 306–17.

M

Nausea & Vomiting Control 1618

Definition: Personal actions to control nausea, retching, and vomiting symptoms

OUTCOME TARGET RATING: Maintain at_____ Increase to_____

	Never demonstrated	Rarely demonstrated	Sometimes demonstrated	Often demonstrated	Consistently demonstrated	
OUTCOME OVERALL RATING	1	2	3	4	5	
Indicators:						
161801 Recognizes onset of nausea	1	2	3	4	5	NA
161802 Describes causal factors	1	2	3	4	5	NA
161803 Recognizes precipitating stimuli	1	2	3	4	5	NA
161804 Uses diary to monitor symptoms over time	1	2	3	4	5	NA
161805 Uses preventive measures	1	2	3	4	5	NA
161806 Avoids causal factors when possible	1	2	3	4	5	NA
161807 Avoids disagreeable odors	1	2	3	4	5	NA
161808 Uses antiemetic medication as recommended	1	2	3	4	5	NA
161809 Reports failure of antiemetic treatment	1	2	3	4	5	NA
161810 Reports bothersome side effects from antiemetics	1	2	3	4	5	NA
161811 Reports uncontrolled symptoms to health professional	1	2	3	4	5	NA
161812 Reports nausea, retching, and vomiting controlled	1	2	3	4	5	NA

Domain-Health Knowledge & Behavior (IV)   *Class*-Health Behavior (Q)   3rd edition 2004

N

OUTCOME CONTENT REFERENCES:

Brown, J. K., & Hogan, C. M. (1990). Chemotherapy. In S. L. Groenwald, M. H. Frogge, M. Goodman, & C. H. Yarbro (Eds.), *Cancer nursing: Principles and practice* (pp. 230–283). Sudbury, MA: Jones and Bartlett.

Engstrom, C., Hernandez, I., Haywood, J., & Lilenbaum, R. (1999). The efficacy and cost effectiveness of new antiemetic guidelines. *Oncology Nursing Forum*, 26(9), 1453–1458.

Houston, D. (1997). Supportive therapies for cancer chemotherapy patients and the role of the oncology nurse. *Cancer Nursing*, 20(6), 409–413.

Nolte, J. J., Berkery, R., Pizzo, B., Baltzer, L., Grossano, D., Lucarelli, C. D., & Kris, M. G. (1998). Assuring the optimal use of serotonin antagonist antiemetics: The process for development and implementation of institutional antiemetic guidelines at Memorial Sloan-Kettering Cancer Center. *Journal of Clinical Oncology*, 16(2), 771–778.

Rhodes, V. A., McDaniel, R. W., Simms, S. G., & Johnson, M. (1995). Nurses' perceptions of antiemetic effectiveness. *Oncology Nursing Forum*, 22(8), 1243–1252.

Wickham, R. (1999). Nausea and vomiting. In C. H. Yarbro, M. H. Frogge, & M. Goodman (Eds.), *Cancer symptom management* (pp. 228–263). Sudbury, MA: Jones and Bartlett.

Nausea & Vomiting: Disruptive Effects 2106

Definition: Severity of observed or reported disruptive effects of chronic nausea, retching, and vomiting on daily functioning

OUTCOME TARGET RATING: Maintain at_____ Increase to_____

OUTCOME OVERALL RATING	Severe 1	Substantial 2	Moderate 3	Mild 4	None 5	
Indicators:						
210601 Decreased fluid intake	1	2	3	4	5	NA
210602 Decreased food intake	1	2	3	4	5	NA
210603 Decreased urine output	1	2	3	4	5	NA
210604 Altered fluid balance	1	2	3	4	5	NA
210605 Altered serum electrolytes	1	2	3	4	5	NA
210606 Altered acid/base balance	1	2	3	4	5	NA
210625 Loss of appetite	1	2	3	4	5	NA
210626 Intolerance of odors	1	2	3	4	5	NA
210607 Altered nutritional status	1	2	3	4	5	NA
210608 Weight loss	1	2	3	4	5	NA
210609 Malaise	1	2	3	4	5	NA
210610 Lethargy	1	2	3	4	5	NA
210611 Intolerance of movement	1	2	3	4	5	NA
210612 Impaired physical activity	1	2	3	4	5	NA
210613 Interrupted sleep	1	2	3	4	5	NA
210614 Withdrawal from interpersonal relationships	1	2	3	4	5	NA
210615 Impaired role performance	1	2	3	4	5	NA
210616 Impaired work performance	1	2	3	4	5	NA
210617 Interference with leisure activities	1	2	3	4	5	NA
210618 Interference with activities of daily living	1	2	3	4	5	NA
210619 Anxiety	1	2	3	4	5	NA
210620 Depression	1	2	3	4	5	NA
210621 Emotional stress	1	2	3	4	5	NA
210622 Helplessness	1	2	3	4	5	NA
210623 Side effects from antiemetic medication	1	2	3	4	5	NA
210624 Treatment delays due to symptom severity	1	2	3	4	5	NA

Domain-Perceived Health (V) *Class*-Symptom Status (V) *3rd edition 2004; revised 2013*

OUTCOME CONTENT REFERENCES:

Cotanch, P. H. (1988). Measuring nausea and vomiting. In M. Frank-Stromborg (Ed.), *Instruments for clinical nursing research* (pp. 313–321). Norwalk, CT: Appleton & Lange.

Engelking, C., Wickham, R., & Iwamoto, R. (1996). Cancer-related gastrointestinal symptoms: Dilemmas in assessment and management. *Developments in Supportive Cancer Care, 1*(1), 3–10.

Ezzone, S., Baker, C., Rosselet, R., & Terepka, E. (1998). Music as an adjunct to antiemetic therapy. *Oncology Nursing Forum, 25*(9), 1551–1556.

Low, K. G. (1996). Nausea and vomiting in pregnancy: A review of the research. *Journal of Gender, Culture, and Health, 1*(3), 151–172.

Rhodes, V. A., & McDaniel, R. W. (1997). Measuring nausea, vomiting, and retching. In M. Frank-Stromborg & S. J. Olsen (Eds.), *Instruments for clinical health-care research* (2nd ed., pp. 509–517). Sudbury, MA: Jones and Bartlett.

Wickham, R. (1999). Nausea and vomiting. In C. H. Yarbro, M. H. Frogge, & M. Goodman (Eds.), *Cancer symptom management* (pp. 228–263). Sudbury, MA: Jones and Bartlett.

Nausea & Vomiting Severity 2107

Definition: Severity of signs and symptoms of nausea, retching, and vomiting

OUTCOME TARGET RATING: Maintain at_____   Increase to_____

OUTCOME OVERALL RATING	Severe 1	Substantial 2	Moderate 3	Mild 4	None 5	
Indicators:						
210701 Frequency of nausea	1	2	3	4	5	NA
210702 Intensity of nausea	1	2	3	4	5	NA
210703 Distress of nausea	1	2	3	4	5	NA
210704 Frequency of retching	1	2	3	4	5	NA
210705 Intensity of retching	1	2	3	4	5	NA
210706 Distress of retching	1	2	3	4	5	NA
210707 Frequency of vomiting	1	2	3	4	5	NA
210708 Intensity of vomiting	1	2	3	4	5	NA
210709 Distress of vomiting	1	2	3	4	5	NA
210710 Excessive secretion of saliva	1	2	3	4	5	NA
210711 Alteration in taste	1	2	3	4	5	NA
210712 Intolerance of odors	1	2	3	4	5	NA
210713 Weight loss	1	2	3	4	5	NA
210714 Heartburn	1	2	3	4	5	NA
210715 Gastric pain	1	2	3	4	5	NA
210716 Projectile vomiting	1	2	3	4	5	NA
210717 Blood in emesis	1	2	3	4	5	NA
210718 Coffee ground emesis	1	2	3	4	5	NA
210719 Fecal odor of emesis	1	2	3	4	5	NA
210720 Electrolyte imbalance	1	2	3	4	5	NA

Duration of nausea: _____(hours) _____(days) _____(months)
Amount of emesis: _____(cc)

***Domain**-Perceived Health (V)*   ***Class**-Symptom Status (V)*   *3rd edition 2004; revised 2013*

N

OUTCOME CONTENT REFERENCES:
Cotanch, P. H. (1988). Measuring nausea and vomiting. In M. Frank-Stromborg (Ed.), *Instruments for clinical nursing research* (pp. 313–321). Norwalk, CT: Appleton & Lange.
Engstrom, C., Hernandez, I., Haywood, J., & Lilenbaum, R. (1999). The efficacy and cost effectiveness of new antiemetic guidelines. *Oncology Nursing Forum, 26*(9), 1453–1458.
Rhodes, V. A., & McDaniel, R. W. (1997). Measuring nausea, vomiting, and retching. In M. Frank-Stromborg & S. J. Olsen (Eds.), *Instruments for clinical health-care research* (2nd ed., pp. 509–517). Sudbury, MA: Jones and Bartlett.
Rhodes, V. A., & McDaniel, R. W. (1999). The index of nausea, vomiting, and retching: A new format of the index of nausea and vomiting. *Oncology Nursing Forum, 26*(5), 889–894.
Wickham, R. (1999). Nausea and vomiting. In C. H. Yarbro, M. H. Frogge, & M. Goodman (Eds.), *Cancer symptom management* (pp. 228–263). Sudbury, MA: Jones and Bartlett.

Neglect Cessation 2513

Definition: Evidence that the victim is no longer receiving substandard care

OUTCOME TARGET RATING: Maintain at_____ Increase to_____

	None	Limited	Moderate	Substantial	Extensive	
OUTCOME OVERALL RATING	1	2	3	4	5	
Indicators:						
251301 Evidence that physical neglect has ceased	1	2	3	4	5	NA
251302 Evidence that emotional neglect has ceased	1	2	3	4	5	NA
251303 Evidence that financial neglect has ceased	1	2	3	4	5	NA
251304 Evidence that spiritual neglect has ceased	1	2	3	4	5	NA
251305 Evidence that health care neglect has ceased	1	2	3	4	5	NA

Domain-*Family Health (VI)* **Class**-*Family Member Health Status (Z)* 3rd edition 2004

OUTCOME CONTENT REFERENCES:

Aber, J. L., Allen, J. P., Carlson, V., & Cicchetti, D. (1990). The effects of maltreatment on development during early childhood: Recent studies and their theoretical, clinical, and policy implications. In D. Cicchetti & V. Carlson (Eds.), *Child maltreatment: Theory and research on the causes and consequences of child abuse and neglect* (pp. 579–619). New York: Cambridge University Press.

Cicchetti, D., & Carlson, V. (Eds.). (1989). *Child maltreatment: Theory and research on the causes and consequences of child abuse and neglect.* New York: Cambridge University Press.

Cowen, P. S. (2001). Elder mistreatment. In M. Maas, K. Buckwalter, M. Hardy, T. Tripp-Reimer, M. Titler, & J. Specht (Eds.), *Nursing care of older adults: Diagnoses, outcomes & interventions* (pp. 93–114). St. Louis: Mosby.

Fulmer, T., & Ashley, J. (1989). Clinical indicators of elder neglect. *Applied Nursing Research, 2*(4), 161–167.

Hudson, M. F., & Johnson, T. F. (1986). Elder neglect and abuse: A review of the literature [Monograph]. *Annual Review of Nursing Research, 6,* 81–134.

Lobo, M. L., Barnard, K. E., & Coombs, J. B. (1992). Failure to thrive: A parent-infant interaction perspective. *Journal of Pediatric Nursing, 7*(4), 251–261.

Olds, D. L., Henderson, C. R., Chamberlin, R., & Tatelbaum, R. (1986). Preventing child abuse and neglect: A randomized trial of nurse home visitation. *Pediatrics, 78*(1), 65–78.

Silverman, J., & Hudson, M. F. (2000). Elder mistreatment: A guide for medical professionals. *North Carolina Medical Journal, 61*(5), 291–296.

Weinman, M. L., Schreiber, N. B., & Robinson, M. (1992). Adolescent mothers: Were there any gains in a parent education program? *Family and Community Health, 15*(3), 1–10.

Young, L. (1981). *Physical child neglect.* Chicago: The National Committee for Prevention of Child Abuse.

N

Neglect Recovery 2512

Definition: Extent of physical, emotional, and spiritual healing following the cessation of substandard care

OUTCOME TARGET RATING: Maintain at_____ Increase to_____

	None	Limited	Moderate	Substantial	Extensive	
OUTCOME OVERALL RATING	1	2	3	4	5	
Indicators:						
251201 Maintenance of personal hygiene	1	2	3	4	5	NA
251205 Appropriate clothing for weather	1	2	3	4	5	NA
251206 Cleanliness of living environment	1	2	3	4	5	NA
251207 Safety of living environment	1	2	3	4	5	NA

Neglect Recovery—cont'd

		None	Limited	Moderate	Substantial	Extensive	
251209	Provision of supervision required	1	2	3	4	5	NA
251210	Demonstration of interest in life	1	2	3	4	5	NA
251211	Expressions of pride in self	1	2	3	4	5	NA
251212	Expressions of hope	1	2	3	4	5	NA
251213	Timely meeting of emotional needs	1	2	3	4	5	NA
251214	Provision of appropriate health care	1	2	3	4	5	NA
251215	Provision of recommended diet	1	2	3	4	5	NA
251216	Provision of medication regimen	1	2	3	4	5	NA
251217	Use of appropriate equipment or appliance	1	2	3	4	5	NA
251220	Normal development	1	2	3	4	5	NA
251218	Normal growth	1	2	3	4	5	NA
251219	Provision of cognitive stimulation	1	2	3	4	5	NA
251221	Expectations of responsibilities reasonable for age	1	2	3	4	5	NA
251224	Consistency of behavior with social norms	1	2	3	4	5	NA

		Extensive	Substantial	Moderate	Limited	None	
251202	Hunger	1	2	3	4	5	NA
251208	Skin breakdown	1	2	3	4	5	NA
251223	Substance abuse	1	2	3	4	5	NA
251227	Fatigue	1	2	3	4	5	NA
251228	Malnutrition	1	2	3	4	5	NA
251229	Dehydration	1	2	3	4	5	NA
251230	Inappropriate attention-seeking behavior	1	2	3	4	5	NA

Domain-Family Health (VI)   **Class**-Family Member Health Status (Z)   *1st edition 1997; revised 2004, 2008*

N

OUTCOME CONTENT REFERENCES:

Aber, J. L., Allen, J. P., Carlson, V., & Cicchetti, D. (1990). The effects of maltreatment on development during early childhood: Recent studies and their theoretical, clinical, and policy implications. In D. Cicchetti & V. Carlson (Eds.), *Child maltreatment: Theory and research on the causes and consequences of child abuse and neglect* (pp. 579–619). New York: Cambridge University Press.

Cicchetti, D., & Carlson, V. (Eds.). (1989). *Child maltreatment: Theory and research on the causes and consequences of child abuse and neglect.* New York: Cambridge University Press.

Cowen, P. S. (2001). Elder mistreatment. In M. Maas, K. Buckwalter, M. Hardy, T. Tripp-Reimer, M. Titler, & J. Specht (Eds.), *Nursing care of older adults: Diagnoses, outcomes & interventions* (pp. 93–114). St. Louis: Mosby.

Fulmer, T., & Ashley, J. (1989). Clinical indicators of elder neglect. *Applied Nursing Research, 2*(4), 161–167.

Fulmer, T., & Paveza, G. (1998). Neglect in the elderly patient. *Nursing Clinics of North America, 33*(3), 457–466.

Hudson, M. F., & Johnson, T. F. (1986). Elder neglect and abuse: A review of the literature [Monograph]. *Annual Review of Nursing Research, 6,* 81–134.

Lobo, M. L., Barnard, K. E., & Coombs, J. B. (1992). Failure to thrive: A parent-infant interaction perspective. *Journal of Pediatric Nursing, 7*(4), 251–261.

Olds, D. L., Henderson, C. R., Chamberlin, R., & Tatelbaum, R. (1986). Preventing child abuse and neglect: A randomized trial of nurse home visitation. *Pediatrics, 78*(1), 65–78.

Polansky, N. A., Halley, C., & Polansky, N. F. (1977). *Profile of neglect: A survey of the state of knowledge.* Washington, DC: U.S. Department of Health, Education, and Welfare.

Weinman, M. L., Schreiber, N. B., & Robinson, M. (1992). Adolescent mothers: Were there any gains in a parent education program? *Family and Community Health, 15*(3), 1–10.

Young, L. (1981). *Physical child neglect.* Chicago: The National Committee for Prevention of Child Abuse.

Neurological Status 0909

Definition: Ability of the peripheral and central nervous systems to receive, process, and respond to internal and external stimuli

OUTCOME TARGET RATING: Maintain at_____ Increase to_____

OUTCOME OVERALL RATING		Severely compromised 1	Substantially compromised 2	Moderately compromised 3	Mildly compromised 4	Not compromised 5	
Indicators:							
090901	Consciousness	1	2	3	4	5	NA
090902	Central motor control	1	2	3	4	5	NA
090903	Cranial sensory and motor function	1	2	3	4	5	NA
090904	Spinal sensory and motor function	1	2	3	4	5	NA
090905	Autonomic function	1	2	3	4	5	NA
090906	Intracranial pressure	1	2	3	4	5	NA
090907	Communication appropriate to situation	1	2	3	4	5	NA
090908	Pupil size	1	2	3	4	5	NA
090909	Pupil reactivity	1	2	3	4	5	NA
090910	Eye movement pattern	1	2	3	4	5	NA
090911	Breathing pattern	1	2	3	4	5	NA
090913	Sleep-rest pattern	1	2	3	4	5	NA
090917	Blood pressure	1	2	3	4	5	NA
090918	Pulse pressure	1	2	3	4	5	NA
090919	Respiratory rate	1	2	3	4	5	NA
090920	Hyperthermia	1	2	3	4	5	NA
090921	Apical heart rate	1	2	3	4	5	NA
090922	Radial pulse rate	1	2	3	4	5	NA
090923	Cognitive orientation	1	2	3	4	5	NA
090924	Cognitive status	1	2	3	4	5	NA

		Severe	Substantial	Moderate	Mild	None	
090914	Seizure activity	1	2	3	4	5	NA
090915	Headaches	1	2	3	4	5	NA

Domain-*Physiologic Health (II)* **Class**-*Neurocognitive (J)* *1st edition 1997; revised 2004*

OUTCOME CONTENT REFERENCES:
American Nurses' Association Council on Medical-Surgical Nursing Practice and American Association of Neuroscience Nurses. (1986). *Neuroscience nursing practice: Process and outcome criteria for selected diagnoses.* Washington, DC: U.S. Government Printing Office.
Hickey, J. V. (2002). *The clinical practice of neurological and neurosurgical nursing* (5th ed.). Philadelphia: Lippincott Williams & Wilkins.
Mitchell, P. H., Hodges, L. C., Muwaswes, M., & Walleck, C. A. (Eds.). (1988). *AANN's neuroscience nursing: Phenomena and practice.* Norwalk, CT: Appleton & Lange.
Riess, P. C. (1995). *Validity and reliability of the Riess Intracranial Aneurysm Assessment Tool and the Glasgow Coma Scale in the aneurysm population.* Master's thesis. Iowa City, IA: The University of Iowa.
Smeltzer, S. C., & Bare, B. G. (Eds.). (2003). *Brunner and Suddarth's textbook of medical-surgical nursing* (10th ed.). Philadelphia: Lippincott Williams & Wilkins.
+Teasdale, G., & Jennett, B. (1974). Assessment of coma and impaired consciousness: A practical scale. *Lancet, 2*(7872), 81–84.

N

Neurological Status: Autonomic 0910

Definition: Ability of the autonomic nervous system to coordinate visceral and homeostatic functions

OUTCOME TARGET RATING: Maintain at_____   Increase to_____

OUTCOME OVERALL RATING	Severely compromised 1	Substantially compromised 2	Moderately compromised 3	Mildly compromised 4	Not compromised 5	
Indicators:						
091001 Apical heart rate	1	2	3	4	5	NA
091020 Radial pulse rate	1	2	3	4	5	NA
091002 Systolic blood pressure	1	2	3	4	5	NA
091003 Diastolic blood pressure	1	2	3	4	5	NA
091004 Cardiac pump effectiveness	1	2	3	4	5	NA
091005 Vasodilatation response	1	2	3	4	5	NA
091006 Vasoconstriction response	1	2	3	4	5	NA
091007 Perspiration response pattern	1	2	3	4	5	NA
091008 Goose bumps response pattern	1	2	3	4	5	NA
091009 Bowel elimination pattern	1	2	3	4	5	NA
091010 Intestinal motility	1	2	3	4	5	NA
091011 Urinary elimination pattern	1	2	3	4	5	NA
091021 Pupil reactivity	1	2	3	4	5	NA
091013 Thermoregulation	1	2	3	4	5	NA
091014 Peripheral tissue perfusion	1	2	3	4	5	NA
091015 Sexual organ response	1	2	3	4	5	NA

	Severe	Substantial	Moderate	Mild	None	
091016 Bronchospasms	1	2	3	4	5	NA
091017 Intestinal spasms	1	2	3	4	5	NA
091018 Bladder spasms	1	2	3	4	5	NA
091022 Headaches	1	2	3	4	5	NA
091023 Dilated pupils	1	2	3	4	5	NA
091024 Constricted pupils	1	2	3	4	5	NA
091025 Hyperthermia	1	2	3	4	5	NA
091026 Dysreflexia	1	2	3	4	5	NA

Domain-*Physiologic Health (II)*   **Class**-*Neurocognitive (J)*   *1st edition 1997; revised 2004*

N

OUTCOME CONTENT REFERENCES:

McCance, K. L., & Huether, S. E. (2002). *Pathophysiology: The biologic basis for disease in adults and children* (4th ed.). St. Louis: Mosby.

Smeltzer, S. C., & Bare, B. G. (Eds.). (2003). *Brunner and Suddarth's textbook of medical-surgical nursing* (10th ed.). Philadelphia: Lippincott Williams & Wilkins.

Neurological Status: Central Motor Control 0911

Definition: Ability of the central nervous system to coordinate skeletal muscle activity for body movement

OUTCOME TARGET RATING: Maintain at_____ Increase to_____

	Severely compromised	Substantially compromised	Moderately compromised	Mildly compromised	Not compromised	
OUTCOME OVERALL RATING	1	2	3	4	5	
Indicators:						
091101	Balance	1	2	3	4	5	NA
091103	Maintenance of posture	1	2	3	4	5	NA
091104	Infantile reflexes (automatisms)	1	2	3	4	5	NA
091105	Babinski's reflex	1	2	3	4	5	NA
091106	Deep tendon reflexes	1	2	3	4	5	NA
091112	Purposeful movement on command	1	2	3	4	5	NA

		Severe	Substantial	Moderate	Mild	None	
091113	Gait abnormalities	1	2	3	4	5	NA
091107	Spasticity	1	2	3	4	5	NA
091108	Involuntary movements	1	2	3	4	5	NA
091109	Nystagmus	1	2	3	4	5	NA
091110	Seizure activity	1	2	3	4	5	NA

Domain-*Physiologic Health (II)* **Class**-*Neurocognitive (J)* *1st edition 1997; revised 2004*

OUTCOME CONTENT REFERENCES:

American Nurses' Association Council on Medical-Surgical Nursing Practice and American Association of Neuroscience Nurses. (1986). *Neuroscience nursing practice: Process and outcome criteria for selected diagnoses.* Washington, DC: U.S. Government Printing Office.
Bickley, L. (2002). *Bates' guide to physical examination and history taking* (8th ed.). Philadelphia: Lippincott Williams & Wilkins.
Hickey, J. V. (2002). *The clinical practice of neurological and neurosurgical nursing* (5th ed.). Philadelphia: Lippincott Williams & Wilkins.
Mitchell, P. H., Hodges, L. C., Muwaswes, M., & Walleck, C. A. (Eds.). (1988). *AANN's neuroscience nursing: Phenomena and practice.* Norwalk, CT: Appleton & Lange.
Smeltzer, S. C., & Bare, B. G. (Eds.). (2003). *Brunner and Suddarth's textbook of medical-surgical nursing* (10th ed.). Philadelphia: Lippincott Williams & Wilkins.

N

Neurological Status: Consciousness 0912

Definition: Arousal, orientation, and attention to the environment

OUTCOME TARGET RATING: Maintain at_____ Increase to_____

	Severely compromised	Substantially compromised	Moderately compromised	Mildly compromised	Not compromised	
OUTCOME OVERALL RATING	1	2	3	4	5	
Indicators:						
091201	Opens eyes to external stimuli	1	2	3	4	5	NA
091202	Cognitive orientation	1	2	3	4	5	NA
091203	Communication appropriate to situation	1	2	3	4	5	NA
091204	Obeys commands	1	2	3	4	5	NA
091205	Motor responses to noxious stimuli	1	2	3	4	5	NA
091206	Attends to environmental stimuli	1	2	3	4	5	NA

Neurological Status: Consciousness—cont'd

	Severe	Substantial	Moderate	Mild	None	
091207 Seizure activity	1	2	3	4	5	NA
091209 Abnormal flexion	1	2	3	4	5	NA
091210 Abnormal extension	1	2	3	4	5	NA
091211 Stupor	1	2	3	4	5	NA
091212 Trance state	1	2	3	4	5	NA
091213 Delirium	1	2	3	4	5	NA
091214 Coma	1	2	3	4	5	NA

Glasgow Coma Scale score: _____

Domain-*Physiologic Health (II)*   **Class**-*Neurocognitive (J)*   *1st edition 1997; revised 2004, 2008*

OUTCOME CONTENT REFERENCES:
American Nurses' Association Council on Medical-Surgical Nursing Practice and American Association of Neuroscience Nurses. (1986). *Neuroscience nursing practice: Process and outcome criteria for selected diagnoses.* Washington, DC: U.S. Government Printing Office.
Hickey, J. V. (2002). *The clinical practice of neurological and neurosurgical nursing* (5th ed.). Philadelphia: Lippincott Williams & Wilkins.
Mitchell, P. H., Hodges, L. C., Muwaswes, M., & Walleck, C. A. (Eds.). (1988). *AANN's neuroscience nursing: Phenomena and practice.* Norwalk, CT: Appleton & Lange.
Riess, P. C. (1995). *Validity and reliability of the Riess Intracranial Aneurysm Assessment Tool and the Glasgow Coma Scale in the aneurysm population.* Master's thesis. Iowa City, IA: The University of Iowa.
Smeltzer, S. C., & Bare, B. G. (Eds.). (2003). *Brunner and Suddarth's textbook of medical-surgical nursing* (10th ed.). Philadelphia: Lippincott Williams & Wilkins.

Neurological Status: Cranial Sensory/Motor Function   0913

N

Definition: Ability of the cranial nerves to convey sensory and motor impulses

OUTCOME TARGET RATING: Maintain at_____   Increase to_____

	Severely compromised	Substantially compromised	Moderately compromised	Mildly compromised	Not compromised	
OUTCOME OVERALL RATING	1	2	3	4	5	
Indicators:						
091301 Olfaction	1	2	3	4	5	NA
091302 Vision	1	2	3	4	5	NA
091303 Corneal reflex	1	2	3	4	5	NA
091304 Taste	1	2	3	4	5	NA
091305 Hearing	1	2	3	4	5	NA
091317 Speech	1	2	3	4	5	NA
091306 Facial sensation	1	2	3	4	5	NA
091307 Facial muscle movement	1	2	3	4	5	NA
091318 Facial symmetry	1	2	3	4	5	NA
091319 Bilateral muscle strength	1	2	3	4	5	NA
091308 Swallowing	1	2	3	4	5	NA
091309 Gag reflex	1	2	3	4	5	NA
091310 Tongue movement	1	2	3	4	5	NA
091312 Purposeful head movement	1	2	3	4	5	NA
091320 Purposeful shoulder movement	1	2	3	4	5	NA

Continued

Neurological Status: Cranial Sensory/Motor Function—cont'd

	Severe	Substantial	Moderate	Mild	None	
091314 Dizziness	1	2	3	4	5	NA
091315 Pronator drift	1	2	3	4	5	NA
091321 Involuntary head movement	1	2	3	4	5	NA
091322 Involuntary facial movement	1	2	3	4	5	NA
091323 Tics	1	2	3	4	5	NA
091324 Hoarseness	1	2	3	4	5	NA
091325 Nasal tone to voice	1	2	3	4	5	NA
091326 Unilateral facial paralysis	1	2	3	4	5	NA

Domain-*Physiologic Health (II)* **Class**-*Neurocognitive (J)* *1st edition 1997; revised 2004*

OUTCOME CONTENT REFERENCES:

Bickley, L. (2002). *Bates' guide to physical examination and history taking* (8th ed.). Philadelphia: Lippincott Williams & Wilkins.

McCance, K. L., & Huether, S. E. (2002). *Pathophysiology: The biologic basis for disease in adults and children* (4th ed.). St. Louis: Mosby.

Riess, P. C. (1995). *Validity and reliability of the Riess Intracranial Aneurysm Assessment Tool and the Glasgow Coma Scale in the aneurysm population.* Master's thesis. Iowa City, IA: The University of Iowa.

Smeltzer, S. C., & Bare, B. G. (Eds.). (2003). *Brunner and Suddarth's textbook of medical-surgical nursing* (10th ed.). Philadelphia: Lippincott Williams & Wilkins.

Neurological Status: Peripheral   0917

Definition: Ability of the peripheral nervous system to transmit impulses to and from the central nervous system

OUTCOME TARGET RATING: Maintain at_____   Increase to_____

	Severely compromised	Substantially compromised	Moderately compromised	Mildly compromised	Not compromised	
OUTCOME OVERALL RATING	1	2	3	4	5	
Indicators:						
091701 Sensation in upper right extremity	1	2	3	4	5	NA
091702 Sensation in upper left extremity	1	2	3	4	5	NA
091703 Sensation in lower right extremity	1	2	3	4	5	NA
091704 Sensation in lower left extremity	1	2	3	4	5	NA
091705 Sensation equal bilaterally	1	2	3	4	5	NA
091706 Motor function in upper right extremity	1	2	3	4	5	NA
091707 Motor function in upper left extremity	1	2	3	4	5	NA
091708 Motor function in lower right extremity	1	2	3	4	5	NA
091709 Motor function in lower left extremity	1	2	3	4	5	NA
091710 Motor function equal bilaterally	1	2	3	4	5	NA
091711 Skin color in upper right extremity	1	2	3	4	5	NA
091712 Skin color in upper left extremity	1	2	3	4	5	NA

Neurological Status: Peripheral—cont'd

		Severely compromised	Substantially compromised	Moderately compromised	Mildly compromised	Not compromised	
091713	Skin color in lower right extremity	1	2	3	4	5	NA
091714	Skin color in lower left extremity	1	2	3	4	5	NA
091715	Proprioception in upper right extremity	1	2	3	4	5	NA
091716	Proprioception in upper left extremity	1	2	3	4	5	NA
091717	Proprioception in lower right extremity	1	2	3	4	5	NA
091718	Proprioception in lower left extremity	1	2	3	4	5	NA
091719	Proprioception equal bilaterally	1	2	3	4	5	NA
091720	Hot/cold discrimination in upper right extremity	1	2	3	4	5	NA
091721	Hot/cold discrimination in upper left extremity	1	2	3	4	5	NA
091722	Hot/cold discrimination in lower right extremity	1	2	3	4	5	NA
091723	Hot/cold discrimination in lower left extremity	1	2	3	4	5	NA
091724	Hot/cold discrimination equal bilaterally	1	2	3	4	5	NA
091725	Muscle tone in upper right extremity	1	2	3	4	5	NA
091726	Muscle tone in upper left extremity	1	2	3	4	5	NA
091727	Muscle tone in lower right extremity	1	2	3	4	5	NA
091728	Muscle tone in lower left extremity	1	2	3	4	5	NA
091729	Muscle tone equal bilaterally	1	2	3	4	5	NA

		Severe	Substantial	Moderate	Mild	None	
091730	Hyperesthesia in upper right extremity	1	2	3	4	5	NA
091731	Hyperesthesia in upper left extremity	1	2	3	4	5	NA
091732	Hyperesthesia in lower right extremity	1	2	3	4	5	NA
091733	Hyperesthesia in lower left extremity	1	2	3	4	5	NA
091734	Hypoesthesia in upper right extremity	1	2	3	4	5	NA
091735	Hypoesthesia in upper left extremity	1	2	3	4	5	NA
091736	Hypoesthesia in lower right extremity	1	2	3	4	5	NA
091737	Hypoesthesia in lower left extremity	1	2	3	4	5	NA
091738	Pain in upper right extremity	1	2	3	4	5	NA
091739	Pain in upper left extremity	1	2	3	4	5	NA

Continued

N

Neurological Status: Peripheral—*cont'd*

	Severely compromised	Substantially compromised	Moderately compromised	Mildly compromised	Not compromised	
091740	Pain in lower right extremity	1	2	3	4	5	NA
091741	Pain in lower left extremity	1	2	3	4	5	NA
091742	Paresthesia in upper right extremity	1	2	3	4	5	NA
091743	Paresthesia in upper left extremity	1	2	3	4	5	NA
091744	Paresthesia in lower right extremity	1	2	3	4	5	NA
091745	Paresthesia in lower left extremity	1	2	3	4	5	NA

Domain-*Physiologic Health (II)*   **Class**-*Neurocognitive (J)*   *4th edition 2008*

OUTCOME CONTENT REFERENCES:
Huether, S. E., & McCance, K. L. (2000). *Understanding pathophysiology* (2nd ed., p. 344). St Louis: Mosby.
Kidd, P. S., & Wagner, K. D. (2001). *High acuity nursing* (3rd ed., pp. 638–639). Upper Saddle River, NJ: Prentice Hall.
Swearingen, P. L. (Ed.). (2003). *Manual of medical-surgical nursing care: Nursing interventions & collaborative management* (5th ed., p. 207). St. Louis: Mosby.

Neurological Status: Spinal Sensory/Motor Function

0914

Definition: Ability of the spinal nerves to convey sensory and motor impulses

OUTCOME TARGET RATING: Maintain at_____   Increase to_____

	Severely compromised	Substantially compromised	Moderately compromised	Mildly compromised	Not compromised	
OUTCOME OVERALL RATING	1	2	3	4	5	

Indicators:

		Severely compromised	Substantially compromised	Moderately compromised	Mildly compromised	Not compromised	
091401	Head and shoulder movement	1	2	3	4	5	NA
091402	Autonomic function	1	2	3	4	5	NA
091403	Deep tendon reflexes	1	2	3	4	5	NA
091404	Upper body skin sensation	1	2	3	4	5	NA
091409	Lower body skin sensation	1	2	3	4	5	NA
091405	Upper body strength	1	2	3	4	5	NA
091410	Lower body strength	1	2	3	4	5	NA

		Severe	Substantial	Moderate	Mild	None	
091406	Flaccidity	1	2	3	4	5	NA
091407	Pronator drift	1	2	3	4	5	NA
091411	Involuntary movement	1	2	3	4	5	NA
091412	Fasciculation	1	2	3	4	5	NA

Domain-*Physiologic Health (II)*   **Class**-*Neurocognitive (J)*   *1st edition 1997; revised 2004*

OUTCOME CONTENT REFERENCES:
Bickley, L. (2002). *Bates' guide to physical examination and history taking* (8th ed.). Philadelphia: Lippincott Williams & Wilkins.
Riess, P. C. (1995). *Validity and reliability of the Riess Intracranial Aneurysm Assessment Tool and the Glasgow Coma Scale in the aneurysm population.* Master's thesis. Iowa City, IA: The University of Iowa.
Smeltzer, S. C., & Bare, B. G. (Eds.). (2003). *Brunner and Suddarth's textbook of medical-surgical nursing* (10th ed.). Philadelphia: Lippincott Williams & Wilkins.

N

Newborn Adaptation 0118

Definition: Adaptive response to the extrauterine environment by a physiologically mature newborn during the first 28 days

OUTCOME TARGET RATING: Maintain at_____ Increase to_____

		Severe deviation from normal range	Substantial deviation from normal range	Moderate deviation from normal range	Mild deviation from normal range	No deviation from normal range	
OUTCOME OVERALL RATING		1	2	3	4	5	
Indicators:							
011801	Apgar score	1	2	3	4	5	NA
011802	Gestational age index	1	2	3	4	5	NA
011803	Apical heart rate (100-160)	1	2	3	4	5	NA
011804	Respiratory rate (30-60)	1	2	3	4	5	NA
011805	Blood pressure ratio of arm to leg	1	2	3	4	5	NA
011806	Oxygen saturation >90%	1	2	3	4	5	NA
011807	Thermoregulation	1	2	3	4	5	NA
011808	Skin color	1	2	3	4	5	NA
011809	Eyes clear	1	2	3	4	5	NA
011810	Cord drying	1	2	3	4	5	NA
011811	Weight	1	2	3	4	5	NA
011812	Feeding tolerance	1	2	3	4	5	NA
011813	Suck reflex	1	2	3	4	5	NA
011814	Muscle tone	1	2	3	4	5	NA
011815	Smooth, synchronous movement	1	2	3	4	5	NA
011816	Attentiveness to stimuli	1	2	3	4	5	NA
011817	Response to stimuli	1	2	3	4	5	NA
011818	Sustained alertness during interaction	1	2	3	4	5	NA
011819	Interaction with caregiver	1	2	3	4	5	NA
011820	Self-consolability	1	2	3	4	5	NA
011821	Blood glucose	1	2	3	4	5	NA
011822	Coombs test	1	2	3	4	5	NA
011823	Bilirubin level	1	2	3	4	5	NA
011824	Bowel elimination	1	2	3	4	5	NA
011825	Urinary elimination	1	2	3	4	5	NA

Domain-*Functional Health (I)*   **Class**-*Growth & Development (B)*   *2nd edition 2000; revised 2004*

N

OUTCOME CONTENT REFERENCES:

American Academy of Pediatrics & The American College of Obstetricians and Gynecologists. (1997). *Guidelines for perinatal care* (4th ed.). Washington, DC: American College of Obstetricians and Gynecologists.

Association of Women's Health, Obstetricians and Neonatal Nurses. (1998). *Standards & guidelines for the professional nursing practice in the care of women and newborns* (5th ed.). Washington, DC: Author

AWHONN Voice. (1996). Clinical commentary: Physiologic assessment of the healthy newborn. *Journal of Obstetric, Gynecologic, and Neonatal Nursing, 4*(6), 5–6.

Committee on Fetus and Newborn. (1993). Routine evaluation of blood pressure, hematocrit, and glucose in newborns. *Pediatrics, 92*(3), 474–476.

Murray, S. S., McKinney, E. S., & Gorrie, T. M. (2002). *Foundations of maternal-newborn nursing* (3rd ed.). Philadelphia: W. B. Saunders.

Simpson, K. R., & Creehan, P. A. (2001). *AWHONN's perinatal nursing* (2nd ed.). Philadelphia: Lippincott Williams & Wilkins.

Nutritional Status 1004

Definition: Extent to which nutrients are ingested and absorbed to meet metabolic needs

OUTCOME TARGET RATING: Maintain at_____   Increase to_____

		Severe deviation from normal range	Substantial deviation from normal range	Moderate deviation from normal range	Mild deviation from normal range	No deviation from normal range	
OUTCOME OVERALL RATING		1	2	3	4	5	
Indicators:							
100401	Nutrient intake	1	2	3	4	5	NA
100402	Food intake	1	2	3	4	5	NA
100408	Fluid intake	1	2	3	4	5	NA
100403	Energy	1	2	3	4	5	NA
100405	Weight/height ratio	1	2	3	4	5	NA
100411	Hydration	1	2	3	4	5	NA

Domain-*Physiologic Health (II)*   **Class**-*Digestion & Nutrition (K)*   *1st edition 1997; revised 2004, 2013*

OUTCOME CONTENT REFERENCES:

Chang, B. L., Uman, G. C., Linn, L. S., Ware, J. E., & Kane, R. L. (1985). Adherence to healthcare regimens among elderly women. *Nursing Research, 34*(1), 27–31.

Collinsworth, R., & Boyle, K. (1989). Nutritional assessment of the elderly. *Journal of Gerontological Nursing, 15*(12), 17–21.

Curtas, S., Chapman, G., & Meguid, M. (1989). Evaluation of nutritional status. *Nursing Clinics of North America, 24*(2), 301–313.

Folsom, A. R., Kaye, S. A., Sellers, T. A., Hang, C. P., Cerhan, J. R., Potter, J. D., & Prineas, R. J. (1993). Body fat distribution and five year risk of death in older women. *Journal of the American Medical Association, 269*(4), 483–487.

Gianino, S., & St. John, R. E. (1993). Nutritional assessment of the patient in the intensive care unit. *Critical Care Nursing Clinics of North America, 5*(1), 1–16.

+Guigoz, Y., Vallas, B., & Garry, P. J. (1996). Mini Nutritional Assessment: A practical assessment tool for grading the nutritional state of elderly patients. *Facts and Research in Gerontology, 4*(Suppl. 2), 15–59.

Tandy, L., & Malan, S. (2001). Impaired swallowing. In M. Maas, K. Buckwalter, M. Hardy, T. Tripp-Reimer, M. Titler, & J. Specht (Eds.), *Nursing care of older adults: Diagnoses, outcomes & interventions* (pp. 158–171). St. Louis: Mosby.

Wakefield, B. (2001). Altered nutrition: Less than body requirements. In M. Maas, K. Buckwalter, M. Hardy, T. Tripp-Reimer, M. Titler, & J. Specht (Eds.), *Nursing care of older adults: Diagnoses, outcomes & interventions* (pp. 145–157). St. Louis: Mosby.

N

Nutritional Status: Biochemical Measures 1005

Definition: Body fluid components and chemical indices of nutritional status

OUTCOME TARGET RATING: Maintain at_____   Increase to_____

		Severe deviation from normal range	Substantial deviation from normal range	Moderate deviation from normal range	Mild deviation from normal range	No deviation from normal range	
OUTCOME OVERALL RATING		1	2	3	4	5	
Indicators:							
100501	Serum albumin	1	2	3	4	5	NA
100502	Serum prealbumin	1	2	3	4	5	NA
100514	Serum creatinine	1	2	3	4	5	NA
100503	Hematocrit	1	2	3	4	5	NA
100504	Hemoglobin	1	2	3	4	5	NA
100510	Serum transferrin	1	2	3	4	5	NA
100505	Total iron binding capacity	1	2	3	4	5	NA
100506	Lymphocyte count	1	2	3	4	5	NA

Nutritional Status: Biochemical Measures—cont'd

	Severe deviation from normal range	Substantial deviation from normal range	Moderate deviation from normal range	Mild deviation from normal range	No deviation from normal range	
100507	Blood glucose	1	2	3	4	5	NA
100508	Blood cholesterol	1	2	3	4	5	NA
100509	Blood triglycerides	1	2	3	4	5	NA
100511	24-hour urinary creatinine	1	2	3	4	5	NA
100512	Urinary urea nitrogen	1	2	3	4	5	NA

Domain-*Physiologic Health (II)*   **Class**-*Digestion & Nutrition (K)*   *1st edition 1997; revised 2004*

OUTCOME CONTENT REFERENCES:

Chang, B. L., Uman, G. C., Linn, L. S., Ware, J. E., & Kane, R. L. (1985). Adherence to healthcare regimens among elderly women. *Nursing Research*, *34*(1), 27–31.

Collinsworth, R., & Boyle, K. (1989). Nutritional assessment of the elderly. *Journal of Gerontological Nursing*, *15*(12), 17–21.

Curtas, S., Chapman, G., & Meguid, M. (1989). Evaluation of nutritional status. *Nursing Clinics of North America*, *24*(2), 301–313.

Folsom, A. R., Kaye, S. A., Sellers, T. A., Hang, C. P., Cerhan, J. R., Potter, J. D., & Prineas, R. J. (1993). Body fat distribution and five year risk of death in older women. *Journal of the American Medical Association*, *269*(4), 483–487.

Gianino, S., & St. John, R. E. (1993). Nutritional assessment of the patient in the intensive care unit. *Critical Care Nursing Clinics of North America*, *5*(1), 1–16.

Nutritional Status: Energy   1007

Definition: Extent to which nutrients provide cellular energy

OUTCOME TARGET RATING: Maintain at_____   Increase to_____

	Severe deviation from normal range	Substantial deviation from normal range	Moderate deviation from normal range	Mild deviation from normal range	No deviation from normal range	
OUTCOME OVERALL RATING	1	2	3	4	5	
Indicators:						
100701 Stamina	1	2	3	4	5	NA
100702 Endurance	1	2	3	4	5	NA
100703 Hand grip strength	1	2	3	4	5	NA
100708 Muscle tone	1	2	3	4	5	NA
100704 Tissue healing	1	2	3	4	5	NA
100705 Infection resistance	1	2	3	4	5	NA
100706 Growth (children)	1	2	3	4	5	NA

Domain-*Physiologic Health (II)*   **Class**-*Digestion & Nutrition (K)*   *1st edition 1997; revised 2004, 2013*

OUTCOME CONTENT REFERENCES:

Chang, B. L., Uman, G. C., Linn, L. S., Ware, J. E., & Kane, R. L. (1985). Adherence to healthcare regimens among elderly women. *Nursing Research*, *34*(1), 27–31.

Collinsworth, R., & Boyle, K. (1989). Nutritional assessment of the elderly. *Journal of Gerontological Nursing*, *15*(12), 17–21.

Curtas, S., Chapman, G., & Meguid, M. (1989). Evaluation of nutritional status. *Nursing Clinics of North America*, *24*(2), 301–313.

+Dartmouth Primary Care Cooperative Information Project. (1987). *COOP Charts*. Hanover, NH: Department of Community and Family Medicine, Dartmouth Medical School.

Folsom, A. R., Kaye, S. A., Sellers, T. A., Hang, C. P., Cerhan, J. R., Potter, J. D., & Prineas, R. J. (1993). Body fat distribution and 5 year risk of death in older women. *Journal of the American Medical Association*, *269*(4), 483–487.

Gianino, S., & St. John, R. E. (1993). Nutritional assessment of the patient in the intensive care unit. *Critical Care Nursing Clinics of North America*, *5*(1), 1–16.

N

Nutritional Status: Food & Fluid Intake 1008

Definition: Amount of food and fluid taken into the body over a 24-hour period

OUTCOME TARGET RATING: Maintain at_____ Increase to_____

	Not adequate	Slightly adequate	Moderately adequate	Substantially adequate	Totally adequate	
OUTCOME OVERALL RATING	1	2	3	4	5	
Indicators:						
100801 Oral food intake	1	2	3	4	5	NA
100802 Tube feeding intake	1	2	3	4	5	NA
100803 Oral fluid intake	1	2	3	4	5	NA
100804 Intravenous fluid intake	1	2	3	4	5	NA
100805 Parenteral nutrition intake	1	2	3	4	5	NA

Domain-Physiologic Health (II) *Class-Digestion & Nutrition (K)* *1st edition 1997; revised 2004*

OUTCOME CONTENT REFERENCES:
Champagne, M. T., & Ashley, M. L. (1989). Nutritional support in the critically ill elderly patient. *Critical Care Nursing Quarterly, 12*(1), 15–25.
Coyle, E. F. (2004). Fluid and fuel intake during exercise. *Journal of Sports Sciences, 22*(1), 39–55.
Duggal, A., & Lawrence, R. M. (2001). Aspects of food refusal in the elderly: The "hunger strike." *International Journal of Eating Disorders, 30*(2), 213–216.
Gianino, S., & St. John, R. E. (1993). Nutritional assessment of the patient in the intensive care unit. *Critical Care Nursing Clinics of North America, 5*(1), 1–16.
Keithley, J. K., & Kohn, C. L. (1990). Managing nutritional problems in people with AIDS. *Oncology Nursing Forum, 17*(1), 23–27.

Nutritional Status: Nutrient Intake 1009

Definition: Nutrient intake to meet metabolic needs

OUTCOME TARGET RATING: Maintain at_____ Increase to_____

	Not adequate	Slightly adequate	Moderately adequate	Substantially adequate	Totally adequate	
OUTCOME OVERALL RATING	1	2	3	4	5	
Indicators:						
100901 Caloric intake	1	2	3	4	5	NA
100902 Protein intake	1	2	3	4	5	NA
100903 Fat intake	1	2	3	4	5	NA
100904 Carbohydrate intake	1	2	3	4	5	NA
100910 Fiber intake	1	2	3	4	5	NA
100905 Vitamin intake	1	2	3	4	5	NA
100906 Mineral intake	1	2	3	4	5	NA
100907 Iron intake	1	2	3	4	5	NA
100908 Calcium intake	1	2	3	4	5	NA
100911 Sodium intake	1	2	3	4	5	NA

Domain-Physiologic Health (II) *Class-Digestion & Nutrition (K)* *1st edition 1997; revised 2004, 2008*

OUTCOME CONTENT REFERENCES:
Champagne, M. T., & Ashley, M. L. (1989). Nutritional support in the critically ill elderly patient. *Critical Care Nursing Quarterly, 12*(1), 15–25.
Coyle, E. F. (2004). Fluid and fuel intake during exercise. *Journal of Sports Sciences, 22*(1), 39–55.
Gianino, S., & St. John, R. E. (1993). Nutritional assessment of the patient in the intensive care unit. *Critical Care Nursing Clinics of North America, 5*(1), 1–16.
Keithley, J. K., & Kohn, C. L. (1990). Managing nutritional problems in people with AIDS. *Oncology Nursing Forum, 17*(1), 23–27.
Viteri, F. (2010). INCAP studies of hematologic and gastrointestinal function in healthy individuals and those with protein-energy malnutrition and infection. *Food and Nutrition Bulletin, 31*(1), 130–140.

Oral Health   1100

Definition: Condition of the mouth, teeth, gums, and tongue

OUTCOME TARGET RATING: Maintain at_____   Increase to_____

OUTCOME OVERALL RATING	Severely compromised 1	Substantially compromised 2	Moderately compromised 3	Mildly compromised 4	Not compromised 5	
Indicators:						
110001 Cleanliness of mouth	1	2	3	4	5	NA
110002 Cleanliness of teeth	1	2	3	4	5	NA
110003 Cleanliness of gums	1	2	3	4	5	NA
110004 Cleanliness of tongue	1	2	3	4	5	NA
110005 Cleanliness of dentures	1	2	3	4	5	NA
110006 Cleanliness of dental appliances	1	2	3	4	5	NA
110007 Fit of dentures	1	2	3	4	5	NA
110008 Fit of dental appliances	1	2	3	4	5	NA
110009 Moistness of lips	1	2	3	4	5	NA
110010 Moisture of oral mucosa and tongue	1	2	3	4	5	NA
110011 Color of mucosa membranes	1	2	3	4	5	NA
110012 Oral mucosa integrity	1	2	3	4	5	NA
110013 Tongue integrity	1	2	3	4	5	NA
110014 Gum integrity	1	2	3	4	5	NA

	Severe	Substantial	Moderate	Mild	None	
110026 Absence of teeth	1	2	3	4	5	NA
110027 Erosion of enamel	1	2	3	4	5	NA
110017 Halitosis	1	2	3	4	5	NA
110018 Bleeding	1	2	3	4	5	NA
110021 Pain	1	2	3	4	5	NA
110028 Toothache	1	2	3	4	5	NA
110029 Tooth fracture	1	2	3	4	5	NA
110022 Oral mucosa lesions	1	2	3	4	5	NA
110023 Dental caries	1	2	3	4	5	NA
110024 Gingivitis	1	2	3	4	5	NA
110025 Periodontal disease	1	2	3	4	5	NA

Dental Prosthesis: Yes / No

Domain-Physiologic Health (II)   *Class*-Tissue Integrity (L)   *1st edition 1997; revised 2004, 2008, 2013*

OUTCOME CONTENT REFERENCES:
Andrew, L. (2004). Beakers for bottles—a health visitor oral health campaign. *Community Practitioner, 77*(1), 18–22.
Fischman, S. (1993). Self-care: Practical periodontal care in today's practice. *International Dental Journal, 43*(Suppl. 2), 179–183.
Jones, J. A. (1989). Integrating the oral examination into clinical practice. *Hospital Practice, 24*(10A), 23–24, 26–27, 30.
+Kayser-Jones, J., Bird, W. F., Paul, S. M., Long, L. & Schell, E. S. (1995). An instrument to assess the oral health status of nursing home residents. *The Gerontologist, 35*(6), 814–824.
Matteson, M. A., McConnell, E. S., & Linton, A. D. (1997). *Gerontological nursing: Concepts & practice* (2nd ed.). Philadelphia: W. B. Saunders.
Raybould, T. P., Carpenter, A. D., Ferretti, G. A., Brown, A. T., Lillich, T. T., & Henslee, J. (1994). Emergence of gram-negative bacilli in the mouths of bone marrow transplant recipients using chlorhexidine mouth rinse. *Oncology Nursing Forum, 21*(4), 691–696.
Richardson, A. (1987). A process standard for oral care. *Nursing Times, 83*(32), 38–40.
Speedie, G. (1983). Nursology of mouth care: Preventing, comforting and seeking activities related to mouth care. *Journal of Advanced Nursing, 8*(1), 33–40.

Ostomy Self-Care   **1615**

Definition: Personal actions to maintain ostomy for elimination

OUTCOME TARGET RATING: Maintain at_____   Increase to_____

		Never demonstrated	Rarely demonstrated	Sometimes demonstrated	Often demonstrated	Consistently demonstrated	
OUTCOME OVERALL RATING		1	2	3	4	5	
Indicators:							
161501	Describes functioning of ostomy	1	2	3	4	5	NA
161502	Describes purpose of ostomy	1	2	3	4	5	NA
161503	Appears comfortable viewing stoma	1	2	3	4	5	NA
161504	Measures stoma for proper appliance fit	1	2	3	4	5	NA
161520	Maintains skin care around ostomy	1	2	3	4	5	NA
161521	Uses correct irrigation technique	1	2	3	4	5	NA
161507	Empties ostomy bag	1	2	3	4	5	NA
161508	Changes ostomy bag	1	2	3	4	5	NA
161509	Monitors for complications related to stoma	1	2	3	4	5	NA
161510	Monitors amount and consistency of stool	1	2	3	4	5	NA
161511	Follows schedule for changing ostomy bag	1	2	3	4	5	NA
161512	Obtains ostomy supplies	1	2	3	4	5	NA
161513	Avoids flatus-producing food and drink	1	2	3	4	5	NA
161514	Maintains adequate fluid intake	1	2	3	4	5	NA
161515	Follows recommended diet	1	2	3	4	5	NA
161516	Avoids odor-producing foods	1	2	3	4	5	NA
161522	Modifies daily activities to optimize self-care	1	2	3	4	5	NA
161523	Obtains assistance from a health professional	1	2	3	4	5	NA
161519	Expresses acceptance of ostomy	1	2	3	4	5	NA

Domain-*Health Knowledge & Behavior (IV)*   **Class**-*Health Behavior (Q)*   *3rd edition 2004; revised 2008*

OUTCOME CONTENT REFERENCES:

Bryant, D., & Fleischer, I. (2000). Changing an ostomy appliance. *Nursing, 30*(11), 51–53.
Lee, J. (2001). Nurse prescribing in practice: Patient choice in stoma care. *British Journal of Community Nursing, 6*(1), 33–34, 36–37.
Martins, M. L., & Cardoso, M. (2001). Group participative education for persons with an ostomy. *World Council of Enterostomal Therapists Journal, 21*(4), 8–17.
Metcalf, C. (1999). Clinical stoma care: Empowering patients through teaching practical skills. *British Journal of Nursing, 8*(9), 593–600.
Sage, S. J. (1991). Nephrostomy dressing change procedure. *Ostomy Wound Management, 32*(4), 32–33, 35–36.
Secord, C., Jackman, M., Wright, L., & Winton, S. (2001). Adjusting to life with an ostomy. *Canadian Nurse, 97*(1), 29–32.
Thompson, J. (2000). A practical ostomy guide. *RN, 63*(11), 61–68.

O

Pain: Adverse Psychological Response 1306

Definition: Severity of observed or reported adverse cognitive and emotional responses to physical pain

OUTCOME TARGET RATING: Maintain at_____   Increase to_____

OUTCOME OVERALL RATING		Severe 1	Substantial 2	Moderate 3	Mild 4	None 5	
Indicators:							
130601	Slowing of thought processes	1	2	3	4	5	NA
130602	Memory impairment	1	2	3	4	5	NA
130603	Interference with concentration	1	2	3	4	5	NA
130604	Indecision	1	2	3	4	5	NA
130605	Pain distress	1	2	3	4	5	NA
130606	Concern about tolerating the pain	1	2	3	4	5	NA
130607	Concern about burdening others	1	2	3	4	5	NA
130608	Concern about abandonment	1	2	3	4	5	NA
130609	Depression	1	2	3	4	5	NA
130610	Anxiety	1	2	3	4	5	NA
130611	Sadness	1	2	3	4	5	NA
130612	Helplessness	1	2	3	4	5	NA
130613	Hopelessness	1	2	3	4	5	NA
130614	Worthlessness	1	2	3	4	5	NA
130615	Sense of isolation	1	2	3	4	5	NA
130616	Fear of procedures and equipment	1	2	3	4	5	NA
130617	Fear of unbearable pain	1	2	3	4	5	NA
130618	Annoyance with disruptive effects of pain	1	2	3	4	5	NA
130619	Suicidal thoughts	1	2	3	4	5	NA
130620	Pessimistic thoughts	1	2	3	4	5	NA
130621	Bitterness toward others	1	2	3	4	5	NA
130622	Anger over disabling effects of pain	1	2	3	4	5	NA

Domain-Perceived Health (V)   *Class*-Symptom Status (V)   2nd edition 2000; revised 2004

P

OUTCOME CONTENT REFERENCES:

Copp, L. A. (1974). The spectrum of suffering. *American Journal of Nursing, 74*(3), 491–495.

Kalfoss, M. H. (1992). The assessment of psychological distress. *Scandinavian Journal of Caring Science, 6*(1), 23–28.

Price, D. D., & Harkins, S. W. (1992). Psychophysical approaches to pain measurement and assessment. In D. C. Turk & R. Melzack (Eds.), *Handbook of pain assessment* (pp. 111–134). New York: The Guilford Press.

Puntillo, K. A., & Wilkie, D. J. (1991). Assessment of pain in the critically ill. In K. A. Puntillo (Ed.), *Pain in the critically ill* (pp. 45–64). Gaithersburg, MD: Aspen.

Pain Control

1605

Definition: Personal actions to control pain

OUTCOME TARGET RATING: Maintain at_____   Increase to_____

OUTCOME OVERALL RATING	Never demonstrated 1	Rarely demonstrated 2	Sometimes demonstrated 3	Often demonstrated 4	Consistently demonstrated 5	
Indicators:						
160502 Recognizes pain onset	1	2	3	4	5	NA
160501 Describes causal factors	1	2	3	4	5	NA
160510 Uses diary to monitor symptoms over time	1	2	3	4	5	NA
160503 Uses preventive measures	1	2	3	4	5	NA
160504 Uses non-analgesic relief measures	1	2	3	4	5	NA
160505 Uses analgesics as recommended	1	2	3	4	5	NA
160513 Reports changes in pain symptoms to health professional	1	2	3	4	5	NA
160507 Reports uncontrolled symptoms to health professional	1	2	3	4	5	NA
160508 Uses available resources	1	2	3	4	5	NA
160509 Recognizes associated symptoms of pain	1	2	3	4	5	NA
160511 Reports pain controlled	1	2	3	4	5	NA

Domain-*Health Knowledge & Behavior (IV)*   **Class**-*Health Behavior (Q)*   *1st edition 1997; revised 2000, 2004*

P

OUTCOME CONTENT REFERENCES:

Howe, C. J. (1993). A new standard of care for pediatric pain management. *American Journal of Maternal Child Nursing, 18*(6), 325–329.

+Hurley, A. C., Volicer, B. J., Hanrahan, P. A., Houde, S., & Volicer, L. (1992). Assessment of discomfort in advanced Alzheimer's patients. *Research in Nursing and Health, 15*(5), 369–377.

Mobily, P., & Herr, K. A. (2001). Pain. In M. Maas, K. Buckwalter, M. Hardy, T. Tripp-Reimer, M. Titler, & J. Specht (Eds.), *Nursing care of older adults: Diagnoses, outcomes & interventions* (pp. 455–475). St. Louis: Mosby.

Puntillo, K., & Weiss, S. J. (1994). Pain: Its mediators and associated morbidity in critically ill cardiovascular surgical patients. *Nursing Research, 43*(1), 31–36.

Sherbourne, C. D. (1992). Pain measures. In A. L. Stewart & J. E. Ware, Jr. (Eds.), *Measuring functioning and well-being* (pp. 220–234). Durham, NC: Duke University Press.

+Walker, S. N., Sechrist, K. R., & Pender, N. J. (1987). The health-promoting lifestyle profile: Development and psychometric characteristics. *Nursing Research, 36*(2), 76–81.

+Walker, S. N., Sechrist, K. R., & Pender, N. J. (1995). *The health-promoting lifestyle profile II*. Omaha, NE: University of Nebraska at Omaha.

Pain: Disruptive Effects   2101

Definition: Severity of observed or reported disruptive effects of chronic pain on daily functioning

OUTCOME TARGET RATING: Maintain at_____   Increase to_____

OUTCOME OVERALL RATING	Severe 1	Substantial 2	Moderate 3	Mild 4	None 5	
Indicators:						
210127 Discomfort	1	2	3	4	5	NA
210101 Disruption of interpersonal relationships	1	2	3	4	5	NA
210102 Impaired role performance	1	2	3	4	5	NA
210108 Impaired concentration	1	2	3	4	5	NA
210128 Disruption of sense of control	1	2	3	4	5	NA
210110 Impaired mood	1	2	3	4	5	NA
210111 Lack of patience	1	2	3	4	5	NA
210112 Interrupted sleep	1	2	3	4	5	NA
210119 Disruption of routine	1	2	3	4	5	NA
210113 Impaired physical mobility	1	2	3	4	5	NA
210129 Interference with activities of daily living	1	2	3	4	5	NA
210130 Impaired work performance	1	2	3	4	5	NA
210131 Impaired school performance	1	2	3	4	5	NA
210115 Loss of appetite	1	2	3	4	5	NA
210117 Impaired urinary elimination	1	2	3	4	5	NA
210120 Impaired bowel elimination	1	2	3	4	5	NA
210123 Absenteeism from work	1	2	3	4	5	NA
210124 Absenteeism from school	1	2	3	4	5	NA
210122 Difficulty maintaining employment	1	2	3	4	5	NA
210132 Impaired life enjoyment	1	2	3	4	5	NA
210133 Hopelessness	1	2	3	4	5	NA
210134 Impaired physical activity	1	2	3	4	5	NA

Domain-Perceived Health (V)   *Class*-Symptom Status (V)   *1st edition 1997; revised 2004, 2008, 2013*

OUTCOME CONTENT REFERENCES:

Howe, C. J. (1993). A new standard of care for pediatric pain management. *American Journal of Maternal Child Nursing, 18*(6), 325–329.

Mobily, P., & Herr, K. A. (2001). Pain. In M. Maas, K. Buckwalter, M. Hardy, T. Tripp-Reimer, M. Titler, & J. Specht (Eds.), *Nursing care of older adults: Diagnoses, outcomes & interventions* (pp. 455–475). St. Louis: Mosby.

Puntillo, K., & Weiss, S. J. (1994). Pain: Its mediators and associated mobility in critically ill cardiovascular surgical patients. *Nursing Research, 43*(1), 31–36.

Sherbourne, C. D. (1992). Pain measures. In A. L. Stewart & J. E. Ware, Jr. (Eds.), *Measuring functioning and well-being* (pp. 220–234). Durham, NC: Duke University Press.

+Von Korff, M., Ormel, J., Keefe, F. J., & Dworkin, S. F. (1992). Grading the severity of chronic pain. *Pain, 50*(2), 133–149.

P

Pain Level 2102

Definition: Severity of observed or reported pain

OUTCOME TARGET RATING: Maintain at_____ Increase to_____

		Severe	Substantial	Moderate	Mild	None	
OUTCOME OVERALL RATING		1	2	3	4	5	
Indicators:							
210201	Reported pain	1	2	3	4	5	NA
210204	Length of pain episodes	1	2	3	4	5	NA
210221	Rubbing affected area	1	2	3	4	5	NA
210217	Moaning and crying	1	2	3	4	5	NA
210206	Facial expressions of pain	1	2	3	4	5	NA
210208	Restlessness	1	2	3	4	5	NA
210222	Agitation	1	2	3	4	5	NA
210223	Irritability	1	2	3	4	5	NA
210224	Wincing	1	2	3	4	5	NA
210225	Tearing	1	2	3	4	5	NA
210226	Diaphoresis	1	2	3	4	5	NA
210218	Pacing	1	2	3	4	5	NA
210219	Narrowed focus	1	2	3	4	5	NA
210209	Muscle tension	1	2	3	4	5	NA
210215	Loss of appetite	1	2	3	4	5	NA
210227	Nausea	1	2	3	4	5	NA
210228	Food intolerance	1	2	3	4	5	NA

		Severe deviation from normal range	Substantial deviation from normal range	Moderate deviation from normal range	Mild deviation from normal range	No deviation from normal range	
210210	Respiratory rate	1	2	3	4	5	NA
210211	Apical heart rate	1	2	3	4	5	NA
210220	Radial pulse rate	1	2	3	4	5	NA
210212	Blood pressure	1	2	3	4	5	NA
210214	Perspiration	1	2	3	4	5	NA

Site of pain: _____

Domain-Perceived Health (V) *Class*-Symptom Status (V) *1st edition 1997; revised 2004, 2008*

OUTCOME CONTENT REFERENCES:

Herr, K., Coyne, P. J., Key, T., Manworren, R., McCaffery, M., Merkel, S., Pelosi-Kelly, J., & Wild, L. (2006). Pain assessment in the nonverbal patient: Position statement with clinical practice recommendations. *Pain Management Nursing, 7*(2), 44–52.

Howe, C. J. (1993). A new standard of care for pediatric pain management. *American Journal of Maternal Child Nursing, 18*(6), 325–329.

+Hurley, A. C., Volicer, B. J., Hanrahan, P. A., Houde, S., & Volicer, L. (1992). Assessment of discomfort in advanced Alzheimer's patients. *Research in Nursing and Health, 15*(5), 369–377.

Mayer, D. M., Torma, L., Byock, I., & Norris, K. (2001). Speaking the language of pain. *American Journal of Nursing, 101*(2), 44–50.

Melzack, R. (1975). The McGill Pain Questionnaire: Major properties and scoring methods. *Pain, 30*(1), 277–299.

Merkel, S. (2002). Pain assessment in infants and young children: The Finger Span Scale. *American Journal of Nursing, 102*(11), 55–56.

Mobily, P., & Herr, K. A. (2001). Pain. In M. Maas, K. Buckwalter, M. Hardy, T. Tripp-Reimer, M. Titler, & J. Specht (Eds.), *Nursing care of older adults: Diagnoses, outcomes & interventions* (pp. 455–475). St. Louis: Mosby.

Puntillo, K., & Weiss, S. J. (1994). Pain: Its mediators and associated morbidity in critically ill cardiovascular surgical patients. *Nursing Research, 43*(1), 31–36.

Sherbourne, C. D. (1992). Pain measures. In A. L. Stewart, & J. E. Ware, Jr. (Eds.), *Measuring functioning and well-being* (pp. 220–234). Durham, NC: Duke University Press.

+Wong, D., & Baker, C. M. (1988). Pain in children: Comparison of assessment scales. *Pediatric Nursing, 14*(1), 9–17.

P

Parent-Infant Attachment   **1500**

Definition: Parent and infant behaviors that demonstrate an enduring affectionate bond

OUTCOME TARGET RATING: Maintain at_____   Increase to_____

		Never demonstrated	Rarely demonstrated	Sometimes demonstrated	Often demonstrated	Consistently demonstrated	
OUTCOME OVERALL RATING		1	2	3	4	5	
Indicators:							
150001	Practices healthy behaviors during pregnancy	1	2	3	4	5	NA
150002	Assigns specific attributes to fetus	1	2	3	4	5	NA
150003	Prepares for infant prior to birth	1	2	3	4	5	NA
150004	Verbalizes positive feelings toward infant	1	2	3	4	5	NA
150005	Holds infant close	1	2	3	4	5	NA
150006	Touches, strokes, pats infant	1	2	3	4	5	NA
150007	Kisses infant	1	2	3	4	5	NA
150008	Smiles at infant	1	2	3	4	5	NA
150009	Visits nursery	1	2	3	4	5	NA
150011	Uses en face position	1	2	3	4	5	NA
150012	Uses eye contact	1	2	3	4	5	NA
150013	Vocalizes to infant	1	2	3	4	5	NA
150014	Plays with infant	1	2	3	4	5	NA
150015	Responds to infant cues	1	2	3	4	5	NA
150016	Consoles infant	1	2	3	4	5	NA
150024	Holds infant for feeding	1	2	3	4	5	NA
150018	Keeps infant dry, clean, and warm	1	2	3	4	5	NA
150019	Infant looks at parent	1	2	3	4	5	NA
150020	Infant responds to parent's cues	1	2	3	4	5	NA
150021	Infant seeks proximity with parent	1	2	3	4	5	NA

Specify parent: _____

P

Domain-Psychosocial Health (III)   *Class*-Social Interaction (P)   *1st edition 1997; revised 2004, 2008*

OUTCOME CONTENT REFERENCES:

Ainsworth, M. S., & Wittig, B. A. (1969). Attachment and exploratory behavior of one-year olds in a strange situation. In B. M. Foss (Ed.), *Determinants of infant behavior* (pp. 111–133). London: Methuen.

Kennell, J., Jerauld, R., Wolfe, H., Chesler, D., Kreger, N. C., McAlpine, W., Steffa, M., & Klaus, M. H. (1974). Maternal behavior one year after early and extended post-partum contact. *Developmental Medicine and Child Neurology, 16*(2), 172–279.

Koniak-Griffin, D. (1988). The relationship between social support, self-esteem, and maternal-fetal attachment in adolescents. *Research in Nursing and Health, 11*(4), 269–278.

+Müller, M. (1994). A questionnaire to measure mother-to-infant attachment. *Journal of Nursing Measurements, 2*(2), 129–141.

Norr, K. F., Roberts, J. E., & Freese, U. (1989). Early postpartum rooming-in and maternal attachment behaviors in a group of medically indigent primiparas. *Journal of Nurse-Midwifery, 34*(2), 85–91.

Parenting Performance **2211**

Definition: Parental actions to provide a child a nurturing and constructive physical, emotional, and social environment

OUTCOME TARGET RATING: Maintain at_____   Increase to_____

		Never demonstrated	Rarely demonstrated	Sometimes demonstrated	Often demonstrated	Consistently demonstrated	
OUTCOME OVERALL RATING		1	2	3	4	5	
Indicators:							
221101	Provides for child's physical needs	1	2	3	4	5	NA
221122	Provides age-appropriate nutrition	1	2	3	4	5	NA
221102	Eliminates controllable environmental hazards	1	2	3	4	5	NA
221130	Provides preventative health care	1	2	3	4	5	NA
221131	Provides episodic health care	1	2	3	4	5	NA
221123	Provides structure for child	1	2	3	4	5	NA
221104	Stimulates cognitive development	1	2	3	4	5	NA
221105	Stimulates social development	1	2	3	4	5	NA
221106	Stimulates emotional growth	1	2	3	4	5	NA
221107	Nurtures spiritual growth	1	2	3	4	5	NA
221124	Stimulates moral growth	1	2	3	4	5	NA
221125	Imparts values that promote functioning in society	1	2	3	4	5	NA
221126	Provides appropriate supervision for child	1	2	3	4	5	NA
221127	Selects appropriate supplemental caregiver	1	2	3	4	5	NA
221128	Monitors supplemental caregiver	1	2	3	4	5	NA
221108	Uses community resources	1	2	3	4	5	NA
221110	Uses interactions appropriate for child's temperament	1	2	3	4	5	NA
221111	Uses behavior management	1	2	3	4	5	NA
221112	Uses age-appropriate discipline	1	2	3	4	5	NA
221113	Provides for child's special needs	1	2	3	4	5	NA
221114	Interacts positively with child	1	2	3	4	5	NA
221115	Empathizes with child	1	2	3	4	5	NA
221129	Maintains open communication	1	2	3	4	5	NA
221116	Verbalizes positive attributes of child	1	2	3	4	5	NA
221117	Exhibits a loving relationship	1	2	3	4	5	NA
221118	Expresses realistic expectations of parental role	1	2	3	4	5	NA
221119	Expresses satisfaction with parental role	1	2	3	4	5	NA
221120	Expresses positive self-esteem	1	2	3	4	5	NA

Domain-Family Health (VI)   *Class-Parenting (DD)*   *1st edition 1997; revised 2004, 2008, 2013*

OUTCOME CONTENT REFERENCES:

Causby, V., Nixon, C., & Bright, J. M. (1991). Influences on adolescent mother-infant interactions. *Adolescence, 26*(103), 619–630.

+Clarke, M., & Hornick, J. (1984). The development of the Nurturance Inventory: An instrument for assessing parenting practices. *Child Psychiatry & Human Development, 15*(1), 49–63.

Fulton, A. M., Murphy, K. R., & Anderson, S. L. (1991). Increasing adolescent mothers' knowledge of child development: An intervention program. *Adolescence, 26*(101), 73–81.

Greaves, P., Glik, D. C., Kronenfeld, J. J., & Jackson, K. (1994). Determinants of controllable in-home child safety hazards. *Health Education Research, 9*(3), 307–315.

Mercer, R. T., & Ferketich, S. L. (1994). Predictors of maternal role competence by risk status. *Nursing Research, 43*(1), 38–43.

Ohashi, J. P. (1992). Maternal role satisfaction: A new approach to assessing parenting. *Scholarly Inquiry for Nursing Practice: An International Journal, 6*(2), 135–149.

Reece, S. M. (1995). Stress and maternal adaptation in first-time mothers more than 35 years old. *Applied Nursing Research, 8*(2), 61–66.

Thompson, P. J., Powell, M. J., Patterson, R. J., & Ellerbee, S. M. (1995). Adolescent parenting: Outcomes and maternal perceptions. *Journal of Obstetric, Gynecologic, and Neonatal Nursing, 24*(8), 713–718.

Parenting Performance: Adolescent   2903

Definition: Parental actions to provide an adolescent with a safe, nurturing and positive physical, emotional, spiritual, and social environment from 12 years through 17 years

OUTCOME TARGET RATING: Maintain at_____   Increase to_____

		Never demonstrated	Rarely demonstrated	Sometimes demonstrated	Often demonstrated	Consistently demonstrated	
OUTCOME OVERALL RATING		1	2	3	4	5	
Indicators:							
290301	Exhibits a loving relationship	1	2	3	4	5	NA
290302	Maintains open communication with adolescent	1	2	3	4	5	NA
290303	Listens openly, thoughtfully, and without interruption	1	2	3	4	5	NA
290304	Promotes appropriate independence	1	2	3	4	5	NA
290305	Serves as role model for personal integrity	1	2	3	4	5	NA
290306	Encourages balance between individual versus group identity	1	2	3	4	5	NA
290307	Assists adolescent to cope constructively with emotions	1	2	3	4	5	NA
290308	Assists adolescent to evaluate consequences of behavior	1	2	3	4	5	NA
290309	Provides clear, consistent rules of behavior	1	2	3	4	5	NA
290310	Enforces family rules of behavior	1	2	3	4	5	NA
290311	Nurtures spiritual growth	1	2	3	4	5	NA
290312	Nurtures moral growth	1	2	3	4	5	NA
290313	Monitors academic performance	1	2	3	4	5	NA
290314	Communicates with teachers about adolescent's academic performance	1	2	3	4	5	NA
290315	Monitors activity involvement to prevent overcommitment	1	2	3	4	5	NA
290316	Respects need for emancipation from parental controls	1	2	3	4	5	NA
290317	Respects need for privacy	1	2	3	4	5	NA
290318	Discusses developmental changes with adolescent	1	2	3	4	5	NA
290319	Assists adolescent to develop healthy body image	1	2	3	4	5	NA
290320	Assists adolescent to develop positive self-esteem	1	2	3	4	5	NA
290321	Encourages participation in activities that contribute to lifelong fitness	1	2	3	4	5	NA
290322	Provides appropriate nutrition	1	2	3	4	5	NA
290323	Provides opportunities for family activities	1	2	3	4	5	NA
290324	Monitors for signs of eating disorders	1	2	3	4	5	NA
290325	Discusses age-appropriate sex education	1	2	3	4	5	NA
290326	Teaches to identify predatory, abusive sexual advances	1	2	3	4	5	NA

P

Continued

Parenting Performance: Adolescent—*cont'd*

		Never demonstrated	Rarely demonstrated	Sometimes demonstrated	Often demonstrated	Consistently demonstrated	
290327	Teaches to report predatory, abusive sexual advances	1	2	3	4	5	NA
290328	Protects from abuse	1	2	3	4	5	NA
290329	Protects from body mutilation	1	2	3	4	5	NA
290330	Uses strategies to prevent participation in violence	1	2	3	4	5	NA
290331	Assists adolescent to cope with stress	1	2	3	4	5	NA
290332	Discusses hazards of substance use	1	2	3	4	5	NA
290333	Establishes clear rules regarding driving	1	2	3	4	5	NA
290334	Establishes clear rules regarding alcohol use	1	2	3	4	5	NA
290335	Establishes clear rules regarding avoidance of drugs	1	2	3	4	5	NA
290336	Reinforces personal hygiene	1	2	3	4	5	NA
290337	Reinforces oral hygiene behaviors	1	2	3	4	5	NA
290338	Maintains recommended dental checkups	1	2	3	4	5	NA
290339	Maintains recommended schedule of health checkups	1	2	3	4	5	NA
290340	Maintains recommended schedule of immunizations	1	2	3	4	5	NA
290341	Promotes adequate sleep	1	2	3	4	5	NA
290342	Teaches danger of hearing damage from portable music devices	1	2	3	4	5	NA
290343	Discusses implications of body piercing and tattoos	1	2	3	4	5	NA
290344	Teaches strategies to prevent injury	1	2	3	4	5	NA
290345	Recognizes symptoms of depression and potential suicide	1	2	3	4	5	NA
290346	Obtains treatment for depressed adolescent	1	2	3	4	5	NA

Domain-*Family Health (VI)*   **Class**-*Parenting (DD)*   5th edition 2013

OUTCOME CONTENT REFERENCES:

Alati, R., Maloney, E., Hutchinson, D. M., Najman, J. M., Mattick, R. P., Bor, W., & Williams, G. M. (2010). Do maternal parenting practices predict problematic patterns of adolescent alcohol consumption? *Addiction 105*(5), 872–880.

Hockenberry, M., & Wilson, D. (2007). *Wong's nursing care of infants and children* (8th ed.). St. Louis: Elsevier Mosby.

Levin, K., & Currie, C. (2010). Adolescent toothbrushing and the home environment: Sociodemographic factors, family relationships and mealtime routines and disorganization. *Community Dentistry and Oral Epidemiology, 38*(1), 10.

Miller, P., & Plant, M. (2010). Parental guidance about drinking: Relationship with teenage psychoactive substance use. *Journal of Adolescence, 33*(1), 55–68.

Noland, H., Price, J., Dake, J., & Telljohann, S. (2009). Adolescents' sleep behaviors and perceptions of sleep. *Journal of School Health, 79*(5), 224–230.

Roest, A., Dubas, J., & Gerris, J. (2010). Value transmissions between parents and children: Gender and developmental phase as transmission belts. *Journal of Adolescence, 33*(1), 21–31.

P

Parenting Performance: Adolescent Physical Safety   2902

Definition: Parental actions to prevent physical injury in an adolescent from 12 years through 17 years of age

OUTCOME TARGET RATING: Maintain at_____   Increase to_____

		Never demonstrated	Rarely demonstrated	Sometimes demonstrated	Often demonstrated	Consistently demonstrated	
OUTCOME OVERALL RATING		1	2	3	4	5	
Indicators:							
290201	Uses strategies to protect from sun exposure	1	2	3	4	5	NA
290226	Encourages appropriate clothing for activity	1	2	3	4	5	NA
290203	Maintains warning devices	1	2	3	4	5	NA
290204	Practices family fire escape plan	1	2	3	4	5	NA
290205	Maintains smoke-free environment	1	2	3	4	5	NA
290206	Monitors use of sport and recreational equipment	1	2	3	4	5	NA
290207	Uses strategies to encourage use of protective gear during high-risk activities	1	2	3	4	5	NA
290208	Uses strategies to encourage seat belt use	1	2	3	4	5	NA
290209	Uses strategies to encourage safe driving	1	2	3	4	5	NA
290210	Uses strategies to prevent water accidents	1	2	3	4	5	NA
290211	Uses strategies to prevent firearm injuries	1	2	3	4	5	NA
290212	Uses strategies to prevent participation in violence	1	2	3	4	5	NA
290213	Uses strategies to prevent tobacco use	1	2	3	4	5	NA
290214	Uses strategies to prevent alcohol use	1	2	3	4	5	NA
290215	Uses strategies to prevent recreational drug use	1	2	3	4	5	NA
290216	Uses strategies to prevent medication misuse	1	2	3	4	5	NA
290217	Uses strategies to prevent exposure to toxic chemicals	1	2	3	4	5	NA
290218	Uses strategies to prevent exposure to excessive noise	1	2	3	4	5	NA
290228	Uses strategies to postpone sexual activity	1	2	3	4	5	NA
290220	Uses strategies to prevent high-risk sexual activity	1	2	3	4	5	NA
290229	Uses strategies to prevent communicable disease	1	2	3	4	5	NA
290222	Protects from physical abuse	1	2	3	4	5	NA
290223	Protects from sexual abuse	1	2	3	4	5	NA
290224	Monitors for warning signs of self-harm	1	2	3	4	5	NA
290227	Obtains training to prepare for emergencies	1	2	3	4	5	NA

P

Domain-Family Health (VI)   *Class*-Parenting (DD)   *3rd edition 2004; revised 2008, 2013*

OUTCOME CONTENT REFERENCES:

Bernardo, L., Garnder, J. J., & Seibel, K. (2001). Playground injuries in children: A review and Pennsylvania trauma center experience. *Journal of the Society of Pediatrics Nurses, 6*(1), 11–20.

Gresham, L. S., Zirkle, D. L., Tolchin, S., Jones, C., Maroufi, A., & Miranda, J. (2001). Partnering for injury prevention: Evaluation of a curriculum-based intervention program among elementary school children. *Journal of Pediatric Nursing, 16*(2), 79–87.

Hall-Long, B. A., Schell, K., & Corrigan, V. (2001). Youth safety education and injury prevention program. *Pediatric Nursing, 27*(2), 141–148.

Polivka, B. J., & Ryan-Wenger, N. (1999). Health promotion and injury prevention behaviors of elementary school children. *Pediatric Nursing 25*(2), 127–134.

Parenting Performance: Early/Middle Childhood Physical Safety   2901

Definition: Parental actions to avoid physical injury of a child from 3 years through 11 years of age

OUTCOME TARGET RATING: Maintain at_____   Increase to_____

		Never demonstrated	Rarely demonstrated	Sometimes demonstrated	Often demonstrated	Consistently demonstrated	
OUTCOME OVERALL RATING		1	2	3	4	5	
Indicators:							
290101	Selects safe, age-appropriate toys	1	2	3	4	5	NA
290102	Provides supervision around pets and animals	1	2	3	4	5	NA
290103	Provides supervision around water	1	2	3	4	5	NA
290104	Avoids leaving child in motor vehicle unsupervised	1	2	3	4	5	NA
290105	Monitors proper use of car seat/seat belt	1	2	3	4	5	NA
290106	Supervises selection of weather-appropriate clothing	1	2	3	4	5	NA
290107	Protects from sun exposure	1	2	3	4	5	NA
290108	Maintains environment to prevent harmful falls	1	2	3	4	5	NA
290109	Maintains environment to prevent burns, electrical shock, and chemical exposure	1	2	3	4	5	NA
290110	Maintains environment to prevent poisoning	1	2	3	4	5	NA
290111	Practices family fire escape plan	1	2	3	4	5	NA
290112	Keeps medication out of reach	1	2	3	4	5	NA
290113	Maintains warning devices	1	2	3	4	5	NA
290114	Locks or removes doors from unused appliances	1	2	3	4	5	NA
290115	Maintains smoke-free environment	1	2	3	4	5	NA
290116	Ensures home playground equipment meets safety guidelines	1	2	3	4	5	NA
290117	Provides supervision while on playground equipment	1	2	3	4	5	NA
290118	Selects appropriate clothing for activity	1	2	3	4	5	NA
290119	Uses strategies to encourage use of protective helmet	1	2	3	4	5	NA
290120	Uses strategies to encourage use of protective gear during high-risk activities	1	2	3	4	5	NA
290121	Eliminates access to firearms	1	2	3	4	5	NA
290122	Protects from exposure to violence	1	2	3	4	5	NA
290123	Monitors use of sport and recreational equipment	1	2	3	4	5	NA
290124	Uses strategies to prevent tobacco use	1	2	3	4	5	NA
290125	Uses strategies to prevent alcohol use	1	2	3	4	5	NA
290126	Uses strategies to prevent recreational drug use	1	2	3	4	5	NA
290127	Uses strategies to prevent medication misuse	1	2	3	4	5	NA

P

Parenting Performance: Early/Middle Childhood Physical Safety—cont'd

		Never demonstrated	Rarely demonstrated	Sometimes demonstrated	Often demonstrated	Consistently demonstrated	
290128	Uses strategies to prevent exposure to toxic chemicals	1	2	3	4	5	NA
290129	Uses strategies to prevent exposure to excessive noise	1	2	3	4	5	NA
290130	Uses strategies to prevent precocious sexual behavior	1	2	3	4	5	NA
290131	Protects from physical abuse	1	2	3	4	5	NA
290132	Protects from sexual abuse	1	2	3	4	5	NA
290134	Obtains training to prepare for emergencies	1	2	3	4	5	NA

Domain-Family Health (VI)   *Class*-Parenting (DD)   *3rd edition 2004; revised 2008, 2013*

OUTCOME CONTENT REFERENCES:

Bernardo, L., Gardner, J. J., & Seibel, K. (2001). Playground injuries in children: A review and Pennsylvania trauma center experience. *Journal of the Society of Pediatrics Nurses, 6*(1), 1120–.

Gresham, L. S., Zirkle, D. L., Tolchin, S., Jones, C., Maroufi, A., & Miranda, J. (2001). Partnering for injury prevention: Evaluation of a curriculum-based intervention program among elementary school children. *Journal of Pediatric Nursing, 16*(2), 79–87.

Hall-Long, B. A., Schell, K., & Corrigan, V. (2001). Youth safety education and injury prevention program. *Pediatric Nursing, 27*(2), 141–148.

Polivka, B. J., & Ryan-Wenger, N. (1999). Health promotion and injury prevention behaviors of elementary school children. *Pediatric Nursing, 25*(2), 127–134.

U. S. Consumer Product Safety Commission. (1997). *Handbook for public playground safety*. Washington, DC: Author.

Parenting Performance: Infant   **2904**

Definition: Parental actions to provide an infant a safe, nurturing and positive physical, emotional, spiritual and social environment from 28 days to first birthday

OUTCOME TARGET RATING: Maintain at_____   Increase to_____

		Never demonstrated	Rarely demonstrated	Sometimes demonstrated	Often demonstrated	Consistently demonstrated	
OUTCOME OVERALL RATING		1	2	3	4	5	
Indicators:							
290401	Exhibits a loving relationship	1	2	3	4	5	NA
290402	Provides safe, age-appropriate developmental activities	1	2	3	4	5	NA
290403	Interacts with infant to promote trust	1	2	3	4	5	NA
290404	Interacts with infant to promote language development	1	2	3	4	5	NA
290405	Interacts with infant to promote social development	1	2	3	4	5	NA
290406	Provides transitional objects to reduce anxiety	1	2	3	4	5	NA
290407	Responds appropriately to infant temperament	1	2	3	4	5	NA
290408	Provides appropriate sensory/motor stimulation	1	2	3	4	5	NA
290409	Provides appropriate supervision	1	2	3	4	5	NA
290410	Uses a social support system to assist with infant	1	2	3	4	5	NA
290411	Selects appropriate supplemental caregiver	1	2	3	4	5	NA

Continued

P

Parenting Performance: Infant—cont'd

		Never demonstrated	Rarely demonstrated	Sometimes demonstrated	Often demonstrated	Consistently demonstrated	
290412	Monitors supplemental caregiver	1	2	3	4	5	NA
290413	Uses strategies to eliminate risk for abuse	1	2	3	4	5	NA
290414	Protects from abuse	1	2	3	4	5	NA
290415	Sets behavioral limits	1	2	3	4	5	NA
290416	Maintains safe sleep environment	1	2	3	4	5	NA
290417	Provides appropriate weaning	1	2	3	4	5	NA
290418	Allows non-nutritive sucking	1	2	3	4	5	NA
290419	Provides age-appropriate nutrition	1	2	3	4	5	NA
290420	Encourages oral hygiene as primary teeth erupt	1	2	3	4	5	NA
290421	Provides a spiritual environment	1	2	3	4	5	NA
290422	Maintains smoke-free environment	1	2	3	4	5	NA
290423	Maintains recommended well-child checkups	1	2	3	4	5	NA
290424	Maintains recommended immunizations	1	2	3	4	5	NA
290425	Uses strategies to prevent injury	1	2	3	4	5	NA
290426	Protects from sun exposure	1	2	3	4	5	NA
290427	Obtains assistance from a health professional when symptoms occur	1	2	3	4	5	NA

Domain-*Family Health (VI)* **Class**-*Parenting (DD)* *5th edition 2013*

OUTCOME CONTENT REFERENCES:
Hockenberry, M., & Wilson, D. (2007). *Wong's nursing care of infants and children* (8th ed.). St. Louis: Elsevier Mosby.
Knitzer, J. (2008). Giving infants and toddlers a head start: Getting policies in sync with knowledge. *Infants & Young Children, 21*(1), 18–29.
Poobalan, A. S., Aucott, L. S., Ross, L., Smith, W. C., Helms, P. J., & Williams, J. H. (2007). Effects of treating postnatal depression on mother-infant interaction and child development: Systematic review. *British Journal of Psychiatry, 191*(5), 378–386.
Sutton, B. (2005). Scientific foundations for social brain concept. *Psychiatric Annals, 35*(10), 793–802.

P

Parenting Performance: Infant/Toddler Physical Safety   **2900**

Definition: Parental actions to prevent physical injury of a child from birth through 2 years of age

OUTCOME TARGET RATING: Maintain at_____   Increase to_____

		Never demonstrated	Rarely demonstrated	Sometimes demonstrated	Often demonstrated	Consistently demonstrated	
OUTCOME OVERALL RATING		1	2	3	4	5	
Indicators:							
290001	Handles infant/toddler properly	1	2	3	4	5	NA
290002	Uses crib that meets safety regulations	1	2	3	4	5	NA
290003	Positions on back for sleep	1	2	3	4	5	NA
290004	Selects safe, age-appropriate toys	1	2	3	4	5	NA
290005	Keeps sharp, pointed objects out of reach	1	2	3	4	5	NA
290006	Selects foods that prevent choking	1	2	3	4	5	NA
290007	Stores formula/breastmilk safely	1	2	3	4	5	NA
290008	Provides constant supervision around pets and animals	1	2	3	4	5	NA
290009	Provides constant supervision around water	1	2	3	4	5	NA

Parenting Performance: Infant/Toddler Physical Safety—cont'd

		Never demonstrated	Rarely demonstrated	Sometimes demonstrated	Often demonstrated	Consistently demonstrated	
290010	Avoids leaving infant/toddler in motor vehicle unsupervised	1	2	3	4	5	NA
290011	Uses car seat appropriately	1	2	3	4	5	NA
290012	Selects weather-appropriate clothing	1	2	3	4	5	NA
290013	Protects from sun exposure	1	2	3	4	5	NA
290014	Maintains environment to prevent suffocation	1	2	3	4	5	NA
290015	Maintains environment to prevent harmful falls	1	2	3	4	5	NA
290016	Maintains environment to prevent burns, electrical shock, and chemical exposure	1	2	3	4	5	NA
290017	Maintains environment to prevent poisoning	1	2	3	4	5	NA
290018	Keeps medication out of reach	1	2	3	4	5	NA
290019	Maintains smoke-free environment	1	2	3	4	5	NA
290020	Uses strategies to prevent exposure to excessive noise	1	2	3	4	5	NA
290021	Maintains warning devices	1	2	3	4	5	NA
290028	Obtains training to prepare for emergencies	1	2	3	4	5	NA
290023	Ensures home playground equipment meets safety guidelines	1	2	3	4	5	NA
290024	Provides supervision while on playground equipment	1	2	3	4	5	NA
290025	Ensures that infant/toddler wears helmet properly	1	2	3	4	5	NA
290026	Protects from physical abuse	1	2	3	4	5	NA
290027	Protects from sexual abuse	1	2	3	4	5	NA

Domain-*Family Health (VI)*   **Class-***Parenting (DD)*   *3rd edition 2004; revised 2008, 2013*

OUTCOME CONTENT REFERENCES:

Kendrick, D., & Marsh, P. (1998). Babywalkers: Prevalence of use and relationship with other safety practices. *Injury Prevention, 4*(4), 295–298.

Kotch, J., Dufort, V. M., Stewart, P., Fieberg, J., McMurray, M., O'Brien, S., Ngui, E. M., & Brennan, M. (1997). Injuries among children in home and out-of-home care. *Injury Prevention, 3*(4), 267–271.

McBrien, M. (1997). Regency home care pediatric checklist. *Home Care Manager, 1*(2), 17.

Murphy, J. (1999). Pediatric occupant care safety: Clinical implications based on recent literature. *Pediatric Nursing, 25*(2), 137–144, 147–148.

O'Dea, T., Saly, G., & Holte, J. (1998). Safety investigation: Interaction of infant radiant warmers and bilirubin phototherapy lights in the regulation of temperature of newborn infants. *Biomedical Instrument Technology, 32*(4), 355–369.

Showers, J. (1992). "Don't shake the baby": The effectiveness of a prevention program. *Child Abuse & Neglect, 16*(1), 11–18.

Thompson, R., & Emslie, A. (2000). Young children and the risk of accidental injury: Running an audit at nine months. *Community Practitioner, 73*(10), 799–800.

U. S. Consumer Product Safety Commission. (1997). *Handbook for public playground safety.* Washington, DC: Author.

Wong, D., Hockenberry-Eaton, M., Wilson, D., Winkelstein, M. L., & Schwartz, P. (2001). *Wong's essentials of pediatric nursing* (6th ed). St. Louis: Mosby.

P

Parenting Performance: Middle Childhood   **2905**

Definition: Parental actions to provide a child with a safe, nurturing and positive physical, emotional, social, and spiritual environment from 6 years through 11 years

OUTCOME TARGET RATING: Maintain at_____   Increase to_____

OUTCOME OVERALL RATING	Never demonstrated 1	Rarely demonstrated 2	Sometimes demonstrated 3	Often demonstrated 4	Consistently demonstrated 5	
Indicators:						
290501 Exhibits a loving relationship	1	2	3	4	5	NA
290502 Maintains open communication with child	1	2	3	4	5	NA
290503 Promotes appropriate independence	1	2	3	4	5	NA
290504 Encourages safe exploration of environment	1	2	3	4	5	NA
290505 Provides clear, consistent rules of behavior	1	2	3	4	5	NA
290506 Enforces family rules of behavior	1	2	3	4	5	NA
290507 Uses age-appropriate discipline	1	2	3	4	5	NA
290508 Provides for child's special needs	1	2	3	4	5	NA
290509 Monitors school learning environment	1	2	3	4	5	NA
290510 Monitors academic performance	1	2	3	4	5	NA
290511 Communicates with teachers about child's academic performance	1	2	3	4	5	NA
290512 Provides safe after-school activities	1	2	3	4	5	NA
290513 Encourages peer group involvement	1	2	3	4	5	NA
290514 Encourages completion of activities	1	2	3	4	5	NA
290515 Provides opportunities for learning	1	2	3	4	5	NA
290516 Promotes regular physical exercise	1	2	3	4	5	NA
290517 Assist child to maintain optimum weight	1	2	3	4	5	NA
290518 Encourages participation in team activities	1	2	3	4	5	NA
290519 Monitors activities to prevent over-commitment	1	2	3	4	5	NA
290520 Provides opportunities for quiet activities	1	2	3	4	5	NA
290521 Teaches to identify predatory, abusive sexual advances	1	2	3	4	5	NA
290522 Teaches to report predatory, abusive sexual advances	1	2	3	4	5	NA
290523 Protects from abuse	1	2	3	4	5	NA
290524 Prevents exposure to violence	1	2	3	4	5	NA
290525 Maintains sleep routine	1	2	3	4	5	NA
290526 Provides appropriate nutrition	1	2	3	4	5	NA
290527 Discusses prepubescent developmental changes with child	1	2	3	4	5	NA
290528 Discusses age-appropriate sex education	1	2	3	4	5	NA
290529 Accepts child's sexual orientation	1	2	3	4	5	NA
290530 Discusses hazards of substance use	1	2	3	4	5	NA
290531 Assists child to cope with stress	1	2	3	4	5	NA
290532 Nurtures spiritual growth	1	2	3	4	5	NA
290533 Nurtures moral growth	1	2	3	4	5	NA
290534 Promotes respect for others	1	2	3	4	5	NA
290535 Reinforces oral hygiene behaviors	1	2	3	4	5	NA
290536 Maintains recommended dental checkups	1	2	3	4	5	NA
290537 Maintains recommended health checkups	1	2	3	4	5	NA
290538 Maintains recommended immunizations	1	2	3	4	5	NA

P

Parenting Performance: Middle Childhood—cont'd

		Never demonstrated	Rarely demonstrated	Sometimes demonstrated	Often demonstrated	Consistently demonstrated	
290539	Maintains smoke-free environment	1	2	3	4	5	NA
290540	Teaches personal stranger safety	1	2	3	4	5	NA
290541	Uses strategies to prevent injury	1	2	3	4	5	NA
290542	Protects from sun exposure	1	2	3	4	5	NA
290543	Obtains assistance from a health professional for health problems	1	2	3	4	5	NA
290544	Obtains treatment for childhood depression	1	2	3	4	5	NA

Domain-Family Health (VI)   **Class**-Parenting (DD)   5th edition 2013

OUTCOME CONTENT REFERENCES:

American Academy of Pediatrics. (1999). *The complete and authoritative guide: Caring for your school age child ages 5 to 12* (rev. ed.). E. Schor, Ed. New York: Bantam Books.

Cesario, S., & Hughes, L. (2007). Precocious puberty: A comprehensive review of literature. *Journal of Obstetrics, Gynecologic, & Neonatal Nursing, 36*(3), 263–273.

Fowler, J. (1981). *Stages of faith*. San Francisco: Harper and Row.

Hockenberry, M., & Wilson, D. (2007). *Wong's nursing care of infants and children*. (8th ed.). St. Louis: Elsevier Mosby.

Kieckhefer, G., Ward, T., Tsai, S., & Lentz, M. (2008). Nighttime sleep and daytime nap patterns in school age children with and without asthma. *Journal of Developmental & Behavioral Pediatrics, 29*(5), 338–344.

Parenting Performance: Preschooler   2906

Definition: Parental actions to provide a preschooler with a safe, nurturing and positive physical, emotional, spiritual, and social environment from three through five years

OUTCOME TARGET RATING: Maintain at_____   Increase to_____

		Never demonstrated	Rarely demonstrated	Sometimes demonstrated	Often demonstrated	Consistently demonstrated	
OUTCOME OVERALL RATING		1	2	3	4	5	
Indicators:							
290601	Exhibits a loving relationship	1	2	3	4	5	NA
290602	Provides safe, age-appropriate developmental activities	1	2	3	4	5	NA
290603	Interacts with preschooler to promote trust	1	2	3	4	5	NA
290604	Promotes regular physical exercise	1	2	3	4	5	NA
290605	Assist child to maintain optimum eight	1	2	3	4	5	NA
290606	Encourages activities to promote reading	1	2	3	4	5	NA
290607	Maintains open communication with preschooler	1	2	3	4	5	NA
290608	Verbalizes positive attributes of preschooler	1	2	3	4	5	NA
290609	Assists child to cope with fears	1	2	3	4	5	NA
290610	Provides transitional objects to reduce anxiety	1	2	3	4	5	NA
290611	Responds constructively to negative behavior	1	2	3	4	5	NA
290612	Encourages imagination	1	2	3	4	5	NA

P

Continued

Parenting Performance: Preschooler—cont'd

		Never demonstrated	Rarely demonstrated	Sometimes demonstrated	Often demonstrated	Consistently demonstrated	
290613	Teaches family rules of behavior	1	2	3	4	5	NA
290614	Promotes appropriate independence	1	2	3	4	5	NA
290615	Promotes independent dressing	1	2	3	4	5	NA
290616	Promotes independent feeding	1	2	3	4	5	NA
290617	Promotes independent toileting	1	2	3	4	5	NA
290618	Encourages safe exploration of environment	1	2	3	4	5	NA
290619	Nurtures spiritual growth	1	2	3	4	5	NA
290620	Nurtures moral growth	1	2	3	4	5	NA
290621	Encourages interactions with other children	1	2	3	4	5	NA
290622	Monitors preschool learning environment	1	2	3	4	5	NA
290623	Protects from abuse	1	2	3	4	5	NA
290624	Prevents exposure to violence	1	2	3	4	5	NA
290625	Supervises media use	1	2	3	4	5	NA
290626	Monitors supplemental caregiver	1	2	3	4	5	NA
290627	Uses age-appropriate discipline	1	2	3	4	5	NA
290628	Provides for child's special needs	1	2	3	4	5	NA
290629	Maintains safe sleep environment	1	2	3	4	5	NA
290630	Maintains bedtime routine	1	2	3	4	5	NA
290631	Provides age-appropriate nutrition	1	2	3	4	5	NA
290632	Responds constructively to sibling rivalry	1	2	3	4	5	NA
290633	Allows expression of sexual curiosity	1	2	3	4	5	NA
290634	Teaches oral hygiene behaviors	1	2	3	4	5	NA
290635	Maintains recommended dental checkups	1	2	3	4	5	NA
290636	Maintains recommended well-child checkups	1	2	3	4	5	NA
290637	Maintains recommended immunizations	1	2	3	4	5	NA
290638	Maintains smoke-free environment	1	2	3	4	5	NA
290639	Teaches personal stranger safety	1	2	3	4	5	NA
290640	Uses strategies to prevent injury	1	2	3	4	5	NA
290641	Protects from sun exposure	1	2	3	4	5	NA
290642	Obtains assistance from a health professional for health problems	1	2	3	4	5	NA

Domain-Family Health (VI)   **Class**-Parenting (DD)   5th edition 2013

OUTCOME CONTENT REFERENCES:

Hockenberry, M., & Wilson, D. (2007). *Wong's nursing care of infants and children.* (8th ed.). St. Louis: Elsevier Mosby.

Dennis, T. (2006). Emotional self-regulation in preschoolers: The interplay of child approach reactivity, parenting, and control capacities. *Developmental Psychology, 42*(1), 84–97.

Jouriles, E., Brown, A., McDonald, R., Rosefield, D., Leahy, M., & Silver, C. (2008). Intimate partner violence and preschoolers' explicit memory functioning. *Journal of Family Psychology, 22*(3), 420–428.

P

Parenting Performance: Psychosocial Safety   1901

Definition: Parental actions to protect a child from social contacts that might cause harm or injury

OUTCOME TARGET RATING: Maintain at_____   Increase to_____

	Never demonstrated	Rarely demonstrated	Sometimes demonstrated	Often demonstrated	Consistently demonstrated	
OUTCOME OVERALL RATING	1	2	3	4	5	
Indicators:						
190101 Monitors playmates	1	2	3	4	5	NA
190102 Monitors social contacts	1	2	3	4	5	NA
190115 Fosters open communication	1	2	3	4	5	NA
190104 Selects appropriate supplemental caregiver	1	2	3	4	5	NA
190103 Monitors supplemental caregiver	1	2	3	4	5	NA
190105 Recognizes risk for abuse	1	2	3	4	5	NA
190106 Uses strategies to eliminate risk for abuse	1	2	3	4	5	NA
190121 Protects from physical abuse	1	2	3	4	5	NA
190122 Protects from sexual abuse	1	2	3	4	5	NA
190123 Protects from emotional abuse	1	2	3	4	5	NA
190109 Provides required level of supervision	1	2	3	4	5	NA
190112 Uses strategies to prevent high-risk social behavior	1	2	3	4	5	NA
190113 Prevents gang participation	1	2	3	4	5	NA
190116 Fosters mutually interactive communication about sex	1	2	3	4	5	NA
190117 Sets clear rules for behavior	1	2	3	4	5	NA
190119 Maintains structure in child's life	1	2	3	4	5	NA
190120 Maintains daily routine in child's life	1	2	3	4	5	NA

Domain-Family Health (VI)   *Class-Parenting (DD)*   *1st edition 1997; revised 2004, 2008, 2013*

P

OUTCOME CONTENT REFERENCES:

Glick, D., Kronenfeld, J., & Jackson, K. (1993). Safety behaviors among parents of preschoolers. *Health Values, 17*(1), 18–27.

Howell, J. C., & Lynch, J. P. (2000). Youth gangs in schools. *YGS Bulletin*. Washington, DC: U.S. Department of Justice, Office of Justice Programs, Office of Juvenile Justice and Delinquency Prevention.

Jackson, C., & Foshee, V. A. (1998). Violence-related behaviors of adolescents: Relations with responsive and demanding parenting. *Journal of Adolescent Research, 13*(3), 343–359.

Jensen, L. R., Williams, S. D., Thurman, D. J., & Keller, P. A. (1992). Submersion injuries for children less than 5 years in urban Utah. *Western Journal of Medicine, 157*(6), 641–644.

Quan, L., Gore, E. J., Wentz, K., Allen, J., & Novack, A. H. (1989). Ten-year study of pediatric drownings and near-drownings in King County, Washington: Lessons in injury prevention. *Pediatrics, 83*(6), 1035–1040.

Rosenthal, D. A., Feldman, S. S., & Edwards, D. (1998). Mum's the word: Mother's perspectives on communication about sexuality with adolescents. *Journal of Adolescence, 21*(6), 727–743.

Walker, M., Schmidt, L., & Lunghofer, L. (1993). Youth gangs. In M. I. Singer, L. T. Singer, & T. M. Anglin (Eds.), *Handbook for screening adolescents at psychosocial risk* (pp. 504–522). New York: Lexington Books.

Parenting Performance: Toddler   2907

Definition: Parental actions to provide a child with a safe, nurturing and positive physical, emotional, spiritual, and social environment from 1 year through 2 years

OUTCOME TARGET RATING: Maintain at_____   Increase to_____

		Never demonstrated	Rarely demonstrated	Sometimes demonstrated	Often demonstrated	Consistently demonstrated	
OUTCOME OVERALL RATING		1	2	3	4	5	
Indicators:							
290701	Exhibits a loving relationship	1	2	3	4	5	NA
290702	Provides safe, age-appropriate developmental activities	1	2	3	4	5	NA
290703	Interacts with toddler to promote trust	1	2	3	4	5	NA
290704	Interacts with toddler to promote language development	1	2	3	4	5	NA
290705	Encourages activities to promote reading	1	2	3	4	5	NA
290706	Encourages interactions with other children	1	2	3	4	5	NA
290707	Provides appropriate supervision	1	2	3	4	5	NA
290708	Promotes a sense of autonomy	1	2	3	4	5	NA
290709	Promotes beginning independence	1	2	3	4	5	NA
290710	Responds constructively to negative behavior	1	2	3	4	5	NA
290711	Sets realistic expectations for behavior	1	2	3	4	5	NA
290712	Uses a social support system to assist with toddler	1	2	3	4	5	NA
290713	Provides transitional objects to reduce anxiety	1	2	3	4	5	NA
290714	Monitors supplemental caregiver	1	2	3	4	5	NA
290715	Teaches right from wrong	1	2	3	4	5	NA
290716	Nurtures spiritual growth	1	2	3	4	5	NA
290717	Uses strategies to eliminate risk for abuse	1	2	3	4	5	NA
290718	Protects from abuse	1	2	3	4	5	NA
290719	Maintains behavioral limits	1	2	3	4	5	NA
290720	Maintains safe sleep environment	1	2	3	4	5	NA
290721	Maintains bedtime routine	1	2	3	4	5	NA
290722	Provides age-appropriate nutrition	1	2	3	4	5	NA
290723	Offers a variety of foods	1	2	3	4	5	NA
290724	Guides toilet training when ready	1	2	3	4	5	NA
290725	Responds constructively to sibling rivalry	1	2	3	4	5	NA
290726	Allows expression of sexual curiosity	1	2	3	4	5	NA
290727	Teaches oral hygiene behaviors	1	2	3	4	5	NA
290728	Maintains recommended dental checkups	1	2	3	4	5	NA
290729	Maintains recommended well-child checkups	1	2	3	4	5	NA
290730	Maintains recommended immunizations	1	2	3	4	5	NA
290731	Maintains smoke-free environment	1	2	3	4	5	NA
290732	Uses strategies to prevent injury	1	2	3	4	5	NA
290733	Protects from sun exposure	1	2	3	4	5	NA
290734	Obtains assistance from a health professional for health problems	1	2	3	4	5	NA

Domain-Family Health (VI)   *Class*-Parenting (DD)   *5th edition 2013*

OUTCOME CONTENT REFERENCES:
Hockenberry, M., & Wilson, D. (2007). *Wong's nursing care of infants and children* (8th ed.). St. Louis: Elsevier Mosby.
Knitzer, J. (2008). Giving infants and toddlers a head start: Getting policies in sync with knowledge. *Infants & Young Children, 21*(1), 18–29.
U.S. National Library of Medicine and National Institute of Health. (2011). *Toddler development.* Retrieved from http://www.nlm.nih.gov/medlineplus/toddlerdevelopment.html#cat1
Wright, C., Parkinson, K., Shipton, D., & Drewett, R. (2007). How do toddler eating problems relate to their eating behavior, food preferences, and growth? *Pediatrics, 120*(4), 1069–1075.

Participation in Health Care Decisions — 1606

Definition: Personal involvement in selecting and evaluating health care options to achieve desired outcome

OUTCOME TARGET RATING: Maintain at_____   Increase to_____

	Never demonstrated	Rarely demonstrated	Sometimes demonstrated	Often demonstrated	Consistently demonstrated	
OUTCOME OVERALL RATING	1	2	3	4	5	
Indicators:						
160601 Claims decision-making responsibility	1	2	3	4	5	NA
160602 Exhibits self-direction in decision making	1	2	3	4	5	NA
160603 Seeks reputable information	1	2	3	4	5	NA
160604 Defines available options	1	2	3	4	5	NA
160605 Specifies health outcome preferences	1	2	3	4	5	NA
160606 Identifies health outcome priorities	1	2	3	4	5	NA
160607 Identifies barriers to desired outcome achievement	1	2	3	4	5	NA
160608 Uses problem-solving techniques to achieve desired outcomes	1	2	3	4	5	NA
160609 States intent to act on decision	1	2	3	4	5	NA
160610 Identifies available support for achieving desired outcomes	1	2	3	4	5	NA
160611 Seeks health care services to meet desired outcomes	1	2	3	4	5	NA
160612 Negotiates for care preferences	1	2	3	4	5	NA
160613 Monitors barriers to outcome achievement	1	2	3	4	5	NA
160614 Identifies level of outcome achievement	1	2	3	4	5	NA
160615 Evaluates satisfaction with health care outcomes	1	2	3	4	5	NA

Domain-*Health Knowledge & Behavior (IV)*   **Class**-*Health Behavior (Q)*   *1st edition 1997; revised 2004*

P

OUTCOME CONTENT REFERENCES:
Conn, V., Taylor, S., & Casey, B. (1992). Cardiac rehabilitation program participation and outcomes after myocardial infarction. *Rehabilitation Nursing, 17*(2), 58–62.
+Ende, J., Kazis, L., Ash, A., & Moskowitz, M. A. (1989). Measuring patient's desire for autonomy: Decision making and information-seeking preferences among medical patients. *Journal of General Internal Medicine, 4*(1), 23–30.
Hegyvary, S. T. (1993). Patient care outcomes related to management of symptoms. In J. J. Fitzpatrick & J. J. Stevenson (Eds.), *Annual review of nursing research.* (vol. 11, pp. 145–168). New York: Springer.
Weiler, K., & Moorhead, S. A. (2001). Self-determination. In M. Maas, K. Buckwalter, M. Hardy, T. Tripp-Reimer, M. Titler, & J. Specht (Eds.), *Nursing care of older adults: Diagnoses, outcomes & interventions* (pp. 706–718). St. Louis: Mosby.

Perimenopause Symptom Severity 2104

Definition: Severity of reported adverse physical and emotional responses due to declining hormonal levels

OUTCOME TARGET RATING: Maintain at_____   Increase to_____

		Severe	Substantial	Moderate	Mild	None	
OUTCOME OVERALL RATING		1	2	3	4	5	
Indicators:							
210401	Menstrual irregularity	1	2	3	4	5	NA
210402	Abdominal cramps	1	2	3	4	5	NA
210403	Hot flashes	1	2	3	4	5	NA
210404	Night sweats	1	2	3	4	5	NA
210405	Vaginal dryness	1	2	3	4	5	NA
210406	Mood swings	1	2	3	4	5	NA
210407	Menstrual flow	1	2	3	4	5	NA
210408	Insomnia	1	2	3	4	5	NA
210409	Fatigue	1	2	3	4	5	NA
210410	Musculoskeletal pain	1	2	3	4	5	NA
210411	Weight gain	1	2	3	4	5	NA
210412	Decreased libido	1	2	3	4	5	NA
210413	Heart palpitations	1	2	3	4	5	NA
210414	Vertigo	1	2	3	4	5	NA
210415	Memory changes	1	2	3	4	5	NA

Domain-*Perceived Health (V)*   **Class**-*Symptom Status (V)*   *2nd edition 2000; revised 2004, 2013*

OUTCOME CONTENT REFERENCES:
Alexander, L. L., & LaRosa, J. (1994). *New dimensions in women's health.* Sudbury, MA: Jones and Bartlett.
Andrews, G. (2001). *Women's sexual health* (2nd ed.). London: Bailliere Tindall.
Clark, A. J., Flowers, J., Boots, L., & Shettar, S. (1995). Sleep disturbance in mid-life women. *Journal of Advanced Nursing, 22*(3), 562–568.
Dannels, A., & Charlifue, S. (2004). The perimenopause experience for women with spinal cord injuries. *SCI Nursing, 21*(1), 9–113.
Fogel, C. I., & Woods, N. F. (Eds.). (1995). *Women's health care: A comprehensive handbook.* Thousand Oaks, CA: Sage.
Heger, M., Ventskovskey, B. M., Borzenko, I., Kneis, K. C., Rettengberger, R., Kaszkin-Bettag, M., & Heger, P. W. (2006). Efficacy and safety of a special extract of Rheum rhaponticum (ERr 731) in perimenopausal women with climacteric complaints: A 12-week randomized, double-blind, placebo-controlled trial. *Menopause, 13*(5), 744–759.
Logothetis, M. L. (1991). Women's decisions about estrogen replacement therapy. *Western Journal of Nursing Research, 13*(4), 458–474.
Lyndaker, C., & Hulton, L. (2004). The influence of age on symptoms of perimenopause. *Journal of Obstetric, Gynecologic, & Neonatal Nursing, 33*(3), 340–347.
Richards, M., Rubinow, D. R., Daly, R. C., & Schmidt, P. J. (2006). Premenstrual symptoms and perimenopausal depression. *American Journal of Psychiatry, 163*(1), 133–137.
Woods, N. F., & Mitchell, E. S. (1996). Patterns of depressed mood in midlife women: Observations from the Seattle Midlife Women's Health Study. *Research in Nursing and Health, 19*(2), 111–123.

P

Peripheral Artery Disease Severity 2115

Definition: Severity of signs and symptoms of reduced peripheral blood flow due to atherosclerotic arteries in the extremities

OUTCOME TARGET RATING: Maintain at_____   Increase to_____

		Severe	Substantial	Moderate	Mild	None	
OUTCOME OVERALL RATING		1	2	3	4	5	
Indicators:							
211501	Intermittent claudication intensity	1	2	3	4	5	NA
211502	Unrelieved muscle pain with rest	1	2	3	4	5	NA
211503	Impaired skin color in extremities	1	2	3	4	5	NA

Peripheral Artery Disease Severity—cont'd

	Severe	Substantial	Moderate	Mild	None	
211504	Impaired skin temperature in extremities	1	2	3	4	5	NA
211505	Impaired skin sensation in extremities	1	2	3	4	5	NA
211506	Tingling in extremities	1	2	3	4	5	NA
211507	Numbness of extremities	1	2	3	4	5	NA
211508	Hair loss on extremities	1	2	3	4	5	NA
211509	Restless leg syndrome	1	2	3	4	5	NA
211510	Impaired physical mobility	1	2	3	4	5	NA
211511	Restricted walking distance	1	2	3	4	5	NA
211512	Muscle pain in upper extremities	1	2	3	4	5	NA
211513	Muscle pain in buttocks	1	2	3	4	5	NA
211514	Muscle pain in thigh	1	2	3	4	5	NA
211515	Erectile dysfunction	1	2	3	4	5	NA
211516	Thrombus formation	1	2	3	4	5	NA
211517	Skin ulceration	1	2	3	4	5	NA

Domain-Perceived Health (V)   **Class**-Symptom Status (V)   5th edition 2013

OUTCOME CONTENT REFERENCES:

Hirsch, A., Haskal, Z., Hertzer, N., Bakal, C., Creager, M., Halperin, J., et al. (2006). ACC/AHA 2005 practice guidelines for the management of patients with peripheral artery disease (lower extremity, renal, mesenteric, and abdominal aortic. *Circulation, 113*(11), 463–654.

Jude, A. B. (2004). Intermittent claudication in the patient with diabetes. *British Journal of Diabetes & Vascular Disease, 4*(4), 238–242.

Lewis, S., Dirksen, S., Heitkemper, M., Bucher, L., & Camera, I. (2011). *Medical-surgical nursing: Assessment and management of clinical problems* (8th ed., pp. 874–880). St. Louis: Elsevier.

Peripheral Arterial Disease Coalition. (2007). Gaps in public knowledge of peripheral artery disease: The first national PAD public awareness survey. *Circulation, 116*(18), 2086–2094.

P

Personal Autonomy

1614

Definition: Personal actions of a competent individual to exercise governance in life decisions

OUTCOME TARGET RATING: Maintain at_____   Increase to_____

		Never demonstrated	Rarely demonstrated	Sometimes demonstrated	Often demonstrated	Consistently demonstrated	
OUTCOME OVERALL RATING		1	2	3	4	5	
Indicators:							
161401	Makes informed life decisions	1	2	3	4	5	NA
161402	Considers other opinions when making choices	1	2	3	4	5	NA
161403	Expresses independence with decision-making process	1	2	3	4	5	NA
161404	Makes decisions free from undue pressure by parents	1	2	3	4	5	NA
161405	Makes decisions free from undue pressure by spouse	1	2	3	4	5	NA
161406	Makes decisions free from undue pressure by children	1	2	3	4	5	NA

Continued

Personal Autonomy—cont'd

		Never demonstrated	Rarely demonstrated	Sometimes demonstrated	Often demonstrated	Consistently demonstrated	
161407	Makes decisions free from undue pressure by extended family	1	2	3	4	5	NA
161408	Makes decisions free from undue pressure by friends	1	2	3	4	5	NA
161409	Makes decisions free from undue pressure by health provider	1	2	3	4	5	NA
161410	Asserts personal preferences	1	2	3	4	5	NA
161411	Participates in health care decisions	1	2	3	4	5	NA
161412	Expresses satisfaction with life choices	1	2	3	4	5	NA

Domain-*Health Knowledge & Behavior (IV)*   **Class**-*Health Behavior (Q)*   *3rd edition 2004*

OUTCOME CONTENT REFERENCES:

Aveyard, H. (2000). Is there a concept of autonomy that can usefully inform nursing practice? *Journal of Advanced Nursing, 32*(2), 352–358.

Brennan, M. (1997). A concept analysis of consent. *Journal of Advanced Nursing, 25*(3), 477–484.

Dworkin, G. (1988). *The theory and practice of autonomy.* Cambridge: Cambridge University Press.

Valimaki, M., & Leino-Kilpi, H. (1998). Preconditions for and consequences of self-determination: The psychiatric patient's point of view. *Journal of Advanced Nursing, 27*(1), 204–212.

Wiens, A. G. (1993). Patient autonomy: A theoretical framework for nursing. *Journal of Professional Nursing, 9*(2), 95–103.

Personal Health Screening Behavior   **1634**

Definition: Personal actions to obtain recommended screening for early detection of a communicable or undetected disease

OUTCOME TARGET RATING: Maintain at_____   Increase to_____

		Never demonstrated	Rarely demonstrated	Sometimes demonstrated	Often demonstrated	Consistently demonstrated	
OUTCOME OVERALL RATING		1	2	3	4	5	
Indicators:							
163401	Acknowledges disease risk	1	2	3	4	5	NA
163402	Acknowledges need for screening	1	2	3	4	5	NA
163403	Describes timeframes for screening	1	2	3	4	5	NA
163404	Describes benefits of screening	1	2	3	4	5	NA
163405	Describes contraindications to specific screening	1	2	3	4	5	NA
163406	Maintains updated screening record	1	2	3	4	5	NA
163407	Schedules next screening	1	2	3	4	5	NA
163408	Obtains screening at recommended intervals	1	2	3	4	5	NA
163409	Obtains early screening based on family history as recommended by health professional	1	2	3	4	5	NA
163410	Obtains screening based on personal risk factors as recommended by health professional	1	2	3	4	5	NA
163411	Obtains screening for age recommended by experts	1	2	3	4	5	NA
163412	Obtains screening for occupational risk recommended by experts	1	2	3	4	5	NA

P

Personal Health Screening Behavior—cont'd

		Never demonstrated	Rarely demonstrated	Sometimes demonstrated	Often demonstrated	Consistently demonstrated	
163413	Obtains screening for travel recommended by experts	1	2	3	4	5	NA
163414	Obtains genetic screening as recommended by health professional	1	2	3	4	5	NA
163415	Identifies community resources for screening	1	2	3	4	5	NA
163416	Obtains results of screening	1	2	3	4	5	NA
163417	Obtains health care services following abnormal screening results	1	2	3	4	5	NA

Domain-*Health Knowledge & Behavior (IV)*   **Class**-*Health Behavior (Q)*   *5th edition 2013*

OUTCOME CONTENT REFERENCES:

Agency for Healthcare Research and Quality. (2007). Men: Stay healthy at any age—Your checklist for health (pub. No. 07-IP006-A). Rockville, MD: Author.

American Academy of Pediatrics. (1996). Eye examination and vision screening in infants, children, and young adults—Policy statement (reaffirmed 2003, 2007). *Pediatrics, 98*(1), 153–157.

American Academy of Pediatrics. (2005). Lead exposure in children: Prevention, detection, and management—Policy statement (reaffirmed 2009). *Pediatrics, 116*(4), 1036–1046.

American Academy of Pediatrics. (2006). Identifying infants and young children with developmental disorders in the medical home: An algorithm for developmental surveillance and screening—Policy statement (reaffirmed 2010). *Pediatrics, 118*(1), 405–420.

American Association of Clinical Endocrinologists. (2001). Guidelines for screening and managing diabetes in the United States of America. *Pan American Journal of Public Health, 10*(5), 358–360.

Chacko, M. R., Wiemann, C. M., & Smith, P. B. (2004). Chlamydia and gonorrhea screening in asymptomatic young women. *Journal of Pediatric & Adolescent Gynecology, 17*(3), 169–178.

Engberg, M., Christensen, B., Karlsmose, B., Lous, J., & Lauritzen, T. (2002). General health screenings to improve cardiovascular risk profiles: A randomized controlled trial in general practice with 5-year follow-up. *Journal of Family Practice, 51*(6), 546–552.

Floyd, K. (2003). Costs and effectiveness—The impact of economic studies on TB control. *Tuberculosis, 83*(1–3), 187–200.

Geller, A. C. (2002). Screening for melanoma. *Dermatologic Clinics, 20*(4), 629–640.

Kohl, K. S., Markowitz, L. E., & Koumans, E. H. (2003). Developments in the screening for Chlamydia trachomatis: A review. *Obstetrics and Gynecology Clinics of North America, 30*(4), 637–658.

Lavenson, G. S., Jr., Pantera, R. L., Garza, R. M., Neff, T., Rothwell, S. D., & Cisneros, J. (2004). Development and implementation of a rapid, accurate, and cost-effective protocol for national stroke prevention screening. *The American Journal of Surgery, 188*(6), 638–643.

Long, R., Houston, S., & Hershfield, E. (2003). Recommendations for screening and prevention of tuberculosis in patients with HIV and for screening for HIV in patients with tuberculosis and their contacts. *Canadian Medical Association Journal, 169*(8), 789–791.

Luby, J. L., Heffelfinger, A., Koenig-McNaught, A. L., Brown, K., & Spitznagel, E. (2004). The preschool feelings checklist: A brief and sensitive screening measure for depression in young children. *Journal of the American Academy of Child and Adolescent Psychiatry, 43*(6), 708–717.

Menon, U. (2004). Ovarian cancer screening. *Canadian Medical Association Journal, 171*(4), 323–324.

Mignogna, M. D., & Fedele, S. (2005). Oral cancer screening: 5 minutes to save a life. *Lancet, 356*(9475), 1905–1906.

P

Personal Health Status   **2006**

Definition: Overall physical, psychological, social, and spiritual functioning of an adult 18 years or older

OUTCOME TARGET RATING: Maintain at_____   Increase to_____

		Severely compromised	Substantially compromised	Moderately compromised	Mildly compromised	Not compromised	
OUTCOME OVERALL RATING		1	2	3	4	5	
Indicators:							
200601	Physical fitness	1	2	3	4	5	NA
200602	Mobility level	1	2	3	4	5	NA
200603	Energy level	1	2	3	4	5	NA
200604	Comfort level	1	2	3	4	5	NA
200605	Performance of activities of daily living	1	2	3	4	5	NA

Continued

Personal Health Status—cont'd

		Severely compromised	Substantially compromised	Moderately compromised	Mildly compromised	Not compromised	
200606	Performance of instrumental activities of daily living	1	2	3	4	5	NA
200607	Resistance to infection	1	2	3	4	5	NA
200608	Tissue healing	1	2	3	4	5	NA
200609	Sleep-rest pattern	1	2	3	4	5	NA
200610	Gastrointestinal function	1	2	3	4	5	NA
200611	Cardiac function	1	2	3	4	5	NA
200612	Peripheral tissue perfusion	1	2	3	4	5	NA
200613	Neurologic function	1	2	3	4	5	NA
200614	Pulmonary function	1	2	3	4	5	NA
200615	Kidney function	1	2	3	4	5	NA
200626	Sensory function	1	2	3	4	5	NA
200627	Sexual function	1	2	3	4	5	NA
200628	Endocrine function	1	2	3	4	5	NA
200616	Weight	1	2	3	4	5	NA
200617	Nutritional status	1	2	3	4	5	NA
200618	Cognitive status	1	2	3	4	5	NA
200619	Mental health	1	2	3	4	5	NA
200629	Symptom control	1	2	3	4	5	NA
200630	Pain control	1	2	3	4	5	NA
200620	Mood equilibrium	1	2	3	4	5	NA
200621	Spiritual life	1	2	3	4	5	NA
200622	Ability to cope	1	2	3	4	5	NA
200623	Adjustment to chronic conditions	1	2	3	4	5	NA
200631	Ability to communicate	1	2	3	4	5	NA
200624	Ability to express emotions	1	2	3	4	5	NA
200625	Social relationships	1	2	3	4	5	NA

P

Domain-Perceived Health (V)   **Class**-Health & Life Quality (U)   3rd edition 2004; revised 2008

OUTCOME CONTENT REFERENCES:

Bergner, M., Bobbit, R. A., Carter, W. B., & Gilson, B. S. (1981). The sickness impact profile: Development and final revision of a health status measure. *Medical Care, 19*(8), 787–805.

Kline, N. W. (1988). *Psychophysiological process of stress in people with a chronic physical illness* (doctoral dissertation). The University of Michigan, Ann Arbor, MI.

Mossberg, K., & McFarland, C. (2001). A patient-oriented health status measure in outpatient rehabilitation. *American Journal of Physical Medicine & Rehabilitation, 80*(12), 896–902.

Radosevich, D., & Pruitt, M. (1995). *Twelve-Item Health Status Questionnaire*. Bloomington, MN: Health Outcomes Institute.

Ware, J. E., & Sherbourne, C. D. (1992). The MOS 36-item short-form health survey (SF-36). I. Conceptual framework and item selection. *Medical Care, 30*(6), 473–483.

Personal Resiliency 1309

Definition: Positive adaptation and function of an individual following significant adversity or crisis

OUTCOME TARGET RATING: Maintain at_____   Increase to_____

		Never demonstrated	Rarely demonstrated	Sometimes demonstrated	Often demonstrated	Consistently demonstrated	
OUTCOME OVERALL RATING		1	2	3	4	5	
Indicators:							
130901	Verbalizes positive outlook	1	2	3	4	5	NA
130902	Uses effective coping strategies	1	2	3	4	5	NA
130903	Expresses emotions	1	2	3	4	5	NA
130904	Clarifies ambiguous communication	1	2	3	4	5	NA
130905	Communicates clearly and appropriately for age	1	2	3	4	5	NA
130906	Exhibits positive mood	1	2	3	4	5	NA
130907	Exhibits positive self-esteem	1	2	3	4	5	NA
130908	Expresses comfort with solitude	1	2	3	4	5	NA
130909	Expresses self-efficacy	1	2	3	4	5	NA
130910	Takes responsibility for own actions	1	2	3	4	5	NA
130911	Verbalizes an enhanced sense of control	1	2	3	4	5	NA
130912	Seeks emotional support	1	2	3	4	5	NA
130913	Weighs alternatives to problem-solving	1	2	3	4	5	NA
130914	Adapts to adversities as challenges	1	2	3	4	5	NA
130915	Proposes practical, constructive solutions for disputes	1	2	3	4	5	NA
130916	Makes progress toward goals	1	2	3	4	5	NA
130917	Uses strategies to promote safety	1	2	3	4	5	NA
130918	Uses strategies to avoid violent situations	1	2	3	4	5	NA
130919	Avoids drug misuse	1	2	3	4	5	NA
130920	Avoids alcohol misuse	1	2	3	4	5	NA
130921	Removes self from abusive relationships	1	2	3	4	5	NA
130922	Practices safe sex	1	2	3	4	5	NA
130923	Refrains from harming others	1	2	3	4	5	NA
130924	Identifies role models	1	2	3	4	5	NA
130925	Identifies available community resources	1	2	3	4	5	NA
130926	Uses available community resources	1	2	3	4	5	NA
130927	Uses available support groups	1	2	3	4	5	NA
130928	Participates in employment	1	2	3	4	5	NA
130929	Participates in curricular school activities	1	2	3	4	5	NA
130930	Participates in extracurricular school activities	1	2	3	4	5	NA
130931	Participates in community activities	1	2	3	4	5	NA
130932	Participates in leisure activities	1	2	3	4	5	NA
130933	Uses educational and vocational resources	1	2	3	4	5	NA
130934	Verbalizes readiness to learn	1	2	3	4	5	NA

P

***Domain**-Psychosocial Health (III)*   ***Class**-Psychosocial Adaptation (N)*   *4th edition 2008*

OUTCOME CONTENT REFERENCES:

Fergus, S., & Zimmerman, M. A. (2005). Adolescent resilience: A framework for understanding healthy development in the face of risk. *Annual Review of Public Health, 26*(1), 399–419.

Gorman, C., Dale, S. S., Grossman, W., Klarreich, K., McDowell, J., & Whitaker, L. (2005). The importance of resilience. *Time, 165*(3), A52–A55.

Luthar, S. S., & Cicchetti, D. (2000). The construct of resilience: A critical evaluation and guidelines for future work. *Child Development, 71*(3), 543–562.

Luthar, S. S., & Cicchetti, D. (2000). The construct of resilience: Implications for interventions and social policies. *Development and Psychopathology, 12*(4), 857–885.

Masten, A. S. (2001). Ordinary magic. Resilience processes in development. *American Psychologist, 56*(3), 227–238.

Masten, A. S., Hubbard, J. J., Gest, S. D., Tellegen, A., Garmezy, N., & Ramirez, M. (1999). Competence in the context of adversity: Pathways to resilience and maladaptation from childhood to late adolescence. *Development and Psychopathology, 11*(1), 143–169.

Rogers, S. K., Muir, K., & Evenson, C. R. (2003). Signs of resilience: Assets that support deaf adults' success in bridging the deaf and hearing worlds. *American Annals of the Deaf, 148*(3), 222–232.

Sinclair, V. G., & Wallston, K. A. (2004). The development and psychometric evaluation of the brief resilient coping scale. *Assessment, 11*(1), 94–101.

Personal Safety Behavior 1911

Definition: Personal actions to prevent unintentional physical injury to self

OUTCOME TARGET RATING: Maintain at_____   Increase to_____

		Never demonstrated	Rarely demonstrated	Sometimes demonstrated	Often demonstrated	Consistently demonstrated	
OUTCOME OVERALL RATING		1	2	3	4	5	
Indicators:							
191102	Stores food to minimize spoilage	1	2	3	4	5	NA
191103	Prepares food to minimize contamination	1	2	3	4	5	NA
191132	Uses strategies to prevent suffocation	1	2	3	4	5	NA
191133	Uses strategies to prevent aspiration	1	2	3	4	5	NA
191104	Uses protective helmet during high-risk activities	1	2	3	4	5	NA
191134	Uses protective gear during high-risk activities	1	2	3	4	5	NA
191105	Uses seat belt	1	2	3	4	5	NA
191106	Selects appropriate clothing for activity	1	2	3	4	5	NA
191127	Uses strategies to protect from sun exposure	1	2	3	4	5	NA
191128	Uses proper body mechanics	1	2	3	4	5	NA
191107	Uses assistive devices correctly	1	2	3	4	5	NA
191108	Practices safe leisure activities	1	2	3	4	5	NA
191109	Practices safe sexual behaviors	1	2	3	4	5	NA
191135	Practices firearm safety	1	2	3	4	5	NA
191110	Uses tools correctly	1	2	3	4	5	NA
191111	Uses machinery correctly	1	2	3	4	5	NA
191136	Avoids allergens	1	2	3	4	5	NA
191137	Uses strategies to avoid environmental contaminants	1	2	3	4	5	NA
191113	Avoids recreational drug use	1	2	3	4	5	NA
191129	Follows medication precautions	1	2	3	4	5	NA
191117	Avoids tobacco use	1	2	3	4	5	NA
191123	Avoids smoking in bed	1	2	3	4	5	NA
191124	Uses precautions with flammable material	1	2	3	4	5	NA
191118	Avoids alcohol misuse	1	2	3	4	5	NA
191125	Avoids operating motor vehicle when using alcohol	1	2	3	4	5	NA
191130	Avoids operating motor vehicle when using substances that impair function	1	2	3	4	5	NA
191131	Uses strategies to prevent communicable diseases	1	2	3	4	5	NA
191119	Avoids high-risk behaviors	1	2	3	4	5	NA
191120	Observes rules of the road	1	2	3	4	5	NA

Personal Safety Behavior—*cont'd*

	Never demonstrated	Rarely demonstrated	Sometimes demonstrated	Often demonstrated	Consistently demonstrated	
191138 Uses personal emergency response system	1	2	3	4	5	NA
191139 Seeks safety information related to environment	1	2	3	4	5	NA

Domain-Health Knowledge & Behavior (IV) *Class*-Risk Control & Safety (T) *1st edition 1997; revised 2004, 2008, 2013*

OUTCOME CONTENT REFERENCES:
+Hettler, B. (1982). Wellness promotion and risk reduction on a university campus. In M. Faber & A. Reinhardt (Eds.), *Promoting health through risk reduction.* New York: Macmillan.
Sorock, G. S. (1988). Falls among the elderly: Epidemiology and prevention. *American Journal of Preventive Medicine, 4*(5), 252–255.
Weitzel, E. (2001). Unilateral neglect. In M. Maas, K. Buckwalter, M. Hardy, T. Tripp-Reimer, M. Titler, & J. Specht (Eds.), *Nursing care of older adults: Diagnoses, outcomes & interventions* (pp. 492–502). St. Louis: Mosby.

Personal Time Management   1635

Definition: Personal actions to complete commitments within an expected timeframe with minimum stress

OUTCOME TARGET RATING: Maintain at_____   Increase to_____

	Never demonstrated	Rarely demonstrated	Sometimes demonstrated	Often demonstrated	Consistently demonstrated	
OUTCOME OVERALL RATING	1	2	3	4	5	
Indicators:						
163501 Prioritizes commitments	1	2	3	4	5	NA
163502 Sets short-term goals	1	2	3	4	5	NA
163503 Sets long-term goals	1	2	3	4	5	NA
163504 Identifies realistic timeframe for each activity	1	2	3	4	5	NA
163505 Sets time for completion of commitments	1	2	3	4	5	NA
163506 Manages commitments within set timeframe	1	2	3	4	5	NA
163507 Balances competing demands	1	2	3	4	5	NA
163508 Monitors progress of multiple commitments	1	2	3	4	5	NA
163509 Plans activities by the week	1	2	3	4	5	NA
163510 Constructs a to-do list	1	2	3	4	5	NA
163511 Keeps reminders in an organized system	1	2	3	4	5	NA
163512 Delegates activities	1	2	3	4	5	NA
163513 Monitors completion of delegated activities	1	2	3	4	5	NA
163514 Defers activities appropriately	1	2	3	4	5	NA
163515 Minimizes interruptions	1	2	3	4	5	NA
163516 Breaks complex activities into manageable activities	1	2	3	4	5	NA
163517 Uses strategies to prevent feeling overwhelmed	1	2	3	4	5	NA
163518 Uses strategies to reduce anxiety	1	2	3	4	5	NA
163519 Reassesses commitment priorities	1	2	3	4	5	NA
163520 Maintains organization within personal space	1	2	3	4	5	NA
163521 Uses strategies to manage work load	1	2	3	4	5	NA
163522 Reports low level of stress	1	2	3	4	5	NA

Domain-Health Knowledge & Behavior (IV) *Class*-Health Behavior (Q) *5th edition 2013*

OUTCOME CONTENT REFERENCES:
Allen, D. (2001). *Getting things done: The art of stress-free productivity*. London: Penguin Books
Cohen, S., & Williamson, G. M. (1988). Perceived stress in a probability sample of the United States. In S. Spacapan & S. Oskamp (Eds.), *The social psychology of health*. Newbury Park, CA: Sage.
Johnson, S. (September 2004). Organizing your work and time. *Academic Physician & Scientist*, pp. 2–3.

Personal Well-Being   2002

Definition: Extent of positive perception of one's current health status

OUTCOME TARGET RATING: Maintain at_____   Increase to_____

	Not at all satisfied	Somewhat satisfied	Moderately satisfied	Very satisfied	Completely satisfied	
OUTCOME OVERALL RATING	1	2	3	4	5	
Indicators:						
200201 Performance of activities of daily living	1	2	3	4	5	NA
200212 Performance of usual roles	1	2	3	4	5	NA
200202 Psychological health	1	2	3	4	5	NA
200203 Social relationships	1	2	3	4	5	NA
200204 Spiritual life	1	2	3	4	5	NA
200205 Physical health	1	2	3	4	5	NA
200206 Cognitive status	1	2	3	4	5	NA
200207 Ability to cope	1	2	3	4	5	NA
200208 Ability to relax	1	2	3	4	5	NA
200209 Level of happiness	1	2	3	4	5	NA
200210 Ability to express emotions	1	2	3	4	5	NA
200213 Ability to control activities	1	2	3	4	5	NA
200214 Opportunities for health care choice(s)	1	2	3	4	5	NA

Domain-Perceived Health (V)   **Class**-Health & Life Quality (U)   *1st edition 1997; revised 2004, 2008, 2013*

OUTCOME CONTENT REFERENCES:
Davidhizar, R. E., & Giger, J. N. (2001). Powerlessness. In M. Maas, K. Buckwalter, M. Hardy, T. Tripp-Reimer, M. Titler, & J. Specht (Eds.), *Nursing care of older adults: Diagnoses, outcomes & interventions* (pp. 562–570). St. Louis: Mosby.
+Dupuy, H. (1984). The Psychological General Well-Being (PGWB) Index. In N. K. Wenger, M. E. Mattson, C. D. Furberg, & J. Elinson (Eds.), *Assessment of quality of life in clinical trials of cardiovascular therapies* (pp. 170–183, 353–356). Greenwich, CT: Le Jacq.
Ferrell, B., Grant, M., Schmidt, G. M., Rhiner, M., Whitehead, C. P., & Forman, S. J. (1992). The meaning of quality of life for bone marrow transplant survivors. Part 1. *Cancer Nursing, 15*(3), 153–160.
Ferrell, B. R., Dow, K. H., Leigh, S., Ly, J., & Gulasekaram, P. (1995). Quality of life in long-term cancer survivors. *Oncology Nursing Forum, 22*(6), 915–922.
Kozier, B., Erb, G., & Blais, K. (1992). *Concepts and issues in nursing practice* (2nd ed.). Redwood City, CA: Addison-Wesley Nursing.
+Revicki, D. A., Leidy, N. K., & Howland, L. (1996). Evaluating the psychometric characteristics of the Psychological General Well-Being Index with a new response scale. *Quality of Life Research, 5*(4), 419–425.
Stewart, A., Ware, J., Jr., Sherbourne, C., & Wells, K. (1992). Psychological distress/well-being and cognitive functioning measures. In A. Stewart & J. Ware, Jr. (Eds.), *Measuring functioning and well-being: The medical outcomes study approach* (pp. 102–142). Durham, NC: Duke University Press.
Waterman, J. D., Blegen, M., Clinton, P., & Specht, J. P. (2001). Social isolation. In M. Maas, K. Buckwalter, M. Hardy, T. Tripp-Reimer, M. Titler, & J. Specht (Eds.), *Nursing care of older adults: Diagnoses, outcomes & interventions* (pp. 651–663). St. Louis: Mosby.
Whedon, M., & Ferrell, B. R. (1994). Quality of life in adult bone marrow transplant patients: Beyond the first year. *Seminars in Oncology Nursing, 10*(1), 42–57.

Physical Aging 0113

Definition: Normal physiological changes that occur with the natural aging process

OUTCOME TARGET RATING: Maintain at_____   Increase to_____

		Severe deviation from normal range	Substantial deviation from normal range	Moderate deviation from normal range	Mild deviation from normal range	No deviation from normal range	
OUTCOME OVERALL RATING		1	2	3	4	5	
Indicators:							
011318	Memory	1	2	3	4	5	NA
011319	Cognitive status	1	2	3	4	5	NA
011301	Mean body mass	1	2	3	4	5	NA
011302	Bone density	1	2	3	4	5	NA
011303	Cardiac output	1	2	3	4	5	NA
011304	Vital capacity	1	2	3	4	5	NA
011305	Blood pressure	1	2	3	4	5	NA
011306	Skin elasticity	1	2	3	4	5	NA
011307	Muscle strength	1	2	3	4	5	NA
011320	Joint mobility	1	2	3	4	5	NA
011321	Sensory acuity	1	2	3	4	5	NA
011322	Bladder muscle tone	1	2	3	4	5	NA
011324	Bowel control	1	2	3	4	5	NA
011323	Resistance to infection	1	2	3	4	5	NA
011308	Hearing acuity	1	2	3	4	5	NA
011309	Visual acuity	1	2	3	4	5	NA
011310	Olfactory acuity	1	2	3	4	5	NA
011311	Taste acuity	1	2	3	4	5	NA
011312	Basal metabolic rate	1	2	3	4	5	NA
011313	Fat distribution pattern	1	2	3	4	5	NA
011314	Hair distribution pattern	1	2	3	4	5	NA
011315	Menstrual pattern	1	2	3	4	5	NA
011316	Sexual functioning	1	2	3	4	5	NA

Domain-Functional Health (I)   **Class-**Growth & Development (B)   *1st edition 1997; revised 2004, 2013*

P

OUTCOME CONTENT REFERENCES:

Bemben, M. G., & McCalip, G. A. (1999). Strength and power relationships as a function of age. *Journal of Strength & Conditioning Research, 13*(4), 330–338.

Kennedy-Malone, L., Fletcher, K. R., & Plank, L. M. (Eds.). (2000). *Management guidelines for gerontological nurse practitioners* (pp. 3–24, 536–553). Philadelphia: F. A. Davis.

McWhorter, J. W., & Schuerman, S. E. (2002). Balance and aging. *Orthopaedic Physical Therapy Clinics of North America, 11*(1), 111–130.

Rice, F. P. (2001). *Human development: A life-span approach.* Upper Saddle River, NJ: Prentice Hall.

Schuster, C., & Ashburn, S. (1992). *The process of human development: A holistic approach* (3rd ed.). Philadelphia: J. B. Lippincott.

Wong, A. M., Lin, Y., Chou, S., Tang, F., & Wong, P. (2001). Coordination exercise and postural stability in elderly people: Effect of Tai Chi Chuan. *Archives of Physical Medicine & Rehabilitation, 82*(5), 608–612.

Physical Fitness 2004

Definition: Performance of physical activities with vigor

OUTCOME TARGET RATING: Maintain at_____ Increase to_____

	Severely compromised	Substantially compromised	Moderately compromised	Mildly compromised	Not compromised	
OUTCOME OVERALL RATING	1	2	3	4	5	
Indicators:						
200401 Muscle strength	1	2	3	4	5	NA
200402 Muscle endurance	1	2	3	4	5	NA
200403 Joint flexibility	1	2	3	4	5	NA
200404 Performance of physical activities	1	2	3	4	5	NA
200405 Performance of routine exercise	1	2	3	4	5	NA
200406 Cardiovascular function	1	2	3	4	5	NA
200407 Respiratory function	1	2	3	4	5	NA
200408 Aerobic fitness	1	2	3	4	5	NA
200409 Body mass index	1	2	3	4	5	NA
200410 Waist to hip ratio	1	2	3	4	5	NA
200411 Blood pressure	1	2	3	4	5	NA
200412 Target heart rate during exercise	1	2	3	4	5	NA
200414 Resting heart rate	1	2	3	4	5	NA

Domain-Perceived Health (V)   **Class**-Health & Life Quality (U)   2nd edition 2000; revised 2004

OUTCOME CONTENT REFERENCES:

American College of Sports Medicine. (2000). *Guidelines for exercise testing and prescription* (6th ed.). Baltimore: Williams & Wilkins.

Brown, M., Sinacore, D. R., Ehsani, A. A., Binder, E. F., Holloszy, J. O., & Kohrt, W. M. (2000). Low-intensity exercise as a modifier of physical frailty in older adults. *Archives of Physical Medicine & Rehabilitation, 81*(7), 960–965.

Cauderay, M., Narring, F., & Michaud, P. (2000). A cross-sectional survey assessing physical fitness of 9- to 19-year-old girls and boys in Switzerland. *Pediatric Exercise Science, 12*(4), 398–412.

Haskell, W. L., Lee, I., Pate, R. R., Powell, K. E., Blair, S. N., Franklin, B. A., Macera, C. A., Heath, G. W., Thompson, P. D., & Bauman, A. (2007). Physical activity and public health. Updated recommendation for adults from the American College of Sports Medicine and the American Heart Association. *Medicine & Science in Sports & Exercise, 39*(8), 1423–1434.

NIH Consensus Development Panel on Physical Activity and Cardiovascular Health. (1996). Physical activity and cardiovascular health. *Journal of the American Medical Association, 276*(3), 241–246.

U.S. Department of Health and Human Services. (1991). *Healthy people 2000: National health promotion and disease prevention objectives.* (DHHS Pub No [PHS] 91-50012). Washington, DC: U.S. Government Printing Office.

U.S. Department of Health and Human Services. (2000). *Healthy people 2010.* Washington, DC: U.S. Government Printing Office.

P

Physical Injury Severity 1913

Definition: Severity of signs and symptoms of bodily injuries

OUTCOME TARGET RATING: Maintain at_____ Increase to_____

	Severe	Substantial	Moderate	Mild	None	
OUTCOME OVERALL RATING	1	2	3	4	5	
Indicators:						
191301 Skin abrasions	1	2	3	4	5	NA
191302 Bruises	1	2	3	4	5	NA
191303 Lacerations	1	2	3	4	5	NA
191304 Burns	1	2	3	4	5	NA
191305 Extremity sprains	1	2	3	4	5	NA
191306 Back sprains	1	2	3	4	5	NA
191307 Extremity fractures	1	2	3	4	5	NA
191308 Pelvic fractures	1	2	3	4	5	NA

Physical Injury Severity—*cont'd*

	Severe	Substantial	Moderate	Mild	None	
191309	Hip fractures	1	2	3	4	5	NA
191310	Spinal fractures	1	2	3	4	5	NA
191311	Cranial fractures	1	2	3	4	5	NA
191312	Facial fractures	1	2	3	4	5	NA
191313	Dental injuries	1	2	3	4	5	NA
191314	Open head injuries	1	2	3	4	5	NA
191315	Closed head injuries	1	2	3	4	5	NA
191316	Impaired mobility	1	2	3	4	5	NA
191319	Impaired cognition	1	2	3	4	5	NA
191320	Decreased level of consciousness	1	2	3	4	5	NA
191321	Liver contusion	1	2	3	4	5	NA
191322	Ruptured spleen	1	2	3	4	5	NA
191323	Hemorrhage	1	2	3	4	5	NA
191324	Abdominal trauma	1	2	3	4	5	NA

Domain-*Health Knowledge & Behavior (IV)*   **Class**-*Risk Control & Safety (T)*   *1st edition 1997; revised 2004, 2008, 2013*

OUTCOME CONTENT REFERENCES:
Lawrence, J. I., & Maher, P. L. (1992). An interdisciplinary falls consult team: A collaborative approach to patient falls. *Journal of Nursing Care Quality, 6*(3), 21–29.
Llewellyn, J., Martin, B., Shekleton, M., & Firlit, S. (1988). Analysis of falls in the acute surgical and cardiovascular surgical patient. *Applied Nursing Research, 1*(3), 116–121.
+Maas, M., Swanson, E., Buckwalter, K. C., Specht, J. P., Tripp-Reimer, T., Lenth, R., Tranel, D., Reed, D., Broffit, B., Brenneman, D., Peters, J., Rose, D., Kelley, L., Schutte, D. L., & Sun, C. (1999). *Final report: Nursing interventions for Alzheimer's: Family role trials* (NINR R01-NR01689). Rockville, MD: National Institutes of Health.

Physical Maturation: Female   0114

Definition: Normal physical changes in the female that occur with the transition from childhood to adulthood

OUTCOME TARGET RATING: Maintain at_____   Increase to_____

		Severe deviation from normal range	Substantial deviation from normal range	Moderate deviation from normal range	Mild deviation from normal range	No deviation from normal range	
OUTCOME OVERALL RATING		1	2	3	4	5	
Indicators:							
011401	Growth spurt between 9.5-14.5 years of age	1	2	3	4	5	NA
011402	Bone closure	1	2	3	4	5	NA
011403	Voice changes	1	2	3	4	5	NA
011404	Adult hair distribution	1	2	3	4	5	NA
011405	Breast development	1	2	3	4	5	NA
011406	Menstruation onset	1	2	3	4	5	NA
011407	Increased muscle mass	1	2	3	4	5	NA
011408	Decreased body fat	1	2	3	4	5	NA
011409	Increased sebaceous secretions	1	2	3	4	5	NA
011410	Increased perspiration	1	2	3	4	5	NA

Domain-*Functional Health (I)*   **Class**-*Growth & Development (B)*   *1st edition 1997; revised 2004*

P

OUTCOME CONTENT REFERENCES:
Hockenberry, M. J., Wilson, D., Winkelstein, M. L., & Kline, N. E. (2003). *Wong's nursing care of infants and children* (7th ed.). St. Louis: Mosby.
Rice, F. P. (2001). *Human development: A life-span approach.* Upper Saddle River, NJ: Prentice Hall.
Schuster, C., & Ashburn, S. (1992). *The process of human development: A holistic approach* (3rd ed.). Philadelphia: J. B. Lippincott.

Physical Maturation: Male   **0115**

Definition: Normal physical changes in the male that occur with the transition from childhood to adulthood

OUTCOME TARGET RATING: Maintain at_____   Increase to_____

		Severe deviation from normal range	Substantial deviation from normal range	Moderate deviation from normal range	Mild deviation from normal range	No deviation from normal range	
OUTCOME OVERALL RATING		1	2	3	4	5	
Indicators:							
011501	Growth spurt between 10.5-16 years of age	1	2	3	4	5	NA
011502	Bone closure	1	2	3	4	5	NA
011503	Voice changes	1	2	3	4	5	NA
011504	Adult hair distribution	1	2	3	4	5	NA
011505	Testicular descent	1	2	3	4	5	NA
011506	Penis enlargement	1	2	3	4	5	NA
011507	First ejaculation of sperm (wet dream)	1	2	3	4	5	NA
011508	Increased muscle mass	1	2	3	4	5	NA
011509	Decreased body fat	1	2	3	4	5	NA
011510	Increased sebaceous secretions	1	2	3	4	5	NA
011511	Increased perspiration	1	2	3	4	5	NA

Domain-*Functional Health (I)*   **Class**-*Growth & Development (B)*   *1st edition 1997; revised 2004*

OUTCOME CONTENT REFERENCES:
Hockenberry, M. J., Wilson, D., Winkelstein, M. L., & Kline, N. E. (2003). *Wong's nursing care of infants and children* (7th ed.). St. Louis: Mosby.
Rice, F. P. (2001). *Human development: A life-span approach.* Upper Saddle River, NJ: Prentice Hall.
Schuster, C., & Ashburn, S. (1992). *The process of human development: A holistic approach* (3rd ed.). Philadelphia: J. B. Lippincott.

P

Play Participation   **0116**

Definition: Use of activities by a child from 1 year through 11 years of age to promote enjoyment, entertainment, and development

OUTCOME TARGET RATING: Maintain at_____   Increase to_____

		Never demonstrated	Rarely demonstrated	Sometimes demonstrated	Often demonstrated	Consistently demonstrated	
OUTCOME OVERALL RATING		1	2	3	4	5	
Indicators:							
011601	Participates in play activities	1	2	3	4	5	NA
011610	Expresses satisfaction with play activities	1	2	3	4	5	NA
011603	Enjoys play activities	1	2	3	4	5	NA
011604	Uses social skills during play activities	1	2	3	4	5	NA
011605	Uses physical skills during play activities	1	2	3	4	5	NA
011606	Uses imagination during play activities	1	2	3	4	5	NA
011607	Expresses emotions during play activities	1	2	3	4	5	NA
011608	Uses role playing	1	2	3	4	5	NA

Domain-*Functional Health (I)*   **Class**-*Growth & Development (B)*   *1st edition 1997; revised 2004*

OUTCOME CONTENT REFERENCES:

Gillis, A. J. (1989). The effect of play on immobilized children in hospital. *International Journal of Nursing Studies, 26*(3), 261–269.

Gray, E. (1989). The emotional and play needs of the dying child. *Issues in Comprehensive Pediatric Nursing, 12*(2/3), 207–224.

Jack, L. W. (1987). Using play in psychiatric rehabilitation. *Journal of Psychosocial Nursing, 25*(7), 17–20.

Post, C. (1990). Play therapy with an abused child: A case study. *Journal of Child and Adolescent Psychiatric and Mental Health Nursing, 2*(2), 48–51.

Postpartum Maternal Health Behavior   1624

Definition: Personal actions to promote health of a mother in the period following birth of infant

OUTCOME TARGET RATING: Maintain at_____   Increase to_____

		Never demonstrated	Rarely demonstrated	Sometimes demonstrated	Often demonstrated	Consistently demonstrated	
OUTCOME OVERALL RATING		1	2	3	4	5	
Indicators:							
162401	Adapts to maternal role	1	2	3	4	5	NA
162402	Bonds with infant	1	2	3	4	5	NA
162403	Checks uterine fundus	1	2	3	4	5	NA
162404	Monitors lochia changes	1	2	3	4	5	NA
162405	Maintains perineum care	1	2	3	4	5	NA
162406	Maintains care of surgical incision	1	2	3	4	5	NA
162407	Maintains care of episiotomy	1	2	3	4	5	NA
162408	Monitors discomfort from episiotomy	1	2	3	4	5	NA
162409	Monitors for signs and symptoms of infection	1	2	3	4	5	NA
162410	Monitors for signs of postpartum depression	1	2	3	4	5	NA
162411	Monitors for nipple tenderness	1	2	3	4	5	NA
162412	Monitors breasts for engorgement	1	2	3	4	5	NA
162413	Monitors for stress incontinence	1	2	3	4	5	NA
162414	Monitors for development of new health problems	1	2	3	4	5	NA
162415	Uses water-based vaginal lubricant	1	2	3	4	5	NA
162416	Obtains health care when warning signs occur	1	2	3	4	5	NA
162417	Uses effective pain management strategies	1	2	3	4	5	NA
162418	Uses stress management techniques	1	2	3	4	5	NA
162419	Monitors anxiety level	1	2	3	4	5	NA
162420	Monitors comfort status	1	2	3	4	5	NA
162421	Maintains adequate nutrient intake	1	2	3	4	5	NA
162422	Maintains adequate fluid intake	1	2	3	4	5	NA
162423	Participates in regular exercise	1	2	3	4	5	NA
162424	Performs pelvic floor exercises	1	2	3	4	5	NA
162425	Balances activity and rest	1	2	3	4	5	NA
162426	Monitors sleep patterns	1	2	3	4	5	NA
162427	Uses strategies to obtain needed sleep	1	2	3	4	5	NA
162428	Obtains assistance from health professional for depression as needed	1	2	3	4	5	NA
162429	Discusses options for birth control with health professional	1	2	3	4	5	NA
162430	Follows recommendations for sexual activity restrictions	1	2	3	4	5	NA
162431	Obtains assistance from health professional as needed	1	2	3	4	5	NA
162432	Uses family support	1	2	3	4	5	NA
162433	Uses available support groups	1	2	3	4	5	NA
162434	Participates in postpartum checkups	1	2	3	4	5	NA

P

Domain-*Health Knowledge & Behavior (IV)*   **Class**-*Health Behavior (Q)*   *4th edition 2008*

OUTCOME CONTENT REFERENCES:

Borders, N. (2006). After the afterbirth: A critical review of postpartum health relative to method of delivery. *American College of Nurse-Midwives, 51*(4), 242–248.

Geoghegan, A. H. (2006). Not just an option: Postpartum depression screening becomes law in the state of New Jersey. *Nursing Spectrum—New York & New Jersey Edition, 18A*(20), 8–9.

Piejko, E. (2006). The postpartum visit: Why wait 6 weeks? *Australian Family Physician, 35*(9), 674–678.

Wisner, K. L., Chambers, C., & Sit, D. Y. (2006). Postpartum depression: A major public health problem. *Journal of the American Medical Association, 296*(21), 2616–2618.

Post-Procedure Recovery   2303

Definition: Extent to which an individual returns to baseline function following a procedure or minor surgery requiring anesthesia or sedation

OUTCOME TARGET RATING: Maintain at_____   Increase to_____

		Severe deviation from normal range	Substantial deviation from normal range	Moderate deviation from normal range	Mild deviation from normal range	No deviation from normal range	
OUTCOME OVERALL RATING		1	2	3	4	5	
Indicators:							
230301	Patent airway	1	2	3	4	5	NA
230328	Apical heart rate	1	2	3	4	5	NA
230302	Spontaneous respirations	1	2	3	4	5	NA
230303	Respiratory rate	1	2	3	4	5	NA
230304	Depth of inspiration	1	2	3	4	5	NA
230305	Forceful cough	1	2	3	4	5	NA
230306	Oxygen saturation 92-94% room air	1	2	3	4	5	NA
230307	Systolic blood pressure	1	2	3	4	5	NA
230329	Diastolic blood pressure	1	2	3	4	5	NA
230308	Aldrete score	1	2	3	4	5	NA
230309	Gag reflex	1	2	3	4	5	NA
230310	Swallowing ability	1	2	3	4	5	NA
230311	Retains oral fluids	1	2	3	4	5	NA
230312	Answers questions	1	2	3	4	5	NA
230313	Fully awake	1	2	3	4	5	NA
230314	Moves extremities on command	1	2	3	4	5	NA
230315	Ambulation tolerance	1	2	3	4	5	NA
230330	Body temperature	1	2	3	4	5	NA
230318	Voiding	1	2	3	4	5	NA
230317	Urine output	1	2	3	4	5	NA
230325	Fluid balance	1	2	3	4	5	NA
230326	Electrolyte and acid/base balance	1	2	3	4	5	NA
230327	Wound tissue perfusion	1	2	3	4	5	NA
230331	Amount of drainage from wound drains/tubes	1	2	3	4	5	NA
230332	Amount of drainage on dressing	1	2	3	4	5	NA
		Severe	Substantial	Moderate	Mild	None	
230333	Bleeding	1	2	3	4	5	NA
230321	Nausea	1	2	3	4	5	NA
230322	Vomiting	1	2	3	4	5	NA
230323	Shivering	1	2	3	4	5	NA
230324	Pain	1	2	3	4	5	NA

Domain-Physiologic Health (II)   **Class**-Therapeutic Response (AA)   *3rd edition 2004; revised 2008, 2013*

OUTCOME CONTENT REFERENCES:

Aldrete, J. A. (1998). Modifications to the postanesthesia score for use in ambulatory surgery. *Journal of PeriAnesthesia Nursing, 13*(3), 148–155.

Aldrete J. A., & Kroulik, D. (1970). A postanesthetic recovery score. *Anesthesia & Analgesia, 49*(6), 924–934.

American Society of Anesthesiologists Task Force on Sedation and Analgesia by Non-Anesthesiologists. (2002). Practice guidelines for sedation and analgesia by non-anesthesiologists. *Anesthesiology, 96*(4), 1004–1017.

Craney, J. M., & Gorman, L. N. (1997). Conscious sedation and implantable devices. Safe and effective sedation during pacemaker and implantable cardioverter defibrillator placement. *Critical Care Nursing Clinics of North America, 9*(3), 325–334.

Cohen, S. E., Hamilton, C. L., Riley, E. T., Walker, D. S., Macario, A., & Halpern, J. W. (1998). Obstetric postanesthesia care unit stays: Reevaluation of discharge criteria after regional anesthesia. *Anesthesiology, 89*(6), 1559–1565.

Gross, J. B., Bailey, P. L., Caplan, R. A., Connis, R. T., Cote, C. J., Davis, F. G., Epstein, B. S., Kapur, P. A., Zerwas, J. M., & Zuccaro, G. (1996). Practice guidelines for sedation and analgesia by non-anesthesiologists. *Anesthesiology, 84*(2), 459–471.

Piper, S. N., Suttner, S. W., Schmidt, C. C., Maleck, W. H., Kumle, B., & Boldt, J. (1999). Nefopam and clonidine in the prevention of postanaesthetic shivering. *Anaesthesia, 54*(7), 695–699.

Premenstrual Syndrome (PMS) Severity 2105

Definition: Severity of reported and adverse physical and emotional responses due to cyclic hormonal fluctuations

OUTCOME TARGET RATING: Maintain at_____   Increase to_____

OUTCOME OVERALL RATING	Severe 1	Substantial 2	Moderate 3	Mild 4	None 5	
Indicators:						
210501 Abdominal bloating	1	2	3	4	5	NA
210502 Abdominal cramps	1	2	3	4	5	NA
210503 Disrupted bowel patterns	1	2	3	4	5	NA
210504 Decreased urine output	1	2	3	4	5	NA
210505 Acne	1	2	3	4	5	NA
210506 Anxiety	1	2	3	4	5	NA
210507 Backache	1	2	3	4	5	NA
210508 Breast tenderness	1	2	3	4	5	NA
210509 Decreased energy	1	2	3	4	5	NA
210510 Depression	1	2	3	4	5	NA
210511 Fluid retention	1	2	3	4	5	NA
210512 Food cravings	1	2	3	4	5	NA
210513 Headaches	1	2	3	4	5	NA
210514 Insomnia	1	2	3	4	5	NA
210515 Irritability	1	2	3	4	5	NA
210516 Mood swings	1	2	3	4	5	NA
210517 Nausea	1	2	3	4	5	NA
210518 Vertigo	1	2	3	4	5	NA
210519 Vomiting	1	2	3	4	5	NA

P

Domain-*Perceived Health (V)*   **Class**-*Symptom Status (V)*   2nd edition 2000; revised 2004, 2013

OUTCOME CONTENT REFERENCES:

Alexander, L. L., & LaRosa, J. (1994). *New dimensions in women's health.* Sudbury, MA: Jones and Bartlett.

Carter, J., & Verhoef, M. J. (1994). Efficacy of self-help and alternative treatments of premenstrual syndrome. *Women's Health Issues, 4*(3), 130–137.

Fogel, C. I., & Woods, N. F. (Eds.). (1995). *Women's health care: A comprehensive handbook.* Thousand Oaks, CA: Sage.

Freeman, E. W., Kroll, R., Rapkin, A., Pearlstein, T., Brown, C., Parsey, K., Zhang, P., Patel, H., & Foegh, M. (2001). Evaluation of a unique oral contraceptive in the treatment of premenstrual dysphoric disorder. *Journal of Women's Health & Gender-Based Medicine, 10*(6), 561–569.

Lewis, L. L. (1995). One year in the life of a woman with premenstrual syndrome: A case study. *Nursing Research, 44*(2), 111–116.

Mitchell, E. S., Woods, N. F., & Lentz, M. J. (1994). Differentiation of women with three premenstrual symptom patterns. *Nursing Research, 43*(1), 25–30.

Richards, M., Rubinow, D. R., Daly, R. C., & Schmidt, P. J. (2006). Premenstrual symptoms and perimenopausal depression. *American Journal of Psychiatry, 163*(1), 133–137.

Taylor, D. L. (1994). Evaluating therapeutic change in symptom severity at the level of the individual woman experiencing severe PMS. *Image—The Journal of Nursing Scholarship, 26*(1), 25–33.

Woods, N. F., Lentz, M., Mitchell, E., Taylor, D., & Lee, K. (1986). *The daily health diary. The prevalence of PMS: Final report* (NV01054). Washington, DC: Division of Nursing, U.S. Public Health Services, U.S. Department of Health and Human Services.

Woods, N. F., Mitchell, E. S., & Lentz, M. F. (1995). Social pathways to premenstrual symptoms. *Research in Nursing & Health, 18*(3), 225–237.

Prenatal Health Behavior

1607

Definition: Personal actions to promote a healthy pregnancy and a healthy newborn

OUTCOME TARGET RATING: Maintain at_____ Increase to_____

OUTCOME OVERALL RATING	Never demonstrated	Rarely demonstrated	Sometimes demonstrated	Often demonstrated	Consistently demonstrated	
	1	2	3	4	5	
Indicators:						
160701 Maintains healthy preconceptual state	1	2	3	4	5	NA
160702 Uses proper body mechanics	1	2	3	4	5	NA
160703 Keeps appointments for prenatal care	1	2	3	4	5	NA
160704 Maintains healthy weight gain pattern	1	2	3	4	5	NA
160705 Receives proper dental care	1	2	3	4	5	NA
160706 Uses motor vehicle safety devices correctly	1	2	3	4	5	NA
160707 Attends childbirth education classes	1	2	3	4	5	NA
160709 Participates in regular exercise	1	2	3	4	5	NA
160710 Maintains adequate nutrient intake for pregnancy	1	2	3	4	5	NA
160711 Practices safe sex	1	2	3	4	5	NA
160721 Uses medication as prescribed	1	2	3	4	5	NA
160712 Consults health professional about non-prescription medication use	1	2	3	4	5	NA
160713 Avoids environmental hazards	1	2	3	4	5	NA
160714 Avoids exposure to infectious diseases	1	2	3	4	5	NA
160715 Avoids recreational drug use	1	2	3	4	5	NA
160716 Avoids alcohol use	1	2	3	4	5	NA
160717 Avoids tobacco use	1	2	3	4	5	NA
160718 Avoids teratogenic agents	1	2	3	4	5	NA
160719 Avoids abusive situations	1	2	3	4	5	NA

Domain-*Health Knowledge & Behavior (IV)*   **Class**-*Health Behavior (Q)*   *2nd edition 2000; revised 2004*

P

OUTCOME CONTENT REFERENCES:

Bell, R., & O'Neill M. (1994). Exercise and pregnancy: A review. *Birth, 21*(2), 85–95.

Crowell, D. T. (1995). Weight change in the postpartum period. A review of the literature. *Journal of Nurse Midwifery, 40*(5), 418–423.

Freda, M. C., Andersen, H. F., Damus, K., & Merkatz, I. R. (1993). What pregnant women want to know: A comparison of client and provider perceptions. *Journal of Obstetric, Gynecologic, and Neonatal Nursing, 22*(3), 237.

Kearney, M. H., Murphy, S., Irwin, K., & Rosenbaum, M. (1995). Salvaging self: A grounded theory of pregnancy on crack cocaine. *Nursing Research, 44*(4), 208–213.

McFarlane, J., Parker, B., & Soeken, K. (1996). Abuse during pregnancy: Associations with maternal health and infant birth weight. *Nursing Research, 45*(1), 37–42.

Olds, S., London, M. L., & Ladewig, P. W. (1996). *Maternal-newborn nursing: A family-centered approach* (5th ed.). Menlo Park, CA: Addison-Wesley.

Shapiro, H. R. (1993). Prenatal education in the work place. *AWHONN's Clinical Issues in Perinatal & Women's Health Nursing, 4*(1), 113–121.

Summers, L. (1993). Preconception care: An opportunity to maximize health in pregnancy. *Journal of Nurse Midwifery, 38*(4), 188–198.

Pre-Procedure Readiness   1921

Definition: Readiness of a patient to safely undergo a procedure requiring anesthesia or sedation

OUTCOME TARGET RATING: Maintain at_____   Increase to_____

		Not adequate	Slightly adequate	Moderately adequate	Substantially adequate	Totally adequate	
OUTCOME OVERALL RATING		1	2	3	4	5	
Indicators:							
192101	Knowledge of procedure	1	2	3	4	5	NA
192102	Knowledge of pre-procedure routines	1	2	3	4	5	NA
192103	Knowledge of post-procedure routines	1	2	3	4	5	NA
192104	Knowledge of potential risks and complications	1	2	3	4	5	NA
192105	Identification of changes in health status	1	2	3	4	5	NA
192106	Identification of past adverse reaction to anesthetics	1	2	3	4	5	NA
192107	Bowel prep status	1	2	3	4	5	NA
192108	Intake restriction status	1	2	3	4	5	NA
192109	Completion of skin prep	1	2	3	4	5	NA
192110	Knowledge of identification routines	1	2	3	4	5	NA
192111	Participation in marking procedural site	1	2	3	4	5	NA
192112	Completion of required lab work	1	2	3	4	5	NA
192113	Completion of required physical exam	1	2	3	4	5	NA
192114	Provision of signed consent	1	2	3	4	5	NA
192115	Reported personal preparation for procedure	1	2	3	4	5	NA
192116	Modification of regimen	1	2	3	4	5	NA
192117	Reported changes in medication required for procedure	1	2	3	4	5	NA
192118	Discussion of concerns about procedure	1	2	3	4	5	NA
192119	Discussion of questions prior to procedure	1	2	3	4	5	NA
192120	Participation in pre-procedure checklist	1	2	3	4	5	NA

Domain-*Health Knowledge & Behavior (IV)*   **Class**-*Risk Control & Safety (T)*   *4th edition 2008*

OUTCOME CONTENT REFERENCES:

American Organization of Perioperative Nurses. (2006). *Standards, recommended practices and guidelines.* Denver: Author.

Barnes, S. (2001). Preparing for surgery: Providing the details. *Journal of PeriAnesthesia Nursing, 16*(1), 31–32.

Saufl, N. M. (2004). Universal protocol for preventing wrong site, wrong procedure, wrong person surgery. *Journal of PeriAnesthesia Nursing, 19*(5), 348–351.

Smeltzer, S. C., & Bare, B. G. (2004). *Brunner & Suddarth's textbook of medical-surgical nursing* (10th ed.). Philadelphia: Lippincott Williams & Wilkins.

P

Preterm Infant Organization 0117

Definition: Extrauterine integration of physiologic and behavioral function by the infant born 24 to 37 (term) weeks gestation

OUTCOME TARGET RATING: Maintain at_____ Increase to_____

OUTCOME OVERALL RATING		Severely compromised	Substantially compromised	Moderately compromised	Mildly compromised	Not compromised	
		1	2	3	4	5	
Indicators:							
011701	Apical heart rate (120-160)	1	2	3	4	5	NA
011702	Gestational age index	1	2	3	4	5	NA
011703	Respiratory rate (30-60)	1	2	3	4	5	NA
011704	Oxygen saturation > 85%	1	2	3	4	5	NA
011705	Thermoregulation	1	2	3	4	5	NA
011706	Skin color	1	2	3	4	5	NA
011707	Feeding tolerance	1	2	3	4	5	NA
011708	Relaxed muscle tone	1	2	3	4	5	NA
011709	Smooth synchronous movement	1	2	3	4	5	NA
011710	Flexed posture	1	2	3	4	5	NA
011711	Hands brought to mouth	1	2	3	4	5	NA
011712	Deep sleep	1	2	3	4	5	NA
011713	Light sleep	1	2	3	4	5	NA
011714	Quiet-alert	1	2	3	4	5	NA
011715	Active-alert	1	2	3	4	5	NA
011716	Attentiveness to stimuli	1	2	3	4	5	NA
011717	Response to stimuli	1	2	3	4	5	NA
011718	Appropriate time-out signals	1	2	3	4	5	NA
011719	Sustained alertness during interaction	1	2	3	4	5	NA
011720	Interaction with caregiver	1	2	3	4	5	NA
011721	Self-consolability	1	2	3	4	5	NA

Domain-*Functional Health (I)*   **Class**-*Growth & Development (B)*   *2nd edition 2000; revised 2004*

P

OUTCOME CONTENT REFERENCES

D'Apolito, K. (1991). What is an organized infant? *Neonatal Network, 2*(1), 23–29.

Deacon, J., & O'Neill, P. (Eds.). (1999). *Core curriculum for neonatal intensive care nursing* (2nd ed.). Philadelphia: W. B. Saunders.

Jorgensen, K. M. (1993). *Developmental care of the preterm infant*. South Weymouth, MA: Children's Medical Ventures.

Mattson, S., & Smith, J. E. (Eds.). (2000). *Core curriculum for maternal-newborn nursing* (2nd ed.). Philadelphia: W. B. Saunders.

McGrath, J. M., & Conliffe-Torres, S. (1996). Integrating family-centered developmental assessment and intervention into routine care in the neonatal intensive care unit. *Nursing Clinics of North America, 31*(2), 367–385.

National Association of Neonatal Nurses. (1993). *Infant developmental care guidelines*. Petaluma, CA: Author.

Psychomotor Energy

0006

Definition: Personal drive and energy to maintain activities of daily living, nutrition, and personal safety

OUTCOME TARGET RATING: Maintain at_____ Increase to_____

		Never demonstrated	Rarely demonstrated	Sometimes demonstrated	Often demonstrated	Consistently demonstrated	
OUTCOME OVERALL RATING		1	2	3	4	5	
Indicators:							
000601	Exhibits affect that fits situation	1	2	3	4	5	NA
000602	Exhibits concentration	1	2	3	4	5	NA
000603	Maintains personal grooming and hygiene	1	2	3	4	5	NA
000604	Exhibits normal appetite	1	2	3	4	5	NA
000613	Complies with medication regimen	1	2	3	4	5	NA
000614	Complies with therapeutic regimen	1	2	3	4	5	NA
000606	Shows interest in surroundings	1	2	3	4	5	NA
000608	Exhibits stable energy level	1	2	3	4	5	NA
000609	Exhibits ability to accomplish daily tasks	1	2	3	4	5	NA

		Consistently demonstrated	Often demonstrated	Sometimes demonstrated	Rarely demonstrated	Never demonstrated	
000607	Suicide ideation	1	2	3	4	5	NA
000611	Lethargy	1	2	3	4	5	NA
000612	Depression	1	2	3	4	5	NA

Domain-*Functional Health (I)*   **Class**-*Energy Maintenance (A)*   *2nd edition 2000; revised 2004, 2008*

OUTCOME CONTENT REFERENCES:
American Psychiatric Association. (2000). *Diagnostic and statistical manual of mental disorders* (4th ed., text revision). Washington, DC: Author.
Lieberman, H. R. (2006). Mental energy: Assessing the cognition dimension. *Nutrition Reviews, 64*(7), S10–S13.
O'Connor, P. J. (2006). Mental energy: Assessing the mood dimension. *Nutrition Reviews, 64*(7), S7–S9.

P

Psychosocial Adjustment: Life Change

1305

Definition: Adaptive psychosocial response of an individual to a significant life change

OUTCOME TARGET RATING: Maintain at_____ Increase to_____

		Never demonstrated	Rarely demonstrated	Sometimes demonstrated	Often demonstrated	Consistently demonstrated	
OUTCOME OVERALL RATING		1	2	3	4	5	
Indicators:							
130501	Sets realistic goals	1	2	3	4	5	NA
130502	Maintains self-esteem	1	2	3	4	5	NA
130503	Maintains productivity	1	2	3	4	5	NA
130504	Reports feeling useful	1	2	3	4	5	NA
130505	Verbalizes optimism about present	1	2	3	4	5	NA
130506	Verbalizes optimism about future	1	2	3	4	5	NA
130507	Reports feeling empowered	1	2	3	4	5	NA
130508	Identifies multiple coping strategies	1	2	3	4	5	NA

Continued

Psychosocial Adjustment: Life Change—cont'd

	Never demonstrated	Rarely demonstrated	Sometimes demonstrated	Often demonstrated	Consistently demonstrated	
130509 Uses effective coping strategies	1	2	3	4	5	NA
130510 Uses effective financial management strategies	1	2	3	4	5	NA
130513 Uses available social support	1	2	3	4	5	NA
130514 Participates in leisure activities	1	2	3	4	5	NA
130511 Expresses satisfaction with living arrangements	1	2	3	4	5	NA
130512 Reports feeling socially engaged	1	2	3	4	5	NA

Domain-*Psychosocial Health (III)*   **Class**-*Psychosocial Adaptation (N)*   *1st edition 1997; revised 2004*

OUTCOME CONTENT REFERENCES:

Hernan, J. A. (1984). Exploding aging myths through retirement counseling. *Journal of Gerontological Nursing, 10*(4), 31–33.

Johnson, R. A. (2001). Relocation stress syndrome. In M. Maas, K. Buckwalter, M. Hardy, T. Tripp-Reimer, M. Titler, & J. Specht (Eds.), *Nursing care of older adults: Diagnoses, outcomes & interventions* (pp. 619–630). St. Louis: Mosby.

+Liang, J. (1984). Dimensions of the Life Satisfaction Index A: A structural formulation. *Journal of Gerontology, 39*(5), 613–622.

+Neugarten, B. L., Havighurst, R. J., & Tobin, S. (1961). The measurement of life satisfaction. *Journal of Gerontology, 16*(2), 134–143.

Neuhs, H. P. (1991). Ready for retirement? *Geriatric Nursing, 12*(5), 240–241.

Rosenkoetter, M. M. (1985). Is your older client ready for a role change after retirement? *Journal of Gerontological Nursing, 11*(9), 21–24.

Tincher, B. J. V. (1992). Retirement: Perspectives and theory. *Physical & Occupational Therapy in Geriatrics, 11*(1), 55–62.

P

Quality of Life

2000

Definition: Extent of positive perception of current life circumstances

OUTCOME TARGET RATING: Maintain at_____   Increase to_____

OUTCOME OVERALL RATING	Not at all satisfied 1	Somewhat satisfied 2	Moderately satisfied 3	Very satisfied 4	Completely satisfied 5	
Indicators:						
200001 Health status	1	2	3	4	5	NA
200002 Social circumstances	1	2	3	4	5	NA
200003 Environmental circumstances	1	2	3	4	5	NA
200013 Privacy	1	2	3	4	5	NA
200014 Dignity	1	2	3	4	5	NA
200015 Autonomy	1	2	3	4	5	NA
200004 Economic status	1	2	3	4	5	NA
200005 Education level	1	2	3	4	5	NA
200006 Occupation	1	2	3	4	5	NA
200007 Close relationships	1	2	3	4	5	NA
200008 Achievement of life goals	1	2	3	4	5	NA
200009 Ability to cope	1	2	3	4	5	NA
200010 Self-concept	1	2	3	4	5	NA
200011 Pervasive mood	1	2	3	4	5	NA
200016 Independence in activities of daily living	1	2	3	4	5	NA

Domain-*Perceived Health (V)*   **Class**-*Health & Life Quality (U)*   *1st edition 1997; revised 2004, 2008*

OUTCOME CONTENT REFERENCES:

Andrews, F., & Withey, S. (1976). *Social indicators of well-being: Americans' perceptions of life quality*. New York: Plenum Press.

Davidhizar, R. E., & Giger, J. N. (2001). Powerlessness. In M. Maas, K. Buckwalter, M. Hardy, T. Tripp-Reimer, M. Titler, & J. Specht (Eds.), *Nursing care of older adults: Diagnoses, outcomes & interventions* (pp. 562–570). St. Louis: Mosby.

+Diener, E., Emmons, R. A., Larsen, R. J., & Griffin, S. (1985). The Satisfaction with Life Scale. *Journal of Personality Assessment, 49*(1), 71–75.

Gill, L., & Flenstein, A. R. (1994). A critical appraisal of the quality of quality-of-life measurements. *Journal of the American Medical Association, 272*(8), 619–626.

Mezzich, J., Cohen, N., Ruiperez, M., Banzato, C., & Zapata-Vega, M. (2011). The multicultural quality of life index: Presentation and validation. *Journal of Evaluation in Clinical Practice, 17*(2), 357–364.

Padilla, G., Ferrell, B., Grant, M., & Rhiner, M. (1990). Defining the content domain of quality of life for cancer patients with pain. *Cancer Nursing, 13*(2), 108–115.

Ragsdale, D., Kotarba, J., & Morrow, J. (1992). Quality of life of hospitalized persons with AIDS. *Image—The Journal of Nursing Scholarship, 24*(4), 259–265.

Stewart, A., Ware, J., Sherbourne, C., & Wells, K. (1992). Psychological distress/well-being and cognitive functioning measures. In A. Stewart & J. Ware, Jr. (Eds.), *Measuring functioning and well-being: The medical outcomes study approach* (pp. 102–142). Durham, NC: Duke University Press.

Q

Relocation Adaptation 1311

Definition: Adaptive emotional and behavioral response of a cognitively intact individual to a required change in living environment

OUTCOME TARGET RATING: Maintain at_____ Increase to_____

		Never demonstrated	Rarely demonstrated	Sometimes demonstrated	Often demonstrated	Consistently demonstrated	
OUTCOME OVERALL RATING		1	2	3	4	5	
Indicators:							
131101	Recognizes reason for change in living environment	1	2	3	4	5	NA
131102	Participates in decision-making in new environment	1	2	3	4	5	NA
131103	Expresses satisfaction with daily routine	1	2	3	4	5	NA
131104	Expresses satisfaction with level of independence	1	2	3	4	5	NA
131105	Compares care needs with available resources	1	2	3	4	5	NA
131106	Expresses satisfaction with social relationships	1	2	3	4	5	NA
131107	Expresses satisfaction with variety of food	1	2	3	4	5	NA
131108	Expresses satisfaction with food preparation	1	2	3	4	5	NA
131109	Expresses satisfaction with retained personal belongings	1	2	3	4	5	NA
131110	Expresses satisfaction with living arrangements	1	2	3	4	5	NA
131111	Exhibits positive mood	1	2	3	4	5	NA
131112	Appears content	1	2	3	4	5	NA
131113	Respects others' rights	1	2	3	4	5	NA
131114	Maintains positive relationship with family	1	2	3	4	5	NA
131115	Maintains positive relationships with friends	1	2	3	4	5	NA
131116	Maintains positive relationships with others in new environment	1	2	3	4	5	NA
131117	Participates in social activities	1	2	3	4	5	NA

		Consistently demonstrated	Often demonstrated	Sometimes demonstrated	Rarely demonstrated	Never demonstrated	
131118	Agitation	1	2	3	4	5	NA
131119	Anxiety	1	2	3	4	5	NA
131120	Fear	1	2	3	4	5	NA
131121	Worry	1	2	3	4	5	NA
131122	Frustration	1	2	3	4	5	NA
131123	Anger	1	2	3	4	5	NA
131124	Depression	1	2	3	4	5	NA
131125	Withdrawal	1	2	3	4	5	NA
131126	Loneliness	1	2	3	4	5	NA
131127	Boredom	1	2	3	4	5	NA
131128	Apathy	1	2	3	4	5	NA
131129	Suspicion	1	2	3	4	5	NA

Domain-Psychosocial Health (III) **Class**-Psychosocial Adaptation (N) 5th edition 2013

OUTCOME CONTENT REFERENCES:

Bekhet, A., Fouad, R., & Zauszniewski, A. (2010). The role of positive cognitions in Egyptian elders' relocation adjustment. *Western Journal of Nursing Research, 33*(1), 121–135.

Chen, F. (2010). Assisting adults with severe mental illness in transitioning from parental homes to independent living. *Community Mental Health Journal, 46*(4), 372–380.

Hertz, J. E., Koren, M. E., Rossetti, J., & Robertson, J. F. (2008). Early identification of relocation risk in older adults with critical illness. *Critical Care Nursing Quarterly, 31*(1), 59–64.

Hertz, J. E., Rossetti, J., Koren, M. E., & Robertson, J .F. (2005). *Management of relocation in cognitively intact older adults.* Iowa City, IA: The University of Iowa Gerontological Nursing Interventions Research Center.

Lee, G. E. (2010). Predictors of adjustment to nursing home life of elderly residents: A cross-sectional survey. *International Journal of Nursing Studies, 47*(8), 957–964.

Walker, C. A., Cox Curry, L., & Hogstel, M. O. (2007). Relocation stress in older adults transitioning from home to a long-term care facility: Myth or reality? *Journal of Psychosocial Nursing and Mental Health Services, 45*(1), 38–45.

Respiratory Status 0415

Definition: Movement of air in and out of the lungs and exchange of carbon dioxide and oxygen at the alveolar level

OUTCOME TARGET RATING: Maintain at_____   Increase to_____

OUTCOME OVERALL RATING	Severe deviation from normal range 1	Substantial deviation from normal range 2	Moderate deviation from normal range 3	Mild deviation from normal range 4	No deviation from normal range 5	
Indicators:						
041501 Respiratory rate	1	2	3	4	5	NA
041502 Respiratory rhythm	1	2	3	4	5	NA
041503 Depth of inspiration	1	2	3	4	5	NA
041504 Auscultated breath sounds	1	2	3	4	5	NA
041532 Airway patency	1	2	3	4	5	NA
041505 Tidal volume	1	2	3	4	5	NA
041506 Achievement of expected incentive spirometer	1	2	3	4	5	NA
041507 Vital capacity	1	2	3	4	5	NA
041508 Oxygen saturation	1	2	3	4	5	NA
041509 Pulmonary function tests	1	2	3	4	5	NA

	Severe	Substantial	Moderate	Mild	None	
041510 Accessory muscle use	1	2	3	4	5	NA
041511 Chest retraction	1	2	3	4	5	NA
041512 Pursed lips breathing	1	2	3	4	5	NA
041513 Cyanosis	1	2	3	4	5	NA
041514 Dyspnea at rest	1	2	3	4	5	NA
041515 Dyspnea with mild exertion	1	2	3	4	5	NA
041516 Restlessness	1	2	3	4	5	NA
041517 Somnolence	1	2	3	4	5	NA
041518 Diaphoresis	1	2	3	4	5	NA
041519 Impaired cognition	1	2	3	4	5	NA
041520 Accumulation of sputum	1	2	3	4	5	NA
041521 Atelectasis	1	2	3	4	5	NA
041522 Adventitious breath sounds	1	2	3	4	5	NA
041523 Impaired expiration	1	2	3	4	5	NA
041524 Gasping	1	2	3	4	5	NA
041525 Agonal respirations	1	2	3	4	5	NA
041526 Grunting	1	2	3	4	5	NA
041527 Clubbing of fingers	1	2	3	4	5	NA

R

Continued

Respiratory Status—cont'd

		Severe deviation from normal range	Substantial deviation from normal range	Moderate deviation from normal range	Mild deviation from normal range	No deviation from normal range	
041528	Nasal flaring	1	2	3	4	5	NA
041529	Restlessness	1	2	3	4	5	NA
041530	Fever	1	2	3	4	5	NA
041531	Coughing	1	2	3	4	5	NA

Domain-*Physiologic Health (II)*   **Class**-*Cardiopulmonary (E)*   *4th edition 2008; revised 2013*

OUTCOME CONTENT REFERENCES:
Bailey, P. H., Colella, T., & Mossey, S. (2004). COPD-intuition or template: Nurses' stories of acute exacerbations of chronic obstructive pulmonary disease. *Journal of Clinical Nursing, 13*(6), 756–764.
Booker, R. (2005). A spirometer in primary care—As essential as a stethoscope. *Primary Health Care, 15*(5), 33–36.
Loeb, M., McArthur, M., Peeling, R. W., Petric, M., & Simor, A. E. (2000). Surveillance for outbreaks of respiratory tract infections in nursing homes. *Canadian Medical Association Journal, 162*(8), 1133–1137.
Mintz, M. L. (2006). *Disorders of the respiratory tract: Common challenges in primary care*. Totowa, NJ: Humana Press.
Smeltzer, S. C., & Bare, B. G. (2004). *Brunner & Suddarth's textbook of medical-surgical nursing* (10th ed.). Philadelphia: Lippincott Williams & Wilkins.

Respiratory Status: Airway Patency   0410

Definition: Open, clear tracheobronchial passages for air exchange

OUTCOME TARGET RATING: Maintain at_____   Increase to_____

		Severe deviation from normal range	Substantial deviation from normal range	Moderate deviation from normal range	Mild deviation from normal range	No deviation from normal range	
OUTCOME OVERALL RATING		1	2	3	4	5	
Indicators:							
041004	Respiratory rate	1	2	3	4	5	NA
041005	Respiratory rhythm	1	2	3	4	5	NA
041017	Depth of inspiration	1	2	3	4	5	NA
041012	Ability to clear secretions	1	2	3	4	5	NA

		Severe	Substantial	Moderate	Mild	None	
041002	Anxiety	1	2	3	4	5	NA
041011	Fear	1	2	3	4	5	NA
041003	Choking	1	2	3	4	5	NA
041007	Adventitious breath sounds	1	2	3	4	5	NA
041013	Nasal flaring	1	2	3	4	5	NA
041014	Gasping	1	2	3	4	5	NA
041015	Dyspnea at rest	1	2	3	4	5	NA
041016	Dyspnea with mild exertion	1	2	3	4	5	NA
041018	Accessory muscle use	1	2	3	4	5	NA
041019	Coughing	1	2	3	4	5	NA
041020	Accumulation of sputum	1	2	3	4	5	NA
041021	Agonal respirations	1	2	3	4	5	NA

Domain-*Physiologic Health (II)*   **Class**-*Cardiopulmonary (E)*   *2nd edition 2000; revised 2004, 2008*

OUTCOME CONTENT REFERENCES:

Clochesy, J. M., Brey, C., Cardin, S., Whittaker, A. A., & Rudy, E. B. (1996). *Critical care nursing* (2nd ed.). Philadelphia: W. B. Saunders.

Lewis, S. M., Collier, I. C., Heitkemper, M. M., & Dirksen, S. R. (2000). *Medical-surgical nursing: Assessment & management of clinical problems* (5th ed.). St. Louis: Mosby.

McCance, K. L., & Huether, S. E. (2002). *Pathophysiology: The biologic basis for disease in adults and children* (4th ed.). St. Louis: Mosby.

Smeltzer, S. C., & Bare, B. G. (2004). *Brunner & Suddarth's textbook of medical-surgical nursing* (10th ed.). Philadelphia: Lippincott Williams & Wilkins.

Respiratory Status: Gas Exchange 0402

Definition: Alveolar exchange of carbon dioxide and oxygen to maintain arterial blood gas concentrations

OUTCOME TARGET RATING: Maintain at_____   Increase to_____

		Severe deviation from normal range	Substantial deviation from normal range	Moderate deviation from normal range	Mild deviation from normal range	No deviation from normal range	
OUTCOME OVERALL RATING		1	2	3	4	5	
Indicators:							
040208	Partial pressure of oxygen in arterial blood (PaO_2)	1	2	3	4	5	NA
040209	Partial pressure of carbon dioxide in arterial blood ($PaCO_2$)	1	2	3	4	5	NA
040210	Arterial pH	1	2	3	4	5	NA
040211	Oxygen saturation	1	2	3	4	5	NA
040212	End tidal carbon dioxide	1	2	3	4	5	NA
040213	Chest x-ray findings	1	2	3	4	5	NA
040214	Ventilation perfusion balance	1	2	3	4	5	NA
		Severe	Substantial	Moderate	Mild	None	
040203	Dyspnea at rest	1	2	3	4	5	NA
040204	Dyspnea with mild exertion	1	2	3	4	5	NA
040205	Restlessness	1	2	3	4	5	NA
040206	Cyanosis	1	2	3	4	5	NA
040207	Somnolence	1	2	3	4	5	NA
040216	Impaired cognition	1	2	3	4	5	NA

Domain-*Physiologic Health (II)*   **Class**-*Cardiopulmonary (E)*   *1st edition 1997; revised 2000, 2004, 2008*

R

OUTCOME CONTENT REFERENCES:

Ahrens, T. (1993). Changing perspectives in the assessment of oxygenation. *Critical Care Nurse, 13*(4), 78–83.

Berry, B. E., & Pinard, A. E. (2002). Assessing tissue oxygenation. *Critical Care Nurse, 22*(3), 22–36.

Hayden, R. (1992). What keeps oxygenation on track? *American Journal of Nursing, 92*(12), 32–40.

Janson-Bjerklie, S. (1993). Predicting the outcomes of living with asthma. *Research in Nursing and Health, 16*(4), 241–249.

McCarty, K., & Wilkins, R. (1990). Synopsis of clinical findings in respiratory disorders. In R. Wilkins, R. L. Sheldon, & S. J. Krider (Eds.), *Clinical assessment in respiratory care* (2nd ed., pp. 294–302). St. Louis: Mosby.

Morton, P. (1989). Respiratory systems. In P. Morton (Ed.), *Health assessment in nursing* (pp. 243–281). Springhouse, PA: Springhouse.

Patrick, M. (1991). *Medical-surgical nursing: Pathophysiological concepts* (2nd ed.). Philadelphia: J. B. Lippincott.

Potter, P., & Perry, A. (1991). *Oxygenation: Basic nursing theory and practice.* St. Louis: Mosby.

Smeltzer, S. C., & Bare, B. G. (2004). *Brunner & Suddarth's textbook of medical-surgical nursing* (10th ed.). Philadelphia: Lippincott Williams & Wilkins.

Respiratory Status: Ventilation

0403

Definition: Movement of air in and out of the lungs

OUTCOME TARGET RATING: Maintain at_____ Increase to_____

		Severe deviation from normal range	Substantial deviation from normal range	Moderate deviation from normal range	Mild deviation from normal range	No deviation from normal range	
OUTCOME OVERALL RATING		1	2	3	4	5	
Indicators:							
040301	Respiratory rate	1	2	3	4	5	NA
040302	Respiratory rhythm	1	2	3	4	5	NA
040303	Depth of inspiration	1	2	3	4	5	NA
040318	Percussed sounds	1	2	3	4	5	NA
040324	Tidal volume	1	2	3	4	5	NA
040325	Vital capacity	1	2	3	4	5	NA
040326	Chest x-ray findings	1	2	3	4	5	NA
040327	Pulmonary function tests	1	2	3	4	5	NA

		Severe	Substantial	Moderate	Mild	None	
040309	Accessory muscle use	1	2	3	4	5	NA
040310	Adventitious breath sounds	1	2	3	4	5	NA
040311	Chest retraction	1	2	3	4	5	NA
040312	Pursed lips breathing	1	2	3	4	5	NA
040313	Dyspnea at rest	1	2	3	4	5	NA
040314	Dyspnea with exertion	1	2	3	4	5	NA
040315	Orthopnea	1	2	3	4	5	NA
040317	Tactile fremitus	1	2	3	4	5	NA
040329	Asymmetrical chest expansion	1	2	3	4	5	NA
040330	Impaired vocalization	1	2	3	4	5	NA
040331	Accumulation of sputum	1	2	3	4	5	NA
040332	Impaired expiration	1	2	3	4	5	NA
040333	Distorted voice sounds on auscultation	1	2	3	4	5	NA
040334	Atelectasis	1	2	3	4	5	NA

Domain-Physiologic Health (II) *Class*-Cardiopulmonary (E) *1st edition 1997; revised 2004, 2008*

R

OUTCOME CONTENT REFERENCES:

Ahrens, T. (1993). Changing perspectives in the assessment of oxygenation. *Critical Care Nurse, 13*(4), 78–83.

+Guyatt, G. H., Berman, L. B., Townsend, M., Pugsley, S. O., & Chambers, L. W. (1987). A measure of quality of life for clinical trials in chronic lung disease. *Thorax, 42*(10), 773–778.

Hayden, R. (1992). What keeps oxygenation on track? *American Journal of Nursing, 92*(12), 32–40.

Janson-Bjerklie, S. (1993). Predicting the outcomes of living with asthma. *Research in Nursing and Health, 16*(4), 241–249.

Wilkins, R., & Sheldon, R. (2005). *Clinical assessment in respiratory care* (5th ed.). St. Louis: Mosby.

Morton, P. (1989). Respiratory systems. In P. Morton (Ed.), *Health assessment in nursing* (pp. 243–281). Springhouse, PA: Springhouse.

Patrick, M. (1991). *Medical-surgical nursing: Pathophysiological concepts* (2nd ed.). Philadelphia: J. B. Lippincott.

Potter, P., & Perry, A. (1991). *Oxygenation: Basic nursing theory and practice.* St. Louis: Mosby.

Smeltzer, S. C., & Bare, B. G. (2004). *Brunner & Suddarth's textbook of medical-surgical nursing* (10th ed.). Philadelphia: Lippincott Williams & Wilkins.

Wakefield, B. (2001). Ineffective breathing pattern. In M. Maas, K. Buckwalter, M. Hardy, T. Tripp-Reimer, M. Titler, & J. Specht (Eds.), *Nursing care of older adults: Diagnoses, outcomes & interventions* (pp. 313–323). St. Louis: Mosby.

Rest 0003

Definition: Quantity and pattern of diminished activity for mental and physical rejuvenation

OUTCOME TARGET RATING: Maintain at_____ Increase to_____

OUTCOME OVERALL RATING	Severely compromised 1	Substantially compromised 2	Moderately compromised 3	Mildly compromised 4	Not compromised 5	
Indicators:						
000301 Amount of rest	1	2	3	4	5	NA
000302 Rest pattern	1	2	3	4	5	NA
000303 Rest quality	1	2	3	4	5	NA
000304 Physically rested	1	2	3	4	5	NA
000305 Mentally rested	1	2	3	4	5	NA
000308 Emotionally rested	1	2	3	4	5	NA
000309 Energy restored after rest	1	2	3	4	5	NA
000310 Rested appearance	1	2	3	4	5	NA

Domain-Functional Health (I) *Class*-Energy Maintenance (A) *1st edition 1997; revised 2004, 2008*

OUTCOME CONTENT REFERENCES:

Brown, D. R., Morgan, W. P., & Raglin, J. S. (1993). Effects of exercise and rest on the state anxiety and blood pressure of physically challenged college students. *Journal of Sports Medicine and Physical Fitness, 33*(3), 300–305.

Ellis, J. R., & Nowlis, E. A. (1994). *Providing nursing care within the nursing process* (5th ed.). Philadelphia: J. B. Lippincott.

+Lee, K. A., Hicks, G., & Nino-Murcia, G. (1991). Validity and reliability of a scale to assess fatigue. *Psychiatry Research, 36*(3), 291–298.

Potter, P. A., & Perry, A. G. (2001). *Fundamentals of nursing* (5th ed.). St. Louis: Mosby.

Smeltzer, S. C., & Bare, B. G. (Eds.). (2003). *Brunner and Suddarth's textbook of medical-surgical nursing* (10th ed.). Philadelphia: Lippincott Williams & Wilkins.

Risk Control 1902

Definition: Personal actions to understand, prevent, eliminate, or reduce modifiable health threats

OUTCOME TARGET RATING: Maintain at_____ Increase to_____

OUTCOME OVERALL RATING	Never demonstrated 1	Rarely demonstrated 2	Sometimes demonstrated 3	Often demonstrated 4	Consistently demonstrated 5	
Indicators:						
190219 Seeks current information about health risks	1	2	3	4	5	NA
190220 Identifies risk factors	1	2	3	4	5	NA
190201 Acknowledges personal risk factors	1	2	3	4	5	NA
190221 Acknowledges ability to change behavior	1	2	3	4	5	NA
190202 Monitors environmental risk factors	1	2	3	4	5	NA
190203 Monitors personal risk factors	1	2	3	4	5	NA
190204 Develops effective risk control strategies	1	2	3	4	5	NA
190205 Adjusts risk control strategies	1	2	3	4	5	NA
190206 Commits to risk control strategies	1	2	3	4	5	NA
190207 Follows selected risk control strategies	1	2	3	4	5	NA
190208 Modifies lifestyle to reduce risk	1	2	3	4	5	NA
190209 Avoids exposure to health threats	1	2	3	4	5	NA
190210 Participates in screening for health problems	1	2	3	4	5	NA

R

Continued

Risk Control—*cont'd*

		Never demonstrated	Rarely demonstrated	Sometimes demonstrated	Often demonstrated	Consistently demonstrated	
190211	Participates in screening for identified risks	1	2	3	4	5	NA
190212	Obtains recommended immunizations	1	2	3	4	5	NA
190213	Uses health care services congruent with needs	1	2	3	4	5	NA
190214	Uses personal support systems to reduce risk	1	2	3	4	5	NA
190215	Uses community resources to reduce risk	1	2	3	4	5	NA
190216	Recognizes changes in health status	1	2	3	4	5	NA
190217	Monitors changes in general health status	1	2	3	4	5	NA

Domain-*Health Knowledge & Behavior (IV)*   **Class**-*Risk Control & Safety (T)*   *1st edition 1997; revised 2004, 2013*

OUTCOME CONTENT REFERENCES:
+Hettler, B. (1982). Wellness promotion and risk reduction on a university campus. In M. Faber & A. Reinhardt (Eds.), *Promoting health through risk reduction.* New York: Macmillan.
Hughes, E., Kilmer, G., Li, Y., Valluru, B., Brown, J., Colclough, G., Gethers, S., Roberts, H., Elam-Evans, L., & Balluz, L. (2010). Surveillance for certain health behaviors among states and selected local areas-United States, 2008. *Morbidity and Mortality Weekly Report Surveillance Summaries, 59*(SS-10), 1–221.
Kliche, T., Plaumann, M., Nocker, G., Dubben, S., & Walter, U. (2011). Disease prevention and health promotion programs: Benefits, implementation, quality assurance and open questions—A summary of the evidence. *Journal of Public Health, 19*(4), 283–292.
Lemyre, L., Lee, J., Mercier, P., Bouchard, L., & Krewski, D. (2006). The structure of Canadians' health risk perceptions: Environmental, therapeutic and social health risks. *Health, Risk & Society, 8*(2), 185–195.
Oncken, C., McKee, S., Krishnan-Sarin, S., O'Malley, S., & Mazure, C. (2005). Knowledge and perceived risk of smoking-related conditions: A survey of cigarette smokers. *Preventive Medicine, 40*(6), 779–784.
Pincus, H., Pechura, C., Keyser, D., Bachman, J., & Houtsinger, J. (2006). Depression in primary care: Learning lessons in a national quality improvement program. *Administration and Policy in Mental Health and Mental Health Services Research, 33*(1), 2–15.
Ruffin, M., IV, Nease, D., Jr., Sen, A., Pace, W., Wang, C., Acheson, L., Rubinstein, W., & Gramling, R. (2011). Effect of preventive messages tailored to family history on health behaviors: The family healthware impact trials. *Annals of Family Medicine, 9*(1), 3–11.
Simons-Morton, D. G., Mullen, P. D., Mains, D. A., Tabak, E. R., & Green, L. W. (1992). Characteristics of controlled studies of patient education and counseling for preventive health behaviors. *Patient Education and Counseling, 19*(2), 174–204.
U.S. Department of Health and Human Services. (2010). *The guide to clinical preventive services 2010–2011: Recommendations of the U.S. Preventive Services Task Force.* Rockville, MD: Agency for Healthcare Research and Quality.

R

Risk Control: Alcohol Use   1903

Definition: Personal actions to understand, prevent, eliminate, or reduce the threats to health associated with alcohol use

OUTCOME TARGET RATING: Maintain at_____   Increase to_____

		Never demonstrated	Rarely demonstrated	Sometimes demonstrated	Often demonstrated	Consistently demonstrated	
OUTCOME OVERALL RATING		1	2	3	4	5	
Indicators:							
190318	Seeks current information about alcohol use	1	2	3	4	5	NA
190319	Identifies risk factors for alcohol misuse	1	2	3	4	5	NA
190301	Acknowledges personal risk for alcohol misuse	1	2	3	4	5	NA
190302	Acknowledges consequences associated with alcohol misuse	1	2	3	4	5	NA

Risk Control: Alcohol Use—cont'd

		Never demonstrated	Rarely demonstrated	Sometimes demonstrated	Often demonstrated	Consistently demonstrated	
190320	Acknowledges ability to change behavior	1	2	3	4	5	NA
190303	Monitors environment for factors encouraging alcohol misuse	1	2	3	4	5	NA
190304	Monitors personal alcohol use patterns	1	2	3	4	5	NA
190305	Develops effective alcohol use control strategies	1	2	3	4	5	NA
190306	Adjusts alcohol use control strategies	1	2	3	4	5	NA
190307	Commits to alcohol use control strategies	1	2	3	4	5	NA
190308	Follows selected alcohol use control strategies	1	2	3	4	5	NA
190309	Participates in screening for health problems	1	2	3	4	5	NA
190310	Uses health care services congruent with needs	1	2	3	4	5	NA
190311	Uses personal support systems to control alcohol misuse	1	2	3	4	5	NA
190312	Uses support group to control alcohol misuse	1	2	3	4	5	NA
190313	Uses community resources to control alcohol misuse	1	2	3	4	5	NA
190314	Recognizes changes in general health status	1	2	3	4	5	NA
190315	Monitors changes in general health status	1	2	3	4	5	NA
190316	Controls alcohol intake	1	2	3	4	5	NA

Domain-*Health Knowledge & Behavior (IV)*   **Class**-*Risk Control & Safety (T)*   *1st edition 1997; revised 2004, 2013*

OUTCOME CONTENT REFERENCES:

Hides, L., Cotton, S., Berger, G., Gleeson, J., O'Donnell, C., Proffitt, T., McGorry, P., & Lubman, D. (2009). The reliability and validity of the alcohol, smoking and substance involvement screening test (ASSIST) in first-episode psychosis. *Addictive Behaviors, 34*(10), 821–825.

+MacNeil, G. (1991). A short-form scale to measure alcohol abuse. *Research on Social Work Practice, 1*(1), 68–75.

Neushotz, L., & Fitzpatrick, J. (2008). Improving substance abuse screening and intervention in a primary care clinic. *Archives of Psychiatric Nursing, 22*(2), 76–86.

Palmer, R., Corbin, W., & Cronce, J. (2010). Protective strategies: A mediator of risk associated with age of drinking onset. *Addictive Behaviors, 35*(5), 486–491.

Talashek, M. L., Gerace, L. M., & Starr, K. L. (1994). The substance abuse pandemic: Determinants to guide interventions. *Public Health Nursing, 11*(2), 131–139.

U.S. Department of Health and Human Services. (2010). *The guide to clinical preventive services 2010–2011: Recommendations of the U.S. Preventive Services Task Force*. Rockville, MD: Agency for Healthcare Research and Quality.

Weyerer, S., Schäufele, M., Eifflaender-Gorfer, S., Köhler, L., Maier, W., Haller, F., Cvetanovska-Pllashiniku, G., Pentzek, M., Fuchs, A., van den Bussche, H., Zimmermann, T., Eisele, M., Bickel, H., Mösch, E., Wiese, B., Angermeyer, M., & Riedel-Heller, S. (2009). At-risk alcohol drinking in primary care patients aged 75 years and older. *International Journal of Geriatric Psychiatry, 24*(12), 1376–1385.

R

Risk Control: Cancer 1917

Definition: Personal actions to understand, prevent, eliminate, or reduce the threat of cancer

OUTCOME TARGET RATING: Maintain at_____   Increase to_____

OUTCOME OVERALL RATING	Never demonstrated 1	Rarely demonstrated 2	Sometimes demonstrated 3	Often demonstrated 4	Consistently demonstrated 5	
Indicators:						
191701 Seeks current information about cancer prevention	1	2	3	4	5	NA
191713 Identifies risk factors for cancer	1	2	3	4	5	NA
191714 Acknowledges personal risk factors for cancer	1	2	3	4	5	NA
191702 Avoids exposure to carcinogens	1	2	3	4	5	NA
191703 Protects self from carcinogens	1	2	3	4	5	NA
191710 Eliminates tobacco use	1	2	3	4	5	NA
191704 Modifies environment to eliminate exposure to carcinogens	1	2	3	4	5	NA
191705 Follows dietary recommendations	1	2	3	4	5	NA
191706 Performs recommended self-screening for cancer detection	1	2	3	4	5	NA
191707 Participates in recommended cancer screening	1	2	3	4	5	NA
191715 Monitors changes in general health status	1	2	3	4	5	NA
191711 Obtains recommended vaccinations	1	2	3	4	5	NA
191712 Obtains health care services following abnormal screening results	1	2	3	4	5	NA
191716 Uses personal support systems to reduce cancer risk	1	2	3	4	5	NA
191717 Uses community resources to reduce cancer risk	1	2	3	4	5	NA

Domain-Health Knowledge & Behavior (IV)   *Class*-Risk Control & Safety (T)   2nd edition 2000; revised 2004, 2008, 2013

OUTCOME CONTENT REFERENCES:

Begg, C. B. (2001). Risky concepts: Methods in cancer research. The search for cancer risk factors: When can we stop looking? *American Journal of Public Health, 91*(3), 360–364

Bener, A., El Ayoubi, H. R., Basha, B., Joseph, S., & Chouchane, L. (2011). Breast cancer screening barriers: Knowledge, attitudes, and practices of women toward breast cancer. *Breast Journal, 17*(1): 115–116.

Machia, J. (2001). Breast cancer: Risk, prevention, & tamoxifen. *American Journal of Nursing, 101*(4), 26–36.

Nahar, J., Tickle, K., Ali, A., Chen, Y. (2011). Significant cancer prevention factor extraction: An association rule discovery approach. *Journal of Medical Systems, 35*(3), 353–367.

Ozanne, E., Wittenberg, E., Garber, J., & Weeks, J. (2010). Breast cancer prevention: Patient decision making and risk communication in the high risk setting. *Breast Journal, 16*(1), 38–47.

U.S. Department of Health and Human Services. (2010). *The guide to clinical preventive services 2010–2011: Recommendations of the U.S. Preventive Services Task Force.* Rockville, MD: Agency for Healthcare Research and Quality.

R

Risk Control: Cardiovascular Disease   1914

Definition: Personal actions to understand, prevent, eliminate, or reduce the threat of cardiovascular disease

OUTCOME TARGET RATING: Maintain at_____   Increase to_____

OUTCOME OVERALL RATING		Never demonstrated 1	Rarely demonstrated 2	Sometimes demonstrated 3	Often demonstrated 4	Consistently demonstrated 5	
Indicators:							
191418	Seeks current information about cardiovascular disease	1	2	3	4	5	NA
191419	Identifies risk factors for cardiovascular disease	1	2	3	4	5	NA
191401	Acknowledges personal risk for cardiovascular disease	1	2	3	4	5	NA
191402	Acknowledges ability to change behavior	1	2	3	4	5	NA
191403	Eliminates tobacco use	1	2	3	4	5	NA
191420	Eliminates recreational drug use	1	2	3	4	5	NA
191404	Monitors blood pressure	1	2	3	4	5	NA
191405	Monitors radial pulse rate	1	2	3	4	5	NA
191421	Monitors changes in general health status	1	2	3	4	5	NA
191406	Uses strategies to reduce stress	1	2	3	4	5	NA
191407	Uses effective weight control strategies	1	2	3	4	5	NA
191408	Follows heart-healthy diet	1	2	3	4	5	NA
191409	Uses health care services congruent with needs	1	2	3	4	5	NA
191410	Follows non-prescription medication precautions	1	2	3	4	5	NA
191411	Seeks information about strategies to maintain cardiovascular health	1	2	3	4	5	NA
191412	Monitors effects of stimulants	1	2	3	4	5	NA
191413	Participates in cholesterol screening	1	2	3	4	5	NA
191422	Maintains glycemic control	1	2	3	4	5	NA
191414	Uses medication as prescribed	1	2	3	4	5	NA
191415	Participates in regular exercise	1	2	3	4	5	NA
191416	Participates in aerobic exercise	1	2	3	4	5	NA
191423	Uses personal support systems to reduce cardiovascular risk	1	2	3	4	5	NA
191424	Uses community resources to reduce cardiovascular risk	1	2	3	4	5	NA

Domain-Health Knowledge & Behavior (IV)   **Class**-Risk Control & Safety (T)   2nd edition 2000; revised 2004, 2013

OUTCOME CONTENT REFERENCES:

Andersen, L., Riddoch, C., Kriemler, S., & Hills, A. (2011). Physical activity and cardiovascular risk factors in children. *British Journal of Sports Medicine, 45*(11), 871–876.

Cooney, M., Cooney, H., Dudina, A., & Graham, I. (2011). Total cardiovascular disease risk assessment: A review. *Current Opinion in Cardiology, 26*(5), 429–437.

Fair, J., Gulanick, M., & Braun, L. (2009). Cardiovascular risk factors and lifestyle habits among preventive cardiovascular nurses. *Journal of Cardiovascular Nursing, 24*(4), 277–286.

Gomel, M., Oldenburg, B., Simpson, J. M., & Owen, N. (1993). Work-site cardiovascular risk reduction: A randomized trial of health risk assessment, education, counseling, and incentives. *American Journal of Public Health, 83*(9), 1231–1238.

Jemigan, V., Duran, B., Ahn, D., & Winkleby, M. (2010). Changing patterns in health behaviors and risk factors related to cardiovascular disease among American Indians and Alaska Natives. *American Journal of Public Health, 100*(4), 677–683.

King, K., Thomlinson, E., Sanguins, J., & LeBlanc, P. (2006). Men and women managing coronary artery disease risk: Urban-rural contrasts. *Social Science & Medicine, 62*(5), 1091–1102.

Mochari-Greenberger, H., Mills, T., Simpson, S., & Mosca, L. (2010). Knowledge, preventive action, and barriers to cardiovascular disease prevention by race and ethnicity in women: An American Heart Association national survey. *Journal of Women's Health, 19*(7), 1243–1249.

U.S. Department of Health and Human Services. (2010). *The guide to clinical preventive services 2010–2011: Recommendations of the U.S. Preventive Services Task Force.* Rockville, MD: Agency for Healthcare Research and Quality.

Risk Control: Drug Use — 1904

Definition: Personal actions to understand, prevent, eliminate, or reduce the threats to health associated with drug use

OUTCOME TARGET RATING: Maintain at_____ Increase to_____

OUTCOME OVERALL RATING	Never demonstrated 1	Rarely demonstrated 2	Sometimes demonstrated 3	Often demonstrated 4	Consistently demonstrated 5	
Indicators:						
190418 Seeks current information about drug misuse	1	2	3	4	5	NA
190419 Identifies risk factors for drug misuse	1	2	3	4	5	NA
190401 Acknowledges personal risk for drug misuse	1	2	3	4	5	NA
190402 Acknowledges consequences associated with drug misuse	1	2	3	4	5	NA
190420 Acknowledges ability to change behavior	1	2	3	4	5	NA
190403 Monitors environment for factors encouraging drug misuse	1	2	3	4	5	NA
190404 Monitors personal drug use pattern	1	2	3	4	5	NA
190405 Develops effective drug misuse control strategies	1	2	3	4	5	NA
190406 Adjusts drug misuse control strategies	1	2	3	4	5	NA
190407 Commits to drug misuse control strategies	1	2	3	4	5	NA
190408 Follows selected drug misuse control strategies	1	2	3	4	5	NA
190409 Participates in screening for health problems	1	2	3	4	5	NA
190410 Uses health care services congruent with needs	1	2	3	4	5	NA
190411 Uses personal support systems to control drug misuse	1	2	3	4	5	NA
190412 Uses support group to control drug misuse	1	2	3	4	5	NA
190413 Uses community resources to control drug misuse	1	2	3	4	5	NA
190414 Recognizes changes in general health status	1	2	3	4	5	NA
190415 Monitors changes in general health status	1	2	3	4	5	NA
190416 Eliminates adverse drug use	1	2	3	4	5	NA

Domain-*Health Knowledge & Behavior (IV)* **Class**-*Risk Control & Safety (T)* *1st edition 1997; revised 2004, 2013*

OUTCOME CONTENT REFERENCES:

Brown, N. K. (2000). Clinical judgments of high-risk behavior during recovery. *Journal of Psychoactive Drugs, 32*(3), 299–304.

Farhat, T., Iannotti, R., & Simons-Morton, B. (2010). Overweight, obesity, youth and health-risk behaviors. *American Journal of Preventive Medicine, 38*(3), 258–267.

Hides, L., Lubman, D., Devlin, H., Cotton, S., Campbell, A., Gibbie, T., & Hellard, M. (2007). Reliability and validity of the Kessler 10 and patient health questionnaire among injecting drug users. *Australian and New Zealand Journal of Psychiatry, 41*(2), 166–168.

Simons-Morton, D. G., Mullen, P. D., Mains, D. A., Tabek, E. R., & Green, L. W. (1992). Characteristics of controlled studies of patient education and counseling for preventive health behaviors. *Patient Education and Counseling, 19*(2), 174–204.

+Skinner, H. A. (1982). The drug abuse screening test. *Addictive Behaviors, 7*(4), 363–371.

Talashek, M. L., Gerace, L. M., & Starr, K. L. (1994). The substance abuse pandemic: Determinants to guide interventions. *Public Health Nursing, 11*(2), 131–139.

U.S. Department of Health and Human Services. (2010). *The guide to clinical preventive services 2010–2011: Recommendations of the U.S. Preventive Services Task Force.* Rockville, MD: Agency for Healthcare Research and Quality.

Weitzel, E. A. (2001). Risk for poisoning: Drug toxicity. In M. Maas, K. Buckwalter, M. Hardy, T. Tripp-Reimer, M. Titler, & J. Specht (Eds.), *Nursing care of older adults: Diagnoses, outcomes & interventions* (pp. 34–46). St. Louis: Mosby.

Risk Control: Dry Eye 1927

Definition: Personal actions to understand, prevent, eliminate, or reduce the threat of dry eye

OUTCOME TARGET RATING: Maintain at_____   Increase to_____

OUTCOME OVERALL RATING		Never demonstrated 1	Rarely demonstrated 2	Sometimes demonstrated 3	Often demonstrated 4	Consistently demonstrated 5	
Indicators:							
192701	Seeks current information about dry eye	1	2	3	4	5	NA
192702	Identifies risk factors for dry eye	1	2	3	4	5	NA
192703	Identifies incomplete eyelid closure	1	2	3	4	5	NA
192704	Acknowledges personal risk factors for dry eye	1	2	3	4	5	NA
192705	Produces adequate tears	1	2	3	4	5	NA
192706	Acknowledges relationship of age and dry eye	1	2	3	4	5	NA
192707	Acknowledges relationship of gender and dry eye	1	2	3	4	5	NA
192708	Acknowledges relationship of hormones and dry eye	1	2	3	4	5	NA
192709	Acknowledges relationship of autoimmune diseases and dry eye	1	2	3	4	5	NA
192710	Identifies signs and symptoms of dry eye	1	2	3	4	5	NA
192711	Reduces contact lenses wearing time	1	2	3	4	5	NA
192712	Uses eye drops when wearing contact lenses	1	2	3	4	5	NA
192713	Avoids injury to the eye	1	2	3	4	5	NA
192714	Protects ocular surface integrity	1	2	3	4	5	NA
192715	Limits exposure to prolonged air conditioning	1	2	3	4	5	NA
192716	Limits exposure to strong wind	1	2	3	4	5	NA
192717	Limits exposure to direct sunlight	1	2	3	4	5	NA
192718	Limits exposure to air pollution	1	2	3	4	5	NA
192719	Limits exposure to low humidity	1	2	3	4	5	NA
192720	Limits prolonged reading	1	2	3	4	5	NA
192721	Limits prolonged use of computer	1	2	3	4	5	NA
192722	Avoids tobacco use	1	2	3	4	5	NA
192723	Blinks at frequent intervals	1	2	3	4	5	NA
192724	Closes eyelids completely	1	2	3	4	5	NA
192725	Obtains periodic eye exam	1	2	3	4	5	NA
192726	Uses ointments and lubricants as prescribed	1	2	3	4	5	NA
192727	Identifies medications that contribute to dry eye	1	2	3	4	5	NA
192728	Uses devices to protect eyes	1	2	3	4	5	NA
192729	Uses moisture chamber to prevent tear evaporation	1	2	3	4	5	NA

R

Domain-*Health Knowledge & Behavior (IV)*   **Class**-*Risk Control & Safety (T)*   *5th edition 2013*

OUTCOME CONTENT REFERENCES:

Dawson, D. (2005). Development of a new eye care guideline for critically ill patients. *Intensive Critical Care Nursing, 21*(2), 119–122.

Ezra, D. G., Chan, M. P., Solebo, L, Malik, A. P., Crane, E., Coombes, A., & Healy, M. (2009). Randomised trial comparing ocular lubricants and polyacrylamide hydrogel dressings in the prevention of exposure keratopathy in the critically ill. *Intensive Care Medicine, 35*(3), 455–461.

Germano, E. M., Mello, M. J., Sena, D. F., Correia, J. B., & Amorim, M. M. (2009). Incidence and risk factors of corneal epithelial defects in mechanically ventilated children. *Critical Care Medicine, 37*(3), 1097–100.

Joyce, N. (2002). *Eye care for the intensive care patient: A systemic review* (pp. 1–87). South Australia: Joanna Briggs Institute for Evidence Based Nursing and Midwifery.

Kanski, J. J., & Bowling, B. (2011). *Clinical ophthalmology: A systematic approach* (7th ed., pp. 121–130). Edinburgh, Scotland: Elsevier Limited.

Koroloff, N., Boots, R., Lipman, J., Thomas, P., Rickard, C., & Cover, F. (2004). A randomized controlled study of the efficacy of hypromellose and lacri-lube combination versus polyethylene/cling wrap to prevent corneal epithelial breakdown in the semiconscious intensive care patient. *Intensive Care Medicine, 30*(6), 1122–1126.

Rao, S. N. (2008). Progression: The new approach to dry eye. *Review of Ophthalmology,* 55–58.

Rosenberg, J. B., & Eisen, L. A. (2008). Eye care in the intensive care unit: Narrative review and meta-analysis. *Critical Care Medicine, 36*(12), 3151–3155.

Sahai, A., & Malik, P. (2005). Dry eye: Prevalence and attributable risk factors in a hospital-based population. *Indian Journal of Ophthalmology, 53*(2), 87–91.

Sendecka, M., Baryluk, A., Polz-Dacewicz, M. (2004). Prevalence and risk factors of dry eye syndrome. *Przeglad Epidemiologiczny, 58*(1), 227–233.

So, H. M., Lee, C. C., Leung, A. K., Lim, J. M., Chan, C. S., & Yan, W. W. (2008). Comparing the effectiveness of polyethylene covers (Gladwrap) with lanolin (Duraters) eye ointment to prevent corneal abrasions in critically ill patients: A randomized controlled study. *International Journal of Nursing Studies, 45*(11), 1565–1571.

Risk Control: Hearing Impairment 1915

Definition: Personal actions to understand, prevent, eliminate, or reduce threats to hearing function

OUTCOME TARGET RATING: Maintain at_____   Increase to_____

OUTCOME OVERALL RATING		Never demonstrated 1	Rarely demonstrated 2	Sometimes demonstrated 3	Often demonstrated 4	Consistently demonstrated 5	
Indicators:							
191513	Seeks current information about hearing impairment	1	2	3	4	5	NA
191514	Identifies risk factors for hearing impairment	1	2	3	4	5	NA
191515	Acknowledges personal risk factors for hearing impairment	1	2	3	4	5	NA
191501	Monitors symptoms of hearing deterioration	1	2	3	4	5	NA
191502	Protects eardrum integrity	1	2	3	4	5	NA
191503	Avoids trauma to the ear	1	2	3	4	5	NA
191504	Reduces noise exposure	1	2	3	4	5	NA
191516	Seeks assistance in removing excessive cerumen	1	2	3	4	5	NA
191506	Manages ear infections	1	2	3	4	5	NA
191507	Uses hearing protective devices	1	2	3	4	5	NA
191508	Obtains periodic ear examinations	1	2	3	4	5	NA
191509	Obtains periodic hearing tests	1	2	3	4	5	NA
191510	Uses ear medication as prescribed	1	2	3	4	5	NA
191511	Avoids placing objects in ear	1	2	3	4	5	NA

***Domain**-Health Knowledge & Behavior (IV)*   ***Class**-Risk Control & Safety (T)*   *2nd edition 2000; revised 2004, 2013*

OUTCOME CONTENT REFERENCES:

Daniel, E. (2007). Noise and hearing loss: A review. *Journal of School Health, 77*(5), 225–231.

Muhr, P., & Rosenhall, U. (2010). Self-assessed auditory symptoms, noise exposure, and measured auditory function among healthy young Swedish men. *International Journal of Audiology, 49*(4), 317–325.

Phipps, W. J., Monahan, F. D., Sands J. K., Marek, J., & Neighbors, M. (Eds.). (2003). *Medical-surgical nursing: Concepts and clinical practice* (7th ed). St. Louis: Mosby.

Smeltzer, S., Bare, B., Hinkle, J., & Cheever, K. (2010). *Brunner and Suddarth's textbook of medical-surgical nursing* (12th ed.). Philadelphia: Lippincott Williams & Wilkins.

U.S. Department of Health and Human Services. (2010). *The guide to clinical preventive services 2010–2011: Recommendations of the U.S. Preventive Services Task Force.* Rockville, MD: Agency for Healthcare Research and Quality.

Risk Control: Hypertension 1928

Definition: Personal actions to understand, prevent, eliminate, or reduce the threat of high blood pressure

OUTCOME TARGET RATING: Maintain at_____   Increase to_____

		Never demonstrated	Rarely demonstrated	Sometimes demonstrated	Often demonstrated	Consistently demonstrated	
OUTCOME OVERALL RATING		1	2	3	4	5	
Indicators:							
192801	Seeks current information about hypertension	1	2	3	4	5	NA
192802	Identifies risk factors for hypertension	1	2	3	4	5	NA
192803	Acknowledges personal risk factors for hypertension	1	2	3	4	5	NA
192804	Acknowledges ability to change behavior	1	2	3	4	5	NA
192805	Identifies signs and symptoms of hypertension	1	2	3	4	5	NA
192806	Checks blood pressure at recommended intervals	1	2	3	4	5	NA
192807	Monitors health status changes	1	2	3	4	5	NA
192808	Follows dietary recommendations	1	2	3	4	5	NA
192809	Adheres to sodium intake recommendations	1	2	3	4	5	NA
192810	Maintains recommended body weight	1	2	3	4	5	NA
192811	Participates in regular exercise	1	2	3	4	5	NA
192812	Uses relaxation techniques	1	2	3	4	5	NA
192813	Uses strategies to facilitate sleep	1	2	3	4	5	NA
192814	Uses strategies to reduce stress	1	2	3	4	5	NA
192815	Monitors medication effects that influence blood pressure	1	2	3	4	5	NA
192816	Eliminates tobacco use	1	2	3	4	5	NA
192817	Consumes alcohol in moderation	1	2	3	4	5	NA
192818	Consumes caffeine in moderation	1	2	3	4	5	NA
192819	Monitors changes in general health status	1	2	3	4	5	NA
192820	Uses health care services to screen for hypertension	1	2	3	4	5	NA
192821	Uses personal support systems to modify lifestyle	1	2	3	4	5	NA
192822	Uses community resources to reduce hypertension risk	1	2	3	4	5	NA

R

Domain-Health Knowledge & Behavior (IV)   *Class*-Risk Control & Safety (T)   5th edition 2013

OUTCOME CONTENT REFERENCES:

Anglum, A. (2009). Primary care management of childhood adolescent hypertension. *Journal of American Academy Nurse Practitioners, 21*(10), 529–534.

British Columbia: Ministry of Health Services. (2008). *Guidelines and protocols: Hypertension—Detection, diagnosis and management.* Retrieved from http://www.bcguidelines.ca/gpac/guideline_hypertension.html

Chummun, H. (2009). Hypertension—A contemporary approach to nursing care. *British Journal of Nursing, 18*(13), 784–789.

Good, L. B. (2010). Hypertension highlights: Blood pressure targets, global risk factors, and diabetes: The latest data are not encouraging. *Medscape Cardiology.* Retrieved February 7, 2011, from www.medscape.com/viewarticle/715584

National Heart, Lung, and Blood Institute (NHLBI). (2003). JNC 7 express: The seventh report of the Joint National Committee on Prevention, Detection, Evaluation, and Treatment of High Blood Pressure. Bethesda, MD: Author.

Risk Control: Hyperthermia 1922

Definition: Personal actions to understand, prevent, eliminate, or reduce the threat of high body temperature

OUTCOME TARGET RATING: Maintain at_____ Increase to_____

OUTCOME OVERALL RATING	Never demonstrated 1	Rarely demonstrated 2	Sometimes demonstrated 3	Often demonstrated 4	Consistently demonstrated 5	
Indicators:						
192220 Seeks current information about hyperthermia	1	2	3	4	5	NA
192221 Identifies risk factors for hyperthermia	1	2	3	4	5	NA
192201 Acknowledges personal risk factors for hyperthermia	1	2	3	4	5	NA
192202 Identifies signs and symptoms of hyperthermia	1	2	3	4	5	NA
192203 Identifies health conditions that accelerate heat production	1	2	3	4	5	NA
192222 Monitors environment for factors that increase body temperature	1	2	3	4	5	NA
192206 Identifies relationship of age to body temperature	1	2	3	4	5	NA
192207 Modifies living environment to control body temperature	1	2	3	4	5	NA
192223 Monitors changes in general health status	1	2	3	4	5	NA
192208 Modifies fluid intake as appropriate	1	2	3	4	5	NA
192209 Modifies physical activity to control body temperature	1	2	3	4	5	NA
192210 Wears appropriate clothing to protect skin	1	2	3	4	5	NA
192211 Maintains intact skin integument	1	2	3	4	5	NA
192212 Participates in screening for health problems that increase risk	1	2	3	4	5	NA
192213 Performs self-protective actions to control body temperature	1	2	3	4	5	NA
192214 Identifies prescribed medication effects on body temperature	1	2	3	4	5	NA
192215 Avoids strenuous activities to reduce risk	1	2	3	4	5	NA
192216 Avoids alcohol consumption	1	2	3	4	5	NA
192217 Uses community shelters to reduce risk	1	2	3	4	5	NA
192218 Performs outdoor activities at coolest part of day	1	2	3	4	5	NA
192219 Allows for acclimatization to warmer temperatures	1	2	3	4	5	NA

Domain-Health Knowledge & Behavior (IV) **Class**-Risk Control & Safety (T) 4th edition 2008; revised 2013

OUTCOME CONTENT REFERENCES:

DeVaul, R. (2003). Heat stress precautions. *Occupational Health & Safety, 72*(5), 86–88.

Elliott, F. (2006). Take stock to stop heat stress. *Occupational Health & Safety, 75*(5), 98–99.

Jepson, R., Alonso, E., & McFarland, H. (2009). Case study. Overheated dialysate: A case study and review. *Nephrology Nursing Journal, 36*(5), 551–553.

Kare, J., & Shneiderman, A. (2001). Hyperthermia and hypothermia in the older population. *Topics in Emergency Medicine, 23*(3), 39–52.

McLafferty, E. (2010). Prevention and management of hyperthermia during a heat wave. *Nursing Older People, 22*(7), 23–27.

McLaren, C., Null, J., & Quinn, J. (2005). Heat stress from enclosed vehicles: Moderate ambient temperatures cause significant temperature rise in enclosed vehicles. *Pediatrics, 116*(1), 109–112.

Nixdorf-Miller, A., & Hunsaker, D. M., Hunsaker, J. C., III. (2006). Hypothermia and hyperthermia medicolegal investigation of morbidity and mortality from exposure to environmental temperature extremes. *Archives of Pathologic Laboratory Medicine, 130*(9), 1297–1304.

Wood, L. (2004). Heat resistant: How to identify the rationale with which to support the frequency and type of health monitoring of employees, in relation to heat exposure in their working roles. *Occupational Health, 56*(7), 25–30.

R

Risk Control: Hypotension   1933

Definition: Personal actions to understand, prevent, eliminate, or reduce the threat of low blood pressure

OUTCOME TARGET RATING: Maintain at_____   Increase to_____

OUTCOME OVERALL RATING		Never demonstrated 1	Rarely demonstrated 2	Sometimes demonstrated 3	Often demonstrated 4	Consistently demonstrated 5	
Indicators:							
193301	Seeks current information about hypotension	1	2	3	4	5	NA
193302	Identifies risk factors for hypotension	1	2	3	4	5	NA
193303	Identifies signs and symptoms of hypotension	1	2	3	4	5	NA
193304	Identifies signs and symptoms of shock	1	2	3	4	5	NA
193305	Monitors blood pressure at recommended intervals	1	2	3	4	5	NA
193306	Identifies tolerance for low blood pressure	1	2	3	4	5	NA
193307	Develops effective strategies to take medication as prescribed	1	2	3	4	5	NA
193308	Report episodes of lightheadedness or dizziness to health provider	1	2	3	4	5	NA
193309	Monitors frequency of hypotensive episodes	1	2	3	4	5	NA
193310	Monitors for orthostatic hypotension when changing positions	1	2	3	4	5	NA
193311	Avoids standing for long periods of time	1	2	3	4	5	NA
193312	Wears compression stockings	1	2	3	4	5	NA
193313	Maintains hydration	1	2	3	4	5	NA
193314	Eats frequent low-carbohydrate meals	1	2	3	4	5	NA
193315	Includes more sodium in diet	1	2	3	4	5	NA
193316	Includes caffeinated drinks with meals	1	2	3	4	5	NA
193317	Acknowledges risk for hypotension when taking pain medication	1	2	3	4	5	NA
193318	Acknowledges risk for hypotension when taking antidepressants	1	2	3	4	5	NA
193319	Commits to alcohol use control strategies	1	2	3	4	5	NA
193320	Acknowledges higher risk for falls with hypotension medications	1	2	3	4	5	NA

Domain-*Health Knowledge & Behavior (IV)*   **Class**-*Risk Control & Safety (T)*   *5th edition 2013*

R

OUTCOME CONTENT REFERENCES:

Arbogast, S., Alshekhlee, A., Hussain, Z., McNeeley, K., & Chelimksy, T. (2009). Hypotension unawareness in profound orthostatic hypotension. *The American Journal of Medicine, 122*(6), 574–580.

Weiss, A., Chagnac, A., Beloosesky, Y., Weinstein, T., Grinblat, J., & Grossman, E. (2004). Orthostatic hypotension in the elderly: Are the diagnostic criteria adequate? *Journal of Human Hypertension, 18*(5), 301–305.

Risk Control: Hypothermia 1923

Definition: Personal actions to understand, prevent, eliminate, or reduce the threat of low body temperature

OUTCOME TARGET RATING: Maintain at_____ Increase to_____

		Never demonstrated	Rarely demonstrated	Sometimes demonstrated	Often demonstrated	Consistently demonstrated	
OUTCOME OVERALL RATING		1	2	3	4	5	
Indicators:							
192319	Seeks current information about hypothermia	1	2	3	4	5	NA
192320	Identifies risk factors for hypothermia	1	2	3	4	5	NA
192301	Acknowledges personal risk factors for hypothermia	1	2	3	4	5	NA
192302	Identifies signs and symptoms of hypothermia	1	2	3	4	5	NA
192303	Identifies health conditions that decrease heat production	1	2	3	4	5	NA
192304	Identifies conditions that jeopardize ability to conserve heat	1	2	3	4	5	NA
192305	Identifies health conditions that accelerate heat loss	1	2	3	4	5	NA
192321	Monitors environment for factors that decrease body temperature	1	2	3	4	5	NA
192307	Identifies relationship of age to body temperature	1	2	3	4	5	NA
192322	Monitors changes in general health status	1	2	3	4	5	NA
192308	Modifies living environment to promote heat conservation	1	2	3	4	5	NA
192309	Modifies physical activity to maintain body temperature	1	2	3	4	5	NA
192310	Maintains emergency cold weather supplies in vehicle	1	2	3	4	5	NA
192311	Maintains intact skin integument	1	2	3	4	5	NA
192312	Participates in screening for health problems that increase risk	1	2	3	4	5	NA
192313	Performs self-protective actions to control body temperature	1	2	3	4	5	NA
192314	Modifies fluid intake as appropriate	1	2	3	4	5	NA
192315	Wears appropriate clothing to protect skin	1	2	3	4	5	NA
192316	Performs outdoor activities at warmest part of day	1	2	3	4	5	NA
192317	Identifies prescribed medication effects on body temperature	1	2	3	4	5	NA
192318	Allows for acclimatization to colder temperatures	1	2	3	4	5	NA

Domain-*Health Knowledge & Behavior (IV)* **Class**-*Risk Control & Safety (T)* *4th edition 2008; revised 2013*

OUTCOME CONTENT REFERENCES:
Cuddy, M. (2004). The effects of drugs on thermoregulation. *Advanced Practice in Acute Clinical Care, 15*(2), 238–253.
Elliott, F. (2005). Do the prep work. *Occupational Health & Safety, 74*(11), 68, 70.
Kare, J., & Shneiderman, A. (2001). Hyperthermia and hypothermia in the older population. *Topics in Emergency Medicine, 23*(3), 39–52.
Keresztes, P. A., & Brick, K. (2006). Therapeutic hypothermia after cardiac arrest. *Dimensions of Critical Care Nursing, 25*(2), 71–76.
Lynch, S., Dixon, J., & Leary, D. (2010). Reducing the risk of unplanned perioperative hypothermia. *AORN Journal, 92*(5), 553–565.
Neno, R. (2005). Hypothermia: Assessment, treatment and prevention. *Nursing Standard, 19*(20), 47–52.
Nixdorf-Miller, A., Hunsaker, D. M., & Hunsaker, J. C., III. (2006). Hypothermia and hyperthermia medicolegal investigation of morbidity and mortality from exposure to environmental temperature extremes. *Archives of Pathologic Laboratory Medicine, 130*(9), 1297–1304.

Risk Control: Infectious Process   1924

Definition: Personal actions to understand, prevent, eliminate or reduce the threat of acquiring an infection

OUTCOME TARGET RATING: Maintain at_____   Increase to_____

		Never demonstrated	Rarely demonstrated	Sometimes demonstrated	Often demonstrated	Consistently demonstrated	
OUTCOME OVERALL RATING		1	2	3	4	5	
Indicators:							
192425	Seeks current information about infection control	1	2	3	4	5	NA
192426	Identifies risk factors for infection	1	2	3	4	5	NA
192401	Acknowledges personal risk factors for infection	1	2	3	4	5	NA
192402	Acknowledges consequences associated with infection	1	2	3	4	5	NA
192403	Acknowledges behaviors associated with risk for infection	1	2	3	4	5	NA
192404	Identifies infection risk in daily activities	1	2	3	4	5	NA
192405	Identifies signs and symptoms of infection	1	2	3	4	5	NA
192406	Seeks validation of perceived infection risk	1	2	3	4	5	NA
192407	Identifies strategies to protect self from others with infection	1	2	3	4	5	NA
192408	Monitors personal behaviors for factors associated with infection risk	1	2	3	4	5	NA
192409	Monitors environment for factors associated with infection risk	1	2	3	4	5	NA
192410	Monitors time of infectious disease incubation period	1	2	3	4	5	NA
192411	Maintains a clean environment	1	2	3	4	5	NA
192412	Uses strategies to disinfect supplies	1	2	3	4	5	NA
192413	Develops effective infection control strategies	1	2	3	4	5	NA
192414	Uses universal precautions	1	2	3	4	5	NA
192415	Practices hand sanitization	1	2	3	4	5	NA
192416	Practices infection control strategies	1	2	3	4	5	NA
192417	Adjusts infection control strategies	1	2	3	4	5	NA
192420	Monitors changes in general health status	1	2	3	4	5	NA
192421	Takes immediate actions to reduce risk	1	2	3	4	5	NA
192422	Obtains recommended immunizations	1	2	3	4	5	NA
192423	Uses reputable sources of information	1	2	3	4	5	NA
192424	Uses health care services congruent with needs	1	2	3	4	5	NA
192427	Seeks information on health risks prior to travel	1	2	3	4	5	NA

Domain-*Health Knowledge & Behavior (IV)*   **Class**-*Risk Control & Safety (T)*   *4th edition 2008; revised 2013*

OUTCOME CONTENT REFERENCES:
Carruthers, S. (2003). The ins and outs of injection in Western Australia. *Journal of Substance Use, 8,* 11–18.
Grundmann, H., Aires-de-Sousa, M., Boyce, J., & Tiemersma, E. (2006). Emergence and resurgence of meticillin-resistant staphylococcus aureus as a public-health threat. *Lancet, 368,* 874–885.
Krein, S. L., Olmsted, R. N., Hofer, T. P., Kowalski, C., Forman, J., Banaszak, J., & Saint, S. (2006). Translating infection prevention evidence into practice using quantitative and qualitative research. *American Journal of Infection Control, 34,* 507–512.
Nichol, K. L., & Treanor, J. J. (2006). Vaccines for seasonal and pandemic influenza. *Journal of Infectious Diseases, 194*(Suppl. 2), S111–S118.
Veenema, T. G., & Toke, J. (2006). Early detection and surveillance for biopreparedness and emerging infectious diseases. *Online Journal of Issues in Nursing, 11*(1), 3.

R

Risk Control: Lipid Disorder 1929

Definition: Personal actions to understand, prevent, eliminate, or reduce the threat of hyperlipidemia

OUTCOME TARGET RATING: Maintain at_____ Increase to_____

		Never demonstrated	Rarely demonstrated	Sometimes demonstrated	Often demonstrated	Consistently demonstrated	
OUTCOME OVERALL RATING		1	2	3	4	5	
Indicators:							
192901	Seeks current information about lipid disorders	1	2	3	4	5	NA
192902	Identifies risk factors for lipid disorders	1	2	3	4	5	NA
192903	Acknowledges personal risk factors for lipid disorder	1	2	3	4	5	NA
192904	Modifies lifestyle to reduce risk	1	2	3	4	5	NA
192905	Develops effective risk control strategies	1	2	3	4	5	NA
192906	Commits to risk control strategies	1	2	3	4	5	NA
192907	Monitors changes in general health status	1	2	3	4	5	NA
192908	Participates in aerobic exercise	1	2	3	4	5	NA
192909	Follows dietary recommendations	1	2	3	4	5	NA
192910	Maintains recommended body weight	1	2	3	4	5	NA
192911	Avoids tobacco use	1	2	3	4	5	NA
192912	Obtains prescribed laboratory tests	1	2	3	4	5	NA
192913	Uses medication as prescribed	1	2	3	4	5	NA
192914	Uses significant others to support behavior changes	1	2	3	4	5	NA
192915	Uses reputable sources of information	1	2	3	4	5	NA
192916	Uses community resources to identify lipid disorder risk	1	2	3	4	5	NA

Domain-*Health Knowledge & Behavior (IV)* **Class**-*Risk Control & Safety (T)* *5th edition 2013*

OUTCOME CONTENT REFERENCES:
Bertolotti, M. (2009). High protein intake reduces intrahepatocellular lipid deposition in humans. *The American Journal of Clinical Nutrition, 90*(4), 1002–1009.
Gatti, A., Maranghi, M., Bacci, S., Carallo, C., Gnasso, A., Mandosi, E., Fallarino, M., Morano, S., Trischitta, V., & Filetti, S. (2009). Poor glycemic control is an independent risk factor for low HDL cholesterol in patients with type 2 diabetes. *Diabetes Care, 32*(8), 1550–1552.
Lowenstein, C. J., & Cameron, S. J. (2010). High-density lipoprotein metabolism and endothelial function. *Current Opinion in Endocrinology, Diabetes & Obesity, 17*(2), 166–170.
McCauley, K. M. (2007). Modifying women's risk for cardiovascular disease. *JOGNN: Journal of Obstetric, Gynecologic & Neonatal Nursing, 36*(2), 116–124.
Sassen, B., Cornelissen, V., Kiers, H., Wittink, H., Kok, G., & Vanhees, L. (2009). Physical fitness matters more than physical activity in controlling cardiovascular disease risk factors. *European Journal of Cardiovascular Prevention & Rehabilitation, 16*(6), 677–683.

Risk Control: Osteoporosis 1930

Definition: Personal actions to understand, prevent, eliminate, or reduce the threat of osteoporosis

OUTCOME TARGET RATING: Maintain at_____ Increase to_____

		Never demonstrated	Rarely demonstrated	Sometimes demonstrated	Often demonstrated	Consistently demonstrated	
OUTCOME OVERALL RATING:		1	2	3	4	5	
Indicators:							
193001	Seeks current information about osteoporosis	1	2	3	4	5	NA
193002	Identifies risk factors for osteoporosis	1	2	3	4	5	NA
193003	Acknowledges personal risk factors for osteoporosis	1	2	3	4	5	NA

Risk Control: Osteoporosis—cont'd

		Never demonstrated	Rarely demonstrated	Sometimes demonstrated	Often demonstrated	Consistently demonstrated	
193004	Monitors personal risk factors	1	2	3	4	5	NA
193005	Selects foods that provide calcium to meet requirement	1	2	3	4	5	NA
193006	Uses calcium supplements within recommended guidelines	1	2	3	4	5	NA
193007	Uses Vitamin D supplements within recommended guidelines	1	2	3	4	5	NA
193008	Avoids alcohol misuse	1	2	3	4	5	NA
193009	Avoids tobacco use	1	2	3	4	5	NA
193010	Maintains recommended body weight	1	2	3	4	5	NA
193011	Participates in weight-bearing activities appropriate for age	1	2	3	4	5	NA
193012	Obtains periodic prescribed physical examination	1	2	3	4	5	NA
193013	Reports family history of osteoporosis	1	2	3	4	5	NA
193014	Reports history of fractures	1	2	3	4	5	NA
193015	Identifies medications that may reduce bone density	1	2	3	4	5	NA
193016	Reports use of medications that may reduce bone density	1	2	3	4	5	NA
193017	Obtains standardized bone mineral density evaluation	1	2	3	4	5	NA
193018	Follows recommendations based on bone mineral density evaluation	1	2	3	4	5	NA
193019	Takes anti-resorptive medications as prescribed	1	2	3	4	5	NA
193020	Reports side effects of prescribed anti-resorptive medication	1	2	3	4	5	NA
193021	Follows proper procedure for oral bisphosphonate therapy	1	2	3	4	5	NA
193022	Monitors changes in general health status	1	2	3	4	5	NA
193023	Uses personal support systems to reduce osteoporosis risk	1	2	3	4	5	NA
193024	Uses community resources to reduce osteoporosis risk	1	2	3	4	5	NA

Domain-Health Knowledge & Behavior (IV)   **Class**-Risk Control & Safety (T)   5th edition 2013

OUTCOME CONTENT REFERENCES:

Alexander, L., LaRosa, J. H., Bader, H., Garfield, S., & Alexander, W. J. (2010). *New dimensions in women's health* (5th ed.). Boston: Jones & Bartlett.

Daly, R., Ahlborg, H., Ringsberg, K., Gardsell, P., Sembo, I., Karlsson, M. (2008). Association between changes in habitual physical activity and changes in bone density, muscle strength, and functional performance in elderly men and women. *Journal of the American Geriatrics Society, 56*(12), 2252–2260.

International Society for Clinical Densitometry (ISCD). (2004). *Pocket guide to bone mineral density testing.* Retrieved from http://www.iscd.org/visitors/pdfs/ISCD-CANADIANPanelOfficialPositions-BMDcard.pdf

Matheson, E., Mainous, A., & Carnemolla, M. (2009). The association between onion consumption and bone density in perimenopausal and postmenopausal non-Hispanic white women 50 years and older. *Menopause, 16*(4), 756–759.

National Institute of Arthritis and Musculoskeletal and Skin Diseases. (2009). *Bone mass measurement: What the numbers mean.* Retrieved from http://www.niams.nih.gov/Health_Info/Bone/Bone_Health/bone_mass_measure.asp

Papaloannou, A., Morin, S., Cheung, A., Atkinson, S., Brown, J., Feldman, S., et al. (2010). 2010 clinical practice guidelines for the diagnosis and management of osteoporosis in Canada: A summary. *Canadian Medical Association Journal, 182*(17), 1864–1873.

Rosen, H. (2010). *Drugs that affect bone metabolism.* Retrieved from http://www.uptodate.com/contents/drugs-that-affect-bone-metabolism

Vupadhyayula, P. M., Gallagher, J. C., Templin, T., Logsdon, S. M., & Smith, L. M. (2009). Effects of soy protein isolate on bone mineral density and physical performance indices in postmenopausal women—A 2-year randomized, double-blind, placebo-controlled trial. *Menopause, 16*(2), 320–328.

R

Risk Control: Sexually Transmitted Diseases (STD)   1905

Definition: Personal actions to understand, prevent, eliminate, or reduce the threat of acquiring a sexually transmitted disease

OUTCOME TARGET RATING: Maintain at_____   Increase to_____

		Never demonstrated	Rarely demonstrated	Sometimes demonstrated	Often demonstrated	Consistently demonstrated	
OUTCOME OVERALL RATING		1	2	3	4	5	
Indicators:							
190519	Seeks current information about sexually transmitted diseases	1	2	3	4	5	NA
190520	Identifies risk factors for sexually transmitted diseases	1	2	3	4	5	NA
190501	Acknowledges personal risk factors for sexually transmitted disease	1	2	3	4	5	NA
190502	Acknowledges consequences associated with sexually transmitted disease	1	2	3	4	5	NA
190521	Acknowledges ability to change behavior	1	2	3	4	5	NA
190505	Develops effective strategies to reduce sexually transmitted disease exposure	1	2	3	4	5	NA
190522	Limits number of partners	1	2	3	4	5	NA
190509	Inquires of partner's sexually transmitted disease status before sexual activity	1	2	3	4	5	NA
190523	Negotiates safe sexual practices with partner	1	2	3	4	5	NA
190524	Uses a condom	1	2	3	4	5	NA
190525	Practices safe anal sex	1	2	3	4	5	NA
190510	Uses strategies to prevent sexually transmitted disease transmission	1	2	3	4	5	NA
190511	Recognizes signs and symptoms of sexually transmitted disease	1	2	3	4	5	NA
190526	Monitors for signs and symptoms of sexually transmitted disease	1	2	3	4	5	NA
190512	Participates in screening for sexually transmitted disease	1	2	3	4	5	NA
190527	Obtains health care services when necessary	1	2	3	4	5	NA
190528	Uses community resources to reduce sexually transmitted disease risk	1	2	3	4	5	NA
190517	Maintains absence of sexually transmitted disease	1	2	3	4	5	NA

R

Domain-Health Knowledge & Behavior (IV)   *Class-Risk Control & Safety (T)*   *1st edition 1997; revised 2004, 2013*

OUTCOME CONTENT REFERENCES:

+Card, J. J. (Ed.). (1993). *Handbook of adolescent sexuality and pregnancy: Research and evaluation instruments.* Thousand Oaks, CA: Sage.

Jenness, S., Begier, E., Neaigus, A., Murrill, C., Wendel, T., & Hagan, H. (2011). Unprotected anal intercourse and sexually transmitted diseases in high-risk heterosexual women. *American Journal of Public Health, 101*(4), 745–750.

Kalichman, S., Cain, D., Eaton, L., Jooste, S., & Simbayi, L. (2011). Randomized clinical trial of brief risk reduction counseling for sexual transmitted infection clinic patients in Cape Town, South Africa. *American Journal of Public Health, 101*(9), e9–e17.

Marston, C., & King, E. (2006). Factors that shape young people's sexual behaviour: A systematic review. *Lancet, 386*, 1581–1586.

Miller, K. E., & Graves, J. C. (2000). Update on the prevention and treatment of sexually transmitted diseases. *American Family Physician, 61*(2), 379–386.

Rotheram-Borus, M. J., Reid, M. A., & Rosario, M. (1994). Factors mediating changes in sexual HIV risk behaviors among gay and bisexual male adolescents. *American Journal of Public Health, 84*(12), 1938–1946.

Scott-Sheldon, L., Fielder, R., & Carey, M. (2010). Sexual risk reduction interventions for patients attending sexually transmitted disease clinics in the United States: A meta-analytic review, 1986 to early 2009. *Annals of Behavioral Medicine, 40*(2), 191–204.

Simons-Morton, D. G., Mullen, P. D., Mains, D. A., Tabak, E. R., & Green, L. W. (1992). Characteristics of controlled studies of patient education and counseling for preventive health behaviors. *Patient Education and Counseling, 19*(2), 174–204.

U.S. Department of Health and Human Services. (2010). *The guide to clinical preventive services 2010–2011: Recommendations of the U.S. Preventive Services Task Force.* Rockville, MD: Agency for Healthcare Research and Quality.

Risk Control: Stroke 1931

Definition: Personal actions to understand, prevent, eliminate, or reduce the threat of a cerebral vascular accident

OUTCOME TARGET RATING: Maintain at_____   Increase to_____

		Never demonstrated	Rarely demonstrated	Sometimes demonstrated	Often demonstrated	Consistently demonstrated	
OUTCOME OVERALL RATING		1	2	3	4	5	
Indicators:							
193101	Seeks current information about stroke prevention	1	2	3	4	5	NA
193102	Identifies risk factors for stroke	1	2	3	4	5	NA
193103	Acknowledges personal risk factors for stroke	1	2	3	4	5	NA
193104	Acknowledges ability to change behavior	1	2	3	4	5	NA
193105	Acknowledges ability to change modifiable risk factors	1	2	3	4	5	NA
193106	Develops effective risk control strategies	1	2	3	4	5	NA
193107	Commits to risk control strategies	1	2	3	4	5	NA
193108	Monitors blood pressure	1	2	3	4	5	NA
193109	Participates in regular exercise	1	2	3	4	5	NA
193110	Uses effective weight control strategies	1	2	3	4	5	NA
193111	Follows dietary recommendations	1	2	3	4	5	NA
193112	Reduces intake of dietary saturated fat and cholesterol	1	2	3	4	5	NA
193113	Reduces sodium intake	1	2	3	4	5	NA
193114	Participates in screening for dyslipidemia	1	2	3	4	5	NA
193115	Participates in vascular screening	1	2	3	4	5	NA
193116	Maintains glycemic control	1	2	3	4	5	NA
193117	Uses medication as prescribed	1	2	3	4	5	NA
193118	Complies with treatment regimen for comorbid conditions	1	2	3	4	5	NA
193119	Eliminates tobacco use	1	2	3	4	5	NA
193120	Follows alcohol restrictions	1	2	3	4	5	NA
193121	Uses strategies to reduce stress	1	2	3	4	5	NA
193122	Uses health care services congruent with needs	1	2	3	4	5	NA
193123	Recognizes changes in general health status	1	2	3	4	5	NA
193124	Monitors changes in general health status	1	2	3	4	5	NA

Domain-Health Knowledge & Behavior (IV)   *Class*-Risk Control & Safety (T)   5th edition 2013

R

OUTCOME CONTENT REFERENCES:

Brassard, A. (2009). Identification of patients at risk of ischemic events for long-term secondary prevention. *Journal of the American Academy of Nurse Practitioners, 21*(12), 677–689.

Elkind, M. S. (2009). TIA and stroke: Pathophysiology, management, and prevention. *American Health & Drug Benefits, 2*(Suppl. 8), S8–S14.

Furie, K. L., Kasner, S. E., Adams, R. J., Albers, G. W., Bush, R. L., Fagan, S. C., Halperin, J. L., Johnston, S. C., Katzan, I., Kernan, W. N., Mitchell, P. H., Ovbiagele, B., Palesch, Y. Y., Sacco, R. L., Schwamm, L. H., Wassertheil-Smoller, S., Turan, T. N., & Wentworth, D. (2011). Guidelines for the prevention of stroke in patients with stroke or transient ischemic attack: A guideline for healthcare professionals from the American Heart Association/American Stroke Association. *Stroke, 42*(1), 227–276.

Gillham, S., Endacott, R. (2010). Impact of enhanced secondary prevention on health behaviour in patients following minor stroke and transient ischaemic attack: A randomized controlled trial. *Clinical Rehabilitation, 24*(9), 822–830.

Johnson, M., Moorhead, S., Bulechek, G., Butcher, H., Maas, M., Swanson, E. (2012). Stroke. In *NOC and NIC linkages to NANDA-I and clinical conditions: Supporting critical reasoning and quality care* (3rd ed., pp. 352–355). St. Louis: Elsevier Mosby.

Klein-Ritter, D. (2009). An evidence-based review of the AMA/AHA guideline for the primary prevention of ischemic stroke. *Geriatrics, 64*(9), 16–20.

Lewis, S. L., Heitkemper, M. M., Dirksen, S. R., O'Brien, P. G., & Bucher, L. (2007). *Medical-surgical nursing: Assessment and management of clinical problems* (7th ed.). St. Louis: Mosby.

Sit, J. W., Yip, V. Y., Ko, S. K., Gun, A. P., & Lee, J. S. (2007). A quasi-experimental study on a community-based stroke prevention programme for clients with minor stroke. *Journal of Clinical Nursing, 16*(2), 272–281.

Slark, J. (2010). Adherence to secondary prevention strategies after stroke: A review of the literature. *British Journal of Neuroscience Nursing, 6*(6), 282–286.

Risk Control: Sun Exposure 1925

Definition: Personal actions to understand, prevent, or reduce threats to skin and eyes from sun exposure

OUTCOME TARGET RATING: Maintain at_____   Increase to_____

		Never demonstrated	Rarely demonstrated	Sometimes demonstrated	Often demonstrated	Consistently demonstrated	
OUTCOME OVERALL RATING		1	2	3	4	5	
Indicators:							
192516	Seeks current information about control of sun exposure	1	2	3	4	5	NA
192517	Identifies risk of sun exposure	1	2	3	4	5	NA
192501	Acknowledges personal risk factors of sun exposure	1	2	3	4	5	NA
192502	Selects sunscreen with recommended sun protection factor or greater	1	2	3	4	5	NA
192503	Applies appropriate amount of sunscreen	1	2	3	4	5	NA
192504	Reapplies sunscreen as needed	1	2	3	4	5	NA
192505	Avoids sun exposure between 10 a.m. and 3 p.m.	1	2	3	4	5	NA
192506	Monitors length of sun exposure	1	2	3	4	5	NA
192507	Seeks outdoor activities in the shade	1	2	3	4	5	NA
192508	Wears appropriate clothing to protect skin	1	2	3	4	5	NA
192509	Wears hat with 4-inch brim to protect head and face	1	2	3	4	5	NA
192510	Uses ointment to protect lips	1	2	3	4	5	NA
192511	Wears ultraviolet (UV) protection glasses when outdoors	1	2	3	4	5	NA
192512	Avoids use of ultraviolet (UV) devices	1	2	3	4	5	NA
192513	Follows recommendations for regular skin inspection	1	2	3	4	5	NA
192514	Checks medication side effects for photosensitivity	1	2	3	4	5	NA
192515	Uses reputable sources of information	1	2	3	4	5	NA

R

Domain-*Health Knowledge & Behavior (IV)*   **Class**-*Risk Control & Safety (T)*   *4th edition 2008; revised 2013*

OUTCOME CONTENT REFERENCES:

Ascherio, A., Munger, K., & Giovannucci, E. (2011). Sun exposure and vitamin D are independent risk factors for CNS demyelination. *Neurology, 76*(6), 540–548.

Castanedo-Cazares, J. P., Lepe, V., Torres-Alvarez, B., & Moncada, B. (2003). A simple measure for applying sunscreen while on holidays. *Dermatology Online Journal, 9*(3), 23.

Centers for Disease Control and Prevention. (April 26, 2002). Guidelines for school programs to prevent skin cancer. *MMWR Morbidity and Mortality Reports: Recommendations and Reports, 51*(RR04), 1–15. Retrieved September 20, 2005, from http://www.cdc.gov/mmwr/preview/mmwrhtml/rr5104a1.htm

Geller, A., Rutsch, L., Kenausis, K., & Zhang, Z. (2003). Evaluation of the SunWise school program. *Journal of School Nursing, 19*(2), 93–99.

Hatmaker, G. (2003). Development of a skin cancer prevention program. *Journal of School Nursing, 19*(2), 89–92.

Hedges, T., & Scriven, A. (2010). Young park users' attitudes and behavior to sun protection. *Global Health Promotion, 17*(4), 24–31.

Livingston, P. M., White, V., Hayman, J., & Dobbinson, S. (2003). Sun exposure and sun protection behaviours among Australian adolescents: Trends over time. *Preventive Medicine, 37*(6, Pt 1), 577–584.

Scarlett, W. L. (2003). Ultraviolet radiation: Sun exposure, tanning beds, and vitamin D levels. *Journal of the American Osteopathic Association, 103*(8), 371–375.

Risk Control: Thrombus

1932

Definition: Personal actions to understand, prevent, eliminate, or reduce the threat of thrombus formation or embolus

OUTCOME TARGET RATING: Maintain at_____ Increase to_____

OUTCOME OVERALL RATING	Never demonstrated 1	Rarely demonstrated 2	Sometimes demonstrated 3	Often demonstrated 4	Consistently demonstrated 5	
Indicators:						
193201 Seeks current information about embolus prevention	1	2	3	4	5	NA
193202 Identifies risk factors for thrombus formation	1	2	3	4	5	NA
193203 Acknowledges personal risk factors for thrombus formation	1	2	3	4	5	NA
193204 Identifies signs and symptoms of thrombus formation or embolus	1	2	3	4	5	NA
193205 Monitors for signs and symptoms of thrombus formation or embolus	1	2	3	4	5	NA
193206 Monitors environment for factors that increase risk of thrombus formation	1	2	3	4	5	NA
193207 Complies with treatment regimen for comorbid conditions	1	2	3	4	5	NA
193208 Uses medication as prescribed	1	2	3	4	5	NA
193209 Monitors medication side effects	1	2	3	4	5	NA
193210 Uses therapeutic stockings as recommended	1	2	3	4	5	NA
193211 Follows recommendations for physical activity	1	2	3	4	5	NA
193212 Uses effective weight control strategies	1	2	3	4	5	NA
193213 Eliminates tobacco use	1	2	3	4	5	NA
193214 Follows recommended alcohol restrictions	1	2	3	4	5	NA
193215 Follows fluid intake recommendations	1	2	3	4	5	NA
193216 Avoids sitting for long time periods	1	2	3	4	5	NA
193217 Follows activity recommendations for travel	1	2	3	4	5	NA
193218 Shift positions while sitting	1	2	3	4	5	NA
193219 Follows non-prescription medication precautions	1	2	3	4	5	NA
193220 Obtains periodic laboratory tests	1	2	3	4	5	NA
193221 Monitors changes in general health status	1	2	3	4	5	NA

Domain-*Health Knowledge & Behavior (IV)* **Class**-*Risk Control & Safety (T)* *5th edition 2013*

R

OUTCOME CONTENT REFERENCES:

Agnelli, G., & Becattini, C. (2008). Treatment of DVT: How long is enough and how do you predict recurrence. *Journal of Thrombosis and Thrombolysis, 25*(1), 37–44.

Andrews, P. L., & Habashi, N. M. (2010). Detecting, managing, and preventing pulmonary embolism. *American Nurse Today, 5*(9), 21–26.

Farley, A. H., McLafferty, E., Hendry, C. (2009). Pulmonary embolism: Identification, clinical features and management. *Nursing Standard, 23*(28), 49–56.

Findlay, J., Keogh, M., & Cooper, L. (2010). Venous thromboembolism prophylaxis: The role of the nurse. *British Journal of Nursing, 19*(16), 1028–1032.

Fitzgerald, J. (2010). Venous thromboembolism: Have we made headway? *Orthopaedic Nursing, 29*(4), 226–234.

Headley, C. M., & Melander, S. (2011). When it may be a pulmonary embolism. *Nephrology Nursing Journal, 38*(2), 127–152.

Houman Fekrazad, M., Lopes, R. D., Stashenko, G. J., Alexander, J. H., & Garcia, D. (2009). Treatment of venous thromboembolism: Guidelines translated for the clinician. *Journal of Thrombosis and Thrombolysis, 28*(3), 270–275.

Kearon, C., Kahn, S. R., Agnelli, G., Goldhaber, S., Raskob, G. E., Comerota, A. J., American College of Chest Physicians. (2008). Antithrombotic therapy for venous thromboembolic disease: American College of Chest Physicians evidence-based clinical practice guidelines (8th ed.). *Chest, 133*(Suppl. 6), 454S–545S

Lancaster, S. L., Owens, A., Bryant, A. S., Ramey, L. S., Nicholson, J., Gossett, K., Forni, J. T., & Padgett, T. M. (2010). Emergency: Upper-extremity deep vein thrombosis. *American Journal of Nursing, 110*(5), 48–52.

Meetoo, D. (2010). In too deep: Understanding, detecting and managing DVT. *British Journal of Nursing, 19*(16), 1021–1022, 1024–1027.

Mendes-Eastman, S., Shields, M., & Kirkland, L. (2001). Pulmonary embolism: Even your patient is at risk. *Plastic Surgical Nursing, 21*(2), 69–94.

Perry, M. (2008). Knowing the early signs of pulmonary embolism. *Practice Nursing, 19*(12), 620–623.

Yang, J. C. (2005). Prevention and treatment of deep vein thrombosis and pulmonary embolism in critically ill patients. *Critical Care Nursing Quarterly, 28*(1), 72–79.

Yee, C. A. (2010). Conquering pulmonary embolism. *OR Nurse, 4*(5), 18–24.

Risk Control: Tobacco Use   1906

Definition: Personal actions to understand, prevent, eliminate or reduce the threats to health associated with tobacco use

OUTCOME TARGET RATING: Maintain at_____   Increase to_____

		Never demonstrated	Rarely demonstrated	Sometimes demonstrated	Often demonstrated	Consistently demonstrated	
OUTCOME OVERALL RATING		1	2	3	4	5	
Indicators:							
190627	Seeks current information about hazards of tobacco use	1	2	3	4	5	NA
190628	Acknowledges addictive property of tobacco	1	2	3	4	5	NA
190629	Identifies risk factors for tobacco use	1	2	3	4	5	NA
190601	Acknowledges personal risk factors for tobacco use	1	2	3	4	5	NA
190619	Acknowledges personal satisfaction associated with tobacco use	1	2	3	4	5	NA
190630	Acknowledges personal disadvantages associated with tobacco use	1	2	3	4	5	NA
190602	Acknowledges consequences associated with tobacco use	1	2	3	4	5	NA
190631	Acknowledges ability to change behavior	1	2	3	4	5	NA
190603	Monitors environment for factors encouraging tobacco use	1	2	3	4	5	NA
190620	Acknowledges influence of peer pressure	1	2	3	4	5	NA
190621	Uses strategies to prevent tobacco use around peers	1	2	3	4	5	NA
190622	Recognizes social influences to engage in tobacco use	1	2	3	4	5	NA
190623	Recognizes cultural influences to engage in tobacco use	1	2	3	4	5	NA
190610	Uses health care services congruent with needs	1	2	3	4	5	NA
190612	Uses personal support systems to prevent tobacco use	1	2	3	4	5	NA
190613	Uses support group to prevent tobacco use	1	2	3	4	5	NA
190625	Avoids situations that encourage tobacco use	1	2	3	4	5	NA
190626	Uses reputable sources of information	1	2	3	4	5	NA
190614	Uses community resources to prevent tobacco use	1	2	3	4	5	NA

Domain-Health Knowledge & Behavior (IV)   *Class-Risk Control & Safety (T)*   *1st edition 1997; revised; 2004, 2008, 2013*

R

OUTCOME CONTENT REFERENCES:

DiNapoli, P. (2009). Early initiation of tobacco use in adolescent girls: Key sociostructural influences. *Applied Nursing Research, 22*(2), 126–132.

+Fagerstrom, K. O. (1978). Measuring degree of physical dependence in tobacco smoking with reference to individualization of treatment. *Addiction Behavior, 3,* 235–241.

Hirdes, J. P., & Maxwell, M. A. (1994). Smoking cessation and quality of life outcomes among older adults in the Campbell's survey on well-being. *Canadian Journal of Public Health, 85*(2), 99–102.

Hu, M., Griesler, P., Schaffran, C., & Kandel, D. (2011). Risk and protective factors for nicotine dependence in adolescence. *Journal of Child Psychology & Psychiatry, 52*(10), 1063–1072.

Klesges, R., Sherrill-Mittleman, D., Ebbert, J., Talcott, W., & DeBon, M. (2010). Tobacco use harm reduction, elimination, and escalation in a large military cohort. *American Journal of Public Health, 100*(12), 2487–2492.

Smith, K., Wakefield, M., Terry-McElrath, Y., Chaloupla, F., Flay, B., Johnston, L., Saba, A., & Siebel, C. (2008). Relation between newspaper coverage of tobacco issues and smoking attitudes and behavior among American teens. *Tobacco Control, 17*(10), 17–24.

Sussman, S., Dent, C. W., Stacy, A. W., Sun, P., Craig, S., Simon, T. R., Burton, D., & Flay, B. R. (1993). Project towards no tobacco use: 1-year behavioral outcomes. *American Journal of Public Health, 83*(9), 1245–1250.

Talashek, M. L., Gerace, L. M., & Starr, K. L. (1994). The substance abuse pandemic: Determinants to guide interventions. *Public Health Nursing, 11*(2), 131–139.

U.S. Department of Health and Human Services. (2010). *The guide to clinical preventive services 2010–2011: Recommendations of the U.S. Preventive Services Task Force.* Rockville, MD: Agency for Healthcare Research and Quality.

Windsor, R. A., Lowe, J. B., Perkins, L. L., Smith-Yoder, D., Artz, L., Crawford, M., Amburgy, K., & Boyd, N. R. (1993). Health education for pregnant smokers: Its behavioral impact and cost benefit. *American Journal of Public Health, 83*(2), 201–206.

Risk Control: Unintended Pregnancy 1907

Definition: Personal actions to understand, prevent, or reduce the possibility of unintended pregnancy

OUTCOME TARGET RATING: Maintain at_____   Increase to_____

		Never demonstrated	Rarely demonstrated	Sometimes demonstrated	Often demonstrated	Consistently demonstrated	
OUTCOME OVERALL RATING		1	2	3	4	5	
Indicators:							
190717	Seeks current information about family planning strategies	1	2	3	4	5	NA
190718	Identifies risk factors for unintended pregnancy	1	2	3	4	5	NA
190701	Acknowledges personal risk factors for unintended pregnancy	1	2	3	4	5	NA
190703	Acknowledges consequences associated with unintended pregnancy	1	2	3	4	5	NA
190705	Understands physiological processes of conception	1	2	3	4	5	NA
190719	Monitors changes in general health status	1	2	3	4	5	NA
190706	Develops effective pregnancy prevention strategies	1	2	3	4	5	NA
190707	Adjusts pregnancy prevention strategies	1	2	3	4	5	NA
190708	Commits to pregnancy prevention strategies	1	2	3	4	5	NA
190709	Follows selected pregnancy prevention strategies	1	2	3	4	5	NA
190710	Uses personal support systems to enhance prevention strategies	1	2	3	4	5	NA
190711	Uses available community resources	1	2	3	4	5	NA
190712	Identifies personal contraceptive method	1	2	3	4	5	NA
190713	Obtains contraceptive supplies and devices	1	2	3	4	5	NA
190714	Uses contraceptive methods correctly	1	2	3	4	5	NA
190715	Uses health care services congruent with needs	1	2	3	4	5	NA

Domain-*Health Knowledge & Behavior (IV)*   **Class**-*Risk Control & Safety (T)*   *1st edition 1997; revised 2004, 2013*

OUTCOME CONTENT REFERENCES:

+Card, J. J. (Ed.). (1993). *Handbook of adolescent sexuality and pregnancy: Research and evaluation instruments.* Thousand Oaks, CA: Sage.

Finer, L. (2010). Unintended pregnancy among U.S. adolescents: Accounting for sexual activity. *Journal of Adolescent Health, 47*(3), 312–314.

Moos, M., Bartholomew, N., & Lohr, K. (2003). Counseling in the clinical setting to prevent unintended pregnancy: An evidence-based research agenda. *Contraception, 67*(2), 115–132.

Secor-Turner, M., Sieving, R., Eisenberg, M., & Skay, C. (2011). Associations between sexually experienced adolescents' sources of information and sexual risk outcomes. *Sex Education, 11*(4), 489–500.

Sieving, R., McMorris, B., Beckman, K., Pettingell, S., Secor-Turner, M., Kugler, K., Garwick, A., Resnick, M., & Bearinger, L. (2011). Prime time: 12-month health outcomes of a clinic-based intervention to prevent pregnancy risk behavior. *Journal of Adolescent Health, 49*(2), 172-179.

U.S. Department of Health and Human Services. (2010). *The guide to clinical preventive services 2010–2011: Recommendations of the U.S. Preventive Services Task Force.* Rockville, MD: Agency for Healthcare Research and Quality.

Risk Control: Visual Impairment

1916

Definition: Personal actions to understand, prevent, eliminate, or reduce threats to visual function

OUTCOME TARGET RATING: Maintain at_____   Increase to_____

OUTCOME OVERALL RATING	Never demonstrated 1	Rarely demonstrated 2	Sometimes demonstrated 3	Often demonstrated 4	Consistently demonstrated 5	
Indicators:						
191613 Seeks current information about visual impairment	1	2	3	4	5	NA
191614 Identifies risk factors for visual impairment	1	2	3	4	5	NA
191615 Acknowledges personal risk factors for visual impairment	1	2	3	4	5	NA
191601 Monitors symptoms of vision deterioration	1	2	3	4	5	NA
191602 Monitors environment for eye hazards	1	2	3	4	5	NA
191616 Monitors changes in general health status	1	2	3	4	5	NA
191603 Avoids trauma to the eye	1	2	3	4	5	NA
191604 Uses adequate lighting for activity	1	2	3	4	5	NA
191605 Takes breaks from activity causing eye strain	1	2	3	4	5	NA
191606 Monitors for symptoms of eye disease	1	2	3	4	5	NA
191607 Uses eye medication as prescribed	1	2	3	4	5	NA
191608 Uses devices to protect eyes	1	2	3	4	5	NA
191617 Wears ultraviolet (UV) protection glasses when outdoors	1	2	3	4	5	NA
191609 Obtains eye exams	1	2	3	4	5	NA
191611 Obtains glaucoma screening	1	2	3	4	5	NA
191612 Obtains macular degeneration screening	1	2	3	4	5	NA

Domain-*Health Knowledge & Behavior (IV)*   **Class**-*Risk Control & Safety (T)*   *2nd edition 2000; revised 2004, 2013*

OUTCOME CONTENT REFERENCES:

Bener, A., Al-Mahdi, H., Vachhani, P., Al-Nufal, M., & Ali, A. (2010). Do excessive internet use, television viewing and poor lifestyle habits affect low vision in school children? *Journal of Child Health Care, 14*(4), 375–385.

Horowitz, A., Brennan, M., & Reinhardt, J. (2005). Prevalence and risk factors for self-reported visual impairment among middle-aged and older adults. *Research on Aging, 27*(3), 307–326.

Moskowitz, A. (2007). Study: Half of U.S. adults at high risk for vision loss not receiving eye exams. *Ocular Surgery News, 25*(9), 27.

Phipps, W. J., Monahan, F. D., Sands, J. K., Marek, J., & Neighbors, M. (Eds.). (2003). *Medical-surgical nursing: Concepts and clinical practice* (7th ed.). St. Louis: Mosby.

Sharts-Hopko, N. (2010). Lifestyle strategies for the prevention of vision loss. *Holistic Nursing Practice, 24*(5), 284–291.

Smeltzer, S., Bare, B., Hinkle, J., & Cheever, K. (2010). *Brunner and Suddarth's textbook of medical-surgical nursing* (12th ed., pp. 325–326). Philadelphia: Lippincott Williams & Wilkins.

U.S. Department of Health and Human Services. (2010). *The guide to clinical preventive services 2010–2011: Recommendations of the U.S. Preventive Services Task Force.* Rockville, MD: Agency for Healthcare Research and Quality.

Risk Detection 1908

Definition: Personal actions to identify personal health threats

OUTCOME TARGET RATING: Maintain at_____ Increase to_____

OUTCOME OVERALL RATING	Never demonstrated 1	Rarely demonstrated 2	Sometimes demonstrated 3	Often demonstrated 4	Consistently demonstrated 5	
Indicators:						
190801 Recognizes signs and symptoms that indicate risks	1	2	3	4	5	NA
190802 Identifies potential health risks	1	2	3	4	5	NA
190803 Seeks validation of perceived risks	1	2	3	4	5	NA
190804 Performs self-examinations at recommended intervals	1	2	3	4	5	NA
190805 Participates in screening at recommended intervals	1	2	3	4	5	NA
190806 Acquires knowledge of family history	1	2	3	4	5	NA
190807 Maintains updated knowledge of family history	1	2	3	4	5	NA
190808 Maintains updated knowledge of personal history	1	2	3	4	5	NA
190809 Uses resources to stay informed about personal risks	1	2	3	4	5	NA
190813 Monitors changes in general health status	1	2	3	4	5	NA
190810 Uses health care services congruent with needs	1	2	3	4	5	NA
190812 Obtains information about changes in health recommendations	1	2	3	4	5	NA

Domain-*Health Knowledge & Behavior (IV)* **Class**-*Risk Control & Safety (T)* *1st edition 1997; revised 2004, 2013*

OUTCOME CONTENT REFERENCES:

Fries, J., Koop, C., Sokolov, J., Beadle, C., & Wright, D. (1998). Beyond health promotion: Reducing need and demand for medical care: Health care reforms to improve health while reducing costs. *Health Affairs, 17*(2), 70–84.

+Hettler, B. (1982). Wellness promotion and risk reduction on a university campus. In M. Faber & A. Reinhardt (Eds.), *Promoting health through risk reduction* (pp. 207–238). New York: Macmillan.

Simons-Morton, D. G., Mullen, P. D., Mains, D. A., Tabak, E. R., & Green, L. W. (1992). Characteristics of controlled studies of patient education and counseling for preventive health behaviors. *Patient Education and Counseling, 19*(2), 174–204.

U.S. Department of Health and Human Services. (2010). *The guide to clinical preventive services 2010–2011: Recommendations of the U.S. Preventive Services Task Force.* Rockville, MD: Agency for Healthcare Research and Quality.

R

Role Performance 1501

Definition: Congruence of an individual's role behavior with role expectations

OUTCOME TARGET RATING: Maintain at_____ Increase to_____

		Not adequate	Slightly adequate	Moderately adequate	Substantially adequate	Totally adequate	
OUTCOME OVERALL RATING		1	2	3	4	5	
Indicators:							
150107	Description of role changes with illness or disability	1	2	3	4	5	NA
150117	Description of role changes with death of family member	1	2	3	4	5	NA
150108	Description of role changes with elderly dependents	1	2	3	4	5	NA
150109	Description of role changes with new family member	1	2	3	4	5	NA
150110	Description of role changes when family member leaves home	1	2	3	4	5	NA
150111	Reported strategies for role change(s)	1	2	3	4	5	NA
150101	Performance of role expectations	1	2	3	4	5	NA
150102	Knowledge of role transition periods	1	2	3	4	5	NA
150103	Performance of family role behaviors	1	2	3	4	5	NA
150115	Performance of parental role behaviors	1	2	3	4	5	NA
150113	Performance of intimate role behaviors	1	2	3	4	5	NA
150104	Performance of community role behaviors	1	2	3	4	5	NA
150105	Performance of work role behaviors	1	2	3	4	5	NA
150106	Performance of friendship role behaviors	1	2	3	4	5	NA
150112	Reported comfort with role expectations	1	2	3	4	5	NA
150116	Reported comfort with role change(s)	1	2	3	4	5	NA

Domain-*Psychosocial Health (III)*   **Class**-*Social Interaction (P)*   *1st edition 1997; revised 2004, 2013*

OUTCOME CONTENT REFERENCES:

Knutson, A. L. (1965). *The individual, society, and health behavior*. New York: Sage.

Moorhead, S. A. (1985). Role supplementation. In G. M. Bulechek, & J. C. McCloskey (Eds.), *Nursing interventions: Treatments for nursing diagnoses* (pp. 152–159). Philadelphia: W. B. Saunders.

+Weissman, M. M., & Bothwell, S. (1976). Assessment of social adjustment by patient self-report. *Archives of General Psychiatry, 33*(9), 1111–1115.

R

Safe Health Care Environment 1934

Definition: Physical and system arrangements to minimize factors that might cause physical harm or injury in the health care facility

OUTCOME TARGET RATING: Maintain at_____ Increase to_____

OUTCOME OVERALL RATING	Not adequate 1	Slightly adequate 2	Moderately adequate 3	Substantially adequate 4	Totally adequate 5	
Indicators:						
193401 Provision of lighting	1	2	3	4	5	NA
193402 Placement of handrails	1	2	3	4	5	NA
193403 Use of personal alarm system	1	2	3	4	5	NA
193404 Nurse call system within reach	1	2	3	4	5	NA
193405 Bed in low position	1	2	3	4	5	NA
193406 Arrangement of furniture to reduce risks based on patient needs	1	2	3	4	5	NA
193407 Room temperature regulation	1	2	3	4	5	NA
193408 Elimination of harmful noise levels	1	2	3	4	5	NA
193409 Provision of assistive devices in accessible locations	1	2	3	4	5	NA
193410 Equipment safety alarms on and working	1	2	3	4	5	NA
193411 Provision of equipment that meets safety standards	1	2	3	4	5	NA
193412 Provision of safe play area	1	2	3	4	5	NA
193413 Provision of age-appropriate toys	1	2	3	4	5	NA
193414 Use of electrical outlet covers	1	2	3	4	5	NA
193415 Safe storage of hazardous materials	1	2	3	4	5	NA
193416 Falls prevention policy	1	2	3	4	5	NA
193417 Computerized physician order entry	1	2	3	4	5	NA
193418 High alert medication policy	1	2	3	4	5	NA
193419 Point of care bedside medication charting	1	2	3	4	5	NA
193420 Medication reconciliation activity	1	2	3	4	5	NA
193421 Allergy alert system	1	2	3	4	5	NA
193422 Safe storage of medication	1	2	3	4	5	NA
193423 Error reporting system including near miss	1	2	3	4	5	NA
193424 Patient safety program	1	2	3	4	5	NA
193425 Use of evidence-based practice protocols	1	2	3	4	5	NA
193426 Care management systems in place	1	2	3	4	5	NA
193427 Evaluation of physical restraints use and reassessment policy	1	2	3	4	5	NA
193428 Evaluation of chemical restraints use and reassessment policy	1	2	3	4	5	NA

Domain-*Health Knowledge & Behavior (IV)* **Class**-*Risk Control & Safety (T)* 5th edition 2013

S

OUTCOME CONTENT REFERENCES:

Alexander, J., Weiner, B., Baker, L., Shortell, S., Becker, M. (2006). Care management implementation and patient safety. *Journal of Patient Safety*, *2*(2), 83–93.

Kerfoot, K., Papala, K., Ebright, P. & Rogers, S. (2006). The power of collaboration with patient safety programs: Building safe passage for patients, nurses, and clinical staff. *JONA: Journal of Nursing Administration*, *36*(12) 582–588.

Kilbridge, P., Classen, D., Bates, D., & Denham, C. (2006). The national quality forum safe practice standard for computerized physician order entry: Updating a critical patient safety practice. *Journal of Patient Safety*, *2*(4), 183–190.

Richardson, W. (2006). Innovations in patient safety management: Bedside nurses' assessment of near misses. *Topics in Emergency Medicine*, *28*(2) 154–160.

Young, B., & Hatlie, M. (Eds.). (2004). *The patient safety handbook* (pp. 591–631). Sudbury, MA: Jones and Bartlett.

Safe Home Environment 1910

| Definition: Physical arrangements to minimize environmental factors that might cause physical injury in the home |

OUTCOME TARGET RATING: Maintain at_____ Increase to_____

		Not adequate	Slightly adequate	Moderately adequate	Substantially adequate	Totally adequate	
OUTCOME OVERALL RATING		1	2	3	4	5	
Indicators:							
191026	Building maintenance	1	2	3	4	5	NA
191027	Exterior lighting	1	2	3	4	5	NA
191028	Interior lighting	1	2	3	4	5	NA
191029	Availability of clean water	1	2	3	4	5	NA
191037	Safe food storage	1	2	3	4	5	NA
191038	Safe food preparation	1	2	3	4	5	NA
191030	Cleanliness of dwelling	1	2	3	4	5	NA
191031	Elimination of pests	1	2	3	4	5	NA
191032	Space to move safely in dwelling	1	2	3	4	5	NA
191033	Locks on windows	1	2	3	4	5	NA
191034	Locks on doors	1	2	3	4	5	NA
191002	Placement of handrails	1	2	3	4	5	NA
191023	Carbon monoxide detector maintenance	1	2	3	4	5	NA
191003	Smoke detector maintenance	1	2	3	4	5	NA
191039	Availability of emergency response system	1	2	3	4	5	NA
191005	Accessibility of telephone	1	2	3	4	5	NA
191040	Accessibility of bathroom	1	2	3	4	5	NA
191024	Safe storage of medication	1	2	3	4	5	NA
191007	Proper disposal of medication	1	2	3	4	5	NA
191008	Accessibility of assistive devices	1	2	3	4	5	NA
191041	Equipment maintained to meet safety standards	1	2	3	4	5	NA
191010	Safe storage of firearms	1	2	3	4	5	NA
191011	Safe storage of hazardous materials	1	2	3	4	5	NA
191012	Safe disposal of hazardous materials	1	2	3	4	5	NA
191025	Safe storage of matches/lighters	1	2	3	4	5	NA
191042	Elimination of mold	1	2	3	4	5	NA
191043	Elimination of radon	1	2	3	4	5	NA
191036	Elimination of toxic fumes	1	2	3	4	5	NA
191035	Elimination of tobacco smoke	1	2	3	4	5	NA
191013	Arrangement of furniture to reduce risks	1	2	3	4	5	NA
191014	Safety of play area	1	2	3	4	5	NA
191015	Removal of doors from unused appliances	1	2	3	4	5	NA
191016	Correction of lead hazard risks	1	2	3	4	5	NA
191017	Safety of age-appropriate toys	1	2	3	4	5	NA
191018	Use of electrical outlet covers	1	2	3	4	5	NA
191019	Room temperature regulation	1	2	3	4	5	NA
191020	Elimination of harmful noise levels	1	2	3	4	5	NA
191021	Placement of window guards	1	2	3	4	5	NA

S

Domain-*Health Knowledge & Behavior (IV)*   **Class**-*Risk Control & Safety (T)*   *1st edition 1997; revised 2004, 2008, 2013*

OUTCOME CONTENT REFERENCES:

Black, S. (2002). Safe home. *Nursing Standard, 16*(25), 16–17.

Halperin, S. F., Bass, J. L., & Mehta, K. A., (1983). Knowledge of accident prevention among parents of young children in nine Massachusetts towns. *Public Health Reports, 98*(6), 548–552.

Head, B. J. (2001). Impaired home maintenance management. In M. Maas, K. Buckwalter, M. Hardy, T. Tripp-Reimer, M. Titler, & J. Specht (Eds.), *Nursing care of older adults: Diagnoses, outcomes & interventions* (pp. 64–74). St. Louis: Mosby.

Mayhew, M. S. (1991). Strategies for promoting safety and preventing injury. *Nursing Clinics of North America, 26*(1), 885–893.

+Tymchuk, A. J. (1997). Home dangers and precautions: Interview/observation. *The UCLA Parent/Child Health & Wellness Project.*

Wasserman, R. C., Dameron, D. O., Brozicevic, M. M., & Aronson, R. A. (1989). Injury hazards in home day care. *The Journal of Pediatrics, 114*(4), 591–593.

Weitzel, E. (2001). Unilateral neglect. In M. Maas, K. Buckwalter, M. Hardy, T. Tripp-Reimer, M. Titler, & J. Specht (Eds.), *Nursing care of older adults: Diagnoses, outcomes & interventions* (pp. 492–502). St. Louis: Mosby.

Safe Wandering   1926

Definition: Safe, socially acceptable moving about without apparent purpose in an individual with cognitive impairment

OUTCOME TARGET RATING: Maintain at_____   Increase to_____

	Never demonstrated	Rarely demonstrated	Sometimes demonstrated	Often demonstrated	Consistently demonstrated	
OUTCOME OVERALL RATING	1	2	3	4	5	
Indicators:						
192601 Moves about without harming self	1	2	3	4	5	NA
192602 Moves about without harming others	1	2	3	4	5	NA
192603 Sits for more than 5 minutes at a time	1	2	3	4	5	NA
192604 Paces a given route	1	2	3	4	5	NA
192605 Appears content in environment	1	2	3	4	5	NA
192606 Remains in secure area when unaccompanied	1	2	3	4	5	NA
192607 Moves about only in own and public space	1	2	3	4	5	NA
192608 Uses own toileting facilities	1	2	3	4	5	NA
192609 Performs purposeful activities	1	2	3	4	5	NA
192610 Locates landmarks in familiar setting	1	2	3	4	5	NA
192611 Can be redirected from unsafe activities	1	2	3	4	5	NA
192612 Distracts easily	1	2	3	4	5	NA
192613 Dresses appropriately	1	2	3	4	5	NA

	Consistently demonstrated	Often demonstrated	Sometimes demonstrated	Rarely demonstrated	Never demonstrated	
192614 Falls	1	2	3	4	5	NA
192615 Appears agitated	1	2	3	4	5	NA
192616 Bumps into obstacles while moving	1	2	3	4	5	NA
192617 States wants to go home	1	2	3	4	5	NA
192618 Attempts to elope from secure area	1	2	3	4	5	NA
192619 Gets lost in secure area	1	2	3	4	5	NA
192620 Invades others' space	1	2	3	4	5	NA
192621 Upsets others in environment	1	2	3	4	5	NA
192622 Disrupts group activities	1	2	3	4	5	NA

Domain-*Health Knowledge & Behavior (IV)*   **Class**-*Risk Control & Safety (T)*   4th edition 2008

S

OUTCOME CONTENT REFERENCES:

Algase, D. L., Beattie, E. R. A., Song, J. A., Milke, D., Duffield, C., & Cowan, B. (2004). Validation of the Algase Wandering Scale (Version 2) in a cross cultural sample. *Aging & Mental Health, 8*(2), 133–142.

Algase, D. L., Son, G., Beattie, E., Song, J., Leitsch, S., & Yao, L. (2004). The interrelatedness of wandering and wayfinding in a community sample of persons with dementia. *Dementia and Geriatric Cognitive Disorders, 17*(3), 231–239.

Aud, M. A. (2004). Dangerous wandering: Elopements of older adults with dementia from long-term care facilities. *American Journal of Alzheimer's Disease and Other Dementias, 19*(6), 361–368.

Kelley, L. S., Buckwalter, K. C., & Maas, M. L. (1999). Access to health care resources for family caregivers of elderly persons with dementia. *Nursing Outlook, 47*(1), 8–14.

Kiely, D. K., Morris, J. N., & Algase, D. L. (2000). Resident characteristics associated with wandering in nursing homes. *International Journal of Geriatric Psychiatry, 15*(11), 1013–1020.

Maas, M., Reed, D., Park, M., Specht, J., Schutte, D., Kelley, L., et al. (2004). Outcomes of family involvement in care intervention for caregivers of individuals with dementia. *Nursing Research, 53*(2), 76–86.

Williams-Burgess, C., Ugeriza, D., & Gabbai, M. (1996). Agitation in older persons with dementia: A research synthesis. *Online Journal of Knowledge Synthesis for Nursing, E3*(1), 97.

Seizure Self-Control   1620

Definition: Personal actions to reduce or minimize the occurrence of seizure episodes

OUTCOME TARGET RATING: Maintain at_____ Increase to_____

		Never demonstrated	Rarely demonstrated	Sometimes demonstrated	Often demonstrated	Consistently demonstrated	
OUTCOME OVERALL RATING		1	2	3	4	5	
Indicators:							
162001	Describes precipitating seizure factors	1	2	3	4	5	NA
162002	Uses medication as prescribed	1	2	3	4	5	NA
162016	Obtains needed medication	1	2	3	4	5	NA
162004	Contacts health professional when medication side effects occur	1	2	3	4	5	NA
162006	Avoids seizure triggers/risk factors	1	2	3	4	5	NA
162017	Obtains medical attention immediately if seizure frequency increases	1	2	3	4	5	NA
162008	Uses effective stress reduction techniques to decrease seizure activity	1	2	3	4	5	NA
162009	Maintains positive attitude toward seizure disorder	1	2	3	4	5	NA
162010	Maintains role performance	1	2	3	4	5	NA
162011	Maintains social relationships	1	2	3	4	5	NA
162012	Maintains sleep-wake pattern	1	2	3	4	5	NA
162013	Follows prescribed physical exercise program	1	2	3	4	5	NA
162015	Implements safety practices in environment	1	2	3	4	5	NA

Domain-*Health Knowledge & Behavior (IV)* **Class**-*Health Behavior (Q)* *3rd edition 2004; revised 2008, 2013*

OUTCOME CONTENT REFERENCES:

Dilorio, C., Faherty, B., & Manteuffel, B. (1993). Learning needs of persons with epilepsy: A comparison of perceptions of persons with epilepsy, nurses and physicians. *Journal of Neuroscience Nursing, 25*(1), 22–29.

Santilli, N. (Ed.). (1996). *Managing seizure disorders: A handbook for health care professionals.* Philadelphia: J. B. Lippincott.

S

Self-Awareness

1215

Definition: Acknowledges one's strengths, limitations, values, feelings, attitudes, thoughts, and behaviors in relationship to the environment and others

OUTCOME TARGET RATING: Maintain at_____ Increase to_____

		Never demonstrated	Rarely demonstrated	Sometimes demonstrated	Often demonstrated	Consistently demonstrated	
OUTCOME OVERALL RATING		1	2	3	4	5	
Indicators:							
121501	Differentiates self from environment	1	2	3	4	5	NA
121502	Differentiates self from others	1	2	3	4	5	NA
121503	Recognizes personal physical abilities	1	2	3	4	5	NA
121504	Recognizes personal mental abilities	1	2	3	4	5	NA
121505	Recognizes personal emotional abilities	1	2	3	4	5	NA
121506	Recognizes personal physical limitations	1	2	3	4	5	NA
121507	Recognizes personal mental limitations	1	2	3	4	5	NA
121508	Recognizes personal emotional limitations	1	2	3	4	5	NA
121509	Recognizes personal behavioral patterns	1	2	3	4	5	NA
121510	Recognizes personal values	1	2	3	4	5	NA
121511	Recognizes subjective response to others	1	2	3	4	5	NA
121512	Recognizes subjective response to situations	1	2	3	4	5	NA
121513	Maintains awareness of internal signals to situations	1	2	3	4	5	NA
121514	Maintains awareness of external signals to situations	1	2	3	4	5	NA
121515	Maintains awareness of thoughts	1	2	3	4	5	NA
121516	Maintains awareness of feelings	1	2	3	4	5	NA
121517	Reflects on thoughts for self-discovery	1	2	3	4	5	NA
121518	Reflects on feelings for self-discovery	1	2	3	4	5	NA
121519	Reflects on intentions for self-discovery	1	2	3	4	5	NA
121520	Expresses feelings to others	1	2	3	4	5	NA
121521	Reflects on interactions with others	1	2	3	4	5	NA
121522	Expresses needs to others	1	2	3	4	5	NA
121523	Accepts ownership of thoughts	1	2	3	4	5	NA
121524	Accepts ownership of feelings	1	2	3	4	5	NA
121525	Accepts ownership of behaviors	1	2	3	4	5	NA
121526	Remembers oneself in the past	1	2	3	4	5	NA
121527	Imagines oneself in the future	1	2	3	4	5	NA

Domain-*Psychosocial Health (III)* **Class**-*Psychological Well-Being (M)* 5th edition 2013

S

OUTCOME CONTENT REFERENCES:

Engin, E., & Cam, O. (2009). Effect of self-awareness education on the self-efficacy and sociotropy-autonomy characteristics of nursing in a psychiatry clinic. *Archives of Psychiatric Nursing, 23*(2), 148–156.

Herwig, U., Kaffenberger, T., Jancke, L., & Bruhl. (2010). Self-related awareness and emotion regulation. *NeuroImage, 50*(2), 734–741.

Leary, M. R. & Buttermore, N. R. (2003). The evolution of the human self: Tracing the natural history of self-awareness. *Journal for the Theory of Social Behaviour* (*33*)4, 365–404.

Miller, J. (2008). Exploring self-awareness in mental health practice. *Mental Health Practice, 12*(3), 31–35.

Murdock, N. L., & Wang, C. (2008). Humanistic theories. In F. T. L. Leong (Ed.), *The encyclopedia of counseling.* Thousand Oaks, CA: Sage.

Prigatano, G. P. (2009). Anosognosia: Clinical and ethical considerations. *Current Opinion in Neurology, 22*(6), 606–611.

Rochat, P. (2003). Five levels of self-awareness as they unfold early in life. *Consciousness and Cognition, 12*(4), 717–731.

Stuart, G. (2009). *Principles and practice of psychiatric nursing* (9th ed.). St. Louis: Elsevier Mosby.

Townsend, M. (2006). *Psychiatric mental health nursing: Concepts of care in evidence-based practice* (5th ed.). Philadelphia: F. A. Davis.

Williamson, C., Alcantar, O., Rothlind, J., Cahn-Weiner, D., Miller, B. L., & Rosen, H. J. (2010). Standardised measurement of self-awareness deficits in FTD and AD. *Journal of Neurology, Neurosurgery, and Psychiatry, 81*(2), 140–145.

Self-Care Status 0313

Definition: Personal actions to perform basic personal care activities and instrumental activities of daily living

OUTCOME TARGET RATING: Maintain at_____ Increase to_____

	Severely compromised	Substantially compromised	Moderately compromised	Mildly compromised	Not compromised	
OUTCOME OVERALL RATING	1	2	3	4	5	
Indicators:						
031301 Bathes self	1	2	3	4	5	NA
031302 Dresses self	1	2	3	4	5	NA
031303 Prepares food and fluid for eating	1	2	3	4	5	NA
031304 Feeds self	1	2	3	4	5	NA
031305 Maintains personal cleanliness	1	2	3	4	5	NA
031306 Maintains oral hygiene	1	2	3	4	5	NA
031307 Toilets self independently	1	2	3	4	5	NA
031315 Manages own non-parenteral medication	1	2	3	4	5	NA
031309 Manages own parenteral medication	1	2	3	4	5	NA
031310 Performs household tasks	1	2	3	4	5	NA
031311 Manages household finances	1	2	3	4	5	NA
031312 Arranges for own transportation	1	2	3	4	5	NA
031313 Obtains required household items	1	2	3	4	5	NA
031314 Recognizes safety needs in the home	1	2	3	4	5	NA

Domain-Functional Health (I) **Class**-Self-Care (D) *3rd edition 2004; revised 2008, 2013*

OUTCOME CONTENT REFERENCES:

Armer, J. M., Conn, V. S., Decker, S. A., & Tripp-Reimer, T. (2001). Self-care deficit. In M. Maas, K. Buckwalter, M. Hardy, T. Tripp-Reimer, M. Titler, & J. Specht (Eds.), *Nursing care of older adults: Diagnoses, outcomes & interventions* (pp. 366–384). St. Louis: Mosby.

Head, B. J. (2001). Impaired home maintenance management. In M. Maas, K. Buckwalter, M. Hardy, T. Tripp-Reimer, M. Titler, & J. Specht (Eds.), *Nursing care of older adults: Diagnoses, outcomes & interventions* (pp. 64–74). St. Louis: Mosby.

Hickey, T. (1988). Self-care behavior of older adults. *Family and Community Health, 11*(3), 22–35.

Katz, S., & Akpom, C. A. (1976). A measure of primary sociobiological functions. *International Journal of Health Services, 6*(3), 493–507.

Katz, S., Ford, A. B., Moskowitz, R. W., Jackson, B. A., & Jaffe, M. W. (1963). Studies of illness in the aged. The Index of ADL: A standardized measure of biological and psychosocial function. *Journal of the American Medical Association, 185*(12), 914–919.

Klein, R. M., & Bell, B. (1982). Self-care skills: Behavioral measurement with Klein-Bell ADL Scale. *Archives of Physical Medicine and Rehabilitation, 63*(7), 335–338.

Leenerts, M. H., Teel, C. S., & Pendleton, M. K. (2002). Building a model of self-care for health promotion in aging. *Journal of Nursing Scholarship, 34*(4), 355–361.

Resnick, B. (2001). Motivating older adults to engage in self-care. *Patient Care for the Nurse Practitioner, 4*(9), 13–14, 16, 19.

S

Self-Care: Activities of Daily Living (ADL) 0300

Definition: Personal actions to perform the most basic physical tasks and personal care activities independently with or without assistive device

OUTCOME TARGET RATING: Maintain at_____ Increase to_____

	Severely compromised	Substantially compromised	Moderately compromised	Mildly compromised	Not compromised	
OUTCOME OVERALL RATING	1	2	3	4	5	
Indicators:						
030001 Eating	1	2	3	4	5	NA
030002 Dressing	1	2	3	4	5	NA
030003 Toileting	1	2	3	4	5	NA
030004 Bathing	1	2	3	4	5	NA
030005 Grooming	1	2	3	4	5	NA
030006 Hygiene	1	2	3	4	5	NA
030007 Oral hygiene	1	2	3	4	5	NA
030008 Walking	1	2	3	4	5	NA
030009 Wheelchair mobility	1	2	3	4	5	NA
030010 Transfer performance	1	2	3	4	5	NA
030012 Positions self	1	2	3	4	5	NA

Domain-Functional Health (I)   **Class**-Self-Care (D)   1st edition 1997; revised 2004, 2013

OUTCOME CONTENT REFERENCES:

Armer, J. M., Conn, V. S., Decker, S. A., & Tripp-Reimer, T. (2001). Self-care deficit. In M. Maas, K. Buckwalter, M. Hardy, T. Tripp-Reimer, M. Titler, & J. Specht (Eds.), *Nursing care of older adults: Diagnoses, outcomes & interventions* (pp. 366–384). St. Louis: Mosby.

Hickey, T. (1988). Self-care behavior of older adults. *Family and Community Health, 11*(3), 22–35.

Katz, S., & Akpom, C. A. (1976). A measure of primary sociobiological functions. *International Journal of Health Services, 6*(3), 493–507.

+Katz, S., Ford, A. B., Moskowitz, R. W., Jackson, B. A., & Jaffe, M. W. (1963). Studies of illness in the aged. The Index of ADL: A standardized measure of biological and psychosocial function. *Journal of the American Medical Association, 185*(12), 914–919.

Klein, R. M., & Bell, B. (1982). Self-care skills: Behavioral measurement with Klein-Bell ADL Scale. *Archives of Physical Medicine and Rehabilitation, 63*(7), 335–338.

Leenerts, M. H., Teel, C. S., & Pendleton, M. K. (2002). Building a model of self-care for health promotion in aging. *Journal of Nursing Scholarship, 34*(4), 355–361.

Resnick, B. (2001). Motivating older adults to engage in self-care. *Patient Care for the Nurse Practitioner, 4*(9), 13–14, 16, 19.

Weitzel, E. (2001). Unilateral neglect. In M. Maas, K. Buckwalter, M. Hardy, T. Tripp-Reimer, M. Titler, & J. Specht (Eds.), *Nursing care of older adults: Diagnoses, outcomes & interventions* (pp. 492–502). St. Louis: Mosby.

Self-Care: Bathing 0301

S

Definition: Personal actions to cleanse own body independently with or without assistive device

OUTCOME TARGET RATING: Maintain at_____ Increase to_____

	Severely compromised	Substantially compromised	Moderately compromised	Mildly compromised	Not compromised	
OUTCOME OVERALL RATING	1	2	3	4	5	
Indicators:						
030101 Gets in and out of bathroom	1	2	3	4	5	NA
030102 Gets bath supplies	1	2	3	4	5	NA
030103 Obtains bath water	1	2	3	4	5	NA
030104 Turns on water	1	2	3	4	5	NA
030105 Regulates water temperature	1	2	3	4	5	NA
030106 Regulates water flow	1	2	3	4	5	NA

Continued

Self-Care: Bathing—cont'd

	Severely compromised	Substantially compromised	Moderately compromised	Mildly compromised	Not compromised	
030107 Bathes at sink	1	2	3	4	5	NA
030108 Bathes in tub	1	2	3	4	5	NA
030109 Bathes in shower	1	2	3	4	5	NA
030113 Washes face	1	2	3	4	5	NA
030114 Washes upper body	1	2	3	4	5	NA
030115 Washes lower body	1	2	3	4	5	NA
030116 Cleans perineal area	1	2	3	4	5	NA
030111 Dries body	1	2	3	4	5	NA

Domain-Functional Health (I)   **Class**-Self-Care (D)   *1st edition 1997; revised 2004, 2013*

OUTCOME CONTENT REFERENCES:

Armer, J. M., Conn, V. S., Decker, S. A., & Tripp-Reimer, T. (2001). Self-care deficit. In M. Maas, K. Buckwalter, M. Hardy, T. Tripp-Reimer, M. Titler, & J. Specht (Eds.), *Nursing care of older adults: Diagnoses, outcomes & interventions* (pp. 366–384). St. Louis: Mosby.

+*Guide for the Uniform Data Set for Medical Rehabilitation* (including the FIM™ instrument) (version 5.1). (1997). Buffalo, NY: University at Buffalo.

Gulick, E. E. (1990). The self-administered ADL scale for persons with multiple sclerosis. In C. F. Waltz, & O. L. Strickland (Eds.), *Measurement of nursing outcomes* (pp. 128–147). New York: Springer.

Hickey, T. (1988). Self-care behavior of older adults. *Family and Community Health*, 11(3), 22–35.

Klein, R. M., & Bell, B. (1982). Self-care skills: Behavioral measurement with Klein-Bell ADL Scale. *Archives of Physical Medicine and Rehabilitation*, 63(7), 335–338.

Leenerts, M. H., Teel, C. S., & Pendleton, M. K. (2002). Building a model of self-care for health promotion in aging. *Journal of Nursing Scholarship*, 34(4), 355–361.

McKeighten, R. J., Mehmert, P. A., & Dickel, C. A. (1990). Bathing/hygiene self-care deficit: Defining characteristics and related factors across age groups and diagnosis-related groups in an acute care setting. *Nursing Diagnosis*, 1(4), 155–161.

Resnick, B. (2001). Motivating older adults to engage in self-care. *Patient Care for the Nurse Practitioner*, 4(9), 13–14, 16, 19.

Shillam, L. L., & Beeman, C., & Loshin, P. (1983). Effect of occupational therapy intervention on bathing independence of disabled persons. *The American Journal of Occupational Therapy*, 37(11), 744–748.

Self-Care: Dressing   0302

Definition: Personal actions to dress self independently with or without assistive device

OUTCOME TARGET RATING: Maintain at_____   Increase to_____

	Severely compromised	Substantially compromised	Moderately compromised	Mildly compromised	Not compromised	
OUTCOME OVERALL RATING	1	2	3	4	5	
Indicators:						
030201 Selects clothing	1	2	3	4	5	NA
030215 Gets clothing from drawer	1	2	3	4	5	NA
030216 Gets clothing from closet	1	2	3	4	5	NA
030203 Picks up clothing	1	2	3	4	5	NA
030204 Puts clothing on upper body	1	2	3	4	5	NA
030205 Puts clothing on lower body	1	2	3	4	5	NA
030206 Buttons clothing	1	2	3	4	5	NA
030207 Uses fasteners	1	2	3	4	5	NA
030208 Uses zippers	1	2	3	4	5	NA
030209 Puts on socks	1	2	3	4	5	NA
030210 Puts on shoes	1	2	3	4	5	NA
030213 Ties shoes	1	2	3	4	5	NA
030211 Removes clothes from upper body	1	2	3	4	5	NA
030214 Removes clothes from lower body	1	2	3	4	5	NA

Domain-Functional Health (I)   **Class**-Self-Care (D)   *1st edition 1997; revised 2004, 2008, 2013*

S

OUTCOME CONTENT REFERENCES:

Armer, J. M., Conn, V. S., Decker, S. A., & Tripp-Reimer, T. (2001). Self-care deficit. In M. Maas, K. Buckwalter, M. Hardy, T. Tripp-Reimer, M. Titler, & J. Specht (Eds.), *Nursing care of older adults: Diagnoses, outcomes & interventions* (pp. 366–384). St. Louis: Mosby.

Beck, C. (1988). Measurement of dressing performance in persons with dementia. *American Journal of Alzheimer's Care and Related Disorders and Research, 3*(3), 21–25.

Cole, S. L. (1992). Dress for success: A nurse's knowledge of simple clothing adaptations and dressing aids may make the difference between rehabilitation success and failure. *Geriatric Nursing, 13*(4), 217–221.

Cook, E. A., Luschen, L., & Sikes, S. (1991). Dressing training for an elderly woman with cognitive and perceptual impairments. *The American Journal of Occupational Therapy, 45*(7), 652–654.

Dudgeon, B. J., DeLisa, J. A., & Miller, R. M. (1984). Optokinetic nystagmus and upper extremity dressing independence after stroke. *Archives of Physical Medicine & Rehabilitation, 66*(3), 164–167.

Ford, L. J. (1975). Teaching dressing skills to a severely retarded child. *The American Journal of Occupational Therapy, 2*(29), 87–92.

+*Guide for the Uniform Data Set for Medical Rehabilitation* (including the FIM™ instrument) (version 5.1). (1997). Buffalo, NY: University at Buffalo.

Hickey, T. (1988). Self-care behavior of older adults. *Family and Community Health, 11*(3), 22–35.

Leenerts, M. H., Teel, C. S., & Pendleton, M. K. (2002). Building a model of self-care for health promotion in aging. *Journal of Nursing Scholarship, 34*(4), 355–361.

Panikoff, L. B. (1983). Recovery trends of functional skills in the head injured adult. *The American Journal of Occupational Therapy, 37*(11), 735–743.

Resnick, B. (2001). Motivating older adults to engage in self-care. *Patient Care for the Nurse Practitioner, 4*(9), 13–14, 16, 19.

Runge, M. (1967). Self-dressing techniques for patients with spinal cord injury. *The American Journal of Occupational Therapy, 21*(6), 367–375.

Self-Care: Eating 0303

Definition: Personal actions to prepare and ingest food and fluid independently with or without assistive device

OUTCOME TARGET RATING: Maintain at_____ Increase to_____

		Severely compromised	Substantially compromised	Moderately compromised	Mildly compromised	Not compromised	
OUTCOME OVERALL RATING		1	2	3	4	5	
Indicators:							
030301	Prepares food for ingestion	1	2	3	4	5	NA
030302	Opens containers	1	2	3	4	5	NA
030316	Cuts up food	1	2	3	4	5	NA
030303	Uses utensils	1	2	3	4	5	NA
030304	Gets food onto the utensil	1	2	3	4	5	NA
030305	Picks up cup or glass	1	2	3	4	5	NA
030306	Brings food to mouth with fingers	1	2	3	4	5	NA
030307	Brings food to mouth with container	1	2	3	4	5	NA
030308	Brings food to mouth with utensil	1	2	3	4	5	NA
030309	Drinks from a cup or glass	1	2	3	4	5	NA
030310	Places food in mouth	1	2	3	4	5	NA
030311	Manipulates food in mouth	1	2	3	4	5	NA
030312	Chews food	1	2	3	4	5	NA
030313	Swallows food	1	2	3	4	5	NA
030317	Swallows fluid	1	2	3	4	5	NA
030314	Completes a meal	1	2	3	4	5	NA

Domain-*Functional Health (I)* **Class**-*Self-Care (D)* *1st edition 1997; revised 2004, 2013*

S

OUTCOME CONTENT REFERENCES:

Armer, J. M., Conn, V. S., Decker, S. A., & Tripp-Reimer, T. (2001). Self-care deficit. In M. Maas, K. Buckwalter, M. Hardy, T. Tripp-Reimer, M. Titler, & J. Specht (Eds.), *Nursing care of older adults: Diagnoses, outcomes & interventions* (pp. 366–384). St. Louis: Mosby.

Athlin, E., Norberg, A., Axelson, K., Moller, A., & Nordstrom, G. (1989). Aberrant eating behavior in elderly parkinsonian patients with and without dementia: Analysis of video-recorded meals. *Research in Nursing and Health, 12*(1), 41–51.

+*Guide for the Uniform Data Set for Medical Rehabilitation* (including the FIM™ instrument) (version 5.1). (1997). Buffalo, NY: University at Buffalo.

Hickey, T. (1988). Self-care behavior of older adults. *Family and Community Health, 11*(3), 22–35.

Leenerts, M. H., Teel, C. S., & Pendleton, M. K. (2002). Building a model of self-care for health promotion in aging. *Journal of Nursing Scholarship, 34*(4), 355–361.

Luiselli, J. K. (1993). Training self-feeding skills in children who are deaf and blind. *Behavior Modification, 17*(4), 457–473.

Piazza, C. C., Anderson, C., & Fisher, W. (1993). Teaching self-feeding skills to patients with Rett Syndrome. *Developmental Medicine and Child Neurology, 35*(11), 991–996.

Resnick, B. (2001). Motivating older adults to engage in self-care. *Patient Care for the Nurse Practitioner, 4*(9), 13–14, 16, 19.

Tandy, L., & Malan, S. (2001). Impaired swallowing. In M. Maas, K. Buckwalter, M. Hardy, T. Tripp-Reimer, M. Titler, & J. Specht (Eds.), *Nursing care of older adults: Diagnoses, outcomes & interventions* (pp. 158–171). St. Louis: Mosby.

Self-Care: Hygiene 0305

Definition: Personal actions to maintain own personal cleanliness and kempt appearance independently with or without assistive device

OUTCOME TARGET RATING: Maintain at_____ Increase to_____

OUTCOME OVERALL RATING	Severely compromised 1	Substantially compromised 2	Moderately compromised 3	Mildly compromised 4	Not compromised 5	
Indicators:						
030501 Washes hands	1	2	3	4	5	NA
030503 Cleans perineal area	1	2	3	4	5	NA
030515 Wears protective pads	1	2	3	4	5	NA
030504 Cleans ears	1	2	3	4	5	NA
030505 Keeps nose blown and clean	1	2	3	4	5	NA
030506 Maintains oral hygiene	1	2	3	4	5	NA
030508 Shampoos hair	1	2	3	4	5	NA
030509 Combs or brushes hair	1	2	3	4	5	NA
030510 Shaves	1	2	3	4	5	NA
030511 Applies makeup	1	2	3	4	5	NA
030512 Cares for fingernails	1	2	3	4	5	NA
030516 Cares for toenails	1	2	3	4	5	NA
030513 Uses a mirror	1	2	3	4	5	NA
030514 Maintains neat appearance	1	2	3	4	5	NA
030517 Maintains body hygiene	1	2	3	4	5	NA

Domain-Functional Health (I)   **Class**-Self-Care (D)   *1st edition 1997; revised 2004, 2008, 2013*

OUTCOME CONTENT REFERENCES:

Armer, J. M., Conn, V. S., Decker, S. A., & Tripp-Reimer, T. (2001). Self-care deficit. In M. Maas, K. Buckwalter, M. Hardy, T. Tripp-Reimer, M. Titler, & J. Specht (Eds.), *Nursing care of older adults: Diagnoses, outcomes & interventions* (pp. 366–384). St. Louis: Mosby.

Cole, G. (1991). Hygiene and care of the patient's environment. In G. Cole (Ed.), *Basic nursing skills and concepts* (pp. 261–290). St. Louis: Mosby.

+*Guide for the Uniform Data Set for Medical Rehabilitation* (including the FIM™ instrument) (version 5.1). (1997). Buffalo, NY: University at Buffalo.

Hallstrom, R., & Beck, S. L. (1993). Implementation of the AORN skin shaving standard: Evaluation of a planned change. *AORN Journal, 58*(3), 498–506.

Hickey, T. (1988). Self-care behavior of older adults. *Family and Community Health, 11*(3), 22–35.

Leenerts, M. H., Teel, C. S., & Pendleton, M. K. (2002). Building a model of self-care for health promotion in aging. *Journal of Nursing Scholarship, 34*(4), 355–361.

McKeighten, R. J., Mehmert, P. A., & Dickel, C. A. (1990). Bathing/hygiene self-care deficit: Defining characteristics and related factors across age groups and diagnosis-related groups in an acute care setting. *Nursing Diagnosis, 1*(4), 155–161.

Ney, D. F. (1993). Cerumen impaction, ear hygiene practices, and hearing acuity. *Geriatric Nursing—American Journal of Care for the Aging, 14*(2), 70–73.

Resnick, B. (2001). Motivating older adults to engage in self-care. *Patient Care for the Nurse Practitioner, 4*(9), 13–14, 16, 19.

Wong, S. E., Flanagan, S. G., Kuehnel, T. G., Liberman, R. P., Hunnicut, R., & Adams-Badgett, J. (1988). Training chronic mental patients to independently practice personal grooming skills. *Hospital and Community Psychiatry, 39*(8), 874–879.

S

Self-Care: Instrumental Activities of Daily Living (IADL) 0306

Definition: Personal actions to perform activities needed to function in the home or community independently with or without assistive device

OUTCOME TARGET RATING: Maintain at_____ Increase to_____

		Severely compromised	Substantially compromised	Moderately compromised	Mildly compromised	Not compromised	
OUTCOME OVERALL RATING		1	2	3	4	5	
Indicators:							
030601	Shops for groceries	1	2	3	4	5	NA
030602	Shops for clothing	1	2	3	4	5	NA
030603	Shops for household supplies	1	2	3	4	5	NA
030604	Prepares meals	1	2	3	4	5	NA
030605	Serves meals	1	2	3	4	5	NA
030606	Operates phone	1	2	3	4	5	NA
030607	Handles written communication	1	2	3	4	5	NA
030608	Opens containers	1	2	3	4	5	NA
030609	Performs housework	1	2	3	4	5	NA
030610	Performs household repairs	1	2	3	4	5	NA
030611	Performs yard work	1	2	3	4	5	NA
030612	Manages money	1	2	3	4	5	NA
030613	Manages business affairs	1	2	3	4	5	NA
030614	Travels on public transportation	1	2	3	4	5	NA
030615	Drives own car	1	2	3	4	5	NA
030616	Does own laundry	1	2	3	4	5	NA
030617	Manages own non-parenteral medication	1	2	3	4	5	NA
030619	Manages own parenteral medication	1	2	3	4	5	NA

Domain-Functional Health (I)   **Class**-Self-Care (D)   1st edition 1997; revised 2004, 2008, 2013

OUTCOME CONTENT REFERENCES:
Armer, J. M., Conn, V. S., Decker, S. A., & Tripp-Reimer, T. (2001). Self-care deficit. In M. Maas, K. Buckwalter, M. Hardy, T. Tripp-Reimer, M. Titler, & J. Specht (Eds.), *Nursing care of older adults: Diagnoses, outcomes & interventions* (pp. 366–384). St. Louis: Mosby.
Fillenbaum, G. G., & Smyer, M. A. (1981). The development, validity, and reliability of the OARS Multidimensional Functional Assessment Questionnaire. *Journal of Gerontology, 36*(4), 428–434.
Head, B. J. (2001). Impaired home maintenance management. In M. Maas, K. Buckwalter, M. Hardy, T. Tripp-Reimer, M. Titler, & J. Specht (Eds.), *Nursing care of older adults: Diagnoses, outcomes & interventions* (pp. 64–74). St. Louis: Mosby.
Hickey, T. (1988). Self-care behavior of older adults. *Family and Community Health, 11*(3), 22–35.
Jette, A. M. (1980). Functional status index: Reliability of a chronic disease evaluation instrument. *Archives of Physical Medicine & Rehabilitation, 61*(9), 395–401.
+Katz, S., Ford, A. B., Moskowitz, R. W., Jackson, B. A., & Jaffe, M. W. (1963). Studies of illness in the aged. The Index of ADL: A standardized measure of biological and psychosocial function. *Journal of the American Medical Association, 185*(12), 914–919.
Lawton, M. P. (1983). Assessment of behaviors required to maintain residence in the community. In T. Crook, S. Ferris, & R. Bartus (Eds.), *Assessment in geriatric psychopharmacology* (pp. 119–135). New Canaan, CT: Mark Powley Associates.
Lawton, M. P., & Brody, E. M. (1969). Assessment of older people: Self-maintaining and instrumental activities of daily living. *Gerontologist, 9*(3), 179–186.
Leenerts, M. H., Teel, C. S., & Pendleton, M. K. (2002). Building a model of self-care for health promotion in aging. *Journal of Nursing Scholarship, 34*(4), 355–361.
Linn, M. W., & Linn, B. S. (1982). The Rapid Disability Rating Scale-2. *Journal of the American Geriatric Society, 30*(6), 378–382.
Meenan, R. F., Gertman, P. M., & Mason, J. H. (1980). Measuring health status in arthritis: The arthritis impact measurement scales. *Arthritis Rheumatism, 23*(2), 146–152.
Pearlman, R. (1987). Development of a functional assessment questionnaire for geriatric patients: The Comprehensive Older Persons' Evaluation (COPE). *Journal of Chronic Disease, 40*(56), 85S–94S.
Resnick, B. (2001). Motivating older adults to engage in self-care. *Patient Care for the Nurse Practitioner, 4*(9), 13–14, 16, 19.
Shanas, E., Townsend, P., Wedderburn, D., Friis, H., Milhoj, P., & Stehouwer, J. (1968). *Old people in three industrial societies.* New York: Atherton Press.

S

Self-Care: Non-Parenteral Medication   0307

Definition: Personal actions to administer oral and topical medications to meet therapeutic goals independently with or without assistive device

OUTCOME TARGET RATING: Maintain at_____   Increase to_____

		Severely compromised	Substantially compromised	Moderately compromised	Mildly compromised	Not compromised	
OUTCOME OVERALL RATING		1	2	3	4	5	
Indicators:							
030701	Identifies medication	1	2	3	4	5	NA
030702	Administers correct dose	1	2	3	4	5	NA
030716	Monitors therapeutic effects	1	2	3	4	5	NA
030717	Adjusts medication to achieve therapeutic effects	1	2	3	4	5	NA
030705	Follows medication precautions	1	2	3	4	5	NA
030706	Monitors medication side effects	1	2	3	4	5	NA
030707	Uses memory aids	1	2	3	4	5	NA
030708	Performs self-monitoring activities	1	2	3	4	5	NA
030709	Uses monitoring equipment accurately	1	2	3	4	5	NA
030710	Maintains required supplies	1	2	3	4	5	NA
030718	Uses medication as prescribed	1	2	3	4	5	NA
030712	Stores medication properly	1	2	3	4	5	NA
030713	Disposes of medication properly	1	2	3	4	5	NA
030714	Obtains required laboratory tests	1	2	3	4	5	NA
030719	Understands implications of test results	1	2	3	4	5	NA

Domain-Functional Health (I)   Class-Self-Care (D)   1st edition 1997; revised 2004, 2008, 2013

OUTCOME CONTENT REFERENCES:

Armer, J. M., Conn, V. S., Decker, S. A., & Tripp-Reimer, T. (2001). Self-care deficit. In M. Maas, K. Buckwalter, M. Hardy, T. Tripp-Reimer, M. Titler, & J. Specht (Eds.), *Nursing care of older adults: Diagnoses, outcomes & interventions* (pp. 366–384). St. Louis: Mosby.

Barry, K. (1993). Patient self-medication: An innovative approach to medication teaching. *Journal of Nursing Care Quality, 8*(1), 75–82.

Felsenthal, G., Glomski, N., & Jones, D. (1986). Medication education program in an inpatient geriatric rehabilitation unit. *Archives of Physical Medication and Rehabilitation, 67*(1), 27–29.

Hickey, T. (1988). Self-care behavior of older adults. *Family and Community Health, 11*(3), 22–35.

Leenerts, M. H., Teel, C. S., & Pendleton, M. K. (2002). Building a model of self-care for health promotion in aging. *Journal of Nursing Scholarship, 34*(4), 355–361.

Lorish, D. D., Richards, B., & Brown, S. (1990). Perspective of the patient with rheumatoid arthritis on issues related to missed medication. *Arthritis Care and Research, 3*(2), 78–84.

Resnick, B. (2001). Motivating older adults to engage in self-care. *Patient Care for the Nurse Practitioner, 4*(9), 13–14, 16, 19.

S

Self-Care: Oral Hygiene 0308

Definition: Personal actions to care for own mouth and teeth independently with or without assistive device

OUTCOME TARGET RATING: Maintain at_____ Increase to_____

		Severely compromised	Substantially compromised	Moderately compromised	Mildly compromised	Not compromised	
OUTCOME OVERALL RATING		1	2	3	4	5	
Indicators:							
030801	Brushes teeth	1	2	3	4	5	NA
030802	Flosses teeth	1	2	3	4	5	NA
030810	Uses mouthwash	1	2	3	4	5	NA
030803	Cleans mouth, gums, and tongue	1	2	3	4	5	NA
030804	Cleans dentures or dental appliances	1	2	3	4	5	NA
030806	Uses fluoridation	1	2	3	4	5	NA
030807	Obtains regular dental care	1	2	3	4	5	NA

Domain-Functional Health (I)   **Class**-Self-Care (D)   *1st edition 1997; revised 2004, 2013*

OUTCOME CONTENT REFERENCES:

Armer, J. M., Conn, V. S., Decker, S. A., & Tripp-Reimer, T. (2001). Self-care deficit. In M. Maas, K. Buckwalter, M. Hardy, T. Tripp-Reimer, M. Titler, & J. Specht (Eds.), *Nursing care of older adults: Diagnoses, outcomes & interventions* (pp. 366–384). St. Louis: Mosby.

Fischman, S. (1993). Self-care: Practical periodontal care in today's practice. *International Dental Journal, 43*(2, Suppl. 1), 179–183.

Hickey, T. (1988). Self-care behavior of older adults. *Family and Community Health, 11*(3), 22–35.

Horowitz, L. G. (1990). Dental patient education: Self-care to healthy human development. *Patient Education and Counseling, 15*(1), 65–71.

Leenerts, M. H., Teel, C. S., & Pendleton, M. K. (2002). Building a model of self-care for health promotion in aging. *Journal of Nursing Scholarship, 34*(4), 355–361.

+Niederman, R., & Sullivan, T. M. (1981). Oral hygiene skill achievement index I. *Journal of Periodontology, 52*(3), 143–149.

+Niederman, R., Sullivan, T. M., Weiss, D., Morhart, R., Robbins, W., & Maier, D. (1981). Oral hygiene skill achievement index II. *Journal of Periodontology. 52*(3), 150–154.

Rayant, G. A., & Sheiham, A. (1980). An analysis of factors affecting compliance with tooth-cleaning recommendations. *Journal of Clinical Periodontology, 7*(4), 289–299.

Resnick, B. (2001). Motivating older adults to engage in self-care. *Patient Care for the Nurse Practitioner, 4*(9), 13–14, 16, 19.

Richardson, A. (1987). A process standard for oral care. *Nursing Times, 83*(32), 38–40.

Self-Care: Parenteral Medication 0309

Definition: Personal actions to administer parenteral medications to meet therapeutic goals independently with or without assistive device

OUTCOME TARGET RATING: Maintain at_____ Increase to_____

		Severely compromised	Substantially compromised	Moderately compromised	Mildly compromised	Not compromised	
OUTCOME OVERALL RATING		1	2	3	4	5	
Indicators:							
030901	Identifies medication	1	2	3	4	5	NA
030902	Administers correct dose	1	2	3	4	5	NA
030918	Monitors therapeutic effects	1	2	3	4	5	NA
030919	Adjusts medication to achieve therapeutic effects	1	2	3	4	5	NA
030905	Follows medication precautions	1	2	3	4	5	NA
030906	Monitors medication side effects	1	2	3	4	5	NA
030907	Uses memory aids	1	2	3	4	5	NA

Continued

S

Self-Care: Parenteral Medication—cont'd

		Severely compromised	Substantially compromised	Moderately compromised	Mildly compromised	Not compromised	
030908	Performs self-monitoring activities	1	2	3	4	5	NA
030909	Uses monitoring equipment accurately	1	2	3	4	5	NA
030910	Maintains required supplies	1	2	3	4	5	NA
030921	Uses medication as prescribed	1	2	3	4	5	NA
030912	Stores medication properly	1	2	3	4	5	NA
030913	Disposes of medication properly	1	2	3	4	5	NA
030920	Disposes of syringes and needles properly	1	2	3	4	5	NA
030914	Maintains asepsis	1	2	3	4	5	NA
030915	Monitors injection sites	1	2	3	4	5	NA
030916	Obtains required laboratory tests	1	2	3	4	5	NA

Domain-*Functional Health (I)*   **Class**-*Self-Care (D)*   *1st edition 1997; revised 2004, 2008, 2013*

OUTCOME CONTENT REFERENCES:

Armer, J. M., Conn, V. S., Decker, S. A., & Tripp-Reimer, T. (2001). Self-care deficit. In M. Maas, K. Buckwalter, M. Hardy, T. Tripp-Reimer, M. Titler, & J. Specht (Eds.), *Nursing care of older adults: Diagnoses, outcomes & interventions* (pp. 366–384). St. Louis: Mosby.

Gilbert, D. N., Dworkin, R. J., Raber, S. R., & Leggett, J. E. (1997). Outpatient parenteral antimicrobial-drug therapy. *New England Journal of Medicine, 337*(12), 829–838.

Hickey, T. (1988). Self-care behavior of older adults. *Family and Community Health, 11*(3), 22–35.

Leenerts, M. H., Teel, C. S., & Pendleton, M. K. (2002). Building a model of self-care for health promotion in aging. *Journal of Nursing Scholarship, 34*(4), 355–361.

Resnick, B. (2001). Motivating older adults to engage in self-care. *Patient Care for the Nurse Practitioner, 4*(9), 13–14, 16, 19.

Robinson, J., Gould, M. A., Burrows-Hudson, S., Baltz, P., Currier, H., Piwkiewicz, D., et al. (1991). A care plan for self-administration of epoetin alpha. *ANNA Journal, 18*(6), 573–580.

Sarisley, C. (1987). Designing a teaching program for outpatient antibiotic therapy. *Journal of Nursing Staff Development, 3*(3), 128–135.

Self-Care: Toileting   0310

Definition: Personal actions to toilet self independently with or without assistive device

OUTCOME TARGET RATING: Maintain at_____ Increase to_____

		Severely compromised	Substantially compromised	Moderately compromised	Mildly compromised	Not compromised	
OUTCOME OVERALL RATING		1	2	3	4	5	
Indicators:							
031001	Responds to full bladder in timely manner	1	2	3	4	5	NA
031002	Responds to urge to have a bowel movement in timely manner	1	2	3	4	5	NA
031013	Gets in and out of bathroom	1	2	3	4	5	NA
031004	Removes clothing	1	2	3	4	5	NA
031005	Positions self on toilet or commode	1	2	3	4	5	NA
031014	Gets to toilet between urge and passage of urine	1	2	3	4	5	NA
031015	Gets to toilet between urge and evacuation of stool	1	2	3	4	5	NA
031006	Empties bladder	1	2	3	4	5	NA
031011	Empties bowel	1	2	3	4	5	NA
031007	Wipes self after urinating	1	2	3	4	5	NA

S

Self-Care: Toileting—*cont'd*

		Severely compromised	Substantially compromised	Moderately compromised	Mildly compromised	Not compromised	
031012	Wipes self after bowel movement	1	2	3	4	5	NA
031008	Gets up from toilet or commode	1	2	3	4	5	NA
031009	Adjusts clothing after toileting	1	2	3	4	5	NA

Domain-*Functional Health (I)*   **Class**-*Self-Care (D)*   *1st edition 1997; revised 2004, 2008, 2013*

OUTCOME CONTENT REFERENCES:

Armer, J. M., Conn, V. S., Decker, S. A., & Tripp-Reimer, T. (2001). Self-care deficit. In M. Maas, K. Buckwalter, M. Hardy, T. Tripp-Reimer, M. Titler, & J. Specht (Eds.), *Nursing care of older adults: Diagnoses, outcomes & interventions* (pp. 366–384). St. Louis: Mosby.

Burgio, K. L., Burgio, L. D., McCormick, K. A., & Engel, B. T. (1991). Assessing toileting skills and habits in an adult day care center. *Journal of Gerontological Nursing, 17*(12), 32–35.

+*Guide for the Uniform Data Set for Medical Rehabilitation* (including the FIM™ instrument) (version 5.1). (1997). Buffalo, NY: University at Buffalo.

Hickey, T. (1988). Self-care behavior of older adults. *Family and Community Health, 11*(3), 22–35.

+Katz, S., Ford, A. B., Moskowitz, R. W., Jackson, B. A., & Jaffe, M. W. (1963). Studies of illness in the aged. The Index of ADL: A standardized measure of biological and psychosocial function. *Journal of the American Medical Association, 185*(12), 914–919.

Leenerts, M. H., Teel, C. S., & Pendleton, M. K. (2002). Building a model of self-care for health promotion in aging. *Journal of Nursing Scholarship, 34*(4), 355–361.

Okamoto, G. A., Sousa, J., Telzrow, R. W., Holm, R. A., McCartin, R., & Shurtleff, D. B. (1984). Toileting skills in children with myelomeningocele: Rates of learning. *Archives of Physical Medicine and Rehabilitation, 65*(4), 182–185.

Resnick, B. (2001). Motivating older adults to engage in self-care. *Patient Care for the Nurse Practitioner, 4*(9), 13–14, 16, 19.

Seim, H. C. (1989). Toilet training in first children. *The Journal of Family Practice, 29*(6), 633–636.

Self-Direction of Care   1613

Definition: Care recipient actions taken to direct others who assist with or perform physical tasks and personal health care

OUTCOME TARGET RATING: Maintain at_____   Increase to_____

		Never demonstrated	Rarely demonstrated	Sometimes demonstrated	Often demonstrated	Consistently demonstrated	
OUTCOME OVERALL RATING		1	2	3	4	5	
Indicators:							
161301	Sets health care goals	1	2	3	4	5	NA
161302	Describes appropriate care	1	2	3	4	5	NA
161311	Obtains needed resources	1	2	3	4	5	NA
161304	Instructs others in appropriate care behaviors	1	2	3	4	5	NA
161305	Evaluates the care given by others	1	2	3	4	5	NA
161306	Determines that care is completed appropriately	1	2	3	4	5	NA
161307	Expresses confidence in problem solving	1	2	3	4	5	NA
161308	Takes corrective action when care is not appropriate	1	2	3	4	5	NA
161309	Instructs others in appropriate health maintenance activities	1	2	3	4	5	NA

S

Domain-*Health Knowledge & Behavior (IV)*   **Class**-*Health Behavior (Q)*   *2nd edition 2000; revised 2004, 2008*

OUTCOME CONTENT REFERENCES:

Edwards, P. A. (Ed.). (2000). *The specialty practice of rehabilitation nursing: A core curriculum* (4th ed.). Glenview, IL: Association of Rehabilitation Nurses.

Orem, D. E. (1985). A concept of self-care for the rehabilitation client. *Rehabilitation Nursing, 10*(3), 33–36.

Rehabilitation Nursing Foundation. (1995). *Twenty-one rehabilitation nursing diagnoses: A guide to interventions and outcomes.* Glenview, IL: Author.

Self-Esteem   1205

Definition: Personal judgment of self-worth

OUTCOME TARGET RATING: Maintain at_____   Increase to_____

OUTCOME OVERALL RATING	Never positive 1	Rarely positive 2	Sometimes positive 3	Often positive 4	Consistently positive 5	
Indicators:						
120501 Verbalizations of self-acceptance	1	2	3	4	5	NA
120502 Acceptance of self-limitations	1	2	3	4	5	NA
120503 Maintenance of erect posture	1	2	3	4	5	NA
120504 Maintenance of eye contact	1	2	3	4	5	NA
120505 Description of self	1	2	3	4	5	NA
120506 Regard for others	1	2	3	4	5	NA
120507 Open communication	1	2	3	4	5	NA
120508 Fulfillment of personally significant roles	1	2	3	4	5	NA
120509 Maintenance of grooming and hygiene	1	2	3	4	5	NA
120510 Balance of participation and listening in groups	1	2	3	4	5	NA
120511 Confidence level	1	2	3	4	5	NA
120512 Acceptance of compliments from others	1	2	3	4	5	NA
120513 Expected response from others	1	2	3	4	5	NA
120514 Acceptance of constructive criticism	1	2	3	4	5	NA
120515 Willingness to confront others	1	2	3	4	5	NA
120521 Description of success in work	1	2	3	4	5	NA
120522 Description of success in school	1	2	3	4	5	NA
120517 Description of success in social groups	1	2	3	4	5	NA
120518 Description of pride in self	1	2	3	4	5	NA
120519 Feelings about self-worth	1	2	3	4	5	NA

Domain-*Psychosocial Health (III)*   **Class**-*Psychological Well-Being (M)*   *1st edition 1997; revised 2008*

OUTCOME CONTENT REFERENCES:

Bonham, P., & Cheney, A. (1982). Concept of self: A framework for nursing assessment. In P. L. Chinn (Ed.), *Advances in nursing theory development* (pp. 173–189). Rockville, MD: Aspen.

Coopersmith, S. (1967). *The antecedents of self-esteem.* San Francisco: W. H. Freeman.

Crandall, R. (1973). The measurement of self-esteem and related constructs. In J. P. Robinson & P. R. Shaver (Eds.), *Measures of social psychological attitudes.* Ann Arbor, MI: Institute for Social Research, University of Michigan.

Fitts, W. (1965). *Manual for the Tennessee Self-Concept Scale.* Nashville, TN: Counselor Recordings & Tests.

Groh, C. J., & Whall, A. L. (2001). Self-esteem disturbance. In M. Maas, K. Buckwalter, M. Hardy, T. Tripp-Reimer, M. Titler, & J. Specht (Eds.), *Nursing care of older adults: Diagnoses, outcomes & interventions* (pp. 593–600). St. Louis: Mosby.

Larson, J. (1989). Validation of the defining characteristics of disturbance in self-esteem in patients with anorexia nervosa. In R. Carroll-Johnson (Ed.) *Classification of nursing diagnoses: Proceedings of the eighth conference* (North American Nursing Diagnosis Association) (pp. 307–312). Philadelphia: J. B. Lippincott.

+Nugent, W. R., & Thomas, J. W. (1993). Validation of a clinical measure of self-esteem. *Research on Social Work Practice, 3*(2), 191–207.

Roid, G., & Fitts, W. (1988). *Tennessee Self-Concept Scale: Revised manual.* Los Angeles: Western Psychological Services.

Rosenberg, M. (1965). *Society & the adolescent self-image.* Princeton, NJ: Princeton University Press.

Stanwyck, D. (1983). Self-esteem through the life span. *Family and Community Health, 6*(2), 11–28.

S

Self-Management: Acute Illness   3100

Definition: Personal actions to manage a reversible illness, its treatment, and to prevent complications

OUTCOME TARGET RATING: Maintain at_____   Increase to_____

		Never demonstrated	Rarely demonstrated	Sometimes demonstrated	Often demonstrated	Consistently demonstrated	
OUTCOME OVERALL RATING		1	2	3	4	5	
Indicators:							
310001	Monitors signs and symptoms of illness	1	2	3	4	5	NA
310002	Follows recommended precautions	1	2	3	4	5	NA
310003	Monitors for signs and symptoms of complications	1	2	3	4	5	NA
310004	Obtains required laboratory test	1	2	3	4	5	NA
310005	Identifies cultural beliefs that impact treatment	1	2	3	4	5	NA
310006	Discusses cultural beliefs that impact treatment with health provider	1	2	3	4	5	NA
310007	Follows recommended treatment	1	2	3	4	5	NA
310008	Performs prescribed procedure	1	2	3	4	5	NA
310009	Uses treatment devices correctly	1	2	3	4	5	NA
310010	Monitors treatment therapeutic effects	1	2	3	4	5	NA
310011	Monitors treatment side effects	1	2	3	4	5	NA
310012	Uses strategies to reduce transmission of illness to others	1	2	3	4	5	NA
310013	Follows medication regimen	1	2	3	4	5	NA
310014	Monitors medication therapeutic effects	1	2	3	4	5	NA
310015	Monitors medication side effects	1	2	3	4	5	NA
310016	Monitors medication adverse effects	1	2	3	4	5	NA
310017	Seeks assistance for self-care	1	2	3	4	5	NA
310018	Adjusts activity level during illness	1	2	3	4	5	NA
310019	Adjusts diet during illness	1	2	3	4	5	NA
310020	Avoids behaviors that potentiate illness	1	2	3	4	5	NA
310021	Uses strategies to cope with illness	1	2	3	4	5	NA
310022	Uses strategies to enhance comfort	1	2	3	4	5	NA
310023	Uses strategies to maintain adequate sleep	1	2	3	4	5	NA
310024	Balances activity and rest	1	2	3	4	5	NA
310025	Monitors changes in illness	1	2	3	4	5	NA
310026	Uses reputable sources of information	1	2	3	4	5	NA
310027	Obtains advice from health provider as needed	1	2	3	4	5	NA
310028	Uses health care services congruent with needs	1	2	3	4	5	NA
310029	Schedules appointments with health professional as needed	1	2	3	4	5	NA

Domain-Health Knowledge & Behavior (IV)   *Class*-Health Management (FF)   *5th edition 2013*

OUTCOME CONTENT REFERENCES:
Jones, R., White, P., Armstrong, D., Ashworth, M., & Peters, M. (2010). *Managing acute illness.* London: The King's Fund.
Scruggs, B. (2009). Chronic health care: It is so much different than acute health care – or it should be. *Home Health Care Management & Practice, 22*(1), 43–48.
Starnino, V., Mariscal, S., Holter, M., Davidson, L., Cook, K., Fukui, S., et al. (2010). Outcomes of an illness self-management group using wellness recovery action planning. *Psychiatric Rehabilitation Journal, 34*(1), 57–60.

S

Self-Management: Anticoagulation Therapy   3101

Definition: Personal actions to manage therapy to maintain blood clotting time within a prescribed range and prevent complications

OUTCOME TARGET RATING: Maintain at_____ Increase to_____

		Never demonstrated	Rarely demonstrated	Sometimes demonstrated	Often demonstrated	Consistently demonstrated	
OUTCOME OVERALL RATING		1	2	3	4	5	
Indicators:							
310101	Seeks information about anticoagulation therapy	1	2	3	4	5	NA
310102	Seeks information about actions of anticoagulation agent	1	2	3	4	5	NA
310103	Participates in health care decisions	1	2	3	4	5	NA
310104	Uses medication as prescribed	1	2	3	4	5	NA
310105	Seeks information about potential complications	1	2	3	4	5	NA
310106	Seeks information about laboratory test for clotting time	1	2	3	4	5	NA
310107	Obtains laboratory tests	1	2	3	4	5	NA
310108	Monitors for signs and symptoms of thromboembolism	1	2	3	4	5	NA
310109	Monitors for signs and symptoms of bleeding	1	2	3	4	5	NA
310110	Monitors for signs and symptoms of atrial fibrillation	1	2	3	4	5	NA
310111	Monitors for signs and symptoms of stroke	1	2	3	4	5	NA
310112	Monitors for signs and symptoms of transient ischemic attack	1	2	3	4	5	NA
310113	Reports symptoms of complications	1	2	3	4	5	NA
310114	Notifies health professionals of anticoagulation therapy	1	2	3	4	5	NA
310115	Uses strategies to reduce venous stasis	1	2	3	4	5	NA
310116	Uses strategies to prevent internal bleeding	1	2	3	4	5	NA
310117	Uses strategies to prevent physical injuries	1	2	3	4	5	NA
310118	Monitors vital signs	1	2	3	4	5	NA
310119	Follows dietary restrictions	1	2	3	4	5	NA
310120	Avoids substances that interact with anticoagulant agent	1	2	3	4	5	NA
310121	Eliminates alcohol use	1	2	3	4	5	NA
310122	Eliminates tobacco use	1	2	3	4	5	NA
310123	Discusses non-prescription medication use with health provider	1	2	3	4	5	NA
310124	Develops plan for medical emergencies	1	2	3	4	5	NA
310125	Informs caregiver about management of anticoagulation therapy	1	2	3	4	5	NA
310126	Shares plan for immediate treatment with family caregiver	1	2	3	4	5	NA

S

Domain-Health Knowledge & Behavior (IV)   *Class-Health Management (FF)*   *5th edition 2013*

OUTCOME CONTENT REFERENCES:

Findlay, J., Keogh, M., & Cooper, L. (2010). Venous thromboembolism prophylaxis: The role of the nurse. *British Journal of Nursing, 19*(16), 1028–1032.

Fitzgerald, J. (2010). Venous thromboembolism: Have we made headway? *Orthopaedic Nursing, 29*(4), 226–234.

Headley, C. M., & Melander, S. (2011). When it may be a pulmonary embolism. *Nephrology Nursing Journal, 38*(2), 127–152.

Houman Fekrazad, M., Lopes, R. D., Stashenko, G. J., Alexander, J. H., & Garcia, D. (2009). Treatment of venous thromboembolism: Guidelines translated for the clinician. *Journal of Thrombosis and Thrombolysis, 28*(3), 270–275.

Lancaster, S. L., Owens, A., Bryant, A. S., Ramey, L. S., Nicholson, J., Gossett, K., et al. (2010). Emergency: Upper-extremity deep vein thrombosis. *AJN: American Journal of Nursing, 110*(5), 48–52.

Lankshear, A., Harden, J., & Simms, J. (2010). Safe practice for patients receiving anticoagulant therapy. *Nursing Standard, 24*(20), 47–56.

Long, E., Pitfield, A. F., & Kissoon, N. (2011). Anticoagulation therapy: Indications, monitoring, and complications. *Pediatric Emergency Care, 27*(1), 55–61.

Shaughnessy, K. (2007). Massive pulmonary embolism. *Critical Care Nurse, 27*(1), 39–40, 42–51.

Thomson, R., Parkin, D., Eccles, M., Sudlow, M., & Robinson, A. (2000). Decision analysis and guidelines for anticoagulant therapy to prevent stroke in patients with atrial fibrillation. *Lancet, 355*(9208), 956–962.

Winans, A., Rudd, K., & Triller, D. (2010). Assessing anticoagulation knowledge in patients new to warfarin. *The Annals of Pharmacotherapy, 44*(7–8), 1152–1157.

Yee, C. A. (2010). Conquering pulmonary embolism. *OR Nurse, 4*(5), 18–24.

Self-Management: Asthma **0704**

Definition: Personal actions to manage asthma, its treatment, and to prevent complications

OUTCOME TARGET RATING: Maintain at_____ Increase to_____

OUTCOME OVERALL RATING	Never demonstrated 1	Rarely demonstrated 2	Sometimes demonstrated 3	Often demonstrated 4	Consistently demonstrated 5	
Indicators:						
070418 Describes causal factors	1	2	3	4	5	NA
070419 Recognizes onset of asthma	1	2	3	4	5	NA
070401 Initiates action to avoid personal triggers	1	2	3	4	5	NA
070402 Initiates action to manage personal triggers	1	2	3	4	5	NA
070426 Shares acute asthma management with relevant individual(s)	1	2	3	4	5	NA
070427 Shares emergency plan with relevant individual(s)	1	2	3	4	5	NA
070428 Follows emergency plan for acute attacks	1	2	3	4	5	NA
070429 Adjusts life routine for optimal health	1	2	3	4	5	NA
070403 Makes appropriate environmental modifications	1	2	3	4	5	NA
070420 Uses diary to monitor symptoms over time	1	2	3	4	5	NA
070430 Obtains early treatment for infection	1	2	3	4	5	NA
070405 Participates in age-appropriate activities	1	2	3	4	5	NA
070406 Sleeps through the night with no cough or wheeze	1	2	3	4	5	NA
070431 Reports energy restored after rest	1	2	3	4	5	NA
070432 Maintains access to medication	1	2	3	4	5	NA
070433 Monitors medication side effects	1	2	3	4	5	NA
070409 Reports symptom control with minimal medication use	1	2	3	4	5	NA
070410 Monitors peak flow routinely	1	2	3	4	5	NA
070411 Monitors peak flow when symptoms occur	1	2	3	4	5	NA

S

Continued

Self-Management: Asthma—cont'd

		Never demonstrated	Rarely demonstrated	Sometimes demonstrated	Often demonstrated	Consistently demonstrated	
070412	Makes appropriate medication choices	1	2	3	4	5	NA
070434	Uses inhalers, spacers, and nebulizers correctly	1	2	3	4	5	NA
070414	Self-manages exacerbations	1	2	3	4	5	NA
070415	Reports uncontrolled symptoms	1	2	3	4	5	NA
070435	Uses support group	1	2	3	4	5	NA
070421	Reports asthma controlled	1	2	3	4	5	NA

		Consistently demonstrated (4 + occurrences)	Often demonstrated (3 occurrences)	Sometimes demonstrated (2 occurrences)	Rarely demonstrated (1 occurrence)	Never demonstrated (no occurrence)	
070422	Emergency visits related to asthma within the last year	1	2	3	4	5	NA
070423	Hospitalizations related to asthma within the last year	1	2	3	4	5	NA
070424	School absences related to asthma within the school year	1	2	3	4	5	NA
070425	Work absences related to asthma within the last year	1	2	3	4	5	NA

Domain-*Health Knowledge & Behavior (IV)*   **Class**-*Health Management (FF)*   *2nd edition 2000; revised 2004, 2008, 2013*

OUTCOME CONTENT REFERENCES:

Cross, S. (1997). Revised guidelines on asthma management. *Professional Nurse, 12*(6), 408–410.

Gallagher, C. (2002). Childhood asthma: Tools that help parents manage it. *American Journal of Nursing, 102*(8), 71–83.

Le, J. T., Pearlman, D. S., Nickals, R., Lowenthal, M., & Rosenthal, R. (1998). Algorithm for the diagnosis and management of asthma: A practice parameter update. *Annals of Allergy, Asthma and Immunology, 81*(5 pt 1), 415–420.

National Heart, Lung, and Blood Institute. National Asthma Education Program. (2007). *Expert panel report 3: Guidelines for the diagnosis and management of asthma* (NIH Publication No. 07-4051). Bethesda, MD: U.S. Department of Health and Human Services.

Perry, C. S., & Toole, K. A. (2000). Impact of school nurse case management on asthma control in school-aged children. *Journal of School Health, 70*(7), 303–304.

Rhee, H., Belyea, M., & Brasch, J. (2010). Family support and asthma outcomes in adolescents: Barriers to adherence as a mediator. *Journal of Adolescent Health, 47*(5), 472–478.

Tettersell, M. J. (1993). Asthma patients' knowledge in relation to compliance with drug therapy. *Journal of Advanced Nursing, 18*(1), 103–113.

Yawn, B. P. (2005). Asthma. In D. L. Huber (Ed.), *Disease management: A guide for case managers* (pp. 100–131). St. Louis: Elsevier Saunders.

Yoos, H. L., Philipson, E., McMullen, A. (2003). Asthma management across the life span: The child with asthma. *Nursing Clinics of North America, 38*(4), 635–652.

S

Self-Management: Cardiac Disease   1617

Definition: Personal actions to manage heart disease, its treatment, and to prevent disease progression and complications

OUTCOME TARGET RATING: Maintain at_____   Increase to_____

		Never demonstrated	Rarely demonstrated	Sometimes demonstrated	Often demonstrated	Consistently demonstrated	
OUTCOME OVERALL RATING		1	2	3	4	5	
Indicators:							
161701	Accepts diagnosis	1	2	3	4	5	NA
161702	Seeks information about methods to maintain cardiovascular health	1	2	3	4	5	NA
161703	Participates in health care decisions	1	2	3	4	5	NA
161704	Participates in prescribed cardiac rehabilitation	1	2	3	4	5	NA
161705	Performs treatment regimen as prescribed	1	2	3	4	5	NA
161706	Monitors symptom onset	1	2	3	4	5	NA
161707	Monitors symptom persistence	1	2	3	4	5	NA
161708	Monitors symptom severity	1	2	3	4	5	NA
161709	Monitors symptom frequency	1	2	3	4	5	NA
161710	Reports symptoms of worsening disease	1	2	3	4	5	NA
161711	Reports signs and symptoms of depression	1	2	3	4	5	NA
161712	Uses diary to monitor symptoms over time	1	2	3	4	5	NA
161713	Uses preventive measures to reduce risk of complications	1	2	3	4	5	NA
161714	Uses symptom relief methods	1	2	3	4	5	NA
161744	Obtains health care when warning signs occur	1	2	3	4	5	NA
161716	Monitors pulse rate and rhythm	1	2	3	4	5	NA
161717	Monitors blood pressure	1	2	3	4	5	NA
161718	Limits sodium intake	1	2	3	4	5	NA
161719	Limits fat and cholesterol intake	1	2	3	4	5	NA
161720	Follows recommended diet	1	2	3	4	5	NA
161721	Follows fluid restrictions	1	2	3	4	5	NA
161722	Monitors effects of stimulants	1	2	3	4	5	NA
161723	Monitors body weight	1	2	3	4	5	NA
161724	Uses effective weight control strategies	1	2	3	4	5	NA
161725	Maintains optimum weight	1	2	3	4	5	NA
161726	Follows recommendations for alcohol use	1	2	3	4	5	NA
161727	Participates in smoking cessation regimen	1	2	3	4	5	NA
161728	Participates in recommended exercise	1	2	3	4	5	NA
161729	Uses energy conservation techniques	1	2	3	4	5	NA
161730	Balances activity and rest	1	2	3	4	5	NA
161731	Performs usual life routine	1	2	3	4	5	NA
161732	Follows recommendations for sexual activity	1	2	3	4	5	NA
161733	Obtains required medication	1	2	3	4	5	NA
161734	Uses medication as prescribed	1	2	3	4	5	NA
161735	Monitors prescribed medication therapeutic effects	1	2	3	4	5	NA

Continued

S

Self-Management: Cardiac Disease—cont'd

		Never demonstrated	Rarely demonstrated	Sometimes demonstrated	Often demonstrated	Consistently demonstrated	
161736	Uses only non-prescription medication approved by health professional	1	2	3	4	5	NA
161737	Uses stress management strategies	1	2	3	4	5	NA
161746	Obtains influenza seasonal vaccine	1	2	3	4	5	NA
161747	Obtains pneumonia vaccine	1	2	3	4	5	NA
161739	Uses health care services congruent with needs	1	2	3	4	5	NA
161740	Participates in screening for cholesterol	1	2	3	4	5	NA
161741	Reports need for financial assistance	1	2	3	4	5	NA
161742	Keeps appointments with health professional	1	2	3	4	5	NA
161743	Maintains plan for medical emergencies	1	2	3	4	5	NA
161745	Adjusts life routine for optimal health	1	2	3	4	5	NA

Domain-Health Knowledge & Behavior (IV)   **Class**-Health Management (FF)   *3rd edition 2004; revised 2008, 2013*

OUTCOME CONTENT REFERENCES:

Chen, A., Yehle, K., Plake, K., Murawski, M., & Mason, H. (2011). Health literacy and self-care of patients with heart failure. *Journal of Cardiovascular Nursing, 26*(6), 446–451.

Dunbar, S. B., Jacobson, L. H., & Deaton, C. (1998). Heart failure: Strategies to enhance patient self-management. *AACN Clinical Issues: Advanced Practice in Acute & Critical Care, 9*(2), 244–256.

Dusseldorp, E., Van Elderan, T., Maes, S., Meulman, J., & Kraaij, V. (1999). A meta-analysis of psychoeducational programs for coronary heart disease patients. *Health Psychology, 18*(5), 506–519.

Jessup, M., Abraham, W., Casey, D., Feldman, A., Francis, G., Ganiats, T., et al. (2009). 2009 focused update: ACCF/AHA guidelines for the diagnosis and management of heart failure in adults: A report of the American College of Cardiology Foundation/American Heart Association Task Force on Practice Guidelines. *Journal of the American College of Cardiology, 53*(15), 1343–1382.

Johnson, J., & Pearson, V. (2000). The effects of a structured education course on stroke survivors living in the community…including commentary by Phipps, M. *Rehabilitation Nursing, (25),* 59–65.

National Institutes of Health, National Heart, Lung, and Blood Institute (NHLBI), & National High Blood Pressure Education Program. (2004). *The seventh report of the Joint National Committee on Prevention, Detection, Evaluation, & Treatment of High Blood Pressure* (NIH Publication No. 04-5230). Bethesda, MD: Author.

S

Self-Management: Chronic Disease 3102

Definition: Personal actions to manage a chronic disease, its treatment, and to prevent disease progression and complications

OUTCOME TARGET RATING: Maintain at_____   Increase to_____

		Never demonstrated	Rarely demonstrated	Sometimes demonstrated	Often demonstrated	Consistently demonstrated	
OUTCOME OVERALL RATING		1	2	3	4	5	
Indicators:							
310201	Accepts diagnosis	1	2	3	4	5	NA
310202	Seeks information about disease	1	2	3	4	5	NA
310203	Monitors signs and symptoms of disease	1	2	3	4	5	NA
310204	Follows recommended precautions	1	2	3	4	5	NA
310205	Seeks information about methods to prevent complications	1	2	3	4	5	NA
310206	Monitors for signs and symptoms of complications	1	2	3	4	5	NA
310207	Reports signs and symptoms of complications	1	2	3	4	5	NA
310208	Uses symptom relief strategies	1	2	3	4	5	NA
310209	Identifies cultural beliefs that impact treatment	1	2	3	4	5	NA
310210	Discusses cultural beliefs that impact treatment with health provider	1	2	3	4	5	NA
310211	Follows recommended treatment	1	2	3	4	5	NA
310212	Performs prescribed procedure	1	2	3	4	5	NA
310213	Uses treatment devices correctly	1	2	3	4	5	NA
310214	Monitors treatment therapeutic effects	1	2	3	4	5	NA
310215	Monitors treatment side effects	1	2	3	4	5	NA
310216	Alters roles to meet treatment requirements	1	2	3	4	5	NA
310217	Obtains required laboratory tests	1	2	3	4	5	NA
310218	Follows medication regimen	1	2	3	4	5	NA
310219	Monitors medication therapeutic effects	1	2	3	4	5	NA
310220	Monitors medication side effects	1	2	3	4	5	NA
310221	Monitors medication adverse effects	1	2	3	4	5	NA
310222	Uses only non-prescription medication approved by health professional	1	2	3	4	5	NA
310223	Seeks assistance for self-care	1	2	3	4	5	NA
310224	Follows recommended diet	1	2	3	4	5	NA
310225	Follows recommended activity level	1	2	3	4	5	NA
310226	Participates in recommended exercises	1	2	3	4	5	NA
310227	Eliminates tobacco use	1	2	3	4	5	NA
310228	Uses stress management strategies	1	2	3	4	5	NA
310229	Maintains optimum weight	1	2	3	4	5	NA
310230	Monitors vital signs	1	2	3	4	5	NA
310231	Avoids behaviors that potentiate disease progression	1	2	3	4	5	NA
310232	Uses strategies to prevent complications	1	2	3	4	5	NA
310233	Adjusts life routine for optimal health	1	2	3	4	5	NA
310234	Uses strategies to cope with effects of disease	1	2	3	4	5	NA

Continued

S

Self-Management: Chronic Disease—cont'd

		Never demonstrated	Rarely demonstrated	Sometimes demonstrated	Often demonstrated	Consistently demonstrated	
310235	Uses strategies to enhance comfort	1	2	3	4	5	NA
310236	Uses strategies to control pain	1	2	3	4	5	NA
310237	Uses strategies to maintain adequate sleep	1	2	3	4	5	NA
310238	Balances activity and rest	1	2	3	4	5	NA
310239	Obtains influenza seasonal vaccine	1	2	3	4	5	NA
310240	Obtains pneumonia vaccine	1	2	3	4	5	NA
310241	Participates in prescribed educational program	1	2	3	4	5	NA
310242	Monitors changes in disease	1	2	3	4	5	NA
310243	Uses reputable sources of information	1	2	3	4	5	NA
310244	Participates in health care decisions	1	2	3	4	5	NA
310245	Uses case manager to coordinate care	1	2	3	4	5	NA
310246	Uses health care services congruent with needs	1	2	3	4	5	NA
310247	Develops plan for medical emergencies	1	2	3	4	5	NA
310248	Obtains advice from health professional as needed	1	2	3	4	5	NA
310249	Keeps appointments with health professional	1	2	3	4	5	NA
310250	Uses support group	1	2	3	4	5	NA
310251	Uses available community resources	1	2	3	4	5	NA

Domain-*Health Knowledge & Behavior (IV)*   **Class**-*Health Management (FF)*   *5th edition 2013*

OUTCOME CONTENT REFERENCES:

Elzen, H., Slaets, J., Snijders, T., & Steverink, N. (2007). Evaluation of the chronic disease self-management program (CDSMP) among chronically ill older people in the Netherlands. *Social Science & Medicine, 64*(9), 1832–1841.

Kralik, D., Koch, T., Price, K., & Howard, N. (2004). Chronic illness self-management: Taking action to create order. *Journal of Clinical Nursing, 13*(2), 259–267.

Scruggs, B. (2009). Chronic health care: It is so much different than acute health care – or it should be. *Home Health Care Management & Practice, 22*(1), 43–48.

Swendeman, D., Ingram, B., & Rotheram-Borus, J. (2009). Common elements in self-management of HIV and other chronic illnesses: An integrative framework. *AIDS Care, 21*(10), 1321–1334.

Yukawa, K., Yamazaki, Y., Yonekura, Y., Togari, T., Abbott, F., Homma, M., et al. (2010). Effectiveness of chronic disease self-management program in Japan: Preliminary report of a longitudinal study. *Nursing & Health Sciences, 12*(4), 456–463.

S

Self-Management: Chronic Obstructive Pulmonary Disease

3103

Definition: Personal actions to manage chronic obstructive pulmonary disease, its treatment, and to prevent disease progression and complications

OUTCOME TARGET RATING: Maintain at_____   Increase to_____

		Never demonstrated	Rarely demonstrated	Sometimes demonstrated	Often demonstrated	Consistently demonstrated	
OUTCOME OVERALL RATING		1	2	3	4	5	
Indicators:							
310301	Accepts diagnosis	1	2	3	4	5	NA
310302	Seeks information about methods to prevent progression of disease	1	2	3	4	5	NA
310303	Seeks information about methods to prevent complications	1	2	3	4	5	NA
310304	Participates in health care decisions	1	2	3	4	5	NA
310305	Performs treatment regimen as prescribed	1	2	3	4	5	NA
310306	Avoids environmental risk factors	1	2	3	4	5	NA
310307	Participates in pulmonary rehabilitation	1	2	3	4	5	NA
310308	Monitors pulse rate and rhythm	1	2	3	4	5	NA
310309	Monitors respiratory rate and rhythm	1	2	3	4	5	NA
310310	Monitors body temperature	1	2	3	4	5	NA
310311	Monitors oxygen saturation	1	2	3	4	5	NA
310312	Monitors food intake effects on breathing	1	2	3	4	5	NA
310313	Monitors fluid intake effects on breathing	1	2	3	4	5	NA
310314	Monitors symptom onset	1	2	3	4	5	NA
310315	Monitors symptom persistence	1	2	3	4	5	NA
310316	Monitors symptom severity	1	2	3	4	5	NA
310317	Monitors symptom frequency	1	2	3	4	5	NA
310318	Monitors disease progression	1	2	3	4	5	NA
310319	Reports symptoms of worsening disease	1	2	3	4	5	NA
310320	Obtains health care when warning signs occur	1	2	3	4	5	NA
310321	Uses symptom relief methods	1	2	3	4	5	NA
310322	Obtains required medication	1	2	3	4	5	NA
310323	Uses medication as prescribed	1	2	3	4	5	NA
310324	Monitors prescribed medication therapeutic effects	1	2	3	4	5	NA
310325	Monitors medication side effects	1	2	3	4	5	NA
310326	Uses oxygen correctly	1	2	3	4	5	NA
310327	Participates in smoking cessation regimen	1	2	3	4	5	NA
310328	Participates in recommended exercise	1	2	3	4	5	NA
310329	Uses energy conservation techniques	1	2	3	4	5	NA
310330	Balances activity and rest	1	2	3	4	5	NA
310331	Uses strategies to cope with functional changes	1	2	3	4	5	NA
310332	Monitors for signs and symptoms of depression	1	2	3	4	5	NA
310333	Uses relaxation techniques	1	2	3	4	5	NA

Continued

S

Self-Management: Chronic Obstructive Pulmonary Disease—cont'd

		Never demonstrated	Rarely demonstrated	Sometimes demonstrated	Often demonstrated	Consistently demonstrated	
310334	Adjusts life routine for optimal health	1	2	3	4	5	NA
310335	Obtains influenza seasonal vaccine	1	2	3	4	5	NA
310336	Obtains pneumonia vaccine	1	2	3	4	5	NA
310337	Uses health care services congruent with needs	1	2	3	4	5	NA
310338	Reports need for financial assistance	1	2	3	4	5	NA
310339	Keeps appointments with health professional	1	2	3	4	5	NA
310340	Maintains plan for medical emergencies	1	2	3	4	5	NA
310341	Uses available community resources	1	2	3	4	5	NA

***Domain-**Health Knowledge & Behavior (IV)* ***Class-**Health Management (FF)* *5th edition 2013*

OUTCOME CONTENT REFERENCES:

Bourbeau, J. (2008). Clinical decision processes and patient engagement in self-management. *Disease Management & Health Outcomes, 16*(6), 327–333.

Chen, K.-H., Chen, M.-L., Lee, S., Cho, H.-Y., & Weng, L.-C. (2008). Self-management behaviours for patients with chronic obstructive pulmonary disease: A qualitative study. *Journal of Advanced Nursing, 64*(6), 595–604.

Gallagher, R., Donoghue, J., Chenoweth, L., Stein-Parbury, J. (2008). Self-management in older patients with chronic illness. *International Journal of Nursing Practice, 14*(5), 373–382.

Hibbard, J. H., Greene J., Tusler, M. (2009). Improving the outcomes of disease management by tailoring care to the patient's level of activation. *The American Journal of Managed Care, 15*(6), 353–360.

Horsley, Liz. (2008). ACP guideline recommends diagnosis and management strategies for copd. *American Family Physician, 78*(3), 401–402.

Kuebler, K. K., Buchsel, P. C., Balkstra, C. R. (2008) Differentiating chronic obstructive pulmonary disease from asthma. *Journal of the American Academy of Nurse Practitioners, 20*(9), 445–454.

Kuzma, A. M., Meli, Y., Meldrum, C., Jellen, P., Butler-Lebair, M., Koczen-Doyle, D., et al. (2008). Multidisciplinary care of the patient with chronic obstructive pulmonary disease. *Proceedings Of The American Thoracic Society, 5*(4), 567–571.

Kyung, K. A., Chin, P. A., (2007). The effect of a pulmonary rehabilitation programme on older patients with chronic pulmonary disease. *Journal of Clinical Nursing, 17*(1), 118–125.

Lewis, S., Dirksen, S., Heitkemper, M., Bucher, L., & Camera, I. (2011). *Medical-surgical nursing: Assessment and management of clinical problems* (8th ed.). St. Louis: Mosby.

Ries, Andrew L. (2008). Pulmonary rehabilitation: Summary of an evidence-based guideline. *Respiratory Care, 53*(9), 1203–1207.

Rosser, B. A., Eccleaton, C. E. (2009). Promoting self-management through technology: Smart Solutions for long-term health conditions, *Journal of Integrated Care, 17*(6), 10–19.

Self-Management: Coronary Artery Disease   3104

Definition: Personal actions to manage coronary artery disease, its treatment, and to prevent disease progression and complications

OUTCOME TARGET RATING: Maintain at_____   Increase to_____

		Never demonstrated	Rarely demonstrated	Sometimes demonstrated	Often demonstrated	Consistently demonstrated	
OUTCOME OVERALL RATING		1	2	3	4	5	
Indicators:							
310401	Accepts diagnosis	1	2	3	4	5	NA
310402	Seeks information about methods to manage disease	1	2	3	4	5	NA
310403	Participates in health care decisions	1	2	3	4	5	NA
310404	Participates in prescribed cardiac rehabilitation	1	2	3	4	5	NA
310405	Performs treatment regimen as prescribed	1	2	3	4	5	NA
310406	Monitors heart rate and rhythm	1	2	3	4	5	NA

S

Self-Management: Coronary Artery Disease—cont'd

		Never demonstrated	Rarely demonstrated	Sometimes demonstrated	Often demonstrated	Consistently demonstrated	
310407	Monitors blood pressure	1	2	3	4	5	NA
310408	Monitors for pain	1	2	3	4	5	NA
310409	Monitors for shortness of breath	1	2	3	4	5	NA
310410	Monitors symptom onset	1	2	3	4	5	NA
310411	Monitors symptom persistence	1	2	3	4	5	NA
310412	Monitors symptom severity	1	2	3	4	5	NA
310413	Monitors symptom frequency	1	2	3	4	5	NA
310414	Reports symptoms of worsening disease	1	2	3	4	5	NA
310415	Uses diary to monitor symptoms over time	1	2	3	4	5	NA
310416	Uses symptom relief methods	1	2	3	4	5	NA
310417	Uses preventive strategies to reduce risk of complications	1	2	3	4	5	NA
310418	Obtains health care for change in symptoms	1	2	3	4	5	NA
310419	Uses medication as prescribed	1	2	3	4	5	NA
310420	Monitors medication therapeutic effects	1	2	3	4	5	NA
310421	Monitors medication side effects	1	2	3	4	5	NA
310422	Avoids stopping medication suddenly	1	2	3	4	5	NA
310423	Uses only non-prescription medication approved by health professional	1	2	3	4	5	NA
310424	Follows prescribed diet	1	2	3	4	5	NA
310425	Monitors effects of stimulants	1	2	3	4	5	NA
310426	Uses effective weight control strategies	1	2	3	4	5	NA
310427	Maintains optimum weight	1	2	3	4	5	NA
310428	Follows recommendations for alcohol use	1	2	3	4	5	NA
310429	Eliminates tobacco use	1	2	3	4	5	NA
310430	Avoids secondhand smoke	1	2	3	4	5	NA
310431	Participates in recommended exercise	1	2	3	4	5	NA
310432	Follows recommendations for sexual activity	1	2	3	4	5	NA
310433	Uses stress management strategies	1	2	3	4	5	NA
310434	Uses anger management techniques	1	2	3	4	5	NA
310435	Obtains influenza seasonal vaccine	1	2	3	4	5	NA
310436	Obtains pneumonia vaccine	1	2	3	4	5	NA
310437	Uses health care services congruent with needs	1	2	3	4	5	NA
310438	Participates in screening for cholesterol	1	2	3	4	5	NA
310439	Participates in screening for blood glucose level	1	2	3	4	5	NA
310440	Uses social support	1	2	3	4	5	NA
310441	Keeps appointments with health professional	1	2	3	4	5	NA
310442	Maintains plan for medical emergencies	1	2	3	4	5	NA
310443	Adapts life routine for optimal health	1	2	3	4	5	NA

Domain-Health Knowledge & Behavior (IV)   **Class**-Health Management (FF)   5th edition 2013

S

OUTCOME CONTENT REFERENCES:

Alm-Roijer, C., Stagmo, M., Uden, G., & Erhardt, L. (2004). Better knowledge improves adherence to lifestyle changes and medication in patients with coronary heart disease. *European Journal of Cardiovascular Nursing, 3*(4), 321–330.

Arnetz, J., Winblad, U., Hoglund, A., Lindahl, B., Spangberg, K., Wallentin, L., et al. (2010). Is patient involvement during hospitalization for acute myocardial infarction associated with post-discharge treatment outcome? *Health Expectations, 13*(3), 298–311.

Kang, Y., Yang, I., & Kim, N. (2010). Correlates of health behaviors in patients with coronary artery disease. *Asian Nursing Research, 4*(1), 45–55.

National Heart, Lung, and Blood Institute. (2011). Coronary artery disease. Retrieved from http://www.nhlbi.nih.gov/health/dci/Diseases/Cad/CAD_WhatIs.html

Pope, C. A., Muhlestein, J. B., May, H. T., Renlund, D. G., Anderson, J. L., & Horne, B. D. (2006). Ischemic heart disease events triggered by short-term exposure to fine particulate air pollution. *Circulation, 114*(23), 2443–2448.

Smeltzer, S., Bare, B., Hinkle, J., & Cheever, K. (2008). *Brunner and Suddarth's textbook of medical-surgical nursing* (11th ed., pp. 859–912). Philadelphia: Lippincott Williams & Wilkins.

Tokunaga-Nakawatase, Y., Taru, C., & Miyawaki, I. (2011). Development of an evaluation scale for self-management behavior related to physical activity of patients with coronary heart disease. *European Journal of Cardiovascular Nursing,* doi:10.1016/j.ejcnurse.2011.01.001.

Self-Management: Diabetes 1619

Definition: Personal actions to manage diabetes, its treatment, and to prevent complications

OUTCOME TARGET RATING: Maintain at_____ Increase to_____

OUTCOME OVERALL RATING	Never demonstrated 1	Rarely demonstrated 2	Sometimes demonstrated 3	Often demonstrated 4	Consistently demonstrated 5	
Indicators:						
161901 Accepts diagnosis	1	2	3	4	5	NA
161902 Seeks information about methods to prevent complications	1	2	3	4	5	NA
161903 Performs preventive foot care practices	1	2	3	4	5	NA
161904 Obtains dilated vision examination as recommended	1	2	3	4	5	NA
161905 Adjusts medication when acutely ill	1	2	3	4	5	NA
161906 Reports non-healing breaks in skin to primary care provider	1	2	3	4	5	NA
161907 Participates in health care decisions	1	2	3	4	5	NA
161908 Participates in prescribed educational program	1	2	3	4	5	NA
161909 Performs treatment regimen as prescribed	1	2	3	4	5	NA
161910 Performs correct procedure for blood glucose testing	1	2	3	4	5	NA
161911 Monitors blood glucose	1	2	3	4	5	NA
161912 Treats symptoms of hyperglycemia	1	2	3	4	5	NA
161913 Treats symptoms of hypoglycemia	1	2	3	4	5	NA
161914 Monitors frequency of hypoglycemia episodes	1	2	3	4	5	NA
161915 Reports symptoms of complications	1	2	3	4	5	NA
161916 Uses diary to monitor blood glucose level over time	1	2	3	4	5	NA
161917 Uses preventive measures to reduce risk for complications	1	2	3	4	5	NA
161941 Obtains health care if blood glucose levels fluctuate outside of recommendations	1	2	3	4	5	NA
161919 Monitors urinary glucose and ketones	1	2	3	4	5	NA
161920 Follows recommended diet	1	2	3	4	5	NA
161921 Follows recommended activity level	1	2	3	4	5	NA
161922 Monitors body weight	1	2	3	4	5	NA

Self-Management: Diabetes—*cont'd*

		Never demonstrated	Rarely demonstrated	Sometimes demonstrated	Often demonstrated	Consistently demonstrated	
161923	Uses effective weight control strategies	1	2	3	4	5	NA
161924	Maintains optimum weight	1	2	3	4	5	NA
161925	Follows recommendations for alcohol use	1	2	3	4	5	NA
161926	Participates in smoking cessation regimen	1	2	3	4	5	NA
161927	Participates in recommended exercise	1	2	3	4	5	NA
161928	Performs usual life routine	1	2	3	4	5	NA
161929	Uses correct procedure for insulin administration	1	2	3	4	5	NA
161930	Stores insulin correctly	1	2	3	4	5	NA
161931	Obtains required medication	1	2	3	4	5	NA
161932	Uses medication as prescribed	1	2	3	4	5	NA
161933	Monitors medication therapeutic effects	1	2	3	4	5	NA
161934	Rotates injection sites	1	2	3	4	5	NA
161935	Uses only non-prescription medication approved by health professional	1	2	3	4	5	NA
161945	Obtains influenza seasonal vaccine	1	2	3	4	5	NA
161946	Obtains pneumonia vaccine	1	2	3	4	5	NA
161937	Uses health care services congruent with needs	1	2	3	4	5	NA
161938	Reports need for financial assistance	1	2	3	4	5	NA
161939	Keeps appointments with health professional	1	2	3	4	5	NA
161940	Maintains plan for medical emergencies	1	2	3	4	5	NA
161943	Obtains preconception counseling	1	2	3	4	5	NA
161944	Monitors for signs and symptoms of depression	1	2	3	4	5	NA
161942	Adjusts life routine for optimal health	1	2	3	4	5	NA

Domain-Health Knowledge & Behavior (IV)   **Class**-Health Management (FF)   3rd edition 2004; revised 2008, 2013

OUTCOME CONTENT REFERENCES:

American Diabetes Association. (1998). Standards of medical care for patients with diabetes mellitus. *Diabetes Care, 21*(Suppl. 1), S23–S31.

American Diabetes Association. (1998). Testing of glycemia in diabetes. *Diabetes Care, 21*(Suppl. 1), S69–S71.

Cryer, P. E. (2001). Hypoglycemia risk reduction in Type I Diabetes. *Experimental & Clinical Endocrinology & Diabetes, 109*(Suppl. 2), S412–S423.

Dalewitz, J., Khan, N., & Hershey, C. O. (2000). Barriers to control blood glucose in diabetes mellitus. *American Journal of Medical Quality, 15*(1), 16–25.

Funnell, M. M., Hunt, C., Kulkarni, K., Rubin, R. R., & Yarborough, P. C. (Eds.). (1998). *A core curriculum for Association of Diabetes educators.* Chicago: American Association of Diabetes Educators.

Kelley, D. B. (Ed.). (1998). *Intensive diabetes management.* (2nd ed.). Alexandria, VA: American Diabetes Association.

Lebovitz, H. E. (Ed.). (1998). *Therapy for diabetes mellitus and related disorders* (3rd ed.). Alexandria, VA: American Diabetes Association.

Lewis, S. M., Collier, I. C., Heitkemper, M. M., & Dirksen, S. R. (2000). *Medical-surgical nursing: Assessment & management of clinical problems* (5th ed.). St. Louis: Mosby.

McCance, K. L., & Huether, S. E. (2002). *Pathophysiology: The biologic basis for disease in adults and children* (4th ed.). St. Louis: Mosby.

Miller, D. K., & Fain, J. A. (2006). Diabetes self-management education. *Nursing Clinics of North America, 41*(4), 655–666.

S

Self-Management: Dysrhythmia   3105

Definition: Personal actions to manage cardiac dysrhythmia, its treatment, and to prevent disease progression and complications

OUTCOME TARGET RATING: Maintain at_____ Increase to_____

		Never demonstrated	Rarely demonstrated	Sometimes demonstrated	Often demonstrated	Consistently demonstrated	
OUTCOME OVERALL RATING		1	2	3	4	5	
Indicators:							
310501	Accepts diagnosis	1	2	3	4	5	NA
310502	Seeks information about methods to manage dysrhythmia	1	2	3	4	5	NA
310503	Participates in health care decisions	1	2	3	4	5	NA
310504	Performs treatment regimen as prescribed	1	2	3	4	5	NA
310505	Monitors radial pulse rate and rhythm	1	2	3	4	5	NA
310506	Monitors for heart palpitations	1	2	3	4	5	NA
310507	Monitors blood pressure	1	2	3	4	5	NA
310508	Monitors factors that precede dysrhythmia onset	1	2	3	4	5	NA
310509	Monitors symptom persistence	1	2	3	4	5	NA
310510	Monitors symptom severity	1	2	3	4	5	NA
310511	Monitors symptom frequency	1	2	3	4	5	NA
310512	Reports significant change in radial pulse immediately	1	2	3	4	5	NA
310513	Reports redness or pain at site	1	2	3	4	5	NA
310514	Reports painful shocks	1	2	3	4	5	NA
310515	Reports increase in severity or frequency of dysrhythmia	1	2	3	4	5	NA
310516	Monitors effects of stimulants	1	2	3	4	5	NA
310517	Uses diary to monitor symptoms over time	1	2	3	4	5	NA
310518	Uses preventive measures to reduce episodes of dysrhythmia	1	2	3	4	5	NA
310519	Obtains health care when warning signs occur	1	2	3	4	5	NA
310520	Obtains required medication	1	2	3	4	5	NA
310521	Uses medication as prescribed	1	2	3	4	5	NA
310522	Follows schedule for taking medications	1	2	3	4	5	NA
310523	Monitors prescribed medication therapeutic effects	1	2	3	4	5	NA
310524	Monitors medication side effects	1	2	3	4	5	NA
310525	Uses only non-prescription medication approved by health professional	1	2	3	4	5	NA
310526	Uses anxiety reducing techniques	1	2	3	4	5	NA
310527	Performs usual life routine	1	2	3	4	5	NA
310528	Follows recommendations for alcohol use	1	2	3	4	5	NA
310529	Participates in smoking cessation regimen	1	2	3	4	5	NA
310530	Participates in physical activities that do not cause dysrhythmia	1	2	3	4	5	NA
310531	Follows recommendations for sexual activity	1	2	3	4	5	NA

S

Self-Management: Dysrhythmia—cont'd

		Never demonstrated	Rarely demonstrated	Sometimes demonstrated	Often demonstrated	Consistently demonstrated	
310532	Reports need for financial assistance	1	2	3	4	5	NA
310533	Keeps appointments with health professional	1	2	3	4	5	NA
310534	Maintains plan for medical emergencies	1	2	3	4	5	NA
310535	Follows recommendations for site care immediately post surgery	1	2	3	4	5	NA
310536	Wears loose-fitting clothes over implant site	1	2	3	4	5	NA
310537	Carries medical identification bracelet	1	2	3	4	5	NA
310538	Avoids contact activities that could cause trauma to site	1	2	3	4	5	NA
310539	Avoids devices that can disrupt pacemaker or defibrillator function	1	2	3	4	5	NA
310540	Follows manufacturer's instructions for device	1	2	3	4	5	NA
310541	Follows maintenance schedule for device	1	2	3	4	5	NA
310542	Notifies health professional of pacemaker or defibrillator prior to procedures	1	2	3	4	5	NA

Domain-Health Knowledge & Behavior (IV)   **Class**-Health Management (FF)   5th edition 2013

OUTCOME CONTENT REFERENCES:

National Heart, Lung, and Blood Institute. (2009). *Implantable cardioverter defibrillator*. Retrieved from http://www.nhlbi.nih.gov/health/dci/Diseases/icd/icd_whatis.html

National Heart, Lung, and Blood Institute. (2011). *Arrhythmia*. Retrieved from http://www.nhlbi.nih.gov/health/dci/Diseases/arr/arr_whatis.html

Xu, W., Sun, G., Lin, Z., Chen, M., Yang, B., Chen, H., et al. (2010). Knowledge, attitude, and behavior in patients with atrial fibrillation undergoing radiofrequency catheter ablation. *Journal of Interventional Cardiac Electrophysiology*, 28(3), 199–207.

Self-Management: Heart Failure

3106

Definition: Personal actions to manage heart failure, its treatment, and to prevent disease progression and complications

OUTCOME TARGET RATING: Maintain at_____   Increase to_____

		Never demonstrated	Rarely demonstrated	Sometimes demonstrated	Often demonstrated	Consistently demonstrated	
OUTCOME OVERALL RATING		1	2	3	4	5	
Indicators:							
310601	Accepts diagnosis	1	2	3	4	5	NA
310602	Seeks information about heart failure management	1	2	3	4	5	NA
310603	Participates in health care decisions	1	2	3	4	5	NA
310604	Obtains required laboratory tests	1	2	3	4	5	NA
310605	Monitors heart rate and rhythm	1	2	3	4	5	NA

Continued

S

Self-Management: Heart Failure—cont'd

		Never demonstrated	Rarely demonstrated	Sometimes demonstrated	Often demonstrated	Consistently demonstrated	
310606	Monitors respiratory rate	1	2	3	4	5	NA
310607	Monitors for shortness of breath	1	2	3	4	5	NA
310608	Monitors blood pressure	1	2	3	4	5	NA
310609	Monitors for edema	1	2	3	4	5	NA
310610	Monitors for complications of edema	1	2	3	4	5	NA
310611	Obtains assistance for an exacerbation	1	2	3	4	5	NA
310612	Performs treatment regimen as prescribed	1	2	3	4	5	NA
310613	Follows prescribed diet	1	2	3	4	5	NA
310614	Follows sodium intake recommendations	1	2	3	4	5	NA
310615	Follows fluid restrictions	1	2	3	4	5	NA
310616	Limits alcohol use	1	2	3	4	5	NA
310617	Eliminates tobacco use	1	2	3	4	5	NA
310618	Avoids smoke	1	2	3	4	5	NA
310619	Monitors body weight	1	2	3	4	5	NA
310620	Uses effective weight control strategies	1	2	3	4	5	NA
310621	Maintains optimum weight	1	2	3	4	5	NA
310622	Elevates legs when sitting	1	2	3	4	5	NA
310623	Applies elastic stockings correctly	1	2	3	4	5	NA
310624	Follows recommendations for physical activity	1	2	3	4	5	NA
310625	Uses energy conservation techniques	1	2	3	4	5	NA
310626	Balances activity and rest	1	2	3	4	5	NA
310627	Manages basic activities of daily living	1	2	3	4	5	NA
310628	Manages instrumental activities of daily living	1	2	3	4	5	NA
310629	Obtains influenza seasonal vaccine	1	2	3	4	5	NA
310630	Obtains pneumonia vaccine	1	2	3	4	5	NA
310631	Uses pulse oximetry monitor correctly	1	2	3	4	5	NA
310632	Uses oxygen correctly	1	2	3	4	5	NA
310633	Uses medication as prescribed	1	2	3	4	5	NA
310634	Monitors prescribed medication therapeutic effects	1	2	3	4	5	NA
310635	Monitors side effects of medication	1	2	3	4	5	NA
310636	Uses only non-prescription medication approved by health professional	1	2	3	4	5	NA
310637	Uses stress management strategies	1	2	3	4	5	NA
310638	Reports signs and symptoms of depression	1	2	3	4	5	NA
310639	Obtains assistance for depression	1	2	3	4	5	NA
310640	Obtains support from family	1	2	3	4	5	NA

S

Self-Management: Heart Failure—cont'd

		Never demonstrated	Rarely demonstrated	Sometimes demonstrated	Often demonstrated	Consistently demonstrated	
310641	Uses support group	1	2	3	4	5	NA
310642	Keeps appointments with health professional	1	2	3	4	5	NA
310643	Adjusts life routine for optimal health	1	2	3	4	5	NA

Domain-*Health Knowledge & Behavior (IV)*   **Class**-*Health Management (FF)*   *5th edition 2013*

OUTCOME CONTENT REFERENCES:

Chen, A., Yehle, K., Plake, K., Murawski, M., & Mason, H. (2011). Health literacy and self-care of patients with heart failure. *Journal of Cardiovascular Nursing*, 26(6), 446–451.

Jessup, M., Abraham, W., Casey, D., Feldman, A., Francis, G., Ganiats, T., et al. (2009). 2009 focused update: ACCF/AHA guidelines for the diagnosis and management of heart failure in adults: A report of the American College of Cardiology Foundation/American Heart Association Task Force on Practice Guidelines. *Journal of the American College of Cardiology*, 53(15), 1343–1382.

Lainscak, M., Blue, L., Clark, A. L., Dahlström, U., Dickstein, K., Ekman, I., et al. (2011). Self-care management of heart failure: Practical recommendations from the Patient Care Committee of the Heart Failure Association of the European Society of Cardiology. *European Journal of Heart Failure*, 13(2), 115–126.

Smeltzer, S., Bare, B., Hinkle, J., & Cheever, K. (2008). *Brunner and Suddarth's textbook of medical-surgical nursing* (11th ed., pp. 945–972). Philadelphia: Lippincott Williams & Wilkins.

Self-Management: Hypertension 3107

Definition: Personal actions to manage high blood pressure, its treatment, and to prevent complications

OUTCOME TARGET RATING: Maintain at_____   Increase to_____

		Never demonstrated	Rarely demonstrated	Sometimes demonstrated	Often demonstrated	Consistently demonstrated	
	OUTCOME OVERALL RATING	1	2	3	4	5	
Indicators:							
310701	Monitors blood pressure	1	2	3	4	5	NA
310702	Performs correct procedure for blood pressure measurement	1	2	3	4	5	NA
310703	Checks calibration of home blood pressure device	1	2	3	4	5	NA
310704	Maintains target blood pressure	1	2	3	4	5	NA
310705	Uses medication as prescribed	1	2	3	4	5	NA
310706	Monitors medication therapeutic effects	1	2	3	4	5	NA
310707	Monitors medication adverse effects	1	2	3	4	5	NA
310708	Monitors medication side effects	1	2	3	4	5	NA
310709	Uses only non-prescription medication approved by health professional	1	2	3	4	5	NA
310710	Participates in recommended exercises	1	2	3	4	5	NA
310711	Uses strategies for weight reduction	1	2	3	4	5	NA
310712	Maintains optimum body weight	1	2	3	4	5	NA
310713	Follows recommended diet	1	2	3	4	5	NA
310714	Limits sodium intake	1	2	3	4	5	NA
310715	Limits high calorie fluids	1	2	3	4	5	NA
310716	Limits high calorie snacks	1	2	3	4	5	NA

Continued

S

Self-Management: Hypertension—cont'd

		Never demonstrated	Rarely demonstrated	Sometimes demonstrated	Often demonstrated	Consistently demonstrated	
310717	Decreases food portions	1	2	3	4	5	NA
310718	Limits caffeine consumption	1	2	3	4	5	NA
310719	Uses stress management strategies	1	2	3	4	5	NA
310720	Uses relaxation techniques	1	2	3	4	5	NA
310721	Participates in smoking cessation regimen	1	2	3	4	5	NA
310722	Eliminates tobacco use	1	2	3	4	5	NA
310723	Follows recommendations for alcohol use	1	2	3	4	5	NA
310724	Uses strategies to maintain adequate sleep	1	2	3	4	5	NA
310725	Uses diary to monitor blood pressure over time	1	2	3	4	5	NA
310726	Monitors for complications of hypertension	1	2	3	4	5	NA
310727	Contacts health provider when not in target range	1	2	3	4	5	NA
310728	Keeps appointments with health professional	1	2	3	4	5	NA
310729	Uses support group	1	2	3	4	5	NA
310730	Uses reputable sources of information	1	2	3	4	5	NA
310731	Uses available community resources	1	2	3	4	5	NA
310732	Seeks financial resources	1	2	3	4	5	NA
310733	Uses social support	1	2	3	4	5	NA

Domain-Health Knowledge & Behavior (IV)   **Class**-Health Management (FF)   5th edition 2013

OUTCOME CONTENT REFERENCES:

Anglum, A. (2009). Primary care management of childhood adolescent hypertension. *Journal of the American Academy of Nurse Practitioners*, *21*(10), 529–534.

British Columbia: Ministry of Health Services. (2008). *Guidelines and protocols: Hypertension—Detection, diagnosis and management*. Retrieved from http://www.bcguidelines.ca/gpac/guideline_hypertension.html

Chummun, H. (2009). Hypertension—A contemporary approach to nursing care. *British Journal of Nursing, 18*(13), 784–789.

Clark, C., Smith, L., Taylor, R., & Campbell, J. (2010). Nurse led interventions to improve control of blood pressure in people with hypertension: Systematic review and meta-analysis. *BMJ, 341*(7771), 491.

DeSimone, M. E., & Crowe, A. (2009). Nonpharmacological approaches in the management of hypertension. *Journal of the American Academy of Nurse Practitioners, 21*(4), 189–196.

Good, L. B. (2010). Hypertension highlights: Blood pressure targets, global risk factors, and diabetes: The latest data are not encouraging. *Medscape Cardiology*. Retrieved February 7, 2011, from www.medscape.com/viewarticle/715584

National Heart, Lung, and Blood Institute (NHLBI). (2003). JNC 7 express: The seventh report of the Joint National Committee on Prevention, Detection, Evaluation, and Treatment of High Blood Pressure. Bethesda, MD: Author.

S

Self-Management: Kidney Disease

3108

Definition: Personal actions to manage kidney disease, its treatment, and to prevent disease progression and complications

OUTCOME TARGET RATING: Maintain at_____   Increase to_____

		Never demonstrated	Rarely demonstrated	Sometimes demonstrated	Often demonstrated	Consistently demonstrated	
OUTCOME OVERALL RATING		1	2	3	4	5	
Indicators:							
310801	Accepts diagnosis	1	2	3	4	5	NA
310802	Seeks information about methods to maintain kidney function	1	2	3	4	5	NA
310803	Participates in health care decisions	1	2	3	4	5	NA
310804	Performs treatment regimen as prescribed	1	2	3	4	5	NA
310805	Monitors symptom persistence	1	2	3	4	5	NA
310806	Monitors symptom severity	1	2	3	4	5	NA
310807	Monitors symptom frequency	1	2	3	4	5	NA
310808	Reports symptoms of worsening disease	1	2	3	4	5	NA
310809	Monitors weight	1	2	3	4	5	NA
310810	Monitors intake and output	1	2	3	4	5	NA
310811	Monitors blood pressure	1	2	3	4	5	NA
310812	Monitors for signs and symptoms of fluid excess	1	2	3	4	5	NA
310813	Monitors for edema	1	2	3	4	5	NA
310814	Monitors for disequilibrium syndrome	1	2	3	4	5	NA
310815	Reports shortness of breath	1	2	3	4	5	NA
310816	Obtains needed medication	1	2	3	4	5	NA
310817	Uses medication as prescribed	1	2	3	4	5	NA
310818	Uses only non-prescription medication approved by health professional	1	2	3	4	5	NA
310819	Reports side effects of medication	1	2	3	4	5	NA
310820	Monitors prescribed medication therapeutic effects	1	2	3	4	5	NA
310821	Follows recommended diet	1	2	3	4	5	NA
310822	Follows fluid restrictions	1	2	3	4	5	NA
310823	Uses strategies to control nausea	1	2	3	4	5	NA
310824	Uses strategies to prevent infection	1	2	3	4	5	NA
310825	Obtains influenza seasonal vaccine	1	2	3	4	5	NA
310826	Obtains pneumonia vaccine	1	2	3	4	5	NA
310827	Obtains adequate sleep	1	2	3	4	5	NA
310828	Balances activity and rest	1	2	3	4	5	NA
310829	Monitors for activity tolerance	1	2	3	4	5	NA
310830	Uses strategies to conserve energy	1	2	3	4	5	NA
310831	Uses strategies to relieve dry skin	1	2	3	4	5	NA
310832	Assesses fistula bruit daily	1	2	3	4	5	NA
310833	Performs correct procedure for care of dialysis access site	1	2	3	4	5	NA

Continued

S

Self-Management: Kidney Disease—*cont'd*

		Never demonstrated	Rarely demonstrated	Sometimes demonstrated	Often demonstrated	Consistently demonstrated	
310834	Monitors blood clotting time	1	2	3	4	5	NA
310835	Uses strategies to prevent bleeding	1	2	3	4	5	NA
310836	Uses precautions with shunt arm	1	2	3	4	5	NA
310837	Keeps appointments with health professional	1	2	3	4	5	NA
310838	Maintains plans for medical emergencies	1	2	3	4	5	NA
310839	Uses support group	1	2	3	4	5	NA
310840	Uses available community resources	1	2	3	4	5	NA
310841	Uses federal health care resources	1	2	3	4	5	NA

Domain-*Health Knowledge & Behavior (IV)*   **Class**-*Health Management (FF)*   5th edition 2013

OUTCOME CONTENT REFERENCES:
Ali, B., & Gray-Vickrey, P. (2011). Limiting the damage from acute kidney injury. *Nursing, 41*(3), 22–31.
Baird, M. S., & Bethel, S. (Eds.). (2005). *Manual of critical care nursing*. St. Louis: Elsevier Mosby.
LeMone, P., Burke, K., & Bauldoff, G. (2011). *Medical-surgical nursing: Critical thinking in patient care* (5th ed.). Upper Saddle River, NJ: Pearson Education.
National Kidney Foundation. (2002). KDOQI clinical practice guidelines for chronic kidney disease: Evaluation, classification, and stratification. *American Journal of Kidney Disease, 39*(Suppl. 2), S1–S266.
Tangri, N., Stevens, L., Griffith, J., Tighiouart, H., Djurdjev, O., Naimark, D., et al. (2011). A predictive model for progression of chronic kidney disease to kidney failure. *JAMA: The Journal of the American Medical Association, 305*(15), 1553–1559.

Self-Management: Lipid Disorder   3109

Definition: Personal actions to manage hyperlipidemia, its treatment, and to prevent complications

OUTCOME TARGET RATING: Maintain at_____   Increase to_____

		Never demonstrated	Rarely demonstrated	Sometimes demonstrated	Often demonstrated	Consistently demonstrated	
OUTCOME OVERALL RATING		1	2	3	4	5	
Indicators							
310901	Seeks information about methods to manage disorder	1	2	3	4	5	NA
310902	Participates in health care decisions	1	2	3	4	5	NA
310903	Discusses benefits of medication with health professional	1	2	3	4	5	NA
310904	Obtains required laboratory tests	1	2	3	4	5	NA
310905	Monitors lipid levels	1	2	3	4	5	NA
310906	Adapts life routine for optimal health	1	2	3	4	5	NA
310907	Uses effective weight control strategies	1	2	3	4	5	NA
310908	Maintains optimum weight	1	2	3	4	5	NA
310909	Follows recommended diet	1	2	3	4	5	NA
310910	Limits fat and cholesterol intake	1	2	3	4	5	NA
310911	Participates in recommended aerobic exercise	1	2	3	4	5	NA
310912	Follows recommendations for alcohol use	1	2	3	4	5	NA

S

Self-Management: Lipid Disorder—cont'd

		Never demonstrated	Rarely demonstrated	Sometimes demonstrated	Often demonstrated	Consistently demonstrated	
310913	Eliminates tobacco use	1	2	3	4	5	NA
310914	Avoids secondhand smoke	1	2	3	4	5	NA
310915	Uses medication as prescribed	1	2	3	4	5	NA
310916	Monitors medication therapeutic effects	1	2	3	4	5	NA
310917	Monitors medication adverse effects	1	2	3	4	5	NA
310918	Monitors medication side effects	1	2	3	4	5	NA
310919	Avoids stopping medication suddenly	1	2	3	4	5	NA
310920	Uses only non-prescription medication approved by health professional	1	2	3	4	5	NA
310921	Monitors changes in general health	1	2	3	4	5	NA
310922	Uses health care services congruent with needs	1	2	3	4	5	NA
310923	Keeps appointments with health professional	1	2	3	4	5	NA
310924	Uses significant others to support behavior changes	1	2	3	4	5	NA
310925	Uses available community resources	1	2	3	4	5	NA

Domain-*Health Knowledge & Behavior (IV)* **Class**-*Health Management (FF)* *5th edition 2013*

OUTCOME CONTENT REFERENCES:

Bertolotti, M. (2009). High protein intake reduces intrahepatocellular lipid deposition in humans. *The American Journal of Clinical Nutrition, 90*(4), 1002–1009.

Elpers, M. (2008). Common obstacles in lipid management. *Critical Care Nursing Clinics of North America, 20*(3), 287–295.

Gatti, A., Maranghi, M., Bacci, S., Carallo, C., Gnasso, A., Mandosi, E., et al. (2009). Poor glycemic control is an independent risk factor for low HDL cholesterol in patients with type 2 diabetes. *Diabetes Care, 32*(8), 1550–1552.

Iughetti, L., Bruzzi, P., & Predieri, B. (2010). Evaluation and management of hyperlipidemia in children and adolescents. *Current Opinion in Pediatrics, 22*(4), 485–493.

Lowenstein, C. J., & Cameron, S. J. (2010). High-density lipoprotein metabolism and endothelial function. *Current Opinion in Endocrinology, Diabetes & Obesity, 17*(2), 166–170.

S

Self-Management: Multiple Sclerosis 1631

Definition: Personal actions to manage multiple sclerosis and to prevent relapses and complications

OUTCOME TARGET RATING: Maintain at_____ Increase to_____

		Never demonstrated	Rarely demonstrated	Sometimes demonstrated	Often demonstrated	Consistently demonstrated	
OUTCOME OVERALL RATING		1	2	3	4	5	
Indicators:							
163101	Accepts diagnosis	1	2	3	4	5	NA
163102	Seeks information about methods to maintain musculoskeletal health	1	2	3	4	5	NA
163103	Participates in health care decisions	1	2	3	4	5	NA
163104	Performs treatment regimen as prescribed	1	2	3	4	5	NA
163105	Identifies symptoms of disease progression	1	2	3	4	5	NA
163106	Identifies ways to cope with functional changes	1	2	3	4	5	NA
163107	Monitors symptom onset	1	2	3	4	5	NA
163108	Monitors symptom persistence	1	2	3	4	5	NA
163109	Monitors symptom severity	1	2	3	4	5	NA
163110	Monitors symptom frequency	1	2	3	4	5	NA
163111	Reports symptoms of worsening disease	1	2	3	4	5	NA
163112	Reports signs and symptoms of mood changes	1	2	3	4	5	NA
163113	Obtains health care when warning signs occur	1	2	3	4	5	NA
163114	Uses symptom relief methods	1	2	3	4	5	NA
163115	Obtains required medication	1	2	3	4	5	NA
163116	Uses medication as prescribed	1	2	3	4	5	NA
163117	Monitors prescribed medication therapeutic effects	1	2	3	4	5	NA
163118	Monitors medication side effects	1	2	3	4	5	NA
163119	Uses correct procedure for injection administration	1	2	3	4	5	NA
163120	Rotates injection sites	1	2	3	4	5	NA
163121	Stores medication correctly	1	2	3	4	5	NA
163122	Uses preventive measures to reduce medication side effects	1	2	3	4	5	NA
163123	Follows recommended diet	1	2	3	4	5	NA
163124	Uses strategies to control fatigue	1	2	3	4	5	NA
163125	Balances activity and rest	1	2	3	4	5	NA
163126	Participates in recommended exercise	1	2	3	4	5	NA
163127	Uses energy conservation techniques	1	2	3	4	5	NA
163128	Adjusts life routine for optimal health	1	2	3	4	5	NA
163129	Uses stress management strategies	1	2	3	4	5	NA

S

Self-Management: Multiple Sclerosis—cont'd

		Never demonstrated	Rarely demonstrated	Sometimes demonstrated	Often demonstrated	Consistently demonstrated	
163130	Uses alterative treatment techniques	1	2	3	4	5	NA
163139	Obtains influenza seasonal vaccine	1	2	3	4	5	NA
163140	Obtains pneumonia vaccine	1	2	3	4	5	NA
163132	Obtains required liver function tests	1	2	3	4	5	NA
163133	Uses strategies to enhance bladder function	1	2	3	4	5	NA
163134	Uses strategies to enhance bowel function	1	2	3	4	5	NA
163135	Avoids extremes of temperatures	1	2	3	4	5	NA
163136	Keeps appointments with health professional	1	2	3	4	5	NA
163137	Maintains plan for medical emergencies	1	2	3	4	5	NA
163138	Uses available community resources	1	2	3	4	5	NA

Domain *Health Knowledge & Behavior (IV)* **Class**-*Health Management (FF)* *4th edition 2008; revised 2013*

OUTCOME CONTENT REFERENCES:

Denis, L., Namey, M., Costello, K., Frenette, J., Gagnon, N., Harris, C., et al. (2004). Long-term treatment optimization in individuals with multiple sclerosis using disease-modifying therapies: A nursing approach. *Journal of Neuroscience Nursing. 36*(1), 10–22.

Embrey, N., Lowndes, C., & Warner, R. (2003). Benchmarking best practice in relapse management of multiple sclerosis. *Nursing Standard. 17*(22), 38–42.

Jarrett, L. (2003). Attitudes to long-term care in multiple sclerosis. *Nursing Standard, 17*(17), 39–43.

National Multiple Sclerosis Society. http://www.nmss.org.

Ozuna, J. M. (2004). Nursing management: Chronic neurologic problems. In S. M. Lewis, M. M. Heitkemper, & S. R. Dirksen, (Eds.), *Medical-surgical nursing: Assessment and management of clinical problems* (6th ed., pp. 1549–1580). St. Louis: Mosby.

Ward, N., & Winters, S. (2003). Multiple sclerosis. Results of a fatigue management programme in multiple sclerosis. *British Journal of Nursing. 12*(18),1075–1080.

Self-Management: Osteoporosis 3110

Definition: Personal actions to manage osteoporosis, its treatment, and to prevent disease progression and complications

OUTCOME TARGET RATING: Maintain at_____ Increase to_____

S

		Never demonstrated	Rarely demonstrated	Sometimes demonstrated	Often demonstrated	Consistently demonstrated	
OUTCOME OVERALL RATING		1	2	3	4	5	
Indicators:							
311001	Uses medication as prescribed	1	2	3	4	5	NA
311002	Monitors medication side effects	1	2	3	4	5	NA
311003	Follows treatment regimen	1	2	3	4	5	NA
311004	Discusses non-prescription medication use with health provider	1	2	3	4	5	NA
311005	Follows recommendations for calcium supplements	1	2	3	4	5	NA
311006	Follows recommendations for vitamin D supplements	1	2	3	4	5	NA

Continued

Self-Management: Osteoporosis—*cont'd*

		Never demonstrated	Rarely demonstrated	Sometimes demonstrated	Often demonstrated	Consistently demonstrated	
311007	Follows recommended diet	1	2	3	4	5	NA
311008	Eliminates tobacco use	1	2	3	4	5	NA
311009	Follows recommendations for alcohol use	1	2	3	4	5	NA
311010	Participates in weight-bearing exercises	1	2	3	4	5	NA
311011	Participates in muscle-strengthening exercises	1	2	3	4	5	NA
311012	Uses fall prevention strategies	1	2	3	4	5	NA
311013	Reports a fall to health professional	1	2	3	4	5	NA
311014	Reports a fracture to health professional	1	2	3	4	5	NA
311015	Keeps appointment with health professional	1	2	3	4	5	NA
311016	Uses available community resources	1	2	3	4	5	NA

Domain-Health Knowledge & Behavior (IV) **Class**-Health Management (FF) 5th edition 2013

OUTCOME CONTENT REFERENCES:

Alexander, L., LaRosa, J. H., Bader, H., Garfield, S., & Alexander, W. J. (2010). *New dimensions in women's health* (5th ed.). Boston: Jones & Bartlett.

Bhalla, A. (2010). Management of osteoporosis in a pre-menopausal woman. *Best Practice & Research Clinical Rheumatology, 24*(3), 313–327.

Daly, R., Ahlborg, H., Ringsberg, K., Gardsell, P., Sembo, I., Karlsson, M. (2008). Association between changes in habitual physical activity and changes in bone density, muscle strength, and functional performance in elderly men and women. *Journal of the American Geriatrics Society, 56*(12), 2252–2260.

Gates, B., & Das, S. (2011). Management of osteoporosis in elderly men. *Maturitas, 69*(2), 113–119.

International Society for Clinical Densitometry (ISCD). (2004). *Pocket guide to bone mineral density testing.* Retrieved from http://www.iscd.org/visitors/pdfs/ISCD-CANADIANPanelOfficialPositions-BMDcard.pdf

Matheson, E., Mainous, A., & Carnemolla, M. (2009). The association between onion consumption and bone density in perimenopausal and postmenopausal non-Hispanic white women 50 years and older. *Menopause, 16*(4), 756–759.

Papaloannou, A., Morin, S., Cheung, A., Atkinson, S., Brown, J., Feldman, S., et al. (2010). 2010 clinical practice guidelines for the diagnosis and management of osteoporosis in Canada: A summary. *Canadian Medical Association Journal, 182*(17), 1864–1873.

Self-Management: Peripheral Artery Disease

3111

Definition: Personal actions to manage peripheral artery disease, its treatment, and to prevent disease progression

OUTCOME TARGET RATING: Maintain at_____ Increase to_____

		Never demonstrated	Rarely demonstrated	Sometimes demonstrated	Often demonstrated	Consistently demonstrated	
OUTCOME OVERALL RATING		1	2	3	4	5	
Indicators:							
311101	Monitors signs and symptoms of peripheral artery disease	1	2	3	4	5	NA
311102	Monitors signs and symptoms of claudication	1	2	3	4	5	NA
311103	Seeks information about peripheral artery disease	1	2	3	4	5	NA
311104	Seeks information about claudication	1	2	3	4	5	NA
311105	Uses medication as prescribed	1	2	3	4	5	NA

S

Self-Management: Peripheral Artery Disease—cont'd

		Never demonstrated	Rarely demonstrated	Sometimes demonstrated	Often demonstrated	Consistently demonstrated	
311106	Participates in prescribed exercise	1	2	3	4	5	NA
311107	Uses effective weight control strategies	1	2	3	4	5	NA
311108	Maintains optimum weight	1	2	3	4	5	NA
311109	Eliminates tobacco use	1	2	3	4	5	NA
311110	Monitors blood cholesterol	1	2	3	4	5	NA
311111	Limits fat and cholesterol intake	1	2	3	4	5	NA
311112	Monitors blood pressure	1	2	3	4	5	NA
311113	Monitors for symptoms of thromboembolism	1	2	3	4	5	NA
311114	Controls blood glucose level	1	2	3	4	5	NA
311115	Monitors for signs and symptoms of worsening peripheral artery disease	1	2	3	4	5	NA
311116	Monitors sensation in lower extremities	1	2	3	4	5	NA
311117	Monitors temperature in lower extremities	1	2	3	4	5	NA
311118	Monitors color in lower extremities	1	2	3	4	5	NA
311119	Monitors muscle strength in lower extremities	1	2	3	4	5	NA
311120	Monitors changes in general health	1	2	3	4	5	NA
311121	Discusses treatment options with health provider	1	2	3	4	5	NA
311122	Schedules appointments at regular intervals	1	2	3	4	5	NA
311123	Keeps appointments with health professional	1	2	3	4	5	NA
311124	Develops plan for medical emergencies	1	2	3	4	5	NA

***Domain**-Health Knowledge & Behavior (IV)*   ***Class**-Health Management (FF)*   *5th edition 2013*

OUTCOME CONTENT REFERENCES:

Hirsch, A., Haskal, Z., Hertzer, N., Bakal, C., Creager, M., Halperin, J., et al. (2006). ACC/AHA 2005 practice guidelines for the management of patients with peripheral artery disease (lower extremity, renal, mesenteric, and abdominal aortic. *Circulation, 113*(11), e463–e654.

Hirsch, A., Murphy, T., Lovell, M., Twillman, G., Treat-Jacobson, D., Harwood, E., et.al. (2007). Gaps in public knowledge of peripheral artery disease: The first national PAD public awareness survey. *Circulation, 116*(18), 2086–2094.

Lewis, S., Dirksen, S., Heitkemper, M., Bucher, L., & Camera, I. (2011). *Medical-surgical nursing: Assessment and management of clinical problems* (8th ed., pp. 874–880). St. Louis: Elsevier Mosby.

S

Sensory Function   2405

Definition: Ability to correctly sense skin stimulation, sounds, proprioception, taste and smell, and visual images

OUTCOME TARGET RATING: Maintain at_____ Increase to_____

	Severely compromised	Substantially compromised	Moderately compromised	Mildly compromised	Not compromised	
OUTCOME OVERALL RATING	1	2	3	4	5	
Indicators:						
240501 Skin stimulation perception	1	2	3	4	5	NA
240502 Hearing acuity	1	2	3	4	5	NA
240507 Head position perception	1	2	3	4	5	NA
240508 Body position perception	1	2	3	4	5	NA
240504 Odor discrimination	1	2	3	4	5	NA
240505 Taste discrimination	1	2	3	4	5	NA
240506 Visual acuity	1	2	3	4	5	NA

Domain-Physiologic Health (II)   **Class**-Sensory (Y)   *3rd edition 2004; revised 2008, 2013*

OUTCOME CONTENT REFERENCES:

Chung, J. (2006). Measuring sensory processing patterns of older Chinese people: Psychometric validation of the adult sensory profile. *Aging & Mental Health*, *10*(6), 648–655.

LeMone, P., Burke, K., & Bauldoff, G. (2011). *Medical-surgical nursing: Critical thinking in patient care* (5th ed., p. 258). Upper Saddle River, NJ: Pearson Education.

Smeltzer, S., Bare, B., Hinkle, J., & Cheever, K. (2010). *Brunner and Suddarth's textbook of medical-surgical nursing* (12th ed., pp. 325–326). Philadelphia: Lippincott Williams & Wilkins.

Swanson, E. A., & Drury, J. (2001). Sensory/perceptual alterations. In M. Maas, K. Buckwalter, M. Hardy, T. Tripp-Reimer, M. Titler, & J. Specht (Eds.), *Nursing care of older adults: Diagnoses, outcomes & interventions* (pp. 476–491). St. Louis: Mosby.

Sensory Function: Hearing   2401

Definition: Ability to correctly sense sounds

OUTCOME TARGET RATING: Maintain at_____ Increase to_____

	Severely compromised	Substantially compromised	Moderately compromised	Mildly compromised	Not compromised	
OUTCOME OVERALL RATING	1	2	3	4	5	
Indicators:						
240101 Auditory acuity (left)	1	2	3	4	5	NA
240102 Auditory acuity (right)	1	2	3	4	5	NA
240103 Air conduction of sound (left)	1	2	3	4	5	NA
240112 Air conduction of sound (right)	1	2	3	4	5	NA
240104 Bone conduction of sound (left)	1	2	3	4	5	NA
240113 Bone conduction of sound (right)	1	2	3	4	5	NA
240105 Ratio of air and bone conduction	1	2	3	4	5	NA
240107 Auditory discrimination of discrete sounds	1	2	3	4	5	NA
240108 Hears a whisper six inches from left ear (voice test)	1	2	3	4	5	NA
240114 Hears a whisper six inches from right ear (voice test)	1	2	3	4	5	NA
240109 Turns to sound	1	2	3	4	5	NA
240110 Responds to auditory stimuli	1	2	3	4	5	NA

S

Sensory Function: Hearing—cont'd

		Severe	Substantial	Moderate	Mild	None	
240106	Tinnitus (left)	1	2	3	4	5	NA
240115	Tinnitus (right)	1	2	3	4	5	NA
240116	Loss of high pitch tones	1	2	3	4	5	NA
240117	Loss of ability to distinguish conversation from background environmental noise	1	2	3	4	5	NA

Assistive device: Yes / No

Domain-*Physiologic Health (II)*   **Class**-*Sensory (Y)*   *2nd edition 2000; revised 2004, 2008, 2013*

OUTCOME CONTENT REFERENCES:

May, J. J. (2000). Occupational hearing loss. *American Journal of Industrial Medicine, 37*(1), 112–120.

LeMone, P., Burke, K., & Bauldoff, G. (2011). *Medical-surgical nursing: Critical thinking in patient care* (5th ed., p. 258). Upper Saddle River, NJ: Pearson Education.

Sataloff, J., & Roberts, B. (1999). Differential diagnosis in occupation hearing loss compensation claims. *Journal of Occupation Hearing Loss, 2*(4), 183–189.

Smeltzer, S., Bare, B., Hinkle, J., & Cheever, K. (2010). *Brunner and Suddarth's textbook of medical-surgical nursing* (12th ed., pp. 325–326). Philadelphia: Lippincott Williams & Wilkins.

Swanson, E. A., & Drury, J. (2001). Sensory/perceptual alterations. In M. Maas, K. Buckwalter, M. Hardy, T. Tripp-Reimer, M. Titler, & J. Specht (Eds.), *Nursing care of older adults: Diagnoses, outcomes & interventions* (pp. 476–491). St. Louis: Mosby.

Sensory Function: Proprioception   **2402**

Definition: Ability to correctly sense position and movement of the head and body

OUTCOME TARGET RATING: Maintain at_____   Increase to_____

		Severely compromised	Substantially compromised	Moderately compromised	Mildly compromised	Not compromised	
OUTCOME OVERALL RATING		1	2	3	4	5	
Indicators:							
240201	Head position discrimination	1	2	3	4	5	NA
240202	Head movement discrimination	1	2	3	4	5	NA
240214	Upper limb movement discrimination (right)	1	2	3	4	5	NA
240215	Upper limb movement discrimination (left)	1	2	3	4	5	NA
240216	Lower limb movement discrimination (right)	1	2	3	4	5	NA
240217	Lower limb movement discrimination (left)	1	2	3	4	5	NA
240218	Upper limb position discrimination (right)	1	2	3	4	5	NA
240219	Upper limb position discrimination (left)	1	2	3	4	5	NA
240220	Lower limb position discrimination (right)	1	2	3	4	5	NA
240221	Lower limb position discrimination (left)	1	2	3	4	5	NA
240212	Trunk movement discrimination	1	2	3	4	5	NA
240213	Trunk position discrimination	1	2	3	4	5	NA
240205	Sense of balance	1	2	3	4	5	NA

S

Continued

Sensory Function: Proprioception—cont'd

		Severe	Substantial	Moderate	Mild	None	
240206	Vertigo	1	2	3	4	5	NA
240207	Lightheadedness	1	2	3	4	5	NA
240208	Nystagmus	1	2	3	4	5	NA

Domain-Physiologic Health (II)   *Class*-Sensory (Y)   *2nd edition 2000; revised 2004, 2013*

OUTCOME CONTENT REFERENCES:
Boerboom, A., Huizinga, M., Kaan, W., Stewart, R., Hof, A., Bulstra, S., et al. (2008). Validation of a method to measure the proprioception of the knee. *Gait & Posture, 28*(4), 610–614.
LeMone, P., Burke, K., & Bauldoff, G. (2011). *Medical-surgical nursing: Critical thinking in patient care* (5th ed., p. 258). Upper Saddle River, NJ: Pearson Education.
Smeltzer, S., Bare, B., Hinkle, J., & Cheever, K. (2010). *Brunner and Suddarth's textbook of medical-surgical nursing* (12th ed., pp. 325–326). Philadelphia: Lippincott Williams & Wilkins.
Swanson, E. A., & Drury, J. (2001). Sensory/perceptual alterations. In M. Maas, K. Buckwalter, M. Hardy, T. Tripp-Reimer, M. Titler, & J. Specht (Eds.), *Nursing care of older adults: Diagnoses, outcomes & interventions* (pp. 476–491). St. Louis: Mosby.

Sensory Function: Tactile   2400

Definition: Ability to correctly sense stimulation of the skin

OUTCOME TARGET RATING: Maintain at_____   Increase to_____

		Severely compromised	Substantially compromised	Moderately compromised	Mildly compromised	Not compromised	
OUTCOME OVERALL RATING		1	2	3	4	5	
Indicators:							
240013	Sharp discrimination	1	2	3	4	5	NA
240014	Dull discrimination	1	2	3	4	5	NA
240002	2-point discrimination	1	2	3	4	5	NA
240003	Vibration discrimination	1	2	3	4	5	NA
240015	Temperature discrimination	1	2	3	4	5	NA
240016	Light touch	1	2	3	4	5	NA
240007	Noxious stimulus discrimination	1	2	3	4	5	NA
240017	Pressure discrimination	1	2	3	4	5	NA

		Severe	Substantial	Moderate	Mild	None	
240008	Paresthesia	1	2	3	4	5	NA
240009	Hyperparesthesia	1	2	3	4	5	NA
240011	Tingling	1	2	3	4	5	NA
240012	Loss of sensation	1	2	3	4	5	NA

Domain-Physiologic Health (II)   *Class*-Sensory (Y)   *2nd edition 2000; revised 2004, 2013*

OUTCOME CONTENT REFERENCES:
LeMone, P., Burke, K., & Bauldoff, G. (2011). *Medical-surgical nursing: Critical thinking in patient care* (5th ed., p. 258). Upper Saddle River, NJ: Pearson Education.
McPoil, T., & Cornwall, M. (2006). Plantar tactile sensory thresholds in healthy men and women. *Foot, 16*(4), 192–397.
Smeltzer, S., Bare, B., Hinkle, J., & Cheever, K. (2010). *Brunner and Suddarth's textbook of medical-surgical nursing* (12th ed., pp. 325–326). Philadelphia: Lippincott Williams & Wilkins.
Swanson, E. A., & Drury, J. (2001). Sensory/perceptual alterations. In M. Maas, K. Buckwalter, M. Hardy, T. Tripp-Reimer, M. Titler, & J. Specht (Eds.), *Nursing care of older adults: Diagnoses, outcomes & interventions* (pp. 476–491). St. Louis: Mosby.

S

Sensory Function: Taste & Smell   2403

Definition: Ability to correctly sense chemicals that are inhaled or dissolved in saliva

OUTCOME TARGET RATING: Maintain at_____   Increase to_____

	Severely compromised	Substantially compromised	Moderately compromised	Mildly compromised	Not compromised	
OUTCOME OVERALL RATING	1	2	3	4	5	
Indicators:						
240301 Odor discrimination	1	2	3	4	5	NA
240304 Sweet flavor recognition	1	2	3	4	5	NA
240305 Salty flavor recognition	1	2	3	4	5	NA
240306 Bitter flavor recognition	1	2	3	4	5	NA
240307 Sour flavor recognition	1	2	3	4	5	NA
	Severe	**Substantial**	**Moderate**	**Mild**	**None**	
240302 Odor distortion	1	2	3	4	5	NA
240308 Taste distortion	1	2	3	4	5	NA
240310 Metallic taste	**1**	**2**	**3**	**4**	**5**	NA
240311 Hemianosmia	1	2	3	4	5	NA

Domain-*Physiologic Health (II)*   **Class**-*Sensory (Y)*   *2nd edition 2000; revised 2004, 2013*

OUTCOME CONTENT REFERENCES:

LeMone, P., Burke, K., & Bauldoff, G. (2011). *Medical-surgical nursing: Critical thinking in patient care* (5th ed., p. 258). Upper Saddle River, NJ: Pearson Education.
Pelletier, C. (2002). Beyond the tongue map: Evaluating taste and smell perception. *ASHA Leader, 7*(19), 6–7, 20.
Smeltzer, S., Bare, B., Hinkle, J., & Cheever, K. (2010). *Brunner and Suddarth's textbook of medical-surgical nursing* (12th ed., pp. 325–326). Philadelphia: Lippincott Williams & Wilkins.
Swanson, E. A., & Drury, J. (2001). Sensory/perceptual alterations. In M. Maas, K. Buckwalter, M. Hardy, T. Tripp-Reimer, M. Titler, & J. Specht (Eds.), *Nursing care of older adults: Diagnoses, outcomes & interventions* (pp. 476–491). St. Louis: Mosby.

Sensory Function: Vision   2404

Definition: Ability to correctly sense visual images

OUTCOME TARGET RATING: Maintain at_____   Increase to_____

	Severely compromised	Substantially compromised	Moderately compromised	Mildly compromised	Not compromised	
OUTCOME OVERALL RATING	1	2	3	4	5	
Indicators:						
240401 Central visual acuity (left)	1	2	3	4	5	NA
240421 Central visual acuity (right)	1	2	3	4	5	NA
240402 Peripheral visual acuity (left)	1	2	3	4	5	NA
240422 Peripheral visual acuity (right)	1	2	3	4	5	NA
240403 Central visual fields (left)	1	2	3	4	5	NA
240423 Central visual fields (right)	1	2	3	4	5	NA
240404 Peripheral visual fields (left)	1	2	3	4	5	NA
240424 Peripheral visual fields (right)	1	2	3	4	5	NA
240416 Response to visual stimuli	1	2	3	4	5	NA
	Severe	**Substantial**	**Moderate**	**Mild**	**None**	
240405 Hemianopia	1	2	3	4	5	NA
240406 Floaters	1	2	3	4	5	NA

S

Continued

Sensory Function: Vision—cont'd

		Severe	Substantial	Moderate	Mild	None	
240407	Flashes of light	1	2	3	4	5	NA
240408	Halos around lights	1	2	3	4	5	NA
240409	Spiderwebs	1	2	3	4	5	NA
240410	Double vision	1	2	3	4	5	NA
240411	Blurred vision	1	2	3	4	5	NA
240412	Distorted vision	1	2	3	4	5	NA
240413	Color vision distortions	1	2	3	4	5	NA
240414	Night blindness	1	2	3	4	5	NA
240415	Day blindness	1	2	3	4	5	NA
240417	Headaches	1	2	3	4	5	NA
240418	Dizziness	1	2	3	4	5	NA
240419	Eye strain	1	2	3	4	5	NA

Assistive device: Yes / No

Domain-Physiologic Health (II)   *Class*-Sensory (Y)   2nd edition 2000; revised 2004, 2013

OUTCOME CONTENT REFERENCES:

LeMone, P., Burke, K., & Bauldoff, G. (2011). *Medical-surgical nursing: Critical thinking in patient care* (5th ed., p. 258). Upper Saddle River, NJ: Pearson Education.

Smeltzer, S., Bare, B., Hinkle, J., & Cheever, K. (2010). *Brunner and Suddarth's textbook of medical-surgical nursing* (12th ed., pp. 325–326). Philadelphia: Lippincott Williams & Wilkins.

Swanson, E. A., & Drury, J. (2001). Sensory/perceptual alterations. In M. Maas, K. Buckwalter, M. Hardy, T. Tripp-Reimer, M. Titler, & J. Specht (Eds.), *Nursing care of older adults: Diagnoses, outcomes & interventions* (pp. 476–491). St. Louis: Mosby.

Sexual Functioning

0119

Definition: Integration of physical, socioemotional, and intellectual aspects of sexual expression and performance

OUTCOME TARGET RATING: Maintain at_____   Increase to_____

		Never demonstrated	Rarely demonstrated	Sometimes demonstrated	Often demonstrated	Consistently demonstrated	
OUTCOME OVERALL RATING		1	2	3	4	5	
Indicators:							
011901	Attains sexual arousal	1	2	3	4	5	NA
011902	Sustains penile/clitoral erection through orgasm	1	2	3	4	5	NA
011903	Sustains arousal through orgasm	1	2	3	4	5	NA
011904	Uses assistive device as needed	1	2	3	4	5	NA
011905	Adapts sexual techniques as needed	1	2	3	4	5	NA
011906	Refrains from substance use that adversely affects sexual function	1	2	3	4	5	NA
011927	Uses hormone replacement therapy as needed	1	2	3	4	5	NA
011907	Expresses ability to perform sexually despite physical imperfections	1	2	3	4	5	NA
011908	Expresses comfort with sexual expression	1	2	3	4	5	NA

S

Sexual Functioning—cont'd

	Never demonstrated	Rarely demonstrated	Sometimes demonstrated	Often demonstrated	Consistently demonstrated	
011909 Expresses self-esteem	1	2	3	4	5	NA
011910 Expresses comfort with body	1	2	3	4	5	NA
011911 Expresses sexual interest	1	2	3	4	5	NA
011912 Expresses ability to be intimate	1	2	3	4	5	NA
011913 Expresses willingness to be sexual	1	2	3	4	5	NA
011914 Reports available consenting partner	1	2	3	4	5	NA
011915 Expresses respect for partner	1	2	3	4	5	NA
011916 Expresses acceptance of partner	1	2	3	4	5	NA
011917 Expresses knowledge of partner's sexual capabilities	1	2	3	4	5	NA
011918 Expresses knowledge of personal sexual capabilities	1	2	3	4	5	NA
011919 Expresses knowledge of partner's sexual needs	1	2	3	4	5	NA
011920 Expresses knowledge of personal sexual needs	1	2	3	4	5	NA
011921 Communicates comfortably with partner	1	2	3	4	5	NA
011922 Communicates sexual needs with partner	1	2	3	4	5	NA
011923 Communicates sexual preferences with partner	1	2	3	4	5	NA
011924 Performs sexually if environment conducive	1	2	3	4	5	NA
011925 Performs sexually without coercion of partner	1	2	3	4	5	NA

Domain-Functional Health (I)   **Class-**Growth & Development (B)   *2nd edition 2000; revised 2004, 2008*

OUTCOME CONTENT REFERENCES:

Arcos, B. (2004). Female sexual function and response. *Journal of the American Osteopathic Association, 104*(1), 516–520.

Clark, J. C. (1993). Psychosocial responses of the patient: Altered sexual health. In S. I. Groenwald, M. H. Frogge, M. Goodman, & C. H. Yarbro (Eds.), *Cancer nursing principles and practice* (3rd ed., pp. 449–467). Sudbury, MA: Jones and Bartlett.

Dobkin, P. L., & Bradley, I. (1991). Assessment of sexual dysfunction in oncology patients: Review, critique, and suggestions. *Journal of Psychosocial Oncology, 9*(1), 43–71.

Dunning, P. (1993). Sexuality and women with diabetes. *Patient Education and Counseling, 21*(1–2), 5–14.

Kralik, D., Koch, T., & Telford, K. (2001). Constructions of sexuality for midlife women living with chronic illness. *Journal of Advanced Nursing, 35*(2), 180–187.

Masters, W. H., & Johnson, V. E. (1970). *Human sexual inadequacy.* Boston: Little, Brown and Company.

Tuttle, B. (1984). Adult sexual response. In L. P. Higgins & J. W. Hawkins (Eds.), *Human sexuality across the life span: Implications for nursing practice* (pp. 39–76). Monterey, CA: Wadsworth Health Sciences.

S

Sexual Identity

1207

Definition: Acknowledgment and acceptance of own sexual identity

OUTCOME TARGET RATING: Maintain at_____   Increase to_____

OUTCOME OVERALL RATING		Never demonstrated	Rarely demonstrated	Sometimes demonstrated	Often demonstrated	Consistently demonstrated	
		1	2	3	4	5	
Indicators:							
120701	Affirms self as a sexual being	1	2	3	4	5	NA
120702	Exhibits clear sense of sexual orientation	1	2	3	4	5	NA
120703	Exhibits comfort with sexual orientation	1	2	3	4	5	NA
120704	Integrates sexual orientation into life roles	1	2	3	4	5	NA
120706	Uses healthy coping behaviors to resolve sexual identity issues	1	2	3	4	5	NA
120707	Challenges negative images of sexual self	1	2	3	4	5	NA
120708	Seeks social support	1	2	3	4	5	NA
120709	Reports healthy intimate relationships	1	2	3	4	5	NA
120710	Reports healthy sexual functioning	1	2	3	4	5	NA
120711	Describes risks associated with sexual activity	1	2	3	4	5	NA
120712	Uses precautions to minimize risks associated with sexual activity	1	2	3	4	5	NA
120713	Describes personal sexual value system	1	2	3	4	5	NA
120714	Sets personal sexual boundaries	1	2	3	4	5	NA

Domain-Psychosocial Health (III)   *Class*-Psychological Well-Being (M)   2nd edition 2000; revised 2004, 2008

OUTCOME CONTENT REFERENCES:

Bohan, J. S. (1996). *Psychology and sexual orientation: Coming to terms.* New York: Routledge.

Cain, R. (1991). Stigma management and gay identity development. *Social Work, 36*(1), 67–73.

Cass, V. E. (1984). Homosexual identity formation: Testing a theoretical model. *The Journal of Sex Research, 20*(2), 143–167.

Eliason, M. J. (1996). *Who cares? Institutional barriers to health care for lesbian, gay, and bisexual persons.* New York: NLN Press.

Kinsey, A. C., Pomeroy, W. B., & Martin, C. E. (1948). *Sexual behavior in the human male.* Philadelphia: W. B. Saunders.

Nass, G., Libby, R., & Fischer, M. P. (1989). *Sexual choices: An introduction to human sexuality* (2nd ed.). Monterey, CA: Wadsworth Health Sciences.

Troiden, R. R. (1989). The formation of homosexual identities. *Journal of Homosexuality, 17*(1–2), 43–73.

Tuttle, B. (1984). Adult sexual response. In L. P. Higgins & J. W. Hawkins (Eds.), *Human sexuality across the life span: Implications for nursing practice* (pp. 39–76). Monterey, CA: Wadsworth Health Sciences.

S

Shock Severity: Anaphylactic   0417

Definition: Severity of signs and symptoms of blood flow inadequate to perfuse tissues due to vasodilation and capillary permeability with a rapid-onset systemic hypersensitivity reaction

OUTCOME TARGET RATING: Maintain at_____   Increase to_____

OUTCOME OVERALL RATING	Severe 1	Substantial 2	Moderate 3	Mild 4	None 5	
Indicators:						
041701 Decreased systolic blood pressure	1	2	3	4	5	NA
041702 Decreased diastolic blood pressure	1	2	3	4	5	NA
041703 Increased heart rate	1	2	3	4	5	NA
041704 Arrhythmias	1	2	3	4	5	NA
041705 Rhinitis	1	2	3	4	5	NA
041706 Respiratory wheezes	1	2	3	4	5	NA
041707 Respiratory stridor	1	2	3	4	5	NA
041708 Laryngospasm	1	2	3	4	5	NA
041709 Bronchospasm	1	2	3	4	5	NA
041710 Dyspnea	1	2	3	4	5	NA
041711 Decrease in arterial oxygen	1	2	3	4	5	NA
041712 Warm, flushed skin	1	2	3	4	5	NA
041713 Edema of the lips, eyelids, tongue	1	2	3	4	5	NA
041714 Angioedema	1	2	3	4	5	NA
041715 Edema of hands and feet	1	2	3	4	5	NA
041716 Edema of genitalia	1	2	3	4	5	NA
041717 Parathesias	1	2	3	4	5	NA
041718 Pruritus	1	2	3	4	5	NA
041719 Abdominal cramps	1	2	3	4	5	NA
041720 Vomiting	1	2	3	4	5	NA
041721 Diarrhea	1	2	3	4	5	NA
041722 Decreased urine output	1	2	3	4	5	NA
041723 Panic	1	2	3	4	5	NA
041724 Decreased level of consciousness	1	2	3	4	5	NA

Domain-*Physiologic Health (II)*   **Class-***Cardiopulmonary (E)*   *5th edition 2013*

OUTCOME CONTENT REFERENCES:

LeMone, P., Burke, K., & Bauldoff, G. (2011). *Medical-surgical nursing: Critical thinking in patient care* (5th ed., pp. 260–261). Upper Saddle River, NJ: Pearson Education.

Limsuwan, T., & Demoly, P. (2010). Acute symptoms of drug hypersensitivity (urticaria, angioedema, anaphylaxis, anaphylactic shock). *Medical Clinics of North America*, 94(4), 691–710.

Smeltzer, S., Bare, B., Hinkle, J., & Cheever, K. (2010). *Brunner and Suddarth's textbook of medical-surgical nursing* (12th ed., pp. 327–332). Philadelphia: Lippincott Williams & Wilkins.

Wilmot, L. (2010). Shock: Early recognition and management. *Journal of Emergency Nursing*, 36(2), 134–139.

Younker, J., & Soar, J. (2010). Recognition and treatment of anaphylaxis. *Nursing in Critical Care*, 15(2), 94–98.

S

Shock Severity: Cardiogenic 0418

Definition: Severity of signs and symptoms of blood flow inadequate to perfuse tissues due to the heart's inability to contract and pump blood

OUTCOME TARGET RATING: Maintain at_____ Increase to_____

		Severe	Substantial	Moderate	Mild	None	
OUTCOME OVERALL RATING		1	2	3	4	5	
Indicators:							
041801	Decreased pulse pressure	1	2	3	4	5	NA
041802	Decreased mean arterial pressure	1	2	3	4	5	NA
041803	Decreased systolic blood pressure	1	2	3	4	5	NA
041804	Decreased diastolic blood pressure	1	2	3	4	5	NA
041805	Prolonged capillary refill time	1	2	3	4	5	NA
041806	Increased central venous pressure	1	2	3	4	5	NA
041807	Increased heart rate	1	2	3	4	5	NA
041808	Weak, thready pulse	1	2	3	4	5	NA
041809	Arrhythmias	1	2	3	4	5	NA
041810	Chest pain	1	2	3	4	5	NA
041811	Increased respiratory rate	1	2	3	4	5	NA
041812	Crackles in lungs	1	2	3	4	5	NA
041813	Pulmonary edema	1	2	3	4	5	NA
041814	Decreased arterial oxygen	1	2	3	4	5	NA
041815	Increased arterial carbon dioxide	1	2	3	4	5	NA
041816	Cyanosis	1	2	3	4	5	NA
041817	Cold, moist skin	1	2	3	4	5	NA
041818	Pallor	1	2	3	4	5	NA
041819	Distention of veins in neck	1	2	3	4	5	NA
041820	Dependent edema	1	2	3	4	5	NA
041821	Decreased urine output	1	2	3	4	5	NA
041822	Restlessness	1	2	3	4	5	NA
041823	Anxiety	1	2	3	4	5	NA
041824	Feelings of doom	1	2	3	4	5	NA
041825	Decreased level of consciousness	1	2	3	4	5	NA
041826	Metabolic acidosis	1	2	3	4	5	NA

Domain-*Physiologic Health (II)* **Class**-*Cardiopulmonary (E)* *5th edition 2013*

OUTCOME CONTENT REFERENCES:
Garretson, G., & Malberti, S. (2007). Understanding hypovolaemic, cardiogenic, and septic shock. *Nursing Standard, 21*(50), 46–55.
Josephson, L. (2008). Cardiogenic shock. *Dimensions of Critical Care Nursing, 27*(4), 160–170.
Kelley, D. (2005). Hypovolemic shock: An overview. *Critical Care Nursing Quarterly, 28*(1), 2–19.
LeMone, P., Burke, K., & Bauldoff, G. (2011). *Medical-surgical nursing: Critical thinking in patient care* (5th ed., p. 258). Upper Saddle River, NJ: Pearson Education.
Scottish Intercollegiate Guidelines Network (SIGN). (2007). Acute coronary Syndromes. A national clinical guideline. Edinburgh: Author.
Smeltzer, S., Bare, B., Hinkle, J., & Cheever, K. (2010). *Brunner and Suddarth's textbook of medical-surgical nursing* (12th ed., pp. 325–326). Philadelphia: Lippincott Williams & Wilkins.
Wilmot, L. (2010). Shock: Early recognition and management. *Journal of Emergency Nursing, 36*(2), 134–139.

S

Shock Severity: Hypovolemic

0419

Definition: Severity of signs and symptoms of blood flow inadequate to perfuse tissues due to a severe decrease in intravascular fluid volume

OUTCOME TARGET RATING: Maintain at_____ Increase to_____

OUTCOME OVERALL RATING	Severe 1	Substantial 2	Moderate 3	Mild 4	None 5	
Indicators:						
041901 Decreased pulse pressure	1	2	3	4	5	NA
041902 Decreased mean arterial pressure	1	2	3	4	5	NA
041903 Decreased systolic blood pressure	1	2	3	4	5	NA
041904 Decreased diastolic blood pressure	1	2	3	4	5	NA
041905 Delayed capillary refill	1	2	3	4	5	NA
041906 Increased heart rate	1	2	3	4	5	NA
041907 Weak, thready pulse	1	2	3	4	5	NA
041908 Arrhythmias	1	2	3	4	5	NA
041909 Chest pain	1	2	3	4	5	NA
041910 Increased respiratory rate	1	2	3	4	5	NA
041911 Shallow respirations	1	2	3	4	5	NA
041912 Crackles in lungs	1	2	3	4	5	NA
041913 Decreased arterial oxygen	1	2	3	4	5	NA
041914 Increased arterial carbon dioxide	1	2	3	4	5	NA
041915 Cold, clammy skin	1	2	3	4	5	NA
041916 Pallor	1	2	3	4	5	NA
041917 Prolonged coagulation times	1	2	3	4	5	NA
041918 Hypoactive bowel sounds	1	2	3	4	5	NA
041919 Thirst	1	2	3	4	5	NA
041920 Decreased urine output	1	2	3	4	5	NA
041921 Confusion	1	2	3	4	5	NA
041922 Lethargy	1	2	3	4	5	NA
041923 Decreased level of consciousness	1	2	3	4	5	NA
041924 Sluggish pupil response	1	2	3	4	5	NA
041925 Metabolic acidosis	1	2	3	4	5	NA
041926 Hyperkalemia	1	2	3	4	5	NA

Domain-Physiologic Health (II)   **Class**-Cardiopulmonary (E)   5th edition 2013

OUTCOME CONTENT REFERENCES:

Garretson, G., & Malberti, S. (2007). Understanding hypovolaemic, cardiogenic, and septic shock. *Nursing Standard, 21*(50), 46–55.

LeMone, P., Burke, K., & Bauldoff, G. (2011). *Medical-surgical nursing: Critical thinking in patient care* (5th ed., pp. 253–267). Upper Saddle River, NJ: Pearson Education.

Smeltzer, S., Bare, B., Hinkle, J., & Cheever, K. (2010). *Brunner and Suddarth's textbook of medical-surgical nursing* (12th ed., pp. 322–324). Philadelphia: Lippincott Williams & Wilkins.

Wilmot, L. (2010). Shock: Early recognition and management. *Journal of Emergency Nursing, 36*(2), 134–139.

S

Shock Severity: Neurogenic   0420

Definition: Severity of signs and symptoms of blood flow inadequate to perfuse tissues due to sustained vasodilation resulting from a parasympathetic-sympathetic system imbalance

OUTCOME TARGET RATING: Maintain at_____ Increase to_____

		Severe	Substantial	Moderate	Mild	None	
OUTCOME OVERALL RATING		1	2	3	4	5	
Indicators:							
042001	Bounding pulse	1	2	3	4	5	NA
042002	Decreased heart rate	1	2	3	4	5	NA
042003	Decreased systolic blood pressure	1	2	3	4	5	NA
042004	Decreased diastolic blood pressure	1	2	3	4	5	NA
042005	Increased heart rate	1	2	3	4	5	NA
042006	Arrhythmias	1	2	3	4	5	NA
042007	Respiratory changes	1	2	3	4	5	NA
042008	Decreased arterial oxygen	1	2	3	4	5	NA
042009	Warm, dry skin	1	2	3	4	5	NA
042010	Cold, clammy skin	1	2	3	4	5	NA
042011	Decreased body temperature	1	2	3	4	5	NA
042012	Decreased urine output	1	2	3	4	5	NA
042013	Hypoactive bowel sounds	1	2	3	4	5	NA
042014	Restlessness	1	2	3	4	5	NA
042015	Anxiety	1	2	3	4	5	NA
042016	Lethargy	1	2	3	4	5	NA
042017	Decreased level of consciousness	1	2	3	4	5	NA
042018	Dilated pupils	1	2	3	4	5	NA
042019	Sluggish pupil response	1	2	3	4	5	NA

Domain-Physiologic Health (II)   *Class*-Cardiopulmonary (E)   5th edition 2013

OUTCOME CONTENT REFERENCES:

Guly, H., Bouamra, O., & Lecky, F. (2007). The incidence of neurogenic shock in patients with isolated spinal cord injury in the emergency department. *Resuscitation, 76*(1), 57–62.

King, K., & Olson, D. (2007). What you should know about neurogenic shock. *American Nurse Today, 2*(2), 36, 38.

LeMone, P., Burke, K., & Bauldoff, G. (2011). *Medical-surgical nursing: Critical thinking in patient care* (5th ed., pp. 259–260). Upper Saddle River, NJ: Pearson Education.

Smeltzer, S., Bare, B., Hinkle, J., & Cheever, K. (2010). *Brunner and Suddarth's textbook of medical-surgical nursing* (12th ed., p. 328). Philadelphia: Lippincott Williams & Wilkins.

Wilmot, L. (2010). Shock: Early recognition and management. *Journal of Emergency Nursing, 36*(2), 134–139.

S

Shock Severity: Septic   0421

Definition: Severity of signs and symptoms of blood flow inadequate to perfuse tissues due to vasodilation resulting from the release of endotoxins with widespread infection

OUTCOME TARGET RATING: Maintain at_____ Increase to_____

		Severe	Substantial	Moderate	Mild	None	
OUTCOME OVERALL RATING		1	2	3	4	5	
Indicators:							
042101	Decreased systolic blood pressure	1	2	3	4	5	NA
042102	Decreased diastolic blood pressure	1	2	3	4	5	NA
042103	Increased heart rate	1	2	3	4	5	NA
042104	Weak, thready pulse	1	2	3	4	5	NA

Shock Severity: Septic—cont'd

		Severe	Substantial	Moderate	Mild	None	
042105	Arrhythmias	1	2	3	4	5	NA
042106	Increased respiratory rate	1	2	3	4	5	NA
042107	Increased depth of respirations	1	2	3	4	5	NA
042108	Shallow respirations	1	2	3	4	5	NA
042109	Dyspnea	1	2	3	4	5	NA
042110	Decreased arterial oxygen	1	2	3	4	5	NA
042111	Increased body temperature	1	2	3	4	5	NA
042112	Chills	1	2	3	4	5	NA
042113	Warm, flushed skin	1	2	3	4	5	NA
042114	Decreased body temperature	1	2	3	4	5	NA
042115	Cold, clammy skin	1	2	3	4	5	NA
042116	Pallor	1	2	3	4	5	NA
042117	Intravascular clotting	1	2	3	4	5	NA
042118	Decreased urine output	1	2	3	4	5	NA
042119	Hypoactive bowel sounds	1	2	3	4	5	NA
042120	Nausea	1	2	3	4	5	NA
042121	Vomiting	1	2	3	4	5	NA
042122	Diarrhea	1	2	3	4	5	NA
042123	Confusion	1	2	3	4	5	NA
042124	Lethargy	1	2	3	4	5	NA
042125	Decreased level of consciousness	1	2	3	4	5	NA
042126	Metabolic acidosis	1	2	3	4	5	NA

Domain-*Physiologic Health (II)*   **Class**-*Cardiopulmonary (E)*   *5th edition 2013*

OUTCOME CONTENT REFERENCES:

Chen, W., Kuo, C. (2007). Characteristics of heart rate variability can predict impending septic shock in emergency department patients with sepsis. *Academic Emergency Medicine, 14*(5), 392–397.

Garretson, G., & Malberti, S. (2007). Understanding hypovolaemic, cardiogenic, and septic shock. *Nursing Standard, 21*(50), 46–55.

LeMone, P., Burke, K., & Bauldoff, G. (2011). *Medical-surgical nursing: Critical thinking in patient care* (5th ed., p. 259). Upper Saddle River, NJ: Pearson Education.

Smeltzer, S., Bare, B., Hinkle, J., & Cheever, K. (2010). *Brunner and Suddarth's textbook of medical-surgical nursing* (12th ed., pp. 328–331). Philadelphia: Lippincott Williams & Wilkins.

Wilmot, L. (2010). Shock: Early recognition and management. *Journal of Emergency Nursing, 36*(2), 134–139.

Skeletal Function   0211

S

Definition: Ability of the bones to support the body and facilitate movement

OUTCOME TARGET RATING: Maintain at_____   Increase to_____

		Severely compromised	Substantially compromised	Moderately compromised	Mildly compromised	Not compromised	
OUTCOME OVERALL RATING		1	2	3	4	5	
Indicators:							
021101	Bone integrity	1	2	3	4	5	NA
021102	Bone density	1	2	3	4	5	NA
021103	Joint movement	1	2	3	4	5	NA
021104	Weight bearing	1	2	3	4	5	NA
021105	Skeletal alignment	1	2	3	4	5	NA
021106	Joint stability	1	2	3	4	5	NA

Domain-*Functional Health (I)*   **Class**-*Mobility (C)*   *2nd edition 2000; revised 2004*

OUTCOME CONTENT REFERENCES:
Bouxsein, M. L., Myers, E. R., & Hayes, W. C. (1996). Biomechanics of age-related fractures. In R. Marcus, D. Feldman, & J. Kelsey (Eds.), *Osteoporosis.* San Diego: Academic Press.
Carter, D. R., Van Der Meulen, M. C. H., & Beaupre, G. S. (1996). Skeletal development: Mechanical consequences of growth, aging, and disease. In R. Marcus, D. Feldman, & J. Kelsey (Eds.), *Osteoporosis.* San Diego: Academic Press.
Krahl, H., Michaelis, U., Peiper, H., Quack, G., & Montag, M. (1994) Stimulation of bone growth through sports: A radiologic investigation of the upper extremities in professional tennis players. *The American Journal of Sports Medicine, 22*(6), 751–758.
Melton, L. J. (1997). Epidemiology of spinal osteoporosis. *Spine, 22*(Suppl. 24), 2S–11S.
Mourad, L. (1991). *Orthopedic disorders.* St. Louis: Mosby.
Sowers, M. (1997). Clinical epidemiology and osteoporosis: Measures and their interpretation. *Epidemiology and Clinical Decision Making, 26*(1), 219–231.
Vincente-Rodriguez, G. (2006). How does exercise affect bone development during growth? *Sports Medicine, 36*(7), 561–569.

Sleep 0004

Definition: Natural periodic suspension of consciousness during which the body is restored

OUTCOME TARGET RATING: Maintain at_____   Increase to_____

OUTCOME OVERALL RATING	Severely compromised 1	Substantially compromised 2	Moderately compromised 3	Mildly compromised 4	Not compromised 5	
Indicators:						
000401 Hours of sleep	1	2	3	4	5	NA
000402 Observed hours of sleep	1	2	3	4	5	NA
000403 Sleep pattern	1	2	3	4	5	NA
000404 Sleep quality	1	2	3	4	5	NA
000405 Sleep efficiency	1	2	3	4	5	NA
000407 Sleep routine	1	2	3	4	5	NA
000418 Sleeps through the night consistently	1	2	3	4	5	NA
000408 Feelings of rejuvenation after sleep	1	2	3	4	5	NA
000410 Wakeful at appropriate times	1	2	3	4	5	NA
000419 Comfortable bed	1	2	3	4	5	NA
000420 Comfortable temperature in room	1	2	3	4	5	NA
000411 Electroencephalogram findings	1	2	3	4	5	NA
000412 Electromyogram findings	1	2	3	4	5	NA
000413 Electro-oculogram findings	1	2	3	4	5	NA

	Severe	Substantial	Moderate	Mild	None	
000421 Difficulty getting to sleep	1	2	3	4	5	NA
000406 Interrupted sleep	1	2	3	4	5	NA
000409 Inappropriate napping	1	2	3	4	5	NA
000416 Sleep apnea	1	2	3	4	5	NA
000417 Dependence on sleep aids	1	2	3	4	5	NA
000422 Nightmares	1	2	3	4	5	NA
000423 Nocturia	1	2	3	4	5	NA
000424 Snoring	1	2	3	4	5	NA
000425 Pain	1	2	3	4	5	NA

Domain-*Functional Health (I)*   **Class**-*Energy Maintenance (A)*   *1st edition 1997; revised 2000, 2004, 2008*

OUTCOME CONTENT REFERENCES:
+Buysse, D. J., Reynolds, C. F., III, Monk, T. H., Berman, S. R., & Kupfer, D. J. (1989). The Pittsburgh Sleep Quality Index: A new instrument for psychiatric practice and research. *Psychiatry Research, 28*(2), 193–213.
Ellis, J. R., & Nowlis, E. A. (1994). *Providing nursing care within the nursing process* (5th ed.). Philadelphia: J. B. Lippincott.
Hoch, C. C., Reynolds, C. F., & Houck, P. (1988). Sleep patterns in Alzheimer, depressed, and healthy elderly. *Western Journal of Nursing Research, 10*(3), 239–256.

S

Mead-Bennet, E. (1989). The relationship of primigravid sleep experience and select moods on the first postpartum day. *Journal of Obstetric, Gynecologic, & Neonatal Nursing*, 19(2), 146–152.

Noland, H., Price, J., Dake, J., & Telljohann, S. (2009). Adolescents' sleep behaviors and perceptions of sleep. *Journal of School Health*, 79(5), 224–230.

Paulsen, V. M., & Shaver, J. L. (1991). Stress, support, psychological states and sleep. *Social Science and Medicine*, 32(11), 1237–1243.

Porth, C. M. (2002). *Pathophysiology: Concepts of altered health states* (6th ed.). Philadelphia: Lippincott Williams & Wilkins.

Potter, P. A., & Perry, A. G. (2001). *Fundamentals of nursing* (5th ed.). St. Louis: Mosby.

Redeker, N. S. (2000). Sleep in acute care settings: An integrative review. *Journal of Nursing Scholarship*, 32(1), 31–38.

Schoenfelder, D. P., & Culp, K. R. (2001). Sleep pattern disturbance. In M. Maas, K. Buckwalter, M. Hardy, T. Tripp-Reimer, M. Titler, & J. Specht (Eds.), *Nursing care of older adults: Diagnoses, outcomes & interventions* (pp. 401–413). St. Louis: Mosby.

Topf, M. (1992). Effects of personal control over hospital noise on sleep. *Research in Nursing and Health*, 15(1), 19–28.

Topf, M., & Davis, J. E. (1993). Critical care unit noise and rapid eye movement sleep. *Heart & Lung*, 22(3), 252–258.

Williams, P. D., White, M. A., Powell, G. M., Alexander, D. J., & Conlon, M. (1988). Activity level in hospitalized children during sleep onset latency. *Computers in Nursing*, 6(2), 70–76.

Smoking Cessation Behavior   1625

Definition: Personal actions to eliminate tobacco use

OUTCOME TARGET RATING: Maintain at_____   Increase to_____

		Never demonstrated	Rarely demonstrated	Sometimes demonstrated	Often demonstrated	Consistently demonstrated	
OUTCOME OVERALL RATING		1	2	3	4	5	
Indicators:							
162501	Expresses willingness to stop smoking	1	2	3	4	5	NA
162502	Expresses belief in the ability to stop smoking	1	2	3	4	5	NA
162503	Identifies benefits of smoking cessation	1	2	3	4	5	NA
162504	Identifies negative consequences of tobacco use	1	2	3	4	5	NA
162505	Develops effective strategies to eliminate tobacco use	1	2	3	4	5	NA
162506	Identifies barriers to tobacco elimination	1	2	3	4	5	NA
162507	Adjusts tobacco elimination strategies as needed	1	2	3	4	5	NA
162508	Commits to tobacco elimination strategies	1	2	3	4	5	NA
162509	Follows selected tobacco elimination strategies	1	2	3	4	5	NA
162510	Participates in screening for associated health problems	1	2	3	4	5	NA
162511	Uses strategies to cope with withdrawal symptoms	1	2	3	4	5	NA
162512	Uses behavior modification strategies	1	2	3	4	5	NA
162513	Uses effective coping strategies	1	2	3	4	5	NA
162514	Obtains assistance from health professional	1	2	3	4	5	NA
162515	Uses personal support system	1	2	3	4	5	NA
162516	Uses reputable sources of information	1	2	3	4	5	NA
162517	Uses nicotine replacement therapy	1	2	3	4	5	NA
162518	Uses alternative therapies	1	2	3	4	5	NA

Continued

S

Smoking Cessation Behavior—cont'd

		Never demonstrated	Rarely demonstrated	Sometimes demonstrated	Often demonstrated	Consistently demonstrated	
162519	Identifies emotional states that affect tobacco use	1	2	3	4	5	NA
162520	Adjusts lifestyle to promote tobacco elimination	1	2	3	4	5	NA
162521	Uses prescribed medication as recommended	1	2	3	4	5	NA
162522	Uses non-prescription medication as recommended	1	2	3	4	5	NA
162523	Uses available support groups	1	2	3	4	5	NA
162524	Uses available community resources	1	2	3	4	5	NA
162525	Participates in counseling	1	2	3	4	5	NA
162526	Participates in telephone counseling	1	2	3	4	5	NA
162527	Monitors for signs of depression	1	2	3	4	5	NA
162528	Eliminates tobacco use	1	2	3	4	5	NA
162529	Commits to tobacco abstinence	1	2	3	4	5	NA

Domain-Health Knowledge & Behavior (IV)   *Class*-Health Behavior (Q)   4th edition 2008

OUTCOME CONTENT REFERENCES:

American Cancer Society. (2006). *Guide to quitting smoking.* Retrieved February 20, 2007, from http://www.cancer.org/docroot/PED/content/PED_10_13X_Guide_for_Quitting_Smoking.asp

Anderson, N. R. (2006). The role of the home healthcare nurse in smoking cessation: Guidelines for successful intervention. *Home Healthcare Nurse, 24*(7), 424–431.

Giarelli, E. (2006). Smoking cessation for women: Evidence of the effectiveness of nursing interventions. *Clinical Journal of Oncology Nursing, 10*(5), 667–671.

Higgins, S. T., Heil, S. H., Dumeer, A. M., Thomas, C. S., Solomon, L. J., & Bernstein, I. M. (2006). Smoking status in the initial weeks of quitting as a predictor of smoking-cessation outcomes in pregnant women. *Drug and Alcohol Dependence, 85*(2), 138–141.

Kassel, J. D., & Yates, M. (2002). Is there a role for assessment in smoking cessation treatment? *Behaviour Research and Therapy, 40*(12), 1457–1470.

McEwen, A., Hajek, P., McRobbie, H., & West, R. (2006). *Manual of smoking cessation: A guide for counselors and practitioners.* Malden, MA: Blackwell.

Molyneux, A., Lewis, S., Coleman, T., McNeill, A., Godfrey, C., Madeley, R., et al. (2006). Designing smoking cessation services for school-age smokers: A survey and qualitative study. *Nicotine & Tobacco Research, 8*(4), 539–546.

Price, J. H., Jordan, T. R., & Dake, J. A. (2006). Perceptions and use of smoking cessation in nurse-midwives practice. *Journal of Midwifery & Women's Health, 51*(3), 208–215.

Scheibmeir, M. S., & O'Connell, K. A. (2002). Promoting smoking cessation in adults. *Nursing Clinics of North America, 37*(2), 331–340.

Schofield, I. (2006). Supporting older people to quit smoking. *Nursing Older People, 18*(6), 29–33.

S

Social Anxiety Level   1216

Definition: Severity of irrational avoidance, apprehension, and distress in anticipation of or during social situations

OUTCOME TARGET RATING: Maintain at_____ Increase to_____

	Severe	Substantial	Moderate	Mild	None	
OUTCOME OVERALL RATING	1	2	3	4	5	
Indicators:						
121601 Avoidance of social situations	1	2	3	4	5	NA
121602 Avoidance of unfamiliar people	1	2	3	4	5	NA
121603 Avoidance of leaving home	1	2	3	4	5	NA
121604 Anxious anticipation of social situations	1	2	3	4	5	NA
121605 Anxious anticipation of encountering unfamiliar people	1	2	3	4	5	NA
121606 Activation of sympathetic nervous system responses	1	2	3	4	5	NA
121607 Negative self-perceptions of social skills	1	2	3	4	5	NA
121608 Negative self-perceptions of acceptance by others	1	2	3	4	5	NA
121609 Fear of scrutiny by others	1	2	3	4	5	NA
121610 Fear of interacting with members of the opposite sex	1	2	3	4	5	NA
121611 Fear of interacting with superiors	1	2	3	4	5	NA
121612 Discomfort during social encounters	1	2	3	4	5	NA
121613 Discomfort with changing routine	1	2	3	4	5	NA
121614 Concern about judgment of others after social encounters	1	2	3	4	5	NA
121615 Panic symptoms in social situations	1	2	3	4	5	NA
121616 Interference with role functioning	1	2	3	4	5	NA
121617 Interference with relationships	1	2	3	4	5	NA

Domain-Psychosocial Health (III)   *Class*-Psychological Well-Being (M)   5th edition 2013

OUTCOME CONTENT REFERENCES

Alfano, C. A., Pina, A. A., Villalta, I. K., Beidel, D. C., Ammerman, R. T., & Crosby, L. E. (2009). Mediators and moderators of outcome in the behavioral treatment of childhood social phobia. *Journal of the American Academy of Child and Adolescent Psychiatry, 48*(9), 945–953.

American Psychiatric Association. (2000). *Diagnostic and statistical manual of mental disorders* (4th ed., text revision) Washington, DC: Author.

Borge, F., Hoffart, A., & Sexton, H. (2010). Predictors of outcome in residential cognitive and interpersonal treatment for social phobia: Do cognitive and social dysfunction moderate treatment outcome? *Journal of Behavior Therapy and Experimental Psychiatry, 41*(3), 212–219.

Kneisl, C. R., Wilson, H. S., & Trigoboff, E. (2004). *Contemporary psychiatric-mental health nursing.* Upper Saddle River, NJ: Prentice Hall.

Mohr, W. K. (2006). *Psychiatric-mental health nursing* (6th ed.). Philadelphia: Lippincott, Williams, & Wilkins.

Stuart, G. W. (2009). *Principles and practice of psychiatric nursing* (9th ed.). St. Louis: Elsevier Mosby.

S

Social Interaction Skills 1502

Definition: Personal behaviors that promote effective relationships

OUTCOME TARGET RATING: Maintain at_____   Increase to_____

		Never demonstrated	Rarely demonstrated	Sometimes demonstrated	Often demonstrated	Consistently demonstrated	
OUTCOME OVERALL RATING		1	2	3	4	5	
Indicators:							
150201	Uses disclosure as appropriate	1	2	3	4	5	NA
150202	Exhibits receptiveness	1	2	3	4	5	NA
150203	Cooperates with others	1	2	3	4	5	NA
150204	Exhibits sensitivity to others	1	2	3	4	5	NA
150205	Uses assertive behaviors as appropriate	1	2	3	4	5	NA
150206	Uses confrontation as appropriate	1	2	3	4	5	NA
150207	Exhibits consideration	1	2	3	4	5	NA
150208	Exhibits genuineness	1	2	3	4	5	NA
150209	Exhibits warmth	1	2	3	4	5	NA
150210	Exhibits poise	1	2	3	4	5	NA
150211	Appears relaxed	1	2	3	4	5	NA
150212	Engages others	1	2	3	4	5	NA
150213	Exhibits trust	1	2	3	4	5	NA
150214	Uses compromise as appropriate	1	2	3	4	5	NA
150216	Uses conflict resolution strategies	1	2	3	4	5	NA

Domain-*Psychosocial Health (III)*   **Class**-*Social Interaction (P)*   *1st edition 1997; revised 2004*

OUTCOME CONTENT REFERENCES:

Cutting, A. L., & Dunn, J. (2006). Conversations with siblings and with friends: Links between relationship quality and social understanding. *British Journal of Developmental Psychology, 24*(1), 73–87.

Erickson, D. H., Beiser, M., Iacono, W. G., Fleming, J. A. E., & Lin, T. (1989). The role of social relationships in the course of first-episode schizophrenia and affective psychosis. *American Journal of Psychiatry, 146*(11), 1456–1461.

Gotcher, J. M. (1992). Interpersonal communication and psychosocial adjustment. *Journal of Psychosocial Oncology, 10*(3), 21–39.

Heltsley, M. E., & Powers, R. C. (1975). Social interaction and perceived adequacy of interaction of the rural aged. *The Gerontologist, 15*(6), 533–536.

Levin, J., & Levin, W. C. (1981). Willingness to interact with an old person. *Research on Aging, 3*(2), 211–217.

Nussbaum, J. F. (1983). Relational closeness of elderly interaction: Implications for life satisfaction. *Western Journal of Speech Communication, 47*(3), 229–243.

+Ruehlman, L. S., & Karoly, P. (1991). With a little flak from my friends: Development and preliminary validation of the Test of Negative Social Exchange (TENSE). *Psychological Assessment: A Journal of Consulting and Clinical Psychology, 3*(1), 97–104.

Richter, G., & Richter, J. (1989). Social relationships reflected by depressive inpatients. *Acta Psychiatrica Scandinavica, 80*(6), 573–578.

Sheppard, M. (1993). Client satisfaction, extended intervention and interpersonal skills in community mental health. *Journal of Advanced Nursing, 18*(2), 246–259.

Waterman, J. D., Blegen, M., Clinton, P., & Specht, J. P. (2001). Social isolation. In M. Maas, K. Buckwalter, M. Hardy, T. Tripp-Reimer, M. Titler, & J. Specht (Eds.), *Nursing care of older adults: Diagnoses, outcomes & interventions* (pp. 651–663). St. Louis: Mosby.

Webb, L., Delaney, J. J., & Young, L. R. (1989). Age, interpersonal attraction, and social interaction. *Research on Aging, 11*(1), 107–123.

S

Social Involvement   1503

Definition: Social interactions with persons, groups, or organizations

OUTCOME TARGET RATING: Maintain at_____ Increase to_____

OUTCOME OVERALL RATING		Never demonstrated 1	Rarely demonstrated 2	Sometimes demonstrated 3	Often demonstrated 4	Consistently demonstrated 5	
Indicators:							
150301	Interacts with close friends	1	2	3	4	5	NA
150302	Interacts with neighbors	1	2	3	4	5	NA
150303	Interacts with family members	1	2	3	4	5	NA
150304	Interacts with members of work group(s)	1	2	3	4	5	NA
150305	Participates as member of church	1	2	3	4	5	NA
150306	Participates in active church work	1	2	3	4	5	NA
150307	Participates in organized activity	1	2	3	4	5	NA
150308	Participates as officer in organization	1	2	3	4	5	NA
150309	Participates as a volunteer	1	2	3	4	5	NA
150311	Participates in leisure activities with others	1	2	3	4	5	NA
150313	Participates in team sports	1	2	3	4	5	NA

Domain-*Psychosocial Health (III)*   **Class**-*Social Interaction (P)*   *1st edition 1997; revised 2004*

OUTCOME CONTENT REFERENCES:

Cutting, A. L., & Dunn, J. (2006). Conversations with siblings and with friends: Links between relationship quality and social understanding. *British Journal of Developmental Psychology, 24*(1), 73–87.

Erickson, D. H., Beiser, M., Iacono, W. G., Fleming, J. A. E., & Lin, T. (1989). The role of social relationships in the course of first-episode schizophrenia and affective psychosis. *American Journal of Psychiatry, 146*(11), 1456–1461.

Gotcher, J. M. (1992). Interpersonal communication and psychosocial adjustment. *Journal of Psychosocial Oncology, 10*(3), 21–39.

Heltsley, M. E., & Powers, R. C. (1975). Social interaction and perceived adequacy of interaction of the rural aged. *The Gerontologist, 15*(6), 533–536.

Jylha, M., & Aro, S. (1989). Social ties and survival among the elderly in Tampere, Finland. *International Journal of Epidemiology, 18*(1) 158–164.

Levin, J., & Levin, W. C. (1981). Willingness to interact with an old person. *Research on Aging, 3*(2), 211–217.

Nussbaum, J. F. (1983). Relational closeness of elderly interaction: Implications for life satisfaction. *Western Journal of Speech Communication, 47*(3), 229–243.

Richter, G., & Richter, J. (1989). Social relationships reflected by depressive inpatients. *Acta Psychiatrica Scandinavica, 80*(6), 573–578.

Rohrer, J. E., Arif, A. A., Pierce, J. R., Jr., & Blackburn, C. (2004). Unsafe neighborhoods, social group activity, and self-rated health. *Journal of Public Health Management, 10*(2), 124–129.

Sheppard, M. (1993). Client satisfaction, extended intervention and interpersonal skills in community mental health. *Journal of Advanced Nursing, 18*(2), 246–259.

Waterman, J. D., Blegen, M., Clinton, P., & Specht, J. P. (2001). Social isolation. In M. Maas, K. Buckwalter, M. Hardy, T. Tripp-Reimer, M. Titler, & J. Specht (Eds.), *Nursing care of older adults: Diagnoses, outcomes & interventions* (pp. 651–663). St. Louis: Mosby.

Webb, L., Delaney, J. J., & Young, L. R. (1989). Age, interpersonal attraction, and social interaction. *Research on Aging, 11*(1), 107–123.

S

Social Support 1504

Definition: Reliable assistance from others

OUTCOME TARGET RATING: Maintain at_____ Increase to_____

		Not adequate	Slightly adequate	Moderately adequate	Substantially adequate	Totally adequate	
OUTCOME OVERALL RATING		1	2	3	4	5	
Indicators:							
150408	Willingness to call on others for assistance	1	2	3	4	5	NA
150401	Money available from others when needed	1	2	3	4	5	NA
150412	Assistance offered by others	1	2	3	4	5	NA
150402	Time provided by others	1	2	3	4	5	NA
150403	Labor provided by others	1	2	3	4	5	NA
150404	Information provided by others	1	2	3	4	5	NA
150405	Emotional assistance provided by others	1	2	3	4	5	NA
150406	Confidant relationship(s)	1	2	3	4	5	NA
150407	Persons who can help as needed	1	2	3	4	5	NA
150409	Assistive social network	1	2	3	4	5	NA
150410	Supportive social contacts	1	2	3	4	5	NA
150411	Stable social network	1	2	3	4	5	NA

Domain-*Psychosocial Health (III)*   **Class**-*Social Interaction (P)*   *1st edition 1997; revised 2004, 2008*

OUTCOME CONTENT REFERENCES:

Akister, J., & Johnson, K. (2002). Parenting issues that may be addressed through a confidential helpline. *Health & Social Care in the Community, 10*(2), 106–111.

Bisconti, T. L., Bergeman, C. S., & Boker, S. M. (2006). Social support as a predictor of variability: An examination of the adjustment trajectories of recent widows. *Psychology and Aging, 21*(3), 590–599.

Dimond, M., & Jones, S. L. (1983). Social support: A review and theoretical integration. In P. L. Chinn (Ed.), *Advances in nursing theory development* (pp. 235–249). Rockville, MD: Aspen.

Gleeson-Kreig, J., Bernal, H., & Woolley, S. (2002). The role of social support in the self-management of diabetes mellitus among a Hispanic population. *Public Health Nursing, 19*(3), 215–222.

Hutchison, C. (1999). Social support: Factors to consider when designing studies that measure social support. *Journal of Advanced Nursing, 29*(6), 1520–1526.

Martire, L. M., Schulz, R., Mittelmark, M. B., & Newsom, J. T. (1999). Stability and change in older adults' social contact and social support: The cardiovascular health study. *Journals of Gerontology Series B-Psychological Sciences & Social Sciences, 54*(5), S302–311.

+Sarason, I. G., Sarason, B. R., Shearin, E. N., & Pierce, G. R. (1987). A brief measure of social support: Practical and theoretical implications. *Journal of Social and Personal Relationships, 4*(4), 497–510.

Tilden, V. P. (1985). Issues of conceptualization and measurement of social support in the construction of nursing theory. *Research in Nursing and Health, 8*(2), 199–206.

Travis, S., & Hunt, P. (2001). Supportive and palliative care networks: A new model for integrated care. *International Journal of Palliative Nursing, 7*(10), 501–504.

van Tilburg, T. (1998). Losing and gaining in old age: Changes in personal network size and social support in a four-year longitudinal study. *Journals of Gerontology Series B-Psychological Sciences & Social Sciences, 53*(6), S313–S323.

Warren, B. J. (1997). Depression, stressful life events, social support, and self-esteem in middle class African American women. *Archives of Psychiatric Nursing, 11*(3), 107–117.

Waterman, J. D., Blegen, M., Clinton, P., & Specht, J. P. (2001). Social isolation. In M. Maas, K. Buckwalter, M. Hardy, T. Tripp-Reimer, M. Titler, & J. Specht (Eds.), *Nursing care of older adults: Diagnoses, outcomes & interventions* (pp. 651–663). St. Louis: Mosby.

Wellisch, D., Kagawa-Singer, M., Reid, S. L., & Lin, Y., Nishikawa-Lee, S., & Wellisch, M. (1999). An exploratory study of social support: A cross-cultural comparison of Chinese, Japanese, and Anglo-American breast cancer patients. *Psycho-Oncology, 8*(3), 207–219.

Spiritual Health   2001

Definition: Connectedness with self, others, higher power, all life, nature, and the universe that transcends and empowers the self

OUTCOME TARGET RATING: Maintain at_____   Increase to_____

OUTCOME OVERALL RATING	Severely compromised 1	Substantially compromised 2	Moderately compromised 3	Mildly compromised 4	Not compromised 5	
Indicators:						
200101 Quality of faith	1	2	3	4	5	NA
200102 Quality of hope	1	2	3	4	5	NA
200103 Meaning and purpose in life	1	2	3	4	5	NA
200104 Achievement of spiritual world view	1	2	3	4	5	NA
200105 Feelings of peacefulness	1	2	3	4	5	NA
200106 Ability to love	1	2	3	4	5	NA
200107 Ability to forgive	1	2	3	4	5	NA
200109 Ability to pray	1	2	3	4	5	NA
200110 Ability to worship	1	2	3	4	5	NA
200108 Spiritual experiences	1	2	3	4	5	NA
200122 Spiritual contentment	1	2	3	4	5	NA
200111 Participation in spiritual rites and passages	1	2	3	4	5	NA
200113 Participation in meditation	1	2	3	4	5	NA
200115 Participation in spiritual reading	1	2	3	4	5	NA
200112 Interaction with spiritual leaders	1	2	3	4	5	NA
200114 Expression through music	1	2	3	4	5	NA
200119 Expression through art	1	2	3	4	5	NA
200120 Expression through writing	1	2	3	4	5	NA
200116 Connectedness with inner self	1	2	3	4	5	NA
200117 Connectedness with others	1	2	3	4	5	NA
200121 Interaction with others to share thoughts, feelings, and beliefs	1	2	3	4	5	NA

Domain-Perceived Health (V)   *Class*-Health & Life Quality (U)   *1st edition 1997; revised 2004*

OUTCOME CONTENT REFERENCES:
Burkhardt, M. A. (1989). Spirituality: An analysis of the concept. *Holistic Nursing Practice, 3*(3), 69–77.
Burkhart, L., & Solari-Twadell, P. A. (2001). Spirituality and religiousness: Differentiating the diagnoses through a review of the nursing literature. *Nursing Diagnosis: The International Journal of Nursing Language and Classification, 12*(2), 45–54.
Emblen, J. D. (1992). Religion and spirituality defined according to current use in nursing literature. *Journal of Professional Nursing, 8*(1), 41–47.
Haase, J. E., Britt, T., Coward, D. D., Leidy, N. K., & Penn, P. E. (1992). Simultaneous concept analysis of spiritual perspective, hope, acceptance and self-transcendence. *Image—The Journal of Nursing Scholarship, 24*(2), 141–146.
Labun, E. (1988). Spiritual care: An element in nursing care planning. *Journal of Advanced Nursing, 13*(3), 314–320.
LeMone, P. (2001). Spiritual distress. In M. Maas, K. Buckwalter, M. Hardy, T. Tripp-Reimer, M. Titler, & J. Specht (Eds.), *Nursing care of older adults: Diagnoses, outcomes & interventions* (pp. 782–793). St. Louis: Mosby.
Pender, N., Murdaugh, C., & Parsons, M. A. (2001). *Health promotion in nursing practice* (4th ed.). Upper Saddle River, NJ: Prentice Hall.
Reed, P. G. (1992). An emerging paradigm for the investigation of spirituality in nursing. *Research in Nursing and Health, 15*(5), 349–357.
+Roberts, K. T., & Aspy, C. B. (1993). Development of the Serenity Scale. *Journal of Nursing Measurement, 1*(2), 145–164.

S

Stress Level 1212

Definition: Severity of manifested physical or mental tension resulting from factors that alter an existing equilibrium

OUTCOME TARGET RATING: Maintain at_____ Increase to_____

		Severe	Substantial	Moderate	Mild	None	
OUTCOME OVERALL RATING		1	2	3	4	5	
Indicators:							
121201	Increased blood pressure	1	2	3	4	5	NA
121202	Increased radial pulse rate	1	2	3	4	5	NA
121203	Increased respiratory rate	1	2	3	4	5	NA
121204	Dilated pupils	1	2	3	4	5	NA
121205	Increased muscle tension in neck, shoulders and back	1	2	3	4	5	NA
121206	Tension headache	1	2	3	4	5	NA
121207	Sweaty palms	1	2	3	4	5	NA
121208	Dry mouth and throat	1	2	3	4	5	NA
121209	Diarrhea	1	2	3	4	5	NA
121210	Urinary frequency	1	2	3	4	5	NA
121211	Change in food intake	1	2	3	4	5	NA
121212	Upset stomach	1	2	3	4	5	NA
121213	Restlessness	1	2	3	4	5	NA
121214	Sleep disturbance	1	2	3	4	5	NA
121235	Interruption of thought process	1	2	3	4	5	NA
121215	Forgetfulness	1	2	3	4	5	NA
121216	Frequent cognitive mistakes	1	2	3	4	5	NA
121217	Diminished attention to detail	1	2	3	4	5	NA
121218	Inability to concentrate on tasks	1	2	3	4	5	NA
121219	Emotional outbursts	1	2	3	4	5	NA
121220	Irritability	1	2	3	4	5	NA
121221	Depression	1	2	3	4	5	NA
121222	Anxiety	1	2	3	4	5	NA
121223	Suspiciousness	1	2	3	4	5	NA
121224	Oppressive thoughts	1	2	3	4	5	NA
121225	Flashback episodes	1	2	3	4	5	NA
121226	Dissociation	1	2	3	4	5	NA
121227	Compulsive behavior	1	2	3	4	5	NA
121228	Increased alcohol use	1	2	3	4	5	NA
121229	Increased psychotropic medication use	1	2	3	4	5	NA
121230	Increased smoking	1	2	3	4	5	NA
121231	Absenteeism	1	2	3	4	5	NA
121232	Decreased productivity	1	2	3	4	5	NA
121233	Increased frequency of accidents	1	2	3	4	5	NA
121234	Change in libido	1	2	3	4	5	NA
121236	Hair loss	1	2	3	4	5	NA

Domain-Psychosocial Health (III)   *Class-Psychological Well-Being (M)*   *3rd edition 2004; revised 2008, 2013*

OUTCOME CONTENT REFERENCES:

American Psychiatric Association. (2000). *Diagnostic and statistical manual of mental disorders* (4th ed., text revision). Washington DC: Author.

Campbell, R. J. (1989). *Psychiatric dictionary* (6th ed.). New York: Oxford University.

Curtis, R., Groarke, A.,. Coughlan, R., & Gsel, A. (2004). The influence of disease severity, perceived stress, social support and coping in patients with chronic illness: A 1 year follow up. *Psychology, Health & Medicine, 9*(4), 456–475.

Lazarus, R. S., & Folkman, S. (1984). *Stress, appraisal, and coping.* New York: Springer.

Richardson, C. G., & Ratner, P. A. (2005). Sense of coherence as a moderator of the effects of stressful life events of health. *Journal of Epidemiology & Community Health, 59*(11), 979–984.

Stanhope, M., & Lancaster, J. (1988). *Community health nursing: Process and practice for promoting health* (2nd ed.). St. Louis: Mosby.

Tasman, A., Kay, J., & Lieberman, J. A. (1997). *Psychiatry* (vol. 2). Philadelphia: Saunders.

Student Health Status   2005

Definition: Overall physical, psychological, and social functioning of a school-age child

OUTCOME TARGET RATING: Maintain at_____   Increase to_____

		Severely compromised	Substantially compromised	Moderately compromised	Mildly compromised	Not compromised	
OUTCOME OVERALL RATING		1	2	3	4	5	
Indicators:							
200501	Physical health	1	2	3	4	5	NA
200502	Mental health	1	2	3	4	5	NA
200503	School attendance	1	2	3	4	5	NA
200504	Readiness to learn	1	2	3	4	5	NA
200505	Academic performance at grade level or higher	1	2	3	4	5	NA
200506	Standardized test performance at grade level or higher	1	2	3	4	5	NA
200507	Progression to graduation on expected schedule	1	2	3	4	5	NA
200508	Return to class after visit to health office	1	2	3	4	5	NA
200509	Physician office visits minimized	**1**	**2**	**3**	**4**	**5**	NA
200510	Emergency room visits minimized	1	2	3	4	5	NA
200511	Reports to the health office for medications at appropriate time	1	2	3	4	5	NA
200512	Participation in mandated screenings	1	2	3	4	5	NA
200513	Family follow-up of referrals	1	2	3	4	5	NA
200514	Participation in self-care activities	1	2	3	4	5	NA
200516	Financial resources for health care	1	2	3	4	5	NA
200517	Participation in curricular school activities	1	2	3	4	5	NA
200518	Participation in extracurricular school activities	1	2	3	4	5	NA
200519	Participation in physical activities	1	2	3	4	5	NA
200520	Growth	1	2	3	4	5	NA
200521	Development	1	2	3	4	5	NA
200522	Optimum weight	1	2	3	4	5	NA
200523	Healthy dietary habits	1	2	3	4	5	NA
200524	Postponement of sexual activity	1	2	3	4	5	NA

		Severe	Substantial	Moderate	Mild	None	
200527	Alcohol use	1	2	3	4	5	NA
200528	Recreational drug use	1	2	3	4	5	NA
200533	Performance-enhancing drug use	1	2	3	4	5	NA
200529	Tobacco use	1	2	3	4	5	NA
200530	Occurrence of accidents	1	2	3	4	5	NA
200531	Disruptive behavior	1	2	3	4	5	NA
200534	Eating disorder	1	2	3	4	5	NA
200532	Occurrence of sexually transmitted disease	1	2	3	4	5	NA
200535	Risk for pregnancy	1	2	3	4	5	NA

S

Domain-Perceived Health (V)   *Class*-Health & Life Quality (U)   *3rd edition 2004; revised 2008, 2013*

OUTCOME CONTENT REFERENCES:

Council of Chief State School Officers. (1998). *Incorporating health-related indicators in education accountability systems*. Washington, DC: Author.

Howard, M. (1991). *How to help your teenager postpone sexual involvement*. Lexington, NY: Continuum.

Marx, E., & Wooley, S. F. (Eds). (1998). *Health is academic: A guide to coordinated school health programs*. New York: Teachers College Columbia University.

Miller, B., Card, J., Paikoff, R. J., & Peterson, J. (1992). *Preventing adolescent pregnancy*. Newbury Park, CA: Sage.

Novello, A. C., DeGraw, C., & Kleinman, D. V. (1992). Healthy children ready to learn: An essential collaboration between health and education. *Public Health Reports, 107*(1), 3–10.

Tyson, H. (1999). A load off the teachers' backs: Coordinated school health programs. *Phi Delta Kappan, 80*(5), K1–K8.

Washington State Office of Superintendent of Public Instruction. (2001). *School nurse outcome measures*. Olympia, WA: Author.

Substance Addiction Consequences   1407

Definition: Severity of change in health status and social functioning due to substance addiction

OUTCOME TARGET RATING: Maintain at_____   Increase to_____

OUTCOME OVERALL RATING		Severe 1	Substantial 2	Moderate 3	Mild 4	None 5	
Indicators:							
140701	Sustained decrease in physical activity	1	2	3	4	5	NA
140702	Chronic impaired motor function	1	2	3	4	5	NA
140703	Chronic decreased endurance	1	2	3	4	5	NA
140704	Chronic fatigue	1	2	3	4	5	NA
140723	Chronic hygiene problems	1	2	3	4	5	NA
140705	Chronic impaired cognitive function	1	2	3	4	5	NA
140706	Chronic impaired breathing	1	2	3	4	5	NA
140707	Prolonged recovery from illnesses	1	2	3	4	5	NA
140718	Absenteeism from work	1	2	3	4	5	NA
140719	Absenteeism from school	1	2	3	4	5	NA
140720	Difficulty maintaining role performance	1	2	3	4	5	NA
140709	Difficulty maintaining employment	1	2	3	4	5	NA
140710	Difficulty maintaining adequate housing	1	2	3	4	5	NA
140711	Difficulty supporting self financially	1	2	3	4	5	NA
140721	Difficulty maintaining social interactions	1	2	3	4	5	NA
140722	Risk for infection from sharing needles	1	2	3	4	5	NA

		Severe (4 + occurrences)	Substantial (3 occurrences)	Moderate (2 occurrences)	Mild (1 occurrence)	None (no occurrence)	
140712	Traffic accidents within the last year	1	2	3	4	5	NA
140717	Traffic tickets within the last year	1	2	3	4	5	NA
140713	Arrests within the last year	1	2	3	4	5	NA
140714	Emergency room visits within the last year	1	2	3	4	5	NA
140715	Hospitalizations within the last year	1	2	3	4	5	NA

Domain-Perceived Health (V)   *Class*-Symptom Status (V)   1st edition 1997; revised 2004, 2008, 2013

OUTCOME CONTENT REFERENCES:

Carruthers, S. (2003). The ins and outs of injection in Western Australia. *Journal of Substance Use, 8*(1), 11–18.

Leri, F., Bruneau, J., & Stewart, J. (2003). Understanding polydrug use: Review of heroin and cocaine co-use. *Addiction, 98*(1), 7–22.

McCuster, J., Stoddard, A. M., Zapka, J. G., & Lewis, B. F. (1993). Behavioral outcomes of AIDS educational interventions for drug users in short term treatment. *American Journal of Public Health, 83*(10), 1463–1466.

+McLellan, A. T., Luborsky, L., Woody, G. E., & O'Brien, C. P. (1980). An improved diagnostic evaluation instrument for substance abuse patients. *Journal of Nervous and Mental Disease, 168*(1), 26–33.

Millson, P. E., Challacombe, L., Villeneuve, P. J., Fischer, B., Strike, C. J., Myers, T., et al. (2004). Self-perceived health among Canadian opiate users: A comparison to the general population and to other chronic disease populations. *Canadian Journal of Public Health, 95*(2), 99–103.

Simons-Morton, D. G., Mullen, P. D., Mains, D. A., Tabak, E. R., & Green, L. W. (1992). Characteristics of controlled studies of patient education and counseling for preventive health behaviors. *Patient Education and Counseling, 19*(2), 174–204.

Talashek, M. L., Gerace, L. M., & Starr, K. L. (1994). The substance abuse pandemic: Determinants to guide interventions. *Public Health Nursing, 11*(2), 131–139.

Substance Withdrawal Severity 2108

Definition: Severity of signs and symptoms of withdrawal from addictive drugs, tobacco, or alcohol

OUTCOME TARGET RATING: Maintain at_____ Increase to_____

OUTCOME OVERALL RATING	Severe	Substantial	Moderate	Mild	None	
	1	2	3	4	5	
Indicators:						
210801 Substance-seeking behavior	1	2	3	4	5	NA
210802 Substance cravings	1	2	3	4	5	NA
210803 Irritability	1	2	3	4	5	NA
210804 Agitation	1	2	3	4	5	NA
210805 Emotional outbursts	1	2	3	4	5	NA
210806 Depression	1	2	3	4	5	NA
210807 Hyperreflexia	1	2	3	4	5	NA
210808 Myoclonus	1	2	3	4	5	NA
210809 Fasciculations	1	2	3	4	5	NA
210810 Muscle pain	1	2	3	4	5	NA
210811 Tremors	1	2	3	4	5	NA
210812 Change in vital signs	1	2	3	4	5	NA
210813 Dysrhythmia	1	2	3	4	5	NA
210814 Change in appetite	1	2	3	4	5	NA
210815 Nausea	1	2	3	4	5	NA
210816 Vomiting	1	2	3	4	5	NA
210817 Abdominal pain	1	2	3	4	5	NA
210818 Diarrhea	1	2	3	4	5	NA
210819 Rhinorrhea	1	2	3	4	5	NA
210820 Lacrimation	1	2	3	4	5	NA
210821 Pupil change	1	2	3	4	5	NA
210822 Goose bumps	1	2	3	4	5	NA
210823 Hot and cold flashes	1	2	3	4	5	NA
210824 Photophobia	1	2	3	4	5	NA
210825 Paresthesias	1	2	3	4	5	NA
210826 Abnormal sensitivity to sound	1	2	3	4	5	NA
210827 Headaches	1	2	3	4	5	NA
210828 Yawning	1	2	3	4	5	NA
210829 Impaired concentration	1	2	3	4	5	NA
210830 Disorientation	1	2	3	4	5	NA
210831 Difficulty sleeping	1	2	3	4	5	NA
210832 Hallucinations	1	2	3	4	5	NA
210833 Seizures	1	2	3	4	5	NA
210834 Fever	1	2	3	4	5	NA
210835 Chills	1	2	3	4	5	NA
210836 Flushing	1	2	3	4	5	NA

Continued

S

Substance Withdrawal Severity—cont'd

		Severe	Substantial	Moderate	Mild	None	
210837	Diaphoresis	1	2	3	4	5	NA
210838	Fatigue	1	2	3	4	5	NA
210839	Weakness	1	2	3	4	5	NA
210840	Alcohol level in blood	1	2	3	4	5	NA
210841	Substance level in blood	1	2	3	4	5	NA
210842	Substance level in urine	1	2	3	4	5	NA

Identify substance(s): _____

Domain-*Perceived Health (V)* **Class**-*Symptom Status (V)* *4th edition 2008; revised 2013*

OUTCOME CONTENT REFERENCES:
Boyd, M. A. (Ed.). (2005). *Psychiatric nursing contemporary practice* (3rd ed.). Philadelphia: Lippincott Williams & Wilkins.
Olmedo, R., & Hoffman, R. S. (2000). Withdrawal symptoms. *Emergency Medical Clinics of North America*, *18*(2), 273–288.

Suffering Severity

2003

Definition: Severity of signs and symptoms of long-term anguish due to a distressing event, injury, or loss

OUTCOME TARGET RATING: Maintain at_____ Increase to_____

		Severe	Substantial	Moderate	Mild	None	
OUTCOME OVERALL RATING		1	2	3	4	5	
Indicators:							
200301	Self-absorption	1	2	3	4	5	NA
200302	Depression	1	2	3	4	5	NA
200303	Sadness	1	2	3	4	5	NA
200304	Powerlessness	1	2	3	4	5	NA
200305	Grief	1	2	3	4	5	NA
200306	Guilt	1	2	3	4	5	NA
200307	Hopelessness	1	2	3	4	5	NA
200308	Helplessness	1	2	3	4	5	NA
200309	Worthlessness	1	2	3	4	5	NA
200314	Vulnerability	1	2	3	4	5	NA
200315	Spiritual distress	1	2	3	4	5	NA
200316	Despair	1	2	3	4	5	NA
200319	Loneliness	1	2	3	4	5	NA
200310	Fear of reoccurrence	1	2	3	4	5	NA
200311	Fear of unbearable pain	1	2	3	4	5	NA
200312	Fear of unknown circumstances	1	2	3	4	5	NA
200313	Fear of being alone	1	2	3	4	5	NA
200317	Bitterness toward others	1	2	3	4	5	NA

Domain-*Perceived Health (V)* **Class**-*Symptom Status (V)* *2nd edition 2000; revised 2004, 2013*

OUTCOME CONTENT REFERENCES:
Ankri, J., Adrieu, S., Beaufils, B., Grand, A., & Henrard, J. C. (2005). Beyond the global score of the Zarit Burden Interview: Useful dimensions for clinicians. *International Journal of Geriatric Psychiatry*, *20*(3), 254–260.
Cherny, N. I., Coyle, N., & Foley, K. M. (1994). The treatment of suffering when patients request elective death. *Journal of Palliative Care*, *10*(2), 71–79.
Copp, L. A. (1974). The spectrum of suffering. *American Journal of Nursing*, *74*(3), 491–495.
Duffy, M. E. (1992). A theoretical and empirical review of the concept of suffering. In P. L. Starck & J. P. McGovern (Eds.), *The hidden dimension of illness: Human suffering* (Pub. No. 15-2451, pp. 291–303). New York: National League for Nursing Press.

Fochtman, D. (2006). The concept of suffering in children and adolescents with cancer. *Journal of Pediatric Oncology Nursing, 23*(2), 92–102.

Hall, P. (2006). Mothers' experiences of postnatal depression: An interpretative phenomenological analysis. *Community Practitioner, 79*(8), 256–260.

Jacob, S. R., & Scandrett-Hobdon, S. (1994). Mothers grieving the death of a child: Case reports of maternal grief. *The Nurse Practitioner, 19*(7), 60–65.

Mako, C., Galek, K., & Poppito, S. R. (2006). Spiritual pain among patients with advanced cancer in palliative care. *Journal of Palliative Medicine, 9*(5), 1106–1113.

Mount, B. M. (1984). Psychological and social aspects of cancer pain. In P. D. Wall & R. Melzack (Eds.), *Textbook of pain* (pp. 460–471). New York: Churchill Livingstone.

Price, D. D., & Harkins, S. W. (1992). Psychophysical approaches to pain measurement and assessment. In D. C. Turk & R. Melzack (Eds.), *Handbook of pain assessment* (pp. 111–134). New York: The Guilford Press.

Steeves, R. H., Kahn, D. L., & Benoliel, J. Q. (1990). Nurses' interpretation of the suffering of their patients. *Western Journal of Nursing Research, 12*(6), 714–731.

Suicide Self-Restraint   1408

Definition: Personal actions to refrain from gestures and attempts at killing self

OUTCOME TARGET RATING: Maintain at_____   Increase to_____

		Never demonstrated	Rarely demonstrated	Sometimes demonstrated	Often demonstrated	Consistently demonstrated	
OUTCOME OVERALL RATING		1	2	3	4	5	
Indicators:							
140801	Expresses feelings	1	2	3	4	5	NA
140815	Expresses sense of hope	1	2	3	4	5	NA
140802	Maintains connectedness in relationships	1	2	3	4	5	NA
140823	Obtains assistance as needed	1	2	3	4	5	NA
140804	Verbalizes suicidal ideas	1	2	3	4	5	NA
140805	Control impulses	1	2	3	4	5	NA
140806	Refrains from gathering means for suicide	1	2	3	4	5	NA
140807	Refrains from giving away possessions	1	2	3	4	5	NA
140816	Refrains from inflicting serious injury	1	2	3	4	5	NA
140809	Refrains from using non-prescribed mood altering substances	1	2	3	4	5	NA
140810	Discloses plan for suicide if present	1	2	3	4	5	NA
140811	Upholds suicide contract	1	2	3	4	5	NA
140812	Maintains self-control without supervision	1	2	3	4	5	NA
140813	Refrains from attempting suicide	1	2	3	4	5	NA
140824	Obtains treatment for depression	1	2	3	4	5	NA
140825	Obtains treatment for substance abuse	1	2	3	4	5	NA
140819	Reports adequate pain control for chronic pain	1	2	3	4	5	NA
140826	Uses suicide prevention resources	1	2	3	4	5	NA
140827	Uses social support group	1	2	3	4	5	NA
140821	Uses available mental health care services	1	2	3	4	5	NA
140822	Plans for future	1	2	3	4	5	NA

Domain-Psychosocial Health (III)   **Class**-Self-Control (O)   *1st edition 1997; revised 2000, 2004, 2008*

S

OUTCOME CONTENT REFERENCES:

Aubert, P., Daigle, M. S., & Daigle, J. (2004). Cultural traits and immigration: Hostility and suicidality in Chinese Canadian students. *Transcultural Psychiatry, 41*(4), 514–532.

Conwell, Y. (1997). Management of suicidal behavior in the elderly. *The Psychiatric Clinics of North America, 20*(3), 667–683.

Cugino, A., Markovich, E. I., Rosenblatt, S., Jarjoura, D., Blend, D., & Whittier, F. C. (1992). Searching for a pattern: Repeat suicide attempts. *Journal of Psychosocial Nursing, 30*(3), 23–25.

Forster, P. (1994). Accurate assessment of short-term suicide risk in a crisis. *Psychiatric Annals, 24*(11), 571–578.

Hirschfeld, R. M. A., & Russell, J. M. (1997). Assessment and treatment of suicidal patients. *The New England Journal of Medicine, 337*(13), 910–915.

Ingram, T. N. (2001). Risk for violence: Self-directed or directed at others. In M. Maas, K. Buckwalter, M. Hardy, T. Tripp-Reimer, M. Titler, & J. Specht (Eds.), *Nursing care of older adults: Diagnoses, outcomes & interventions* (pp. 696–705). St. Louis: Mosby.

+Ivanoff, A., Joon Jang, S., Smyth, N. J., & Linehan, M. M. (1994). Fewer reasons for staying alive when you are thinking of killing yourself: The Brief Reasons for Living Inventory. *Journal of Psychopathology and Behavioral Assessment, 16*(1), 1–13.

Josepho, S. A., & Plutchek, R. (1994). Stress, coping, and suicide risk in psychiatric inpatients. *Suicide and Life-Threatening Behavior, 24*(1), 48–57.

+Linehan, M. M., Goodstein, J. L., Nielsen, S. L., & Chiles, J. A. (1983). Reasons for staying alive when you are thinking of killing yourself: The Reasons for Living Inventory. *Journal of Consulting and Clinical Psychology, 51*(2), 276–286, 484–485.

Lipshitz, A. (1995). Suicide prevention in young adults (age 18–30). *Suicide and Life-Threatening Behavior, 25*(1), 155–169.

Mellick, E., Buckwalter, K. C., & Stolley, J. M. (1992). Suicide among elderly white men: Development of a profile. *Journal of Psychosocial Nursing, 30*(2), 29–34.

Robie, D., Edgemon-Hill, E. J., Phelps, B., Schmitz, C., & Laughlin, J. A. (1999). Suicide prevention protocol: One hospital's nursing protocol for identification and intervention. *American Journal of Nursing, 99*(12), 53, 55, 57.

Valente, S. M., & Trainor, D. (1998). Rational suicide among patients who are terminally ill. *Official Journal of the Association of Operating Room Nurses, 68*(2), 252–255, 257–258, 260–264.

Surgical Recovery: Convalescence 2304

Definition: Extent of physiologic, psychological, and role function following discharge from postanesthesia care to the final post-operative clinic visit

OUTCOME TARGET RATING: Maintain at_____ Increase to_____

		Severe deviation from normal range	Substantial deviation from normal range	Moderate deviation from normal range	Mild deviation from normal range	No deviation from normal range	
OUTCOME OVERALL RATING		1	2	3	4	5	
Indicators:							
230401	Systolic blood pressure	1	2	3	4	5	NA
230402	Diastolic blood pressure	1	2	3	4	5	NA
230403	Hemodynamic stability	1	2	3	4	5	NA
230404	Body temperature	1	2	3	4	5	NA
230405	Radial pulse rate	1	2	3	4	5	NA
230406	Radial pulse rhythm	1	2	3	4	5	NA
230407	Respiratory rate	1	2	3	4	5	NA
230408	Depth of inspiration	1	2	3	4	5	NA
230409	Urine output	1	2	3	4	5	NA
230410	Bowel sounds	1	2	3	4	5	NA
230411	Bowel elimination	1	2	3	4	5	NA
230412	Electrolyte balance	1	2	3	4	5	NA
230413	Fluid intake	1	2	3	4	5	NA
230414	Hydration	1	2	3	4	5	NA
230415	Food intake	1	2	3	4	5	NA
230416	Blood glucose level	1	2	3	4	5	NA
230417	Tissue integrity	1	2	3	4	5	NA
230418	Neurovascular integrity	1	2	3	4	5	NA
230419	Wound healing	1	2	3	4	5	NA
230420	Ambulation	1	2	3	4	5	NA
230421	Cognition	1	2	3	4	5	NA
230422	Concentration	1	2	3	4	5	NA
230423	Sleep	1	2	3	4	5	NA
230424	Performance of prescribed exercise	1	2	3	4	5	NA
230425	Performance of prescribed wound care	1	2	3	4	5	NA
230426	Adjustment to body changes due to surgery	1	2	3	4	5	NA

S

Surgical Recovery: Convalescence—cont'd

	Severe deviation from normal range	Substantial deviation from normal range	Moderate deviation from normal range	Mild deviation from normal range	No deviation from normal range	
230427	Use of prescribed assistive devices	1	2	3	4	5	NA
230428	Performance of self-care activities	1	2	3	4	5	NA
230429	Resumption of normal activities	1	2	3	4	5	NA
230430	Resumption of normal role function	1	2	3	4	5	NA

		Severe	Substantial	Moderate	Mild	None	NA
230431	Atelectasis	1	2	3	4	5	NA
230432	Pneumonia	1	2	3	4	5	NA
230433	Pain	1	2	3	4	5	NA
230434	Drainage on dressing	1	2	3	4	5	NA
230435	Drainage from drains	1	2	3	4	5	NA
230436	Wound infection	1	2	3	4	5	NA
230437	Wound dehiscence	1	2	3	4	5	NA
230438	Thrombophlebitis	1	2	3	4	5	NA
230439	Pulmonary embolus	1	2	3	4	5	NA
230440	Nausea	1	2	3	4	5	NA
230441	Vomiting	1	2	3	4	5	NA
230442	Paralytic ileus	1	2	3	4	5	NA
230443	Constipation	1	2	3	4	5	NA
230444	Fatigue	1	2	3	4	5	NA
230445	Anxiety	1	2	3	4	5	NA
230446	Depression	1	2	3	4	5	NA

Domain-*Physiologic Health (II)*   **Class**-*Therapeutic Response (AA)*   *5th edition 2013*

OUTCOME CONTENT REFERENCES:

Capasso, V. A., Codner, C., Nuzzo-Meuller, G., Cox, E. M., & Bouvier, S. (2006). Peripheral arterial sheath removal program: A performance improvement initiative. *Journal of Vascular Nursing, 24*(4), 127–132.

Douglas, M. & Rowed, S. (2005). The implementation of a postoperative care process on a neurosurgical unit. *Journal of Neuroscience Nursing, 37*(6), 329–333.

Galli, B., Munver, R., Sawczuk, I., & Kochis, E. (2005). Laparoscopic radical nephrectomy in renal cell carcinoma. *Urologic Nursing, 25*(2), 83–86, 133.

Gilmartin, J. (2007). Contemporary day surgery: Patients' experience of discharge and recovery. *Journal of Clinical Nursing, 16*(6), 1109–1117.

Hodgins, M. J., Ouellet, L. L., Pond, S., Knorr, S., & Geldart, G. (2008). Effect of telephone follow-up on surgical orthopedic recovery. *Applied Nursing Research, 21*(4), 218–226.

Montin, L., Leino-Kilpi, H., & Suominen, T., & Lepisto, J. (2008). A systematic review of empirical studies between 1966 and 2005 of patient outcomes of total hip arthroplasty and related factors. *Journal of Clinical Nursing, 17*(1), 40–45.

Oakes, C. L., Ellington, K. J., Oakes, K. J., Olson, R. L., Neill, K. M. & Vacchiano, C. A. (2002). Assessment of postanesthesia short-term quality of life: A pilot study. *AANA Journal, 70*(4), 27–273.

Pasero, C., & Belden, J. (2006). Evidence-based perianesthesia care: Accelerated postoperative recovery programs. *Journal of PeriAnesthesia Nursing 21*(3), 168–176.

Pop, R. S., Manworren, R. C., Guzzetta, C. E., & Hynan, L. S. (2007). Perianesthesia nurses' pain management after tonsillectomy and adenoidectomy: Pediatric patient outcomes. *Journal of PeriAnesthesia Nursing, 22*(2), 91–101.

Richards, N. M. (2007). Outcomes in special populations undergoing cardiac surgery: Octogenarians, women and adults with congenital heart disease. *Critical Care Nursing Clinics of North America, 19*(4), 467–485.

Slusarz, R.; Beuth, W., & Ksiazkiewicz, B. (2009). Postsurgical examination of functional outcome of patients having undergone surgical treatment of intracranial aneurysm. *Scandinavian Journal of Caring Science, 23*(1), 130–139.

S

Surgical Recovery: Immediate Post-Operative   2305

Definition: Extent to which an individual achieves physiological baseline function following major surgery requiring anesthesia

OUTCOME TARGET RATING: Maintain at_____   Increase to_____

		Severe deviation from normal range	Substantial deviation from normal range	Moderate deviation from normal range	Mild deviation from normal range	No deviation from normal range	
OUTCOME OVERALL RATING		1	2	3	4	5	
Indicators:							
230501	Patent airway	1	2	3	4	5	NA
230502	Systolic blood pressure	1	2	3	4	5	NA
230503	Diastolic blood pressure	1	2	3	4	5	NA
230504	Pulse pressure	1	2	3	4	5	NA
230505	Body temperature	1	2	3	4	5	NA
230506	Apical heart rate	1	2	3	4	5	NA
230507	Apical heart rhythm	1	2	3	4	5	NA
230508	Radial pulse rate	1	2	3	4	5	NA
230509	Depth of inspiration	1	2	3	4	5	NA
230510	Respiratory rate	1	2	3	4	5	NA
230511	Respiratory rhythm	1	2	3	4	5	NA
230512	Oxygen saturation	1	2	3	4	5	NA
230513	Level of consciousness	1	2	3	4	5	NA
230514	Cognitive orientation	1	2	3	4	5	NA
230515	Urine output	1	2	3	4	5	NA
230516	Bowel sounds	1	2	3	4	5	NA
230517	Gag reflex	1	2	3	4	5	NA
230518	Tissue integrity						
230519	Peripheral sensation	1	2	3	4	5	NA
230520	Drainage from wound drains/tubes	1	2	3	4	5	NA

		Severe	Substantial	Moderate	Mild	None	NA
230521	Bleeding	1	2	3	4	5	NA
230522	Pain	1	2	3	4	5	NA
230523	Drainage on dressing	1	2	3	4	5	NA
230524	Wound site swelling	1	2	3	4	5	NA
230525	Intracranial pressure	1	2	3	4	5	NA
230526	Nausea	1	2	3	4	5	NA
230527	Vomiting	1	2	3	4	5	NA
230528	Headache	1	2	3	4	5	NA
230529	Sore throat	1	2	3	4	5	NA
230530	Hyperglycemia	1	2	3	4	5	NA
230531	Hypoglycemia	1	2	3	4	5	NA

Domain-*Physiologic Health (II)*   **Class**-*Therapeutic Response (AA)*   *5th edition 2013*

OUTCOME CONTENT REFERENCES:
Capasso, V. A., Codner, C., Nuzzo-Meuller, G., Cox, E. M. & Bouvier, S. (2006). Peripheral arterial sheath removal program: A performance improvement initiative. *Journal of Vascular Nursing, 24*(4), 127–132.
Douglas, M., & Rowed, S. (2005). The implementation of a postoperative care process on a neurosurgical unit. *Journal of Neuroscience Nursing, 37*(6), 329–333.
Galli, B., Munver, R., Sawczuk, I., & Kochis, E. (2005). Laparoscopic radical nephrectomy in renal cell carcinoma. *Urologic Nursing, 25*(2), 83–86, 133.
Gilmartin, J. (2007). Contemporary day surgery: Patients' experience of discharge and recovery. *Journal of Clinical Nursing, 16*(6), 1109–1117.
Hodgins, M. J., Ouellet, L. L., Pond, S., Knorr, S., & Geldart, G. (2008). Effect of telephone follow-up on surgical orthopedic recovery. *Applied Nursing Research, 21*(4), 218–226.

Montin, L., Leino-Kilpi, H., & Suominen, T., & Lepisto, J. (2008). A systematic review of empirical studies between 1966 and 2005 of patient outcomes of total hip arthroplasty and related factors. *Journal of Clinical Nursing*, *17*(1), 40–45.

Oakes, C. L., Ellington, K. J., Oakes, K. J., Olson, R. L., Neill, K. M., & Vacchiano, C. A. (2002). Assessment of postanesthesia short-term quality of life: A pilot study. *AANA Journal*, *70*(4), 27–273.

Pasero, C., & Belden, J. (2006). Evidence-based perianesthesia care: Accelerated postoperative recovery programs. *Journal of PeriAnesthesia Nursing 21*(3), 168–176.

Pop, R. S., Manworren, R. C., Guzzetta, C. E., & Hynan, L. S. (2007). Perianesthesia nurses' pain management after tonsillectomy and adenoidectomy: Pediatric patient outcomes. *Journal of PeriAnesthesia Nursing*, *22*(2), 91–101.

Richards, N. M. (2007). Outcomes in special populations undergoing cardiac surgery: Octogenarians, women and adults with congenital heart disease. *Critical Care Nursing Clinics of North America*, *19*(4), 467–485.

Slusarz, R.; Beuth, W., & Ksiazkiewicz, B. (2009). Postsurgical examination of functional outcome of patients having undergone surgical treatment of intracranial aneurysm. *Scandinavian Journal of Caring Science*, *23*(1), 130–139.

Swallowing Status   1010

Definition: Safe passage of fluids and/or solids from the mouth to the stomach

OUTCOME TARGET RATING: Maintain at_____   Increase to_____

OUTCOME OVERALL RATING	Severely compromised 1	Substantially compromised 2	Moderately compromised 3	Mildly compromised 4	Not compromised 5	
Indicators:						
101001 Maintains food in mouth	1	2	3	4	5	NA
101002 Handles oral secretions	1	2	3	4	5	NA
101003 Saliva production	1	2	3	4	5	NA
101004 Chewing ability	1	2	3	4	5	NA
101005 Delivery of bolus to hypopharynx is timed with swallow reflex	1	2	3	4	5	NA
101006 Ability to clear oral cavity	1	2	3	4	5	NA
101007 Timely bolus formation	1	2	3	4	5	NA
101008 Number of swallows appropriate for bolus size/texture	1	2	3	4	5	NA
101009 Meal duration with respect to amount consumed	1	2	3	4	5	NA
101010 Timely swallow reflex	1	2	3	4	5	NA
101015 Maintains neutral head and trunk position	1	2	3	4	5	NA
101016 Food acceptance	1	2	3	4	5	NA
101018 Swallow study findings	1	2	3	4	5	NA

	Severe	Substantial	Moderate	Mild	None	
101011 Changes in voice quality	1	2	3	4	5	NA
101012 Choking	1	2	3	4	5	NA
101020 Coughing	1	2	3	4	5	NA
101021 Gagging	1	2	3	4	5	NA
101013 Increased swallow effort	1	2	3	4	5	NA
101014 Gastric reflux	1	2	3	4	5	NA
101017 Discomfort with swallowing	1	2	3	4	5	NA

Domain-*Physiologic Health (II)*   **Class**-*Digestion & Nutrition (K)*   *2nd edition 2000; revised 2004*

OUTCOME CONTENT REFERENCES:

Arvedson, J., & Brodsky, L. (Eds.). (2002). *Pediatric swallowing and feeding: Assessment and management* (2nd ed.). San Diego: Singular.

Bosch, J., Van Dyke, D., Smith, S., & Poulton, S. (1997). The role of medical condition in the exacerbation of self-injurious behavior: An exploratory study. *Mental Retardation*, *35*(2), 124–130.

Christensen, J. R. (1989). Developmental approach to pediatric neurogenic dysphagia. *Dysphagia*, *3*(3), 131–134.

Feinberg, M. (1997). The effects of medication on swallowing. In B. Sonies (Ed.), *Dysphagia: A continuum of care* (pp. 107–120). Gaithersburg, MD: Aspen.

Hendrix, T. R. (1993). Art and science of history taking in the patient with difficulty swallowing. *Dysphagia*, *8*(2), 69–73.

S

The Joanna Briggs Institute for Evidence Based Nursing and Midwifery. (2000). Identification and nursing management of dysphagia in adults with neurological impairment. *Best Practice*, 4(2). Australia: Blackwell Science-Asia.

Kramer, S. S., & Eicher, P. M. (1993). The evaluation of pediatric feeding abnormalities. *Dysphagia*, 8(3), 215–24.

Langmore, S. (2000). *Endoscopic evaluation and treatment of swallowing disorders*. New York: Thieme Medical.

Lespargot, A., Langevin, M., Muller, S., & Guillemont, S. (1993). Swallowing disturbances associated with drooling in cerebral-palsied children. *Developmental Medicine and Child Neurology*, 35(4), 298–304.

Morris, S. E. (1989). Development of oral-motor skills in the neurologically impaired child receiving non-oral feedings. *Dysphagia*, 3(3), 135–154.

Ramsay, M., Gisel, E. G., & Boutry, M. (1993). Non-organic failure to thrive: Growth failure secondary to feeding skills disorder. *Developmental Medicine and Child Neurology*, 35(4), 285–297.

Tuchman, D., & Walter, R. (Eds.). (1994). *Disorders of feeding and swallowing in infants and children*. San Diego: Singular.

Wolf, L. S., & Glass, R. P. (1992). *Feeding and swallowing disorders in infancy*. Tucson: Therapy Skill Builders.

Swallowing Status: Esophageal Phase   1011

Definition: Safe passage of fluids and/or solids from the pharynx to the stomach

OUTCOME TARGET RATING: Maintain at_____   Increase to_____

OUTCOME OVERALL RATING	Severely compromised 1	Substantially compromised 2	Moderately compromised 3	Mildly compromised 4	Not compromised 5	
Indicators:						
101106 Maintains neutral head and neck position	1	2	3	4	5	NA
101114 Food acceptance	1	2	3	4	5	NA
101115 Volume acceptance	1	2	3	4	5	NA
101116 Swallow study findings: esophageal phase	1	2	3	4	5	NA

	Severe	Substantial	Moderate	Mild	None	
101101 Choking with swallowing	1	2	3	4	5	NA
101118 Coughing with swallowing	1	2	3	4	5	NA
101102 Gastric reflux	1	2	3	4	5	NA
101103 Epigastric pain	1	2	3	4	5	NA
101104 Discomfort with swallowing	1	2	3	4	5	NA
101108 Nighttime coughing	1	2	3	4	5	NA
101109 Nighttime vomiting	1	2	3	4	5	NA
101119 Nighttime choking	1	2	3	4	5	NA
101110 Repetitive swallowing	1	2	3	4	5	NA
101111 Hematemesis	1	2	3	4	5	NA
101112 Acidic breath odor	1	2	3	4	5	NA
101113 Bruxism	1	2	3	4	5	NA

Domain-Physiologic Health (II)   *Class*-Digestion & Nutrition (K)   *2nd edition 2000; revised 2004*

OUTCOME CONTENT REFERENCES:

Arvedson, J., & Brodsky, L. (Eds.). (2002). *Pediatric swallowing and feeding: Assessment and management* (2nd ed.). San Diego: Singular.

Bosch, J., Van Dyke, D., Smith, S., & Poulton, S. (1997). The role of medical condition in the exacerbation of self-injurious behavior: An exploratory study. *Mental Retardation*, 35(2), 124–130.

Christensen, J. R. (1989). Developmental approach to neurogenic pediatric dysphagia. *Dysphagia*, 3(3), 131–134.

Feinberg, M. (1997). The effects of medication on swallowing. In B. Sonies (Ed.), *Dysphagia: A continuum of care* (pp. 107–120). Gaithersburg, MD: Aspen.

Hendrix, T. R. (1993). Art and science of history taking in the patient with difficulty swallowing. *Dysphagia*, 8(2), 69–73.

Kramer, S., & Eicher, P. M. (1993). The evaluation of pediatric feeding abnormalities. *Dysphagia*, 8(3), 215–224.

Langmore, S. (2000). *Endoscopic evaluation and treatment of swallowing disorders*. New York: Thieme Medical.

Lespargot, A., Langevin, M., Muller, S., & Guillemont, S. (1993). Swallowing disturbances associated with drooling in cerebral-palsied children. *Developmental Medicine and Child Neurology*, 35(4), 298–304.

Morris, S. (1989). Development of oral-motor skills in the neurologically impaired child receiving non-oral feedings. *Dysphagia*, 3(3), 135–154.

Ramsay, M., Gisel, E. G., & Boutry, M. (1993). Non-organic failure to thrive: Growth failure secondary to feeding skills disorder. *Developmental Medicine and Child Neurology*, 35(4), 285–297.

Tuchman, D., & Walter, R. (Eds.). (1994). *Disorders of feeding and swallowing in infants and children*. San Diego: Singular.

Wolf, L. S., & Glass, R. P. (1992). *Feeding and swallowing disorders in infancy*. Tucson: Therapy Skill Builders.

Swallowing Status: Oral Phase   1012

Definition: Preparation, containment and posterior movement of fluids and/or solids in the mouth

OUTCOME TARGET RATING: Maintain at_____   Increase to_____

OUTCOME OVERALL RATING		Severely compromised	Substantially compromised	Moderately compromised	Mildly compromised	Not compromised	
		1	2	3	4	5	
Indicators:							
101201	Maintains food in mouth	1	2	3	4	5	NA
101202	Handles oral secretions	1	2	3	4	5	NA
101203	Bolus formation	1	2	3	4	5	NA
101204	Timely bolus formation	1	2	3	4	5	NA
101205	Chewing ability	1	2	3	4	5	NA
101206	Delivery of bolus to hypopharynx timed with swallow reflex	1	2	3	4	5	NA
101207	Ability to clear oral cavity	1	2	3	4	5	NA
101209	Lip closure	1	2	3	4	5	NA
101210	Number of swallows appropriate for bolus size/texture	1	2	3	4	5	NA
101211	Nippling efficiency	1	2	3	4	5	NA
101212	Rate of food consumption	1	2	3	4	5	NA
101214	Gag reflex						NA
101215	Swallow study findings: oral phase	1	2	3	4	5	NA

		Severe	Substantial	Moderate	Mild	None	
101208	Coughing before swallowing	1	2	3	4	5	NA
101217	Choking before swallowing	1	2	3	4	5	NA
101218	Gagging before swallowing	1	2	3	4	5	NA
101213	Nasal reflux	1	2	3	4	5	NA

Domain-*Physiologic Health (II)*   **Class**-*Digestion & Nutrition (K)*   *2nd edition 2000; revised 2004*

OUTCOME CONTENT REFERENCES:
Arvedson, J., & Brodsky, L. (Eds.). (2002). *Pediatric swallowing and feeding: Assessment and management* (2nd ed.). San Diego: Singular.
Bosch, J., Van Dyke, D., Smith, S., & Poulton, S. (1997). The role of medical condition in the exacerbation of self-injurious behavior: An exploratory study. *Mental Retardation, 35*(2), 124–130.
Christensen, J. R. (1989). Developmental approach to neurogenic pediatric dysphagia. *Dysphagia, 3*(3), 131–134.
Feinberg, M. (1997). The effects of medication on swallowing. In B. Sonies (Ed.), *Dysphagia: A continuum of care* (pp. 107–120). Gaithersburg, MD: Aspen.
Hendrix, T. R. (1993). Art and science of history taking in the patient with difficulty swallowing. *Dysphagia, 8*(2), 69–73.
Kramer, S., & Eicher, P. M. (1993). The evaluation of pediatric feeding abnormalities. *Dysphagia, 8*(3), 215–224.
Langmore, S. (2000). *Endoscopic evaluation and treatment of swallowing disorders.* New York: Thieme Medical.
Lespargot, A., Langevin, M., Muller, S., & Guillemont, S. (1993). Swallowing disturbances associated with drooling in cerebral-palsied children. *Developmental Medicine and Child Neurology, 35*(4), 298–304.
Morris, S. (1989). Development of oral-motor skills in the neurologically impaired child receiving non-oral feedings. *Dysphagia, 3*(3), 135–154.
Ramsay, M., Gisel, E. G., & Boutry, M. (1993). Non-organic failure to thrive: Growth failure secondary to feeding skills disorder. *Developmental Medicine and Child Neurology, 35*(4), 285–297.
Tuchman, D., & Walter, R. (Eds.). (1994). *Disorders of feeding and swallowing in infants and children.* San Diego: Singular.
Wolf, L. S., & Glass, R. P. (1992). *Feeding and swallowing disorders in infancy.* Tucson: Therapy Skill Builders.

S

Swallowing Status: Pharyngeal Phase 1013

Definition: Safe passage of fluids and/or solids from the mouth to the esophagus

OUTCOME TARGET RATING: Maintain at _____ Increase to _____

		Severely compromised	Substantially compromised	Moderately compromised	Mildly compromised	Not compromised	
OUTCOME OVERALL RATING		1	2	3	4	5	
Indicators:							
101301	Timely swallow reflex	1	2	3	4	5	NA
101304	Number of swallows appropriate for bolus size/texture	1	2	3	4	5	NA
101305	Maintains neutral head and neck position	1	2	3	4	5	NA
101307	Laryngeal elevation	1	2	3	4	5	NA
101311	Food acceptance	1	2	3	4	5	NA
101312	Swallow study findings: pharyngeal phase	1	2	3	4	5	NA
		Severe	**Substantial**	**Moderate**	**Mild**	**None**	
101302	Changes in voice quality	1	2	3	4	5	NA
101303	Choking	1	2	3	4	5	NA
101314	Coughing	1	2	3	4	5	NA
101315	Gagging	1	2	3	4	5	NA
101306	Increased swallow effort	1	2	3	4	5	NA
101310	Nasal reflux	1	2	3	4	5	NA
101316	Aspirations	1	2	3	4	5	NA

Domain-Physiologic Health (II) **Class**-*Digestion & Nutrition (K)* 2nd edition 2000; revised 2004

OUTCOME CONTENT REFERENCES:

Arvedson, J., & Brodsky, L. (Eds.). (2002). Pediatric swallowing and feeding: Assessment and management (2nd ed.). San Diego: Singular.

Bosch, J., Van Dyke, D., Smith, S., & Poulton, S. (1997). The role of medical condition in the exacerbation of self-injurious behavior: An exploratory study. *Mental Retardation, 35*(2), 124–130.

Christensen, J. R. (1989). Developmental approach to neurogenic pediatric dysphagia. *Dysphagia, 3*(3), 131–134.

Feinberg, M. (1997). The effects of medication on swallowing. In B. Sonies (Ed.), *Dysphagia: A continuum of care* (pp. 107–120). Gaithersburg, MD: Aspen.

Hendrix, T. R. (1993). Art and science of history taking in the patient with difficulty swallowing. *Dysphagia, 8*(2), 69–73.

Kramer, S., & Eicher, P. M. (1993). The evaluation of pediatric feeding abnormalities. *Dysphagia, 8*(3), 215–24.

Langmore, S. (2000). *Endoscopic evaluation and treatment of swallowing disorders.* New York: Thieme Medical.

Lespargot, A., Langevin, M., Muller, S., & Guillemont, S. (1993). Swallowing disturbances associated with drooling in cerebral-palsied children. *Developmental Medicine and Child Neurology, 35*(4), 298–304.

Morris, S. (1989). Development of oral-motor skills in the neurologically impaired child receiving non-oral feedings. *Dysphagia, 3*(3), 135–154.

Ramsay, M., Gisel, E. G., & Boutry, M. (1993). Non-organic failure to thrive: Growth failure secondary to feeding skills disorder. *Developmental Medicine and Child Neurology, 35*(4), 285–297.

Tuchman, D., & Walter, R. (Eds.). (1994). *Disorders of feeding and swallowing in infants and children.* San Diego: Singular.

Wolf, L. S., & Glass, R. P. (1992). *Feeding and swallowing disorders in infancy.* Tucson: Therapy Skill Builders.

S

Symptom Control 1608

Definition: Personal actions to minimize perceived adverse changes in physical and emotional functioning

OUTCOME TARGET RATING: Maintain at_____   Increase to_____

	Never demonstrated	Rarely demonstrated	Sometimes demonstrated	Often demonstrated	Consistently demonstrated	
OUTCOME OVERALL RATING	1	2	3	4	5	
Indicators:						
160801 Monitors symptom onset	1	2	3	4	5	NA
160802 Monitors symptom persistence	1	2	3	4	5	NA
160803 Monitors symptom severity	1	2	3	4	5	NA
160804 Monitors symptom frequency	1	2	3	4	5	NA
160805 Monitors symptom variation	1	2	3	4	5	NA
160806 Uses preventive measures	1	2	3	4	5	NA
160807 Uses symptom relief measures	1	2	3	4	5	NA
160813 Obtains health care when warning signs occur	1	2	3	4	5	NA
160809 Uses available resources	1	2	3	4	5	NA
160810 Uses diary to monitor symptoms over time	1	2	3	4	5	NA
160811 Reports symptoms controlled	1	2	3	4	5	NA

Domain-*Health Knowledge & Behavior (IV)*   **Class**-*Health Behavior (Q)*   *1st edition 1997; revised 2000, 2004, 2008*

OUTCOME CONTENT REFERENCES:

Coleman, C. L., Holzemer, W. L., Eller, L. S., Corless, I., Reynolds, N., Nokes, K. M., et al. (2006). Gender differences in use of prayer as a self-care strategy for managing symptoms in African Americans living with HIV/AIDS. *Journal of the Association of Nurses in AIDS Care, 17*(4), 16–23.

Hegyvary, S. T. (1993). Patient care outcomes related to management of symptoms. In J. J. Fitzpatrick & J. S. Stevenson (Eds.), *Annual review of nursing research* (Vol. 11, pp. 145–168). New York: Springer.

Kercsmar, C. M., Dearborn, D. G., Schluchter, M., Xue, L., Kirchner, H. L., Sobolewski, J., et al. (2006). Reduction in asthma morbidity in children as a result of home remediation aimed at moisture sources. *Environmental Health Perspectives, 114*(10), 1574–1580.

Kim, S. H., Oh, E. G., & Lee, W. H. (2006). Symptom experience, psychological distress, and quality of life in Korean patients with liver cirrhosis: A cross-sectional survey. *International Journal of Nursing Studies, 43*(8), 1047–1056.

+McCorkle, R., & Benoliel, J. Q. (1983). Symptom distress, current concerns, and mood disturbances after diagnosis of life-threatening disease. *Social Science Medicine, 17*(7), 431–438.

+McCorkle, R., & Young, K. (1978). Development of a Symptom Distress Scale. *Cancer Nursing, 1*(5), 373–378.

Segrin, T., Dorros, S. M., Meek, P., & Lopez, A. M. (2007). Depression and anxiety in women with breast cancer and their partners. *Nursing Research, 56*(1), 44–53.

Sherbourne, C. D., Allen, H. M., Kamberg, C. J., & Wells, K. B. (1992). Physical/psychophysiological symptoms measure. In A. L. Stewart & J. E. Ware, Jr. (Eds.), *Measuring functioning and well-being* (pp. 261–272). Durham, NC: Duke University Press.

Strauss, A. L., Corbin, J., Fagerhaugh, S., Glaser, B. G., Maines, D., Suczek, B., et al. (1984). Symptom control. In *Chronic illness and the quality of life.* (2nd ed., pp. 49–59). St. Louis: Mosby.

White, M. A., & Grilo, C. M. (2007). Symptom severity in obese women with binge eating disorder as a function of smoking history. *International Journal of Eating Disorders, 40*(1), 77–81.

Williams, P. D., Piamjariyakul, U., Ducey, K., Badura, J., Boltz, K. D., Olberding, K., et al. (2006). Cancer treatment, symptom monitoring, and self-care in adults: Pilot study. *Cancer Nursing, 29*(5), 347–355.

S

Symptom Severity   **2103**

Definition: Severity of adverse physical, emotional, and social responses

OUTCOME TARGET RATING: Maintain at_____ Increase to_____

OUTCOME OVERALL RATING	Severe 1	Substantial 2	Moderate 3	Mild 4	None 5	
Indicators:						
210301 Symptom intensity	1	2	3	4	5	NA
210302 Symptom frequency	1	2	3	4	5	NA
210303 Symptom persistence	1	2	3	4	5	NA
210304 Associated discomfort	1	2	3	4	5	NA
210305 Associated restlessness	1	2	3	4	5	NA
210306 Associated fear	1	2	3	4	5	NA
210307 Associated anxiety	1	2	3	4	5	NA
210308 Impaired physical mobility	1	2	3	4	5	NA
210309 Impaired role performance	1	2	3	4	5	NA
210310 Impaired interpersonal relationships	1	2	3	4	5	NA
210311 Impaired mood	1	2	3	4	5	NA
210312 Impaired life enjoyment	1	2	3	4	5	NA
210313 Inadequate sleep	1	2	3	4	5	NA
210316 Sleep deficit	1	2	3	4	5	NA
210314 Loss of appetite	1	2	3	4	5	NA

Domain-*Perceived Health (V)* **Class**-*Symptom Status (V)* *1st edition 1997; revised 2004, 2013*

OUTCOME CONTENT REFERENCES:

Banes, S., Gott, M., Payne, S., Parker, C., Seamark, D., Gariballa, S., et al (2006). Prevalence of symptoms in a community-based sample of heart failure patients. *Journal of Pain & Symptom Management, 32*(3), 208–216.

Docherty, S. L., Sandelowski, M., & Preisser, J. S. (2006). Three months in the symptom life of a teenage girl undergoing treatment for cancer. *Research in Nursing & Health, 29*(4), 294–310.

Hartford, M., Karlson, B. W., Sjolin, M., Holmberg, S., & Herlitz, J. (1993). Symptoms, thoughts, and environmental factors in suspected acute myocardial infarction. *Heart & Lung, 22*(1), 64–70.

Hegyvary, S. T. (1993). Patient care outcomes related to management of symptoms. In J. J. Fitzpatrick & J. S. Stevenson (Eds.), *Annual review of nursing research,* (Vol. 11, pp. 145–168). New York: Springer.

+McCorkle, R., & Benoliel, J. Q. (1983). Symptom distress, current concerns, and mood disturbances after diagnosis of life-threatening disease. *Social Science Medicine, 17*(7), 431–438.

+McCorkle, R., & Young, K. (1978). Development of a Symptom Distress Scale. *Cancer Nursing, 1*(5), 373–378.

Payne, J. K., Piper, B. F., Rabinowitz, I. & Zimmerman, M. B. (2006). Biomarkers, fatigue, sleep, and depressive symptoms in women with breast cancer: A pilot study. *Oncology Nursing Forum, 33*(4), 775–783.

Sherbourne, C. D., Allen, H. M., Kamberg, C. J., & Wells, K. B. (1992). Physical/psychophysiologic symptoms measure. In A. L. Stewart & J. E. Ware, Jr. (Eds.), *Measuring functioning and well-being* (pp. 261–272). Durham, NC: Duke University Press.

Strauss, A. L., Corbin, J., Fagerhaugh, S., Glaser, B. G., Maines, D., Suczek, B., et al. (1984). Symptom control. In *Chronic illness and the quality of life* (2nd ed., pp. 49–59). St. Louis: Mosby.

S

Systemic Toxin Clearance: Dialysis   2302

Definition: Clearance of toxins from the body with peritoneal dialysis or hemodialysis

OUTCOME TARGET RATING: Maintain at_____   Increase to_____

OUTCOME OVERALL RATING	Severe deviation from normal range	Substantial deviation from normal range	Moderate deviation from normal range	Mild deviation from normal range	No deviation from normal range	
	1	2	3	4	5	
Indicators:						
230212 Urea reduction ratio (URR) $\geq$ 65%	1	2	3	4	5	NA
230216 Blood pressure	1	2	3	4	5	NA
230214 Serum potassium	1	2	3	4	5	NA
230217 Serum sodium	1	2	3	4	5	NA
230220 Serum creatinine	1	2	3	4	5	NA
230221 Serum calcium	1	2	3	4	5	NA
230222 Serum bicarbonate	1	2	3	4	5	NA
230223 Serum magnesium	1	2	3	4	5	NA
230224 Serum phosphorous	1	2	3	4	5	NA
230225 Creatinine clearance	1	2	3	4	5	NA
230226 Blood urea nitrogen to creatinine ratio	1	2	3	4	5	NA

	Severe	Substantial	Moderate	Mild	None	
230203 Nausea	1	2	3	4	5	NA
230204 Vomiting	1	2	3	4	5	NA
230205 Weakness	1	2	3	4	5	NA
230206 Malaise	1	2	3	4	5	NA
230207 Anorexia	1	2	3	4	5	NA
230208 Insomnia	1	2	3	4	5	NA
230209 Edema	1	2	3	4	5	NA
230210 Dizziness	1	2	3	4	5	NA
230211 Pruritus	1	2	3	4	5	NA
230218 Ascites	1	2	3	4	5	NA
230219 Muscle cramps	1	2	3	4	5	NA
230227 Anemia	1	2	3	4	5	NA
230228 Weight gain	1	2	3	4	5	NA
230229 Impaired concentration	1	2	3	4	5	NA

Domain-Physiologic Health (II)   **Class**-Therapeutic Response (AA)   2nd edition 2000; revised 2004, 2008

S

OUTCOME CONTENT REFERENCES:

Broscious, S. K., & Castagnola, J. (2006). Chronic kidney disease: Acute manifestations and role of critical care nurses. *Critical Care Nurse, 26*(4), 17–28.

Brundage, D. J. (1992). *Renal disorders.* St. Louis: Mosby.

Gutch, C. F., Stoner, M. H., & Corea, A. L. (1999). *Review of hemodialysis for nurses and dialysis personnel* (6th ed). St. Louis: Mosby.

Guzman, N. J., & Peterson, J. C. (1993). In C. C. Tisher & C. S. Wilcox (Eds.), *House officers series: Nephrology* (2nd ed., pp. 60–87). Baltimore, MD: Williams & Wilkins.

Lancaster, L. E. (Ed.). (1995). *ANNA's core curriculum for nephrology nurses* (section X, 3rd ed.). Pitman, NJ: Anthony J. Janetti.

Smeltzer, S. C., & Bare, B. G. (2004). *Brunner & Suddarth's textbook of medical-surgical nursing* (10th ed.). Philadelphia: Lippincott Williams & Wilkins.

Thermoregulation 0800

Definition: Balance among heat production, heat gain, and heat loss

OUTCOME TARGET RATING: Maintain at_____   Increase to_____

		Severely compromised	Substantially compromised	Moderately compromised	Mildly compromised	Not compromised	
OUTCOME OVERALL RATING		1	2	3	4	5	
Indicators:							
080009	Presence of goose bumps when cold	1	2	3	4	5	NA
080010	Sweating when hot	1	2	3	4	5	NA
080011	Shivering when cold	1	2	3	4	5	NA
080017	Apical heart rate	1	2	3	4	5	NA
080012	Radial pulse rate	1	2	3	4	5	NA
080013	Respiratory rate	1	2	3	4	5	NA
080015	Reported thermal comfort	1	2	3	4	5	NA

		Severe	Substantial	Moderate	Mild	None	
080001	Increased skin temperature	1	2	3	4	5	NA
080018	Decreased skin temperature	1	2	3	4	5	NA
080019	Hyperthermia	1	2	3	4	5	NA
080020	Hypothermia	1	2	3	4	5	NA
080003	Headache	1	2	3	4	5	NA
080004	Muscle aches	1	2	3	4	5	NA
080005	Irritability	1	2	3	4	5	NA
080006	Drowsiness	1	2	3	4	5	NA
080007	Skin color changes	1	2	3	4	5	NA
080008	Muscle twitching	1	2	3	4	5	NA
080014	Dehydration	1	2	3	4	5	NA
080021	Heat cramps	1	2	3	4	5	NA
080022	Heat stroke	1	2	3	4	5	NA
080023	Frost bite	1	2	3	4	5	NA

Domain-*Physiologic Health (II)*   **Class**-*Metabolic Regulation (I)*   *1st edition 1997; revised 2004, 2008*

OUTCOME CONTENT REFERENCES:

Ainslie, P. N., Campbell, I. T., Lambert, J. P., MacLaren, D. P. M., & Reilly, R. (2005). Physiological and metabolic aspects of very prolonged exercise with particular reference to hill walking. *Sports Medicine, 35*(7), 619–647.

Ballester, J. M., & Harchelroad, F. P. (1999). Hyperthermia: How to recognize and prevent heat-related illnesses. *Geriatrics, 54*(7), 20–24.

Caruso, C., Hadley, B., Shuklou, R., & Frame, P. (1992). Cooling effects and comfort of four cooling blanket temperatures in humans with fever. *Nursing Research, 41*(2), 68–72.

Charkoudian, N. (2003). Skin blood flow in adult human thermoregulation: How it works, when it does not, and why. *Mayo Clinic Proceedings, 78*(5), 603–612.

Elliott, F. (2005). Do the prep work. *Occupational Health & Safety, 74*(11), 68, 70.

Erickson, R., & Kerklin, S. (1992). Comparison of methods for core temperature measurement. *Heart & Lung, 21*(3), 297.

Finke, C. (1991). Measurement of the thermoregulatory response: A review. *Focus on Critical Care, 18*(5), 408–412.

Franceschl, V. (1991). Accuracy and feasibility of measuring oral temperature in critically ill adults. *Focus on Critical Care, 18*(3), 221–228.

Holtzclaw, B. J. (2001). Risk for altered body temperature. In M. Maas, K. Buckwalter, M. Hardy, T. Tripp-Reimer, M. Titler, & J. Specht (Eds.), *Nursing care of older adults: Diagnoses, outcomes & interventions* (pp. 201–216). St. Louis: Mosby.

Murphy, K. (1992). Acetaminophen and ibuprofen: Finer control and overdose. *Pediatric Nursing, 18*(4), 428–431.

Parker, R. J., & Davidson, A. C. (2005). Hypothyroidism—An unexpected diagnosis following emergency treatment for heatstroke. *International Journal of Clinical Practice, 59*(Suppl. 147), 31–33.

Segatore, M. (1992). Fever after traumatic brain injury. *American Association of Neuroscience Nurse, 24*(2), 104–109.

Stewart, G., & Webster, D. (1992). Re-evaluation of the tympanic thermometer in the emergency department. *Annals of Emergency Medicine, 21*(2), 158–161.

Summers, S., Dudgeon, N., Byram, K., & Zingsheim, K. (1990). The effects of two warming methods on core and surface temperatures, hemoglobin oxygen saturation, blood pressure, and perceived comfort of hypothermic postanesthesia patients. *Journal of Post Anesthesia Nursing, 5*(5), 354–364.

Watson, G., Casa, D. J., Fiala, K. A., Hile, A., Roti, M. W., Healey, J. C., et al. (2006). Creatine use and exercise heat tolerance in dehydrated men. *Journal of Athletic Training, 41*(1), 18–29.

T

Thermoregulation: Newborn 0801

Definition: Balance among heat production, heat gain, and heat loss during the first 28 days of life

OUTCOME TARGET RATING: Maintain at_____ Increase to_____

		Severely compromised	Substantially compromised	Moderately compromised	Mildly compromised	Not compromised	
OUTCOME OVERALL RATING		1	2	3	4	5	
Indicators:							
080106	Weight gain	1	2	3	4	5	NA
080107	Non-shivering thermogenesis	1	2	3	4	5	NA
080108	Assumes heat retention posture with hypothermia	1	2	3	4	5	NA
080109	Assumes heat dissipation posture with hyperthermia	1	2	3	4	5	NA
080110	Weaning from Isolette to crib	1	2	3	4	5	NA
080113	Acid/base balance	1	2	3	4	5	NA

		Severe	Substantial	Moderate	Mild	None	
080116	Temperature instability	1	2	3	4	5	NA
080117	Hyperthermia	1	2	3	4	5	NA
080118	Hypothermia	1	2	3	4	5	NA
080119	Irregular respirations	1	2	3	4	5	NA
080120	Tachypnea	1	2	3	4	5	NA
080103	Restlessness	1	2	3	4	5	NA
080104	Lethargy	1	2	3	4	5	NA
080105	Skin color changes	1	2	3	4	5	NA
080111	Dehydration	1	2	3	4	5	NA
080112	Blood glucose instability	1	2	3	4	5	NA
080114	Hyperbilirubinemia	1	2	3	4	5	NA

Domain-*Physiologic Health (II)* **Class**-*Metabolic Regulation (I)* *1st edition 1997; revised 2004*

OUTCOME CONTENT REFERENCES:

Bliss-Holtz, J. (1992). Temperature relationships in cold-stressed infants. *Neonatal Network, 11*(2), 72.

Bohnhorst, B., Heyne, T., Peter, C. S., & Poets, C. F. (2001). Skin-to-skin (kangaroo) care, respiratory control, and thermoregulation. *Journal of Pediatrics, 138*(2), 193–197.

Deacon, J., & O'Neill, P. (Eds.). (1999). *Core curriculum for neonatal intensive care nursing* (2nd ed.). Philadelphia: W. B. Saunders.

Greer, P. (1988). Head coverings for newborns under radiant warmers. *Journal of Obstetric, Gynecologic, and Neonatal Nursing, 17*(4), 265–270.

Keeling, E. B. (1992). Thermoregulation and axillary temperature measurements in neonates: A review of the literature. *Maternal-Child Nursing Journal, 20*(3–4), 124–140.

Konrad, C. (1980). *Nursing interventions to assess and control fever in infants and small children.* Unpublished master's thesis, The University of Iowa, Iowa City.

Mattson, S., & Smith, J. E. (Eds.). (2000). *Core curriculum for maternal-newborn nursing* (2nd ed.). Philadelphia: W. B. Saunders.

Truman, P. (2006). Jaundice in the preterm infant. *Paediatric Nursing, 18*(5), 20–22.

T

Tissue Integrity: Skin & Mucous Membranes   **1101**

Definition: Structural intactness and normal physiological function of skin and mucous membranes

OUTCOME TARGET RATING: Maintain at_____   Increase to_____

		Severely compromised	Substantially compromised	Moderately compromised	Mildly compromised	Not compromised	
OUTCOME OVERALL RATING		1	2	3	4	5	
Indicators:							
110101	Skin temperature	1	2	3	4	5	NA
110102	Sensation	1	2	3	4	5	NA
110103	Elasticity	1	2	3	4	5	NA
110104	Hydration	1	2	3	4	5	NA
110106	Perspiration	1	2	3	4	5	NA
110108	Texture	1	2	3	4	5	NA
110109	Thickness	1	2	3	4	5	NA
110111	Tissue perfusion	1	2	3	4	5	NA
110112	Hair growth on skin	1	2	3	4	5	NA
110113	Skin integrity	1	2	3	4	5	NA
		Severe	Substantial	Moderate	Mild	None	
110105	Abnormal pigmentation	1	2	3	4	5	NA
110115	Skin lesions	1	2	3	4	5	NA
110116	Mucous membrane lesions	1	2	3	4	5	NA
110117	Scar tissue	1	2	3	4	5	NA
110118	Skin cancers	1	2	3	4	5	NA
110119	Skin flaking	1	2	3	4	5	NA
110120	Skin scaling	1	2	3	4	5	NA
110121	Erythema	1	2	3	4	5	NA
110122	Blanching	1	2	3	4	5	NA
110123	Necrosis	1	2	3	4	5	NA
110124	Induration	1	2	3	4	5	NA
110125	Corneal abrasion	1	2	3	4	5	NA

Domain-*Physiologic Health (II)*   **Class**-*Tissue Integrity (L)*   *1st edition 1997; revised 2004, 2013*

OUTCOME CONTENT REFERENCES:
+Bergstrom, N., Braden, B. J., Laguzza, A., & Holman, V. (1987). The Braden Scale for predicting pressure sore risk. *Nursing Research, 36*(4), 205–210.
Cohen, I. K., Diegelmann, R. F., & Lindblad, W. L. (1992). *Wound healing: Biochemical and clinical aspects.* Philadelphia: W. B. Saunders.
Hardy, M. D. (2001). Impaired skin integrity: Dry skin. In M. Maas, K. Buckwalter, M. Hardy, T. Tripp-Reimer, M. Titler, & J. Specht (Eds.), *Nursing care of older adults: Diagnoses, outcomes & interventions* (pp. 137–144). St. Louis: Mosby.
Lazarus, G. S., Cooper, D. M., Knighton, D. R., Margohs, D. J., Pecoraro, R. E., Rodeheaver, G., et al. (1994). Definitions and guidelines for assessment of wounds and evaluation of healing. *Archives of Dermatology, 130*(4), 489–493.
Maklebust, J., & Sieggreen, M. (1996). *Pressure ulcers: Guidelines for prevention and nursing management* (2nd ed.). Springhouse, PA: Springhouse.
Potter, P. A., & Perry, A. G. (2001). *Fundamentals of nursing* (5th ed.). St. Louis: Mosby.
Van Rijswijk, L. (1993). Full-thickness leg ulcers: Patient demographics and predictors of healing. *The Journal of Family Practice, 36*(6), 625–632.

T

Tissue Perfusion 0422

Definition: Adequacy of the blood flow through body organs to function at the cellular level

OUTCOME TARGET RATING: Maintain at_____   Increase to_____

		Severe deviation from normal range	Substantial deviation from normal range	Moderate deviation from normal range	Mild deviation from normal range	No deviation from normal range	
OUTCOME OVERALL RATING		1	2	3	4	5	
Indicators:							
042201	Blood flow through the liver vasculature	1	2	3	4	5	NA
042202	Blood flow through the kidney vasculature	1	2	3	4	5	NA
042203	Blood flow through the gastrointestinal tract vasculature	1	2	3	4	5	NA
042204	Blood flow through the spleen vasculature	1	2	3	4	5	NA
042205	Blood flow through the pancreas vasculature	1	2	3	4	5	NA
042206	Blood flow through the coronary vasculature	1	2	3	4	5	NA
042207	Blood flow through the pulmonary vasculature	1	2	3	4	5	NA
042208	Blood flow through the cerebral vasculature	1	2	3	4	5	NA
042209	Blood flow through the peripheral vessels	1	2	3	4	5	NA
042210	Blood flow through the vasculature at the cellular level	1	2	3	4	5	NA

Domain-*Physiologic Health (II)*   **Class**-*Cardiopulmonary (E)*   *5th edition 2013*

OUTCOME CONTENT REFERENCES:

Kelechi, T. J., & Michel, Y. (2007). A descriptive study of skin temperature, tissue perfusion, and tissue oxygen in patients with chronic venous disease. *Biological Research for Nursing, 9*(1), 70–80.

Maar, S. P. (2008). Searching for the holy grail: A review of markers of tissue perfusion in pediatric critical care. *Pediatric Emergency Care, 24*(12), 883–887.

Santos, F., de Melo, R., & Lopes, M. (2010). Characterization of health status with regard to tissue integrity and tissue perfusion in patients with venous ulcers according to the nursing outcomes classification. *Journal of Vascular Nursing, 28*(1), 14–20.

T

Tissue Perfusion: Abdominal Organs   **0404**

Definition: Adequacy of blood flow through the small vessels of the abdominal viscera to maintain organ function

OUTCOME TARGET RATING: Maintain at_____   Increase to_____

		Severe deviation from normal range	Substantial deviation from normal range	Moderate deviation from normal range	Mild deviation from normal range	No deviation from normal range	
OUTCOME OVERALL RATING		1	2	3	4	5	
Indicators:							
040424	Diastolic blood pressure	1	2	3	4	5	NA
040425	Systolic blood pressure	1	2	3	4	5	NA
040426	Mean blood pressure	1	2	3	4	5	NA
040402	Urine output	1	2	3	4	5	NA
040403	Electrolyte and acid/base balance	1	2	3	4	5	NA
040405	Bowel sounds	1	2	3	4	5	NA
040418	Urine specific gravity	1	2	3	4	5	NA
040419	Blood urea nitrogen	1	2	3	4	5	NA
040420	Plasma creatinine	1	2	3	4	5	NA
040421	Liver function test findings	1	2	3	4	5	NA
040422	Pancreatic enzymes	1	2	3	4	5	NA
		Severe	Substantial	Moderate	Mild	None	
040407	Abnormal thirst	1	2	3	4	5	NA
040408	Abdominal pain	1	2	3	4	5	NA
040409	Nausea	1	2	3	4	5	NA
040410	Vomiting	1	2	3	4	5	NA
040411	Malabsorption deficiencies	1	2	3	4	5	NA
040412	Chronic gastritis	1	2	3	4	5	NA
040413	Abdominal distention	1	2	3	4	5	NA
040414	Ascites	1	2	3	4	5	NA
040415	Gastrointestinal varices	1	2	3	4	5	NA
040416	Constipation	1	2	3	4	5	NA
040417	Diarrhea	1	2	3	4	5	NA
040427	Altered fluid balance	1	2	3	4	5	NA
040428	Loss of appetite	1	2	3	4	5	NA

Domain-Physiologic Health (II)   **Class-**Cardiopulmonary (E)   *1st edition 1997; revised 2004, 2008*

T

OUTCOME CONTENT REFERENCES:
Lewis, S. M., Collier, I. C., Heitkemper, M. M., & Dirksen, S. R. (2000). *Medical-surgical nursing: Assessment & management of clinical problems* (5th ed.). St. Louis: Mosby.
McCance, K. L., & Huether, S. E. (2002). *Pathophysiology: The biologic basis for disease in adults and children* (4th ed.). St. Louis: Mosby.
Smeltzer, S. C., & Bare, B. G. (2004). *Brunner & Suddarth's textbook of medical surgical nursing* (10th ed.). Philadelphia: Lippincott Williams & Wilkins.

Tissue Perfusion: Cardiac 0405

Definition: Adequacy of blood flow through the coronary vasculature to maintain heart function

OUTCOME TARGET RATING: Maintain at_____   Increase to_____

	Severe deviation from normal range	Substantial deviation from normal range	Moderate deviation from normal range	Mild deviation from normal range	No deviation from normal range	
OUTCOME OVERALL RATING	1	2	3	4	5	
Indicators:						
040515 Apical heart rate	1	2	3	4	5	NA
040516 Radial pulse rate	1	2	3	4	5	NA
040517 Systolic blood pressure	1	2	3	4	5	NA
040518 Diastolic blood pressure	1	2	3	4	5	NA
040519 Mean blood pressure	1	2	3	4	5	NA
040501 Ejection fraction	1	2	3	4	5	NA
040502 Pulmonary wedge pressure	1	2	3	4	5	NA
040503 Cardiac index	1	2	3	4	5	NA
040509 Electrocardiogram findings	1	2	3	4	5	NA
040510 Cardiac enzymes	1	2	3	4	5	NA
040511 Coronary angiogram findings	1	2	3	4	5	NA
040512 Exercise stress test findings	1	2	3	4	5	NA
040513 Thallium scan findings	1	2	3	4	5	NA

	Severe	Substantial	Moderate	Mild	None	
040504 Angina	1	2	3	4	5	NA
040520 Arrhythmia	1	2	3	4	5	NA
040521 Tachycardia	1	2	3	4	5	NA
040522 Bradycardia	1	2	3	4	5	NA
040505 Profuse diaphoresis	1	2	3	4	5	NA
040506 Nausea	1	2	3	4	5	NA
040507 Vomiting	1	2	3	4	5	NA

Domain-Physiologic Health (II)   *Class*-Cardiopulmonary (E)   *1st edition 1997; revised 2000, 2004, 2008*

OUTCOME CONTENT REFERENCES:
Lewis, S. M., Collier, I. C., Heitkemper, M. M., & Dirksen, S. R. (2000). *Medical-surgical nursing: Assessment & management of clinical problems* (5th ed.). St. Louis: Mosby.
McCance, K. L., & Huether, S. E. (2002). *Pathophysiology: The biologic basis for disease in adults and children* (4th ed.). St. Louis: Mosby.
Smeltzer, S. C., & Bare, B. G. (2004). *Brunner & Suddarth's textbook of medical surgical nursing* (10th ed.). Philadelphia: Lippincott Williams & Wilkins.

T

Tissue Perfusion: Cellular 0416

Definition: Adequacy of blood flow through the vasculature to maintain function at the cellular level

OUTCOME TARGET RATING: Maintain at_____ Increase to_____

		Severe deviation from normal range	Substantial deviation from normal range	Moderate deviation from normal range	Mild deviation from normal range	No deviation from normal range	
OUTCOME OVERALL RATING		1	2	3	4	5	
Indicators:							
041601	Systolic blood pressure	1	2	3	4	5	NA
041602	Diastolic blood pressure	1	2	3	4	5	NA
041603	Mean arterial blood gases	1	2	3	4	5	NA
041604	Oxygen saturation	1	2	3	4	5	NA
041605	Fluid balance	1	2	3	4	5	NA
041606	Apical heart rate	1	2	3	4	5	NA
041607	Heart rhythm	1	2	3	4	5	NA
041608	Electrolyte and acid/base balance	1	2	3	4	5	NA
041609	Capillary refill	1	2	3	4	5	NA
041610	Urine output	1	2	3	4	5	NA
041611	Creatinine clearance	1	2	3	4	5	NA
		Severe	Substantial	Moderate	Mild	None	
041612	Agitation	1	2	3	4	5	NA
041613	Necrosis	1	2	3	4	5	NA
041614	Nausea	1	2	3	4	5	NA
041615	Vomiting	1	2	3	4	5	NA
041616	Pain	1	2	3	4	5	NA
041617	Decreased level of consciousness	1	2	3	4	5	NA
041618	Pale cool skin	1	2	3	4	5	NA
041619	Skin breakdown	1	2	3	4	5	NA

Domain-*Physiologic Health (II)*   **Class**-*Cardiopulmonary (E)*   *4th edition 2008*

OUTCOME CONTENT REFERENCES:

Bridges, E. J., & Dukes, M. S. (2005). Cardiovascular aspects of septic shock: Pathophysiology, monitoring, and treatment. *Critical Care Nursing, 25*(2), 14–36.

Goodrich, D. (2006). Continuous central venous oximetry monitoring. *Critical Care Nursing Clinics, 18*(2), 203–209.

O'Donnell, J. M., & Nacul, F. (Eds.). (2001). *Surgical intensive care medicine* (pp. 411–425). Boston: Kluwer Academic.

Swearingen, P. L., & Keen, J. H. (Eds.). (2001). *Manual of critical care nursing: Nursing interventions and collaborative management* (4th ed., pp. 593–604). St. Louis: Mosby.

T

Tissue Perfusion: Cerebral   0406

Definition: Adequacy of blood flow through the cerebral vasculature to maintain brain function

OUTCOME TARGET RATING: Maintain at_____   Increase to_____

		Severe deviation from normal range	Substantial deviation from normal range	Moderate deviation from normal range	Mild deviation from normal range	No deviation from normal range	
OUTCOME OVERALL RATING		1	2	3	4	5	
Indicators:							
040602	Intracranial pressure	1	2	3	4	5	NA
040613	Systolic blood pressure	1	2	3	4	5	NA
040614	Diastolic blood pressure	1	2	3	4	5	NA
040617	Mean blood pressure	1	2	3	4	5	NA
040615	Cerebral angiogram findings	1	2	3	4	5	NA

		Severe	Substantial	Moderate	Mild	None	
040603	Headache	1	2	3	4	5	NA
040604	Carotid bruit	1	2	3	4	5	NA
040605	Restlessness	1	2	3	4	5	NA
040606	Listlessness	1	2	3	4	5	NA
040607	Unexplained anxiety	1	2	3	4	5	NA
040608	Agitation	1	2	3	4	5	NA
040609	Vomiting	1	2	3	4	5	NA
040610	Hiccoughs	1	2	3	4	5	NA
040611	Syncope	1	2	3	4	5	NA
040616	Fever	1	2	3	4	5	NA
040618	Impaired cognition	1	2	3	4	5	NA
040619	Decreased level of consciousness	1	2	3	4	5	NA
040620	Impaired neurological reflexes	1	2	3	4	5	NA

Domain-Physiologic Health (II)   *Class*-Cardiopulmonary (E)   *1st edition 1997; revised 2004, 2008*

OUTCOME CONTENT REFERENCES:
Lewis, S. M., Collier, I. C., Heitkemper, M. M., & Dirksen, S. R. (2000). *Medical-surgical nursing: Assessment & management of clinical problems* (5th ed.). St. Louis: Mosby.
McCance, K. L., & Huether, S. E. (2002). *Pathophysiology: The biologic basis for disease in adults and children* (4th ed.). St. Louis: Mosby.
Smeltzer, S. C., & Bare, B. G. (2004). *Brunner & Suddarth's textbook of medical surgical nursing* (10th ed.). Philadelphia: Lippincott Williams & Wilkins.

T

Tissue Perfusion: Peripheral   **0407**

Definition: Adequacy of blood flow through the small vessels of the extremities to maintain tissue function

OUTCOME TARGET RATING: Maintain at_____   Increase to_____

		Severe deviation from normal range	Substantial deviation from normal range	Moderate deviation from normal range	Mild deviation from normal range	No deviation from normal range	
OUTCOME OVERALL RATING		1	2	3	4	5	
Indicators:							
040715	Capillary refill fingers	1	2	3	4	5	NA
040716	Capillary refill toes	1	2	3	4	5	NA
040710	Extremity skin temperature	1	2	3	4	5	NA
040730	Carotid pulse strength (right)	1	2	3	4	5	NA
040731	Carotid pulse strength (left)	1	2	3	4	5	NA
040732	Brachial pulse strength (right)	1	2	3	4	5	NA
040733	Brachial pulse strength (left)	1	2	3	4	5	NA
040734	Radial pulse strength (right)	1	2	3	4	5	NA
040735	Radial pulse strength (left)	1	2	3	4	5	NA
040736	Femoral pulse strength (right)	1	2	3	4	5	NA
040737	Femoral pulse strength (left)	1	2	3	4	5	NA
040738	Pedal pulse strength (right)	1	2	3	4	5	NA
040739	Pedal pulse strength (left)	1	2	3	4	5	NA
040727	Systolic blood pressure	1	2	3	4	5	NA
040728	Diastolic blood pressure	1	2	3	4	5	NA
040740	Mean blood pressure	1	2	3	4	5	NA

		Severe	Substantial	Moderate	Mild	None	
040711	Extremity bruits	1	2	3	4	5	NA
040712	Peripheral edema	1	2	3	4	5	NA
040713	Localized extremity pain	1	2	3	4	5	NA
040729	Necrosis	1	2	3	4	5	NA
040741	Numbness	1	2	3	4	5	NA
040742	Tingling	1	2	3	4	5	NA
040743	Pallor	1	2	3	4	5	NA
040744	Muscle weakness	1	2	3	4	5	NA
040745	Muscle cramps	1	2	3	4	5	NA
040746	Skin breakdown	1	2	3	4	5	NA
040747	Rubor	1	2	3	4	5	NA
040748	Paresthesia	1	2	3	4	5	NA

Domain-*Physiologic Health (II)*   **Class**-*Cardiopulmonary (E)*   *1st edition 1997; revised 2004, 2008*

T

OUTCOME CONTENT REFERENCES:
Cohen, I. K., Diegelmann, R. F., & Lindblad, W. L. (1992). *Wound healing: Biochemical and clinical aspects*. Philadelphia: W. B. Saunders.
Lazarus, G. S., Cooper, D. M., Knighton, D. R., Margohs, D. J., Pecoraro, R. E., Rodeheaver, G., et al. (1994). Definitions and guidelines for assessment of wounds and evaluation of healing. *Archives of Dermatology, 130*(4), 489–493.
Maklebust, J., & Sieggreen, M. (1996). *Pressure ulcers: Guidelines for prevention and nursing management* (2nd ed.). Springhouse, PA: Springhouse.
Potter, P. A., & Perry, A. G. (2001). *Fundamentals of nursing* (5th ed.). St. Louis: Mosby.
Smeltzer, S. C., & Bare, B. G. (2004). *Brunner & Suddarth's textbook of medical surgical nursing* (10th ed.). Philadelphia: Lippincott Williams & Wilkins.
Van Rijswijk, L. (1993). Full-thickness leg ulcers: Patient demographics and predictors of healing. *The Journal of Family Practice, 36*(6), 625–632.

Tissue Perfusion: Pulmonary

0408

Definition: Adequacy of blood flow through pulmonary vasculature to perfuse alveoli/capillary unit

OUTCOME TARGET RATING: Maintain at_____   Increase to_____

	Severe deviation from normal range	Substantial deviation from normal range	Moderate deviation from normal range	Mild deviation from normal range	No deviation from normal range	
OUTCOME OVERALL RATING	1	2	3	4	5	
Indicators:						
040810 Ventilation-perfusion scan	1	2	3	4	5	NA
040811 Pulmonary artery pressure (PAP)	1	2	3	4	5	NA
040814 Respiratory rhythm	1	2	3	4	5	NA
040815 Respiratory rate	1	2	3	4	5	NA
040816 Systolic blood pressure	1	2	3	4	5	NA
040817 Diastolic blood pressure	1	2	3	4	5	NA
040822 Mean blood pressure	1	2	3	4	5	NA
040818 Partial pressure of oxygen in arterial blood (PaO_2)	1	2	3	4	5	NA
040819 Partial pressure of carbon dioxide in arterial blood ($PaCO_2$)	1	2	3	4	5	NA
040820 Arterial pH	1	2	3	4	5	NA
040821 Oxygen saturation	1	2	3	4	5	NA

	Severe	Substantial	Moderate	Mild	None	
040805 Chest pain	1	2	3	4	5	NA
040806 Pleural friction rub	1	2	3	4	5	NA
040807 Hemoptysis	1	2	3	4	5	NA
040808 Unexplained anxiety	1	2	3	4	5	NA
040823 Shortness of breath	1	2	3	4	5	NA
040824 Impaired gas exchange	1	2	3	4	5	NA

Domain-*Physiologic Health (II)*   **Class**-*Cardiopulmonary (E)*   *1st edition 1997; revised 2004, 2008*

OUTCOME CONTENT REFERENCES:

Lewis, S. M., Collier, I. C., Heitkemper, M. M., & Dirksen, S. R. (2000). *Medical-surgical nursing: Assessment & management of clinical problems* (5th ed.). St. Louis: Mosby.

McCance, K. L., & Huether, S. E. (2002). *Pathophysiology: The biologic basis for disease in adults and children* (4th ed.). St. Louis: Mosby.

Smeltzer, S. C., & Bare, B. G. (2004). *Brunner & Suddarth's textbook of medical surgical nursing* (10th ed.). Philadelphia: Lippincott Williams & Wilkins.

T

Transfer Performance 0210

Definition: Ability to change body location independently with or without assistive device

OUTCOME TARGET RATING: Maintain at_____ Increase to_____

		Severely compromised	Substantially compromised	Moderately compromised	Mildly compromised	Not compromised	
OUTCOME OVERALL RATING		1	2	3	4	5	
Indicators:							
021009	Transfers from one surface to another while lying	1	2	3	4	5	NA
021001	Transfers from bed to chair	1	2	3	4	5	NA
021002	Transfers from chair to bed	1	2	3	4	5	NA
021003	Transfers from chair to chair	1	2	3	4	5	NA
021004	Transfers from wheelchair to vehicle	1	2	3	4	5	NA
021005	Transfers from vehicle to wheelchair	1	2	3	4	5	NA
021007	Transfers from wheelchair to toilet	1	2	3	4	5	NA
021008	Transfers from toilet to wheelchair	1	2	3	4	5	NA

Domain-*Functional Health (I)*   **Class**-*Mobility (C)*   *1st edition 1997; revised 2004, 2008*

OUTCOME CONTENT REFERENCES:

+*Guide for the Uniform Data Set for Medical Rehabilitation* (including the FIM™ instrument) (version 5.1). (1997). Buffalo, NY: University at Buffalo.

Kane, R. L., & Kane, R. A. (2000). *Assessing older persons: Measures, meaning, and practical applications.* New York: Oxford University Press.

Mikulic, M. A., Griffith, E. R., & Jebsen, R. H. (1976). Clinical application of a standardized mobility test. *Archives of Physical Medicine and Rehabilitation, 57*(3), 143–146.

T

Urinary Continence   0502

Definition: Control of elimination of urine from the bladder

OUTCOME TARGET RATING: Maintain at_____   Increase to_____

		Never demonstrated	Rarely demonstrated	Sometimes demonstrated	Often demonstrated	Consistently demonstrated	
OUTCOME OVERALL RATING		1	2	3	4	5	
Indicators:							
050201	Recognizes urge to void	1	2	3	4	5	NA
050202	Maintains predictable pattern of voiding	1	2	3	4	5	NA
050203	Responds to urge in timely manner	1	2	3	4	5	NA
050204	Voids in appropriate receptacle	1	2	3	4	5	NA
050205	Gets to toilet between urge and passage of urine	1	2	3	4	5	NA
050218	Maintains barrier-free environment for independent toileting	1	2	3	4	5	NA
050206	Voids >150 milliliters each time	1	2	3	4	5	NA
050208	Starts and stops stream	1	2	3	4	5	NA
050209	Empties bladder completely	1	2	3	4	5	NA
050215	Ingests adequate amount of fluid	1	2	3	4	5	NA
050216	Manages clothing independently	1	2	3	4	5	NA
050217	Toilets independently	1	2	3	4	5	NA
050219	Identifies medication that interferes with urinary control	1	2	3	4	5	NA

		Consistently demonstrated	Often demonstrated	Sometimes demonstrated	Rarely demonstrated	Never demonstrated	
050207	Urine leakage between voidings	1	2	3	4	5	NA
050210	Post void residual >100-200 milliliters	1	2	3	4	5	NA
050211	Urine leakage with increased abdominal pressure (e.g., sneezing, laughing, lifting)	1	2	3	4	5	NA
050212	Wets clothing during day	1	2	3	4	5	NA
050213	Wets clothing or bedding during night	1	2	3	4	5	NA
050214	Urinary tract infection	1	2	3	4	5	NA

Domain-Physiologic Health (II)   *Class*-Elimination (F)   *1st edition 1997; revised 2004*

U

OUTCOME CONTENT REFERENCES:

Lewthwaite, B., & Girouard, L. (2006). Urinary drainage following continence surgery: Development of Canadian best practice guidelines. *Urologic Nursing, 26*(1), 33–39.

+Morris, J. N., Hawes, C., Fries, B. E., Phillips, C. D., Mor, V., Katz, S., et al. (1990). Designing the national resident assessment instrument for nursing homes. *Gerontologist 30*(3), 293–307.

+O'Donnell, P. D., & Calandro, V. J. (1991). Incontinence Management Scale for elderly inpatient men. *Urology, 37*(3), 220–223.

Palmer, M. H., McCormick, K. A., Langford, A., Langlais, J., & Alvaran, M. (1992). Continence outcomes: Documentation on medical records in the nursing home environment. *Journal of Nursing Care Quality, 6*(3), 36–43.

Specht, J. P., & Maas, M. L. (2001). Urinary incontinence: Functional, iatrogenic, overflow, reflex, stress, total, and urge. In M. Maas, K. Buckwalter, M. Hardy, T. Tripp-Reimer, M. Titler, & J. Specht (Eds.), *Nursing care of older adults: Diagnoses, outcomes & interventions* (pp. 252–278). St. Louis: Mosby.

Viktrup, L., Summers, K. H., & Dennett, S. L. (2004). Clinical practice guidelines for the initial management of urinary incontinence in women: A European-focused review. *BJU International Journal, 94*(Suppl. 1), 14–22.

Urinary Elimination   0503

Definition: Collection and discharge of urine

OUTCOME TARGET RATING: Maintain at_____   Increase to_____

		Severely compromised	Substantially compromised	Moderately compromised	Mildly compromised	Not compromised	
OUTCOME OVERALL RATING		1	2	3	4	5	
Indicators:							
050301	Elimination pattern	1	2	3	4	5	NA
050302	Urine odor	1	2	3	4	5	NA
050303	Urine amount	1	2	3	4	5	NA
050304	Urine color	1	2	3	4	5	NA
050306	Urine clarity	1	2	3	4	5	NA
050307	Fluid intake	1	2	3	4	5	NA
050313	Empties bladder completely	1	2	3	4	5	NA
050314	Recognition of urge	1	2	3	4	5	NA

		Severe	Substantial	Moderate	Mild	None	
050305	Visible urine particles	1	2	3	4	5	NA
050329	Visible blood in urine	1	2	3	4	5	NA
050309	Pain with urination	1	2	3	4	5	NA
050330	Burning with urination	1	2	3	4	5	NA
050310	Hesitancy with urination	1	2	3	4	5	NA
050331	Urinary frequency	1	2	3	4	5	NA
050311	Urgency with urination	1	2	3	4	5	NA
050332	Urinary retention	1	2	3	4	5	NA
050333	Nocturia	1	2	3	4	5	NA
050312	Urinary incontinence	1	2	3	4	5	NA
050334	Stress incontinence	1	2	3	4	5	NA
050335	Urge incontinence	1	2	3	4	5	NA
050336	Functional incontinence	1	2	3	4	5	NA

Domain-Physiologic Health (II)   **Class**-Elimination (F)   *1st edition 1997; revised 2004*

OUTCOME CONTENT REFERENCES:

Anonymous. (2006). In brief: Kegels hold up as urinary continence treatment. *Harvard Women's Health Watch, 13*(9), 7.

Anonymous. (2006). Promoting urinary continence in older people. *Nursing Older People, 18*(3), 35–36.

Borello-France, D. F., Zyczynski, H. M., Downey, P. A., Rause, C. R., & Wister, J. A. (2006). Effect of pelvic-floor muscle exercise position on continence and quality-of-life outcomes in women with stress urinary incontinence. *Physical Therapy, 86*(7), 974–986.

Brundage, D. J., & Linton, A. D. (1997). Age related changes in the genitourinary system. In M. A. Matteson, E. S. McConnell, & A. D. Linton (Eds.), *Gerontological nursing: Concepts in practice* (2nd ed.). Philadelphia: W. B. Saunders.

Burns, P. A. (2006). A nurse led continence service reduced symptoms of incontinence, frequency, urgency, and nocturia. *Evidence-Based Nursing, 9*(3), 85.

Morton, P. G. (1989). *Health assessment in nursing.* Springhouse, PA: Springhouse.

Palmer, M. H., McCormick, K. A., Langford, A., Langlais, J., & Alvaran, M. (1992). Continence outcomes: Documentation on medical records in the nursing home environment. *Journal of Nursing Care Quality, 6*(3), 36–43.

Potter, P. A., & Perry, A. G. (2001). *Fundamentals of nursing* (5th ed.). St. Louis: Mosby.

Vision Compensation Behavior 1611

Definition: Personal actions to compensate for visual impairment

OUTCOME TARGET RATING: Maintain at_____ Increase to_____

		Never demonstrated	Rarely demonstrated	Sometimes demonstrated	Often demonstrated	Consistently demonstrated	
OUTCOME OVERALL RATING		1	2	3	4	5	
Indicators:							
161101	Monitors symptoms of vision deterioration	1	2	3	4	5	NA
161102	Positions self to advantage vision	1	2	3	4	5	NA
161103	Reminds others to use techniques that advantage vision	1	2	3	4	5	NA
161104	Uses adequate lighting for activity being performed	1	2	3	4	5	NA
161105	Wears eyeglasses correctly	1	2	3	4	5	NA
161106	Wears contact lenses correctly	1	2	3	4	5	NA
161107	Cares for eyewear correctly	1	2	3	4	5	NA
161108	Uses vision assistive devices	1	2	3	4	5	NA
161109	Uses computer assistive devices	1	2	3	4	5	NA
161113	Uses animal assistance	1	2	3	4	5	NA
161110	Uses support services for low-vision	1	2	3	4	5	NA
161111	Uses Braille	1	2	3	4	5	NA

Domain-*Health & Knowledge Behavior (IV)* **Class**-*Health Behavior (Q)* *2nd edition 2000; revised 2004*

OUTCOME CONTENT REFERENCES:
Burrell, L. O. (Ed). (1992). *Adult nursing in hospital and community settings.* Norwalk, CT: Appleton & Lange.
Phipps, W. J., Monahan, F. D., Sands J. K., Marek, J., & Neighbors, M. (Eds.). (2003). *Medical-surgical nursing: Concepts and clinical practice* (7th ed). St. Louis: Mosby.
Smeltzer, S. C., & Bare, B. G. (Eds.). (2003). *Brunner and Suddarth's textbook of medical-surgical nursing* (10th ed.). Philadelphia: Lippincott Williams & Wilkins.

V

Vital Signs 0802

Definition: Extent to which temperature, pulse, respiration, and blood pressure are within normal range

OUTCOME TARGET RATING: Maintain at_____   Increase to_____

	Severe deviation from normal range	Substantial deviation from normal range	Moderate deviation from normal range	Mild deviation from normal range	No deviation from normal range	
OUTCOME OVERALL RATING	1	2	3	4	5	
Indicators:						
080201 Body temperature	1	2	3	4	5	NA
080202 Apical heart rate	1	2	3	4	5	NA
080208 Apical heart rhythm	1	2	3	4	5	NA
080203 Radial pulse rate	1	2	3	4	5	NA
080204 Respiratory rate	1	2	3	4	5	NA
080210 Respiratory rhythm	1	2	3	4	5	NA
080205 Systolic blood pressure	1	2	3	4	5	NA
080206 Diastolic blood pressure	1	2	3	4	5	NA
080209 Pulse pressure	1	2	3	4	5	NA
080211 Depth of inspiration	1	2	3	4	5	NA

Domain-*Physiologic Health (II)*   **Class**-*Metabolic Regulation (I)*   *1st edition 1997; revised 2004, 2008*

OUTCOME CONTENT REFERENCES:
Caruso, C., Hadley, B., Shukla, R., & Frame, P. (1992). Cooling effects and comfort of four cooling blanket temperatures in humans with fever. *Nursing Research*, *41*(2), 68–72.
Finke, C. (1991). Measurement of the thermoregulatory response: A review. *Focus on Critical Care*, *18*(5), 408–412.
Summers, S., Dudgeon, N., Byram, K., & Zingsheim, K. (1990). The effects of two warming methods on core and surface temperatures, hemoglobin oxygen saturation, blood pressure, and perceived comfort of hypothermic postanesthesia patients. *Journal of Post Anesthesia Nursing*, *5*(5), 354–364.
Thomas, S. A., Liehr, P., DeKeyser, F., Frazier, L., & Friedmann, E. (2002). A review of nursing research on blood pressure. *Journal of Nursing Scholarship*, *34*(4), 313–321.

V

Weight: Body Mass 1006

Definition: Extent to which body weight, muscle, and fat are congruent to height, frame, gender and age

OUTCOME TARGET RATING: Maintain at_____ Increase to_____

		Severe deviation from normal range	Substantial deviation from normal range	Moderate deviation from normal range	Mild deviation from normal range	No deviation from normal range	
OUTCOME OVERALL RATING		1	2	3	4	5	
Indicators:							
100601	Weight	1	2	3	4	5	NA
100602	Triceps skinfold thickness	1	2	3	4	5	NA
100603	Subscapular skinfold thickness	1	2	3	4	5	NA
100604	Waist/hip circumference ratio (women)	1	2	3	4	5	NA
100605	Neck/waist circumference ratio (men)	1	2	3	4	5	NA
100606	Body fat percentage	1	2	3	4	5	NA
100607	Head circumference percentile (child)	1	2	3	4	5	NA
100608	Height percentile (child)	1	2	3	4	5	NA
100609	Weight percentile (child)	1	2	3	4	5	NA

Domain-*Physiologic Health (II)* **Class**-*Metabolic Regulation (I)* *1st edition 1997; revised 2004*

OUTCOME CONTENT REFERENCES:

Collinsworth, R., & Boyle, K. (1989). Nutritional assessment of the elderly. *Journal of Gerontological Nursing, 15*(12), 17–21.

Curtas, S., Chapman, G., & Meguid, M. (1989). Evaluation of nutritional status. *Nursing Clinics of North America, 24*(2), 301–313.

Flegal, K. M., Tabak, C. J., & Ogden, C. L. (2006). Overweight in children: Definitions and interpretation. *Health Education Research, 21*(6), 755–760.

Folsom, A. R., Kaye, S. A., Sellers, T. A., Hang, C. P., Cerhan, J. R., Potter, J. D., et al. (1993). Body fat distribution and five-year risk of death in older women. *Journal of the American Medical Association, 269*(4), 483–487.

Gianino, S., & St. John, R. E. (1993). Nutritional assessment of the patient in the intensive care unit. *Critical Care Nursing Clinics of North America, 5*(1), 1–16.

Koo, W. W., & Hockman, E. M. (2006). Post hospital discharge feeding for preterm infants: Effects of standard compared with enriched milk formula on growth, bone mass, and body composition. *American Journal of Clinical Nutrition, 84*(6), 1357–1364.

Moscicki, A., Ellenberg, J. H., Murphy, D. A., & Jiahong, X. (2006). Associations among body composition, androgen levels, and human immunodeficiency virus status in adolescents. *Journal of Adolescent Health, 39*(2), 164–173.

Yang, F., Lu, J. H., Lei, S. F., Chen, X. D., Liu, M. Y., Jian, W. X., et al. (2006). Receiver-operating characteristic analysis of body mass index, waist circumference and waist-to-hip ratio for obesity: Screening in young adults in central south of China. *Clinical Nutrition, 25*(6), 1030–1039.

W

Weight Gain Behavior 1626

Definition: Personal actions to gain weight following voluntary or involuntary significant weight loss

OUTCOME TARGET RATING: Maintain at_____ Increase to_____

		Never demonstrated	Rarely demonstrated	Sometimes demonstrated	Often demonstrated	Consistently demonstrated	
OUTCOME OVERALL RATING		1	2	3	4	5	
Indicators:							
162601	Obtains assistance for weight from health professional	1	2	3	4	5	NA
162602	Identifies cause of weight loss	1	2	3	4	5	NA
162603	Receives proper dental care	1	2	3	4	5	NA
162604	Sets achievable weight gain goals	1	2	3	4	5	NA
162605	Selects a healthy target weight	1	2	3	4	5	NA
162606	Commits to a healthy eating plan	1	2	3	4	5	NA
162607	Identifies caloric intake requirements	1	2	3	4	5	NA
162608	Maintains an adequate supply of nutritious food and fluid	1	2	3	4	5	NA
162609	Obtains financial assistance for purchasing food	1	2	3	4	5	NA
162610	Prepares food to enhance swallowing	1	2	3	4	5	NA
162611	Uses flavor enhancers	1	2	3	4	5	NA
162612	Obtains assistance with food preparation	1	2	3	4	5	NA
162613	Identifies food and fluid preferences and dislikes	1	2	3	4	5	NA
162614	Identifies food allergies	1	2	3	4	5	NA
162615	Uses vitamin/mineral supplements	1	2	3	4	5	NA
162616	Drinks eight glasses of water daily	1	2	3	4	5	NA
162617	Recognizes signs and symptoms of electrolyte imbalance	1	2	3	4	5	NA
162618	Obtains treatment for electrolyte imbalance	1	2	3	4	5	NA
162619	Monitors appetite level	1	2	3	4	5	NA
162620	Uses prescribed medication to increase appetite	1	2	3	4	5	NA
162621	Uses prescribed medication to enhance weight gain	1	2	3	4	5	NA
162622	Uses nutrient supplements	1	2	3	4	5	NA
162623	Selects high-protein, high-calorie food and fluid	1	2	3	4	5	NA
162624	Eats nutritious food and fluid between meals	1	2	3	4	5	NA
162625	Maintains fluid balance	1	2	3	4	5	NA
162626	Maintains adequate sleep	1	2	3	4	5	NA
162627	Uses diary to monitor food and fluid intake	1	2	3	4	5	NA
162628	Administers enteral tube feedings as recommended	1	2	3	4	5	NA
162629	Administers parenteral nutrition as recommended	1	2	3	4	5	NA
162630	Monitors exercise for caloric requirements	1	2	3	4	5	NA

W

Weight Gain Behavior—*cont'd*

		Never demonstrated	Rarely demonstrated	Sometimes demonstrated	Often demonstrated	Consistently demonstrated	
162631	Uses personal support system to enhance weight gain	1	2	3	4	5	NA
162632	Participates in support groups	1	2	3	4	5	NA
162633	Participates in nutritional monitoring	1	2	3	4	5	NA
162634	Monitors body mass index	1	2	3	4	5	NA
162635	Monitors body weight	1	2	3	4	5	NA

Target weight: _____ kg/lb

Domain-Health Knowledge & Behavior (IV) **Class**-Health Behavior (Q) 4th edition 2008

OUTCOME CONTENT REFERENCES:

Ferguson, M., Cook, A., Bender, S., Rimmasch, H., & Voss, A. (2001). Diagnosing and treating involuntary weight loss. *MEDSURG Nursing*, *10*(4), 165–177.

Huffman, G. B. (2002). Evaluating and treating unintentional weight loss in the elderly. *American Family Physician*, *65*(4), 640–650.

Martin, H., & Ammerman, S. D. (2002). Adolescents with eating disorders: Primary care screening, identification, and early intervention. *Nursing Clinics of North America*, *37*(3), 537–551.

NIH Technology Assessment Conference Panel. Methods for voluntary weight loss and control. *Annals of Internal Medicine*, *119*(7), 764–770.

National Institute for Health and Clinical Excellence. (2006). *Nutrition support in adults: Oral nutrition support, enteral tube feeding and parenteral nutrition.* London: Author.

Orphanidou, C. I., McCargar, L. J., Birmingham, C. L., & Belzberg, A. S. (1997). Changes in body composition and fat distribution after short-term weight gain in patients with anorexia nervosa. *American Journal of Clinical Nutrition*, *65*(4), 1034–1041.

Wolfe, B. E., & Gimby, L. B. (2003). Caring for the hospitalized patient with an eating disorder. *Nursing Clinics of North America*, *38*(1), 75–99.

Yaari, S., & Goldbourt, U. (1998). Voluntary and involuntary weight loss: Associations with long-term mortality in 9,228 middle-aged and elderly men. *American Journal of Epidemiology*, *148*(6), 546–555.

Yeh, S., DeGuzman, B., & Kramer, T. (2002). Reversal of COPD-associated weight loss using the anabolic agent oxandrolone. *Chest*, *122*(2), 421–428.

Weight Loss Behavior 1627

Definition: Personal actions to lose weight through diet, exercise, and behavior modification

OUTCOME TARGET RATING: Maintain at_____ Increase to_____

		Never demonstrated	Rarely demonstrated	Sometimes demonstrated	Often demonstrated	Consistently demonstrated	
OUTCOME OVERALL RATING		1	2	3	4	5	
Indicators:							
162701	Obtains information on weight loss strategies from health professional	1	2	3	4	5	NA
162702	Selects a healthy target weight	1	2	3	4	5	NA
162703	Commits to a healthy eating plan	1	2	3	4	5	NA
162704	Selects nutritious food and fluid	1	2	3	4	5	NA
162705	Controls food portion	1	2	3	4	5	NA
162706	Establishes an exercise routine	1	2	3	4	5	NA
162707	Caloric expenditure exceeds caloric intake	1	2	3	4	5	NA
162708	Controls preoccupation with food	1	2	3	4	5	NA
162709	Identifies emotional states that affect food and fluid intake	1	2	3	4	5	NA
162710	Identifies social situations that affect food and fluid intake	1	2	3	4	5	NA

W

Continued

Weight Loss Behavior—cont'd

		Never demonstrated	Rarely demonstrated	Sometimes demonstrated	Often demonstrated	Consistently demonstrated	
162711	Plans for situations that affect food and fluid intake	1	2	3	4	5	NA
162712	Uses behavior modification strategies	1	2	3	4	5	NA
162713	Uses self-talk motivation	1	2	3	4	5	NA
162714	Avoids high-caloric food and fluid	1	2	3	4	5	NA
162715	Drinks eight glasses of water daily	1	2	3	4	5	NA
162716	Includes vitamins in weight loss plan	1	2	3	4	5	NA
162717	Uses appetite suppressants as prescribed	1	2	3	4	5	NA
162718	Uses weight loss medication as prescribed	1	2	3	4	5	NA
162719	Uses personal support system to enhance weight loss	1	2	3	4	5	NA
162720	Participates in weight loss support group	1	2	3	4	5	NA
162721	Manages setbacks by resuming weight loss efforts	1	2	3	4	5	NA
162722	Monitors body weight	1	2	3	4	5	NA
162723	Monitors body mass index	1	2	3	4	5	NA
162724	Uses diary to monitor food and fluid intake	1	2	3	4	5	NA
162725	Uses diary to monitor exercise over time	1	2	3	4	5	NA
162726	Maintains progress toward target weight	1	2	3	4	5	NA
162727	Uses commercial diet products safely	1	2	3	4	5	NA

Target weight: _____ kg/lb

Domain-Health Knowledge & Behavior (IV)   **Class**-Health Behavior (Q)   4th edition 2008

OUTCOME CONTENT REFERENCES:

Budd, G. M., & Volpe, S. L. (2006). School-based obesity prevention: Research, challenges, and recommendations. *Journal of School Health, 76*(10), 485–495.

Dennis, K. E. (2004). Weight management in women. *Nursing Clinics of North America, 39*(1), 231–241.

Fabricatore, A. N. (2007). Behavior therapy and cognitive-behavioral therapy of obesity: Is there a difference? *Journal of the American Dietetic Association, 107*(1), 92–99.

National Institutes of Health. (2000). *The practical guide: Identification, evaluation, and treatment of overweight and obesity in adults.* Bethesda, MD: U.S. Department of Health and Human Services.

Patel, S. R., Malhotra, A., White, D. P., Gottlieb, D. J., & Hu, F. B. (2006). Association between reduced sleep and weight gain in women. *American Journal of Epidemiology, 164*(10), 947–954.

Tyler, D. O., Allan, J. D., & Alcozer, F. R. (1997). Weight loss methods used by African American and Euro-American women. *Research in Nursing & Health, 20*(5), 413–423.

W

Weight Maintenance Behavior   1628

Definition: Personal actions to maintain optimum body weight

OUTCOME TARGET RATING: Maintain at_____ Increase to_____

		Never demonstrated	Rarely demonstrated	Sometimes demonstrated	Often demonstrated	Consistently demonstrated	
OUTCOME OVERALL RATING		1	2	3	4	5	
Indicators:							
162801	Monitors body weight	1	2	3	4	5	NA
162802	Maintains optimal daily caloric intake	1	2	3	4	5	NA
162803	Balances exercise with caloric intake	1	2	3	4	5	NA
162804	Selects nutritious meals	1	2	3	4	5	NA
162805	Selects nutritious snacks	1	2	3	4	5	NA
162806	Drinks eight glasses of water daily	1	2	3	4	5	NA
162807	Uses nutrient supplements as needed	1	2	3	4	5	NA
162808	Eats in response to hunger	1	2	3	4	5	NA
162809	Maintains recommended eating pattern	1	2	3	4	5	NA
162810	Retains ingested foods	1	2	3	4	5	NA
162811	Maintains fluid balance	1	2	3	4	5	NA
162812	Obtains assistance from health professional	1	2	3	4	5	NA
162813	Uses personal support systems	1	2	3	4	5	NA
162814	Identifies social situations that affect food and fluid intake	1	2	3	4	5	NA
162815	Identifies emotional states that affect food and fluid intake	1	2	3	4	5	NA
162816	Plans for situations that affect food and fluid intake	1	2	3	4	5	NA
162817	Controls preoccupation with food	1	2	3	4	5	NA
162818	Controls preoccupation with weight	1	2	3	4	5	NA
162819	Expresses realistic body image	1	2	3	4	5	NA
162820	Maintains adequate sleep	1	2	3	4	5	NA
162821	Maintains optimum weight	1	2	3	4	5	NA

Target weight: _____ kg/lb

Domain-*Health Knowledge & Behavior (IV)*   **Class**-*Health Behavior (Q)*   *4th edition 2008*

OUTCOME CONTENT REFERENCES:

American Psychiatric Association. (1993). Practice guideline for eating disorders. *American Journal of Psychiatry, 150*(2), 212–223.

Bruce, B., & Wilfley, D. (1996). Binge eating among the overweight population: A serious and prevalent problem. *Journal of the American Dietetic Association, 96*(1), 58–62.

Chang, B. L., Uman, G. C., Linn, L. S., Ware, J. E., & Kane, R. L. (1985). Adherence to health care regimens among elderly women. *Nursing Research, 34*(1) 27–31.

Curtas, S., Chapman, G., & Meguid, M. (1989). Evaluation of nutritional status. *Nursing Clinics of North America, 24*(2), 301–313.

Farrow, J. (1992). The adolescent male with an eating disorder. *Pediatric Annals, 21*(11), 769–774.

Fisher, M., Golden, N. H., Katzman, D. K., Kreipe, R. E., Rees, J., Schebendach, J., et al. (1995). Eating disorders in adolescents: A background paper. *Journal of Adolescent Health, 16*(6), 420–437.

Halmi, K. (1994). A multimodal model for understanding and treating eating disorders. *Journal of Women's Health, 3*(6), 487–493.

Hawks, S. R., & Richins, P. (1994). Toward a new paradigm for the management of obesity. *Journal of Health Education, 25*(3), 147–153.

National Heart, Lung and Blood Institute. (2005). *Aim for a healthy weight* (NIH Publication No. 05-5213). Bethesda, MD: U.S. Department of Health and Human Services.

Wilson, P., Herman, J., & Chubon, S. J. (1991). Eating strategies used by persons with head and neck cancer during and after radiotherapy. *Cancer Nursing, 14*(2), 98–104.

Yates, A. (1992). Biologic considerations in the etiology of eating disorders. *Pediatric Annuals, 21*(11), 739–744.

W

Will to Live

1206

Definition: Desire, determination, and effort to survive

OUTCOME TARGET RATING: Maintain at_____   Increase to_____

OUTCOME OVERALL RATING		Severely compromised	Substantially compromised	Moderately compromised	Mildly compromised	Not compromised	
		1	2	3	4	5	
Indicators:							
120601	Expression of determination to live	1	2	3	4	5	NA
120602	Expression of hope	1	2	3	4	5	NA
120603	Expression of optimism	1	2	3	4	5	NA
120604	Expression of sense of control	1	2	3	4	5	NA
120605	Expression of feelings	1	2	3	4	5	NA
120617	Interest in one's illness	1	2	3	4	5	NA
120618	Interest in one's treatment	1	2	3	4	5	NA
120608	Use of strategies to compensate for problems associated with disease	1	2	3	4	5	NA
120613	Use of treatments to lengthen life	1	2	3	4	5	NA
120609	Use of strategies to enhance health	1	2	3	4	5	NA
120610	Use of strategies to lengthen life	1	2	3	4	5	NA
		Severe	**Substantial**	**Moderate**	**Mild**	**None**	
120614	Depression	1	2	3	4	5	NA
120615	Suicidal thoughts	1	2	3	4	5	NA
120616	Pessimistic thoughts	1	2	3	4	5	NA

Domain-*Psychosocial Health (III)*   **Class**-*Psychological Well-Being (M)*   *1st edition 1997; revised 2004, 2008*

OUTCOME CONTENT REFERENCES:

Chochinov, H. M., Hack, T., Hassard, T., Kristjanson, L. J., McClement, S., & Harlos, M. (2005). Dignity therapy: A novel psychotherapeutic intervention for patients near the end of life. *Journal of Clinical Oncology, 23*(24), 5520–5525.

Dickerson, S. S., Boehmke, M., Ogle, C., & Brown, J. K. (2006). Seeking and managing hope: Patients' experiences using the Internet for cancer care. *Oncology Nursing Forum, 33*(1), E8–E17.

Gaskins, S., & Brown, K. (1992). Psychosocial responses among individuals with human immunodeficiency virus infection. *Applied Nursing Research, 5*(3), 111–121.

Greer, S., Morris, T., & Pettingale, K. (1979). Psychological response to breast cancer: Effect on outcome. *The Lancet, 2*(8146), 785–787.

Hagopian, G. (1993). Cognitive strategies used in adapting to a cancer diagnosis. *Oncology Nursing Forum, 20*(5), 759–763.

+Ivanoff, A., Joon Jang, S., Smyth, N. J., & Linehan, M. M. (1994). Fewer reasons for staying alive when you are thinking of killing yourself: The Brief Reasons for Living Inventory. *Journal of Psychopathology and Behavioral Assessment, 16*(1), 1–13.

Katz, R., & Lowe, L. (1989). The "will to live" as perceived by nurses and physicians. *Issues in Mental Health Nursing, 10*(1), 15–22.

+Linehan, M. M., Goodstein, J. L., Nielsen, S. L., & Chiles, J. A. (1983). Reasons for staying alive when you are thinking of killing yourself: The Reasons for Living Inventory. *Journal of Consulting and Clinical Psychology, 51*(2), 276–286, 484–485.

Lipman, M. M. (2005). Office visit: Creating a will to live by. *Consumer Reports on Health, 17*(6), 11.

Richardson, A. (2004). Creating a culture of compassion: Developing supportive care for people with cancer. *European Journal of Oncology Nursing, 8*(4), 293–305.

Weisman, A. (1972). *On death and denying: A psychiatric study of terminality.* New York: Behavioral Publications.

W

Wound Healing: Primary Intention 1102

Definition: Extent of regeneration of cells and tissues following intentional closure

OUTCOME TARGET RATING: Maintain at_____   Increase to_____

	None	Limited	Moderate	Substantial	Extensive	
OUTCOME OVERALL RATING	1	2	3	4	5	
Indicators:						
110201 Skin approximation	1	2	3	4	5	NA
110213 Wound edge approximation	1	2	3	4	5	NA
110214 Scar formation	1	2	3	4	5	NA

	Extensive	Substantial	Moderate	Limited	None	
110202 Purulent drainage	1	2	3	4	5	NA
110203 Serous drainage	1	2	3	4	5	NA
110204 Sanguineous drainage	1	2	3	4	5	NA
110205 Serosanguineous drainage	1	2	3	4	5	NA
110206 Sanguineous drainage from drain	1	2	3	4	5	NA
110207 Serosanguineous drainage from drain	1	2	3	4	5	NA
110208 Surrounding skin erythema	1	2	3	4	5	NA
110215 Surrounding skin bruising	1	2	3	4	5	NA
110209 Periwound edema	1	2	3	4	5	NA
110210 Increased skin temperature	1	2	3	4	5	NA
110211 Foul wound odor	1	2	3	4	5	NA

Location of wound (# from picture): _____

Domain-*Physiologic Health (II)*   **Class**-*Tissue Integrity (L)*   *1st edition 1997; revised 2004*

1. Front of head
2. Right ear
3. Left ear
4. Front of neck
5. Right chest
6. Left chest
7. Sternum
8. Right upper quadrant
9. Left upper quadrant
10. Right lower quadrant
11. Left lower quadrant
12. Abdominal midline
13. Navel
14. Pubic and perineal area
15. Right trochanter (hip)
16. Left trochanter (hip)
17. Right anterior thigh
18. Right knee
19. Right lower anterior leg
20. Right ankle (inner/outer)
21. Right foot
22. Right toes

23. Left anterior thigh
24. Left knee
25. Left lower anterior leg
26. Left ankle (inner/outer)
27. Left foot
28. Left toes
29. Right upper interior arm
30. Right interior forearm
31. Right wrist
32. Right palm
33. Right fingers _____(specify)
34. Left upper interior arm
35. Left interior forearm
36. Left wrist
37. Left palm
38. Left fingers _____(specify)
39. Back of head
40. Back of neck
41. Left scapula
42. Right scapula
43. Spine
44. Left back

45. Right back
46. Left buttock
47. Right buttock
48. Sacrum
49. Left posterior thigh
50. Left lower posterior leg
51. Left heel
52. Left bottom foot
53. Right posterior thigh
54. Right lower posterior leg
55. Right heel
56. Right bottom foot
57. Left upper posterior arm
58. Left elbow
59. Left posterior forearm
60. Left dorsal hand
61. Right upper posterior arm
62. Right elbow
63. Right posterior forearm
64. Right dorsal hand

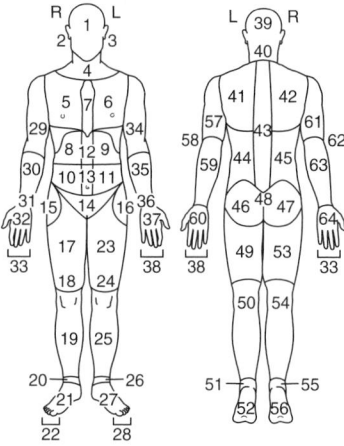

OUTCOME CONTENT REFERENCES:
Cohen, I. K., Diegelmann, R. F., & Lindblad, W. L. (1992). *Wound healing: Biochemical and clinical aspects.* Philadelphia: W. B. Saunders.
+Holden-Lund, C. (1988). Effects of relaxation with guided imagery on surgical stress and wound healing. *Research in Nursing & Health, 11*(4), 235–244.
Lazarus, G. S., Cooper, D. M., Knighton, D. R., Margohs, D. J., Pecoraro, R. E., Rodeheaver, G., et al. (1994). Definitions and guidelines for assessment of wounds and evaluation of healing. *Archives of Dermatology, 130*(4), 489–493.
Potter, P. A., & Perry, A. G. (2001). *Fundamentals of nursing* (5th ed.). St. Louis: Mosby.

W

Wound Healing: Secondary Intention　　1103

Definition: Extent of regeneration of cells and tissues in an open wound

OUTCOME TARGET RATING: Maintain at_____　　Increase to_____

		None	Limited	Moderate	Substantial	Extensive	
OUTCOME OVERALL RATING		1	2	3	4	5	
Indicators:							
110301	Granulation	1	2	3	4	5	
110320	Scar formation	1	2	3	4	5	
110321	Decreased wound size	1	2	3	4	5	

		Extensive	Substantial	Moderate	Limited	None	
110303	Purulent drainage	1	2	3	4	5	NA
110304	Serous drainage	1	2	3	4	5	NA
110305	Sanguineous drainage	1	2	3	4	5	NA
110306	Serosanguineous drainage	1	2	3	4	5	NA
110307	Surrounding skin erythema	1	2	3	4	5	NA
110322	Wound inflammation	1	2	3	4	5	NA
110308	Periwound edema	1	2	3	4	5	NA
110310	Blistered skin	1	2	3	4	5	NA
110311	Macerated skin	1	2	3	4	5	NA
110312	Necrosis	1	2	3	4	5	NA
110313	Sloughing	1	2	3	4	5	NA
110314	Tunneling	1	2	3	4	5	NA
110315	Undermining	1	2	3	4	5	NA
110316	Sinus tract formation	1	2	3	4	5	NA
110317	Foul wound odor	1	2	3	4	5	NA

Location of wound (# from picture): _____

Domain-*Physiologic Health (II)*　　**Class**-*Tissue Integrity (L)*　　*1st edition 1997; revised 2004*

1. Front of head
2. Right ear
3. Left ear
4. Front of neck
5. Right chest
6. Left chest
7. Sternum
8. Right upper quadrant
9. Left upper quadrant
10. Right lower quadrant
11. Left lower quadrant
12. Abdominal midline
13. Navel
14. Pubic and perineal area
15. Right trochanter (hip)
16. Left trochanter (hip)
17. Right anterior thigh
18. Right knee
19. Right lower anterior leg
20. Right ankle (inner/outer)
21. Right foot
22. Right toes
23. Left anterior thigh
24. Left knee
25. Left lower anterior leg
26. Left ankle (inner/outer)
27. Left foot
28. Left toes
29. Right upper interior arm
30. Right interior forearm
31. Right wrist
32. Right palm
33. Right fingers _____(specify)
34. Left upper interior arm
35. Left interior forearm
36. Left wrist
37. Left palm
38. Left fingers _____(specify)
39. Back of head
40. Back of neck
41. Left scapula
42. Right scapula
43. Spine
44. Left back
45. Right back
46. Left buttock
47. Right buttock
48. Sacrum
49. Left posterior thigh
50. Left lower posterior leg
51. Left heel
52. Left bottom foot
53. Right posterior thigh
54. Right lower posterior leg
55. Right heel
56. Right bottom foot
57. Left upper posterior arm
58. Left elbow
59. Left posterior forearm
60. Left dorsal hand
61. Right upper posterior arm
62. Right elbow
63. Right posterior forearm
64. Right dorsal hand

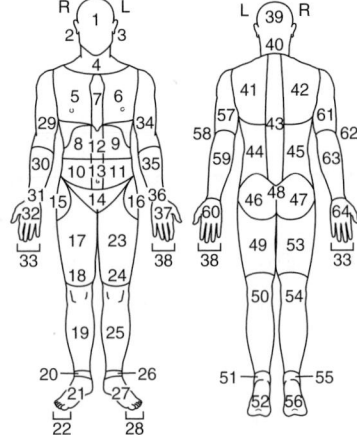

W

OUTCOME CONTENT REFERENCES:

Cohen, I. K., Diegelmann, R. F., & Lindblad, W. L. (1992). *Wound healing: Biochemical and clinical aspects.* Philadelphia: W. B. Saunders.

Flanagan, M. (1994). Assessment criteria. *Nursing Times, 90*(35), 76–88.

Frantz, R. A. (2001). Impaired skin integrity: Pressure ulcer. In M. Maas, K. Buckwalter, M. Hardy, T. Tripp-Reimer, M. Titler, & J. Specht (Eds.), *Nursing care of older adults: Diagnoses, outcomes & interventions* (pp. 121–136). St. Louis: Mosby.

Frantz, R. A., & Gardner, S. (1994). Elderly skin care: Principles of chronic wound care. *Journal of Gerontological Nursing, 20*(9), 35–44.

Lazarus, G. S., Cooper, D. M., Knighton, D. R., Margohs, D. J., Pecoraro, R. E., Rodeheaver, G., et al. (1994). Definitions and guidelines for assessment of wounds and evaluation of healing. *Archives of Dermatology, 130*(4), 489–493.

Maklebust, J., & Sieggreen, M. (1996). *Pressure ulcers: Guidelines for prevention and nursing management* (2nd ed.). Springhouse, PA: Springhouse.

Potter, P. A., & Perry, A. G. (2001). *Fundamentals of nursing* (5th ed.). St. Louis: Mosby.

+Thomas, D. R., Rodeheaver, G. T., Bartolucci, A. A., Frantz, R. A., Sussman, C., Ferrell, B. A., Cuddigan, J., Stotts, N. A., & Makleburt, J. (1997). Pressure ulcer scale for healing: Derivation and validation of the PUSH tool. *Advances in Wound Care, 10*(5) 96–101.

Van Rijswijk, L. (1993). Full-thickness leg ulcers: Patient demographics and predictors of healing. *The Journal of Family Practice, 36*(6), 625–632.

W

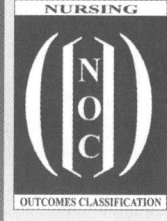

PART FOUR

NOC Linkages: Health Patterns and NANDA International

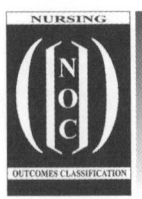

NOC Linkages—Health Patterns

This section provides updated linkages among the Health Patterns identified by Gordon[1,2] and the NOC outcomes developed to date at three levels of abstraction: individual, family, and community. These linkages were first published in the second edition of NOC. Early work by Gordon[1] suggests the importance of the nurse assessing 11 health concepts utilizing patterns of behavior over time rather than isolated patient events. This approach examines the *sequence of behavior* over time incorporating a broad view of behavior as physiological, psychological, or sociological in nature. The patterns were proposed by Gordon to serve as a means of identifying nursing diagnoses during the early development of patient problem statements that were standardized for use in clinical practice and provide a structured framework for the assessment of a client. For example, the nurse can use an interview approach and perform a physical exam for each patient receiving nursing care to assess each of the 11 health patterns.

Due to the popularity and long history of use of these health patterns in nursing, linkages among the NOC outcomes and the 11 health patterns were developed to assist nurses who routinely use the health patterns as an assessment structure in practice. In addition, many educational institutions use the patterns as a tool to teach the assessment phase of the nursing process to nursing students. These linkages provide another way of identifying relevant outcomes for nurses using the NOC in education, practice, and research.

Each outcome is placed under a specific pattern based on the pattern name and definition developed by Gordon. Outcomes that describe the actual health status of a more general nature were placed in the Health Perception–Health Management Pattern when they did not fit into the more specific pattern. Many of these outcomes would be assessed primarily by physical exam rather than by interviewing the client about his or her perceptions of health.

Thirty-six outcomes could not be placed in this structure and appear as a list at the end of the linkages. Linkages of the NOC to the 11 health patterns are important for: (1) assisting individuals in learning and using the NOC, (2) improving diagnostic reasoning skills in nursing, (3) identifying new outcomes for development of the NOC, especially as the family and community level outcomes are further developed, and (4) emphasizing the effectiveness of nursing interventions with the current emphasis in health care on outcomes. Current use of this pattern focus by nurses is predominant in the United States and internationally.

References

1. Gordon, M. (1994). *Nursing diagnosis: Process and application* (3rd ed.). New York: McGraw-Hill.
2. Gordon, M. (2011). *Manual of nursing diagnosis* (12th ed.). Sudbury, MA: Jones & Bartlett Learning.

NURSING OUTCOMES CLASSIFICATION (NOC) ORGANIZED BY THE ELEVEN HEALTH PATTERNS

Health Perception–Health Management Pattern:

This pattern describes the client's perceived pattern of health and well-being and how health is managed across time. It includes general perceptions about health, general health management, prevention practices, potential or actual noncompliance, motivation for health promotion, and unrealistic health or illness perceptions. At the family level general perceptions of the family's health status are the focus of this pattern. Assessment of this pattern may reveal the influential member of the family for health-related decisions. At the community level general concerns about community health problems and services are assessed. This may include objective data from mortality and morbidity statistics, accident rates, and violence statistics, for example.

Individual Level:

Acceptance: Health Status
Adherence Behavior
Adherence Behavior: Healthy Diet
Aspiration Prevention
Burn Recovery
Cardiopulmonary Status
Caregiver Emotional Health
Caregiver Home Care Readiness
Caregiver Performance: Direct Care
Caregiver Performance: Indirect Care
Caregiver Physical Health
Caregiver Well-Being
Child Development: 1 Month
Child Development: 2 Months
Child Development: 4 Months
Child Development: 6 Months
Child Development: 12 Months
Child Development: 2 Years
Child Development: 3 Years
Child Development: 4 Years
Child Development: 5 Years
Child Development: Middle Childhood
Child Development: Adolescence
Compliance Behavior
Compliance Behavior: Prescribed Activity
Compliance Behavior: Prescribed Diet
Compliance Behavior: Prescribed Medication
Development: Late Adulthood
Development: Middle Adulthood
Development: Young Adulthood
Discharge Readiness: Independent Living
Discharge Readiness: Supported Living
Fall Prevention Behavior
Falls Occurrence
Fatigue: Disruptive Effects
Fetal Status: Antepartum
Fetal Status: Intrapartum
Health Promoting Behavior
Health Seeking Behavior
Immune Status

Immunization Behavior
Infection Severity
Infection Severity: Newborn
Lifestyle Balance
Maternal Status: Antepartum
Maternal Status: Intrapartum
Maternal Status: Postpartum
Medication Response
Motivation
Pain Control
Pain: Disruptive Effects
Participation in Health Care Decisions
Personal Health Screening Behavior
Personal Health Status
Personal Safety Behavior
Personal Time Management
Personal Well-Being
Physical Aging
Physical Injury Severity
Postpartum Maternal Health Behavior
Post-Procedure Recovery
Prenatal Health Behavior
Pre-Procedure Readiness
Preterm Infant Organization
Quality of Life
Respiratory Status
Respiratory Status: Ventilation
Risk Control
Risk Control: Alcohol Use
Risk Control: Cancer
Risk Control: Cardiovascular Disease
Risk Control: Drug Use
Risk Control: Dry Eye
Risk Control: Hearing Impairment
Risk Control: Hypertension
Risk Control: Hyperthermia
Risk Control: Hypotension
Risk Control: Hypothermia
Risk Control: Infectious Process
Risk Control: Lipid Disorder

Individual Level—cont'd:

Risk Control: Osteoporosis
Risk Control: Sexually Transmitted Diseases (STD)
Risk Control: Stroke
Risk Control: Sun Exposure
Risk Control: Thrombus
Risk Control: Tobacco Use
Risk Control: Unintended Pregnancy
Risk Control: Visual Impairment
Risk Detection
Safe Home Environment
Seizure Self-Control
Self-Care: Non-Parenteral Medication
Self-Care: Parenteral Medication
Self-Direction of Care
Self-Management: Acute Illness
Self-Management: Anticoagulation Therapy
Self-Management: Asthma
Self-Management: Cardiac Disease
Self-Management: Chronic Disease
Self-Management: Chronic Obstructive Pulmonary Disease
Self-Management: Coronary Artery Disease
Self-Management: Diabetes

Self-Management: Dysrhythmia
Self-Management: Heart Failure
Self-Management: Hypertension
Self-Management: Kidney Disease
Self-Management: Lipid Disorder
Self-Management: Multiple Sclerosis
Self-Management: Osteoporosis
Self-Management: Peripheral Artery Disease
Student Health Status
Substance Withdrawal Severity
Surgical Recovery: Convalescence
Surgical Recovery: Immediate Post-Operative
Symptom Control
Tissue Perfusion
Tissue Perfusion: Abdominal Organs
Tissue Perfusion: Cardiac
Tissue Perfusion: Cellular
Tissue Perfusion: Peripheral
Tissue Perfusion: Pulmonary
Vital Signs
Will to Live

Family Level:

Family Health Status

Family Participation in Professional Care

Community Level:

Community Disaster Readiness
Community Disaster Response
Community Health Status
Community Immune Status

Community Risk Control: Chronic Disease
Community Risk Control: Communicable Disease
Community Risk Control: Lead Exposure
Community Risk Control: Violence

Nutrition-Metabolic Pattern:

This pattern describes the pattern of food and fluid consumption relative to metabolic need. Physical exam for this pattern focuses on the skin, bony prominences, hair, oral mucous membranes, teeth, height and weight for life stage, and body temperature. At the family level assessment focuses on patterns of food consumption and identifies who makes decisions about the nutritional intake of family members while the community assessment focuses on geographic neighborhoods.

Individual Level:

Appetite
Blood Glucose Level
Bottle Feeding Establishment: Infant
Bottle Feeding Performance
Breastfeeding Establishment: Infant
Breastfeeding Establishment: Maternal
Breastfeeding Maintenance
Breastfeeding Weaning
Burn Healing
Cup Feeding Establishment: Infant
Cup Feeding Performance

Dry Eye Severity
Eating Disorder Self-Control
Electrolyte & Acid/Base Balance
Electrolyte Balance
Fluid Balance
Fluid Overload Severity
Gastrointestinal Function
Growth
Hydration
Hypercalcemia Severity
Hyperchloremia Severity

Individual Level—cont'd:

Hyperglycemia Severity
Hyperkalemia Severity
Hypermagnesemia Severity
Hypernatremia Severity
Hyperphosphatemia Severity
Hypocalcemia Severity
Hypochloremia Severity
Hypoglycemia Severity
Hypokalemia Severity
Hypomagnesemia Severity
Hyponatremia Severity
Hypophosphatemia Severity
Infant Nutritional Status
Liver Function
Metabolic Acidosis Severity
Metabolic Alkalosis Severity
Nausea & Vomiting Control
Nausea & Vomiting: Disruptive Effects
Nausea & Vomiting Severity
Nutritional Status

Nutritional Status: Biochemical Measures
Nutritional Status: Energy
Nutritional Status: Food & Fluid Intake
Nutritional Status: Nutrient Intake
Oral Health
Respiratory Status: Airway Patency
Swallowing Status
Swallowing Status: Esophageal Phase
Swallowing Status: Oral Phase
Swallowing Status: Pharyngeal Phase
Thermoregulation
Thermoregulation: Newborn
Tissue Integrity: Skin & Mucous Membranes
Weight: Body Mass
Weight Gain Behavior
Weight Loss Behavior
Weight Maintenance Behavior
Wound Healing: Primary Intention
Wound Healing: Secondary Intention

Family Level

Family Risk Control: Obesity

Community Level

Community Risk Control: Obesity

Elimination Pattern:

This pattern describes patterns of excretory function (e.g., bowel, bladder, and skin) at the individual level. Physical examination includes gross screening of specimens and prostheses such as ostomy bags. The nurse identifies patterns of urinary or bowel incontinence and difficulty with urination and constipation. At the family and community levels the focus is on waste disposal and related hygiene practices.

Individual Level:

Bowel Continence
Bowel Elimination
Kidney Function
Ostomy Self-Care

Systemic Toxin Clearance: Dialysis
Urinary Continence
Urinary Elimination

NOC currently has no outcomes focused on the elimination pattern at the family or community level.

Activity-Exercise Pattern:

This pattern focuses on exercise, activity, leisure, and recreation and includes perceived capabilities for movement, self-care, and home management. Physical examination includes gait, posture, muscle tone, absence of body part, and the use of assistive devices. At the family and community levels patterns of activity are assessed. This includes recreational and cultural activities and public transportation.

Individual Level:

Activity Tolerance
Ambulation
Ambulation: Wheelchair
Balance

Body Mechanics Performance
Body Positioning: Self-Initiated
Bone Healing
Cardiac Pump Effectiveness

Individual Level—cont'd:

Circulation Status
Coordinated Movement
Elopement Occurrence
Elopement Propensity Risk
Endurance
Energy Conservation
Exercise Participation
Fatigue Level
Gait
Hyperactivity Level
Immobility Consequences: Physiological
Immobility Consequences: Psycho-Cognitive
Joint Movement
Joint Movement: Ankle
Joint Movement: Elbow
Joint Movement: Fingers
Joint Movement: Hip
Joint Movement: Knee
Joint Movement: Neck
Joint Movement: Passive
Joint Movement: Shoulder
Joint Movement: Spine

Joint Movement: Wrist
Leisure Participation
Mechanical Ventilation Weaning Response: Adult
Mobility
Neurological Status: Autonomic
Neurological Status: Consciousness
Physical Fitness
Play Participation
Psychomotor Energy
Respiratory Status: Gas Exchange
Safe Wandering
Self-Care Status
Self-Care: Activities of Daily Living (ADL)
Self-Care: Bathing
Self-Care: Dressing
Self-Care: Eating
Self-Care: Hygiene
Self-Care: Instrumental Activities of Daily Living (IADL)
Self-Care: Oral Hygiene
Self-Care: Toileting
Skeletal Function
Transfer Performance

NOC currently has no outcomes focused on the activity-exercise pattern at the family or community level.

Cognitive-Perceptual Pattern:

This pattern describes sensory, perceptual, and cognitive function. The areas of concern are the adequacy of language skills, memory, problem solving, and decision-making skills and the sensory functions of vision, hearing, touch, taste, and smell. In addition, pain perception and compensation for sensory loss are included. The focus of the family and community pattern is on how decisions are made.

Individual Level:

Abstract Thinking
Cognition
Cognitive Orientation
Concentration
Decision-Making
Delirium Level
Dementia Level
Distorted Thought Self-Control
Hearing Compensation Behavior
Heedfulness of Affected Side
Information Processing
Knowledge: Acute Illness Management
Knowledge: Anticoagulation Therapy Management
Knowledge: Arthritis Management
Knowledge: Asthma Management
Knowledge: Body Mechanics
Knowledge: Bottle Feeding
Knowledge: Breastfeeding
Knowledge: Cancer Management
Knowledge: Cancer Threat Reduction

Knowledge: Cardiac Disease Management
Knowledge: Child Physical Safety
Knowledge: Chronic Disease Management
Knowledge: Chronic Obstructive Pulmonary Disease Management
Knowledge: Conception Prevention
Knowledge: Coronary Artery Disease Management
Knowledge: Cup Feeding
Knowledge: Dementia Management
Knowledge: Depression Management
Knowledge: Diabetes Management
Knowledge: Disease Process
Knowledge: Dysrhythmia Management
Knowledge: Eating Disorder Management
Knowledge: Energy Conservation
Knowledge: Fall Prevention
Knowledge: Fertility Promotion
Knowledge: Health Behavior
Knowledge: Health Promotion
Knowledge: Health Resources
Knowledge: Healthy Diet

Individual Level—cont'd:

Knowledge: Healthy Lifestyle
Knowledge: Heart Failure Management
Knowledge: Hypertension Management
Knowledge: Infant Care
Knowledge: Infection Management
Knowledge: Inflammatory Bowel Disease Management
Knowledge: Kidney Disease Management
Knowledge: Labor & Delivery
Knowledge: Lipid Disorder Management
Knowledge: Medication
Knowledge: Multiple Sclerosis Management
Knowledge: Osteoporosis Management
Knowledge: Ostomy Care
Knowledge: Pain Management
Knowledge: Parenting
Knowledge: Peripheral Artery Disease Management
Knowledge: Personal Safety
Knowledge: Pneumonia Management
Knowledge: Postpartum Maternal Health
Knowledge: Preconception Maternal Health
Knowledge: Pregnancy
Knowledge: Pregnancy & Postpartum Sexual Functioning
Knowledge: Prescribed Activity
Knowledge: Prescribed Diet
Knowledge: Preterm Infant Care

Knowledge: Sexual Functioning
Knowledge: Stress Management
Knowledge: Stroke Management
Knowledge: Stroke Prevention
Knowledge: Substance Use Control
Knowledge: Thrombus Prevention
Knowledge: Time Management
Knowledge: Treatment Procedure
Knowledge: Treatment Regimen
Knowledge: Weight Management
Memory
Neurological Status
Neurological Status: Central Motor Control
Neurological Status: Cranial Sensory/Motor Function
Neurological Status: Peripheral
Neurological Status: Spinal Sensory/Motor Function
Pain Level
Sensory Function
Sensory Function: Hearing
Sensory Function: Proprioception
Sensory Function: Tactile
Sensory Function: Taste & Smell
Sensory Function: Vision
Tissue Perfusion: Cerebral
Vision Compensation Behavior

Community Level:

Community Competence

NOC currently has no outcomes focused on the cognitive-perceptual pattern at the family level.

Sleep-Rest Pattern:

This pattern describes sleep, rest, and relaxation at the individual, family, and community levels. The family and community levels focus on disturbances such as noise, family schedules, and patterns of relaxation focused on group activities.

Individual Level:

Rest

Sleep

NOC currently has no outcomes focused on the sleep-rest pattern at the family or community level.

Self Perception–Self Concept Pattern:

This pattern describes the self-concept pattern and perceptions of self, including body image, social self, self-competency, and subjective mood states. Negative evaluations of self include discomfort, change, loss, and threat. At the family and community level the focus is on status in the community, competency, and image.

Individual Level:

Anxiety Level
Body Image
Comfort Status
Comfort Status: Environment

Comfort Status: Physical
Comfort Status: Psychospiritual
Comfort Status: Sociocultural
Depression Level

Individual Level—cont'd:

Dignified Life Closure
Discomfort Level
Hope
Identity
Loneliness Severity
Mood Equilibrium
Pain: Adverse Psychological Response

Personal Autonomy
Self-Awareness
Self-Esteem
Social Anxiety Level
Suffering Severity
Symptom Severity

Family Level:

Family Functioning

Community Level:

Community Health Screening Effectiveness

Community Program Effectiveness

Role-Relationship Pattern:

This pattern describes patterns of role-engagements and relationships. This pattern includes family roles, work or student roles, and social roles. Loss, change, and threat are some of the major challenges included in this pattern.

At the family level the dynamics of the family are the focus and center on supportive and close relationships or on the negative relationships that include abuse and violence.

Individual Level:

Abuse Cessation
Abuse Protection
Abusive Behavior Self-Restraint
Caregiver-Patient Relationship
Communication
Communication: Expressive
Communication: Receptive
Neglect Cessation
Neglect Recovery
Parent-Infant Attachment
Parenting Performance
Parenting Performance: Adolescent
Parenting Performance: Adolescent Physical Safety

Parenting Performance: Early/Middle Childhood Physical Safety
Parenting Performance: Infant
Parenting Performance: Infant/Toddler Physical Safety
Parenting Performance: Middle Childhood
Parenting Performance: Preschooler
Parenting Performance: Psychosocial Safety
Parenting Performance: Toddler
Role Performance
Social Interaction Skills
Social Involvement
Social Support

Family Level:

Family Integrity
Family Social Climate

Family Support During Treatment

Community Level:

Community Violence Level

Sexuality-Reproductive Pattern:

This pattern describes the client's patterns of satisfaction and dissatisfaction with sexuality and reproductive patterns. At

the family level the focus is on the couple while the community level focuses on attitudes toward sexuality.

Individual Level:

Abuse Recovery: Sexual
Perimenopause Symptom Severity
Physical Maturation: Female
Physical Maturation: Male

Premenstrual Syndrome (PMS) Severity
Sexual Functioning
Sexual Identity

NOC currently has no outcomes focused on the sexuality-reproductive pattern at the family or community level.

Coping–Stress Tolerance Pattern:

This pattern describes general coping patterns and the effectiveness of the pattern in terms of stress tolerance. At the family level similar patterns are the focus. The community level focuses on such problem areas as unemployment, racial or ethnic tensions, drug abuse, or accident rates.

Individual Level:

Abuse Recovery
Abuse Recovery: Emotional
Abuse Recovery: Financial
Abuse Recovery: Physical
Adaptation to Physical Disability
Aggression Self-Restraint
Agitation Level
Alcohol Abuse Cessation Behavior
Anger Self-Restraint
Anxiety Self-Control
Caregiver Adaptation to Patient Institutionalization
Caregiver Lifestyle Disruption
Caregiver Role Endurance
Caregiver Stressors
Child Adaptation to Hospitalization
Comfortable Death
Coping

Depression Self-Control
Drug Abuse Cessation Behavior
Fear Level
Fear Level: Child
Fear Self-Control
Grief Resolution
Guilt Resolution
Impulse Self-Control
Mutilation Self-Restraint
Newborn Adaptation
Personal Resiliency
Psychosocial Adjustment: Life Change
Relocation Adaptation
Smoking Cessation Behavior
Stress Level
Substance Addiction Consequences
Suicide Self-Restraint

Family Level:

Family Coping
Family Normalization

Family Resiliency

Community Level:

Community Grief Response

Community Resiliency

Value-Belief Pattern:

This pattern describes patterns of values, beliefs (including spiritual), or goals that guide choices and decisions. This pattern provides guidelines for behavior at the individual, family, and community levels.

Individual Level:

Health Beliefs
Health Beliefs: Perceived Ability to Perform
Health Beliefs: Perceived Control
Health Beliefs: Perceived Resources

Health Beliefs: Perceived Threat
Health Orientation
Spiritual Health

Community Level

Community Risk Control: Unhealthy Cultural Traditions

NOC currently has no outcomes focused on the value-belief pattern at the family level.

Outcomes Not Placed Within a Pattern

Acute Respiratory Acidosis Severity
Acute Respiratory Alkalosis Severity
Allergic Response: Localized
Allergic Response: Systemic
Blood Coagulation
Blood Loss Severity
Blood Transfusion Reaction
Client Satisfaction
Client Satisfaction: Access to Care Resources
Client Satisfaction: Caring
Client Satisfaction: Case Management
Client Satisfaction: Communication
Client Satisfaction: Continuity of Care
Client Satisfaction: Cultural Needs Fulfillment
Client Satisfaction: Functional Assistance
Client Satisfaction: Pain Management
Client Satisfaction: Physical Care
Client Satisfaction: Physical Environment

Client Satisfaction: Protection of Rights
Client Satisfaction: Psychological Care
Client Satisfaction: Safety
Client Satisfaction: Symptom Control
Client Satisfaction: Teaching
Client Satisfaction: Technical Aspects of Care
Hemodialysis Access
Hypertension Severity
Hypotension Severity
Immune Hypersensitivity Response
Mechanical Ventilation Response: Adult
Peripheral Artery Disease Severity
Safe Health Care Environment
Shock Severity: Anaphylactic
Shock Severity: Cardiogenic
Shock Severity: Hypovolemic
Shock Severity: Neurogenic
Shock Severity: Septic

NOC Linkages—NANDA International Diagnoses

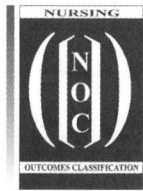

As the classifications of nursing terminologies become more complete, the sheer number of possible combinations of nursing diagnoses, nursing interventions, and nursing outcomes can be overwhelming to the nurse planning care for patients, regardless of the setting. In 2012, a new book focused on NOC and NIC linkages[1] was published structured on both nursing diagnoses and frequent clinical conditions experienced by patients. This book is an excellent resource for nurses using all three terminologies. Although there are outcomes identified for each NANDA International diagnosis in this book, it is not an extensive list of outcomes that might be selected to best meet the needs of the patient. This section contains suggested linkages between the NANDA-I classification[2] published in 2012 and the current edition of NOC. The 490 NOC outcomes in this edition are linked to 216 nursing diagnoses.

A linkage is an association or relationship that exists between a patient, family, or community problem (nursing diagnosis) and a desired outcome (resolution or improvement of the problem). The change in an outcome is usually a result of an intervention by a nurse or other health care provider. Treatments chosen for a diagnosis vary depending on the expertise of the nurse, the outcome selected, the time interval of the patient-nurse interaction, and preferences of the patient. Outcomes are measured prior to intervention and at designated intervals post intervention. In general, linkages of diagnoses and outcomes assist the nurse to select an outcome for a specific patient problem based on the definition of the problem, the defining characteristics, and the related factors of the diagnosis. This process facilitates assessment of the patient's condition, enhances clinical decision-making, and strengthens the nurse's diagnostic reasoning. The linkages also assist in the development of standardized care plans for specific populations that can be individualized by the nurse for each patient. Linkages also enhance and support efforts to computerize nursing data in an electronic health record or care-planning software. The linkage work supports the continuing refinement of the NOC classification by helping to identify missing outcomes for future development.

The linkages of outcomes to nursing diagnoses identified in this section are options the nurse may select during the care-planning process. Other outcomes may also be appropriate for a specific clinical problem and need to be considered by the nurse. The linkages are primarily based on expert judgment at this point, but as research and clinical data become available, new linkages from actual use in practice are included and the linkages are refined. Research is needed in this area to validate the linkages provided between NANDA-I diagnoses and NOC outcomes. This research and clinical validation needs to include a variety of patient populations (patients with both acute and chronic illnesses), patients across the lifespan (from birth to death), and patients receiving care in a variety of settings (acute care to home care).

The nursing diagnoses are divided into the three main types of diagnoses provided in the NANDA-I classification: *actual nursing diagnoses* (where the patient has the problem), *risk nursing diagnoses* (where the patient has a high probability of developing the problem), and *health-promotion nursing diagnoses* (where the patient can improve his or her health and well-being). For an *actual nursing diagnosis*, three categories of outcomes are provided. The first category provides outcomes to measure resolution of the nursing diagnosis. The second category provides additional outcomes to measure the defining characteristics identified for the nursing diagnosis. The third category identifies outcomes associated with the related factors or intermediate outcomes. Dividing the outcomes by the components of each NANDA-I actual diagnosis assists the nurse to choose outcomes that can measure the overall outcome as well as the defining characteristic or the impact of the related factors for each diagnosis. For a *risk nursing diagnosis* two categories of outcomes are provided. The first category provides outcomes to assess and measure actual occurrence of the diagnosis. The second category of outcomes is associated with the risk factors. This allows the nurse to assess a potential problem and measure the key risk factors for a patient at risk for developing the diagnosis. For a *health-promoting diagnosis* only one category of outcomes is needed. This type of diagnosis provides only defining characteristics in the NANDA-I classification. Each diagnosis has a list of outcomes focused on measuring the identified defining characteristics.

References

1. Johnson, M., Moorhead, S., Bulechek, G., Butcher, H., Maas, M., & Swanson, E. (2012). *NOC and NIC linkages to NANDA-I and clinical conditions: Supporting critical reasoning and quality care.* St. Louis: Elsevier.
2. *Nursing diagnoses—Definitions and classification 2012-2014.* Copyright © 2012, 1994-2012 by NANDA International. Used by arrangement with Blackwell Publishing Limited, a company of John Wiley and Sons, Inc.

Actual Nursing Diagnoses

Activity Intolerance

Definition: Insufficient physiological or psychological energy to endure or complete required or desired daily activities

Outcomes to Measure Resolution of Diagnosis

Activity Tolerance
Endurance

Psychomotor Energy

Additional Outcomes to Measure Defining Characteristics

Cardiac Pump Effectiveness
Cardiopulmonary Status
Discomfort Level
Energy Conservation
Fatigue: Disruptive Effects
Fatigue Level

Respiratory Status: Gas Exchange
Rest
Self-Care Status
Self-Care: Activities of Daily Living (ADL)
Self-Care: Instrumental Activities of Daily Living (IADL)
Vital Signs

Outcomes Associated with Related Factors or Intermediate Outcomes

Ambulation
Ambulation: Wheelchair
Client Satisfaction: Functional Assistance
Compliance Behavior: Prescribed Activity
Exercise Participation
Immobility Consequences: Physiological
Mobility
Nutritional Status: Energy

Personal Health Status
Physical Fitness
Respiratory Status
Self-Management: Asthma
Self-Management: Cardiac Disease
Self-Management: Multiple Sclerosis
Self-Management: Osteoporosis

Activity Planning, Ineffective

Definition: Inability to prepare for a set of actions fixed in time and under certain conditions

Outcomes to Measure Resolution of Diagnosis

Decision-Making

Personal Time Management

Additional Outcomes to Measure Defining Characteristics

Adherence Behavior
Agitation Level
Anxiety Level
Community Competence
Community Disaster Readiness
Community Health Screening Effectiveness
Community Program Effectiveness
Compliance Behavior
Compliance Behavior: Prescribed Activity
Compliance Behavior: Prescribed Diet

Compliance Behavior: Prescribed Medication
Fear Level
Guilt Resolution
Health Beliefs: Perceived Resources
Lifestyle Balance
Motivation
Personal Resiliency
Social Anxiety Level
Social Support

Outcomes Associated with Related Factors or Intermediate Outcomes

Abstract Thinking
Cognition
Health Beliefs: Perceived Ability to Perform
Health Beliefs: Perceived Control
Health Orientation

Information Processing
Knowledge: Time Management
Personal Health Screening Behavior
Self-Awareness
Self-Esteem

Airway Clearance, Ineffective

Definition: Inability to clear secretions or obstructions from the respiratory tract to maintain a clear airway

Outcomes to Measure Resolution of Diagnosis
Respiratory Status: Airway Patency

Additional Outcomes to Measure Defining Characteristics

Agitation Level
Anxiety Level
Aspiration Prevention
Mechanical Ventilation Response: Adult
Respiratory Status

Respiratory Status: Gas Exchange
Respiratory Status: Ventilation
Symptom Control
Vital Signs

Outcomes Associated with Related Factors or Intermediate Outcomes

Allergic Response: Systemic
Immune Hypersensitivity Response
Infection Severity
Infection Severity: Newborn
Knowledge: Asthma Management
Knowledge: Chronic Obstructive Pulmonary Disease
    Management
Knowledge: Pneumonia Management

Mechanical Ventilation Weaning Response: Adult
Neurological Status: Cranial Sensory/Motor Function
Neurological Status: Spinal Sensory/Motor Function
Risk Control: Infectious Process
Risk Control: Tobacco Use
Self-Management: Asthma
Self-Management: Chronic Obstructive Pulmonary Disease
Smoking Cessation Behavior

Anxiety

Definition: Vague, uneasy feeling of discomfort or dread accompanied by an autonomic response (the source often non-specific or unknown to the individual); a feeling of apprehension caused by anticipation of danger. It is an alerting signal that warns of impending danger and enables the individual to take measures to deal with threat

Outcomes to Measure Resolution of Diagnosis
Anxiety Level

Social Anxiety Level

Additional Outcomes to Measure Defining Characteristics

Agitation Level
Anxiety Self-Control
Bowel Continence
Concentration
Coping
Decision-Making
Delirium Level
Distorted Thought Self-Control
Elopement Propensity Risk
Fatigue Level
Fear Level

Fear Level: Child
Hyperactivity Level
Information Processing
Nausea & Vomiting Control
Nausea & Vomiting Severity
Neurological Status: Autonomic
Safe Wandering
Sensory Function: Tactile
Sleep
Urinary Continence
Vital Signs

Continued

Anxiety—cont'd

Outcomes Associated with Related Factors or Intermediate Outcomes

Abuse Recovery

Acceptance: Health Status

Adaptation to Physical Disability

Aggression Self-Restraint

Child Adaptation to Hospitalization

Client Satisfaction: Caring

Client Satisfaction: Continuity of Care

Client Satisfaction: Psychological Care

Comfort Status

Comfort Status: Environment

Comfort Status: Physical

Comfort Status: Psychospiritual

Comfort Status: Sociocultural

Dementia Level

Grief Resolution

Immunization Behavior

Impulse Self-Control

Infection Severity

Lifestyle Balance

Mutilation Self-Restraint

Neglect Recovery

Parent-Infant Attachment

Personal Well-Being

Psychosocial Adjustment: Life Change

Relocation Adaptation

Self-Awareness

Self-Esteem

Sexual Identity

Social Interaction Skills

Spiritual Health

Stress Level

Substance Withdrawal Severity

Symptom Control

Autonomic Dysreflexia

Definition: Life-threatening, uninhibited sympathetic response of the nervous system to a noxious stimulus after a spinal cord injury at T7 or above

Outcomes to Measure Resolution of Diagnosis

Neurological Status: Autonomic

Shock Severity: Neurogenic

Additional Outcomes to Measure Defining Characteristics

Cardiopulmonary Status

Hydration

Hypertension Severity

Hypotension Severity

Neurological Status

Neurological Status: Cranial Sensory/Motor Function

Neurological Status: Peripheral

Pain Level

Respiratory Status

Risk Control: Hypothermia

Sensory Function: Tactile

Sensory Function: Vision

Vital Signs

Outcomes Associated with Related Factors or Intermediate Outcomes

Bowel Elimination

Caregiver Performance: Direct Care

Circulation Status

Knowledge: Disease Process

Knowledge: Hypertension Management

Knowledge: Treatment Regimen

Self-Management: Chronic Disease

Sensory Function

Symptom Severity

Tissue Integrity: Skin & Mucous Membranes

Urinary Elimination

Body Image, Disturbed

Definition: Confusion in mental picture of one's physical self

Outcomes to Measure Resolution of Diagnosis
Body Image

Additional Outcomes to Measure Defining Characteristics

Adaptation to Physical Disability	Identity
Anger Self-Restraint	Lifestyle Balance
Fear Level	Self-Awareness
Fear Level: Child	Self-Esteem
Heedfulness of Affected Side	Social Anxiety Level

Outcomes Associated with Related Factors or Intermediate Outcomes

Abuse Recovery: Emotional	Physical Injury Severity
Abuse Recovery: Physical	Psychosocial Adjustment: Life Change
Abuse Recovery: Sexual	Sexual Functioning
Burn Recovery	Sexual Identity
Comfort Status: Psychospiritual	Surgical Recovery: Convalescence
Coping	Weight: Body Mass
Distorted Thought Self-Control	Weight Gain Behavior
Loneliness Severity	Weight Loss Behavior
Ostomy Self-Care	

Bowel Incontinence

Definition: Change in normal bowel habits characterized by involuntary passage of stool

Outcomes to Measure Resolution of Diagnosis
Bowel Continence

Additional Outcomes to Measure Defining Characteristics

Bowel Elimination	Tissue Integrity: Skin & Mucous Membranes

Outcomes Associated with Related Factors or Intermediate Outcomes

Cognition	Medication Response
Delirium Level	Mobility
Dementia Level	Neurological Status: Autonomic
Fluid Overload Severity	Neurological Status: Spinal Sensory/Motor Function
Gastrointestinal Function	Nutritional Status: Food & Fluid Intake
Infection Severity	Ostomy Self-Care
Knowledge: Health Behavior	Physical Aging
Knowledge: Healthy Diet	Safe Home Environment
Knowledge: Medication	Self-Care: Non-Parenteral Medication
Knowledge: Ostomy Care	Self-Care: Toileting
Knowledge: Prescribed Diet	Stress Level

Breast Milk, Insufficient

Definition: Low production of maternal breast milk

Outcomes to Measure Resolution of Diagnosis

Breastfeeding Establishment: Maternal

Infant Nutritional Status

Additional Outcomes to Measure Defining Characteristics

Breastfeeding Establishment: Infant

Outcomes Associated with Related Factors or Intermediate Outcomes

Alcohol Abuse Cessation Behavior

Blood Loss Severity

Eating Disorder Self-Control

Fluid Balance

Hydration

Maternal Status: Postpartum

Medication Response

Nutritional Status: Food & Fluid Intake

Nutritional Status: Nutrient Intake

Risk Control: Alcohol Use

Risk Control: Tobacco Use

Smoking Cessation Behavior

Breastfeeding, Ineffective

Definition: Dissatisfaction or difficulty a mother, infant, or child experiences with the breastfeeding process

Outcomes to Measure Resolution of Diagnosis

Breastfeeding Establishment: Infant

Breastfeeding Establishment: Maternal

Additional Outcomes to Measure Defining Characteristics

Breastfeeding Maintenance

Breastfeeding Weaning

Fluid Balance

Infant Nutritional Status

Nutritional Status: Food & Fluid Intake

Outcomes Associated with Related Factors or Intermediate Outcomes

Anxiety Level

Anxiety Self-Control

Child Development: 1 Month

Child Development: 2 Months

Cognition

Family Integrity

Family Normalization

Family Social Climate

Fatigue Level

Hydration

Knowledge: Breastfeeding

Knowledge: Infant Care

Pain Level

Parent-Infant Attachment

Parenting Performance: Infant

Postpartum Maternal Health Behavior

Social Support

Swallowing Status

Breastfeeding, Interrupted

Definition: Break in the continuity of the breastfeeding process as a result of inability or inadvisability to put baby to breast for feeding

Outcomes to Measure Resolution of Diagnosis
Breastfeeding Maintenance

Additional Outcomes to Measure Defining Characteristics

Breastfeeding Establishment: Maternal
Infant Nutritional Status

Knowledge: Breastfeeding
Parent-Infant Attachment

Outcomes Associated with Related Factors or Intermediate Outcomes

Bottle Feeding Performance
Breastfeeding Weaning
Cup Feeding Performance
Fatigue Level
Infection Severity
Infection Severity: Newborn
Medication Response
Parenting Performance

Parenting Performance: Infant
Personal Health Status
Postpartum Maternal Health Behavior
Preterm Infant Organization
Risk Control: Alcohol Use
Risk Control: Drug Use
Role Performance

Breathing Pattern, Ineffective

Definition: Inspiration and/or expiration that does not provide adequate ventilation

Outcomes to Measure Resolution of Diagnosis

Mechanical Ventilation Weaning Response: Adult
Respiratory Status

Respiratory Status: Ventilation

Additional Outcomes to Measure Defining Characteristics

Allergic Response: Systemic
Respiratory Status: Airway Patency

Respiratory Status: Gas Exchange
Shock Severity: Anaphylactic

Outcomes Associated with Related Factors or Intermediate Outcomes

Acute Respiratory Acidosis Severity
Acute Respiratory Alkalosis Severity
Anxiety Level
Cognition
Energy Conservation
Fatigue: Disruptive Effects
Fatigue Level
Neurological Status: Autonomic

Neurological Status: Spinal Sensory/Motor Function
Pain Level
Preterm Infant Organization
Self-Management: Asthma
Self-Management: Chronic Obstructive Pulmonary Disease
Smoking Cessation Behavior
Weight: Body Mass

Cardiac Output, Decreased

Definition: Inadequate blood pumped by the heart to meet metabolic demands of the body

Outcomes to Measure Resolution of Diagnosis

Cardiac Pump Effectiveness

Circulation Status

Additional Outcomes to Measure Defining Characteristics

Agitation Level

Anxiety Level

Cardiopulmonary Status

Endurance

Fatigue Level

Fluid Overload Severity

Kidney Function

Respiratory Status

Respiratory Status: Gas Exchange

Respiratory Status: Ventilation

Tissue Perfusion

Tissue Perfusion: Abdominal Organs

Tissue Perfusion: Cardiac

Tissue Perfusion: Cellular

Tissue Perfusion: Cerebral

Tissue Perfusion: Peripheral

Tissue Perfusion: Pulmonary

Urinary Elimination

Vital Signs

Weight: Body Mass

Outcomes Associated with Related Factors or Intermediate Outcomes

Knowledge: Cardiac Disease Management

Knowledge: Coronary Artery Disease Management

Knowledge: Dysrhythmia Management

Knowledge: Heart Failure Management

Neurological Status: Autonomic

Self-Management: Cardiac Disease

Self-Management: Coronary Artery Disease

Self-Management: Dysrhythmia

Self-Management: Heart Failure

Caregiver Role Strain

Definition: Difficulty in performing family/significant other caregiver role

Outcomes to Measure Resolution of Diagnosis

Caregiver Home Care Readiness

Caregiver Performance: Direct Care

Caregiver Performance: Indirect Care

Caregiver Role Endurance

Additional Outcomes to Measure Defining Characteristics

Anger Self-Restraint

Bottle Feeding Performance

Caregiver Adaptation to Patient Institutionalization

Caregiver Emotional Health

Caregiver Lifestyle Disruption

Caregiver-Patient Relationship

Caregiver Physical Health

Caregiver Stressors

Caregiver Well-Being

Coping

Cup Feeding Performance

Depression Level

Depression Self-Control

Family Functioning

Family Social Climate

Grief Resolution

Guilt Resolution

Knowledge: Time Management

Parenting Performance

Parenting Performance: Adolescent

Parenting Performance: Infant

Parenting Performance: Middle Childhood

Parenting Performance: Preschooler

Parenting Performance: Toddler

Personal Resiliency

Personal Time Management

Postpartum Maternal Health Behavior

Role Performance

Caregiver Role Strain—cont'd

Outcomes Associated with Related Factors or Intermediate Outcomes

Anxiety Level
Dementia Level
Drug Abuse Cessation Behavior
Elopement Propensity Risk
Energy Conservation
Family Coping
Family Participation in Professional Care
Family Resiliency
Family Support During Treatment
Fatigue Level
Knowledge: Health Resources

Knowledge: Medication
Knowledge: Treatment Regimen
Leisure Participation
Lifestyle Balance
Psychomotor Energy
Safe Home Environment
Social Involvement
Social Support
Stress Level
Substance Withdrawal Severity

Childbearing Process, Ineffective

Definition: Pregnancy and childbirth process and care of the newborn that does not match the environmental context, norms, and expectations

Outcomes to Measure Resolution of Diagnosis

Fetal Status: Antepartum
Fetal Status: Intrapartum
Maternal Status: Antepartum

Maternal Status: Intrapartum
Maternal Status: Postpartum
Parent-Infant Attachment

Additional Outcomes to Measure Defining Characteristics

Bottle Feeding Performance
Breastfeeding Establishment: Maternal
Child Development: 1 Month
Cup Feeding Performance
Growth
Infant Nutritional Status

Knowledge: Pregnancy
Parenting Performance
Parenting Performance: Infant
Prenatal Health Behavior
Social Support

Outcomes Associated with Related Factors or Intermediate Outcomes

Abuse Protection
Alcohol Abuse Cessation Behavior
Anxiety Level
Drug Abuse Cessation Behavior
Knowledge: Bottle Feeding
Knowledge: Breastfeeding
Knowledge: Cup Feeding
Knowledge: Healthy Lifestyle
Knowledge: Infant Care
Knowledge: Labor & Delivery

Knowledge: Medication
Knowledge: Preconception Maternal Health
Knowledge: Prescribed Diet
Lifestyle Balance
Parenting Performance: Psychosocial Safety
Personal Health Status
Personal Time Management
Risk Detection
Smoking Cessation Behavior
Surgical Recovery: Immediate Post Operative

Comfort, Impaired

Definition: Perceived lack of ease, relief, and transcendence in physical, psychospiritual, environmental, cultural, and social dimensions

Outcomes to Measure Resolution of Diagnosis

Comfort Status
Comfort Status: Environment
Comfort Status: Physical

Comfort Status: Psychospiritual
Comfort Status: Sociocultural

Additional Outcomes to Measure Defining Characteristics

Agitation Level
Anxiety Level
Client Satisfaction: Physical Environment
Fatigue Level
Fear Level
Pain: Disruptive Effects

Pain Level
Sleep
Stress Level
Symptom Control
Tissue Perfusion

Outcomes Associated with Related Factors or Intermediate Outcomes

Medication Response
Personal Autonomy
Relocation Adaptation
Safe Home Environment

Self-Management: Acute Illness
Social Support
Symptom Severity

Communication, Impaired Verbal

Definition: Decreased, delayed, or absent ability to receive, process, transmit, and/or use a system of symbols

Outcomes to Measure Resolution of Diagnosis

Communication
Communication: Expressive

Communication: Receptive

Additional Outcomes to Measure Defining Characteristics

Cognitive Orientation
Comfort Status: Sociocultural
Information Processing

Respiratory Status
Sensory Function: Vision

Outcomes Associated with Related Factors or Intermediate Outcomes

Adaptation to Physical Disability
Child Development: 3 Years
Child Development: 4 Years
Child Development: 5 Years
Child Development: Middle Childhood
Client Satisfaction: Communication
Cognition
Delirium Level
Dementia Level
Distorted Thought Self-Control
Medication Response

Mood Equilibrium
Neurological Status
Neurological Status: Cranial Sensory/Motor Function
Self-Awareness
Self-Esteem
Sensory Function: Hearing
Social Anxiety Level
Social Support
Stress Level
Tissue Perfusion: Cerebral

Community Coping, Ineffective

Definition: Pattern of community activities for adaptation and problem-solving that is unsatisfactory for meeting the demands or needs of the community

Outcomes to Measure Resolution of Diagnosis

Community Competence

Community Disaster Response

Community Program Effectiveness

Additional Outcomes to Measure Defining Characteristics

Community Risk Control: Chronic Disease

Community Risk Control: Communicable Disease

Community Risk Control: Lead Exposure

Community Risk Control: Obesity

Community Risk Control: Unhealthy Cultural Traditions

Community Risk Control: Violence

Community Violence Level

Outcomes Associated with Related Factors or Intermediate Outcomes

Community Disaster Readiness

Community Grief Response

Community Health Screening Effectiveness

Community Health Status

Community Immune Status

Community Resiliency

Community Health, Deficient

Definition: Presence of one or more health problems or factors that deter wellness or increase the risk of health problems experienced by an aggregate

Outcomes to Measure Resolution of Diagnosis

Community Health Status

Additional Outcomes to Measure Defining Characteristics

Community Grief Response

Community Immune Status

Community Risk Control: Chronic Disease

Community Risk Control: Communicable Disease

Community Risk Control: Lead Exposure

Community Risk Control: Obesity

Community Risk Control: Unhealthy Cultural Traditions

Community Risk Control: Violence

Community Violence Level

Outcomes Associated with Related Factors or Intermediate Outcomes

Community Competence

Community Health Screening Effectiveness

Community Program Effectiveness

Confusion, Acute

Definition: Abrupt onset of reversible disturbances of consciousness, attention, cognition, and perception that develop over a short period of time

Outcomes to Measure Resolution of Diagnosis

Cognitive Orientation	Delirium Level

Additional Outcomes to Measure Defining Characteristics

Abstract Thinking	Information Processing
Agitation Level	Memory
Cognition	Motivation
Concentration	Neurological Status: Consciousness
Distorted Thought Self-Control	Psychomotor Energy

Outcomes Associated with Related Factors or Intermediate Outcomes

Alcohol Abuse Cessation Behavior	Physical Aging
Blood Glucose Level	Sleep
Dementia Level	Substance Withdrawal Severity
Drug Abuse Cessation Behavior	Tissue Perfusion: Cerebral
Fatigue Level	

Confusion, Chronic

Definition: Irreversible, longstanding, and/or progressive deterioration of intellect and personality characterized by decreased ability to interpret environmental stimuli and decreased capacity for intellectual thought processes, and manifested by disturbances of memory, orientation, and behavior

Outcomes to Measure Resolution of Diagnosis

Cognitive Orientation	Dementia Level

Additional Outcomes to Measure Defining Characteristics

Abstract Thinking	Identity
Cognition	Information Processing
Concentration	Memory
Decision-Making	Neurological Status: Consciousness
Distorted Thought Self-Control	Social Interaction Skills

Outcomes Associated with Related Factors or Intermediate Outcomes

Knowledge: Dementia Management	Physical Injury Severity
Knowledge: Stroke Management	Risk Control: Stroke
Knowledge: Stroke Prevention	Tissue Perfusion: Cerebral

Constipation

Definition: Decrease in normal frequency of defecation accompanied by difficult or incomplete passage of stool and/or passage of excessively hard, dry stool

Outcomes to Measure Resolution of Diagnosis

Bowel Elimination

Ostomy Self-Care

Additional Outcomes to Measure Defining Characteristics

Appetite	Gastrointestinal Function
Bowel Continence	Nausea & Vomiting Severity
Comfort Status: Physical	Pain Level
Discomfort Level	Stress Level
Fatigue Level	Symptom Severity

Outcomes Associated with Related Factors or Intermediate Outcomes

Adherence Behavior: Healthy Diet	Maternal Status: Antepartum
Cognition	Medication Response
Compliance Behavior: Prescribed Activity	Mobility
Compliance Behavior: Prescribed Diet	Neurological Status: Spinal Sensory/Motor Function
Delirium Level	Nutritional Status: Food & Fluid Intake
Dementia Level	Oral Health
Depression Level	Physical Aging
Electrolyte Balance	Physical Fitness
Exercise Participation	Self-Care: Eating
Fluid Balance	Self-Care: Non-Parenteral Medication
Hydration	Self-Care: Oral Hygiene
Knowledge: Healthy Diet	Self-Care: Toileting
Knowledge: Medication	Symptom Control
Knowledge: Prescribed Diet	Weight: Body Mass

Constipation, Perceived

Definition: Self-diagnosis of constipation combined with abuse of laxatives, enemas, and/or suppositories to ensure a daily bowel movement

Outcomes to Measure Resolution of Diagnosis

Bowel Elimination

Knowledge: Health Behavior

Additional Outcomes to Measure Defining Characteristics

Health Beliefs	Medication Response
Health Beliefs: Perceived Threat	Stress Level

Outcomes Associated with Related Factors or Intermediate Outcomes

Anxiety Level	Knowledge: Healthy Diet
Delirium Level	Knowledge: Medication
Dementia Level	Self-Care: Non-Parenteral Medication
Distorted Thought Self-Control	

Contamination

Definition: Exposure to environmental contaminants in doses sufficient to cause adverse health effects

Outcomes to Measure Resolution of Diagnosis
Personal Safety Behavior

Additional Outcomes to Measure Defining Characteristics

Allergic Response: Localized	Kidney Function
Allergic Response: Systemic	Liver Function
Gastrointestinal Function	Neurological Status
Immune Hypersensitivity Response	Respiratory Status
Immune Status	Tissue Integrity: Skin & Mucous Membranes

Outcomes Associated with Related Factors or Intermediate Outcomes

Community Disaster Response	Risk Control: Cancer
Community Health Status	Risk Control: Infectious Process
Community Immune Status	Risk Control: Tobacco Use
Community Risk Control: Communicable Disease	Risk Detection
Community Risk Control: Lead Exposure	Safe Home Environment
Knowledge: Cancer Threat Reduction	Self-Care: Hygiene
Nutritional Status	Self-Management: Chronic Disease
Nutritional Status: Nutrient Intake	Smoking Cessation Behavior
Personal Health Status	

Coping, Defensive

Definition: Repeated projection of falsely positive self-evaluation based on a self-protective pattern that defends against underlying perceived threats to positive self-regard

Outcomes to Measure Resolution of Diagnosis
Coping

Additional Outcomes to Measure Defining Characteristics

Acceptance: Health Status	Compliance Behavior: Prescribed Activity
Adaptation to Physical Disability	Compliance Behavior: Prescribed Diet
Adherence Behavior	Compliance Behavior: Prescribed Medication
Adherence Behavior: Healthy Diet	Identity
Aggression Self-Restraint	Participation in Health Care Decisions
Anxiety Level	Role Performance
Child Development: Adolescence	Social Interaction Skills
Comfort Status	Social Involvement
Compliance Behavior	

Outcomes Associated with Related Factors or Intermediate Outcomes

Grief Resolution	Quality of Life
Guilt Resolution	Relocation Adaptation
Impulse Self-Control	Self-Awareness
Lifestyle Balance	Self-Esteem
Motivation	Social Support
Personal Health Screening Behavior	Stress Level
Personal Resiliency	Substance Withdrawal Severity
Psychosocial Adjustment: Life Change	

Coping, Ineffective

Definition: Inability to form a valid appraisal of the stressors, inadequate choices of practiced responses, and/or inability to use available resources

Outcomes to Measure Resolution of Diagnosis

Coping

Stress Level

Additional Outcomes to Measure Defining Characteristics

Abusive Behavior Self-Restraint
Acceptance: Health Status
Adaptation to Physical Disability
Aggression Self-Restraint
Agitation Level
Alcohol Abuse Cessation Behavior
Anger Self-Restraint
Anxiety Level
Caregiver Adaptation to Patient Institutionalization
Child Adaptation to Hospitalization
Concentration
Decision-Making
Drug Abuse Cessation Behavior
Impulse Self-Control

Information Processing
Personal Resiliency
Psychosocial Adjustment: Life Change
Risk Control
Risk Control: Alcohol Use
Risk Control: Drug Use
Risk Control: Tobacco Use
Role Performance
Sleep
Smoking Cessation Behavior
Social Support
Substance Withdrawal Severity
Suicide Self-Restraint

Outcomes Associated with Related Factors or Intermediate Outcomes

Abuse Recovery
Anxiety Self-Control
Caregiver Stressors
Cognition
Dementia Level
Depression Level
Depression Self-Control
Energy Conservation
Fatigue Level
Fear Level
Grief Resolution
Guilt Resolution
Health Beliefs: Perceived Threat

Knowledge: Health Resources
Knowledge: Stress Management
Lifestyle Balance
Mutilation Self-Restraint
Parent-Infant Attachment
Personal Well-Being
Quality of Life
Relocation Adaptation
Self-Awareness
Self-Esteem
Social Interaction Skills
Stress Level

Death Anxiety

Definition: Vague, uneasy feeling of discomfort or dread generated by perceptions of a real or imagined threat to one's existence

Outcomes to Measure Resolution of Diagnosis

Comfortable Death
Dignified Life Closure

Hope
Spiritual Health

Additional Outcomes to Measure Defining Characteristics

Anxiety Level
Comfort Status: Psychospiritual
Coping
Depression Level

Fear Level
Fear Level: Child
Psychosocial Adjustment: Life Change
Suffering Severity

Outcomes Associated with Related Factors or Intermediate Outcomes

Acceptance: Health Status
Anxiety Self-Control
Caregiver-Patient Relationship
Comfort Status
Depression Self-Control
Development: Late Adulthood
Discomfort Level
Fear Self-Control

Grief Resolution
Guilt Resolution
Health Beliefs: Perceived Threat
Pain Control
Personal Autonomy
Personal Resiliency
Social Support
Stress Level

Decisional Conflict

Definition: Uncertainty about course of action to be taken when choice among competing actions involves risk, loss, or challenge to values and beliefs

Outcomes to Measure Resolution of Diagnosis

Decision-Making

Additional Outcomes to Measure Defining Characteristics

Cognition
Information Processing
Participation in Health Care Decisions

Personal Autonomy
Stress Level
Vital Signs

Outcomes Associated with Related Factors or Intermediate Outcomes

Anxiety Level
Anxiety Self-Control
Coping
Depression Level
Family Coping
Family Functioning
Family Social Climate
Guilt Resolution
Health Beliefs

Knowledge: Disease Process
Knowledge: Treatment Regimen
Lifestyle Balance
Personal Resiliency
Psychosocial Adjustment: Life Change
Self-Awareness
Social Support
Stress Level

Denial, Ineffective

Definition: Conscious or unconscious attempt to disavow the knowledge or meaning of an event to reduce anxiety and/or fear, but leading to the detriment of health

Outcomes to Measure Resolution of Diagnosis

Acceptance: Health Status
Adaptation to Physical Disability
Anxiety Level

Fear Level
Fear Level: Child

Additional Outcomes to Measure Defining Characteristics

Anxiety Self-Control
Compliance Behavior
Compliance Behavior: Prescribed Activity
Compliance Behavior: Prescribed Medication
Family Resiliency
Fear Self-Control

Health Beliefs
Health Beliefs: Perceived Control
Health Beliefs: Perceived Threat
Knowledge: Disease Process
Personal Resiliency
Symptom Severity

Outcomes Associated with Related Factors or Intermediate Outcomes

Coping
Distorted Thought Self-Control
Health Orientation
Health Seeking Behavior
Hope
Mood Equilibrium

Personal Autonomy
Psychosocial Adjustment: Life Change
Self-Awareness
Social Support
Stress Level
Symptom Control

Dentition, Impaired

Definition: Disruption in tooth development/eruption patterns or structural integrity of individual teeth

Outcomes to Measure Resolution of Diagnosis
Oral Health

Additional Outcomes to Measure Defining Characteristics
Pain Level

Outcomes Associated with Related Factors or Intermediate Outcomes

Alcohol Abuse Cessation Behavior
Health Beliefs: Perceived Resources
Knowledge: Health Behavior
Knowledge: Health Resources
Knowledge: Healthy Diet
Medication Response

Nausea & Vomiting Control
Nausea & Vomiting Severity
Nutritional Status: Nutrient Intake
Risk Control: Tobacco Use
Self-Care: Oral Hygiene
Smoking Cessation Behavior

Diarrhea

Definition: Passage of loose, unformed stools

Outcomes to Measure Resolution of Diagnosis

Bowel Continence   Bowel Elimination

Additional Outcomes to Measure Defining Characteristics

Discomfort Level   Symptom Severity
Pain Level

Outcomes Associated with Related Factors or Intermediate Outcomes

Adherence Behavior: Healthy Diet   Knowledge: Inflammatory Bowel Disease Management
Alcohol Abuse Cessation Behavior   Knowledge: Medication
Anxiety Level   Knowledge: Prescribed Diet
Anxiety Self-Control   Medication Response
Compliance Behavior: Prescribed Diet   Nutritional Status: Biochemical Measures
Electrolyte & Acid/Base Balance   Nutritional Status: Food & Fluid Intake
Fluid Balance   Ostomy Self-Care
Gastrointestinal Function   Self-Care: Non-Parenteral Medication
Hydration   Self-Management: Acute Illness
Infection Severity   Self-Management: Chronic Disease
Infection Severity: Newborn   Stress Level
Knowledge: Disease Process   Symptom Control
Knowledge: Healthy Diet

Diversional Activity, Deficient

Definition: Decreased stimulation from (or interest or engagement in) recreational or leisure activities

Outcomes to Measure Resolution of Diagnosis

Leisure Participation   Play Participation

Additional Outcomes to Measure Defining Characteristics

Loneliness Severity   Social Involvement
Motivation

Outcomes Associated with Related Factors or Intermediate Outcomes

Child Adaptation to Hospitalization   Relocation Adaptation
Client Satisfaction: Physical Environment

Energy Field, Disturbed

Definition: Disruption of the flow of energy surrounding a person's being that results in disharmony of the body, mind, and/or spirit

Outcomes to Measure Resolution of Diagnosis
Personal Health Status

Personal Well-Being

Spiritual Health

Additional Outcomes to Measure Defining Characteristics
Sensory Function: Hearing

Sensory Function: Proprioception

Sensory Function: Tactile

Sensory Function: Taste & Smell

Sensory Function: Vision

Outcomes Associated with Related Factors or Intermediate Outcomes
Anxiety Level

Child Development: Adolescence

Development: Late Adulthood

Development: Middle Adulthood

Development: Young Adulthood

Fear Level

Grief Resolution

Immobility Consequences: Psycho-Cognitive

Knowledge: Acute Illness Management

Knowledge: Chronic Disease Management

Maternal Status: Antepartum

Maternal Status: Intrapartum

Medication Response

Mobility

Pain Level

Physical Injury Severity

Self-Management: Acute Illness

Self-Management: Chronic Disease

Suffering Severity

Surgical Recovery: Immediate Post-Operative

Environmental Interpretation Syndrome, Impaired

Definition: Consistent lack of orientation to person, place, time, or circumstances over more than 3 to 6 months, necessitating a protective environment

Outcomes to Measure Resolution of Diagnosis
Cognitive Orientation

Additional Outcomes to Measure Defining Characteristics
Abstract Thinking

Cognition

Concentration

Decision-Making

Information Processing

Memory

Role Performance

Safe Wandering

Social Interaction Skills

Outcomes Associated with Related Factors or Intermediate Outcomes
Dementia Level

Depression Level

Depression Self-Control

Knowledge: Chronic Disease Management

Knowledge: Dementia Management

Neurological Status

Self-Management: Chronic Disease

Failure to Thrive, Adult

Definition: Progressive functional deterioration of a physical and cognitive nature. The individual's ability to live with multisystem diseases, cope with ensuing problems, and manage his or her care is remarkably diminished

Outcomes to Measure Resolution of Diagnosis
Personal Health Status
Self-Management: Acute Illness

Self-Management: Chronic Disease

Additional Outcomes to Measure Defining Characteristics
Appetite
Bowel Continence
Cognition
Concentration
Decision-Making
Delirium Level
Dementia Level
Depression Level
Eating Disorder Self-Control
Endurance
Fatigue Level
Gastrointestinal Function
Hydration
Infection Severity
Information Processing
Leisure Participation
Memory
Nausea & Vomiting Severity

Nutritional Status
Nutritional Status: Food & Fluid Intake
Nutritional Status: Nutrient Intake
Personal Resiliency
Psychosocial Adjustment: Life Change
Risk Control: Infectious Process
Safe Home Environment
Self-Care: Activities of Daily Living (ADL)
Self-Care: Instrumental Activities of Daily Living (IADL)
Social Interaction Skills
Social Involvement
Suffering Severity
Urinary Continence
Weight: Body Mass
Weight Gain Behavior
Weight Maintenance Behavior
Will to Live

Outcomes Associated with Related Factors or Intermediate Outcomes
Depression Self-Control
Knowledge: Depression Management
Mood Equilibrium

Physical Aging
Stress Level

Family Coping, Compromised

Definition: A usually supportive primary person (family member, significant other, or close friend) who provides insufficient, ineffective, or compromised support, comfort, assistance, or encouragement that may be needed by the client to manage or master adaptive tasks related to his or her health challenge

Outcomes to Measure Resolution of Diagnosis
Caregiver Performance: Direct Care
Caregiver Performance: Indirect Care
Family Coping

Family Normalization
Family Support During Treatment

Outcomes to Measure Defining Characteristics
Anxiety Level
Bottle Feeding Performance
Caregiver Emotional Health
Caregiver Lifestyle Disruption
Client Satisfaction: Access to Care Resources

Client Satisfaction: Caring
Client Satisfaction: Communication
Client Satisfaction: Cultural Needs Fulfillment
Client Satisfaction: Functional Assistance
Client Satisfaction: Pain Management

Family Coping, Compromised—cont'd

Client Satisfaction: Physical Care
Cup Feeding Performance
Fear Level

Grief Resolution
Guilt Resolution
Loneliness Severity

Outcomes Associated with Related Factors or Intermediate Outcomes

Abuse Cessation
Anxiety Self-Control
Caregiver Adaptation to Patient Institutionalization
Caregiver Home Care Readiness
Caregiver-Patient Relationship
Caregiver Physical Health
Caregiver Role Endurance
Caregiver Stressors
Cognition
Family Functioning
Family Integrity
Family Participation in Professional Care
Family Resiliency
Family Social Climate
Fatigue: Disruptive Effects
Knowledge: Bottle Feeding
Knowledge: Chronic Disease Management

Knowledge: Cup Feeding
Knowledge: Disease Process
Knowledge: Health Resources
Knowledge: Infant Care
Knowledge: Medication
Knowledge: Pain Management
Knowledge: Parenting
Knowledge: Prescribed Diet
Knowledge: Stress Management
Lifestyle Balance
Neglect Cessation
Parent-Infant Attachment
Parenting Performance
Relocation Adaptation
Social Involvement
Social Support
Stress Level

Family Coping, Disabled

Definition: Behavior of primary person (family member, significant other, or close friend) that disables his or her capacities and the client's capacities to effectively address tasks essential to either person's adaptation to the health challenge

Outcomes to Measure Resolution of Diagnosis

Caregiver Performance: Direct Care
Caregiver Performance: Indirect Care
Family Coping

Family Normalization
Family Support During Treatment

Additional Outcomes to Measure Defining Characteristics

Abuse Cessation
Abuse Recovery
Anxiety Level
Adaptation to Physical Disability
Aggression Self-Restraint
Agitation Level
Anger Self-Restraint

Caregiver-Patient Relationship
Caregiver Well-Being
Depression Level
Depression Self-Control
Family Resiliency
Neglect Cessation
Neglect Recovery

Outcomes Associated with Related Factors or Intermediate Outcomes

Adherence Behavior: Healthy Diet
Caregiver Emotional Health
Caregiver Stressors
Compliance Behavior
Compliance Behavior: Prescribed Activity
Compliance Behavior: Prescribed Diet
Compliance Behavior: Prescribed Medication

Coping
Family Functioning
Family Social Climate
Fatigue: Disruptive Effects
Guilt Resolution
Knowledge: Chronic Disease Management
Knowledge: Disease Process

Continued

Family Coping, Disabled—cont'd

Knowledge: Health Resources
Knowledge: Infant Care
Knowledge: Medication
Knowledge: Pain Management
Knowledge: Parenting
Knowledge: Prescribed Diet
Knowledge: Stress Management

Lifestyle Balance
Personal Resiliency
Psychosocial Adjustment: Life Change
Social Anxiety Level
Social Support
Stress Level

Family Processes, Dysfunctional

Definition: Psychosocial, spiritual, and physiological functions of the family unit are chronically disorganized, which leads to conflict, denial of problems, resistance to change, ineffective problem-solving, and a series of self-perpetuating crises

Outcomes to Measure Resolution of Diagnosis

Family Functioning
Family Integrity

Family Normalization

Additional Outcomes to Measure Defining Characteristics

Abuse Recovery
Alcohol Abuse Cessation Behavior
Aggression Self-Restraint
Agitation Level
Anger Self-Restraint
Cognition
Communication
Concentration
Decision-Making
Dementia Level
Depression Level
Depression Self-Control
Dignified Life Closure
Family Coping
Family Resiliency
Family Social Climate

Family Support During Treatment
Grief Resolution
Guilt Resolution
Identity
Lifestyle Balance
Loneliness Severity
Parenting Performance
Role Performance
Self-Esteem
Social Anxiety Level
Social Interaction Skills
Social Involvement
Social Support
Substance Addiction Consequences
Substance Withdrawal Severity

Outcomes Associated with Related Factors or Intermediate Outcomes

Adaptation to Physical Disability
Compliance Behavior
Coping
Family Health Status

Knowledge: Healthy Lifestyle
Knowledge: Substance Use Control
Stress Level

Family Processes, Interrupted

Definition: Change in family relationships and/or functioning

Outcomes to Measure Resolution of Diagnosis
Caregiver Adaptation to Patient Institutionalization
Caregiver Home Care Readiness
Family Functioning

Family Normalization
Family Resiliency

Additional Outcomes to Measure Defining Characteristics
Family Coping
Family Social Climate
Family Support During Treatment
Parenting Performance
Parenting Performance: Adolescent
Parenting Performance: Infant

Parenting Performance: Middle Childhood
Parenting Performance: Preschooler
Parenting Performance: Toddler
Social Interaction Skills
Social Involvement
Social Support

Outcomes Associated with Related Factors or Intermediate Outcomes
Abuse Protection
Adaptation to Physical Disability
Coping
Family Health Status

Family Participation in Professional Care
Parent-Infant Attachment
Psychosocial Adjustment: Life Change
Role Performance

Family Therapeutic Regimen Management, Ineffective

Definition: A pattern of regulating and integrating into family processes a program for treatment of illness and the sequelae that is unsatisfactory for meeting specific health goals

Outcomes to Measure Resolution of Diagnosis
Family Normalization

Family Participation in Professional Care

Additional Outcomes to Measure Defining Characteristics
Caregiver Home Care Readiness
Caregiver Performance: Direct Care
Caregiver Performance: Indirect Care
Child Adaptation to Hospitalization

Family Risk Control: Obesity
Family Support During Treatment
Symptom Severity

Outcomes Associated with Related Factors or Intermediate Outcomes
Caregiver Role Endurance
Decision-Making
Family Health Status
Family Integrity
Family Resiliency

Family Social Climate
Knowledge: Acute Illness Management
Knowledge: Chronic Disease Management
Knowledge: Treatment Regimen

Fatigue

Definition: An overwhelming sustained sense of exhaustion and decreased capacity for physical and mental work at the usual level

Outcomes to Measure Resolution of Diagnosis

Fatigue: Disruptive Effects

Fatigue Level

Additional Outcomes to Measure Defining Characteristics

Activity Tolerance	Personal Well-Being
Concentration	Psychomotor Energy
Depression Level	Rest
Endurance	Role Performance
Energy Conservation	Self-Awareness
Exercise Participation	Self-Care Status
Guilt Resolution	Self-Care: Activities of Daily Living (ADL)
Mood Equilibrium	Self-Care: Instrumental Activities of Daily Living (IADL)
Motivation	Sexual Functioning
Personal Health Status	Sleep

Outcomes Associated with Related Factors or Intermediate Outcomes

Anxiety Level	Mobility
Anxiety Self-Control	Nutritional Status: Nutrient Intake
Blood Glucose Level	Pain Level
Comfort Status: Environment	Physical Fitness
Depression Self-Control	Self-Management: Chronic Disease
Lifestyle Balance	Stress Level
Maternal Status: Antepartum	

Fear

Definition: Response to perceived threat that is consciously recognized as a danger

Outcomes to Measure Resolution of Diagnosis

Fear Level

Fear Self-Control

Fear Level: Child

Additional Outcomes to Measure Defining Characteristics

Aggression Self-Restraint	Impulse Self-Control
Agitation Level	Information Processing
Anxiety Level	Memory
Anxiety Self-Control	Nausea & Vomiting Control
Bowel Elimination	Nausea & Vomiting Severity
Cognition	Self-Esteem
Concentration	Social Anxiety Level
Decision-Making	Vital Signs
Fatigue Level	

Outcomes Associated with Related Factors or Intermediate Outcomes

Abuse Recovery	Delirium Level
Caregiver Performance: Direct Care	Dementia Level
Child Adaptation to Hospitalization	Discomfort Level
Coping	Family Support During Treatment

Fear—cont'd

Health Beliefs: Perceived Threat
Neglect Recovery
Pain Level
Personal Resiliency
Psychosocial Adjustment: Life Change

Relocation Adaptation
Social Support
Spiritual Health
Stress Level

Fluid Volume, Deficient

Definition: Decreased intravascular, interstitial, and/or intracellular fluid. This refers to dehydration, water loss alone without change in sodium

Outcomes to Measure Resolution of Diagnosis
Fluid Balance

Hydration

Additional Outcomes to Measure Defining Characteristics
Delirium Level
Hypotension Severity
Thermoregulation
Thermoregulation: Newborn
Tissue Integrity: Skin & Mucous Membranes

Tissue Perfusion: Peripheral
Urinary Elimination
Vital Signs
Weight: Body Mass

Outcomes Associated with Related Factors or Intermediate Outcomes
Appetite
Blood Loss Severity
Bowel Elimination
Burn Recovery
Electrolyte Balance
Gastrointestinal Function

Hypernatremia Severity
Hyponatremia Severity
Kidney Function
Nausea & Vomiting Severity
Nutritional Status: Food & Fluid Intake

Fluid Volume, Excess

Definition: Increased isotonic fluid retention

Outcomes to Measure Resolution of Diagnosis
Fluid Balance

Additional Outcomes to Measure Defining Characteristics
Agitation Level
Anxiety Level
Cardiopulmonary Status
Delirium Level
Electrolyte Balance
Hypertension Severity

Respiratory Status
Respiratory Status: Gas Exchange
Respiratory Status: Ventilation
Urinary Elimination
Vital Signs
Weight: Body Mass

Outcomes Associated with Related Factors or Intermediate Outcomes
Cardiac Pump Effectiveness
Compliance Behavior: Prescribed Diet
Electrolyte & Acid/Base Balance
Fluid Overload Severity
Hypernatremia Severity
Kidney Function

Knowledge: Heart Failure Management
Knowledge: Hypertension Management
Nutritional Status: Food & Fluid Intake
Nutritional Status: Nutrient Intake
Self-Management: Heart Failure
Self-Management: Hypertension

Gas Exchange, Impaired

Definition: Excess or deficit in oxygenation and/or carbon dioxide elimination at the alveolar-capillary membrane

Outcomes to Measure Resolution of Diagnosis

Mechanical Ventilation Response: Adult

Respiratory Status: Gas Exchange

Additional Outcomes to Measure Defining Characteristics

Cognition

Cognitive Orientation

Delirium Level

Electrolyte & Acid/Base Balance

Energy Conservation

Sensory Function: Vision

Symptom Severity

Tissue Perfusion

Tissue Perfusion: Abdominal Organs

Tissue Perfusion: Cardiac

Tissue Perfusion: Cellular

Tissue Perfusion: Peripheral

Tissue Perfusion: Pulmonary

Vital Signs

Outcomes Associated with Related Factors or Intermediate Outcomes

Allergic Response: Systemic

Knowledge: Chronic Obstructive Pulmonary Disease
    Management

Knowledge: Pneumonia Management

Respiratory Status

Respiratory Status: Ventilation

Self-Management: Asthma

Self-Management: Chronic Obstructive Pulmonary Disease

Gastrointestinal Motility, Dysfunctional

Definition: Increased, decreased, ineffective, or lack of peristaltic activity within the gastrointestinal system

Outcomes to Measure Resolution of Diagnosis

Bowel Elimination

Gastrointestinal Function

Additional Outcomes to Measure Defining Characteristics

Discomfort Level

Electrolyte & Acid/Base Balance

Nausea & Vomiting Severity

Pain Level

Symptom Control

Outcomes Associated with Related Factors or Intermediate Outcomes

Adherence Behavior: Healthy Diet

Anxiety Level

Anxiety Self-Control

Compliance Behavior: Prescribed Activity

Compliance Behavior: Prescribed Diet

Exercise Participation

Fluid Balance

Hydration

Infection Severity

Knowledge: Chronic Disease Management

Knowledge: Disease Process

Knowledge: Healthy Diet

Knowledge: Inflammatory Bowel Disease Management

Knowledge: Medication

Knowledge: Prescribed Diet

Knowledge: Stress Management

Medication Response

Mobility

Nutritional Status: Biochemical Measures

Nutritional Status: Food & Fluid Intake

Ostomy Self-Care

Physical Aging

Self-Care: Non-Parenteral Medication

Self-Management: Chronic Disease

Stress Level

Surgical Recovery: Convalescence

Surgical Recovery: Immediate Post-Operative

Grieving

Definition: A normal complex process that includes emotional, physical, spiritual, social, and intellectual responses and behaviors by which individuals, families, and communities incorporate an actual, anticipated, or perceived loss into their daily lives

Outcomes to Measure Resolution of Diagnosis

Community Grief Response
Family Resiliency

Grief Resolution

Additional Outcomes to Measure Defining Characteristics

Anger Self-Restraint
Comfort Status: Psychospiritual
Comfortable Death
Coping
Dignified Life Closure
Family Coping
Family Functioning
Guilt Resolution

Hope
Pain Control
Pain Level
Psychosocial Adjustment: Life Change
Sleep
Spiritual Health
Suffering Severity

Outcomes Associated with Related Factors or Intermediate Outcomes

Adaptation to Physical Disability
Burn Recovery
Caregiver Adaptation to Patient Institutionalization
Community Resiliency
Depression Level
Depression Self-Control

Family Normalization
Heedfulness of Affected Side
Knowledge: Depression Management
Personal Resiliency
Relocation Adaptation
Role Performance

Grieving, Complicated

Definition: A disorder that occurs after the death of a significant other, in which the experience of distress accompanying bereavement fails to follow normative expectations and manifests in functional impairment

Outcomes to Measure Resolution of Diagnosis

Depression Level

Grief Resolution

Additional Outcomes to Measure Defining Characteristics

Anger Self-Restraint
Anxiety Level
Anxiety Self-Control
Comfort Status: Psychospiritual
Coping
Depression Self-Control
Discomfort Level
Fatigue Level
Guilt Resolution

Knowledge: Depression Management
Personal Resiliency
Personal Well-Being
Psychosocial Adjustment: Life Change
Role Performance
Self-Care Status
Sleep
Social Involvement

Outcomes Associated with Related Factors or Intermediate Outcomes

Appetite
Loneliness Severity
Mood Equilibrium

Personal Health Status
Self-Esteem
Social Support

Growth and Development, Delayed

Definition: Deviations from age-group norms

Outcomes to Measure Resolution of Diagnosis

Child Development: 1 Month
Child Development: 2 Months
Child Development: 4 Months
Child Development: 6 Months
Child Development: 12 Months
Child Development: 2 Years
Child Development: 3 Years
Child Development: 4 Years

Child Development: 5 Years
Child Development: Adolescence
Child Development: Middle Childhood
Development: Late Adulthood
Development: Middle Adulthood
Development: Young Adulthood
Growth

Additional Outcomes to Measure Defining Characteristics

Abstract Thinking
Abusive Behavior Self-Restraint
Aggression Self-Restraint
Anger Self-Restraint
Anxiety Self-Control
Depression Self-Control
Fear Self-Control
Impulse Self-Control
Mood Equilibrium

Physical Aging
Physical Maturation: Female
Physical Maturation: Male
Preterm Infant Organization
Psychomotor Energy
Self-Care: Activities of Daily Living (ADL)
Self-Care: Instrumental Activities of Daily Living (IADL)
Weight: Body Mass

Outcomes Associated with Related Factors or Intermediate Outcomes

Abuse Recovery
Abuse Recovery: Emotional
Abuse Recovery: Physical
Adaptation to Physical Disability
Caregiver-Patient Relationship
Child Adaptation to Hospitalization
Community Risk Control: Lead Exposure
Knowledge: Parenting
Neglect Recovery
Parent-Infant Attachment

Parenting Performance
Parenting Performance: Adolescent
Parenting Performance: Infant
Parenting Performance: Middle Childhood
Parenting Performance: Preschooler
Parenting Performance: Toddler
Personal Autonomy
Personal Resiliency
Psychosocial Adjustment: Life Change

Health Behavior, Risk-Prone

Definition: Impaired ability to modify lifestyle/behaviors in a manner that improves health status

Outcomes to Measure Resolution of Diagnosis

Health Beliefs: Perceived Control

Lifestyle Balance

Personal Resiliency

Additional Outcomes to Measure Defining Characteristics

Acceptance: Health Status

Adaptation to Physical Disability

Adherence Behavior

Adherence Behavior: Healthy Diet

Child Adaptation to Hospitalization

Compliance Behavior

Compliance Behavior: Prescribed Activity

Compliance Behavior: Prescribed Diet

Compliance Behavior: Prescribed Medication

Health Beliefs: Perceived Ability to Perform

Health Beliefs: Perceived Threat

Health Seeking Behavior

Health Promoting Behavior

Motivation

Mutilation Self-Restraint

Participation in Health Care Decisions

Personal Autonomy

Psychosocial Adjustment: Life Change

Risk Control

Self-Management: Acute Illness

Self-Management: Anticoagulation Therapy

Self-Management: Asthma

Self-Management: Cardiac Disease

Self-Management: Chronic Disease

Self-Management: Chronic Obstructive Pulmonary Disease

Self-Management: Coronary Artery Disease

Self-Management: Diabetes

Self-Management: Dysrhythmia

Self-Management: Heart Failure

Self-Management: Hypertension

Self-Management: Kidney Disease

Self-Management: Lipid Disorder

Self-Management: Multiple Sclerosis

Self-Management: Osteoporosis

Self-Management: Peripheral Artery Disease

Suicide Self-Restraint

Weight Gain Behavior

Weight Loss Behavior

Outcomes Associated with Related Factors or Intermediate Outcomes

Alcohol Abuse Cessation Behavior

Cognition

Coping

Health Beliefs: Perceived Resources

Health Orientation

Information Processing

Mood Equilibrium

Risk Control: Alcohol Use

Risk Control: Tobacco Use

Self-Awareness

Self-Esteem

Smoking Cessation Behavior

Social Support

Stress Level

Substance Withdrawal Severity

Health Maintenance, Ineffective

Definition: Inability to identify, manage, and/or seek out help to maintain health

Outcomes to Measure Resolution of Diagnosis

Knowledge: Health Promotion

Health Promoting Behavior

Additional Outcomes to Measure Defining Characteristics

Adherence Behavior

Adherence Behavior: Healthy Diet

Compliance Behavior

Compliance Behavior: Prescribed Activity

Compliance Behavior: Prescribed Diet

Compliance Behavior: Prescribed Medication

Health Orientation

Health Seeking Behavior

Knowledge: Acute Illness Management

Knowledge: Anticoagulation Therapy Management

Knowledge: Arthritis Management

Knowledge: Asthma Management

Knowledge: Cancer Management

Knowledge: Cancer Threat Reduction

Knowledge: Cardiac Disease Management

Knowledge: Chronic Disease Management

Knowledge: Chronic Obstructive Pulmonary Disease
Management

Knowledge: Coronary Artery Disease Management

Knowledge: Dementia Management

Knowledge: Depression Management

Knowledge: Diabetes Management

Knowledge: Disease Process

Knowledge: Dysrhythmia Management

Knowledge: Eating Disorder Management

Knowledge: Energy Conservation

Knowledge: Fall Prevention

Knowledge: Health Behavior

Knowledge: Health Resources

Knowledge: Healthy Diet

Knowledge: Healthy Lifestyle

Knowledge: Heart Failure Management

Knowledge: Hypertension Management

Knowledge: Infection Management

Knowledge: Inflammatory Bowel Disease Management

Knowledge: Kidney Disease Management

Knowledge: Lipid Disorder Management

Knowledge: Multiple Sclerosis Management

Knowledge: Osteoporosis Management

Knowledge: Pain Management

Knowledge: Peripheral Artery Disease Management

Knowledge: Personal Safety

Knowledge: Pneumonia Management

Knowledge: Preconception Maternal Health

Knowledge: Prescribed Activity

Knowledge: Prescribed Diet

Knowledge: Stress Management

Knowledge: Stroke Management

Knowledge: Stroke Prevention

Knowledge: Substance Use Control

Knowledge: Thrombus Prevention

Knowledge: Treatment Regimen

Knowledge: Weight Management

Lifestyle Balance

Motivation

Participation in Health Care Decisions

Personal Health Status

Psychosocial Adjustment: Life Change

Risk Detection

Self-Care Status

Self-Direction of Care

Self-Management: Acute Illness

Self-Management: Anticoagulation Therapy

Self-Management: Asthma

Self-Management: Cardiac Disease

Self-Management: Chronic Disease

Self-Management: Chronic Obstructive Pulmonary Disease

Self-Management: Coronary Artery Disease

Self-Management: Diabetes

Self-Management: Dysrhythmia

Self-Management: Heart Failure

Self-Management: Hypertension

Self-Management: Kidney Disease

Self-Management: Lipid Disorder

Self-Management: Multiple Sclerosis

Self-Management: Osteoporosis

Self-Management: Peripheral Artery Disease

Social Support

Health Maintenance, Ineffective—cont'd

Outcomes Associated with Related Factors or Intermediate Outcomes

Abstract Thinking

Client Satisfaction: Access to Care Resources

Cognition

Communication

Coordinated Movement

Coping

Decision-Making

Delirium Level

Dementia Level

Family Coping Grief Resolution

Guilt Resolution

Health Beliefs: Perceived Resources

Information Processing

Spiritual Health

Home Maintenance, Impaired

Definition: Inability to independently maintain a safe growth-promoting immediate environment

Outcomes to Measure Resolution of Diagnosis

Safe Home Environment

Self-Care: Instrumental Activities of Daily Living (IADL)

Additional Outcomes to Measure Defining Characteristics

Comfort Status: Environment

Family Social Climate

Personal Safety Behavior

Role Performance

Self-Care Status

Outcomes Associated with Related Factors or Intermediate Outcomes

Caregiver Emotional Health

Caregiver Physical Health

Cognition

Discharge Readiness: Independent Living

Family Functioning

Fatigue: Disruptive Effects

Knowledge: Health Behavior

Knowledge: Health Resources

Knowledge: Personal Safety

Mobility

Personal Health Status

Self-Management: Acute Illness

Self-Management: Chronic Disease

Social Support

Hopelessness

Definition: Subjective state in which an individual sees limited or no alternatives or personal choices available and is unable to mobilize energy on own behalf

Outcomes to Measure Resolution of Diagnosis

Hope

Psychomotor Energy

Additional Outcomes to Measure Defining Characteristics

Acceptance: Health Status

Appetite

Comfort Status: Psychospiritual

Communication

Depression Level

Mood Equilibrium

Motivation

Participation in Health Care Decisions

Personal Resiliency

Sleep

Will to Live

Continued

Hopelessness—*cont'd*

Outcomes Associated with Related Factors or Intermediate Outcomes

Adaptation to Physical Disability

Coping

Depression Self-Control

Fatigue Level

Fear Self-Control

Grief Resolution

Immobility Consequences: Psycho-Cognitive

Neglect Recovery

Pain: Adverse Psychological Response

Pain: Disruptive Effects

Physical Aging

Play Participation

Quality of Life

Relocation Adaptation

Self-Care: Activities of Daily Living (ADL)

Self-Management: Chronic Disease

Social Involvement

Spiritual Health

Stress Level

Suffering Severity

Symptom Severity

Hyperthermia

Definition: Body temperature elevated above normal range

Outcomes to Measure Resolution of Diagnosis

Thermoregulation

Thermoregulation: Newborn

Additional Outcomes to Measure Defining Characteristics

Neurological Status

Neurological Status: Autonomic

Vital Signs

Outcomes Associated with Related Factors or Intermediate Outcomes

Blood Transfusion Reaction

Comfort Status: Physical

Discomfort Level

Hydration

Infection Severity

Infection Severity: Newborn

Knowledge: Acute Illness Management

Medication Response

Physical Injury Severity

Risk Control: Hyperthermia

Self-Management: Acute Illness

Hypothermia

Definition: Body temperature below normal range

Outcomes to Measure Resolution of Diagnosis

Thermoregulation

Thermoregulation: Newborn

Additional Outcomes to Measure Defining Characteristics

Hypertension Severity

Tissue Perfusion: Peripheral

Vital Signs

Outcomes Associated with Related Factors or Intermediate Outcomes

Comfort Status: Physical

Medication Response

Neurological Status: Autonomic

Nutritional Status: Nutrient Intake

Physical Aging

Physical Injury Severity

Risk Control: Alcohol Use

Risk Control: Hypothermia

Self-Management: Acute Illness

Impulse Control, Ineffective

Definition: A pattern of performing rapid, unplanned reactions to internal or external stimuli without regard for the negative consequences of these reactions to the impulsive individual or to others

Outcomes to Measure Resolution of Diagnosis

Impulse Self-Control
Mutilation Self-Restraint

Suicide Self-Restraint

Additional Outcomes to Measure Defining Characteristics

Abusive Behavior Self-Restraint
Aggression Self-Restraint
Agitation Level
Anger Self-Restraint

Hyperactivity Level
Risk Control: Sexually Transmitted Diseases (STD)
Risk Control: Unintended Pregnancy
Social Interaction Skills

Outcomes Associated with Related Factors or Intermediate Outcomes

Body Image
Child Development: 2 Years
Child Development: 3 Years
Child Development: 4 Years
Child Development: 5 Years
Child Development: Middle Childhood
Child Development: Adolescence
Cognition
Coping
Dementia Level
Development: Late Adulthood
Development: Middle Adulthood
Development: Young Adulthood
Discomfort Level
Distorted Thought Self-Control
Drug Abuse Cessation Behavior
Fatigue: Disruptive Effects

Fatigue Level
Guilt Resolution
Hope
Loneliness Severity
Mood Equilibrium
Personal Autonomy
Personal Health Status
Relocation Adaptation
Self-Awareness
Self-Esteem
Sleep
Smoking Cessation Behavior
Social Involvement
Stress Level
Substance Addiction Consequences
Symptom Severity

Infant Behavior, Disorganized

Definition: Disintegrated physiological and neurobehavioral responses of infant to the environment

Outcomes to Measure Resolution of Diagnosis

Newborn Adaptation

Preterm Infant Organization

Additional Outcomes to Measure Defining Characteristics

Appetite
Bottle Feeding Establishment: Infant
Breastfeeding Establishment: Infant
Child Development: 1 Month
Coordinated Movement

Cup Feeding Establishment: Infant
Parent-Infant Attachment
Sleep
Vital Signs

Outcomes Associated with Related Factors or Intermediate Outcomes

Bottle Feeding Performance
Breastfeeding Maintenance

Child Development: 2 Months
Cup Feeding Performance

Continued

Infant Behavior, Disorganized—cont'd

Discomfort Level
Infant Nutritional Status
Knowledge: Bottle Feeding
Knowledge: Breastfeeding
Knowledge: Cup Feeding
Knowledge: Infant Care
Knowledge: Preterm Infant Care
Neurological Status

Neurological Status: Cranial Sensory/Motor Function
Nutritional Status: Food & Fluid Intake
Pain Level
Parenting Performance: Infant
Parenting Performance: Infant/Toddler Physical Safety
Safe Home Environment
Sensory Function

Infant Feeding Pattern, Ineffective

Definition: Impaired ability of an infant to suck or coordinate the suck/swallow response resulting in inadequate oral nutrition for metabolic needs

Outcomes to Measure Resolution of Diagnosis
Bottle Feeding Establishment: Infant

Breastfeeding Establishment: Infant

Additional Outcomes to Measure Defining Characteristics
Breastfeeding Maintenance
Cup Feeding Establishment: Infant
Hydration

Infant Nutritional Status
Swallowing Status

Outcomes Associated with Related Factors or Intermediate Outcomes
Aspiration Prevention
Breastfeeding Establishment: Maternal
Gastrointestinal Function
Neurological Status
Neurological Status: Cranial Sensory/Motor Function

Newborn Adaptation
Preterm Infant Organization
Swallowing Status: Esophageal Phase
Swallowing Status: Oral Phase
Swallowing Status: Pharyngeal Phase

Insomnia

Definition: A disruption in amount and quality of sleep that impairs functioning

Outcomes to Measure Resolution of Diagnosis
Sleep

Additional Outcomes to Measure Defining Characteristics
Abstract Thinking
Concentration
Endurance
Fatigue: Disruptive Effects
Fatigue Level
Leisure Participation

Mood Equilibrium
Personal Health Status
Personal Well-Being
Quality of Life
Student Health Status

Outcomes Associated with Related Factors or Intermediate Outcomes
Anxiety Level
Bowel Elimination
Comfort Status: Environment
Depression Level

Discomfort Level
Exercise Participation
Fear Level
Fear Level: Child

Insomnia—cont'd

Grief Resolution
Medication Response
Nausea & Vomiting: Disruptive Effects
Pain Level
Parenting Performance: Infant
Parenting Performance: Middle Childhood
Parenting Performance: Preschooler

Parenting Performance: Toddler
Perimenopause Symptom Severity
Premenstrual Syndrome (PMS) Severity
Respiratory Status: Ventilation
Role Performance
Stress Level
Urinary Continence

Intracranial Adaptive Capacity, Decreased

Definition: Intracranial fluid dynamic mechanisms that normally compensate for increases in intracranial volumes are compromised, resulting in repeated disproportionate increases in intracranial pressure (ICP) in response to a variety of noxious and non-noxious stimuli

Outcomes to Measure Resolution of Diagnosis
Neurological Status: Autonomic
Neurological Status: Consciousness

Seizure Self-Control

Additional Outcomes to Measure Defining Characteristics
Cognition
Neurological Status

Tissue Perfusion: Cerebral

Outcomes Associated with Related Factors or Intermediate Outcomes
Bowel Elimination
Cognitive Orientation
Communication
Electrolyte & Acid/Base Balance
Fluid Balance
Hypotension Severity

Hydration
Neurological Status: Central Motor Control
Neurological Status: Cranial Sensory/Motor Function
Neurological Status: Spinal Sensory/Motor Function
Respiratory Status
Urinary Elimination

Knowledge, Deficient

Definition: Absence or deficiency of cognitive information related to a specific topic

Outcomes to Measure Resolution of Diagnosis

Knowledge: Acute Illness Management
Knowledge: Anticoagulation Therapy Management
Knowledge: Arthritis Management
Knowledge: Asthma Management
Knowledge: Body Mechanics
Knowledge: Bottle Feeding
Knowledge: Breastfeeding
Knowledge: Cancer Management
Knowledge: Cancer Threat Reduction
Knowledge: Cardiac Disease Management
Knowledge: Child Physical Safety
Knowledge: Chronic Disease Management
Knowledge: Chronic Obstructive Pulmonary Disease Management
Knowledge: Conception Prevention
Knowledge: Coronary Artery Disease Management
Knowledge: Cup Feeding
Knowledge: Dementia Management
Knowledge: Depression Management
Knowledge: Diabetes Management
Knowledge: Disease Process
Knowledge: Dysrhythmia Management
Knowledge: Eating Disorder Management
Knowledge: Energy Conservation
Knowledge: Fall Prevention
Knowledge: Fertility Promotion
Knowledge: Health Behavior
Knowledge: Health Promotion
Knowledge: Health Resources
Knowledge: Healthy Diet
Knowledge: Healthy Lifestyle
Knowledge: Heart Failure Management

Knowledge: Hypertension Management
Knowledge: Infant Care
Knowledge: Infection Management
Knowledge: Inflammatory Bowel Disease Management
Knowledge: Kidney Disease Management
Knowledge: Labor & Delivery
Knowledge: Lipid Disorder Management
Knowledge: Medication
Knowledge: Multiple Sclerosis Management
Knowledge: Osteoporosis Management
Knowledge: Ostomy Care
Knowledge: Pain Management
Knowledge: Parenting
Knowledge: Peripheral Artery Disease Management
Knowledge: Personal Safety
Knowledge: Pneumonia Management
Knowledge: Postpartum Maternal Health
Knowledge: Preconception Maternal Health
Knowledge: Pregnancy
Knowledge: Pregnancy & Postpartum Sexual Functioning
Knowledge: Prescribed Activity
Knowledge: Prescribed Diet
Knowledge: Preterm Infant Care
Knowledge: Sexual Functioning
Knowledge: Stress Management
Knowledge: Stroke Management
Knowledge: Stroke Prevention
Knowledge: Substance Use Control
Knowledge: Thrombus Prevention
Knowledge: Time Management
Knowledge: Treatment Procedure
Knowledge: Treatment Regimen
Knowledge: Weight Management

Additional Outcomes to Measure Defining Characteristics

Adherence Behavior
Adherence Behavior: Healthy Diet
Agitation Level
Compliance Behavior
Compliance Behavior: Prescribed Activity

Compliance Behavior: Prescribed Diet
Compliance Behavior: Prescribed Medication
Health Seeking Behavior
Motivation
Participation in Health Care Decisions

Outcomes Associated with Related Factors or Intermediate Outcomes

Abstract Thinking
Client Satisfaction: Teaching
Cognition
Communication: Receptive
Concentration

Delirium Level
Dementia Level
Information Processing
Memory
Motivation

Latex Allergy Response

Definition: A hypersensitive reaction to natural latex rubber products

Outcomes to Measure Resolution of Diagnosis

Allergic Response: Localized

Allergic Response: Systemic

Additional Outcomes to Measure Defining Characteristics

Anxiety Level

Cardiopulmonary Status

Discomfort Level

Hypotension Severity

Nausea & Vomiting Severity

Pain Level

Respiratory Status

Shock Severity: Anaphylactic

Symptom Severity

Tissue Integrity: Skin & Mucous Membranes

Outcomes Associated with Related Factors or Intermediate Outcomes

Immune Hypersensitivity Response

Lifestyle, Sedentary

Definition: Reports a habit of life that is characterized by a low physical activity level

Outcomes to Measure Resolution of Diagnosis

Exercise Participation

Additional Outcomes to Measure Defining Characteristics

Activity Tolerance

Compliance Behavior: Prescribed Activity

Endurance

Lifestyle Balance

Personal Health Status

Physical Fitness

Outcomes Associated with Related Factors or Intermediate Outcomes

Health Beliefs: Perceived Resources

Health Promoting Behavior

Knowledge: Health Behavior

Knowledge: Health Promotion

Knowledge: Healthy Lifestyle

Knowledge: Time Management

Leisure Participation

Motivation

Social Support

Memory, Impaired

Definition: Inability to remember or recall bits of information or behavioral skills

Outcomes to Measure Resolution of Diagnosis
Memory

Additional Outcomes to Measure Defining Characteristics

Cognition

Cognitive Orientation

Concentration

Information Processing

Personal Time Management

Outcomes Associated with Related Factors or Intermediate Outcomes

Cardiac Pump Effectiveness

Cardiopulmonary Status

Circulation Status

Electrolyte & Acid/Base Balance

Electrolyte Balance

Hydration

Neurological Status

Respiratory Status

Respiratory Status: Gas Exchange

Respiratory Status: Ventilation

Tissue Perfusion: Cerebral

Mobility: Bed, Impaired

Definition: Limitation of independent movement from one bed position to another

Outcomes to Measure Resolution of Diagnosis
Body Positioning: Self-Initiated

Additional Outcomes to Measure Defining Characteristics

Body Mechanics Performance

Coordinated Movement

Outcomes Associated with Related Factors or Intermediate Outcomes

Cardiopulmonary Status

Cognition

Discomfort Level

Endurance

Energy Conservation

Joint Movement

Joint Movement: Ankle

Joint Movement: Elbow

Joint Movement: Fingers

Joint Movement: Hip

Joint Movement: Knee

Joint Movement: Neck

Joint Movement: Passive

Joint Movement: Shoulder

Joint Movement: Spine

Joint Movement: Wrist

Knowledge: Body Mechanics

Medication Response

Neurological Status: Central Motor Control

Neurological Status: Spinal Sensory/Motor Function

Pain Level

Physical Fitness

Respiratory Status

Skeletal Function

Weight: Body Mass

Mobility: Physical, Impaired

Definition: Limitation in independent, purposeful physical movement of the body or of one or more extremities

Outcomes to Measure Resolution of Diagnosis

Ambulation
Ambulation: Wheelchair

Mobility

Additional Outcomes to Measure Defining Characteristics

Adaptation to Physical Disability
Balance
Body Mechanics Performance
Body Positioning: Self-Initiated
Coordinated Movement

Gait
Joint Movement
Joint Movement: Passive
Respiratory Status
Transfer Performance

Outcomes Associated with Related Factors or Intermediate Outcomes

Activity Tolerance
Anxiety Level
Cardiopulmonary Status
Cognition
Depression Level
Discomfort Level
Endurance
Energy Conservation
Exercise Participation
Health Orientation
Heedfulness of Affected Side
Immobility Consequences: Physiological
Immobility Consequences: Psycho-Cognitive
Joint Movement: Ankle
Joint Movement: Elbow
Joint Movement: Hip
Joint Movement: Knee

Joint Movement: Shoulder
Joint Movement: Spine
Knowledge: Health Promotion
Knowledge: Prescribed Activity
Medication Response
Motivation
Neurological Status: Central Motor Control
Neurological Status: Spinal Sensory/Motor Function
Nutritional Status: Energy
Nutritional Status: Nutrient Intake
Pain Level
Physical Fitness
Self-Management: Osteoporosis
Sensory Function: Proprioception
Skeletal Function
Weight: Body Mass

Mobility: Wheelchair, Impaired

Definition: Limitation of independent operation of wheelchair within environment

Outcomes to Measure Resolution of Diagnosis

Ambulation: Wheelchair

Additional Outcomes to Measure Defining Characteristics

Balance
Body Mechanics Performance

Coordinated Movement
Transfer Performance

Outcomes Associated with Related Factors or Intermediate Outcomes

Adaptation to Physical Disability
Cognition
Depression Level
Endurance
Immobility Consequences: Physiological
Joint Movement
Joint Movement: Elbow
Joint Movement: Fingers
Joint Movement: Shoulder

Joint Movement: Wrist
Knowledge: Body Mechanics
Neurological Status: Peripheral
Neurological Status: Spinal Sensory/Motor Function
Pain Level
Physical Fitness
Sensory Function: Vision
Weight: Body Mass

Moral Distress

Definition: Response to the inability to carry out one's chosen ethical/moral decision/action

Outcomes to Measure Resolution of Diagnosis

Decision-Making

Spiritual Health

Additional Outcomes to Measure Defining Characteristics

Agitation Level

Anxiety Level

Client Satisfaction: Protection of Rights

Comfort Status: Psychospiritual

Dignified Life Closure

Fear Level

Guilt Resolution

Outcomes Associated with Related Factors or Intermediate Outcomes

Anxiety Self-Control

Client Satisfaction: Cultural Needs Fulfillment

Comfortable Death

Coping

Family Coping

Family Functioning

Family Integrity

Fear Self-Control

Information Processing

Knowledge: Treatment Regimen

Participation in Health Care Decisions

Personal Autonomy

Personal Resiliency

Self-Awareness

Self-Esteem

Stress Level

Nausea

Definition: A subjective phenomenon of an unpleasant feeling in the back of the throat and stomach that may or may not result in vomiting

Outcomes to Measure Resolution of Diagnosis

Appetite

Nausea & Vomiting Control

Nausea & Vomiting: Disruptive Effects

Nausea & Vomiting Severity

Additional Outcomes to Measure Defining Characteristics

Client Satisfaction: Symptom Control

Comfort Status: Physical

Discomfort Level

Maternal Status: Antepartum

Medication Response

Nutritional Status: Food & Fluid Intake

Sensory Function: Taste & Smell

Swallowing Status

Outcomes Associated with Related Factors or Intermediate Outcomes

Anxiety Level

Electrolyte & Acid/Base Balance

Fear Level

Fluid Balance

Gastrointestinal Function

Hydration

Infection Severity

Kidney Function

Liver Function

Pain Level

Suffering Severity

Symptom Control

Symptom Severity

Neonatal Jaundice

Definition: The yellow-orange tint of the neonate's skin and mucous membranes that occurs after 24 hours of life as a result of unconjugated bilirubin in the circulation

Outcomes to Measure Resolution of Diagnosis

Tissue Integrity: Skin & Mucous Membranes

Additional Outcomes to Measure Defining Characteristics

Newborn Adaptation

Outcomes Associated with Related Factors or Intermediate Outcomes

Bottle Feeding Establishment: Infant

Bowel Elimination

Breastfeeding Establishment: Infant

Cup Feeding Establishment: Infant

Preterm Infant Organization

Weight: Body Mass

Noncompliance

Definition: Behavior of person and/or caregiver that fails to coincide with a health-promoting or therapeutic plan agreed on by the person (and/or family and/or community) and health care professional. In the presence of an agreed-upon, health-promoting or therapeutic plan, the person's or caregiver's behavior is fully or partially nonadherent and may lead to clinically ineffective or partially ineffective outcomes

Outcomes to Measure Resolution of Diagnosis

Compliance Behavior

Compliance Behavior: Prescribed Activity

Compliance Behavior: Prescribed Diet

Compliance Behavior: Prescribed Medication

Continued

Noncompliance—*cont'd*

Additional Outcomes to Measure Defining Characteristics

Anxiety Self-Control
Bottle Feeding Performance
Breastfeeding Maintenance
Caregiver Performance: Direct Care
Caregiver Performance: Indirect Care
Community Risk Control: Obesity
Cup Feeding Performance
Eating Disorder Self-Control
Ostomy Self-Care
Personal Health Screening Behavior
Self-Care: Non-Parenteral Medication
Self-Care: Parenteral Medication
Self-Management: Acute Illness
Self-Management: Anticoagulation Therapy
Self-Management: Asthma
Self-Management: Cardiac Disease

Self-Management: Chronic Disease
Self-Management: Chronic Obstructive Pulmonary Disease
Self-Management: Coronary Artery Disease
Self-Management: Diabetes
Self-Management: Dysrhythmia
Self-Management: Heart Failure
Self-Management: Hypertension
Self-Management: Kidney Disease
Self-Management: Lipid Disorder
Self-Management: Multiple Sclerosis
Self-Management: Osteoporosis
Self-Management: Peripheral Artery Disease
Smoking Cessation Behavior
Symptom Control
Weight Gain Behavior
Weight Loss Behavior

Outcomes Associated with Related Factors or Intermediate Outcomes

Acceptance: Health Status
Adaptation to Physical Disability
Adherence Behavior
Alcohol Abuse Cessation Behavior
Anxiety Level
Caregiver Home Care Readiness
Caregiver-Patient Relationship
Caregiver Stressors
Client Satisfaction
Client Satisfaction: Case Management
Client Satisfaction: Communication
Client Satisfaction: Safety
Depression Level
Depression Self-Control
Drug Abuse Cessation Behavior
Fall Prevention Behavior
Family Coping
Family Participation in Professional Care
Family Resiliency
Health Beliefs
Health Beliefs: Perceived Ability to Perform
Health Beliefs: Perceived Control
Health Beliefs: Perceived Resources
Health Beliefs: Perceived Threat
Health Orientation
Immunization Behavior
Knowledge: Disease Process
Knowledge: Health Behavior

Knowledge: Health Promotion
Knowledge: Treatment Regimen
Motivation
Participation in Health Care Decisions
Postpartum Maternal Health Behavior
Risk Control
Risk Control: Alcohol Use
Risk Control: Cancer
Risk Control: Cardiovascular Disease
Risk Control: Drug Use
Risk Control: Hearing Impairment
Risk Control: Hypertension
Risk Control: Hyperthermia
Risk Control: Hypotension
Risk Control: Hypothermia
Risk Control: Infectious Process
Risk Control: Lipid Disorder
Risk Control: Osteoporosis
Risk Control: Sexually Transmitted Diseases (STD)
Risk Control: Sun Exposure
Risk Control: Thrombus
Risk Control: Tobacco Use
Risk Control: Unintended Pregnancy
Risk Control: Visual Impairment
Risk Detection
Social Support
Will to Live

Nutrition: Imbalanced, Less than Body Requirements

Definition: Intake of nutrients insufficient to meet metabolic needs

Outcomes to Measure Resolution of Diagnosis

Infant Nutritional Status

Nutritional Status

Nutritional Status: Nutrient Intake

Additional Outcomes to Measure Defining Characteristics

Appetite

Bowel Elimination

Breastfeeding Establishment: Infant

Cup Feeding Establishment: Infant

Discomfort Level

Knowledge: Healthy Diet

Nutritional Status: Biochemical Measures

Nutritional Status: Energy

Nutritional Status: Food & Fluid Intake

Oral Health

Pain Level

Sensory Function: Taste & Smell

Swallowing Status

Tissue Perfusion: Peripheral

Weight: Body Mass

Outcomes Associated with Related Factors or Intermediate Outcomes

Adherence Behavior: Healthy Diet

Compliance Behavior: Prescribed Diet

Depression Level

Eating Disorder Self-Control

Fatigue: Disruptive Effects

Gastrointestinal Function

Health Beliefs

Health Beliefs: Perceived Resources

Knowledge: Eating Disorder Management

Knowledge: Inflammatory Bowel Disease Management

Knowledge: Prescribed Diet

Knowledge: Weight Management

Nausea & Vomiting Severity

Prenatal Health Behavior

Self-Care: Eating

Swallowing Status: Oral Phase

Swallowing Status: Pharyngeal Phase

Nutrition: Imbalanced, More than Body Requirements

Definition: Intake of nutrients that exceeds metabolic needs

Outcomes to Measure Resolution of Diagnosis

Infant Nutritional Status

Nutritional Status: Food & Fluid Intake

Nutritional Status: Nutrient Intake

Additional Outcomes to Measure Defining Characteristics

Anxiety Level

Eating Disorder Self-Control

Exercise Participation

Nutritional Status

Weight: Body Mass

Outcomes Associated with Related Factors or Intermediate Outcomes

Adherence Behavior: Healthy Diet

Compliance Behavior: Prescribed Activity

Compliance Behavior: Prescribed Diet

Knowledge: Healthy Diet

Knowledge: Weight Management

Weight Loss Behavior

Oral Mucous Membrane, Impaired

Definition: Disruption of the lips and/or soft tissue of the oral cavity

Outcomes to Measure Resolution of Diagnosis

Oral Health

Tissue Integrity: Skin & Mucous Membranes

Additional Outcomes to Measure Defining Characteristics

Pain Level

Sensory Function: Taste & Smell

Swallowing Status: Oral Phase

Outcomes Associated with Related Factors or Intermediate Outcomes

Allergic Response: Localized

Blood Coagulation

Depression Level

Hydration

Immune Status

Infection Severity

Infection Severity: Newborn

Knowledge: Cancer Management

Knowledge: Health Promotion

Knowledge: Health Resources

Knowledge: Infection Management

Medication Response

Nausea & Vomiting Severity

Nutritional Status

Nutritional Status: Food & Fluid Intake

Nutritional Status: Nutrient Intake

Physical Injury Severity

Risk Control: Alcohol Use

Risk Control: Drug Use

Risk Control: Infectious Process

Risk Control: Tobacco Use

Self-Care: Oral Hygiene

Stress Level

Pain, Acute

Definition: Unpleasant sensory and emotional experience arising from actual or potential tissue damage or described in terms of such damage (International Association for the Study of Pain); sudden or slow onset of any intensity from mild to severe with an anticipated or predictable end and a duration of <6 months

Outcomes to Measure Resolution of Diagnosis

Pain Control

Pain Level

Additional Outcomes to Measure Defining Characteristics

Anxiety Level

Appetite

Client Satisfaction: Pain Management

Client Satisfaction: Symptom Control

Comfort Status

Comfort Status: Physical

Discomfort Level

Mobility

Nausea & Vomiting Severity

Pain: Adverse Psychological Response

Pain: Disruptive Effects

Sleep

Symptom Control

Symptom Severity

Vital Signs

Outcomes Associated with Related Factors or Intermediate Outcomes

Burn Recovery

Gastrointestinal Function

Kidney Function

Knowledge: Acute Illness Management

Knowledge: Inflammatory Bowel Disease Management

Knowledge: Pain Management

Medication Response

Neurological Status

Physical Injury Severity

Self-Management: Acute Illness

Stress Level

Surgical Recovery: Convalescence

Surgical Recovery: Immediate Post-Operative

Tissue Integrity: Skin & Mucous Membranes

Tissue Perfusion

Tissue Perfusion: Abdominal Organs

Tissue Perfusion: Cardiac

Tissue Perfusion: Cellular

Tissue Perfusion: Peripheral

Wound Healing: Primary Intention

Wound Healing: Secondary Intention

Pain, Chronic

Definition: Unpleasant sensory and emotional experience arising from actual or potential tissue damage or described in terms of such damage (International Association for the Study of Pain); sudden or slow onset of any intensity from mild to severe, constant or recurring without an anticipated or predictable end and a duration of >6 months

Outcomes to Measure Resolution of Diagnosis

Pain: Adverse Psychological Response

Pain Control

Pain: Disruptive Effects

Pain Level

Additional Outcomes to Measure Defining Characteristics

Agitation Level

Anxiety Level

Appetite

Client Satisfaction: Pain Management

Client Satisfaction: Symptom Control

Comfort Status

Comfort Status: Physical

Depression Level

Depression Self-Control

Fatigue Level

Fatigue: Disruptive Effects

Fear Level

Mobility

Personal Well-Being

Psychomotor Energy

Quality of Life

Continued

Pain, Chronic—cont'd

Rest	Suffering Severity
Sleep	Symptom Control
Social Involvement	Symptom Severity
Stress Level	Vital Signs

Outcomes Associated with Related Factors or Intermediate Outcomes

Adaptation to Physical Disability	Self-Care Status
Burn Recovery	Self-Management: Chronic Disease
Knowledge: Arthritis Management	Social Anxiety Level
Knowledge: Pain Management	Wound Healing: Secondary Intention
Psychosocial Adjustment: Life Change	

Parental Role Conflict

Definition: Parental experience of role confusion and conflict in response to crisis

Outcomes to Measure Resolution of Diagnosis
Parenting Performance

Additional Outcomes to Measure Defining Characteristics

Anxiety Level	Parenting Performance: Adolescent
Anxiety Self-Control	Parenting Performance: Infant
Family Functioning	Parenting Performance: Middle Childhood
Family Health Status	Parenting Performance: Preschooler
Family Social Climate	Parenting Performance: Toddler
Fear Level	Psychosocial Adjustment: Life Change
Guilt Resolution	

Outcomes Associated with Related Factors or Intermediate Outcomes

Adaptation to Physical Disability	Child Adaptation to Hospitalization
Alcohol Abuse Cessation Behavior	Drug Abuse Cessation Behavior
Caregiver Adaptation to Patient Institutionalization	Family Normalization
Caregiver Home Care Readiness	Family Participation in Professional Care
Caregiver Lifestyle Disruption	Family Resiliency
Caregiver Performance: Direct Care	Parent-Infant Attachment
Caregiver Performance: Indirect Care	Role Performance
Caregiver Physical Health	Stress Level
Caregiver Stressors	

Parenting, Impaired

Definition: Inability of the primary caretaker to create, maintain, or regain an environment that promotes the optimum growth and development of the child

Outcomes to Measure Resolution of Diagnosis

Parenting Performance
Parenting Performance: Adolescent
Parenting Performance: Infant

Parenting Performance: Middle Childhood
Parenting Performance: Preschooler
Parenting Performance: Toddler

Additional Outcomes to Measure Defining Characteristics

Abuse Cessation
Abuse Recovery
Abusive Behavior Self-Restraint
Breastfeeding Establishment: Maternal
Breastfeeding Maintenance
Caregiver Home Care Readiness
Caregiver Performance: Direct Care
Caregiver Performance: Indirect Care
Child Development: 1 Month
Child Development: 2 Months
Child Development: 4 Months
Child Development: 6 Months
Child Development: 12 Months
Child Development: 2 Years

Child Development: 3 Years
Child Development: 4 Years
Child Development: 5 Years
Child Development: Middle Childhood
Child Development: Adolescence
Family Functioning
Family Social Climate
Neglect Cessation
Neglect Recovery
Parent-Infant Attachment
Parenting Performance: Psychosocial Safety
Role Performance
Safe Home Environment
Social Involvement

Outcomes Associated with Related Factors or Intermediate Outcomes

Abuse Protection
Adaptation to Physical Disability
Alcohol Abuse Cessation Behavior
Anxiety Level
Anxiety Self-Control
Cognition
Coping
Depression Level
Depression Self-Control
Drug Abuse Cessation Behavior
Family Integrity
Fatigue Level
Health Beliefs: Perceived Resources
Knowledge: Bottle Feeding
Knowledge: Breastfeeding
Knowledge: Child Physical Safety
Knowledge: Cup Feeding

Knowledge: Infant Care
Knowledge: Parenting
Knowledge: Preterm Infant Care
Motivation
Parenting Performance: Adolescent Physical Safety
Parenting Performance: Early/Middle Childhood Physical
   Safety
Parenting Performance: Infant/Toddler Physical Safety
Personal Resiliency
Psychosocial Adjustment: Life Change
Self-Esteem
Smoking Cessation Behavior
Social Interaction Skills
Social Support
Stress Level
Substance Addiction Consequences
Substance Withdrawal Severity

Personal Identity, Disturbed

Definition: Inability to maintain an integrated and complete perception of self

Outcomes to Measure Resolution of Diagnosis

Identity

Self-Awareness

Additional Outcomes to Measure Defining Characteristics

Body Image

Comfort Status: Psychospiritual

Comfort Status: Sociocultural

Coping

Distorted Thought Self-Control

Role Performance

Sexual Identity

Outcomes Associated with Related Factors or Intermediate Outcomes

Anger Self-Restraint

Anxiety Level

Anxiety Self-Control

Community Risk Control: Unhealthy Cultural Traditions

Delirium Level

Dementia Level

Depression Level

Depression Self-Control

Dignified Life Closure

Drug Abuse Cessation Behavior

Family Functioning

Family Integrity

Family Normalization

Family Resiliency

Family Social Climate

Family Support During Treatment

Guilt Resolution

Impulse Self-Control

Personal Autonomy

Personal Resiliency

Physical Maturation: Female

Physical Maturation: Male

Psychosocial Adjustment: Life Change

Self-Esteem

Social Anxiety Level

Substance Addiction Consequences

Post-Trauma Syndrome

Definition: Sustained maladaptive response to a traumatic, overwhelming event

Outcomes to Measure Resolution of Diagnosis

Mood Equilibrium

Personal Resiliency

Personal Well-Being

Additional Outcomes to Measure Defining Characteristics

Aggression Self-Restraint

Agitation Level

Anger Self-Restraint

Anxiety Level

Anxiety Self-Control

Comfort Status: Psychospiritual

Concentration

Coping

Depression Level

Depression Self-Control

Distorted Thought Self-Control

Drug Abuse Cessation Behavior

Fear Level

Fear Level: Child

Fear Self-Control

Grief Resolution

Guilt Resolution

Hope

Identity

Impulse Self-Control

Social Anxiety Level

Substance Addiction Consequences

Substance Withdrawal Severity

Symptom Severity

Post-Trauma Syndrome—*cont'd*

Outcomes Associated with Related Factors or Intermediate Outcomes

Abuse Cessation
Abuse Protection
Abuse Recovery
Abuse Recovery: Emotional
Abuse Recovery: Financial
Abuse Recovery: Physical
Abuse Recovery: Sexual
Abusive Behavior Self-Restraint
Adaptation to Physical Disability
Body Image
Burn Recovery
Family Resiliency
Health Beliefs: Perceived Threat

Lifestyle Balance
Mutilation Self-Restraint
Personal Safety Behavior
Psychosocial Adjustment: Life Change
Quality of Life
Risk Detection
Self-Esteem
Sexual Functioning
Sleep
Social Support
Suffering Severity
Suicide Self-Restraint
Will to Live

Powerlessness

Definition: The lived experience of lack of control over a situation, including a perception that one's actions do not significantly affect an outcome

Outcomes to Measure Resolution of Diagnosis

Health Beliefs: Perceived Ability to Perform

Health Beliefs: Perceived Control

Additional Outcomes to Measure Defining Characteristics

Acceptance: Health Status
Adaptation to Physical Disability
Anger Self-Restraint
Caregiver-Patient Relationship
Depression Level
Depression Self-Control
Guilt Resolution
Health Beliefs
Health Beliefs: Perceived Resources

Hope
Participation in Health Care Decisions
Personal Autonomy
Personal Resiliency
Role Performance
Self-Awareness
Self-Esteem
Self-Management: Acute Illness

Outcomes Associated with Related Factors or Intermediate Outcomes

Abuse Recovery
Anxiety Level
Anxiety Self-Control
Client Satisfaction
Client Satisfaction: Access to Care Resources
Client Satisfaction: Case Management
Client Satisfaction: Pain Management
Client Satisfaction: Protection of Rights
Decision-Making
Fatigue Level
Health Orientation
Information Processing

Knowledge: Disease Process
Knowledge: Health Resources
Knowledge: Medication
Knowledge: Personal Safety
Knowledge: Treatment Regimen
Lifestyle Balance
Self-Direction of Care
Self-Management: Chronic Disease
Social Interaction Skills
Social Involvement
Social Support
Stress Level

Protection, Ineffective

Definition: Decrease in the ability to guard self from internal or external threats such as illness or injury

Outcomes to Measure Resolution of Diagnosis

Health Promoting Behavior   Risk Control

Additional Outcomes to Measure or Defining Characteristics

Blood Coagulation   Knowledge: Personal Safety
Bone Healing   Mobility
Burn Healing   Neurological Status: Peripheral
Burn Recovery   Respiratory Status
Cognition   Sleep
Cognitive Orientation   Stress Level
Community Immune Status   Symptom Control
Delirium Level   Thermoregulation
Eating Disorder Self-Control   Thermoregulation: Newborn
Fatigue Level   Wound Healing: Primary Intention
Immunization Behavior   Wound Healing: Secondary Intention

Outcomes Associated with Related Factors or Intermediate Outcomes

Alcohol Abuse Cessation Behavior   Physical Aging
Drug Abuse Cessation Behavior   Preterm Infant Organization
Immune Hypersensitivity Response   Risk Control: Stroke
Immune Status   Risk Control: Thrombus
Knowledge: Cancer Management   Risk Detection
Knowledge: Health Promotion   Self-Management: Anticoagulation Therapy
Medication Response   Smoking Cessation Behavior
Newborn Adaptation   Substance Withdrawal Severity
Nutritional Status   Tissue Integrity: Skin & Mucous Membranes

Rape-Trauma Syndrome

Definition: Sustained maladaptive response to a forced, violent sexual penetration against the victim's will and consent

Outcomes to Measure Resolution of Diagnosis
Abuse Recovery: Sexual

Additional Outcomes to Measure Defining Characteristics

Abuse Protection	Guilt Resolution
Abuse Recovery: Emotional	Mood Equilibrium
Abuse Recovery: Physical	Personal Autonomy
Agitation Level	Personal Health Status
Alcohol Abuse Cessation Behavior	Personal Resiliency
Anger Self-Restraint	Quality of Life
Anxiety Level	Self-Awareness
Anxiety Self-Control	Self-Esteem
Comfort Status: Psychospiritual	Sexual Functioning
Depression Level	Sleep
Depression Self-Control	Substance Addiction Consequences
Fear Level	Substance Withdrawal Severity
Fear Self-Control	Suicide Self-Restraint

Outcomes Associated with Related Factors or Intermediate Outcomes

Abuse Cessation	Hope
Abuse Recovery	Identity
Family Coping	Social Support
Family Support During Treatment	

Relationship, Ineffective

Definition: A pattern of mutual partnership that is insufficient to provide for each other's needs

Outcomes to Measure Resolution of Diagnosis

Caregiver-Patient Relationship	Parenting Performance: Infant
Caregiver Performance: Direct Care	Parenting Performance: Infant/Toddler Physical Safety
Caregiver Performance: Indirect Care	Parenting Performance: Middle Childhood
Parenting Performance	Parenting Performance: Preschooler
Parenting Performance: Adolescent	Parenting Performance: Psychosocial Safety
Parenting Performance: Adolescent Physical Safety	Parenting Performance: Toddler
Parenting Performance: Early/Middle Childhood Physical Safety	

Additional Outcomes to Measure Defining Characteristics

Adaptation to Physical Disability	Development: Middle Adulthood
Caregiver Adaptation to Patient Institutionalization	Development: Young Adulthood
Caregiver Home Care Readiness	Personal Resiliency
Caregiver Role Endurance	Psychosocial Adjustment: Life Change
Caregiver Stressors	Role Performance
Child Development: Adolescence	Social Interaction Skills
Child Development: Middle Childhood	Social Support
Development: Late Adulthood	

Continued

Relationship, Ineffective—cont'd

Outcomes Associated with Related Factors or Intermediate Outcomes

Abuse Cessation

Abuse Recovery

Acceptance: Health Status

Alcohol Abuse Cessation Behavior

Cognition

Coping

Delirium Level

Dementia Level

Drug Abuse Cessation Behavior

Identity

Neglect Cessation

Neglect Recovery

Smoking Cessation Behavior

Stress Level

Substance Addiction Consequences

Substance Withdrawal Severity

Religiosity, Impaired

Definition: Impaired ability to exercise reliance on beliefs and/or participate in rituals of a particular faith tradition

Outcomes to Measure Resolution of Diagnosis

Spiritual Health

Additional Outcomes to Measure Defining Characteristics

Comfort Status: Psychospiritual

Community Risk Control: Unhealthy Cultural Traditions

Hope

Personal Autonomy

Outcomes Associated with Related Factors or Intermediate Outcomes

Acceptance: Health Status

Anxiety Level

Client Satisfaction: Cultural Needs Fulfillment

Comfort Status: Sociocultural

Comfortable Death

Coping

Development: Late Adulthood

Development: Middle Adulthood

Development: Young Adulthood

Dignified Life Closure

Fear Level

Lifestyle Balance

Personal Health Status

Personal Resiliency

Personal Well-Being

Psychosocial Adjustment: Life Change

Quality of Life

Self-Awareness

Social Involvement

Social Support

Stress Level

Suffering Severity

Relocation Stress Syndrome

Definition: Physiological and/or psychosocial disturbance following transfer from one environment to another

Outcomes to Measure Resolution of Diagnosis
Caregiver Adaptation to Patient Institutionalization
Child Adaptation to Hospitalization

Relocation Adaptation

Additional Outcomes to Measure Defining Characteristics
Agitation Level
Anger Self-Restraint
Anxiety Level
Anxiety Self-Control
Coping
Delirium Level
Depression Level
Depression Self-Control
Fear Level
Fear Level: Child

Fear Self-Control
Hope
Identity
Loneliness Severity
Personal Autonomy
Personal Resiliency
Psychosocial Adjustment: Life Change
Self-Esteem
Sleep
Symptom Severity

Outcomes Associated with Related Factors or Intermediate Outcomes
Caregiver Home Care Readiness
Caregiver Performance: Direct Care
Decision-Making
Dementia Level
Discharge Readiness: Independent Living
Discharge Readiness: Supported Living
Elopement Propensity Risk

Family Participation in Professional Care
Grief Resolution
Quality of Life
Safe Wandering
Social Support
Stress Level

Resilience, Impaired Individual

Definition: Decreased ability to sustain a pattern of positive responses to an adverse situation or crisis

Outcomes to Measure Resolution of Diagnosis
Personal Resiliency

Additional Outcomes to Measure Defining Characteristics
Coping
Depression Level
Depression Self-Control
Guilt Resolution
Knowledge: Depression Management
Loneliness Severity

Personal Health Status
Role Performance
Self-Esteem
Social Anxiety Level
Social Involvement

Outcomes Associated with Related Factors or Intermediate Outcomes
Cognition
Community Violence Level
Drug Abuse Cessation Behavior
Family Social Climate
Impulse Self-Control
Knowledge: Parenting

Lifestyle Balance
Mood Equilibrium
Stress Level
Substance Addiction Consequences
Substance Withdrawal Severity
Suffering Severity

Role Performance, Ineffective

Definition: Patterns of behavior and self-expression that do not match the environmental context, norms, and expectations

Outcomes to Measure Resolution of Diagnosis

Caregiver Performance: Direct Care
Caregiver Performance: Indirect Care

Parenting Performance
Role Performance

Additional Outcomes to Measure Defining Characteristics

Abuse Recovery
Acceptance: Health Status
Adaptation to Physical Disability
Anxiety Level
Anxiety Self-Control
Bottle Feeding Performance
Caregiver Lifestyle Disruption
Caregiver Role Endurance
Cognition
Coping
Cup Feeding Performance
Depression Level
Hope
Knowledge: Bottle Feeding
Knowledge: Child Physical Safety
Knowledge: Cup Feeding
Knowledge: Parenting

Lifestyle Balance
Motivation
Parenting Performance: Adolescent
Parenting Performance: Adolescent Physical Safety
Parenting Performance: Early/Middle Childhood Physical Safety
Parenting Performance: Infant
Parenting Performance: Infant/Toddler Physical Safety
Parenting Performance: Middle Childhood
Parenting Performance: Preschooler
Parenting Performance: Psychosocial Safety
Parenting Performance: Toddler
Personal Resiliency
Personal Time Management
Psychosocial Adjustment: Life Change
Social Interaction Skills
Social Involvement

Outcomes Associated with Related Factors or Intermediate Outcomes

Abuse Cessation
Adaptation to Physical Disability
Agitation Level
Body Image
Caregiver Adaptation to Patient Institutionalization
Caregiver Home Care Readiness
Depression Self-Control
Elopement Propensity Risk
Family Functioning
Fatigue Level

Information Processing
Memory
Pain Level
Psychomotor Energy
Relocation Adaptation
Self-Esteem
Social Anxiety Level
Social Support
Stress Level
Substance Addiction Consequences

Self-Care Deficit: Bathing

Definition: Impaired ability to perform or complete bathing activities for self

Outcomes to Measure Resolution of Diagnosis

Self-Care: Bathing

Self-Care: Hygiene

Additional Outcomes to Measure Defining Characteristics

Ambulation

Ambulation: Wheelchair

Body Mechanics Performance

Mobility

Outcomes Associated with Related Factors or Intermediate Outcomes

Adaptation to Physical Disability

Anxiety Level

Client Satisfaction: Physical Environment

Cognition

Comfort Status: Environment

Delirium Level

Dementia Level

Discomfort Level

Endurance

Fatigue Level

Heedfulness of Affected Side

Knowledge: Body Mechanics

Motivation

Neurological Status: Peripheral

Neurological Status: Spinal/Sensory Motor Function

Pain Level

Psychomotor Energy

Safe Home Environment

Sensory Function: Proprioception

Sensory Function: Vision

Skeletal Function

Self-Care Deficit: Dressing

Definition: Impaired ability to perform or complete dressing activities for self

Outcomes to Measure Resolution of Diagnosis

Self-Care: Dressing

Additional Outcomes to Measure Defining Characteristics

Balance

Body Mechanics Performance

Body Positioning: Self-Initiated

Decision-Making

Joint Movement

Mobility

Outcomes Associated with Related Factors or Intermediate Outcomes

Adaptation to Physical Disability

Anxiety Level

Client Satisfaction: Physical Environment

Cognition

Comfort Status: Environment

Coordinated Movement

Delirium Level

Dementia Level

Discomfort Level

Endurance

Fatigue: Disruptive Effects

Fatigue Level

Heedfulness of Affected Side

Joint Movement: Elbow

Joint Movement: Fingers

Joint Movement: Shoulder

Joint Movement: Wrist

Motivation

Neurological Status: Central Motor Control

Neurological Status: Peripheral

Pain Level

Psychomotor Energy

Sensory Function: Proprioception

Sensory Function: Vision

Skeletal Function

Vision Compensation Behavior

Self-Care Deficit: Feeding

Definition: Impaired ability to perform or complete self-feeding activities

Outcomes to Measure Resolution of Diagnosis
Self-Care: Eating

Additional Outcomes to Measure Defining Characteristics

Nutritional Status: Food & Fluid Intake   Swallowing Status

Outcomes Associated with Related Factors or Intermediate Outcomes

Adaptation to Physical Disability   Joint Movement: Fingers
Anxiety Level   Joint Movement: Shoulder
Aspiration Prevention   Joint Movement: Wrist
Client Satisfaction: Physical Environment   Motivation
Cognition   Neurological Status: Central Motor Control
Comfort Status: Environment   Neurological Status: Peripheral
Coordinated Movement   Pain Level
Delirium Level   Psychomotor Energy
Dementia Level   Sensory Function: Vision
Discomfort Level   Skeletal Function
Fatigue Level   Vision Compensation Behavior
Joint Movement: Elbow

Self-Care Deficit: Toileting

Definition: Impaired ability to perform or complete toileting activities for self

Outcomes to Measure Resolution of Diagnosis

Ostomy Self-Care   Self-Care: Toileting

Additional Outcomes to Measure Defining Characteristics

Ambulation   Coordinated Movement
Ambulation: Wheelchair   Self-Care: Dressing
Balance   Self-Care: Hygiene
Body Positioning: Self-Initiated

Outcomes Associated with Related Factors or Intermediate Outcomes

Anxiety Level   Mobility
Client Satisfaction: Physical Environment   Neurological Status: Central Motor Control
Cognition   Neurological Status: Peripheral
Comfort Status: Environment   Pain Level
Delirium Level   Sensory Function: Proprioception
Dementia Level   Sensory Function: Vision
Discomfort Level   Skeletal Function
Endurance   Transfer Performance
Fatigue Level   Vision Compensation Behavior
Joint Movement

Self-Esteem: Chronic Low

Definition: Longstanding negative self-evaluating/feelings about self or self-capabilities

Outcomes to Measure Resolution of Diagnosis
Self-Esteem

Additional Outcomes to Measure Defining Characteristics

Depression Level	Personal Resiliency
Guilt Resolution	Self-Awareness
Personal Autonomy	Social Involvement

Outcomes Associated with Related Factors or Intermediate Outcomes

Abuse Recovery	Grief Resolution
Abuse Recovery: Emotional	Hope
Abuse Recovery: Sexual	Loneliness Severity
Acceptance: Health Status	Mood Equilibrium
Adaptation to Physical Disability	Motivation
Body Image	Psychosocial Adjustment: Life Change
Comfort Status: Psychospiritual	Quality of Life
Comfort Status: Sociocultural	Role Performance
Depression Self-Control	Social Anxiety Level
Distorted Thought Self-Control	Social Interaction Skills
Family Integrity	Spiritual Health
Family Normalization	Stress Level
Family Resiliency	Suffering Severity
Family Social Climate	Symptom Severity

Self-Esteem: Situational Low

Definition: Development of a negative perception of self-worth in response to a current situation

Outcomes to Measure Resolution of Diagnosis
Self-Esteem

Additional Outcomes to Measure Defining Characteristics

Adaptation to Physical Disability	Psychosocial Adjustment: Life Change
Guilt Resolution	Self-Awareness
Personal Resiliency	

Outcomes Associated with Related Factors or Intermediate Outcomes

Abuse Recovery	Eating Disorder Self-Control
Abuse Recovery: Emotional	Grief Resolution
Abuse Recovery: Physical	Heedfulness of Affected Side
Abuse Recovery: Sexual	Lifestyle Balance
Anxiety Level	Neglect Recovery
Body Image	Parenting Performance
Burn Recovery	Personal Autonomy
Coping	Role Performance
Development: Late Adulthood	Social Anxiety Level
Development: Middle Adulthood	Stress Level
Development: Young Adulthood	

Self-Health Management, Ineffective

Definition: Pattern of regulating and integrating into daily living a therapeutic regimen for treatment of illness and its sequelae that is unsatisfactory for meeting specific health goals

Outcomes to Measure Resolution of Diagnosis

Self-Management: Acute Illness
Self-Management: Chronic Disease

Symptom Control

Additional Outcomes to Measure Defining Characteristics

Adherence Behavior
Adherence Behavior: Healthy Diet
Compliance Behavior
Compliance Behavior: Prescribed Activity
Compliance Behavior: Prescribed Diet
Compliance Behavior: Prescribed Medication
Exercise Participation
Motivation
Participation in Health Care Decisions
Postpartum Maternal Health Behavior
Prenatal Health Behavior
Risk Control
Seizure Self-Control
Self-Care: Non-Parenteral Medication
Self-Care: Parenteral Medication

Self-Direction of Care
Self-Management: Anticoagulation Therapy
Self-Management: Asthma
Self-Management: Cardiac Disease
Self-Management: Chronic Obstructive Pulmonary Disease
Self-Management: Coronary Artery Disease
Self-Management: Diabetes
Self-Management: Dysrhythmia
Self-Management: Heart Failure
Self-Management: Hypertension
Self-Management: Kidney Disease
Self-Management: Lipid Disorder
Self-Management: Multiple Sclerosis
Self-Management: Osteoporosis
Self-Management: Peripheral Artery Disease

Outcomes Associated with Related Factors or Intermediate Outcomes

Client Satisfaction: Case Management
Coping
Decision-Making
Discharge Readiness: Independent Living
Family Coping
Family Functioning
Family Normalization
Family Participation in Professional Care
Family Support During Treatment
Health Beliefs
Health Beliefs: Perceived Ability to Perform
Health Beliefs: Perceived Control
Health Beliefs: Perceived Resources
Health Beliefs: Perceived Threat
Health Orientation
Knowledge: Acute Illness Management
Knowledge: Anticoagulation Therapy Management
Knowledge: Arthritis Management
Knowledge: Asthma Management
Knowledge: Cancer Management
Knowledge: Cancer Threat Reduction
Knowledge: Cardiac Disease Management
Knowledge: Chronic Disease Management
Knowledge: Chronic Obstructive Pulmonary Disease
   Management
Knowledge: Coronary Artery Disease Management
Knowledge: Dementia Management
Knowledge: Depression Management
Knowledge: Diabetes Management

Knowledge: Disease Process
Knowledge: Dysrhythmia Management
Knowledge: Eating Disorder Management
Knowledge: Health Behavior Knowledge: Health Promotion
Knowledge: Health Resources
Knowledge: Healthy Diet
Knowledge: Healthy Lifestyle
Knowledge: Heart Failure Management
Knowledge: Hypertension Management
Knowledge: Infection Management
Knowledge: Inflammatory Bowel Disease Management
Knowledge: Kidney Disease Management
Knowledge: Lipid Disorder Management
Knowledge: Multiple Sclerosis Management
Knowledge: Osteoporosis Management
Knowledge: Pain Management
Knowledge: Peripheral Artery Disease Management
Knowledge: Pneumonia Management
Knowledge: Prescribed Activity
Knowledge: Prescribed Diet
Knowledge: Stress Management
Knowledge: Stroke Management
Knowledge: Stroke Prevention
Knowledge: Treatment Procedure
Knowledge: Treatment Regimen
Knowledge: Weight Management
Personal Autonomy
Social Support

Self-Mutilation

Definition: Deliberate self-injurious behavior causing tissue damage with the intent of causing non-fatal injury to attain relief of tension

Outcomes to Measure Resolution of Diagnosis
Mutilation Self-Restraint

Additional Outcomes to Measure Defining Characteristics

Burn Healing	Wound Healing: Primary Intention
Tissue Integrity: Skin & Mucous Membranes	

Outcomes Associated with Related Factors or Intermediate Outcomes

Abuse Recovery	Eating Disorder Self-Control
Abuse Recovery: Emotional	Family Integrity
Abuse Recovery: Physical	Family Social Climate
Abuse Recovery: Sexual	Grief Resolution
Alcohol Abuse Cessation Behavior	Guilt Resolution
Anxiety Level	Identity
Body Image	Impulse Self-Control
Child Development: Adolescence	Loneliness Severity
Child Development: Middle Childhood	Mood Equilibrium
Coping	Personal Resiliency
Depression Level	Risk Control: Drug Use
Development: Late Adulthood	Self-Esteem
Development: Middle Adulthood	Sexual Identity
Development: Young Adulthood	Social Interaction Skills
Distorted Thought Self-Control	Social Support
Drug Abuse Cessation Behavior	Stress Level

Self-Neglect

Definition: A constellation of culturally framed behaviors involving one or more self-care activities in which there is a failure to maintain a socially accepted standard of health and well-being

Outcomes to Measure Resolution of Diagnosis

Personal Health Status	Self-Care Status
Personal Well-Being	

Additional Outcomes to Measure Defining Characteristics

Adherence Behavior	Self-Care: Activities of Daily Living (ADL)
Adherence Behavior: Healthy Diet	Self-Care: Bathing
Comfort Status: Environment	Self-Care: Dressing
Compliance Behavior	Self-Care: Hygiene
Compliance Behavior: Prescribed Activity	Self-Care: Instrumental Activities of Daily Living (IADL)
Compliance Behavior: Prescribed Diet	Self-Care: Oral Hygiene
Compliance Behavior: Prescribed Medication	Self-Care: Toileting
Safe Home Environment	

Continued

Self-Neglect—cont'd

Outcomes Associated with Related Factors or Intermediate Outcomes

Abstract Thinking	Health Beliefs: Perceived Ability to Perform
Adaptation to Physical Disability	Health Beliefs: Perceived Control
Cognition	Health Beliefs: Perceived Resources
Coordinated Movement	Health Orientation
Delirium Level	Information Processing
Dementia Level	Knowledge: Healthy Lifestyle
Depression Level	Memory
Distorted Thought Self-Control	Mobility
Drug Abuse Cessation Behavior	Personal Autonomy
Fear Level	Stress Level
Fear Self-Control	Substance Addiction Consequences
Health Beliefs	

Sexual Dysfunction

Definition: The state in which an individual experiences a change in sexual function during the sexual response phases of desire, excitation, and/or orgasm, which is viewed as unsatisfying, unrewarding, or inadequate

Outcomes to Measure Resolution of Diagnosis
Sexual Functioning

Additional Outcomes to Measure Defining Characteristics
Role Performance

Outcomes Associated with Related Factors or Intermediate Outcomes

Abuse Recovery	Knowledge: Pregnancy & Postpartum Sexual Functioning
Abuse Recovery: Emotional	Knowledge: Sexual Functioning
Abuse Recovery: Physical	Physical Aging
Abuse Recovery: Sexual	Physical Injury Severity
Adaptation to Physical Disability	Physical Maturation: Female
Depression Level	Physical Maturation: Male
Fatigue Level	Sexual Identity

Sexuality Pattern, Ineffective

Definition: Expressions of concern regarding own sexuality

Outcomes to Measure Resolution of Diagnosis
Sexual Identity

Additional Outcomes to Measure Defining Characteristics

Psychosocial Adjustment: Life Change	Self-Awareness
Role Performance	

Outcomes Associated with Related Factors or Intermediate Outcomes

Body Image	Risk Control: Sexually Transmitted Diseases (STD)
Fear Level	Risk Control: Unintended Pregnancy
Knowledge: Sexual Functioning	Self-Esteem
Physical Maturation: Female	Social Support
Physical Maturation: Male	Stress Level

Skin Integrity, Impaired

Definition: Altered epidermis and/or dermis

Outcomes to Measure Resolution of Diagnosis
Tissue Integrity: Skin & Mucous Membranes

Additional Outcomes to Measure Defining Characteristics

Allergic Response: Localized
Burn Healing
Hemodialysis Access

Wound Healing: Primary Intention
Wound Healing: Secondary Intention

Outcomes Associated with Related Factors or Intermediate Outcomes

Body Positioning: Self-Initiated
Burn Recovery
Circulation Status
Fluid Balance
Fluid Overload Severity
Immobility Consequences: Physiological
Medication Response
Neurological Status: Peripheral
Nutritional Status
Ostomy Self-Care
Physical Aging
Risk Control: Hyperthermia

Risk Control: Hypothermia
Risk Control: Sun Exposure
Self-Care: Bathing
Self-Care: Hygiene
Sensory Function: Tactile
Thermoregulation
Thermoregulation: Newborn
Tissue Perfusion
Tissue Perfusion: Cellular
Tissue Perfusion: Peripheral
Weight: Body Mass

Sleep Deprivation

Definition: Prolonged periods of time without sleep (sustained natural, periodic suspension of relative consciousness)

Outcomes to Measure Resolution of Diagnosis
Sleep

Additional Outcomes to Measure Defining Characteristics

Aggression Self-Restraint
Agitation Level
Anxiety Level
Concentration
Delirium Level
Distorted Thought Self-Control
Fatigue: Disruptive Effects
Fatigue Level
Information Processing

Memory
Mood Equilibrium
Pain: Disruptive Effects
Pain Level
Psychomotor Energy
Role Performance
Sensory Function: Proprioception
Symptom Severity

Outcomes Associated with Related Factors or Intermediate Outcomes

Abusive Behavior Self-Restraint
Anxiety Self-Control
Comfort Status
Comfort Status: Environment
Comfort Status: Physical
Comfort Status: Psychospiritual
Dementia Level
Discomfort Level
Exercise Participation

Medication Response
Neurological Status: Autonomic
Pain Control
Parenting Performance: Infant
Parenting Performance: Preschooler
Parenting Performance: Toddler
Physical Aging
Stress Level
Urinary Continence

Sleep Pattern, Disturbed

Definition: Time-limited interruptions of sleep amount and quality due to external factors

Outcomes to Measure Resolution of Diagnosis
Sleep

Additional Outcomes to Measure Defining Characteristics

Fatigue: Disruptive Effects	Role Performance
Fatigue Level	

Outcomes Associated with Related Factors or Intermediate Outcomes

Caregiver Lifestyle Disruption	Comfort Status: Environment
Caregiver Stressors	Depression Level
Client Satisfaction: Physical Environment	

Social Interaction, Impaired

Definition: Insufficient or excessive quantity or ineffective quality of social exchange

Outcomes to Measure Resolution of Diagnosis

Social Interaction Skills	Social Involvement

Additional Outcomes to Measure Defining Characteristics

Caregiver-Patient Relationship	Family Normalization
Child Development: Adolescence	Family Resiliency
Child Development: Middle Childhood	Family Social Climate
Development: Late Adulthood	Leisure Participation
Development: Middle Adulthood	Play Participation
Development: Young Adulthood	Social Anxiety Level
Family Functioning	Social Support
Family Integrity	

Outcomes Associated with Related Factors or Intermediate Outcomes

Adaptation to Physical Disability	Immobility Consequences: Psycho-Cognitive
Comfort Status: Sociocultural	Loneliness Severity
Communication	Memory
Distorted Thought Self-Control	Mobility
Family Health Status	Psychomotor Energy
Family Support During Treatment	Role Performance
Fear Level	Self-Awareness
Fear Level: Child	Self-Esteem
Hyperactivity Level	Stress Level
Identity	Student Health Status

Social Isolation

Definition: Aloneness experienced by the individual and perceived as imposed by others and as a negative or threatening state

Outcomes to Measure Resolution of Diagnosis

Loneliness Severity

Social Involvement

Additional Outcomes to Measure Defining Characteristics

Adaptation to Physical Disability

Child Development: Adolescence

Development: Late Adult

Development: Middle Adult

Development: Young Adult

Family Social Climate

Fear Level

Fear Level: Child

Leisure Participation

Personal Well-Being

Play Participation

Role Performance

Social Anxiety Level

Social Interaction Skills

Social Support

Outcomes Associated with Related Factors or Intermediate Outcomes

Aggression Self-Restraint

Anger Self-Restraint

Body Image

Client Satisfaction: Communication

Cognition

Communication

Dementia Level

Grief Resolution

Mobility

Mood Equilibrium

Personal Health Status

Relocation Adaptation

Self-Esteem

Sorrow: Chronic

Definition: Cyclical, recurring, and potentially progressive pattern of pervasive sadness experienced (by a parent, caregiver, individual with chronic illness or disability) in response to continual loss, throughout the trajectory of an illness or disability

Outcomes to Measure Resolution of Diagnosis

Depression Level

Grief Resolution

Suffering Severity

Additional Outcomes to Measure Defining Characteristics

Agitation Level

Anger Self-Restraint

Cognition

Decision-Making

Depression Self-Control

Discomfort Level

Fear Level

Fear Self-Control

Guilt Resolution

Hope

Information Processing

Loneliness Severity

Mood Equilibrium

Personal Well-Being

Self-Esteem

Social Interaction Skills

Social Involvement

Stress Level

Outcomes Associated with Related Factors or Intermediate Outcomes

Acceptance: Health Status

Adaptation to Physical Disability

Caregiver Role Endurance

Caregiver Stressors

Coping

Lifestyle Balance

Personal Resiliency

Physical Aging

Psychosocial Adjustment: Life Change

Quality of Life

Self-Management: Acute Illness

Self-Management: Chronic Disease

Spiritual Health

Spiritual Distress

Definition: Impaired ability to experience and integrate meaning and purpose in life through connectedness with self, others, art, music, literature, nature, and/or a power greater than oneself

Outcomes to Measure Resolution of Diagnosis

Spiritual Health

Additional Outcomes to Measure Defining Characteristics

Acceptance: Health Status	Hope
Anger Self-Restraint	Leisure Participation
Anxiety Self-Control	Self-Awareness
Comfort Status: Psychospiritual	Social Involvement
Coping	Social Support
Depression Level	Suffering Severity
Guilt Resolution	Suicide Self-Restraint

Outcomes Associated with Related Factors or Intermediate Outcomes

Abusive Behavior Self-Restraint	Pain: Disruptive Effects
Adaptation to Physical Disability	Pain Level
Anxiety Level	Personal Resiliency
Client Satisfaction: Cultural Needs Fulfillment	Personal Well-Being
Comfort Status: Sociocultural	Psychosocial Adjustment: Life Change
Comfortable Death	Quality of Life
Dignified Life Closure	Social Anxiety Level
Family Social Climate	Social Interaction Skills
Grief Resolution	Stress Level
Loneliness Severity	Will to Live
Pain Control	

Stress Overload

Definition: Excessive amounts and types of demands that require action

Outcomes to Measure Resolution of Diagnosis

Caregiver Stressors	Stress Level

Additional Outcomes to Measure Defining Characteristics

Abusive Behavior Self-Restraint	Comfort Status: Psychospiritual
Acceptance: Health Status	Coping
Adaptation to Physical Disability	Decision-Making
Aggression Self-Restraint	Discomfort Level
Agitation Level	Family Coping
Anger Self-Restraint	Family Functioning
Anxiety Level	Psychosocial Adjustment: Life Change
Anxiety Self-Control	Role Performance

Outcomes Associated with Related Factors or Intermediate Outcomes

Abuse Protection	Depression Self-Control
Caregiver Adaptation to Patient Institutionalization	Dignified Life Closure
Comfort Status: Sociocultural	Hearing Compensation Behavior
Comfortable Death	Mutilation Self-Restraint
Community Disaster Response	Pain Level
Community Grief Response	Suffering Severity
Community Resiliency	Suicide Self-Restraint
Community Risk Control: Violence	Symptom Control
Community Violence Level	Symptom Severity
Dementia Level	Vision Compensation Behavior

Surgical Recovery, Delayed

Definition: Extension of the number of post-operative days required to initiate and perform activities that maintain life, health, and well-being

Outcomes to Measure Resolution of Diagnosis
Discharge Readiness: Independent Living
Discharge Readiness: Supported Living

Surgical Recovery: Convalescence

Additional Outcomes to Measure Defining Characteristics
Ambulation
Appetite
Body Positioning: Self-Initiated
Discomfort Level
Endurance
Fatigue Level
Mobility
Nausea & Vomiting Severity
Pain Level
Role Performance

Self-Care Status
Self-Care: Activities of Daily Living (ADL)
Self-Care: Bathing
Self-Care: Dressing
Self-Care: Eating
Self-Care: Hygiene
Self-Care: Instrumental Activities of Daily Living (IADL)
Wound Healing: Primary Intention
Wound Healing: Secondary Intention

Outcomes Associated with Related Factors or Intermediate Outcomes
Health Beliefs
Infection Severity
Infection Severity: Newborn
Knowledge: Infection Management
Knowledge: Treatment Regimen
Pain Control

Pain: Disruptive Effects
Post-Procedure Recovery
Safe Health Care Environment
Surgical Recovery: Immediate Post-Operative
Weight: Body Mass

Swallowing, Impaired

Definition: Abnormal functioning of the swallowing mechanism associated with deficits in oral, pharyngeal, or esophageal structure or function

Outcomes to Measure Resolution of Diagnosis
Swallowing Status
Swallowing Status: Esophageal Phase

Swallowing Status: Oral Phase
Swallowing Status: Pharyngeal Phase

Additional Outcomes to Measure Defining Characteristics
Aspiration Prevention
Bottle Feeding Establishment: Infant
Breastfeeding Establishment: Infant
Nausea & Vomiting Severity

Oral Health
Pain Level
Self-Care: Eating

Outcomes Associated with Related Factors or Intermediate Outcomes
Cardiopulmonary Status
Child Development: 1 Month
Child Development: 2 Months
Child Development: 4 Months
Child Development: 6 Months
Child Development: 12 Months
Gastrointestinal Function
Neurological Status: Cranial Sensory/Motor Function

Newborn Adaptation
Nutritional Status: Energy
Nutritional Status: Food & Fluid Intake
Nutritional Status: Nutrient Intake
Physical Injury Severity
Preterm Infant Organization
Respiratory Status: Airway Patency

Thermoregulation, Ineffective

Definition: Temperature fluctuation between hypothermia and hyperthermia

Outcomes to Measure Resolution of Diagnosis

Thermoregulation

Thermoregulation: Newborn

Additional Outcomes to Measure Defining Characteristics

Hypertension Severity

Neurological Status

Respiratory Status

Tissue Perfusion: Peripheral

Vital Signs

Outcomes Associated with Related Factors or Intermediate Outcomes

Burn Healing

Comfort Status: Environment

Newborn Adaptation

Physical Aging

Physical Injury Severity

Preterm Infant Organization

Risk Control: Hypertension

Risk Control: Hyperthermia

Risk Control: Hypotension

Risk Control: Hypothermia

Tissue Integrity, Impaired

Definition: Damage to mucous membrane, corneal, integumentary, or subcutaneous tissues

Outcomes to Measure Resolution of Diagnosis

Tissue Integrity: Skin & Mucous Membranes

Additional Outcomes to Measure Defining Characteristics

Allergic Response: Localized

Burn Healing

Burn Recovery

Dry Eye Severity

Oral Health

Wound Healing: Primary Intention

Wound Healing: Secondary Intention

Outcomes Associated with Related Factors or Intermediate Outcomes

Body Positioning: Self-Initiated

Circulation Status

Fluid Overload Severity

Hydration

Immobility Consequences: Physiological

Infection Severity

Infection Severity: Newborn

Knowledge: Infection Management

Knowledge: Peripheral Artery Disease Management

Knowledge: Treatment Regimen

Mobility

Nutritional Status

Nutritional Status: Nutrient Intake

Ostomy Self-Care

Risk Control: Dry Eye

Risk Control: Infectious Process

Self-Management: Peripheral Artery Disease

Sensory Function: Tactile

Tissue Perfusion: Peripheral

Tissue Perfusion: Peripheral, Ineffective

Definition: Decrease in blood circulation to the periphery that may compromise health

Outcomes to Measure Resolution of Diagnosis
Tissue Perfusion: Peripheral

Additional Outcomes to Measure Defining Characteristics

Ambulation	Tissue Integrity: Skin & Mucous Membranes
Circulation Status	Tissue Perfusion
Coordinated Movement	Tissue Perfusion: Cellular
Fluid Overload Severity	Vital Signs
Pain Level	Wound Healing: Primary Intention
Peripheral Artery Disease Severity	Wound Healing: Secondary Intention
Sensory Function: Tactile	

Outcomes Associated with Related Factors or Intermediate Outcomes

Blood Coagulation	Knowledge: Lipid Disorder Management
Cardiac Pump Effectiveness	Knowledge: Peripheral Artery Disease Management
Exercise Participation	Mobility
Hypertension Severity	Physical Injury Severity
Knowledge: Chronic Disease Management	Self-Management: Diabetes
Knowledge: Diabetes Management	Self-Management: Hypertension
Knowledge: Disease Process	Self-Management: Lipid Disorder
Knowledge: Health Promotion	Self-Management: Peripheral Artery Disease
Knowledge: Healthy Diet	Smoking Cessation Behavior
Knowledge: Hypertension Management	Weight: Body Mass

Transfer Ability, Impaired

Definition: Limitation of independent movement between two nearby surfaces

Outcomes to Measure Resolution of Diagnosis

Body Positioning: Self-Initiated	Transfer Performance

Additional Outcomes to Measure Defining Characteristics

Coordinated Movement	Self-Care: Toileting
Self-Care: Bathing	

Outcomes Associated with Related Factors or Intermediate Outcomes

Balance	Joint Movement: Spine
Client Satisfaction: Physical Environment	Knowledge: Body Mechanics
Cognition	Knowledge: Fall Prevention
Comfort Status: Environment	Neurological Status: Spinal Sensory/Motor Function
Discomfort Level	Pain Level
Endurance	Physical Fitness
Fatigue Level	Sensory Function: Vision
Joint Movement: Hip	Skeletal Function
Joint Movement: Knee	Vision Compensation Behavior
Joint Movement: Shoulder	Weight: Body Mass

Unilateral Neglect

Definition: Impairment in sensory and motor response, mental representation, and spatial attention of the body, and the corresponding environment, characterized by inattention to one side and overattention to the opposite side. Left-side neglect is more severe and persistent than right-side neglect

Outcomes to Measure Resolution of Diagnosis

Heedfulness of Affected Side
Neurological Status: Peripheral

Sensory Function: Proprioception

Additional Outcomes to Measure Defining Characteristics

Adaptation to Physical Disability
Body Mechanics Performance
Body Positioning: Self-Initiated
Communication: Expressive
Communication: Receptive
Coordinated Movement

Memory
Self-Care Status
Self-Care: Activities of Daily Living (ADL)
Self-Care: Dressing
Self-Care: Eating
Self-Care: Hygiene

Outcomes Associated with Related Factors or Intermediate Outcomes

Neurological Status
Physical Injury Severity

Tissue Perfusion: Cerebral

Urinary Elimination, Impaired

Definition: Dysfunction in urine elimination

Outcomes to Measure Resolution of Diagnosis

Urinary Elimination

Additional Outcomes to Measure Defining Characteristics

Symptom Severity

Urinary Continence

Outcomes Associated with Related Factors or Intermediate Outcomes

Hydration
Infection Severity
Infection Severity: Newborn
Kidney Function

Neurological Status: Spinal Sensory/Motor Function
Physical Aging
Symptom Control

Urinary Incontinence: Functional

Definition: Inability of a usually continent person to reach toilet in time to avoid unintentional loss of urine

Outcomes to Measure Resolution of Diagnosis
Urinary Continence

Additional Outcomes to Measure Defining Characteristics

Self-Care: Toileting

Symptom Severity

Outcomes Associated with Related Factors or Intermediate Outcomes

Agitation Level

Ambulation

Ambulation: Wheelchair

Anxiety Level

Balance

Cognition

Coordinated Movement

Delirium Level

Gait

Medication Response

Mobility

Neurological Status: Spinal Sensory/Motor Function

Safe Home Environment

Self-Care: Dressing

Sensory Function: Vision

Stress Level

Symptom Control

Transfer Performance

Urinary Elimination

Urinary Incontinence: Overflow

Definition: Involuntary loss of urine associated with overdistention of the bladder

Outcomes to Measure Resolution of Diagnosis
Urinary Continence

Additional Outcomes to Measure Defining Characteristics
Symptom Severity

Outcomes Associated with Related Factors or Intermediate Outcomes

Bowel Elimination

Knowledge: Disease Process

Knowledge: Medication

Medication Response

Neurological Status: Spinal Sensory/Motor Function

Self-Care: Toileting

Urinary Elimination

Urinary Incontinence: Reflex

Definition: Involuntary loss of urine at somewhat predictable intervals when a specific bladder volume is reached

Outcomes to Measure Resolution of Diagnosis
Urinary Continence

Additional Outcomes to Measure Defining Characteristics

Symptom Severity

Urinary Elimination

Outcomes Associated with Related Factors or Intermediate Outcomes

Cognition

Knowledge: Disease Process

Neurological Status

Neurological Status: Spinal Sensory/Motor Function

Tissue Integrity: Skin & Mucous Membranes

Urinary Incontinence: Stress

Definition: Sudden leakage of urine with activities that increase intra-abdominal pressure

Outcomes to Measure Resolution of Diagnosis
Urinary Continence

Additional Outcomes to Measure Defining Characteristics
Symptom Severity   Urinary Elimination

Outcomes Associated with Related Factors or Intermediate Outcomes
Physical Aging   Symptom Control

Urinary Incontinence: Urge

Definition: Involuntary passage of urine occurring soon after a strong sense of urgency to void

Outcomes to Measure Resolution of Diagnosis
Urinary Continence

Additional Outcomes to Measure Defining Characteristics
Self-Care: Toileting   Urinary Elimination

Outcomes Associated with Related Factors or Intermediate Outcomes
Bowel Elimination   Medication Response
Infection Severity   Nutritional Status: Food & Fluid Intake
Knowledge: Disease Process   Physical Aging
Knowledge: Medication   Symptom Control
Knowledge: Treatment Regimen

Urinary Retention

Definition: Incomplete emptying of the bladder

Outcomes to Measure Resolution of Diagnosis
Urinary Elimination

Additional Outcomes to Measure Defining Characteristics
Comfort Status: Physical   Symptom Severity
Pain Level   Urinary Continence

Outcomes Associated with Related Factors or Intermediate Outcomes
Medication Response   Physical Aging
Neurological Status: Spinal Sensory/Motor Function Symptom Control

Ventilation, Impaired Spontaneous

Definition: Decreased energy reserves resulting in an inability to maintain independent breathing that is adequate to support life

Outcomes to Measure Resolution of Diagnosis

Respiratory Status
Respiratory Status: Gas Exchange

Respiratory Status: Ventilation

Additional Outcomes to Measure Defining Characteristics

Acute Respiratory Acidosis Severity
Agitation Level
Anxiety Level

Discomfort Level
Vital Signs

Outcomes Associated with Related Factors or Intermediate Outcomes

Allergic Response: Systemic
Electrolyte & Acid/Base Balance
Electrolyte Balance
Endurance
Energy Conservation
Fatigue Level

Mechanical Ventilation Response: Adult
Mechanical Ventilation Weaning Response: Adult
Metabolic Acidosis Severity
Metabolic Alkalosis Severity
Post-Procedure Recovery
Surgical Recovery: Immediate Post-Operative

Ventilatory Weaning Response, Dysfunctional

Definition: Inability to adjust to lowered levels of mechanical ventilator support that interrupts and prolongs the weaning process

Outcomes to Measure Resolution of Diagnosis

Mechanical Ventilation Weaning Response: Adult

Additional Outcomes to Measure Defining Characteristics

Agitation Level
Anxiety Level
Discomfort Level
Fatigue Level
Neurological Status: Consciousness
Respiratory Status

Respiratory Status: Gas Exchange
Respiratory Status: Ventilation
Tissue Perfusion: Peripheral
Tissue Perfusion: Pulmonary
Vital Signs

Outcomes Associated with Related Factors or Intermediate Outcomes

Anxiety Self-Control
Client Satisfaction: Physical Environment
Client Satisfaction: Technical Aspects of Care
Comfort Status: Environment
Energy Conservation
Fear Level
Fear Level: Child
Health Beliefs: Perceived Ability to Perform
Hope
Knowledge: Treatment Procedure
Knowledge: Treatment Regimen

Mechanical Ventilation Response: Adult
Motivation
Nutritional Status: Nutrient Intake
Pain Control
Pain Level
Respiratory Status: Airway Patency
Self-Esteem
Sleep
Social Support
Symptom Severity

Walking, Impaired

Definition: Limitation of independent movement within the environment on foot

Outcomes to Measure Resolution of Diagnosis

Ambulation	Mobility

Additional Outcomes to Measure Defining Characteristics

Body Mechanics Performance	Gait
Coordinated Movement	Skeletal Function

Outcomes Associated with Related Factors or Intermediate Outcomes

Activity Tolerance	Joint Movement: Hip
Balance	Joint Movement: Knee
Client Satisfaction: Functional Assistance	Joint Movement: Spine
Client Satisfaction: Physical Environment	Knowledge: Body Mechanics
Client Satisfaction: Safety	Knowledge: Fall Prevention
Cognition	Neurological Status: Central Motor Control
Delirium Level	Neurological Status: Peripheral
Dementia Level	Pain Level
Depression Level	Physical Fitness
Endurance	Safe Home Environment
Fall Prevention Behavior	Sensory Function: Vision
Fatigue Level	Vision Compensation Behavior
Joint Movement: Ankle	Weight: Body Mass

Wandering

Definition: Meandering, aimless, or repetitive locomotion that exposes the individual to harm; frequently incongruent with boundaries, limits, or obstacles

Outcomes to Measure Resolution of Diagnosis

Safe Wandering

Additional Outcomes to Measure Defining Characteristics

Agitation Level	Elopement Propensity Risk
Elopement Occurrence	Hyperactivity Level

Outcomes Associated with Related Factors or Intermediate Outcomes

Anxiety Level	Hydration
Bowel Continence	Medication Response
Client Satisfaction: Communication	Memory
Client Satisfaction: Physical Care	Pain Level
Client Satisfaction: Physical Environment	Relocation Adaptation
Cognition	Rest
Comfort Status: Environment	Safe Home Environment
Communication: Expressive	Sensory Function: Proprioception
Communication: Receptive	Sensory Function: Vision
Delirium Level	Sleep
Dementia Level	Urinary Continence
Depression Level	

Risk Nursing Diagnoses

Activity Intolerance, Risk for

Definition: At risk for experiencing insufficient physiological or psychological energy to endure or complete required or desired daily activities

Outcomes to Assess and Measure Actual Occurrence of the Diagnosis

Activity Tolerance

Psychomotor Energy

Outcomes Associated with Risk Factors

Adaptation to Physical Disability
Body Mechanics Performance
Cardiac Pump Effectiveness
Cardiopulmonary Status
Circulation Status
Coordinated Movement
Endurance
Energy Conservation
Fatigue Level
Health Promoting Behavior
Knowledge: Body Mechanics
Knowledge: Energy Conservation
Knowledge: Prescribed Activity

Nutritional Status: Energy
Physical Fitness
Respiratory Status
Respiratory Status: Gas Exchange
Respiratory Status: Ventilation
Risk Control
Risk Control: Cardiovascular Disease
Risk Detection
Self-Management: Asthma
Self-Management: Cardiac Disease
Self-Management: Multiple Sclerosis
Self-Management: Osteoporosis
Smoking Cessation Behavior

Activity Planning, Risk for Ineffective

Definition: At risk for an inability to prepare for a set of actions fixed in time and under certain conditions

Outcomes to Assess and Measure Actual Occurrence of the Diagnosis

Adherence Behavior
Decision-Making

Personal Time Management
Self-Direction of Care

Outcomes Associated with Risk Factors

Caregiver Home Care Readiness
Community Competence
Community Program Effectiveness
Compliance Behavior
Compliance Behavior: Prescribed Activity
Compliance Behavior: Prescribed Diet
Compliance Behavior: Prescribed Medication
Coping
Exercise Participation

Information Processing
Lifestyle Balance
Personal Autonomy
Risk Control
Risk Detection
Self-Awareness
Self-Care Status
Self-Esteem
Social Support

Adverse Reaction to Iodinated Contrast Media, Risk for

Definition: At risk for any noxious or unintended reaction associated with the use of iodinated contrast media that can occur within seven (7) days after contrast agent injection

Outcomes to Assess and Measure Actual Occurrence of the Diagnosis

Allergic Response: Localized
Allergic Response: Systemic
Immune Hypersensitivity Response

Shock Severity: Anaphylactic
Symptom Severity

Outcomes Associated with Risk Factors

Anxiety Level
Hydration
Knowledge: Medication
Medication Response
Neurological Status: Consciousness

Personal Health Status
Physical Aging
Risk Control
Risk Detection
Self-Management: Chronic Disease

Allergy Response, Risk for

Definition: Risk of an exaggerated immune response or reaction to substances

Outcomes to Assess and Measure Actual Occurrence of the Diagnosis

Allergic Response: Localized
Allergic Response: Systemic
Immune Hypersensitivity Response

Shock Severity: Anaphylactic
Symptom Severity

Outcomes Associated with Risk Factors

Health Beliefs: Perceived Threat
Medication Response
Risk Control

Risk Detection
Safe Home Environment

Aspiration, Risk for

Definition: At risk for entry of gastrointestinal secretions, oropharyngeal secretions, solids, or fluids into tracheobronchial passages

Outcomes to Assess and Measure Actual Occurrence of the Diagnosis

Respiratory Status
Respiratory Status: Airway Patency

Respiratory Status: Gas Exchange
Respiratory Status: Ventilation

Outcomes Associated with Risk Factors

Aspiration Prevention
Body Positioning: Self-Initiated
Cognitive Orientation
Gastrointestinal Function
Immobility Consequences: Physiological
Mechanical Ventilation Response: Adult
Mechanical Ventilation Weaning Response: Adult
Nausea & Vomiting Control
Nausea & Vomiting Severity

Neurological Status: Consciousness
Physical Injury Severity
Post-Procedure Recovery
Risk Control
Risk Detection
Seizure Self-Control
Self-Care: Eating
Self-Care: Non-Parenteral Medication
Surgical Recovery: Convalescence

Aspiration, Risk for—*cont'd*

Surgical Recovery: Immediate Post-Operative
Swallowing Status
Swallowing Status: Esophageal Phase

Swallowing Status: Oral Phase
Swallowing Status: Pharyngeal Phase

Attachment, Risk for Impaired

Definition: At risk for disruption of the interactive process between parent/significant other and child that fosters the development of a protective and nurturing reciprocal relationship

Outcomes to Assess and Measure Actual Occurrence of the Diagnosis
Parent-Infant Attachment

Outcomes Associated with Risk Factors

Anxiety Level
Anxiety Self-Control
Child Development: 1 Month
Child Development: 2 Months
Child Development: 4 Months
Child Development: 6 Months
Child Development: 12 Months
Coping
Knowledge: Parenting
Knowledge: Preterm Infant Care
Parenting Performance

Parenting Performance: Infant
Parenting Performance: Middle Childhood
Parenting Performance: Preschooler
Parenting Performance: Toddler
Preterm Infant Organization
Risk Control
Risk Detection
Social Interaction Skills
Stress Level
Substance Addiction Consequences

Autonomic Dysreflexia, Risk for

Definition: At risk for life-threatening, uninhibited response of the sympathetic nervous system, post-spinal shock, in an individual with a spinal cord injury or lesion at T6 or above (has been demonstrated in patients with injuries at T7 and T8)

Outcomes to Assess and Measure Actual Occurrence of the Diagnosis
Cardiopulmonary Status
Neurological Status: Autonomic

Shock Severity: Neurogenic

Outcomes Associated with Risk Factors

Bone Healing
Bowel Elimination
Burn Recovery
Circulation Status
Gastrointestinal Function
Hypertension Severity
Hypotension Severity
Infection Severity
Medication Response
Pain Level
Risk Control
Risk Control: Hyperthermia

Risk Control: Hypothermia
Risk Control: Infectious Process
Risk Detection
Sensory Function: Tactile
Substance Withdrawal Severity
Symptom Severity
Thermoregulation
Tissue Integrity: Skin & Mucous Membranes
Urinary Elimination
Vital Signs
Wound Healing: Secondary Intention

Bleeding, Risk for

Definition: At risk for a decrease in blood volume that may compromise health

Outcomes to Assess and Measure Actual Occurrence of the Diagnosis

Blood Loss Severity

Circulation Status

Outcomes Associated with Risk Factors

Blood Coagulation

Compliance Behavior: Prescribed Medication

Fall Prevention Behavior

Falls Occurrence

Gastrointestinal Function

Hemodialysis Access

Knowledge: Anticoagulation Therapy Management

Knowledge: Cancer Management

Knowledge: Fall Prevention

Knowledge: Medication

Knowledge: Personal Safety

Knowledge: Treatment Regimen

Liver Function

Maternal Status: Antepartum

Maternal Status: Intrapartum

Maternal Status: Postpartum

Medication Response

Personal Safety Behavior

Physical Injury Severity

Risk Control

Risk Detection

Self-Management: Anticoagulation Therapy

Surgical Recovery: Convalescence

Surgical Recovery: Immediate Post-Operative

Blood Glucose Level, Risk for Unstable

Definition: At risk for variation of blood glucose/sugar levels from the normal range that may compromise health

Outcomes to Assess and Measure Actual Occurrence of the Diagnosis

Blood Glucose Level

Hyperglycemia Severity

Hypoglycemia Severity

Outcomes Associated with Risk Factors

Acceptance: Health Status

Compliance Behavior: Prescribed Activity

Compliance Behavior: Prescribed Diet

Compliance Behavior: Prescribed Medication

Coping

Depression Level

Endurance

Exercise Participation

Knowledge: Diabetes Management

Knowledge: Medication

Knowledge: Prescribed Activity

Knowledge: Prescribed Diet

Knowledge: Treatment Regimen

Knowledge: Weight Management

Maternal Status: Antepartum

Maternal Status: Intrapartum

Maternal Status: Postpartum

Medication Response

Mood Equilibrium

Nutritional Status

Nutritional Status: Biochemical Measures

Nutritional Status: Food & Fluid Intake

Nutritional Status: Nutrient Intake

Personal Health Status

Physical Fitness

Prenatal Health Behavior

Risk Control

Risk Detection

Self-Management: Diabetes

Stress Level

Weight Gain Behavior

Weight Loss Behavior

Weight Maintenance Behavior

Body Temperature, Risk for Imbalanced

Definition: At risk for failure to maintain body temperature within normal range

Outcomes to Assess and Measure Actual Occurrence of the Diagnosis

Thermoregulation

Thermoregulation: Newborn

Outcomes Associated with Risk Factors

Activity Tolerance

Burn Healing

Exercise Participation

Hydration

Immune Status

Infection Severity

Infection Severity: Newborn

Medication Response

Neurological Status: Autonomic

Newborn Adaptation

Physical Aging

Physical Fitness

Post-Procedure Recovery

Risk Control

Risk Control: Hyperthermia

Risk Control: Hypothermia

Risk Control: Infectious Process

Risk Control: Sun Exposure

Risk Detection

Substance Withdrawal Severity

Surgical Recovery: Immediate Post-Operative

Weight Maintenance Behavior

Caregiver Role Strain, Risk for

Definition: At risk for caregiver vulnerability for felt difficulty in performing the family caregiver role

Outcomes to Assess and Measure Actual Occurrence of the Diagnosis

Caregiver Performance: Direct Care
Caregiver Performance: Indirect Care

Caregiver Role Endurance
Parenting Performance

Outcomes Associated with Risk Factors

Abuse Cessation
Abuse Protection
Abusive Behavior Self-Restraint
Caregiver Emotional Health
Caregiver Home Care Readiness
Caregiver Lifestyle Disruption
Caregiver-Patient Relationship
Caregiver Physical Health
Caregiver Stressors
Child Development: 1 Month
Child Development: 2 Months
Child Development: 4 Months
Child Development: 6 Months
Child Development: 12 Months
Child Development: 2 Years
Child Development: 3 Years
Child Development: 4 Years
Child Development: 5 Years
Child Development: Middle Childhood
Child Development: Adolescence
Cognition
Coping
Cup Feeding Performance
Dementia Level
Depression Level
Development: Late Adulthood
Development: Middle Adulthood
Development: Young Adulthood
Discharge Readiness: Independent Living
Discharge Readiness: Supported Living
Drug Abuse Cessation Behavior

Family Coping
Family Functioning
Family Support During Treatment
Fatigue Level
Knowledge: Disease Process
Knowledge: Energy Conservation
Knowledge: Healthy Diet
Knowledge: Infant Care
Knowledge: Medication
Knowledge: Pain Management
Knowledge: Parenting
Knowledge: Prescribed Activity
Knowledge: Prescribed Diet
Knowledge: Treatment Procedure
Knowledge: Treatment Regimen
Leisure Participation
Lifestyle Balance
Mood Equilibrium
Personal Resiliency
Personal Time Management
Preterm Infant Organization
Rest
Risk Control
Risk Control: Drug Use
Risk Detection
Role Performance
Sleep
Social Support
Stress Level
Substance Addiction Consequences
Substance Withdrawal Severity

Childbearing Process, Risk for Ineffective

Definition: Risk for a pregnancy and childbirth process and care of the newborn that does not match the environmental context, norms, and expectations

Outcomes to Assess and Measure Actual Occurrence of the Diagnosis

Maternal Status: Antepartum
Maternal Status: Intrapartum

Maternal Status: Postpartum
Parent-Infant Attachment

Outcomes Associated with Risk Factors

Abuse Protection
Alcohol Abuse Cessation Behavior
Anxiety Level
Caregiver Emotional Health
Cognition
Depression Level
Drug Abuse Cessation Behavior
Fear Level
Hyperglycemia Severity
Hypertension Severity
Hypoglycemia Severity
Knowledge: Diabetes Management
Knowledge: Healthy Diet
Knowledge: Hypertension Management
Knowledge: Infant Care
Knowledge: Labor & Delivery
Knowledge: Medication

Knowledge: Preconception Maternal Health
Knowledge: Pregnancy
Nausea & Vomiting Severity
Nutritional Status: Nutrient Intake
Parenting Performance: Infant
Parenting Performance: Psychosocial Safety
Personal Autonomy
Personal Health Status
Prenatal Health Behavior
Risk Control
Risk Control: Hypertension
Risk Detection
Seizure Self-Control
Self-Management: Diabetes
Self-Management: Hypertension
Smoking Cessation Behavior
Social Support

Confusion, Risk for Acute

Definition: At risk for reversible disturbances of consciousness, attention, cognition, and perception that develop over a short period of time

Outcomes to Assess and Measure Actual Occurrence of the Diagnosis

Cognitive Orientation

Delirium Level

Outcomes Associated with Risk Factors

Alcohol Abuse Cessation Behavior
Cognition
Concentration
Development: Late Adulthood
Dementia Level
Drug Abuse Cessation Behavior
Electrolyte & Acid/Base Balance
Electrolyte Balance
Hydration
Infection Severity
Information Processing
Kidney Function
Knowledge: Stroke Management
Medication Response
Memory
Mobility

Nutritional Status: Nutrient Intake
Pain Level
Physical Aging
Post-Procedure Recovery
Risk Control
Risk Control: Alcohol Use
Risk Control: Drug Use
Risk Control: Infectious Process
Risk Control: Stroke
Risk Detection
Sensory Function
Sleep
Substance Withdrawal Severity
Surgical Recovery: Immediate Post-Operative
Urinary Elimination

Constipation, Risk for

Definition: At risk for a decrease in normal frequency of defecation accompanied by difficult or incomplete passage of stool and/or passage of excessively hard, dry stool

Outcomes to Assess and Measure Actual Occurrence of the Diagnosis
Bowel Elimination

Outcomes Associated with Risk Factors

Adherence Behavior: Healthy Diet
Compliance Behavior: Prescribed Activity
Compliance Behavior: Prescribed Diet
Delirium Level
Dementia Level
Depression Level
Eating Disorder Self-Control
Electrolyte Balance
Exercise Participation
Gastrointestinal Function
Hydration
Immobility Consequences: Physiological
Knowledge: Bottle Feeding
Knowledge: Healthy Diet
Knowledge: Healthy Lifestyle
Knowledge: Medication
Knowledge: Prescribed Diet
Maternal Status: Antepartum
Medication Response
Mobility
Neurological Status
Nutritional Status: Food & Fluid Intake
Nutritional Status: Nutrient Intake
Risk Control
Risk Detection
Self-Care: Non-Parenteral Medication
Self-Care: Oral Hygiene
Self-Care: Toileting
Self-Management: Chronic Disease
Stress Level
Surgical Recovery: Convalescence
Surgical Recovery: Immediate Post-Operative
Weight: Body Mass

Contamination, Risk for

Definition: At risk of exposure to environmental contaminants in doses sufficient to cause adverse health effects

Outcomes to Assess and Measure Actual Occurrence of the Diagnosis

Personal Safety Behavior
Safe Home Environment

Outcomes Associated with Risk Factors

Community Disaster Response
Community Risk Control: Communicable Disease
Community Risk Control: Lead Exposure
Gastrointestinal Function
Immune Status
Kidney Function
Knowledge: Child Physical Safety
Knowledge: Personal Safety
Liver Function
Maternal Status: Antepartum
Neurological Status
Nutritional Status: Nutrient Intake
Personal Health Status
Respiratory Status
Risk Control
Risk Control: Tobacco Use
Risk Detection
Self-Care: Hygiene
Self-Management: Chronic Disease
Smoking Cessation Behavior
Tissue Integrity: Skin & Mucous Membranes

Development, Risk for Delayed

Definition: At risk for delay of 25% or more in one or more of the areas of social or self-regulatory behavior, or in cognitive, language, gross or fine motor skills

Outcomes to Assess and Measure Actual Occurrence of the Diagnosis

Child Development: 1 Month
Child Development: 2 Months
Child Development: 4 Months
Child Development: 6 Months
Child Development: 12 Months
Child Development: 2 Years

Child Development: 3 Years
Child Development: 4 Years
Child Development: 5 Years
Child Development: Middle Childhood
Child Development: Adolescence

Outcomes Associated with Risk Factors

Abstract Thinking
Abuse Protection
Abuse Recovery
Abuse Recovery: Emotional
Abuse Recovery: Physical
Abuse Recovery: Sexual
Abusive Behavior Self-Restraint
Alcohol Abuse Cessation Behavior
Caregiver Emotional Health
Drug Abuse Cessation Behavior
Fetal Status: Antepartum
Fetal Status: Intrapartum
Hearing Compensation Behavior
Hyperactivity Level
Infant Nutritional Status
Infection Severity
Infection Severity: Newborn
Information Processing
Knowledge: Chronic Disease Management
Knowledge: Infant Care
Knowledge: Parenting
Neglect Recovery
Newborn Adaptation
Nutritional Status
Nutritional Status: Nutrient Intake

Parent-Infant Attachment
Parenting Performance
Parenting Performance: Adolescent
Parenting Performance: Adolescent Physical Safety
Parenting Performance: Early/Middle Childhood Physical
  Safety
Parenting Performance: Infant
Parenting Performance: Infant/Toddler Physical Safety
Parenting Performance: Middle Childhood
Parenting Performance: Preschooler
Parenting Performance: Psychosocial Safety
Parenting Performance: Toddler
Play Participation
Prenatal Health Behavior
Preterm Infant Organization
Risk Control
Risk Control: Alcohol Use
Risk Control: Drug Use
Risk Control: Unintended Pregnancy
Risk Detection
Seizure Self-Control
Smoking Cessation Behavior
Social Interaction Skills
Substance Addiction Consequences
Vision Compensation Behavior

Disuse Syndrome, Risk for

Definition: At risk for deterioration of body systems as the result of prescribed or unavoidable musculoskeletal inactivity

Outcomes to Assess and Measure Actual Occurrence of the Diagnosis
Immobility Consequences: Physiological

Outcomes Associated with Risk Factors

Bone Healing	Neurological Status: Spinal/Sensory Motor Function
Burn Recovery	Pain Level
Heedfulness of Affected Side	Risk Control
Neurological Status: Consciousness	Risk Detection

Dry Eye, Risk for

Definition: At risk for eye discomfort or damage to the cornea and conjunctiva due to reduced quantity or quality of tears to moisten the eye

Outcomes to Assess and Measure Actual Occurrence of the Diagnosis
Dry Eye Severity

Outcomes Associated with Risk Factors

Allergic Response: Localized	Risk Control
Immune Hypersensitivity Response	Risk Control: Dry Eye
Mechanical Ventilation Response: Adult	Risk Control: Sun Exposure
Medication Response	Risk Control: Visual Impairment
Neurological Status: Consciousness	Risk Detection
Neurological Status: Cranial Sensory/Motor Function	Smoking Cessation Behavior
Physical Aging	Surgical Recovery: Immediate Post-Operative

Electrolyte, Risk for Imbalance

Definition: At risk for change in serum electrolyte levels that may compromise health

Outcomes to Assess and Measure Actual Occurrence of the Diagnosis

Electrolyte Balance

Hypercalcemia Severity

Hyperchloremia Severity

Hyperkalemia Severity

Hypermagnesemia Severity

Hypernatremia Severity

Hyperphosphatemia Severity

Hypocalcemia Severity

Hypochloremia Severity

Hypokalemia Severity

Hypomagnesemia Severity

Hyponatremia Severity

Hypophosphatemia Severity

Outcomes Associated with Risk Factors

Bowel Elimination

Burn Healing

Burn Recovery

Fluid Balance

Fluid Overload Severity

Gastrointestinal Function

Hydration

Kidney Function

Medication Response

Nausea & Vomiting Severity

Nutritional Status: Biochemical Measures

Risk Control

Risk Detection

Systemic Toxin Clearance: Dialysis

Wound Healing: Secondary Intention

Falls, Risk for

Definition: At risk for increased susceptibility to falling that may cause physical harm

Outcomes to Assess and Measure Actual Occurrence of the Diagnosis

Falls Occurrence

Physical Injury Severity

Outcomes Associated with Risk Factors

Alcohol Abuse Cessation Behavior
Ambulation
Ambulation: Wheelchair
Balance
Blood Glucose Level
Bowel Continence
Circulation Status
Client Satisfaction: Safety
Cognition
Coordinated Movement
Delirium Level
Dementia Level
Endurance
Fall Prevention Behavior
Fatigue Level
Fatigue: Disruptive Effects
Gait
Hearing Compensation Behavior
Heedfulness of Affected Side
Hydration
Hypotension Severity
Knowledge: Child Physical Safety
Knowledge: Fall Prevention
Medication Response
Mobility
Neurological Status: Central Motor Control
Neurological Status: Peripheral

Nutritional Status
Parenting Performance: Early/Middle Childhood Physical Safety
Parenting Performance: Infant/Toddler Physical Safety
Physical Aging
Physical Fitness
Post-Procedure Recovery
Risk Control
Risk Control: Alcohol Use
Risk Detection
Safe Health Care Environment
Safe Home Environment
Safe Wandering
Seizure Self-Control
Self-Care: Toileting
Self-Management: Acute Illness
Sensory Function
Sensory Function: Hearing
Sensory Function: Vision
Skeletal Function
Sleep
Surgical Recovery: Immediate Post-Operative
Transfer Performance
Urinary Continence
Vision Compensation Behavior
Vital Signs

Fluid Volume, Risk for Deficient

Definition: At risk for experiencing decreased intravascular, interstitial, and/or intracellular fluid. This refers to a risk for dehydration, water loss alone without change in sodium

Outcomes to Assess and Measure Actual Occurrence of the Diagnosis

Fluid Balance
Hydration

Outcomes Associated with Risk Factors

Adherence Behavior: Healthy Diet
Blood Glucose Level
Bowel Elimination
Breastfeeding Establishment: Infant
Breastfeeding Maintenance
Burn Healing
Compliance Behavior: Prescribed Diet
Electrolyte & Acid/Base Balance
Gastrointestinal Function
Infection Severity
Infection Severity: Newborn
Knowledge: Healthy Diet
Knowledge: Medication
Knowledge: Prescribed Diet

Medication Response
Nausea & Vomiting Severity
Nutritional Status: Food & Fluid Intake
Risk Control
Risk Control: Hyperthermia
Risk Detection
Swallowing Status
Thermoregulation
Thermoregulation: Newborn
Urinary Elimination
Weight: Body Mass
Weight Gain Behavior
Weight Loss Behavior

Fluid Volume, Risk for Imbalanced

Definition: At risk for a decrease, increase, or rapid shift from one to the other of intravascular, interstitial, and/or intracellular fluid that may compromise health. This refers to body fluid loss, gain, or both

Outcomes to Assess and Measure Actual Occurrence of the Diagnosis

Fluid Balance
Fluid Overload Severity
Hydration

Outcomes Associated with Risk Factors

Burn Healing
Burn Recovery
Cardiac Pump Effectiveness
Gastrointestinal Function
Infection Severity
Infection Severity: Newborn
Kidney Function
Knowledge: Heart Failure Management
Knowledge: Inflammatory Bowel Disease Management
Nausea & Vomiting Severity
Nutritional Status: Food & Fluid Intake

Physical Injury Severity
Post-Procedure Recovery
Risk Control
Risk Control: Hyperthermia
Risk Detection
Surgical Recovery: Immediate Post-Operative
Thermoregulation
Thermoregulation: Newborn
Wound Healing: Primary Intention
Wound Healing: Secondary Intention

Gastrointestinal Motility, Risk for Dysfunctional

Definition: At risk for increased, decreased, ineffective, or lack of peristaltic activity within the gastrointestinal system

Outcomes to Assess and Measure Actual Occurrence of the Diagnosis

Bowel Elimination

Gastrointestinal Function

Outcomes Associated with Risk Factors

Adherence Behavior: Healthy Diet

Anxiety Level

Compliance Behavior: Prescribed Diet

Exercise Participation

Infection Severity

Infection Severity: Newborn

Knowledge: Diabetes Management

Knowledge: Healthy Diet

Knowledge: Inflammatory Bowel Disease Management

Knowledge: Medication

Knowledge: Prescribed Diet

Medication Response

Mobility

Nutritional Status: Food & Fluid Intake

Physical Aging

Physical Fitness

Preterm Infant Organization

Risk Control

Risk Control: Infectious Process

Risk Detection

Self-Management: Chronic Disease

Self-Management: Diabetes

Stress Level

Surgical Recovery: Convalescence

Surgical Recovery: Immediate Post-Operative

Tissue Perfusion: Abdominal Organs

Gastrointestinal Perfusion, Risk for Ineffective

Definition: At risk for decrease in gastrointestinal circulation that may compromise health

Outcomes to Assess and Measure Actual Occurrence of the Diagnosis

Tissue Perfusion

Tissue Perfusion: Abdominal Organs

Outcomes Associated with Risk Factors

Blood Coagulation

Blood Loss Severity

Cardiac Pump Effectiveness

Circulation Status

Gastrointestinal Function

Kidney Function

Knowledge: Coronary Artery Disease Management

Knowledge: Diabetes Management

Knowledge: Inflammatory Bowel Disease Management

Knowledge: Stroke Prevention

Knowledge: Thrombus Prevention

Liver Function

Medication Response

Peripheral Artery Disease Severity

Physical Aging

Physical Injury Severity

Risk Control

Risk Control: Stroke

Risk Detection

Self-Management: Coronary Artery Disease

Self-Management: Diabetes

Self-Management: Peripheral Artery Disease

Smoking Cessation Behavior

Grieving, Complicated, Risk for

Definition: At risk for a disorder that occurs after the death of a significant other, in which the experience of distress accompanying bereavement fails to follow normative expectations and manifests in functional impairment

Outcomes to Assess and Measure Actual Occurrence of the Diagnosis
Grief Resolution

Outcomes Associated with Risk Factors

Anxiety Level
Anxiety Self-Control
Comfort Status: Psychospiritual
Comfort Status: Sociocultural
Coping
Depression Level
Depression Self-Control
Family Coping
Family Normalization
Family Resiliency

Loneliness Severity
Mood Equilibrium
Personal Resiliency
Risk Control
Risk Detection
Self-Esteem
Social Support
Stress Level
Suffering Severity

Growth, Risk for Disproportionate

Definition: At risk for growth above the 97th percentile or below the 3rd percentile for age, crossing two percentile channels

Outcomes to Assess and Measure Actual Occurrence of the Diagnosis

Growth
Physical Maturation: Female

Physical Maturation: Male
Weight: Body Mass

Outcomes Associated with Risk Factors

Abuse Cessation
Abuse Protection
Adherence Behavior: Healthy Diet
Aggression Self-Restraint
Alcohol Abuse Cessation Behavior
Anger Self-Restraint
Appetite
Bottle Feeding Establishment: Infant
Bottle Feeding Performance
Breastfeeding Establishment: Infant
Breastfeeding Maintenance
Community Disaster Response
Community Risk Control: Lead Exposure
Compliance Behavior: Prescribed Diet
Cup Feeding Establishment: Infant
Cup Feeding Performance
Drug Abuse Cessation Behavior
Eating Disorder Self-Control
Infection Severity
Infection Severity: Newborn

Knowledge: Bottle Feeding
Knowledge: Breastfeeding
Knowledge: Cup Feeding
Knowledge: Eating Disorder Management
Knowledge: Health Resources
Knowledge: Infant Care
Knowledge: Preconception Maternal Health
Knowledge: Pregnancy
Knowledge: Preterm Infant Care
Neglect Cessation
Nutritional Status: Food & Fluid Intake
Nutritional Status: Nutrient Intake
Prenatal Health Behavior
Preterm Infant Organization
Risk Control
Risk Detection
Substance Addiction Consequences
Weight Gain Behavior
Weight Loss Behavior

Human Dignity, Risk for Compromised

Definition: At risk for perceived loss of respect and honor

Outcomes to Assess and Measure Actual Occurrence of the Diagnosis

Client Satisfaction: Protection of Rights

Dignified Life Closure

Outcomes Associated with Risk Factors

Bowel Continence

Client Satisfaction

Client Satisfaction: Caring

Client Satisfaction: Communication

Client Satisfaction: Cultural Needs Fulfillment

Client Satisfaction: Physical Care

Client Satisfaction: Psychological Care

Comfort Status: Physical

Comfort Status: Psychospiritual

Comfort Status: Sociocultural

Comfortable Death

Decision-Making

Neglect Recovery

Participation in Health Care Decisions

Personal Autonomy

Personal Well-Being

Risk Control

Risk Detection

Self-Awareness

Self-Esteem

Urinary Continence

Infant Behavior, Risk for Disorganized

Definition: At risk for alteration in integrating and modulation of the physiological and behavioral systems of functioning (i.e., autonomic, motor, state-organization, self-regulatory, and attentional-interactional systems)

Outcomes to Assess and Measure Actual Occurrence of the Diagnosis

Newborn Adaptation

Preterm Infant Organization

Outcomes Associated with Risk Factors

Child Development: 1 Month
Child Development: 2 Months
Child Development: 4 Months
Child Development: 6 Months
Child Development: 12 Months
Comfort Status: Environment
Coordinated Movement
Discomfort Level
Knowledge: Infant Care

Knowledge: Parenting
Knowledge: Preterm Infant Care
Neurological Status
Oral Health
Pain Level
Risk Control
Risk Detection
Sleep
Thermoregulation: Newborn

Infection, Risk for

Definition: At risk for being invaded by pathogenic organisms

Outcomes to Assess and Measure Actual Occurrence of the Diagnosis

Infection Severity

Infection Severity: Newborn

Outcomes Associated with Risk Factors

Burn Healing
Community Risk Control: Communicable Disease
Gastrointestinal Function
Hemodialysis Access
Immobility Consequences: Physiological
Immune Status
Immunization Behavior
Knowledge: Acute Illness Management
Knowledge: Chronic Disease Management
Maternal Status: Antepartum
Maternal Status: Intrapartum
Maternal Status: Postpartum
Medication Response
Nutritional Status
Nutritional Status: Nutrient Intake
Oral Health

Physical Injury Severity
Respiratory Status: Airway Patency
Respiratory Status: Ventilation
Risk Control
Risk Control: Infectious Process
Risk Control: Sexually Transmitted Diseases (STD)
Risk Detection
Self-Management: Chronic Disease
Smoking Cessation Behavior
Surgical Recovery: Convalescence
Surgical Recovery: Immediate Post-Operative
Tissue Integrity: Skin & Mucous Membranes
Weight: Body Mass
Wound Healing: Primary Intention
Wound Healing: Secondary Intention

Injury, Risk for

Definition: At risk for injury as a result of environmental conditions interacting with the individual's adaptive and defensive resources

Outcomes to Assess and Measure Actual Occurrence of the Diagnosis

Falls Occurrence

Physical Injury Severity

Outcomes Associated with Risk Factors

Allergic Response: Systemic
Ambulation
Ambulation: Wheelchair
Balance
Blood Coagulation
Blood Glucose Level
Client Satisfaction: Safety
Cognitive Orientation
Community Immune Status
Community Risk Control: Communicable Disease
Coordinated Movement
Delirium Level
Dementia Level
Elopement Propensity Risk
Fall Prevention Behavior
Gait
Immune Hypersensitivity Response
Immune Status
Immunization Behavior
Information Processing
Knowledge: Body Mechanics
Knowledge: Child Physical Safety

Knowledge: Fall Prevention
Knowledge: Personal Safety
Mobility
Nutritional Status: Nutrient Intake
Parenting Performance: Adolescent Physical Safety
Parenting Performance: Early/Middle Childhood Physical Safety
Parenting Performance: Infant/Toddler Physical Safety
Parenting Performance: Psychosocial Safety
Personal Safety Behavior
Risk Control
Risk Detection
Safe Home Environment
Safe Wandering
Seizure Self-Control
Self-Care Status
Sensory Function
Sensory Function: Hearing
Sensory Function: Vision
Tissue Integrity: Skin & Mucous Membranes
Tissue Perfusion
Transfer Performance

Latex Allergy Response, Risk for

Definition: Risk of hypersensitivity to natural latex rubber products that may compromise health

Outcomes to Assess and Measure Actual Occurrence of the Diagnosis

Allergic Response: Localized
Immune Hypersensitivity Response

Tissue Integrity: Skin & Mucous Membranes

Outcomes Associated with Risk Factors

Allergic Response: Systemic
Compliance Behavior: Prescribed Diet
Knowledge: Health Behavior
Pre-Procedure Readiness

Risk Control
Risk Detection
Self-Management: Asthma

Liver Function, Risk for Impaired

Definition: At risk for a decrease in liver function that may compromise health

Outcomes to Assess and Measure Actual Occurrence of the Diagnosis

Liver Function

Outcomes Associated with Risk Factors

Alcohol Abuse Cessation Behavior
Blood Coagulation
Drug Abuse Cessation Behavior
Electrolyte & Acid/Base Balance
Infection Severity
Knowledge: Medication
Medication Response

Risk Control
Risk Control: Alcohol Use
Risk Control: Drug Use
Risk Control: Infectious Process
Risk Control: Sexually Transmitted Diseases (STD)
Risk Detection

Loneliness, Risk for

Definition: At risk for experiencing discomfort associated with a desire or need for more contact with others

Outcomes to Assess and Measure Actual Occurrence of the Diagnosis

Loneliness Severity

Social Anxiety Level

Outcomes Associated with Risk Factors

Adaptation to Physical Disability
Caregiver Stressors
Development: Late Adulthood
Family Functioning
Family Integrity
Family Social Climate
Grief Resolution
Immobility Consequences: Psycho-Cognitive
Leisure Participation
Neglect Cessation

Parent-Infant Attachment
Personal Resiliency
Play Participation
Psychosocial Adjustment: Life Change
Risk Control
Risk Detection
Social Interaction Skills
Social Involvement
Social Support

Maternal-Fetal Dyad, Risk for Disturbed

Definition: At risk for disruption of the symbiotic maternal-fetal dyad as a result of comorbid or pregnancy-related conditions

Outcomes to Assess and Measure Actual Occurrence of the Diagnosis

Fetal Status: Antepartum

Maternal Status: Antepartum

Maternal Status: Intrapartum

Parent-Infant Attachment

Outcomes Associated with Risk Factors

Abuse Protection

Alcohol Abuse Cessation Behavior

Anxiety Level

Blood Glucose Level

Cardiopulmonary Status

Depression Level

Drug Abuse Cessation Behavior

Fatigue: Disruptive Effects

Fear Level

Hyperglycemia Severity

Hypertension Severity

Hypoglycemia Severity

Knowledge: Asthma Management

Knowledge: Cardiac Disease Management

Knowledge: Chronic Obstructive Pulmonary Disease Management

Knowledge: Diabetes Management

Knowledge: Eating Disorder Management

Knowledge: Health Behavior

Knowledge: Healthy Diet

Knowledge: Healthy Lifestyle

Knowledge: Hypertension Management

Knowledge: Medication

Knowledge: Preconception Maternal Health

Knowledge: Pregnancy

Knowledge: Prescribed Diet

Medication Response

Nausea & Vomiting Severity

Nutritional Status

Prenatal Health Behavior

Risk Control

Risk Control: Hypertension

Risk Detection

Seizure Self-Control

Self-Management: Asthma

Self-Management: Cardiac Disease

Self-Management: Chronic Obstructive Pulmonary Disease

Self-Management: Diabetes

Self-Management: Hypertension

Smoking Cessation Behavior

Stress Level

Symptom Severity

Vital Signs

Neonatal Jaundice, Risk for

Definition: At risk for the yellow-orange tint of the neonate's skin and mucous membranes that occurs after 24 hours of life as a result of unconjugated bilirubin in the circulation

Outcomes to Assess and Measure Actual Occurrence of the Diagnosis
Tissue Integrity: Skin & Mucous Membranes

Outcomes Associated with Risk Factors

Bottle Feeding Establishment: Infant
Bowel Elimination
Breastfeeding Establishment: Infant
Cup Feeding Establishment: Infant
Infant Nutritional Status

Newborn Adaptation
Preterm Infant Organization
Risk Control
Risk Detection
Weight: Body Mass

Nutrition: Imbalanced, Risk for More than Body Requirements

Definition: At risk for an intake of nutrients that exceeds metabolic needs

Outcomes to Assess and Measure Actual Occurrence of the Diagnosis

Infant Nutritional Status
Nutritional Status
Nutritional Status: Food & Fluid Intake

Nutritional Status: Nutrient Intake
Weight: Body Mass

Outcomes Associated with Risk Factors

Adherence Behavior: Healthy Diet
Compliance Behavior: Prescribed Diet
Exercise Participation
Family Risk Control: Obesity
Growth
Knowledge: Healthy Diet
Knowledge: Infant Care
Knowledge: Stress Management

Knowledge: Weight Management
Personal Health Status
Risk Control
Risk Detection
Stress Level
Weight Loss Behavior
Weight Maintenance Behavior

Parenting, Risk for Impaired

Definition: At risk for inability of the primary caretaker to create, maintain, or regain an environment that promotes the optimum growth and development of the child

Outcomes to Assess and Measure Actual Occurrence of the Diagnosis

Parent-Infant Attachment

Parenting Performance

Parenting Performance: Psychosocial Safety

Outcomes Associated with Risk Factors

Abusive Behavior Self-Restraint

Aggression Self-Restraint

Bottle Feeding Performance

Caregiver Emotional Health

Caregiver Physical Health

Caregiver Role Endurance

Caregiver Stressors

Caregiver Well-Being

Child Development: 1 Month

Child Development: 2 Months

Child Development: 4 Months

Child Development: 6 Months

Child Development: 12 Months

Child Development: 2 Years

Child Development: 3 Years

Child Development: 4 Years

Child Development: 5 Years

Child Development: Middle Childhood

Child Development: Adolescence

Cognition

Coping

Cup Feeding Performance

Decision-Making

Depression Level

Depression Self-Control

Distorted Thought Self-Control

Family Coping

Family Health Status

Family Normalization

Family Resiliency

Family Risk Control: Obesity

Family Social Climate

Fatigue Level

Health Beliefs: Perceived Resources

Health Orientation

Hyperactivity Level

Information Processing

Knowledge: Health Resources

Knowledge: Infant Care

Knowledge: Parenting

Knowledge: Preterm Infant Care

Mood Equilibrium

Parenting Performance: Adolescent

Parenting Performance: Infant

Parenting Performance: Middle Childhood

Parenting Performance: Preschooler

Parenting Performance: Toddler

Personal Health Status

Personal Resiliency

Risk Control

Risk Control: Alcohol Use

Risk Control: Drug Use

Risk Control: Tobacco Use

Risk Detection

Role Performance

Safe Home Environment

Self-Esteem

Sleep

Social Interaction Skills

Social Support

Stress Level

Substance Withdrawal Severity

Perioperative Positioning Injury, Risk for

Definition: At risk for inadvertent anatomical and physical changes as a result of posture or equipment used during an invasive/surgical procedure

Outcomes to Assess and Measure Actual Occurrence of the Diagnosis

Physical Injury Severity

Tissue Integrity: Skin & Mucous Membranes

Outcomes Associated with Risk Factors

Aspiration Prevention

Circulation Status

Cognitive Orientation

Delirium Level

Fluid Overload Severity

Immobility Consequences: Physiological

Neurological Status: Spinal Sensory/Motor Function

Pre-Procedure Readiness

Post-Procedure Recovery

Risk Control

Risk Detection

Sensory Function

Surgical Recovery: Immediate Post-Operative

Thermoregulation

Tissue Perfusion

Tissue Perfusion: Cellular

Tissue Perfusion: Peripheral

Weight: Body Mass

Peripheral Neurovascular Dysfunction, Risk for

Definition: At risk for disruption in circulation, sensation, or motion of an extremity

Outcomes to Assess and Measure Actual Occurrence of the Diagnosis

Joint Movement: Ankle

Joint Movement: Elbow

Joint Movement: Fingers

Joint Movement: Hip

Joint Movement: Knee

Joint Movement: Shoulder

Neurological Status: Peripheral

Sensory Function: Tactile

Tissue Perfusion: Peripheral

Outcomes Associated with Risk Factors

Blood Coagulation

Bone Healing

Burn Healing

Burn Recovery

Circulation Status

Immobility Consequences: Physiological

Neurological Status: Spinal Sensory/Motor Function

Physical Injury Severity

Risk Control

Risk Detection

Skeletal Function

Surgical Recovery: Convalescence

Tissue Perfusion: Cellular

Personal Identity, Risk for Disturbed

Definition: Risk for the inability to maintain an integrated and complete perception of self

Outcomes to Assess and Measure Actual Occurrence of the Diagnosis

Identity	Self-Awareness

Outcomes Associated with Risk Factors

Abuse Recovery	Family Normalization
Abuse Recovery: Emotional	Family Resiliency
Abuse Recovery: Sexual	Guilt Resolution
Comfort Status: Psychospiritual	Personal Resiliency
Comfort Status: Sociocultural	Risk Control
Dementia Level	Risk Detection
Depression Level	Role Performance
Depression Self-Control	Self-Esteem
Distorted Thought Self-Control	Sexual Identity
Drug Abuse Cessation Behavior	Spiritual Health
Family Functioning	Substance Addiction Consequences

Poisoning, Risk for

Definition: At risk of accidental exposure to, or ingestion of, drugs or dangerous products in doses sufficient that may compromise health

Outcomes to Assess and Measure Actual Occurrence of the Diagnosis

Personal Health Status	Symptom Severity

Outcomes Associated with Risk Factors

Caregiver Performance: Direct Care	Parenting Performance: Infant/Toddler Physical Safety
Cognition	Personal Safety Behavior
Community Risk Control: Lead Exposure	Risk Control
Delirium Level	Risk Control: Alcohol Use
Knowledge: Child Physical Safety	Risk Control: Drug Use
Knowledge: Medication	Risk Detection
Knowledge: Personal Safety	Safe Home Environment
Mood Equilibrium	Self-Care: Non-Parenteral Medication
Parenting Performance: Adolescent Physical Safety	Self-Care: Parenteral Medication
Parenting Performance: Early/Middle Childhood Physical Safety	Sensory Function: Vision
	Vision Compensation Behavior

Post-Trauma Syndrome, Risk for

Definition: At risk for sustained maladaptive response to a traumatic, overwhelming event

Outcomes to Assess and Measure Actual Occurrence of the Diagnosis

Abuse Recovery

Comfort Status: Psychospiritual

Outcomes Associated with Risk Factors

Abuse Cessation

Abuse Protection

Abuse Recovery: Emotional

Abuse Recovery: Sexual

Grief Resolution

Guilt Resolution

Health Beliefs: Perceived Threat

Impulse Self-Control

Information Processing

Personal Resiliency

Psychosocial Adjustment: Life Change

Relocation Adaptation

Risk Control

Risk Detection

Self-Awareness

Self-Esteem

Social Support

Spiritual Health

Powerlessness, Risk for

Definition: At risk for the lived experience of lack of control over a situation, including a perception that one's actions do not significantly affect an outcome.

Outcomes to Assess and Measure Actual Occurrence of the Diagnosis

Health Beliefs: Perceived Control

Participation in Health Care Decisions

Personal Autonomy

Self-Direction of Care

Outcomes Associated with Risk Factors

Abuse Recovery

Adaptation to Physical Disability

Anxiety Level

Body Image

Coping

Dignified Life Closure

Health Beliefs: Perceived Ability to Perform

Health Beliefs: Perceived Resources

Immobility Consequences: Psycho-Cognitive

Knowledge: Disease Process

Knowledge: Health Resources

Knowledge: Medication

Knowledge: Prescribed Diet

Knowledge: Treatment Procedure

Knowledge: Treatment Regimen

Pain Level

Participation in Health Care Decisions

Personal Autonomy

Personal Resiliency

Physical Injury Severity

Risk Control

Risk Detection

Self-Awareness

Self-Direction of Care

Self-Esteem

Social Support

Spiritual Health

Stress Level

Relationship, Risk for Ineffective

Definition: Risk for a pattern of mutual partnership that is insufficient to provide for each other's needs

Outcome to Assess and Measure Actual Occurrence of the Diagnosis

Caregiver-Patient Relationship

Parent-Infant Attachment

Outcomes Associated with Risk Factors

Abuse Cessation

Abuse Recovery

Abuse Recovery: Emotional

Abuse Recovery: Financial

Abuse Recovery: Physical

Abuse Recovery: Sexual

Adaptation to Physical Disability

Aggression Self-Restraint

Alcohol Abuse Cessation Behavior

Caregiver Adaptation to Patient Institutionalization

Caregiver Performance: Direct Care

Caregiver Performance: Indirect Care

Caregiver Stressors

Cognition

Dementia Level

Development: Late Adulthood

Development: Middle Adulthood

Development: Young Adulthood

Drug Abuse Cessation Behavior

Family Functioning

Family Health Status

Family Integrity

Family Normalization

Family Resiliency

Family Social Climate

Information Processing

Parenting Performance

Parenting Performance: Adolescent

Parenting Performance: Infant

Parenting Performance: Middle Childhood

Parenting Performance: Preschooler

Parenting Performance: Toddler

Psychosocial Adjustment: Life Change

Relocation Adaptation

Risk Control

Risk Control: Alcohol Use

Risk Control: Drug Use

Risk Control: Tobacco Use

Risk Detection

Role Performance

Social Interaction Skills

Social Involvement

Social Support

Stress Level

Substance Addiction Consequences

Substance Withdrawal Severity

Religiosity, Risk for Impaired

Definition: At risk for an impaired ability to exercise reliance on religious beliefs and/or participate in rituals of a particular faith tradition

Outcomes to Assess and Measure Actual Occurrence of the Diagnosis

Comfort Status: Psychospiritual

Spiritual Health

Outcomes Associated with Risk Factors

Acceptance: Health Status

Adaptation to Physical Disability

Anxiety Level

Client Satisfaction: Cultural Needs Fulfillment

Coping

Depression Level

Development: Late Adulthood

Fear Level

Grief Resolution

Hope

Loneliness Severity

Mobility

Pain: Disruptive Effects

Pain Level

Participation in Health Care Decisions

Personal Autonomy

Personal Resiliency

Psychosocial Adjustment: Life Change

Risk Control

Risk Detection

Self-Awareness

Social Involvement

Social Support

Suffering Severity

Relocation Stress Syndrome, Risk for

Definition: At risk for physiological and/or psychosocial disturbance following transfer from one environment to another

Outcomes to Assess and Measure Actual Occurrence of the Diagnosis

Child Adaptation to Hospitalization

Discharge Readiness: Independent Living

Psychosocial Adjustment: Life Change

Relocation Adaptation

Outcomes Associated with Risk Factors

Acceptance: Health Status

Agitation Level

Cognition

Coping

Discharge Readiness: Supported Living

Elopement Propensity Risk

Family Participation in Professional Care

Grief Resolution

Memory

Participation in Health Care Decisions

Personal Autonomy

Personal Health Status

Risk Control

Risk Detection

Self-Direction of Care

Social Support

Stress Level

Renal Perfusion, Risk for Ineffective

Definition: At risk for a decrease in blood circulation to the kidney that may compromise health

Outcomes to Assess and Measure Actual Occurrence of the Diagnosis

Tissue Perfusion

Tissue Perfusion: Abdominal Organs

Outcomes Associated with Risk Factors

Blood Loss Severity

Burn Healing

Burn Recovery

Cardiopulmonary Status

Circulation Status

Drug Abuse Cessation Behavior

Electrolyte & Acid/Base Balance

Fluid Balance

Fluid Overload Severity

Hydration

Hypertension Severity

Hypotension Severity

Immune Hypersensitivity Response

Infection Severity

Kidney Function

Knowledge: Diabetes Management

Knowledge: Heart Failure Management

Knowledge: Hypertension Management

Knowledge: Infection Management

Knowledge: Lipid Disorder Management

Medication Response

Metabolic Acidosis Severity

Nutritional Status: Biochemical Measures

Physical Aging

Physical Injury Severity

Post-Procedure Recovery

Risk Control

Risk Detection

Safe Home Environment

Self-Management: Diabetes

Self-Management: Heart Failure

Self-Management: Hypertension

Self-Management: Lipid Disorder

Smoking Cessation Behavior

Surgical Recovery: Immediate Post-Operative

Vital Signs

Resilience, Risk for Compromised

Definition: At risk for decreased ability to sustain a pattern of positive responses to an adverse situation or crisis

Outcomes to Assess and Measure Actual Occurrence of the Diagnosis

Family Resiliency   Personal Resiliency

Outcomes Associated with Risk Factors

Acceptance: Health Status	Hope
Adaptation to Physical Disability	Pain Level
Anxiety Level	Psychomotor Energy
Client Satisfaction: Case Management	Psychosocial Adjustment: Life Change
Client Satisfaction: Continuity of Care	Risk Control
Client Satisfaction: Symptom Control	Risk Control: Unintended Pregnancy
Dignified Life Closure	Risk Detection
Family Coping	Stress Level
Family Functioning	Suffering Severity
Family Normalization	Symptom Control
Grief Resolution	Symptom Severity

Self-Esteem: Chronic Low, Risk for

Definition: At risk for longstanding negative self-evaluating/feelings about self or self-capabilities

Outcomes to Assess and Measure Actual Occurrence of the Diagnosis

Self-Awareness   Self-Esteem

Outcomes Associated with Risk Factors

Abuse Cessation   Grief Resolution
Abuse Protection   Loneliness Severity
Abuse Recovery   Parent-Infant Attachment
Abuse Recovery: Emotional   Parenting Performance
Acceptance: Health Status   Personal Autonomy
Adaptation to Physical Disability   Personal Resiliency
Comfort Status: Psychospiritual   Psychosocial Adjustment: Life Change
Comfort Status: Sociocultural   Risk Control
Depression Level   Risk Detection
Distorted Thought Self-Control   Sexual Identity
Family Functioning   Social Involvement
Family Integrity   Social Support
Family Resiliency   Spiritual Health
Family Social Climate

Self-Esteem: Situational Low, Risk for

Definition: At risk for developing negative perception of self-worth in response to a current situation

Outcomes to Assess and Measure Actual Occurrence of the Diagnosis

Self-Awareness   Self-Esteem

Outcomes Associated with Risk Factors

Abuse Cessation   Development: Young Adulthood
Abuse Protection   Grief Resolution
Abuse Recovery   Health Beliefs: Perceived Control
Abuse Recovery: Emotional   Neglect Cessation
Abuse Recovery: Financial   Neglect Recovery
Abuse Recovery: Physical   Parenting Performance
Abuse Recovery: Sexual   Personal Autonomy
Acceptance: Health Status   Personal Health Status
Adaptation to Physical Disability   Personal Resiliency
Body Image   Psychosocial Adjustment: Life Change
Burn Recovery   Risk Control
Child Development: Adolescence   Risk Detection
Child Development: Middle Childhood   Role Performance
Coping   Sexual Identity
Development: Late Adulthood   Weight Loss Behavior
Development: Middle Adulthood

Self-Mutilation, Risk for

Definition: At risk for deliberate self-injurious behavior causing tissue damage with the intent of causing non-fatal injury to attain relief of tension

Outcomes to Assess and Measure Actual Occurrence of the Diagnosis
Mutilation Self-Restraint

Outcomes Associated with Risk Factors

Abuse Cessation	Family Integrity
Abuse Protection	Guilt Resolution
Abuse Recovery	Health Beliefs: Perceived Control
Abuse Recovery: Emotional	Identity
Abuse Recovery: Physical	Impulse Self-Control
Abuse Recovery: Sexual	Mood Equilibrium
Agitation Level	Personal Autonomy
Alcohol Abuse Cessation Behavior	Personal Resiliency
Anger Self-Restraint	Risk Control
Anxiety Level	Risk Control: Alcohol Use
Body Image	Risk Control: Drug Use
Child Development: Adolescence	Risk Detection
Child Development: Middle Childhood	Self-Awareness
Coping	Self-Esteem
Decision-Making	Sexual Identity
Depression Level	Social Interaction Skills
Distorted Thought Self-Control	Social Involvement
Drug Abuse Cessation Behavior	Stress Level
Eating Disorder Self-Control	Substance Addiction Consequences
Family Functioning	

Shock, Risk for

Definition: At risk for an inadequate blood flow to the body's tissues, which may lead to life-threatening cellular dysfunction

Outcomes to Assess and Measure Actual Occurrence of the Diagnosis

Shock Severity: Anaphylactic	Shock Severity: Neurogenic
Shock Severity: Cardiogenic	Shock Severity: Septic
Shock Severity: Hypovolemic	Tissue Perfusion: Cellular

Outcomes Associated with Risk Factors

Allergic Response: Systemic	Physical Injury Severity
Blood Loss Severity	Respiratory Status: Gas Exchange
Blood Transfusion Reaction	Risk Control
Circulation Status	Risk Control: Infectious Process
Hemodialysis Access	Risk Detection
Hypotension Severity	Surgical Recovery: Immediate Post-Operative
Infection Severity	Vital Signs
Infection Severity: Newborn	

Skin Integrity, Risk for Impaired

Definition: At risk for alteration in epidermis and/or dermis

Outcomes to Assess and Measure Actual Occurrence of the Diagnosis
Tissue Integrity: Skin & Mucous Membranes

Outcomes Associated with Risk Factors

Allergic Response: Localized
Body Positioning: Self-Initiated
Bowel Continence
Breastfeeding Establishment: Maternal
Circulation Status
Fluid Overload Severity
Hydration
Immobility Consequences: Physiological
Immune Hypersensitivity Response
Immune Status
Infant Nutritional Status
Infection Severity
Infection Severity: Newborn
Medication Response
Mutilation Self-Restraint
Nutritional Status
Nutritional Status: Biochemical Measures

Nutritional Status: Nutrient Intake
Ostomy Self-Care
Physical Aging
Physical Maturation: Female
Physical Maturation: Male
Risk Control
Risk Control: Hyperthermia
Risk Control: Hypothermia
Risk Control: Infectious Process
Risk Control: Sun Exposure
Risk Detection
Sensory Function: Tactile
Tissue Perfusion
Tissue Perfusion: Cellular
Tissue Perfusion: Peripheral
Urinary Continence
Weight: Body Mass

Spiritual Distress, Risk for

Definition: At risk for an impaired ability to experience and integrate meaning and purpose in life though connectedness with self, others, art, music, literature, nature, and/or a power greater than oneself

Outcomes to Assess and Measure Actual Occurrence of the Diagnosis
Spiritual Health

Outcomes Associated with Risk Factors

Acceptance: Health Status
Adaptation to Physical Disability
Anxiety Level
Alcohol Abuse Cessation Behavior
Client Satisfaction: Cultural Needs Fulfillment
Comfort Status: Psychospiritual
Comfort Status: Sociocultural
Comfortable Death
Community Disaster Readiness
Coping
Depression Level
Dignified Life Closure
Drug Abuse Cessation Behavior
Fatigue Level
Grief Resolution
Hope

Loneliness Severity
Mood Equilibrium
Pain: Adverse Psychological Response
Personal Autonomy
Personal Resiliency
Personal Well-Being
Psychosocial Adjustment: Life Change
Risk Control
Risk Detection
Self-Esteem
Social Anxiety Level
Social Interaction Skills
Social Involvement
Stress Level
Suffering Severity

Sudden Infant Death Syndrome, Risk for

Definition: At risk for sudden death of an infant under 1 year of age

Outcomes to Assess and Measure Actual Occurrence of the Diagnosis
No outcomes focused on infant mortality

Outcomes Associated with Risk Factors

Knowledge: Infant Care
Knowledge: Preterm Infant Care
Maternal Status: Antepartum
Newborn Adaptation
Parenting Performance: Infant
Parenting Performance: Infant/Toddler Physical Safety
Prenatal Health Behavior
Preterm Infant Organization

Risk Control
Risk Control: Hyperthermia
Risk Control: Tobacco Use
Risk Detection
Smoking Cessation Behavior
Thermoregulation: Newborn
Weight: Body Mass

Suffocation, Risk for

Definition: At risk of accidental suffocation (inadequate air available for inhalation)

Outcomes to Assess and Measure Actual Occurrence of the Diagnosis

Respiratory Status
Respiratory Status: Airway Patency

Respiratory Status: Ventilation

Outcomes Associated with Risk Factors

Aspiration Prevention
Body Positioning: Self-Initiated
Bottle Feeding Performance
Cognition
Coordinated Movement
Knowledge: Bottle Feeding
Knowledge: Child Physical Safety
Knowledge: Infant Care
Knowledge: Personal Safety
Knowledge: Preterm Infant Care
Neurological Status: Consciousness

Parenting Performance: Infant/Toddler Physical Safety
Personal Safety Behavior
Physical Injury Severity
Post-Procedure Recovery
Risk Control
Risk Detection
Safe Home Environment
Self-Management: Asthma
Sensory Function: Taste & Smell
Smoking Cessation Behavior
Swallowing Status

Suicide, Risk for

Definition: At risk for self-inflicted, life-threatening injury

Outcomes to Assess and Measure Actual Occurrence of the Diagnosis
No outcomes to measure occurrence of suicide

Outcomes Associated with Risk Factors

Abuse Recovery
Abuse Recovery: Emotional
Abuse Recovery: Financial
Abuse Recovery: Physical
Abuse Recovery: Sexual
Adaptation to Physical Disability
Alcohol Abuse Cessation Behavior
Anger Self-Restraint
Child Development: Adolescence
Depression Level
Depression Self-Control
Development: Late Adulthood
Development: Young Adulthood
Drug Abuse Cessation Behavior
Family Functioning
Family Integrity
Grief Resolution
Guilt Resolution
Hope
Impulse Self-Control
Knowledge: Stress Management
Loneliness Severity
Mood Equilibrium
Pain: Adverse Psychological Response
Pain Control
Pain: Disruptive Effects

Pain Level
Personal Autonomy
Personal Resiliency
Personal Well-Being
Psychomotor Energy
Psychosocial Adjustment: Life Change
Relocation Adaptation
Risk Control
Risk Control: Alcohol Use
Risk Control: Drug Use
Risk Detection
Self-Awareness
Self-Esteem
Self-Management: Chronic Disease
Sexual Identity
Social Interaction Skills
Social Involvement
Social Support
Stress Level
Student Health Status
Substance Addiction Consequences
Substance Withdrawal Severity
Suffering Severity
Suicide Self-Restraint
Symptom Control
Will to Live

Thermal Injury, Risk for

Definition: At risk for damage to skin and mucous membranes due to extreme temperatures

Outcomes to Assess and Measure Actual Occurrence of the Diagnosis

Burn Healing

Burn Recovery

Oral Health

Tissue Integrity: Skin & Mucous Membranes

Outcomes Associated with Risk Factors

Bottle Feeding Performance

Cup Feeding Performance

Delirium Level

Dementia Level

Elopement Propensity Risk

Fatigue Level

Heedfulness of Affected Side

Knowledge: Child Physical Safety

Knowledge: Infant Care

Knowledge: Personal Safety

Medication Response

Neurological Status: Cranial Sensory/Motor Function

Parenting Performance: Infant/Toddler Physical Safety

Personal Safety Behavior

Risk Control

Risk Control: Alcohol Use

Risk Control: Drug Use

Risk Control: Hyperthermia

Risk Control: Hypothermia

Risk Control: Sun Exposure

Risk Control: Tobacco Use

Risk Detection

Safe Home Environment

Safe Wandering

Tissue Perfusion: Cardiac, Risk for Decreased

Definition: At risk for a decrease in cardiac (coronary) circulation that may compromise health

Outcomes to Assess and Measure Actual Occurrence of the Diagnosis

Tissue Perfusion

Tissue Perfusion: Cardiac

Outcomes Associated with Risk Factors

Adherence Behavior: Healthy Diet

Alcohol Abuse Cessation Behavior

Cardiac Pump Effectiveness

Circulation Status

Compliance Behavior: Prescribed Diet

Compliance Behavior: Prescribed Medication

Drug Abuse Cessation Behavior

Family Risk Control: Obesity

Hydration

Hypertension Severity

Knowledge: Conception Prevention

Knowledge: Coronary Artery Disease Management

Knowledge: Diabetes Management

Knowledge: Health Behavior

Knowledge: Healthy Diet

Knowledge: Hypertension Management

Knowledge: Lipid Disorder Management

Knowledge: Medication

Knowledge: Prescribed Activity

Knowledge: Prescribed Diet

Knowledge: Substance Use Control

Knowledge: Weight Management

Medication Response

Physical Fitness

Respiratory Status: Gas Exchange

Risk Control

Risk Control: Alcohol Use

Risk Control: Drug Use

Risk Control: Cardiovascular Disease

Risk Control: Hypertension

Risk Control: Lipid Disorder

Risk Control: Tobacco Use

Risk Detection

Self-Management: Cardiac Disease

Self-Management: Coronary Artery Disease

Self-Management: Diabetes

Self-Management: Hypertension

Self-Management: Lipid Disorder

Smoking Cessation Behavior

Surgical Recovery: Immediate Post-Operative

Weight: Body Mass

Tissue Perfusion: Cerebral, Risk for Ineffective

Definition: At risk for a decrease in cerebral tissue circulation that may compromise health

Outcomes to Assess and Measure Actual Occurrence of the Diagnosis

Tissue Perfusion	Tissue Perfusion: Cerebral

Outcomes Associated with Risk Factors

Blood Coagulation	Neurological Status
Cardiac Pump Effectiveness	Physical Injury Severity
Circulation Status	Risk Control
Drug Abuse Cessation Behavior	Risk Control: Drug Use
Hypertension Severity	Risk Control: Stroke
Knowledge: Anticoagulation Therapy Management	Risk Control: Thrombus
Knowledge: Cardiac Disease Management	Risk Detection
Knowledge: Coronary Artery Disease Management	Self-Management: Coronary Artery Disease
Knowledge: Dysrhythmia Management	Self-Management: Dysrhythmia
Knowledge: Heart Failure Management	Self-Management: Heart Failure
Knowledge: Hypertension Management	Self-Management: Hypertension
Knowledge: Lipid Disorder Management	Self-Management: Lipid Disorder
Knowledge: Peripheral Artery Disease Management	Self-Management: Peripheral Artery Disease
Knowledge: Thrombus Prevention	Substance Addiction Consequences
Medication Response	

Tissue Perfusion: Peripheral, Risk for Ineffective

Definition: At risk for a decrease in blood circulation to the periphery that may compromise health

Outcomes to Assess and Measure Actual Occurrence of the Diagnosis

Tissue Perfusion	Tissue Perfusion: Peripheral

Outcomes Associated with Risk Factors

Compliance Behavior: Prescribed Activity	Peripheral Artery Disease Severity
Exercise Participation	Personal Safety Behavior
Hypertension Severity	Physical Aging
Knowledge: Diabetes Management	Risk Control
Knowledge: Disease Process	Risk Control: Hypertension
Knowledge: Health Promotion	Risk Control: Lipid Disorder
Knowledge: Healthy Diet	Risk Control: Thrombus
Knowledge: Healthy Lifestyle	Risk Control: Tobacco Use
Knowledge: Hypertension Management	Risk Detection
Knowledge: Lipid Disorder Management	Self-Management: Diabetes
Knowledge: Prescribed Activity	Self-Management: Hypertension
Knowledge: Substance Use Control	Self-Management: Lipid Disorder
Knowledge: Thrombus Prevention	Self-Management: Peripheral Artery Disease
Knowledge: Weight Management	Smoking Cessation Behavior
Lifestyle Balance	Weight: Body Mass

Trauma, Risk for

Definition: At risk of accidental tissue injury (e.g., wound, burn, fracture)

Outcomes to Assess and Measure Actual Occurrence of the Diagnosis

Bone Healing
Burn Healing
Burn Recovery
Falls Occurrence

Physical Injury Severity
Tissue Integrity: Skin & Mucous Membranes
Wound Healing: Primary Intention
Wound Healing: Secondary Intention

Outcomes Associated with Risk Factors

Abuse Protection
Agitation Level
Alcohol Abuse Cessation Behavior
Balance
Cognition
Community Risk Control: Violence
Community Violence Level
Coordinated Movement
Delirium Level
Dementia Level
Elopement Propensity Risk
Fall Prevention Behavior
Gait
Hearing Compensation Behavior
Knowledge: Child Physical Safety
Knowledge: Fall Prevention
Knowledge: Personal Safety
Neurological Status: Peripheral

Parenting Performance: Adolescent Physical Safety
Parenting Performance: Early/Middle Childhood Physical
   Safety
Parenting Performance: Infant/Toddler Physical Safety
Personal Safety Behavior
Physical Fitness
Risk Control
Risk Control: Alcohol Use
Risk Control: Drug Use
Risk Control: Sun Exposure
Risk Detection
Safe Home Environment
Safe Wandering
Sensory Function: Tactile
Sensory Function: Vision
Skeletal Function
Substance Withdrawal Severity
Vision Compensation Behavior

Urinary Incontinence: Urge, Risk for

Definition: At risk for involuntary loss of urine occurring soon after a strong sensation or urgency to void

Outcomes to Assess and Measure Actual Occurrence of the Diagnosis
Urinary Continence

Outcomes Associated with Risk Factors

Bowel Elimination	Risk Control
Infection Severity	Risk Control: Alcohol Use
Knowledge: Medication	Risk Control: Infectious Process
Knowledge: Treatment Regimen	Risk Detection
Medication Response	Self-Care: Toileting
Neurological Status: Spinal Sensory/Motor Function	Urinary Elimination

Vascular Trauma, Risk for

Definition: At risk for damage to a vein and its surrounding tissues related to the presence of a catheter and/or infused solutions

Outcomes to Assess and Measure Actual Occurrence of the Diagnosis
Hemodialysis Access

Outcomes Associated with Risk Factors

Allergic Response: Localized	Risk Detection
Risk Control	Self-Care: Parenteral Medication

Violence: Other-Directed, Risk for

Definition: At risk for behaviors in which an individual demonstrates that he or she can be physically, emotionally, and/or sexually harmful to others

Outcomes to Assess and Measure Actual Occurrence of the Diagnosis

Abusive Behavior Self-Restraint	Anger Self-Restraint
Aggression Self-Restraint	

Outcomes Associated with Risk Factors

Abuse Cessation	Hyperactivity Level
Abuse Protection	Impulse Self-Control
Abuse Recovery: Emotional	Maternal Status: Antepartum
Abuse Recovery: Physical	Maternal Status: Intrapartum
Abuse Recovery: Sexual	Neurological Status
Agitation Level	Parent-Infant Attachment
Alcohol Abuse Cessation Behavior	Risk Control
Cognition	Risk Control: Alcohol Use
Delirium Level	Risk Control: Drug Use
Dementia Level	Risk Detection
Distorted Thought Self-Control	Stress Level
Drug Abuse Cessation Behavior	Suicide Self-Restraint

Violence: Self-Directed, Risk for

Definition: At risk for behaviors in which an individual demonstrates that he or she can be physically, emotionally, and/or sexually harmful to self

Outcomes to Assess and Measure Actual Occurrence of the Diagnosis

Mutilation Self-Restraint

Suicide Self-Restraint

Outcomes Associated with Risk Factors

Adaptation to Physical Disability

Alcohol Abuse Cessation Behavior

Anger Self-Restraint

Anxiety Level

Child Development: Adolescence

Cognition

Coping

Depression Level

Depression Self-Control

Development: Late Adulthood

Development: Middle Adulthood

Distorted Thought Self-Control

Drug Abuse Cessation Behavior

Eating Disorder Self-Control

Family Functioning

Family Integrity

Guilt Resolution

Hope

Identity

Impulse Self-Control

Loneliness Severity

Mood Equilibrium

Personal Health Status

Personal Well-Being

Quality of Life

Risk Control

Risk Control: Alcohol Use

Risk Control: Drug Use

Risk Detection

Self-Awareness

Sexual Functioning

Sexual Identity

Social Interaction Skills

Social Involvement

Social Support

Substance Addiction Consequences

Will to Live

Health-Promotion Nursing Diagnoses

Breastfeeding, Readiness for Enhanced

Definition: A pattern of proficiency and satisfaction of the mother-infant dyad that is sufficient to support the breastfeeding process and can be strengthened

Outcomes to Measure Defining Characteristics

Anxiety Self-Control
Bowel Elimination
Breastfeeding Establishment: Infant
Breastfeeding Establishment: Maternal
Breastfeeding Maintenance
Breastfeeding Weaning
Child Development: 1 Month
Child Development: 2 Months
Fluid Balance
Growth
Hydration
Infant Nutritional Status

Knowledge: Breastfeeding
Newborn Adaptation
Nutritional Status: Food & Fluid Intake
Parent-Infant Attachment
Parenting Performance: Infant
Postpartum Maternal Health Behavior
Preterm Infant Organization
Rest
Sleep
Social Support
Swallowing Status
Urinary Elimination

Childbearing Process, Readiness for Enhanced

Definition: A pattern of preparing for and maintaining a healthy pregnancy, childbirth process, and care of the newborn that is sufficient for ensuring well-being and can be strengthened

Outcomes to Measure Defining Characteristics

Bottle Feeding Establishment: Infant
Bottle Feeding Performance
Breastfeeding Establishment: Infant
Breastfeeding Establishment: Maternal
Cup Feeding Establishment: Infant
Cup Feeding Performance
Infant Nutritional Status
Health Seeking Behavior
Knowledge: Bottle Feeding
Knowledge: Breastfeeding
Knowledge: Cup Feeding
Knowledge: Healthy Lifestyle
Knowledge: Infant Care
Knowledge: Labor & Delivery
Knowledge: Postpartum Maternal Health

Knowledge: Preconception Maternal Health
Knowledge: Pregnancy
Knowledge: Pregnancy & Postpartum Sexual Functioning
Maternal Status: Antepartum
Maternal Status: Intrapartum
Maternal Status: Postpartum
Motivation
Parent-Infant Attachment
Parenting Performance: Infant
Parenting Performance: Psychosocial Safety
Personal Autonomy
Personal Time Management
Postpartum Maternal Health Behavior
Prenatal Health Behavior
Social Support

Comfort, Readiness for Enhanced

Definition: A pattern of ease, relief, and transcendence in physical, psychospiritual, environmental, and/or social dimensions that is sufficient for well-being and can be strengthened

Outcomes to Measure Defining Characteristics

Abuse Recovery
Anxiety Level
Comfort Status
Comfort Status: Environment
Comfort Status: Physical
Comfort Status: Psychospiritual
Comfort Status: Sociocultural
Comfortable Death
Coping
Dignified Life Closure
Discomfort Level
Grief Resolution
Guilt Resolution
Health Seeking Behavior
Hope
Mood Equilibrium
Motivation

Personal Autonomy
Personal Health Status
Personal Resiliency
Personal Well-Being
Psychosocial Adjustment: Life Change
Quality of Life
Relocation Adaptation
Rest
Risk Control
Risk Detection
Sleep
Social Interaction Skills
Social Involvement
Social Support
Spiritual Health
Stress Level

Communication, Readiness for Enhanced

Definition: A pattern of exchanging information and ideas with others that is sufficient for meeting one's needs and life's goals and can be strengthened

Outcomes to Measure Defining Characteristics

Child Development: Adolescence
Child Development: Middle Childhood
Client Satisfaction: Communication
Communication
Communication: Expressive
Communication: Receptive
Development: Late Adulthood

Development: Middle Adulthood
Development: Young Adulthood
Information Processing
Motivation
Self-Awareness
Social Interaction Skills

Community Coping, Readiness for Enhanced

Definition: A pattern of community activities for adaptation and problem-solving that is sufficient for meeting the demands or needs of the community for the management of current and future problems/stressors and can be strengthened

Outcomes to Measure Defining Characteristics

Community Competence
Community Disaster Readiness
Community Disaster Response
Community Health Screening Effectiveness
Community Program Effectiveness
Community Resiliency
Community Risk Control: Chronic Disease

Community Risk Control: Communicable Disease
Community Risk Control: Lead Exposure
Community Risk Control: Obesity
Community Risk Control: Unhealthy Cultural Traditions
Community Risk Control: Violence
Community Violence Level

Coping, Readiness for Enhanced

Definition: A pattern of cognitive and behavioral efforts to manage demands that is sufficient for well-being and can be strengthened

Outcomes to Measure Defining Characteristics

Acceptance: Health Status
Adaptation to Physical Disability
Caregiver Adaptation to Patient Institutionalization
Caregiver Emotional Health
Caregiver Stressors
Child Adaptation to Hospitalization
Coping
Decision-Making
Family Resiliency
Health Seeking Behavior
Knowledge: Health Resources
Knowledge: Stress Management
Motivation

Personal Autonomy
Personal Resiliency
Personal Time Management
Personal Well-Being
Psychosocial Adjustment: Life Change
Quality of Life
Role Performance
Self-Awareness
Self-Esteem
Social Interaction Skills
Social Support
Spiritual Health
Stress Level

Decision-Making, Readiness for Enhanced

Definition: A pattern of choosing a course of action that is sufficient for meeting short- and long-term health-related goals and can be strengthened

Outcomes to Measure Defining Characteristics

Adaptation to Physical Disability
Adherence Behavior
Adherence Behavior: Healthy Diet
Client Satisfaction: Protection of Rights
Compliance Behavior
Compliance Behavior: Prescribed Activity
Compliance Behavior: Prescribed Diet
Compliance Behavior: Prescribed Medication
Decision-Making
Family Participation in Professional Care
Family Support During Treatment

Health Beliefs
Health Beliefs: Perceived Ability to Perform
Health Beliefs: Perceived Control
Health Seeking Behavior
Lifestyle Balance
Motivation
Participation in Health Care Decisions
Personal Autonomy
Personal Resiliency
Risk Detection
Self-Awareness

Family Coping, Readiness for Enhanced

Definition: A pattern of management of adaptive tasks by primary person (family member, significant other, or close friend) involved with the client's health challenge that is sufficient for health and growth, in regard to self and in relation to the client, and can be strengthened

Outcomes to Measure Defining Characteristics

Caregiver Home Care Readiness
Caregiver Lifestyle Disruption
Caregiver Performance: Direct Care
Caregiver Performance: Indirect Care
Family Coping
Family Functioning
Family Normalization
Family Resiliency

Health Promoting Behavior
Health Seeking Behavior
Knowledge: Health Behavior
Knowledge: Health Promotion
Lifestyle Balance
Parenting Performance
Personal Resiliency

Family Processes, Readiness for Enhanced

Definition: A pattern of family functioning that is sufficient to support the well-being of family members and can be strengthened

Outcomes to Measure Defining Characteristics

Family Coping
Family Functioning
Family Health Status
Family Integrity
Family Normalization
Family Participation in Professional Care
Family Resiliency
Family Social Climate

Family Support During Treatment
Lifestyle Balance
Parenting Performance: Adolescent
Parenting Performance: Infant
Parenting Performance: Middle Childhood
Parenting Performance: Preschooler
Parenting Performance: Toddler

Fluid Balance, Readiness for Enhanced

Definition: A pattern of equilibrium between the fluid volume and chemical composition of body fluids that is sufficient for meeting physical needs and can be strengthened

Outcomes to Measure Defining Characteristics

Fluid Balance
Health Seeking Behavior
Hydration
Kidney Function
Motivation

Nutritional Status: Food & Fluid Intake
Nutritional Status: Nutrient Intake
Tissue Integrity: Skin & Mucous Membranes
Urinary Elimination
Weight Maintenance Behavior

Hope, Readiness for Enhanced

Definition: A pattern of expectations and desires for mobilizing energy on one's own behalf that is sufficient for well-being and can be strengthened

Outcomes to Measure Defining Characteristics

Comfort Status: Psychospiritual
Coping
Decision-Making
Health Beliefs: Perceived Ability to Perform
Health Seeking Behavior
Hope
Lifestyle Balance
Loneliness Severity
Personal Autonomy

Personal Resiliency
Personal Well-Being
Psychomotor Energy
Psychosocial Adjustment Life Change
Quality of Life
Self-Esteem
Spiritual Health
Will to Live

Immunization Status, Readiness for Enhanced

Definition: A pattern of conforming to local, national, and/or international standards of immunization to prevent infectious disease(s) that is sufficient to protect a person, family, or community and can be strengthened

Outcomes to Measure Defining Characteristics

Community Disaster Readiness
Community Immune Status
Community Program Effectiveness
Community Risk Control: Communicable Disease
Health Seeking Behavior

Immune Status
Immunization Behavior
Knowledge: Health Promotion
Risk Control
Risk Control: Infectious Process

Infant Behavior, Organized, Readiness for Enhanced

Definition: A pattern of modulation of the physiological and behavioral systems of functioning (i.e., autonomic, motor, state-organization, self-regulatory, and attentional-interactional systems) in an infant that is sufficient for well-being and can be strengthened

Outcomes to Measure Defining Characteristics

Child Development: 1 Month
Child Development: 2 Months
Child Development: 4 Months
Child Development: 6 Months
Child Development: 12 Months
Coordinated Movement
Discomfort Level
Infant Nutritional Status
Knowledge: Infant Care
Knowledge: Parenting
Knowledge: Preterm Infant Care

Neurological Status
Newborn Adaptation
Pain Level
Parent-Infant Attachment
Preterm Infant Organization
Sensory Function: Hearing
Sensory Function: Vision
Sleep
Thermoregulation: Newborn
Vital Signs

Knowledge, Readiness for Enhanced

Definition: A pattern of cognitive information related to a specific topic, or its acquisition, that is sufficient for meeting health-related goals and can be strengthened

Outcomes to Measure Defining Characteristics

Adherence Behavior
Adherence Behavior: Healthy Diet
Alcohol Abuse Cessation Behavior
Body Mechanics Performance
Client Satisfaction: Teaching
Communication
Communication: Expressive
Communication: Receptive
Drug Abuse Cessation Behavior
Eating Disorder Self-Control
Health Promoting Behavior
Health Seeking Behavior
Hearing Compensation Behavior
Knowledge: Acute Illness Management
Knowledge: Anticoagulation Therapy Management
Knowledge: Arthritis Management
Knowledge: Asthma Management
Knowledge: Body Mechanics
Knowledge: Bottle Feeding
Knowledge: Breastfeeding
Knowledge: Cancer Management
Knowledge: Cancer Threat Reduction
Knowledge: Cardiac Disease Management
Knowledge: Child Physical Safety
Knowledge: Chronic Disease Management
Knowledge: Chronic Obstructive Pulmonary Disease
    Management
Knowledge: Conception Prevention
Knowledge: Coronary Artery Disease Management
Knowledge: Cup Feeding
Knowledge: Dementia Management
Knowledge: Depression Management
Knowledge: Diabetes Management
Knowledge: Disease Process
Knowledge: Dysrhythmia Management
Knowledge: Eating Disorder Management
Knowledge: Energy Conservation
Knowledge: Fall Prevention
Knowledge: Fertility Promotion
Knowledge: Health Behavior
Knowledge: Health Promotion
Knowledge: Health Resources
Knowledge: Healthy Diet
Knowledge: Healthy Lifestyle
Knowledge: Heart Failure Management
Knowledge: Hypertension Management

Knowledge: Infant Care
Knowledge: Infection Management
Knowledge: Inflammatory Bowel Disease Management
Knowledge: Kidney Disease Management
Knowledge: Labor & Delivery
Knowledge: Lipid Disorder Management
Knowledge: Medication
Knowledge: Multiple Sclerosis Management
Knowledge: Osteoporosis Management
Knowledge: Ostomy Care
Knowledge: Pain Management
Knowledge: Parenting
Knowledge: Peripheral Artery Disease Management
Knowledge: Personal Safety
Knowledge: Pneumonia Management
Knowledge: Postpartum Maternal Health
Knowledge: Preconception Maternal Health
Knowledge: Pregnancy
Knowledge: Pregnancy & Postpartum Sexual Functioning
Knowledge: Prescribed Activity
Knowledge: Prescribed Diet
Knowledge: Preterm Infant Care
Knowledge: Sexual Functioning
Knowledge: Stress Management
Knowledge: Stroke Management
Knowledge: Stroke Prevention
Knowledge: Substance Use Control
Knowledge: Thrombus Prevention
Knowledge: Time Management
Knowledge: Treatment Procedure
Knowledge: Treatment Regimen
Knowledge: Weight Management
Lifestyle Balance
Motivation
Pain Control
Participation in Health Care Decisions
Personal Time Management
Postpartum Maternal Health Behavior
Prenatal Health Behavior
Self-Management: Acute Illness
Self-Management: Anticoagulation Therapy
Self-Management: Asthma
Self-Management: Cardiac Disease
Self-Management: Chronic Disease
Self-Management: Chronic Obstructive Pulmonary Disease
Self-Management: Coronary Artery Disease

Continued

Knowledge, Readiness for Enhanced—*cont'd*

Self-Management: Diabetes
Self-Management: Dysrhythmia
Self-Management: Heart Failure
Self-Management: Hypertension
Self-Management: Kidney Disease
Self-Management: Lipid Disorder
Self-Management: Multiple Sclerosis

Self-Management: Osteoporosis
Self-Management: Peripheral Artery Disease
Smoking Cessation Behavior
Vision Compensation Behavior
Weight Gain Behavior
Weight Loss Behavior
Weight Maintenance Behavior

Nutrition, Readiness for Enhanced

Definition: A pattern of nutrient intake that is sufficient for meeting metabolic needs and can be strengthened

Outcomes to Measure Defining Characteristics

Adherence Behavior: Healthy Diet

Compliance Behavior: Prescribed Diet

Health Seeking Behavior

Knowledge: Healthy Diet

Knowledge: Prescribed Diet

Knowledge: Weight Management

Motivation

Nutritional Status

Nutritional Status: Biochemical Measures

Nutritional Status: Energy

Nutritional Status: Food & Fluid Intake

Nutritional Status: Nutrient Intake

Personal Safety Behavior

Weight Maintenance Behavior

Parenting, Readiness for Enhanced

Definition: A pattern of providing an environment for children or other dependent person(s) that is sufficient to nurture growth and development and can be strengthened

Outcomes to Measure Defining Characteristics

Child Development: 1 Month
Child Development: 2 Months
Child Development: 4 Months
Child Development: 6 Months
Child Development: 12 Months
Child Development: 2 Years
Child Development: 3 Years
Child Development: 4 Years
Child Development: 5 Years
Child Development: Middle Childhood
Child Development: Adolescence
Family Functioning
Family Health Status
Family Integrity
Family Normalization
Family Social Climate

Knowledge: Child Physical Safety
Knowledge: Infant Care
Knowledge: Parenting
Knowledge: Preterm Infant Care
Parenting Performance
Parenting Performance: Adolescent
Parenting Performance: Adolescent Physical Safety
Parenting Performance: Early/Middle Childhood Physical Safety
Parenting Performance: Infant
Parenting Performance: Infant/Toddler Physical Safety
Parenting Performance: Middle Childhood
Parenting Performance: Preschooler
Parenting Performance: Psychosocial Safety
Parenting Performance: Toddler

Power, Readiness for Enhanced

Definition: A pattern of participating knowingly in change that is sufficient for well-being and can be strengthened

Outcomes to Measure Defining Characteristics

Adaptation to Physical Disability
Caregiver Adaptation to Patient Institutionalization
Discharge Readiness: Independent Living
Health Beliefs
Health Beliefs: Perceived Ability to Perform
Health Beliefs: Perceived Control
Health Promoting Behavior
Health Seeking Behavior
Knowledge: Health Promotion

Lifestyle Balance
Participation in Health Care Decisions
Personal Autonomy
Personal Resiliency
Personal Well-Being
Psychosocial Adjustment: Life Change
Self-Awareness
Self-Direction of Care

Relationship, Readiness for Enhanced

Definition: A pattern of mutual partnership that is sufficient to provide for each other's needs and can be strengthened

Outcomes to Measure Defining Characteristics

Caregiver-Patient Relationship
Caregiver Performance: Direct Care
Caregiver Performance: Indirect Care
Comfort Status: Sociocultural
Communication
Development: Late Adulthood
Development: Middle Adulthood
Development: Young Adulthood
Lifestyle Balance
Parenting Performance
Parenting Performance: Adolescent
Parenting Performance: Adolescent Physical Safety

Parenting Performance: Early/Middle Childhood Physical Safety
Parenting Performance: Infant
Parenting Performance: Infant/Toddler Physical Safety
Parenting Performance: Middle Childhood
Parenting Performance: Preschooler
Parenting Performance: Psychosocial Safety
Parenting Performance: Toddler
Role Performance
Self-Awareness
Social Interaction Skills

Religiosity, Readiness for Enhanced

Definition: A pattern of reliance on religious beliefs and/or participation in rituals of a particular faith tradition that is sufficient for well-being and can be strengthened

Outcomes to Measure Defining Characteristics

Client Satisfaction: Cultural Needs Fulfillment
Cognition
Community Resiliency
Community Risk Control: Unhealthy Cultural Traditions
Coping
Decision-Making
Dignified Life Closure
Guilt Resolution

Hope
Lifestyle Balance
Personal Autonomy
Personal Well-Being
Quality of Life
Self-Awareness
Social Support
Spiritual Health

Resilience, Readiness for Enhanced

Definition: A pattern of positive responses to an adverse situation or crisis that is sufficient for optimizing human potential and can be strengthened

Outcomes to Measure Defining Characteristics

Depression Self-Control
Drug Abuse Cessation Behavior
Family Integrity
Family Resiliency
Family Social Climate
Health Beliefs
Health Beliefs: Perceived Ability to Perform
Health Beliefs: Perceived Control
Health Beliefs: Perceived Resources
Health Orientation
Health Promoting Behavior
Hope
Impulse Self-Control

Knowledge: Depression Management
Knowledge: Stress Management
Lifestyle Balance
Mood Equilibrium
Participation in Health Care Decisions
Personal Autonomy
Personal Resiliency
Self-Awareness
Self-Esteem
Social Interaction Skills
Social Involvement
Social Support

Self-Care, Readiness for Enhanced

Definition: A pattern of performing activities for oneself that helps to meet health-related goals and can be strengthened

Outcomes to Measure Defining Characteristics

Adherence Behavior
Adherence Behavior: Healthy Diet
Alcohol Abuse Cessation Behavior
Body Mechanics Performance
Compliance Behavior: Prescribed Activity
Compliance Behavior: Prescribed Diet
Compliance Behavior: Prescribed Medication
Discharge Readiness: Independent Living
Drug Abuse Cessation Behavior
Health Beliefs
Health Beliefs: Perceived Ability to Perform
Health Promoting Behavior
Health Seeking Behavior
Immunization Behavior
Participation in Health Care Decisions
Personal Autonomy
Personal Health Screening Behavior
Personal Safety Behavior
Personal Well-Being
Postpartum Maternal Health Behavior
Prenatal Health Behavior
Risk Control: Alcohol Use
Risk Control: Cancer
Risk Control: Cardiovascular Disease
Risk Control: Drug Use
Risk Control: Dry Eye
Risk Control: Hearing Impairment
Risk Control: Hypertension
Risk Control: Hyperthermia
Risk Control: Hypotension
Risk Control: Hypothermia
Risk Control: Infectious Process
Risk Control: Lipid Disorder
Risk Control: Osteoporosis
Risk Control: Sexually Transmitted Diseases (STD)
Risk Control: Stroke
Risk Control: Sun Exposure

Risk Control: Thrombus
Risk Control: Tobacco Use
Risk Control: Unintended Pregnancy
Risk Control: Visual Impairment
Self-Care Status
Self-Care: Activities of Daily Living (ADL)
Self-Care: Bathing
Self-Care: Dressing
Self-Care: Eating
Self-Care: Hygiene
Self-Care: Instrumental Activities of Daily Living (IADL)
Self-Care: Non-Parenteral Medication
Self-Care: Oral Hygiene
Self-Care: Parenteral Medication
Self-Care: Toileting
Self-Direction of Care
Self-Management: Acute Illness
Self-Management: Anticoagulation Therapy
Self-Management: Asthma
Self-Management: Cardiac Disease
Self-Management: Chronic Disease
Self-Management: Chronic Obstructive Pulmonary Disease
Self-Management: Coronary Artery Disease
Self-Management: Diabetes
Self-Management: Dysrhythmia
Self-Management: Heart Failure
Self-Management: Hypertension
Self-Management: Kidney Disease
Self-Management: Lipid Disorder
Self-Management: Multiple Sclerosis
Self-Management: Osteoporosis
Self-Management: Peripheral Artery Disease
Smoking Cessation Behavior
Weight Gain Behavior
Weight Loss Behavior
Weight Maintenance Behavior

Self-Concept, Readiness for Enhanced

Definition: A pattern of perceptions or ideas about the self that is sufficient for well-being and can be strengthened

Outcomes to Measure Defining Characteristics

Abuse Recovery
Acceptance: Health Status
Adaptation to Physical Disability
Body Image
Child Development: Adolescence
Comfort Status: Psychospiritual
Comfort Status: Sociocultural
Development: Late Adulthood
Development: Middle Adulthood
Development: Young Adulthood

Identity
Personal Autonomy
Personal Resiliency
Personal Well-Being
Psychosocial Adjustment: Life Change
Quality of Life
Role Performance
Self-Awareness
Self-Esteem

Self-Health Management, Readiness for Enhanced

Definition: A pattern of regulating and integrating into daily living a therapeutic regimen for treatment of illness and its sequelae that is sufficient for meeting health-related goals and can be strengthened

Outcomes to Measure Defining Characteristics

Adherence Behavior: Healthy Diet
Client Satisfaction: Case Management
Compliance Behavior
Compliance Behavior: Prescribed Activity
Compliance Behavior: Prescribed Diet
Compliance Behavior: Prescribed Medication
Energy Conservation
Exercise Participation
Health Beliefs: Perceived Ability to Perform
Health Beliefs: Perceived Control
Health Beliefs: Perceived Threat
Health Promoting Behavior
Knowledge: Acute Illness Management
Knowledge: Anticoagulation Therapy Management
Knowledge: Arthritis Management
Knowledge: Asthma Management
Knowledge: Cancer Management
Knowledge: Cancer Threat Reduction
Knowledge: Cardiac Disease Management
Knowledge: Chronic Disease Management
Knowledge: Chronic Obstructive Pulmonary Disease
    Management
Knowledge: Coronary Artery Disease Management
Knowledge: Depression Management
Knowledge: Diabetes Management
Knowledge: Disease Process
Knowledge: Dysrhythmia Management
Knowledge: Energy Conservation

Knowledge: Heart Failure Management
Knowledge: Hypertension Management
Knowledge: Infection Management
Knowledge: Kidney Disease Management
Knowledge: Lipid Disorder Management
Knowledge: Medication
Knowledge: Multiple Sclerosis Management
Knowledge: Osteoporosis Management
Knowledge: Pain Management
Knowledge: Peripheral Artery Disease Management
Knowledge: Pregnancy & Postpartum Sexual Functioning
Knowledge: Prescribed Activity
Knowledge: Prescribed Diet
Knowledge: Treatment Procedure
Knowledge: Treatment Regimen
Knowledge: Weight Management
Ostomy Self-Care
Participation in Health Care Decisions
Risk Control: Infectious Process
Self-Care: Non-Parenteral Medication
Self-Care: Parenteral Medication
Self-Management: Anticoagulation Therapy
Self-Management: Asthma
Self-Management: Cardiac Disease
Self-Management: Chronic Disease
Self-Management: Chronic Obstructive Pulmonary Disease
Self-Management: Coronary Artery Disease
Self-Management: Diabetes

Self-Health Management, Readiness for Enhanced—cont'd

Self-Management: Dysrhythmia
Self-Management: Heart Failure
Self-Management: Hypertension
Self-Management: Kidney Disease
Self-Management: Lipid Disorder

Self-Management: Multiple Sclerosis
Self-Management: Osteoporosis
Self-Management: Peripheral Artery Disease
Symptom Control

Sleep, Readiness for Enhanced

Definition: A pattern of natural, periodic suspension of consciousness that provides adequate rest, sustains a desired lifestyle, and can be strengthened

Outcomes to Measure Defining Characteristics

Health Promoting Behavior
Medication Response
Motivation

Rest
Sleep

Spiritual Well-Being, Readiness for Enhanced

Definition: A pattern of experiencing and integrating meaning and purpose in life through connectedness with self, others, art, music, literature, nature, and/or a power greater than oneself that is sufficient for well-being and can be strengthened

Outcomes to Measure Defining Characteristics

Anger Self-Restraint
Client Satisfaction: Cultural Needs Fulfillment
Comfort Status: Sociocultural
Coping
Dignified Life Closure
Grief Resolution
Guilt Resolution
Hope
Lifestyle Balance

Motivation
Personal Health Status
Personal Resiliency
Personal Well-Being
Psychosocial Adjustment: Life Change
Quality of Life
Social Involvement
Spiritual Health

Urinary Elimination, Readiness for Enhanced

Definition: A pattern of urinary functions that is sufficient for meeting eliminatory needs and can be strengthened

Outcomes to Measure Defining Characteristics

Health Seeking Behavior	Nutritional Status: Food & Fluid Intake
Hydration	Risk Control: Infectious Process
Kidney Function	Self-Care: Toileting
Knowledge: Disease Process	Self-Management: Kidney Disease
Knowledge: Infection Management	Urinary Continence
Knowledge: Medication	Urinary Elimination

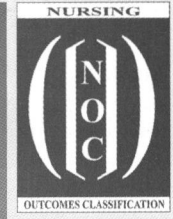

PART FIVE

Core Outcomes
for Nursing Specialties

CORE OUTCOMES FOR NURSING SPECIALTIES

This section provides an alphabetical list of core outcomes for 45 nursing specialty practice areas. Core outcomes are defined as a concise set of outcomes that capture the essence of an area of specialty practice by identifying the outcomes selected most frequently by nurses; it is not a comprehensive list that includes all outcomes used by nurses in that specialty. Core outcomes should also guide curriculum and competency evaluations of nurses preparing for practice in a specific specialty or seeking certification. These outcomes provide a means to measure the effectiveness of practice and are one of the elements that direct the interventions nurses use in the specialty.

EFFORTS TO IDENTIFY CORE OUTCOMES

Initial work to identify specialty core outcomes began after the second edition was published. Information to identify core outcomes was collected from surveys sent to 33 nursing specialty organizations and from individual nurses. Only second edition NOC outcomes were used in the survey, and the survey methodology and results are discussed in the third edition. Since the survey work was completed, 76 new outcomes were added to the third edition, 58 new outcomes were added to the fourth edition, and 107 new outcomes were added to this edition. Several outcomes were not included in the core because they were viewed as a standard of all nursing practice. This included all of the client satisfaction outcomes, the discharge readiness outcomes, and the new outcome *Safe Health Care Environment*. This section also used the higher conceptual level outcomes and did not list all of the more specific outcomes unless they were viewed as foundational to the specialty. For example, *Communication* was used rather than *Communication: Expressive*. For some specialties age factors were important for the core. Six new specialty areas were added to this edition: Diabetes, HIV/AIDS, Infection Control & Epidemiological, Occupational Health, Plastic Surgery, and Transplant.

Refinement of the core outcomes beyond expert opinion is an important next step. When actual data about specialty practice become more widely available, these core outcomes should be validated using clinical data. It is important to debate and analyze these questions: What is a reasonable number of core outcomes for each specialty to address? What methods can be used to maintain and refine current core outcomes for specialty practice? How can nursing organizations be involved in the evolution and continued development of NOC outcomes for specialty practice? Efforts in this direction will allow for continued improvement in the effectiveness efforts involving standardized languages and identifying new outcomes for development.

Air & Surface Transport

Acute Respiratory Acidosis Severity
Acute Respiratory Alkalosis Severity
Agitation Level
Allergic Response: Systemic
Blood Coagulation
Blood Loss Severity
Blood Transfusion Reaction
Cardiopulmonary Status
Circulation Status
Cognition
Cognitive Orientation
Comfort Status
Communication: Expressive
Communication: Receptive
Delirium Level
Electrolyte & Acid/Base Balance
Electrolyte Balance
Fluid Balance
Fluid Overload Severity
Gastrointestinal Function
Hope
Hydration
Hyperglycemia Severity
Hypertension Severity
Hypoglycemia Severity

Hypotension Severity
Immune Hypersensitivity Response
Infection Severity
Infection Severity: Newborn
Kidney Function
Mechanical Ventilation Response: Adult
Medication Response
Metabolic Acidosis Severity
Metabolic Alkalosis Severity
Nausea & Vomiting Severity
Neurological Status
Pain Level
Respiratory Status
Respiratory Status: Airway Patency
Respiratory Status: Gas Exchange
Respiratory Status: Ventilation
Shock Severity: Anaphylactic
Shock Severity: Cardiogenic
Shock Severity: Hypovolemic
Shock Severity: Neurogenic
Shock Severity: Septic
Thermoregulation
Thermoregulation: Newborn
Tissue Perfusion
Vital Signs

Ambulatory Care*

Abuse Recovery
Acceptance: Health Status
Adaptation to Physical Disability
Adherence Behavior
Alcohol Abuse Cessation Behavior
Blood Glucose Level
Compliance Behavior
Compliance Behavior: Prescribed Activity
Compliance Behavior: Prescribed Diet
Compliance Behavior: Prescribed Medication
Drug Abuse Cessation Behavior
Exercise Participation
Family Risk Control: Obesity
Fatigue Level
Fatigue: Disruptive Effects
Health Beliefs: Perceived Ability to Perform
Health Beliefs: Perceived Control
Health Beliefs: Perceived Resources
Health Beliefs: Perceived Threat
Health Orientation
Health Promoting Behavior
Health Seeking Behavior
Hyperglycemia Severity
Hypertension Severity
Hypoglycemia Severity
Knowledge: Health Behavior

Knowledge: Health Promotion
Knowledge: Health Resources
Knowledge: Medication
Knowledge: Treatment Procedure
Knowledge: Treatment Regimen
Lifestyle Balance
Medication Response
Motivation
Nutritional Status
Parenting Performance
Personal Health Screening Behavior
Personal Health Status
Physical Aging
Pre-Procedure Readiness
Self-Care Status
Self-Care: Activities of Daily Living (ADL)
Self-Management: Acute Illness
Self-Management: Chronic Disease
Smoking Cessation Behavior
Surgical Recovery: Convalescence
Vital Signs
Weight Gain Behavior
Weight Loss Behavior
Weight Maintenance Behavior
Weight: Body Mass

*Many of the knowledge outcomes, self-management outcomes, and parenting performance outcomes may be important depending on the focus of the ambulatory care clinic.

Anesthesia

Acute Respiratory Acidosis Severity
Acute Respiratory Alkalosis Severity
Allergic Response: Systemic
Anxiety Level
Aspiration Prevention
Blood Coagulation
Blood Loss Severity
Blood Transfusion Reaction
Cardiac Pump Effectiveness
Cardiopulmonary Status
Circulation Status
Cognition
Cognitive Orientation
Comfort Status
Communication
Communication: Expressive
Communication: Receptive
Delirium Level
Electrolyte & Acid/Base Balance
Electrolyte Balance
Fear Level
Fear Level: Child
Fetal Status: Intrapartum
Fluid Balance
Fluid Overload Severity
Hydration
Hypercalcemia Severity
Hyperchloremia Severity
Hyperglycemia Severity
Hyperkalemia Severity
Hypermagnesemia Severity
Hypernatremia Severity
Hyperphosphatemia Severity
Hypertension Severity
Hypocalcemia Severity
Hypochloremia Severity
Hypoglycemia Severity
Hypokalemia Severity
Hypomagnesemia Severity
Hyponatremia Severity

Hypophosphatemia Severity
Hypotension Severity
Immune Hypersensitivity Response
Knowledge: Treatment Procedure
Mechanical Ventilation Response: Adult
Medication Response
Metabolic Acidosis Severity
Metabolic Alkalosis Severity
Nausea & Vomiting Severity
Neurological Status
Neurological Status: Autonomic
Neurological Status: Consciousness
Neurological Status: Cranial Sensory/Motor Function
Neurological Status: Peripheral
Neurological Status: Spinal Sensory/Motor Function
Pain Level
Participation in Health Care Decisions
Post-Procedure Recovery
Pre-Procedure Readiness
Respiratory Status
Respiratory Status: Airway Patency
Respiratory Status: Gas Exchange
Respiratory Status: Ventilation
Shock Severity: Anaphylactic
Shock Severity: Cardiogenic
Shock Severity: Hypovolemic
Shock Severity: Neurogenic
Surgical Recovery: Immediate Post-Operative
Thermoregulation
Thermoregulation: Newborn
Tissue Integrity: Skin & Mucous Membranes
Tissue Perfusion
Tissue Perfusion: Abdominal Organs
Tissue Perfusion: Cardiac
Tissue Perfusion: Cellular
Tissue Perfusion: Cerebral
Tissue Perfusion: Peripheral
Tissue Perfusion: Pulmonary
Vital Signs

Cardiac Rehabilitation

Acceptance: Health Status
Adherence Behavior
Ambulation
Balance
Cardiac Pump Effectiveness
Cardiopulmonary Status
Circulation Status
Compliance Behavior
Compliance Behavior: Prescribed Activity
Compliance Behavior: Prescribed Diet
Compliance Behavior: Prescribed Medication
Coping
Discomfort Level
Endurance
Energy Conservation
Family Social Climate

Fatigue Level
Fatigue: Disruptive Effects
Fluid Overload Severity
Health Beliefs
Health Beliefs: Perceived Ability to Perform
Health Beliefs: Perceived Control
Health Beliefs: Perceived Resources
Health Orientation
Health Promoting Behavior
Health Seeking Behavior
Hope
Hypercalcemia Severity
Hyperkalemia Severity
Hypertension Severity
Hypocalcemia Severity
Hypokalemia Severity

Cardiac Rehabilitation—cont'd

Knowledge: Anticoagulation Therapy Management
Knowledge: Cardiac Disease Management
Knowledge: Coronary Artery Disease Management
Knowledge: Disease Process
Knowledge: Dysrhythmia Management
Knowledge: Health Behavior
Knowledge: Health Resources
Knowledge: Heart Failure Management
Knowledge: Hypertension Management
Knowledge: Medication
Knowledge: Prescribed Activity
Knowledge: Prescribed Diet
Knowledge: Thrombus Prevention
Knowledge: Weight Management
Lifestyle Balance
Medication Response
Participation in Health Care Decisions
Personal Health Status
Personal Resiliency
Personal Well-Being

Psychosocial Adjustment: Life Change
Quality of Life
Respiratory Status: Gas Exchange
Risk Control: Cardiovascular Disease
Risk Control: Lipid Disorder
Risk Control: Thrombus
Self-Care: Activities of Daily Living (ADL)
Self-Care: Non-Parenteral Medication
Self-Management: Anticoagulation Therapy
Self-Management: Cardiac Disease
Self-Management: Chronic Disease
Self-Management: Coronary Artery Disease
Self-Management: Dysrhythmia
Self-Management: Heart Failure
Smoking Cessation Behavior
Stress Level
Tissue Perfusion: Cardiac
Vital Signs
Weight Maintenance Behavior

Chemical Dependency

Abuse Protection
Abuse Recovery
Abuse Recovery: Emotional
Abuse Recovery: Financial
Abuse Recovery: Physical
Abuse Recovery: Sexual
Agitation Level
Alcohol Abuse Cessation Behavior
Anxiety Level
Comfort Status
Depression Level
Depression Self-Control
Distorted Thought Self-Control
Drug Abuse Cessation Behavior
Family Coping
Family Integrity
Family Support During Treatment
Health Beliefs: Perceived Control
Health Beliefs: Perceived Threat
Health Orientation

Knowledge: Depression Management
Knowledge: Health Resources
Knowledge: Medication
Knowledge: Personal Safety
Liver Function
Medication Response
Pain Level
Pain: Disruptive Effects
Personal Autonomy
Personal Resiliency
Quality of Life
Risk Control: Sexually Transmitted Diseases (STD)
Risk Control: Unintended Pregnancy
Seizure Self-Control
Spiritual Health
Stress Level
Substance Addiction Consequences
Substance Withdrawal Severity
Suffering Severity
Symptom Severity

Community Health

Alcohol Abuse Cessation Behavior
Comfort Status
Community Competence
Community Disaster Readiness
Community Disaster Response
Community Grief Response
Community Health Screening Effectiveness
Community Health Status
Community Immune Status
Community Program Effectiveness
Community Resiliency

Community Risk Control: Chronic Disease
Community Risk Control: Communicable Disease
Community Risk Control: Lead Exposure
Community Risk Control: Obesity
Community Risk Control: Unhealthy Cultural Traditions
Community Risk Control: Violence
Community Violence Level
Compliance Behavior
Coping
Decision-Making
Drug Abuse Cessation Behavior

Continued

Community Health—cont'd

Family Coping
Family Functioning
Family Health Status
Family Integrity
Family Participation in Professional Care
Family Resiliency
Family Risk Control: Obesity
Family Social Climate
Family Support During Treatment
Health Beliefs
Health Orientation
Health Promoting Behavior
Health Seeking Behavior
Immunization Behavior

Knowledge: Acute Illness Management
Knowledge: Chronic Disease Management
Knowledge: Health Behavior
Knowledge: Health Promotion
Knowledge: Health Resources
Knowledge: Parenting
Lifestyle Balance
Personal Resiliency
Personal Well-Being
Quality of Life
Risk Control
Risk Detection
Smoking Cessation Behavior
Spiritual Health

Critical Care

Acute Respiratory Acidosis Severity
Acute Respiratory Alkalosis Severity
Allergic Response: Systemic
Anxiety Level
Blood Coagulation
Blood Loss Severity
Cardiopulmonary Status
Cognitive Orientation
Comfortable Death
Delirium Level
Dignified Life Closure
Electrolyte & Acid/Base Balance
Electrolyte Balance
Family Coping
Family Participation in Professional Care
Family Support During Treatment
Fear Level
Fear Level: Child
Fluid Overload Severity
Hypercalcemia Severity
Hyperchloremia Severity
Hyperglycemia Severity
Hyperkalemia Severity
Hypermagnesemia Severity
Hypernatremia Severity
Hyperphosphatemia Severity
Hypertension Severity
Hypocalcemia Severity
Hypochloremia Severity
Hypoglycemia Severity
Hypokalemia Severity
Hypomagnesemia Severity
Hyponatremia Severity
Hypophosphatemia Severity
Hypotension Severity
Kidney Function
Liver Function

Mechanical Ventilation Response: Adult
Medication Response
Mechanical Ventilation Weaning Response: Adult
Metabolic Acidosis Severity
Metabolic Alkalosis Severity
Nausea & Vomiting Severity
Nausea & Vomiting: Disruptive Effects
Neurological Status: Autonomic
Neurological Status: Consciousness
Neurological Status: Cranial Sensory/Motor Function
Neurological Status: Peripheral
Neurological Status: Spinal Sensory/Motor Function
Newborn Adaptation
Nutritional Status
Pain Level
Pain: Adverse Psychological Response
Pain: Disruptive Effects
Peripheral Artery Disease Severity
Preterm Infant Organization
Respiratory Status
Respiratory Status: Airway Patency
Risk Control: Cardiovascular Disease
Shock Severity: Anaphylactic
Shock Severity: Cardiogenic
Shock Severity: Hypovolemic
Shock Severity: Neurogenic
Shock Severity: Septic
Stress Level
Surgical Recovery: Immediate Post-Operative
Swallowing Status
Symptom Severity
Tissue Perfusion
Tissue Perfusion: Cardiac
Tissue Perfusion: Cellular
Tissue Perfusion: Cerebral
Tissue Perfusion: Pulmonary
Vital Signs

Dermatology

Allergic Response: Localized
Allergic Response: Systemic
Anxiety Level
Body Image
Burn Healing
Burn Recovery
Comfort Status
Compliance Behavior
Compliance Behavior: Prescribed Medication
Coping
Health Beliefs: Perceived Control
Health Promoting Behavior
Health Seeking Behavior
Knowledge: Cancer Management
Knowledge: Cancer Threat Reduction

Knowledge: Disease Process
Knowledge: Medication
Knowledge: Treatment Regimen
Medication Response
Pain Level
Personal Well-Being
Quality of Life
Risk Control: Sun Exposure
Social Anxiety Level
Suffering Severity
Symptom Severity
Tissue Integrity: Skin & Mucous Membranes
Wound Healing: Primary Intention
Wound Healing: Secondary Intention

Diabetes

Acceptance: Health Status
Anxiety Level
Blood Glucose Level
Cognition
Compliance Behavior
Compliance Behavior: Prescribed Diet
Compliance Behavior: Prescribed Medication
Depression Level
Depression Self-Control
Exercise Participation
Fear Level
Gastrointestinal Function
Grief Resolution
Health Promoting Behavior
Hypertension Severity
Immunization Behavior
Kidney Function
Knowledge: Diabetes Management
Knowledge: Hypertension Management
Knowledge: Lipid Disorder Management
Knowledge: Medication
Knowledge: Prescribed Activity
Knowledge: Treatment Procedure
Knowledge: Treatment Regimen
Knowledge: Weight Management

Medication Response
Nutritional Status
Nutritional Status: Food & Fluid Intake
Nutritional Status: Nutrient Intake
Participation in Health Care Decisions
Personal Health Screening Behavior
Personal Health Status
Personal Resiliency
Psychosocial Adjustment: Life Change
Risk Control: Hypertension
Risk Control: Lipid Disorder
Risk Control: Tobacco Use
Self-Management: Diabetes
Self-Management: Hypertension
Self-Management: Lipid Disorder
Sensory Function: Proprioception
Sensory Function: Vision
Social Support
Stress Level
Tissue Integrity: Skin & Mucous Membranes
Weight Loss Behavior
Weight: Body Mass
Wound Healing: Primary Intention
Wound Healing: Secondary Intention

Emergency Care

Acute Respiratory Acidosis Severity
Acute Respiratory Alkalosis Severity
Allergic Response: Systemic
Anxiety Level
Blood Loss Severity
Blood Transfusion Reaction
Cardiopulmonary Status
Community Disaster Readiness
Community Disaster Response
Community Health Status
Community Risk Control: Communicable Disease

Compliance Behavior
Fluid Overload Severity
Health Beliefs
Health Beliefs: Perceived Resources
Health Seeking Behavior
Hyperglycemia Severity
Hypertension Severity
Hypoglycemia Severity
Hypotension Severity
Knowledge: Medication
Knowledge: Personal Safety

Continued

Emergency Care—cont'd

Knowledge: Treatment Procedure
Knowledge: Treatment Regimen
Metabolic Acidosis Severity
Metabolic Alkalosis Severity
Pain Control
Participation in Health Care Decisions
Respiratory Status
Shock Severity: Anaphylactic

Shock Severity: Cardiogenic
Shock Severity: Hypovolemic
Shock Severity: Neurogenic
Shock Severity: Septic
Skeletal Function
Tissue Perfusion
Vital Signs

Gastroenterology

Acceptance: Health Status
Appetite
Aspiration Prevention
Blood Loss Severity
Bowel Elimination
Communication
Decision-Making
Discomfort Level
Electrolyte & Acid/Base Balance
Electrolyte Balance
Gastrointestinal Function
Health Promoting Behavior
Health Seeking Behavior
Hydration
Infant Nutritional Status
Knowledge: Acute Illness Management
Knowledge: Chronic Disease Management
Knowledge: Disease Process
Knowledge: Eating Disorder Management
Knowledge: Health Promotion
Knowledge: Inflammatory Bowel Disease Management
Knowledge: Medication
Knowledge: Ostomy Care
Knowledge: Treatment Regimen
Knowledge: Weight Management

Liver Function
Metabolic Alkalosis Severity
Nausea & Vomiting Control
Nausea & Vomiting Severity
Nausea & Vomiting: Disruptive Effects
Nutritional Status
Nutritional Status: Biochemical Measures
Nutritional Status: Food & Fluid Intake
Nutritional Status: Nutrient Intake
Ostomy Self-Care
Pain Control
Pain Level
Pain: Disruptive Effects
Participation in Health Care Decisions
Respiratory Status: Airway Patency
Self-Care: Non-Parenteral Medication
Sensory Function
Swallowing Status
Swallowing Status: Esophageal Phase
Swallowing Status: Oral Phase
Swallowing Status: Pharyngeal Phase
Symptom Control
Vital Signs
Weight Gain Behavior

Genetics

Cognition
Comfort Status: Psychospiritual
Comfort Status: Sociocultural
Communication
Concentration
Coping
Decision-Making
Family Coping
Family Functioning
Family Integrity
Family Participation in Professional Care
Family Social Climate
Health Beliefs
Health Beliefs: Perceived Control
Health Beliefs: Perceived Threat

Information Processing
Knowledge: Stress Management
Participation in Health Care Decisions
Personal Autonomy
Personal Health Status
Personal Well-Being
Quality of Life
Risk Control: Cancer
Risk Control: Cardiovascular Disease
Risk Detection
Social Support
Spiritual Health
Stress Level
Will to Live

Gerontology

Abstract Thinking
Adherence Behavior: Healthy Diet
Appetite
Balance
Body Mechanics Performance
Bowel Continence
Bowel Elimination
Cardiopulmonary Status
Comfort Status
Communication
Compliance Behavior: Prescribed Diet
Coordinated Movement
Delirium Level
Dementia Level
Depression Level
Development: Late Adulthood
Discomfort Level
Dry Eye Severity
Elopement Occurrence
Elopement Propensity Risk
Endurance
Energy Conservation
Fall Prevention Behavior
Family Social Climate
Fatigue: Disruptive Effects
Gait
Hydration
Hyperglycemia Severity
Hypertension Severity
Hypoglycemia Severity
Knowledge: Acute Illness Management
Knowledge: Anticoagulation Therapy Management
Knowledge: Arthritis Management
Knowledge: Chronic Disease Management
Knowledge: Chronic Obstructive Pulmonary Disease Management
Knowledge: Coronary Artery Disease Management
Knowledge: Dementia Management
Knowledge: Depression Management
Knowledge: Dysrhythmia Management
Knowledge: Fall Prevention
Knowledge: Healthy Diet
Knowledge: Healthy Lifestyle
Knowledge: Inflammatory Bowel Disease Management
Knowledge: Kidney Disease Management
Knowledge: Lipid Disorder Management
Knowledge: Osteoporosis Management

Knowledge: Peripheral Artery Disease Management
Knowledge: Pneumonia Management
Knowledge: Prescribed Diet
Knowledge: Stress Management
Knowledge: Stroke Management
Knowledge: Stroke Prevention
Knowledge: Thrombus Prevention
Knowledge: Weight Management
Neurological Status
Nutritional Status
Oral Health
Peripheral Artery Disease Severity
Personal Health Status
Personal Resiliency
Quality of Life
Respiratory Status: Airway Patency
Rest
Self-Awareness
Self-Care: Hygiene
Self-Care Status
Self-Management: Acute Illness
Self-Management: Anticoagulation Therapy
Self-Management: Chronic Disease
Self-Management: Chronic Obstructive Pulmonary Disease
Self-Management: Coronary Artery Disease
Self-Management: Dysrhythmia
Self-Management: Heart Failure
Self-Management: Hypertension
Self-Management: Kidney Disease
Self-Management: Lipid Disorder
Self-Management: Osteoporosis
Self-Management: Peripheral Artery Disease
Sensory Function
Sensory Function: Hearing
Sensory Function: Proprioception
Sensory Function: Taste & Smell
Sensory Function: Vision
Sleep
Social Involvement
Tissue Integrity: Skin & Mucous Membranes
Tissue Perfusion
Urinary Continence
Urinary Elimination
Vital Signs
Weight: Body Mass

HIV/AIDS

Acceptance: Health Status
Activity Tolerance
Acute Respiratory Acidosis Severity
Acute Respiratory Alkalosis Severity
Adaptation to Physical Disability
Alcohol Abuse Cessation Behavior
Anxiety Level
Anxiety Self-Control
Appetite
Body Image

Bowel Continence
Caregiver Lifestyle Disruption
Caregiver Stressors
Circulation Status
Comfort Status
Comfort Status: Physical
Comfort Status: Psychospiritual
Comfortable Death
Compliance Behavior
Compliance Behavior: Prescribed Activity

Continued

HIV/AIDS—cont'd

Compliance Behavior: Prescribed Diet
Compliance Behavior: Prescribed Medication
Coping
Decision-Making
Depression Level
Depression Self-Control
Dignified Life Closure
Discomfort Level
Electrolyte & Acid/Base Balance
Endurance
Energy Conservation
Family Coping
Family Normalization
Family Support During Treatment
Fatigue Level
Fatigue: Disruptive Effects
Fear Level
Fear Self-Control
Fluid Balance
Gastrointestinal Function
Grief Resolution
Guilt Resolution
Hope
Hydration
Immunization Behavior
Infection Severity
Knowledge: Chronic Disease Management
Knowledge: Depression Management
Knowledge: Disease Process
Knowledge: Energy Conservation
Knowledge: Healthy Diet
Knowledge: Infection Management
Knowledge: Medication
Knowledge: Pain Management
Knowledge: Sexual Functioning
Knowledge: Treatment Procedure
Knowledge: Treatment Regimen
Liver Function
Medication Response
Memory
Metabolic Acidosis Severity
Metabolic Alkalosis Severity
Mood Equilibrium

Nausea & Vomiting Severity
Nausea & Vomiting: Disruptive Effects
Neurological Status: Consciousness
Nutritional Status
Oral Health
Pain Level
Pain: Adverse Psychological Response
Pain: Disruptive Effects
Personal Resiliency
Personal Well-Being
Psychosocial Adjustment: Life Change
Respiratory Status
Respiratory Status: Ventilation
Rest
Risk Control: Cancer
Risk Control: Infectious Process
Risk Detection
Role Performance
Self-Care Status
Self-Care: Activities of Daily Living (ADL)
Self-Care: Instrumental Activities of Daily
     Living (IADL)
Self-Esteem
Sensory Function
Sexual Functioning
Shock Severity: Septic
Sleep
Smoking Cessation Behavior
Social Support
Spiritual Health
Stress Level
Substance Withdrawal Severity
Suffering Severity
Symptom Severity
Thermoregulation
Tissue Integrity: Skin & Mucous Membranes
Tissue Perfusion
Urinary Elimination
Vital Signs
Weight Gain Behavior
Will to Live
Wound Healing: Primary Intention
Wound Healing: Secondary Intention

Home Healthcare

Adherence Behavior: Healthy Diet
Ambulation
Body Mechanics Performance
Bowel Elimination
Burn Recovery
Caregiver Emotional Health
Caregiver Lifestyle Disruption
Caregiver Performance: Direct Care
Caregiver Performance: Indirect Care
Caregiver Physical Health
Caregiver Role Endurance
Caregiver Stressors

Caregiver-Patient Relationship
Comfort Status
Comfortable Death
Compliance Behavior: Prescribed Activity
Compliance Behavior: Prescribed Diet
Compliance Behavior: Prescribed Medication
Dignified Life Closure
Discomfort Level
Endurance
Fall Prevention Behavior
Family Resiliency
Family Support During Treatment

Home Healthcare—*cont'd*

Fatigue Level
Fatigue: Disruptive Effects
Health Beliefs
Health Beliefs: Perceived Ability to Perform
Health Beliefs: Perceived Control
Health Beliefs: Perceived Resources
Health Beliefs: Perceived Threat
Health Orientation
Hyperglycemia Severity
Hypertension Severity
Hypotension Severity
Joint Movement
Knowledge: Acute Illness Management
Knowledge: Anticoagulation Therapy Management
Knowledge: Arthritis Management
Knowledge: Asthma Management
Knowledge: Cancer Management
Knowledge: Cancer Threat Reduction
Knowledge: Cardiac Disease Management
Knowledge: Chronic Disease Management
Knowledge: Chronic Obstructive Pulmonary Disease
  Management
Knowledge: Coronary Artery Disease Management
Knowledge: Dementia Management
Knowledge: Depression Management
Knowledge: Diabetes Management
Knowledge: Disease Process
Knowledge: Dysrhythmia Management
Knowledge: Eating Disorder Management
Knowledge: Fall Prevention
Knowledge: Healthy Diet
Knowledge: Healthy Lifestyle
Knowledge: Heart Failure Management
Knowledge: Hypertension Management
Knowledge: Infection Management
Knowledge: Inflammatory Bowel Disease Management
Knowledge: Kidney Disease Management
Knowledge: Lipid Disorder Management
Knowledge: Medication
Knowledge: Multiple Sclerosis Management
Knowledge: Osteoporosis Management
Knowledge: Pain Management
Knowledge: Peripheral Artery Disease Management
Knowledge: Personal Safety

Knowledge: Pneumonia Management
Knowledge: Prescribed Activity
Knowledge: Stress Management
Knowledge: Stroke Management
Knowledge: Stroke Prevention
Knowledge: Thrombus Prevention
Knowledge: Treatment Procedure
Knowledge: Treatment Regimen
Knowledge: Weight Management
Medication Response
Mobility
Nutritional Status
Peripheral Artery Disease Severity
Personal Health Screening Behavior
Personal Health Status
Personal Resiliency
Risk Control: Infectious Process
Safe Home Environment
Self-Care Status
Self-Care: Activities of Daily Living (ADL)
Self-Care: Bathing
Self-Care: Dressing
Self-Care: Eating
Self-Care: Hygiene
Self-Care: Instrumental Activities of Daily Living (IADL)
Self-Care: Non-Parenteral Medication
Self-Care: Toileting
Self-Management: Acute Illness
Self-Management: Anticoagulation Therapy
Self-Management: Chronic Disease
Self-Management: Chronic Obstructive Pulmonary Disease
Self-Management: Coronary Artery Disease
Self-Management: Dysrhythmia
Self-Management: Heart Failure
Self-Management: Hypertension
Self-Management: Kidney Disease
Self-Management: Lipid Disorder
Self-Management: Osteoporosis
Self-Management: Peripheral Artery Disease
Smoking Cessation Behavior
Spiritual Health
Vital Signs
Weight Maintenance Behavior
Wound Healing: Secondary Intention

Hospice & Palliative Care

Acceptance: Health Status
Comfort Status
Comfortable Death
Communication: Receptive
Community Competence
Community Health Status
Coping
Delirium Level
Development: Late Adulthood
Dignified Life Closure
Fall Prevention Behavior

Falls Occurrence
Family Coping
Family Health Status
Family Integrity
Family Normalization
Family Participation in Professional Care
Family Social Climate
Family Support During Treatment
Fatigue Level
Fatigue: Disruptive Effects
Grief Resolution

Continued

Hospice & Palliative Care—cont'd

Guilt Resolution
Health Beliefs
Knowledge: Chronic Disease Management
Knowledge: Medication
Knowledge: Personal Safety
Medication Response
Oral Health
Pain Level
Pain: Adverse Psychological Response
Pain: Disruptive Effects
Participation in Health Care Decisions
Personal Well-Being
Psychosocial Adjustment: Life Change
Quality of Life
Relocation Adaptation
Safe Home Environment
Self-Awareness
Self-Care Status
Self-Esteem
Social Support
Spiritual Health
Suffering Severity
Symptom Control
Symptom Severity

Infection Control & Epidemiological

Acceptance: Health Status
Activity Tolerance
Acute Respiratory Acidosis Severity
Acute Respiratory Alkalosis Severity
Adaptation to Physical Disability
Anxiety Level
Anxiety Self-Control
Appetite
Blood Glucose Level
Blood Loss Severity
Body Image
Bowel Elimination
Burn Healing
Burn Recovery
Cardiac Pump Effectiveness
Cardiopulmonary Status
Circulation Status
Cognitive Orientation
Comfort Status
Comfort Status: Physical
Comfort Status: Psychospiritual
Comfortable Death
Community Immune Status
Community Program Effectiveness
Community Risk Control: Communicable Disease
Coordinated Movement
Coping
Dignified Life Closure
Discomfort Level
Distorted Thought Self-Control
Electrolyte Balance
Endurance
Energy Conservation
Family Coping
Family Normalization
Family Support During Treatment
Fatigue Level
Fatigue: Disruptive Effects
Fluid Balance
Fluid Overload Severity
Gastrointestinal Function
Health Beliefs: Perceived Ability to Perform
Health Orientation
Health Seeking Behavior
Hope
Hydration
Hypertension Severity
Hypotension Severity
Immobility Consequences: Physiological
Immobility Consequences: Psycho-Cognitive
Immune Status
Immunization Behavior
Infection Severity
Joint Movement
Knowledge: Disease Process
Knowledge: Healthy Diet
Knowledge: Infection Management
Knowledge: Medication
Knowledge: Pain Management
Knowledge: Treatment Procedure
Knowledge: Treatment Regimen
Loneliness Severity
Mechanical Ventilation Response: Adult
Mechanical Ventilation Weaning Response: Adult
Metabolic Acidosis Severity
Metabolic Alkalosis Severity
Mobility
Mood Equilibrium
Nausea & Vomiting Severity
Nausea & Vomiting: Disruptive Effects
Neurological Status
Neurological Status: Consciousness
Nutritional Status
Nutritional Status: Nutrient Intake
Oral Health
Pain Level
Pain: Adverse Psychological Response
Pain: Disruptive Effects
Personal Well-Being
Post-Procedure Recovery
Psychosocial Adjustment: Life Change
Respiratory Status
Respiratory Status: Airway Patency
Respiratory Status: Gas Exchange
Respiratory Status: Ventilation
Rest
Risk Control
Risk Control: Hyperthermia

Infection Control & Epidemiological—cont'd

Risk Control: Hypothermia
Risk Control: Infectious Process
Risk Control: Sexually Transmitted Diseases (STD)
Risk Detection
Role Performance
Safe Home Environment
Self-Care Status
Self-Care: Oral Hygiene
Self-Esteem
Sensory Function
Shock Severity: Anaphylactic
Shock Severity: Cardiogenic
Shock Severity: Hypovolemic
Shock Severity: Neurogenic
Shock Severity: Septic
Sleep
Smoking Cessation Behavior
Social Support
Spiritual Health

Stress Level
Substance Withdrawal Severity
Suffering Severity
Surgical Recovery: Convalescence
Symptom Severity
Thermoregulation
Tissue Integrity: Skin & Mucous Membranes
Tissue Perfusion
Tissue Perfusion: Abdominal Organs
Tissue Perfusion: Cardiac
Tissue Perfusion: Peripheral
Tissue Perfusion: Pulmonary
Urinary Elimination
Vital Signs
Weight Gain Behavior
Weight Maintenance Behavior
Will to Live
Wound Healing: Primary Intention
Wound Healing: Secondary Intention

Intravenous Therapy

Blood Coagulation
Blood Transfusion Reaction
Caregiver Home Care Readiness
Circulation Status
Comfort Status
Communication: Expressive
Communication: Receptive
Electrolyte & Acid/Base Balance
Family Participation in Professional Care
Fluid Balance
Fluid Overload Severity
Hydration
Immobility Consequences: Physiological
Infant Nutritional Status
Infection Severity
Knowledge: Acute Illness Management
Knowledge: Infection Management
Knowledge: Medication
Knowledge: Prescribed Activity

Knowledge: Treatment Procedure
Medication Response
Nutritional Status: Biochemical Measures
Pain Level
Pain: Adverse Psychological Response
Pain: Disruptive Effects
Quality of Life
Risk Control: Infectious Process
Risk Control: Thrombus
Self-Care: Non-Parenteral Medication
Self-Care: Parenteral Medication
Shock Severity: Hypovolemic
Surgical Recovery: Immediate Post-Operative
Symptom Severity
Tissue Perfusion: Cellular
Tissue Perfusion: Peripheral
Urinary Elimination
Vital Signs

Medical-Surgical

Acceptance: Health Status
Acute Respiratory Acidosis Severity
Acute Respiratory Alkalosis Severity
Alcohol Abuse Cessation Behavior
Ambulation
Appetite
Balance
Body Positioning: Self-Initiated
Cardiopulmonary Status
Cognitive Orientation
Comfort Status
Communication

Compliance Behavior: Prescribed Diet
Delirium Level
Dementia Level
Development: Late Adulthood
Development: Middle Adulthood
Discomfort Level
Drug Abuse Cessation Behavior
Electrolyte Balance
Endurance
Family Support During Treatment
Fatigue Level
Fatigue: Disruptive Effects

Continued

Medical-Surgical—*cont'd*

Fluid Overload Severity
Gait
Gastrointestinal Function
Hydration
Hypercalcemia Severity
Hyperchloremia Severity
Hyperglycemia Severity
Hyperkalemia Severity
Hypermagnesemia Severity
Hypernatremia Severity
Hyperphosphatemia Severity
Hypertension Severity
Hypocalcemia Severity
Hypochloremia Severity
Hypoglycemia Severity
Hypokalemia Severity
Hypomagnesemia Severity
Hyponatremia Severity
Hypophosphatemia Severity
Hypotension Severity
Immune Hypersensitivity Response
Infection Severity
Joint Movement
Kidney Function
Knowledge: Arthritis Management
Knowledge: Cancer Management
Knowledge: Cancer Threat Reduction
Knowledge: Cardiac Disease Management
Knowledge: Disease Process
Knowledge: Heart Failure Management
Knowledge: Hypertension Management
Knowledge: Medication
Knowledge: Multiple Sclerosis Management
Knowledge: Weight Management
Liver Function
Metabolic Acidosis Severity

Metabolic Alkalosis Severity
Mobility
Nutritional Status: Food & Fluid Intake
Pain Level
Pain: Adverse Psychological Response
Participation in Health Care Decisions
Physical Aging
Respiratory Status
Respiratory Status: Ventilation
Rest
Risk Control: Hypertension
Risk Control: Lipid Disorder
Risk Control: Osteoporosis
Risk Control: Stroke
Risk Control: Thrombus
Self-Care Status
Self-Care: Activities of Daily Living (ADL)
Self-Care: Instrumental Activities of Daily Living (IADL)
Self-Management: Cardiac Disease
Self-Management: Diabetes
Self-Management: Multiple Sclerosis
Shock Severity: Anaphylactic
Shock Severity: Cardiogenic
Shock Severity: Hypovolemic
Shock Severity: Neurogenic
Shock Severity: Septic
Sleep
Smoking Cessation Behavior
Surgical Recovery: Convalescence
Surgical Recovery: Immediate Post-Operative
Tissue Integrity: Skin & Mucous Membranes
Tissue Perfusion
Transfer Performance
Vital Signs
Wound Healing: Primary Intention
Wound Healing: Secondary Intention

Neonatology

Blood Coagulation
Blood Glucose Level
Bottle Feeding Establishment: Infant
Bowel Elimination
Cardiopulmonary Status
Child Development: 1 Month
Circulation Status
Comfortable Death
Cup Feeding Establishment: Infant
Dignified Life Closure
Electrolyte & Acid/Base Balance
Family Participation In Professional Care
Family Support During Treatment
Fluid Balance
Growth
Hydration
Immune Status
Infection Severity: Newborn
Knowledge: Cup Feeding
Knowledge: Parenting

Knowledge: Preterm Infant Care
Newborn Adaptation
Nutritional Status
Nutritional Status: Biochemical Measures
Nutritional Status: Energy
Nutritional Status: Food & Fluid Intake
Nutritional Status: Nutrient Intake
Parent-Infant Attachment
Parenting Performance
Parenting Performance: Infant
Preterm Infant Organization
Respiratory Status
Respiratory Status: Gas Exchange
Respiratory Status: Ventilation
Thermoregulation
Thermoregulation: Newborn
Tissue Integrity: Skin & Mucous Membranes
Tissue Perfusion
Urinary Elimination
Vital Signs

Nephrology

Adherence Behavior
Body Image
Caregiver Home Care Readiness
Caregiver Lifestyle Disruption
Caregiver Performance: Direct Care
Caregiver Role Endurance
Caregiver Stressors
Caregiver-Patient Relationship
Comfort Status
Compliance Behavior
Delirium Level
Dementia Level
Electrolyte Balance
Fatigue: Disruptive Effects
Fluid Balance
Fluid Overload Severity
Health Beliefs
Health Beliefs: Perceived Control
Health Beliefs: Perceived Threat
Health Promoting Behavior
Health Seeking Behavior
Hypercalcemia Severity
Hyperchloremia Severity
Hyperglycemia Severity
Hyperkalemia Severity
Hypernatremia Severity
Hypertension Severity
Hypotension Severity
Kidney Function
Knowledge: Diabetes Management
Knowledge: Disease Process
Knowledge: Energy Conservation
Knowledge: Health Resources
Knowledge: Hypertension Management
Knowledge: Kidney Disease Management
Knowledge: Personal Safety
Knowledge: Prescribed Activity
Knowledge: Prescribed Diet
Knowledge: Treatment Procedure
Knowledge: Treatment Regimen
Leisure Participation
Loneliness Severity
Medication Response
Mood Equilibrium
Neurological Status
Nutritional Status
Nutritional Status: Biochemical Measures
Nutritional Status: Energy
Nutritional Status: Food & Fluid Intake
Nutritional Status: Nutrient Intake
Pain Level
Pain: Disruptive Effects
Participation in Health Care Decisions
Personal Well-Being
Quality of Life
Risk Control: Cardiovascular Disease
Risk Control: Hypertension
Self-Care: Non-Parenteral Medication
Self-Esteem
Self-Management: Hypertension
Self-Management: Kidney Disease
Sensory Function: Tactile
Social Involvement
Spiritual Health
Suffering Severity
Symptom Control
Symptom Severity
Tissue Perfusion: Cellular
Weight: Body Mass
Wound Healing: Primary Intention

Neuroscience

Abstract Thinking
Activity Tolerance
Adaptation to Physical Disability
Agitation Level
Ambulation
Cognition
Comfort Status
Communication
Communication: Expressive
Communication: Receptive
Coordinated Movement
Coping
Delirium Level
Dementia Level
Elopement Occurrence
Elopement Propensity Risk
Family Coping
Family Normalization
Family Participation in Professional Care
Family Resiliency
Family Support During Treatment
Gait
Heedfulness of Affected Side
Hope
Knowledge: Disease Process
Knowledge: Health Promotion
Knowledge: Multiple Sclerosis Management
Knowledge: Stroke Management
Knowledge: Stroke Prevention
Knowledge: Thrombus Prevention
Knowledge: Treatment Regimen
Medication Response
Mobility
Neurological Status
Neurological Status: Peripheral
Pain Level
Personal Resiliency
Physical Fitness
Psychomotor Energy
Quality of Life
Rest
Risk Control: Stroke

Continued

Neuroscience—cont'd

Risk Control: Thrombus
Safe Wandering
Seizure Self-Control
Self-Management: Multiple Sclerosis
Sensory Function

Shock Severity: Neurogenic
Sleep
Symptom Severity
Thermoregulation

Nurse Practitioner

Abuse Recovery
Adaptation to Physical Disability
Adherence Behavior
Adherence Behavior: Healthy Diet
Alcohol Abuse Cessation Behavior
Allergic Response: Localized
Anxiety Level
Appetite
Blood Glucose Level
Body Mechanics Performance
Bowel Elimination
Cardiac Pump Effectiveness
Cardiopulmonary Status
Circulation Status
Cognition
Cognitive Orientation
Comfort Status
Comfortable Death
Communication: Expressive
Communication: Receptive
Compliance Behavior
Compliance Behavior: Prescribed Diet
Coordinated Movement
Development: Late Adulthood
Development: Middle Adulthood
Development: Young Adulthood
Drug Abuse Cessation Behavior
Family Coping
Family Functioning
Family Health Status
Family Integrity
Family Normalization
Family Participation in Professional Care
Family Resiliency
Family Support During Treatment
Fatigue Level
Fluid Balance
Gastrointestinal Function
Health Beliefs
Health Beliefs: Perceived Ability to Perform
Health Beliefs: Perceived Control
Health Beliefs: Perceived Resources
Health Promoting Behavior
Health Seeking Behavior
Hydration
Identity
Immune Hypersensitivity Response
Immunization Behavior
Infection Severity
Knowledge: Arthritis Management
Knowledge: Asthma Management

Knowledge: Cancer Threat Reduction
Knowledge: Cardiac Disease Management
Knowledge: Diabetes Management
Knowledge: Energy Conservation
Knowledge: Health Behavior
Knowledge: Health Resources
Knowledge: Healthy Diet
Knowledge: Heart Failure Management
Knowledge: Hypertension Management
Knowledge: Infection Management
Knowledge: Medication
Knowledge: Ostomy Care
Knowledge: Personal Safety
Knowledge: Pregnancy & Postpartum Sexual Functioning
Knowledge: Prescribed Activity
Knowledge: Treatment Procedure
Knowledge: Treatment Regimen
Knowledge: Weight Management
Medication Response
Mobility
Mood Equilibrium
Neurological Status
Neurological Status: Autonomic
Neurological Status: Central Motor Control
Neurological Status: Consciousness
Neurological Status: Cranial Sensory/Motor Function
Neurological Status: Spinal Sensory/Motor Function
Nutritional Status
Nutritional Status: Energy
Nutritional Status: Nutrient Intake
Oral Health
Ostomy Self-Care
Pain Level
Pain: Disruptive Effects
Personal Health Status
Personal Resiliency
Personal Safety Behavior
Personal Well-Being
Physical Fitness
Postpartum Maternal Health Behavior
Quality of Life
Respiratory Status
Respiratory Status: Airway Patency
Respiratory Status: Gas Exchange
Respiratory Status: Ventilation
Risk Control
Risk Control: Cancer
Risk Control: Cardiovascular Disease
Risk Control: Drug Use
Risk Control: Tobacco Use
Self-Care: Toileting

Nurse Practitioner—*cont'd*

Self-Esteem
Self-Management: Cardiac Disease
Self-Management: Diabetes
Sensory Function: Hearing
Sensory Function: Proprioception
Sensory Function: Vision
Skeletal Function
Smoking Cessation Behavior
Stress Level
Symptom Severity
Thermoregulation
Tissue Integrity: Skin & Mucous Membranes

Tissue Perfusion: Abdominal Organs
Tissue Perfusion: Cardiac
Tissue Perfusion: Cerebral
Tissue Perfusion: Peripheral
Tissue Perfusion: Pulmonary
Urinary Elimination
Vital Signs
Weight Gain Behavior
Weight Loss Behavior
Weight Maintenance Behavior
Weight: Body Mass

Occupational Health

Acceptance: Health Status
Adaptation to Physical Disability
Adherence Behavior
Alcohol Abuse Cessation Behavior
Allergic Response: Localized
Allergic Response: Systemic
Anger Self-Restraint
Blood Glucose Level
Body Mechanics Performance
Burn Healing
Burn Recovery
Community Disaster Readiness
Community Health Screening Effectiveness
Community Health Status
Community Program Effectiveness
Community Risk Control: Lead Exposure
Community Risk Control: Obesity
Compliance Behavior
Compliance Behavior: Prescribed Activity
Compliance Behavior: Prescribed Diet
Compliance Behavior: Prescribed Medication
Coping
Decision-Making
Depression Level
Depression Self-Control
Drug Abuse Cessation Behavior
Exercise Participation
Family Support During Treatment
Health Beliefs
Health Beliefs: Perceived Ability to Perform
Health Beliefs: Perceived Control
Health Beliefs: Perceived Resources
Health Beliefs: Perceived Threat
Health Orientation
Health Promoting Behavior
Health Seeking Behavior
Hearing Compensation Behavior
Hypertension Severity
Hypoglycemia Severity
Immunization Behavior
Infection Severity
Knowledge: Acute Illness Management
Knowledge: Asthma Management
Knowledge: Body Mechanics

Knowledge: Cancer Management
Knowledge: Cancer Threat Reduction
Knowledge: Chronic Disease Management
Knowledge: Depression Management
Knowledge: Diabetes Management
Knowledge: Disease Process
Knowledge: Health Behavior
Knowledge: Health Promotion
Knowledge: Health Resources
Knowledge: Healthy Diet
Knowledge: Healthy Lifestyle
Knowledge: Hypertension Management
Knowledge: Infection Management
Knowledge: Lipid Disorder Management
Knowledge: Medication
Knowledge: Pain Management
Knowledge: Personal Safety
Knowledge: Stroke Prevention
Knowledge: Substance Use Control
Knowledge: Time Management
Knowledge: Treatment Procedure
Knowledge: Treatment Regimen
Knowledge: Weight Management
Lifestyle Balance
Nutritional Status
Oral Health
Pain Level
Pain: Adverse Psychological Response
Pain: Disruptive Effects
Personal Health Screening Behavior
Personal Safety Behavior
Personal Well-Being
Physical Injury Severity
Psychosocial Adjustment: Life Change
Risk Control
Risk Control: Alcohol Use
Risk Control: Cancer
Risk Control: Cardiovascular Disease
Risk Control: Drug Use
Risk Control: Hearing Impairment
Risk Control: Hypertension
Risk Control: Infectious Process
Risk Control: Lipid Disorder
Risk Control: Stroke

Continued

Occupational Health—*cont'd*

Risk Control: Sun Exposure
Risk Control: Tobacco Use
Risk Control: Visual Impairment
Risk Detection
Role Performance
Self-Management: Acute Illness
Self-Management: Asthma
Self-Management: Chronic Disease
Self-Management: Diabetes
Self-Management: Hypertension
Self-Management: Lipid Disorder
Self-Management: Osteoporosis

Sleep
Smoking Cessation Behavior
Social Support
Stress Level
Substance Addiction Consequences
Substance Withdrawal Severity
Suffering Severity
Weight: Body Mass
Weight Loss Behavior
Weight Maintenance Behavior
Wound Healing: Primary Intention

Oncology

Acceptance: Health Status
Activity Tolerance
Adaptation to Physical Disability
Adherence Behavior
Adherence Behavior: Healthy Diet
Anxiety Level
Anxiety Self-Control
Appetite
Body Image
Comfort Status
Comfortable Death
Communication
Compliance Behavior: Prescribed Diet
Compliance Behavior: Prescribed Medication
Coping
Decision-Making
Dignified Life Closure
Discomfort Level
Electrolyte & Acid/Base Balance
Electrolyte Balance
Endurance
Energy Conservation
Fall Prevention Behavior
Family Coping
Family Participation in Professional Care
Family Support During Treatment
Fatigue Level
Fear Level
Fear Level: Child
Fear Self-Control
Fluid Balance
Grief Resolution
Hope
Hydration
Immobility Consequences: Physiological
Immobility Consequences: Psycho-Cognitive
Infection Severity
Knowledge: Cancer Management
Knowledge: Cancer Threat Reduction
Knowledge: Disease Process
Knowledge: Energy Conservation
Knowledge: Health Behavior
Knowledge: Health Resources
Knowledge: Healthy Diet
Knowledge: Infection Management

Knowledge: Ostomy Care
Knowledge: Pain Management
Knowledge: Prescribed Activity
Knowledge: Treatment Procedure
Knowledge: Treatment Regimen
Lifestyle Balance
Medication Response
Memory
Nausea & Vomiting Control
Nausea & Vomiting Severity
Nausea & Vomiting: Disruptive Effects
Nutritional Status
Ostomy Self-Care
Pain Control
Pain Level
Pain: Adverse Psychological Response
Pain: Disruptive Effects
Participation in Health Care Decisions
Personal Autonomy
Personal Health Status
Personal Resiliency
Personal Well-Being
Psychosocial Adjustment: Life Change
Quality of Life
Risk Control: Cancer
Risk Control: Infectious Process
Self-Awareness
Self-Care Status
Self-Care: Activities of Daily Living (ADL)
Self-Management: Chronic Disease
Sleep
Social Support
Spiritual Health
Stress Level
Suffering Severity
Surgical Recovery: Convalescence
Surgical Recovery: Immediate Post-Operative
Symptom Control
Symptom Severity
Vital Signs
Weight Gain Behavior
Weight Loss Behavior
Weight Maintenance Behavior
Weight: Body Mass
Will to Live

Operating Room

Acute Respiratory Acidosis Severity
Acute Respiratory Alkalosis Severity
Allergic Response: Systemic
Anxiety Level
Aspiration Prevention
Blood Coagulation
Blood Loss Severity
Cardiopulmonary Status
Circulation Status
Cognition
Cognitive Orientation
Comfort Status
Communication
Community Immune Status
Delirium Level
Dry Eye Severity
Electrolyte & Acid/Base Balance
Electrolyte Balance
Family Coping
Family Participation in Professional Care
Fluid Balance
Fluid Overload Severity
Health Beliefs: Perceived Control
Health Beliefs: Perceived Resources
Hydration
Hypercalcemia Severity
Hyperchloremia Severity
Hyperglycemia Severity
Hyperkalemia Severity
Hypermagnesemia Severity
Hypernatremia Severity
Hyperphosphatemia Severity
Hypertension Severity
Hypocalcemia Severity
Hypochloremia Severity
Hypoglycemia Severity
Hypokalemia Severity
Hypomagnesemia Severity
Hyponatremia Severity
Hypophosphatemia Severity
Hypotension Severity

Immobility Consequences: Physiological
Infection Severity
Joint Movement
Kidney Function
Knowledge: Health Promotion
Knowledge: Treatment Regimen
Medication Response
Metabolic Acidosis Severity
Metabolic Alkalosis Severity
Nausea & Vomiting Control
Nausea & Vomiting Severity
Pain Level
Participation in Health Care Decisions
Pre-Procedure Readiness
Psychomotor Energy
Respiratory Status
Respiratory Status: Airway Patency
Respiratory Status: Gas Exchange
Respiratory Status: Ventilation
Risk Control: Thrombus
Seizure Self-Control
Skeletal Function
Sleep
Surgical Recovery: Immediate Post-Operative
Swallowing Status
Swallowing Status: Esophageal Phase
Swallowing Status: Oral Phase
Swallowing Status: Pharyngeal Phase
Symptom Severity
Thermoregulation
Tissue Integrity: Skin & Mucous Membranes
Tissue Perfusion
Tissue Perfusion: Abdominal Organs
Tissue Perfusion: Cardiac
Tissue Perfusion: Cellular
Tissue Perfusion: Cerebral
Tissue Perfusion: Peripheral
Tissue Perfusion: Pulmonary
Vital Signs
Wound Healing: Primary Intention

Ophthalmology

Decision-Making
Dry Eye Severity
Health Beliefs
Knowledge: Disease Process
Knowledge: Health Behavior
Knowledge: Health Resources
Knowledge: Healthy Lifestyle
Knowledge: Hypertension Management
Knowledge: Medication
Knowledge: Multiple Sclerosis Management
Knowledge: Personal Safety
Knowledge: Treatment Regimen
Neurological Status

Neurological Status: Cranial Sensory/Motor Function
Participation in Health Care Decisions
Personal Health Screening Behavior
Physical Aging
Post-Procedure Recovery
Pre-Procedure Readiness
Risk Control
Risk Control: Visual Impairment
Self-Management: Diabetes
Self-Management: Hypertension
Sensory Function: Vision
Surgical Recovery: Immediate Post-Operative
Vision Compensation Behavior

Orthopedics

Adaptation to Physical Disability
Balance
Blood Coagulation
Body Mechanics Performance
Bone Healing
Caregiver Home Care Readiness
Caregiver Lifestyle Disruption
Cognition
Cognitive Orientation
Comfort Status
Communication
Compliance Behavior: Prescribed Activity
Coordinated Movement
Depression Level
Exercise Participation
Fall Prevention Behavior
Gait
Hypercalcemia Severity
Hypocalcemia Severity
Infection Severity
Joint Movement
Joint Movement: Ankle
Joint Movement: Elbow
Joint Movement: Fingers
Joint Movement: Hip
Joint Movement: Knee
Joint Movement: Neck
Joint Movement: Passive
Joint Movement: Shoulder
Joint Movement: Spine
Joint Movement: Wrist

Knowledge: Body Mechanics
Knowledge: Fall Prevention
Knowledge: Infection Management
Mobility
Neurological Status: Consciousness
Neurological Status: Cranial Sensory/Motor Function
Neurological Status: Spinal Sensory/Motor Function
Nutritional Status: Biochemical Measures
Nutritional Status: Food & Fluid Intake
Pain Control
Pain Level
Pain: Adverse Psychological Response
Pain: Disruptive Effects
Participation in Health Care Decisions
Personal Well-Being
Physical Injury Severity
Respiratory Status
Respiratory Status: Airway Patency
Respiratory Status: Gas Exchange
Risk Control: Osteoporosis
Safe Home Environment
Self-Care: Toileting
Self-Management: Osteoporosis
Skeletal Function
Symptom Severity
Tissue Perfusion
Transfer Performance
Vital Signs
Wound Healing: Primary Intention
Wound Healing: Secondary Intention

Otorhinolaryngology & Head-Neck

Abstract Thinking
Acceptance: Health Status
Activity Tolerance
Adaptation to Physical Disability
Ambulation
Appetite
Aspiration Prevention
Blood Loss Severity
Body Image
Comfort Status
Communication
Community Health Status
Community Immune Status
Community Risk Control: Chronic Disease
Community Risk Control: Communicable Disease
Compliance Behavior
Coping
Delirium Level
Electrolyte & Acid/Base Balance
Fluid Balance
Gait
Health Promoting Behavior
Health Seeking Behavior
Hearing Compensation Behavior

Hydration
Immobility Consequences: Physiological
Immobility Consequences: Psycho-Cognitive
Immune Status
Infection Severity
Knowledge: Health Promotion
Knowledge: Health Resources
Knowledge: Infection Management
Knowledge: Treatment Procedure
Knowledge: Treatment Regimen
Medication Response
Mobility
Neurological Status: Cranial Sensory/Motor Function
Nutritional Status
Nutritional Status: Biochemical Measures
Pain Control
Pain Level
Pain: Adverse Psychological Response
Participation in Health Care Decisions
Personal Resiliency
Personal Well-Being
Post-Procedure Recovery
Quality of Life
Respiratory Status

Otorhinolaryngology & Head-Neck—cont'd

Respiratory Status: Airway Patency
Respiratory Status: Gas Exchange
Respiratory Status: Ventilation
Risk Control
Risk Control: Cancer
Risk Control: Hearing Impairment
Risk Control: Tobacco Use
Seizure Self-Control
Self-Care Status
Self-Care: Activities of Daily Living (ADL)
Self-Management: Asthma
Sensory Function
Sensory Function: Hearing
Sensory Function: Taste & Smell

Smoking Cessation Behavior
Spiritual Health
Swallowing Status
Swallowing Status: Esophageal Phase
Swallowing Status: Oral Phase
Swallowing Status: Pharyngeal Phase
Symptom Control
Tissue Integrity: Skin & Mucous Membranes
Tissue Perfusion: Pulmonary
Vital Signs
Will to Live
Wound Healing: Primary Intention
Wound Healing: Secondary Intention

Pain Management

Agitation Level
Ambulation
Anxiety Level
Cognitive Orientation
Comfortable Death
Communication
Delirium Level
Dementia Level
Depression Level
Dignified Life Closure
Electrolyte & Acid/Base Balance
Family Support During Treatment
Fluid Balance
Information Processing
Nausea & Vomiting Severity
Neurological Status: Consciousness
Pain Control
Pain Level
Pain: Adverse Psychological Response
Pain: Disruptive Effects

Personal Resiliency
Respiratory Status
Respiratory Status: Airway Patency
Respiratory Status: Gas Exchange
Respiratory Status: Ventilation
Self-Care Status
Self-Care: Activities of Daily Living (ADL)
Self-Care: Bathing
Self-Care: Dressing
Self-Care: Instrumental Activities of Daily Living (IADL)
Self-Management: Acute Illness
Self-Management: Chronic Disease
Skeletal Function
Stress Level
Surgical Recovery: Convalescence
Surgical Recovery: Immediate Post-Operative
Thermoregulation
Tissue Perfusion: Cardiac
Vital Signs

Parish Nursing

Abuse Recovery
Adaptation to Physical Disability
Adherence Behavior
Anxiety Level
Caregiver Adaptation to Patient Institutionalization
Caregiver Emotional Health
Caregiver Stressors
Caregiver Well-Being
Caregiver-Patient Relationship
Comfort Status: Psychospiritual
Compliance Behavior
Compliance Behavior: Prescribed Diet
Compliance Behavior: Prescribed Medication
Coping
Decision-Making
Dementia Level
Depression Level

Dignified Life Closure
Family Coping
Family Functioning
Family Integrity
Family Normalization
Fear Level
Grief Resolution
Health Beliefs
Health Orientation
Health Promoting Behavior
Health Seeking Behavior
Hope
Knowledge: Acute Illness Management
Knowledge: Cancer Threat Reduction
Knowledge: Chronic Disease Management
Knowledge: Diabetes Management

Continued

Parish Nursing—cont'd

Knowledge: Health Behavior
Knowledge: Health Promotion
Knowledge: Health Resources
Knowledge: Healthy Diet
Knowledge: Healthy Lifestyle
Knowledge: Heart Failure Management
Knowledge: Hypertension Management
Knowledge: Medication
Knowledge: Prescribed Diet
Knowledge: Time Management
Knowledge: Weight Management
Leisure Participation
Lifestyle Balance
Loneliness Severity
Mood Equilibrium
Parenting Performance: Early/Middle Childhood Physical Safety
Parenting Performance: Infant/Toddler Physical Safety
Participation in Health Care Decisions
Personal Health Screening Behavior
Personal Time Management
Personal Well-Being

Physical Fitness
Quality of Life
Relocation Adaptation
Risk Control: Cancer
Risk Control: Cardiovascular Disease
Risk Control: Tobacco Use
Risk Detection
Self-Awareness
Self-Care: Instrumental Activities of Daily Living (IADL)
Self-Care: Non-Parenteral Medication
Self-Esteem
Self-Management: Cardiac Disease
Smoking Cessation Behavior
Social Involvement
Social Support
Spiritual Health
Stress Level
Suffering Severity
Symptom Severity
Weight Loss Behavior
Weight Maintenance Behavior

Pediatrics

Abstract Thinking
Ambulation
Balance
Body Positioning: Self-Initiated
Bottle Feeding Establishment: Infant
Bottle Feeding Performance
Breastfeeding Maintenance
Breastfeeding Weaning
Caregiver Adaptation to Patient Institutionalization
Caregiver Emotional Health
Caregiver Home Care Readiness
Caregiver Lifestyle Disruption
Caregiver Performance: Direct Care
Caregiver Performance: Indirect Care
Caregiver Well-Being
Caregiver Physical Health
Caregiver Role Endurance
Caregiver Stressors
Caregiver-Patient Relationship
Child Adaptation to Hospitalization
Child Development: 1 Month
Child Development: 2 Months
Child Development: 4 Months
Child Development: 6 Months
Child Development: 12 Months
Child Development: 2 Years
Child Development: 3 Years
Child Development: 4 Years
Child Development: 5 Years
Child Development: Adolescence
Child Development: Middle Childhood
Comfort Status
Coping
Cup Feeding Establishment: Infant
Cup Feeding Performance
Exercise Participation

Dignified Life Closure
Family Coping
Family Functioning
Family Health Status
Family Integrity
Family Normalization
Family Participation in Professional Care
Family Resiliency
Family Risk Control: Obesity
Family Social Climate
Family Support During Treatment
Fear Level: Child
Grief Resolution
Growth
Health Promoting Behavior
Health Seeking Behavior
Immobility Consequences: Physiological
Immobility Consequences: Psycho-Cognitive
Immunization Behavior
Infant Nutritional Status
Infection Severity: Newborn
Joint Movement
Knowledge: Acute Illness Management
Knowledge: Asthma Management
Knowledge: Bottle Feeding
Knowledge: Child Physical Safety
Knowledge: Chronic Disease Management
Knowledge: Cup Feeding
Knowledge: Disease Process
Knowledge: Eating Disorder Management
Knowledge: Health Behavior
Knowledge: Healthy Diet
Knowledge: Healthy Lifestyle
Knowledge: Infant Care
Knowledge: Infection Management
Knowledge: Medication

Pediatrics—cont'd

Knowledge: Parenting
Knowledge: Personal Safety
Knowledge: Preterm Infant Care
Knowledge: Treatment Procedure
Knowledge: Treatment Regimen
Medication Response
Mobility
Newborn Adaptation
Nutritional Status
Oral Health
Pain Level
Pain: Adverse Psychological Response
Pain: Disruptive Effects
Parent-Infant Attachment
Parenting Performance
Parenting Performance: Adolescent
Parenting Performance: Adolescent Physical Safety
Parenting Performance: Early/Middle Childhood Physical Safety
Parenting Performance: Infant
Parenting Performance: Infant/Toddler Physical Safety
Parenting Performance: Middle Childhood
Parenting Performance: Preschooler
Parenting Performance: Psychosocial Safety
Parenting Performance: Toddler
Physical Fitness
Physical Injury Severity
Physical Maturation: Female
Physical Maturation: Male
Play Participation
Preterm Infant Organization
Psychosocial Adjustment: Life Change

Respiratory Status: Airway Patency
Respiratory Status: Gas Exchange
Respiratory Status: Ventilation
Risk Control
Risk Control: Alcohol Use
Risk Control: Drug Use
Risk Control: Hyperthermia
Risk Control: Hypothermia
Risk Control: Sexually Transmitted Diseases (STD)
Risk Control: Sun Exposure
Risk Control: Tobacco Use
Risk Control: Unintended Pregnancy
Self-Care: Activities of Daily Living (ADL)
Sexual Functioning
Skeletal Function
Smoking Cessation Behavior
Social Interaction Skills
Social Support
Spiritual Health
Student Health Status
Symptom Severity
Thermoregulation
Thermoregulation: Newborn
Tissue Integrity: Skin & Mucous Membranes
Tissue Perfusion: Pulmonary
Vital Signs
Weight Gain Behavior
Weight Loss Behavior
Weight: Body Mass
Wound Healing: Secondary Intention

Pediatric Oncology

Activity Tolerance
Allergic Response: Systemic
Anxiety Level
Appetite
Blood Loss Severity
Caregiver Performance: Direct Care
Caregiver Performance: Indirect Care
Child Adaptation to Hospitalization
Comfort Status
Comfortable Death
Coping
Depression Level
Discomfort Level
Family Normalization
Family Participation in Professional Care
Family Resiliency
Family Support During Treatment
Fatigue Level
Fatigue: Disruptive Effects
Fear Level
Fear Level: Child
Gastrointestinal Function
Hope
Immune Hypersensitivity Response
Infant Nutritional Status
Kidney Function
Knowledge: Cancer Management

Knowledge: Disease Process
Knowledge: Health Promotion
Knowledge: Healthy Diet
Knowledge: Infection Management
Knowledge: Medication
Knowledge: Treatment Regimen
Liver Function
Nausea & Vomiting Control
Nausea & Vomiting Severity
Pain Level
Pain: Adverse Psychological Response
Parenting Performance
Parenting Performance: Adolescent
Parenting Performance: Infant
Parenting Performance: Middle Childhood
Parenting Performance: Preschooler
Parenting Performance: Toddler
Post-Procedure Recovery
Pre-Procedure Readiness
Skeletal Function
Surgical Recovery: Convalescence
Surgical Recovery: Immediate Post-Operative
Swallowing Status
Swallowing Status: Esophageal Phase
Swallowing Status: Oral Phase
Swallowing Status: Pharyngeal Phase
Will to Live

Perianesthesia

Allergic Response: Systemic
Anxiety Level
Aspiration Prevention
Blood Coagulation
Blood Glucose Level
Blood Loss Severity
Blood Transfusion Reaction
Bowel Elimination
Cardiac Pump Effectiveness
Cardiopulmonary Status
Child Adaptation to Hospitalization
Circulation Status
Comfort Status
Delirium Level
Dementia Level
Discomfort Level
Electrolyte Balance
Fall Prevention Behavior
Fluid Balance
Fluid Overload Severity
Hydration
Hypertension Severity
Hypotension Severity
Immune Hypersensitivity Response
Immune Status
Infection Severity
Kidney Function
Knowledge: Disease Process
Knowledge: Energy Conservation
Knowledge: Infection Management
Knowledge: Medication

Knowledge: Personal Safety
Knowledge: Treatment Procedure
Knowledge: Treatment Regimen
Medication Response
Nausea & Vomiting Severity
Neurological Status: Peripheral
Pain Level
Pain: Adverse Psychological Response
Participation in Health Care Decisions
Post-Procedure Recovery
Prenatal Health Behavior
Pre-Procedure Readiness
Respiratory Status
Respiratory Status: Airway Patency
Respiratory Status: Gas Exchange
Respiratory Status: Ventilation
Shock Severity: Anaphylactic
Shock Severity: Cardiogenic
Shock Severity: Hypovolemic
Shock Severity: Neurogenic
Shock Severity: Septic
Thermoregulation
Thermoregulation: Newborn
Tissue Perfusion
Tissue Perfusion: Abdominal Organs
Tissue Perfusion: Cardiac
Tissue Perfusion: Cellular
Tissue Perfusion: Cerebral
Tissue Perfusion: Pulmonary
Wound Healing: Primary Intention
Wound Healing: Secondary Intention

Perioperative Care

Allergic Response: Systemic
Anxiety Level
Aspiration Prevention
Blood Coagulation
Blood Glucose Level
Blood Loss Severity
Blood Transfusion Reaction
Cardiac Pump Effectiveness
Cardiopulmonary Status
Circulation Status
Communication
Coordinated Movement
Delirium Level
Dementia Level
Discomfort Level
Electrolyte & Acid/Base Balance
Electrolyte Balance
Family Coping
Family Participation in Professional Care
Fluid Balance

Fluid Overload Severity
Gastrointestinal Function
Hemodialysis Access
Hydration
Hypertension Severity
Hypotension Severity
Immune Hypersensitivity Response
Infection Severity
Joint Movement
Joint Movement: Passive
Kidney Function
Knowledge: Infection Management
Knowledge: Medication
Knowledge: Treatment Procedure
Knowledge: Treatment Regimen
Mechanical Ventilation Response: Adult
Medication Response
Nausea & Vomiting Severity
Neurological Status
Neurological Status: Autonomic

Perioperative Care—*cont'd*

Neurological Status: Consciousness
Neurological Status: Cranial Sensory/Motor Function
Neurological Status: Peripheral
Neurological Status: Spinal Sensory/Motor Function
Nutritional Status: Food & Fluid Intake
Pain Level
Personal Resiliency
Physical Injury Severity
Post-Procedure Recovery
Pre-Procedure Readiness
Respiratory Status
Respiratory Status: Airway Patency
Respiratory Status: Gas Exchange
Respiratory Status: Ventilation
Seizure Self-Control
Sensory Function: Tactile
Shock Severity: Anaphylactic
Shock Severity: Cardiogenic

Shock Severity: Hypovolemic
Shock Severity: Neurogenic
Shock Severity: Septic
Skeletal Function
Symptom Severity
Thermoregulation
Thermoregulation: Newborn
Tissue Integrity: Skin & Mucous Membranes
Tissue Perfusion
Tissue Perfusion: Abdominal Organs
Tissue Perfusion: Cardiac
Tissue Perfusion: Cellular
Tissue Perfusion: Cerebral
Tissue Perfusion: Peripheral
Tissue Perfusion: Pulmonary
Urinary Elimination
Vital Signs
Weight: Body Mass

Psychiatric–Mental Health

Abuse Recovery
Acceptance: Health Status
Agitation Level
Alcohol Abuse Cessation Behavior
Anxiety Level
Cognition
Cognitive Orientation
Comfort Status: Psychospiritual
Communication
Concentration
Coping
Decision-Making
Delirium Level
Dementia Level
Depression Level
Depression Self-Control
Distorted Thought Self-Control
Drug Abuse Cessation Behavior
Elopement Occurrence
Elopement Propensity Risk
Fatigue Level
Fear Level
Guilt Resolution
Hope
Identity
Information Processing
Knowledge: Dementia Management
Knowledge: Depression Management
Knowledge: Disease Process
Knowledge: Healthy Lifestyle
Knowledge: Medication

Knowledge: Time Management
Lifestyle Balance
Loneliness Severity
Medication Response
Memory
Mood Equilibrium
Mutilation Self-Restraint
Nutritional Status
Nutritional Status: Food & Fluid Intake
Pain Level
Pain: Adverse Psychological Response
Pain: Disruptive Effects
Participation in Health Care Decisions
Personal Autonomy
Personal Resiliency
Personal Time Management
Psychosocial Adjustment: Life Change
Rest
Self-Care: Activities of Daily Living (ADL)
Self-Esteem
Sleep
Social Anxiety Level
Social Involvement
Social Support
Stress Level
Substance Withdrawal Severity
Suicide Self-Restraint
Symptom Control
Weight Gain Behavior
Weight Loss Behavior
Weight Maintenance Behavior

Plastic Surgery

Anxiety Level
Anxiety Self-Control
Appetite
Blood Glucose Level
Blood Loss Severity
Body Image
Burn Healing
Burn Recovery
Circulation Status
Comfort Status
Comfort Status: Physical
Coping
Discomfort Level
Family Support During Treatment
Fatigue Level
Fatigue: Disruptive Effects
Fluid Balance
Hydration
Immune Status
Infection Severity
Knowledge: Infection Management
Knowledge: Medication
Knowledge: Pain Management
Knowledge: Treatment Procedure
Knowledge: Treatment Regimen
Nausea & Vomiting Severity
Nausea & Vomiting: Disruptive Effects

Neurological Status
Neurological Status: Consciousness
Pain Level
Pain: Adverse Psychological Response
Pain: Disruptive Effects
Personal Well-Being
Post-Procedure Recovery
Psychosocial Adjustment: Life Change
Respiratory Status
Respiratory Status: Airway Patency
Rest
Risk Control
Risk Control: Infectious Process
Risk Detection
Self-Care Status
Self-Esteem
Sensory Function
Shock Severity: Hypovolemic
Sleep
Social Support
Surgical Recovery: Convalescence
Tissue Integrity: Skin & Mucous Membranes
Tissue Perfusion
Vital Signs
Wound Healing: Primary Intention
Wound Healing: Secondary Intention

Radiology

Acceptance: Health Status
Agitation Level
Anxiety Level
Balance
Blood Transfusion Reaction
Body Positioning: Self-Initiated
Cardiac Pump Effectiveness
Cardiopulmonary Status
Circulation Status
Delirium Level
Dementia Level
Discomfort Level
Electrolyte & Acid/Base Balance
Family Support During Treatment
Fatigue Level
Fear Level
Fear Level: Child
Fluid Balance
Hope
Hydration
Immune Hypersensitivity Response
Immune Status

Infection Severity
Joint Movement
Knowledge: Cancer Management
Mobility
Nausea & Vomiting Severity
Neurological Status
Nutritional Status
Nutritional Status: Biochemical Measures
Nutritional Status: Nutrient Intake
Pain Control
Pain: Adverse Psychological Response
Post-Procedure Recovery
Pre-Procedure Readiness
Respiratory Status
Rest
Sleep
Swallowing Status
Thermoregulation
Tissue Integrity: Skin & Mucous Membranes
Tissue Perfusion
Transfer Performance
Vital Signs

Rehabilitation

Adaptation to Physical Disability
Ambulation
Ambulation: Wheelchair
Aspiration Prevention
Balance
Body Mechanics Performance
Body Positioning: Self-Initiated
Bowel Continence
Bowel Elimination
Burn Recovery
Cognition
Cognitive Orientation
Communication
Compliance Behavior: Prescribed Activity
Concentration
Coordinated Movement
Decision-Making
Delirium Level
Dementia Level
Exercise Participation
Fall Prevention Behavior
Fatigue: Disruptive Effects
Gait
Heedfulness of Affected Side
Immobility Consequences: Physiological
Immobility Consequences: Psycho-Cognitive
Joint Movement
Joint Movement: Ankle
Joint Movement: Elbow
Joint Movement: Fingers
Joint Movement: Hip

Joint Movement: Knee
Joint Movement: Neck
Joint Movement: Passive
Joint Movement: Shoulder
Joint Movement: Spine
Joint Movement: Wrist
Knowledge: Arthritis Management
Knowledge: Body Mechanics
Knowledge: Fall Prevention
Knowledge: Ostomy Care
Knowledge: Weight Management
Memory
Mobility
Motivation
Neurological Status
Pain Control
Psychomotor Energy
Psychosocial Adjustment: Life Change
Self-Care Status
Self-Care: Activities of Daily Living (ADL)
Self-Care: Hygiene
Self-Care: Instrumental Activities of Daily Living (IADL)
Self-Care: Non-Parenteral Medication
Self-Care: Oral Hygiene
Self-Care: Toileting
Self-Management: Osteoporosis
Sleep
Swallowing Status
Transfer Performance
Urinary Continence
Urinary Elimination

School Health

Ambulation
Body Image
Cardiopulmonary Status
Child Development: Adolescence
Child Development: Middle Childhood
Cognitive Orientation
Communication
Communication: Expressive
Communication: Receptive
Compliance Behavior: Prescribed Diet
Compliance Behavior: Prescribed Medication
Concentration
Coordinated Movement
Eating Disorder Self-Control
Endurance
Fear Level: Child
Growth
Hope
Hyperactivity Level
Identity
Information Processing
Knowledge: Acute Illness Management

Knowledge: Asthma Management
Knowledge: Chronic Disease Management
Knowledge: Diabetes Management
Knowledge: Eating Disorder Management
Knowledge: Healthy Diet
Knowledge: Healthy Lifestyle
Knowledge: Sexual Functioning
Knowledge: Stress Management
Knowledge: Substance Use Control
Knowledge: Weight Management
Memory
Mood Equilibrium
Neurological Status
Neurological Status: Central Motor Control
Nutritional Status
Oral Health
Personal Autonomy
Personal Health Screening Behavior
Personal Safety Behavior
Personal Time Management
Physical Fitness
Play Participation

Continued

School Health—cont'd

Respiratory Status
Respiratory Status: Airway Patency
Risk Control: Alcohol Use
Risk Control: Sun Exposure
Risk Control: Tobacco Use
Risk Control: Unintended Pregnancy
Safe Home Environment
Self-Awareness
Self-Esteem
Self-Management: Asthma

Self-Management: Diabetes
Sensory Function: Hearing
Sensory Function: Vision
Sleep
Smoking Cessation Behavior
Social Anxiety Level
Social Interaction Skills
Social Involvement
Student Health Status
Vital Signs

Spinal Cord Injury

Activity Tolerance
Adaptation to Physical Disability
Adherence Behavior
Ambulation
Ambulation: Wheelchair
Bowel Continence
Bowel Elimination
Cardiopulmonary Status
Comfort Status
Compliance Behavior
Depression Level
Discomfort Level
Endurance
Energy Conservation
Family Coping
Family Functioning
Family Normalization
Family Social Climate
Grief Resolution
Health Beliefs: Perceived Ability to Perform
Health Beliefs: Perceived Control
Kidney Function
Knowledge: Health Promotion
Knowledge: Health Resources

Knowledge: Medication
Knowledge: Personal Safety
Knowledge: Treatment Procedure
Knowledge: Treatment Regimen
Knowledge: Weight Management
Leisure Participation
Medication Response
Neurological Status
Personal Resiliency
Physical Injury Severity
Psychomotor Energy
Psychosocial Adjustment: Life Change
Risk Control: Hyperthermia
Risk Control: Infectious Process
Self-Care: Activities of Daily Living (ADL)
Self-Care: Instrumental Activities of Daily Living (IADL)
Self-Direction of Care
Sensory Function
Shock Severity: Neurogenic
Skeletal Function
Surgical Recovery: Convalescence
Surgical Recovery: Immediate Post-Operative
Transfer Performance
Urinary Elimination

Transplant

Acceptance: Health Status
Activity Tolerance
Acute Respiratory Acidosis Severity
Acute Respiratory Alkalosis Severity
Adaptation to Physical Disability
Alcohol Abuse Cessation Behavior
Anxiety Level
Anxiety Self-Control
Appetite
Blood Glucose Level
Blood Loss Severity
Blood Transfusion Reaction
Body Image
Bowel Elimination

Cardiac Pump Effectiveness
Cardiopulmonary Status
Circulation Status
Cognitive Orientation
Comfort Status
Comfort Status: Physical
Comfort Status: Psychospiritual
Comfortable Death
Compliance Behavior
Compliance Behavior: Prescribed Activity
Compliance Behavior: Prescribed Diet
Compliance Behavior: Prescribed Medication
Coping
Decision-Making

Transplant—cont'd

Depression Level
Depression Self-Control
Dignified Life Closure
Discomfort Level
Electrolyte & Acid/Base Balance
Endurance
Energy Conservation
Family Support During Treatment
Fatigue Level
Fatigue: Disruptive Effects
Fear Level
Fear Self-Control
Fluid Balance
Fluid Overload Severity
Gastrointestinal Function
Hope
Hydration
Hypertension Severity
Hypoglycemia Severity
Hypotension Severity
Immunization Behavior
Infection Severity
Kidney Function
Knowledge: Cancer Threat Reduction
Knowledge: Chronic Disease Management
Knowledge: Conception Prevention
Knowledge: Depression Management
Knowledge: Diabetes Management
Knowledge: Disease Process
Knowledge: Energy Conservation
Knowledge: Hypertension Management
Knowledge: Infection Management
Knowledge: Lipid Disorder Management
Knowledge: Medication
Knowledge: Pain Management
Knowledge: Prescribed Diet
Knowledge: Sexual Functioning
Knowledge: Stroke Prevention
Knowledge: Treatment Procedure
Knowledge: Treatment Regimen
Liver Function
Mechanical Ventilation Response: Adult
Mechanical Ventilation Weaning Response: Adult
Metabolic Acidosis Severity
Metabolic Alkalosis Severity
Mood Equilibrium
Nausea & Vomiting Severity
Nausea & Vomiting: Disruptive Effects
Neurological Status: Consciousness
Nutritional Status
Oral Health

Pain Level
Pain: Adverse Psychological Response
Pain: Disruptive Effects
Personal Resiliency
Personal Well-Being
Post-Procedure Recovery
Pre-Procedure Readiness
Psychosocial Adjustment: Life Change
Respiratory Status
Respiratory Status: Gas Exchange
Respiratory Status: Ventilation
Rest
Risk Control: Cancer
Risk Control: Hypertension
Risk Control: Infectious Process
Risk Control: Lipid Disorder
Risk Control: Osteoporosis
Risk Control: Stroke
Risk Control: Unintended Pregnancy
Risk Detection
Role Performance
Self-Care Status
Self-Care: Activities of Daily Living (ADL)
Self-Care: Instrumental Activities of Daily Living (IADL)
Self-Esteem
Self-Management: Diabetes
Self-Management: Hypertension
Self-Management: Lipid Disorder
Self-Management: Osteoporosis
Sensory Function
Sexual Functioning
Shock Severity: Cardiogenic
Shock Severity: Hypovolemic
Shock Severity: Septic
Sleep
Smoking Cessation Behavior
Social Support
Spiritual Health
Stress Level
Substance Withdrawal Severity
Suffering Severity
Surgical Recovery: Convalescence
Symptom Severity
Thermoregulation
Tissue Integrity: Skin & Mucous Membranes
Tissue Perfusion
Urinary Elimination
Vital Signs
Will to Live
Wound Healing: Primary Intention

Urology

Acceptance: Health Status
Activity Tolerance
Bowel Continence
Bowel Elimination
Compliance Behavior: Prescribed Diet

Delirium Level
Fatigue Level
Hydration
Hypertension Severity
Kidney Function

Continued

Urology—cont'd

Knowledge: Hypertension Management
Knowledge: Infection Management
Knowledge: Kidney Disease Management
Knowledge: Prescribed Activity
Knowledge: Sexual Functioning
Knowledge: Treatment Procedure
Knowledge: Treatment Regimen
Medication Response
Neurological Status: Central Motor Control
Psychomotor Energy
Psychosocial Adjustment: Life Change

Risk Control: Infectious Process
Self-Care: Toileting
Self-Management: Hypertension
Self-Management: Kidney Disease
Sexual Identity
Sleep
Urinary Continence
Urinary Elimination
Vital Signs
Will to Live

Vascular

Activity Tolerance
Allergic Response: Systemic
Anxiety Level
Blood Glucose Level
Blood Transfusion Reaction
Cardiac Pump Effectiveness
Circulation Status
Cognition
Cognitive Orientation
Communication
Communication: Expressive
Communication: Receptive
Delirium Level
Dignified Life Closure
Distorted Thought Self-Control
Electrolyte & Acid/Base Balance
Exercise Participation
Fear Level
Fluid Balance
Grief Resolution
Hope
Hydration
Immune Hypersensitivity Response
Infection Severity
Kidney Function
Knowledge: Health Promotion
Knowledge: Peripheral Artery Disease Management
Knowledge: Treatment Procedure
Knowledge: Treatment Regimen
Neurological Status

Neurological Status: Peripheral
Neurological Status: Spinal Sensory/Motor Function
Nutritional Status
Pain Control
Pain Level
Pain: Adverse Psychological Response
Participation in Health Care Decisions
Psychomotor Energy
Psychosocial Adjustment: Life Change
Quality of Life
Respiratory Status: Airway Patency
Respiratory Status: Gas Exchange
Respiratory Status: Ventilation
Rest
Risk Control: Sun Exposure
Self-Care: Eating
Self-Management: Peripheral Artery Disease
Sensory Function
Sleep
Spiritual Health
Suffering Severity
Symptom Severity
Thermoregulation
Tissue Integrity: Skin & Mucous Membranes
Tissue Perfusion
Urinary Elimination
Vital Signs
Weight: Body Mass
Wound Healing: Primary Intention
Wound Healing: Secondary Intention

Women's Health, Obstetrics, & Neonatology

Activity Tolerance
Adherence Behavior: Healthy Diet
Blood Coagulation
Bowel Elimination
Breastfeeding Establishment: Infant
Breastfeeding Establishment: Maternal
Breastfeeding Maintenance
Breastfeeding Weaning
Circulation Status

Comfort Status
Community Immune Status
Community Risk Control: Communicable Disease
Community Risk Control: Lead Exposure
Development: Late Adulthood
Development: Middle Adulthood
Development: Young Adulthood
Discomfort Level
Eating Disorder Self-Control

Women's Health, Obstetrics, & Neonatology—cont'd

Family Coping
Family Functioning
Family Health Status
Family Integrity
Family Normalization
Family Participation in Professional Care
Family Social Climate
Fetal Status: Antepartum
Fetal Status: Intrapartum
Health Seeking Behavior
Infection Severity: Newborn
Knowledge: Breastfeeding
Knowledge: Cancer Threat Reduction
Knowledge: Depression Management
Knowledge: Eating Disorder Management
Knowledge: Fertility Promotion
Knowledge: Health Promotion
Knowledge: Healthy Diet
Knowledge: Healthy Lifestyle
Knowledge: Infant Care
Knowledge: Labor & Delivery
Knowledge: Postpartum Maternal Health
Knowledge: Preconception Maternal Health
Knowledge: Pregnancy
Knowledge: Pregnancy & Postpartum Sexual Functioning
Knowledge: Preterm Infant Care
Knowledge: Sexual Functioning

Knowledge: Weight Management
Lifestyle Balance
Medication Response
Newborn Adaptation
Nutritional Status
Pain Level
Parent-Infant Attachment
Parenting Performance: Infant/Toddler Physical Safety
Personal Autonomy
Personal Health Screening Behavior
Personal Time Management
Physical Fitness
Physical Maturation: Female
Postpartum Maternal Health Behavior
Preterm Infant Organization
Respiratory Status: Airway Patency
Respiratory Status: Gas Exchange
Respiratory Status: Ventilation
Rest
Risk Control
Self Esteem
Skeletal Function
Sleep
Thermoregulation: Newborn
Tissue Perfusion
Urinary Continence
Weight: Body Mass

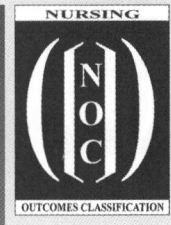

PART SIX

Appendixes

Outcomes: New, Revised, and Retired Since the Fourth Edition

Outcomes New to the Fifth Edition (n=107)

0919 *Abstract Thinking*
0604 *Acute Respiratory Acidosis Severity*
0605 *Acute Respiratory Alkalosis Severity*
1410 *Anger Self-Restraint*
1016 *Bottle Feeding Establishment: Infant*
1017 *Bottle Feeding Performance*
2703 *Community Grief Response*
2807 *Community Health Screening Effectiveness*
2808 *Community Program Effectiveness*
2704 *Community Resiliency*
2809 *Community Risk Control: Obesity*
2810 *Community Risk Control: Unhealthy Cultural Traditions*
1632 *Compliance Behavior: Prescribed Activity*
1018 *Cup Feeding Establishment: Infant*
1019 *Cup Feeding Performance*
0920 *Dementia Level*
2110 *Dry Eye Severity*
1411 *Eating Disorder Self-Control*
0606 *Electrolyte Balance*
1633 *Exercise Participation*
2610 *Family Risk Control: Obesity*
0008 *Fatigue: Disruptive Effects*
0222 *Gait*
1310 *Guilt Resolution*
0607 *Hypercalcemia Severity*
0608 *Hypercholoremia Severity*
2111 *Hyperglycemia Severity*
0609 *Hyperkalemia Severity*
0610 *Hypermagnesemia Severity*
0611 *Hypernatremia Severity*
0612 *Hyperphosphatemia Severity*
2112 *Hypertension Severity*
0613 *Hypocalcemia Severity*
0614 *Hypocholoremia Severity*
2113 *Hypoglycemia Severity*
0615 *Hypokalemia Severity*
0616 *Hypomagnesemia Severity*
0617 *Hyponatremia Severity*
0618 *Hypophosphatemia Severity*
2114 *Hypotension Severity*
1020 *Infant Nutritional Status*
1844 *Knowledge: Acute Illness Management*

1845 *Knowledge: Anticoagulation Therapy Management*
1846 *Knowledge: Bottle Feeding*
1847 *Knowledge: Chronic Disease Management*
1848 *Knowledge: Chronic Obstructive Pulmonary Disease Management*
1849 *Knowledge: Coronary Artery Disease Management*
1850 *Knowledge: Cup Feeding*
1851 *Knowledge: Dementia Management*
1852 *Knowledge: Dysrhythmia Management*
1853 *Knowledge: Eating Disorder Management*
1854 *Knowledge: Healthy Diet*
1855 *Knowledge: Healthy Lifestyle*
1856 *Knowledge: Inflammatory Bowel Disease Management*
1857 *Knowledge: Kidney Disease Management*
1858 *Knowledge: Lipid Disorder Management*
1859 *Knowledge: Osteoporosis Management*
1860 *Knowledge: Peripheral Artery Disease Management*
1861 *Knowledge: Pneumonia Management*
1862 *Knowledge: Stress Management*
1863 *Knowledge: Stroke Management*
1864 *Knowledge: Stroke Prevention*
1865 *Knowledge: Thrombus Prevention*
1866 *Knowledge: Time Management*
2013 *Lifestyle Balance*
0803 *Liver Function*
0619 *Metabolic Acidosis Severity*
0620 *Metabolic Alkalosis Severity*
2903 *Parenting Performance: Adolescent*
2904 *Parenting Performance: Infant*
2905 *Parenting Performance: Middle Childhood*
2906 *Parenting Performance: Preschooler*
2907 *Parenting Performance: Toddler*
2115 *Peripheral Artery Disease Severity*
1634 *Personal Health Screening Behavior*
1635 *Personal Time Management*
1311 *Relocation Adaptation*
1927 *Risk Control: Dry Eye*
1928 *Risk Control: Hypertension*
1933 *Risk Control: Hypotension*
1929 *Risk Control: Lipid Disorder*
1930 *Risk Control: Osteoporosis*
1931 *Risk Control: Stroke*
1932 *Risk Control: Thrombus*

1934 Safe Health Care Environment
1215 Self-Awareness
3100 Self-Management: Acute Illness
3101 Self-Management: Anticoagulation Therapy
3102 Self-Management: Chronic Disease
3103 Self-Management: Chronic Obstructive Pulmonary
    Disease
3104 Self-Management: Coronary Artery Disease
3105 Self-Management: Dysrhythmia
3106 Self-Management: Heart Failure
3107 Self-Management: Hypertension
3108 Self-Management: Kidney Disease

3109 Self-Management: Lipid Disorder
3110 Self-Management: Osteoporosis
3111 Self-Management: Peripheral Artery Disease
0417 Shock Severity: Anaphylactic
0418 Shock Severity: Cardiogenic
0419 Shock Severity: Hypovolemic
0420 Shock Severity: Neurogenic
0421 Shock Severity: Septic
1216 Social Anxiety Level
2304 Surgical Recovery: Convalescence
2305 Surgical Recovery: Immediate Post-Operative
0422 Tissue Perfusion

Outcomes Revised for the Fifth Edition

Label Name Changes (n=20)

Outcomes in this category have minor label name changes.

Fourth Edition Outcome	Label Change for Fifth Edition Outcome
0916 Acute Confusion Level	0916 Delirium Level
1401 Aggression Self-Control	1401 Aggression Self-Restraint
0704 Asthma Self-Management	0704 Self-Management: Asthma
1617 Cardiac Disease Self-Management	1617 Self-Management: Cardiac Disease
2800 Community Health Status: Immunity	2800 Community Immune Status
1619 Diabetes Self-Management	1619 Self-Management: Diabetes
1835 Knowledge: Congestive Heart Failure Management	1835 Knowledge: Heart Failure Management
1802 Knowledge: Diet	1802 Knowledge: Prescribed Diet
1631 Multiple Sclerosis Self-Management	1631 Self-Management: Multiple Sclerosis
1100 Oral Hygiene	1100 Oral Health
2902 Parenting: Adolescent Physical Safety	2902 Parenting Performance: Adolescent Physical Safety
2901 Parenting: Early/Middle Childhood Physical Safety	2901 Parenting Performance: Early/Middle Childhood Physical Safety
2900 Parenting: Infant/Toddler Physical Safety	2900 Parenting Performance: Infant/Toddler Physical Safety
1901 Parenting: Psychosocial Safety	1901 Parenting Performance: Psychosocial Safety
1914 Risk Control: Cardiovascular Health	1914 Risk Control: Cardiovascular Disease
1620 Seizure Control	1620 Seizure Self-Control
1406 Self-Restraint Mutilation	1406 Mutilation Self-Restraint
2400 Sensory Function: Cutaneous	2400 Sensory Function: Tactile
2104 Symptom Severity: Perimenopause	2104 Perimenopause Symptom Severity
2105 Symptom Severity: Premenstrual Syndrome (PMS)	2105 Premenstrual Syndrome (PMS) Severity

Definition Changes (n=96)

Outcomes in this category have minor changes in definition that clarify the concept and improve definition consistency within each scale.

1400 Abusive Behavior Self-Restraint
1300 Acceptance Health Status
1308 Adaptation to Physical Disability
1621 Adherence Behavior: Healthy Diet
1401 Aggression Self-Restraint
0200 Ambulation
0201 Ambulation: Wheelchair
1014 Appetite

0413 Blood Loss Severity
0203 Body Positioning: Self-Initiated
2801 Community Risk Control: Chronic Disease
2803 Community Risk Control: Lead Exposure
1601 Compliance Behavior
1623 Compliance Behavior: Prescribed Medication
0916 Delirium Level
1307 Dignified Life Closure

2600 Family Coping
2602 Family Functioning
2606 Family Health Status
2603 Family Integrity
2604 Family Normalization
2605 Family Participation in Professional Care
2608 Family Resiliency
2601 Family Social Climate
2609 Family Support During Treatment
0603 Fluid Overload Severity
1015 Gastrointestinal Function
1304 Grief Resolution
1105 Hemodialysis Access
0703 Infection Severity
0708 Infection Severity: Newborn
0504 Kidney Function
1831 Knowledge: Arthritis Management
1833 Knowledge: Cancer Management
1830 Knowledge: Cardiac Disease Management
1820 Knowledge: Diabetes Management
1803 Knowledge: Disease Process
1835 Knowledge: Heart Failure Management
1842 Knowledge: Infection Management
1838 Knowledge: Multiple Sclerosis Management
1809 Knowledge: Personal Safety
1811 Knowledge: Prescribed Activity
1802 Knowledge: Prescribed Diet
1203 Loneliness Severity
2106 Nausea & Vomiting: Disruptive Effects
2107 Nausea & Vomiting Severity
1004 Nutritional Status
1007 Nutritional Status: Energy
2900 Parenting Performance: Infant/Toddler Physical Safety
2104 Perimenopause Symptom Severity
1911 Personal Safety Behavior
2002 Personal Well-Being
0113 Physical Aging
1913 Physical Injury Severity
2303 Post-Procedure Recovery
2105 Premenstrual Syndrome (PMS) Severity

1902 Risk Control
1903 Risk Control: Alcohol Use
1917 Risk Control: Cancer
1914 Risk Control: Cardiovascular Disease
1904 Risk Control: Drug Use
1915 Risk Control: Hearing Impairment
1922 Risk Control: Hyperthermia
1923 Risk Control: Hypothermia
1924 Risk Control: Infectious Process
1905 Risk Control: Sexually Transmitted Diseases (STD)
1925 Risk Control: Sun Exposure
1906 Risk Control: Tobacco Use
1907 Risk Control: Unintended Pregnancy
1916 Risk Control: Visual Impairment
1910 Safe Home Environment
0313 Self-Care Status
0300 Self-Care: Activities of Daily Living (ADL)
0301 Self-Care: Bathing
0302 Self-Care: Dressing
0303 Self-Care: Eating
0305 Self-Care: Hygiene
0306 Self-Care: Instrumental Activities of Daily Living (IADL)
0307 Self-Care: Non-Parenteral Medication
0308 Self-Care: Oral Hygiene
0309 Self-Care: Parenteral Medication
0310 Self-Care: Toileting
0704 Self-Management: Asthma
1617 Self-Management: Cardiac Disease
1619 Self-Management: Diabetes
1631 Self-Management: Multiple Sclerosis
2405 Sensory Function
2401 Sensory Function: Hearing
2402 Sensory Function: Proprioception
2400 Sensory Function: Tactile
2403 Sensory Function: Taste & Smell
2404 Sensory Function: Vision
2005 Student Health Status
2108 Substance Withdrawal Severity
2003 Suffering Severity
2103 Symptom Severity

Scale Changes (n=7)

2101 Pain: Disruptive Effects
2405 Sensory Function
2401 Sensory Function: Hearing
2402 Sensory Function: Proprioception

2400 Sensory Function: Tactile
2403 Sensory Function: Taste & Smell
2404 Sensory Function: Vision

Outcomes in the Fourth Edition That Were Retired for This Edition (n=2)

1824 Knowledge: Illness Care

1609 Treatment Behavior: Illness or Injury

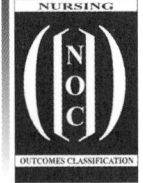

Guidelines for Submission of a New or Revised Outcome

The Nursing-Sensitive Outcomes Classification (NOC) editors are interested in feedback and submission of outcomes for review and potential addition to the NOC. Feedback may be organized in the following manner.

A. GENERAL COMMENTS ABOUT THE CLASSIFICATION

Comments about the classification in general are welcome as are suggestions for outcomes that need to be developed. The outcome suggestions for development can be at the individual, family, or community level.

B. FEEDBACK ON AN OUTCOME

If the submission is a revision of an existing NOC outcome, provide a paragraph briefly describing the rationale for changes and note the changes on a copy of the existing outcome. Suggestions can include changes in the definition, indicators, or scale. Additional indicators and references can be suggested.

C. FEEDBACK ON A MEASUREMENT SCALE(S)

Comments on a particular scale are encouraged. Please briefly explain your suggestion and provide background on your experience in using the scale. Identify the outcome and provide a brief description of the patient population(s) you are using the outcome with.

D. GUIDELINES FOR OUTCOME SUBMISSION

Each submission of a proposed outcome must include a label, a definition, indicators, and a short list of references that support the outcome and document the indicators selected. You also may suggest a scale(s) to use with the outcome. A brief paragraph describing the rationale for adding the outcome to the NOC should be included. The rationale should note how the proposed outcome is different from outcomes already included in the NOC.

General Principles for Developing Outcomes

1. Define the outcome as a variable patient or client state, behavior, or perception that is responsive to nursing intervention(s).
2. Labels should be concise, stated in five or fewer words.
3. Colons can be used to make broader concepts more specific.
4. Labels should describe concepts that can be measured along a continuum.
5. Labels should be neutral and not stated as goals.
6. A set of indicators, more specific than the outcome, must be identified.
7. The definition should clearly define the concept and encompass the indicators and should be consistent with definitions using the same scale.

E. FEEDBACK ON LINKAGES TO NANDA INTERNATIONAL NURSING DIAGNOSES

Comments on linkages to nursing diagnoses are welcome. Please suggest additions or revisions with a brief rationale.

F. FEEDBACK ON CORE OUTCOMES BY SPECIALTY

Comments on core specialty outcomes are welcome. Please send suggestions for additional outcomes as well as any deletions you think are needed.

Comments and suggestions can be sent to: classification-center@uiowa.edu

or by mail to:

The University of Iowa
College of Nursing
Center for Nursing Classification 407
Iowa City, Iowa 52242
Phone: (319) 335-7051

Previous Editions and Translations

Iowa Outcomes Project, Johnson, M., & Maas, M. (Eds.). (1997). *Nursing outcomes classification (NOC)*. St. Louis: Mosby-Year Book. (190 outcomes)

    Translated into Dutch, 1999: Elsevier/Tijidstroom
    Translated into French, 1999: Masson
    Translated into Japanese, 1999: Igaku-Shoin MYW
    Translated into Korean, 1999: Hyun Moon Sa

Iowa Outcomes Project, Johnson, M., Maas, M., & Moorhead, S. (Eds.). (2000). *Nursing outcomes classification (NOC)* (2nd ed.). St. Louis: Mosby. (260 outcomes)

    Translated into German, 2005: Hans Huber
    Translated into Japanese, 2003: Igaku-Shoin MYW
    Translated into Portuguese, 2000: Artmed
    Translated into Spanish, 2001: Ediciones Harcourt

Moorhead, S., Johnson, M., & Maas, M. (Eds.). (2004). *Nursing outcomes classification (NOC)* (3rd ed.). St. Louis: Mosby. (330 outcomes)

    Translated into Chinese, 2005: Elsevier/Singapore
    Translated into Italian, 2007: Casa Editrice Ambrosiana
    Translated into Japanese, 2006: Igaku-Shoin MYW
    Translated into Norwegian, 2007: Akribe
    Translated into Portuguese, 2004: Artmed

Moorhead, S., Johnson, M., Maas, M., & Swanson, E. (Eds.). (2008). *Nursing outcomes classification (NOC)* (4th ed.). St. Louis: Elsevier Mosby. (385 outcomes)

    Translated into Dutch, 2011: Reed Business
    Translated into Japanese, 2010: Igaku-Shoin MYW
    Translated into Portuguese, 2010: Elsevier Editora
    Translated into Spanish, 2009: Elsevier España
    Translated into Taiwanese, 2011: Elsevier Taiwan

COMPANION BOOKS

Johnson, M., Bulechek, G., Dochterman, J., Maas, M., & Moorhead, S. (Eds.). (2001). *Nursing diagnoses, outcomes, and interventions: NANDA, NOC, & NIC linkages*. St. Louis: Mosby.

    Translated into Chinese, 2003: Elsevier (Singapore) Pte Ltd.
    Translated into Italian, 2005: Casa Editrice Ambronsiana
    Translated into Japanese, 2002: Igaku-Shoin MYW
    Translated into Portuguese, 2005: Artmed Editora
    Translated into Spanish, 2002: Ediciones Harcourt

Johnson, M., Bulechek, G., Butcher, H., Dochterman, J. M., Maas, M., Moorhead, S., & Swanson, E. (Eds.). (2006). *NANDA, NOC, & NIC linkages: Nursing diagnoses, outcomes, and interventions* (2nd ed.). St. Louis: Mosby.

    Translated into Simplified Chinese, 2009: Peking University Medical Press
    Translated into Japanese, 2006: Igaku-Shoin MYW
    Translated into Portuguese, 2009: Artmed Editora

Johnson, M., Moorhead, S., Bulechek, G., Butcher, H., Maas, M., & Swanson, E. (2012). *NOC and NIC linkages to NANDA-I and clinical conditions: Supporting critical reasoning and quality care* (3rd ed.). St. Louis: Elsevier Mosby.

Index

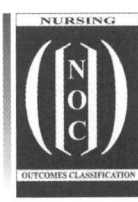

A

Abdomen: bones of, 105f
Ability (term), 7
Abstract Thinking (outcome), 70b
Abstraction: levels of, 3–4, 6–8, 8t
Abuse Cessation (outcome), 71b
Abuse Protection (outcome), 71–72b
Abuse Recovery (outcome), 72b
Abuse Recovery: Emotional (outcome), 73b
Abuse Recovery: Financial (outcome), 74b
Abuse Recovery: Physical (outcome), 75b
Abuse Recovery: Sexual (outcome), 76b
Abusive Behavior Self-Restraint (outcome), 77b
Acceptance: Health Status (outcome), 78b
Activities of daily living (ADLs)
    Self-Care: Activities of Daily Living (ADL) (outcome), 465b
    Self-Care: Instrumental Activities of Daily Living (IADL) (outcome), 469b
Activity-exercise pattern outcomes, 565–566
    individual-level, 565–566
Activity Intolerance (diagnosis), 572b
    definition of, 32–33, 572
    outcomes, 572
Activity Intolerance, Risk for (diagnosis), 643b
    definition of, 643
    outcomes, 643
Activity Planning, Ineffective (diagnosis), 572b
    definition of, 572
    outcomes, 572
Activity Planning, Risk for Ineffective (diagnosis), 643b
    definition of, 643
    outcomes, 643
Activity Tolerance (outcome), 79b
Acute Respiratory Acidosis Severity (outcome), 80b
Acute Respiratory Alkalosis Severity (outcome), 81b
Adaptation to Physical Disability (outcome), 82b
Additional information, 34
Adequate (term), 7
Adherence (term), 7
Adherence Behavior (outcome), 83b
Adherence Behavior: Healthy Diet (outcome), 84b
Adolescence
    Child Development: Adolescence (outcome), 137b
    definition of, 7
    Parenting Performance: Adolescent (outcome), 395–396b
    Parenting Performance: Adolescent Physical Safety (outcome), 397–398b
Adulthood
    late, 7, 196–197b
    middle, 7, 198–199b
    young, 8, 199–200b
Adverse Reaction to Iodinated Contrast Media, Risk for (diagnosis), 644b
    definition of, 644
    outcomes, 644
Aggression Self-Restraint (outcome), 85b

Agitation Level (outcome), 86b
Air & Surface Transport outcomes, 701b
Airway Clearance, Ineffective (diagnosis), 573b
    definition of, 573
    outcomes, 573
Alcohol Abuse Cessation Behavior (outcome), 87–88b
Allergic Response: Localized (outcome), 88b
Allergic Response: Systemic (outcome), 89b
Allergy Response, Risk for (diagnosis), 644b
    definition of, 644
    outcomes, 644
Ambulation (outcome), 90b
Ambulation: Wheelchair (outcome), 91b
Ambulatory Care outcomes, 701b
Anesthesia outcomes, 702b
Anger Self-Restraint (outcome), 91–92b
Anxiety (diagnosis), 573–574b
    definition of, 573
    outcomes, 573, 574
Anxiety Level (outcome), 93b
Anxiety Self-Control (outcome), 94b
Appetite (outcome), 95b
Appropriate (term), 7
Arm bones, 105f
Aspiration, Risk for (diagnosis), 644–645b
    definition of, 644
    outcomes, 644–645
Aspiration Prevention (outcome), 95–96b
Assessment of outcomes, 10–11
Assessments, 5–6
Attachment, Risk for Impaired (diagnosis), 645b
    definition of, 645
    outcomes, 645
Autonomic Dysreflexia (diagnosis), 574b
    definition of, 574
    outcomes, 574
Autonomic Dysreflexia, Risk for (diagnosis), 645b
    definition of, 645
    outcomes, 645
Avoids (term), 7

B

Balance (outcome), 97b
Behavior (term), 7
Behavioral outcomes, 22–31t
Bleeding, Risk for (diagnosis), 646b
    definition of, 646
    outcomes, 646
Blood Coagulation (outcome), 98b
Blood Glucose Level (outcome), 99b
Blood Glucose Level, Risk for Unstable (diagnosis), 646b
    definition of, 646
    outcomes, 646
Blood Loss Severity (outcome), 99–100b

Page numbers followed by *f, t,* and *b* indicate figures, tables, and boxes, respectively.

Blood Transfusion Reaction (outcome), 100b
Body Image (outcome), 101b
Body Image, Disturbed (diagnosis), 575b
  definition of, 575
  outcomes, 575
Body Mechanics Performance (outcome), 102b
Body Positioning: Self-Initiated (outcome), 103b
Body Temperature, Risk for Imbalanced (diagnosis), 647b
  definition of, 647
  outcomes, 647
Bone Healing (outcome), 104b
Bottle Feeding Establishment: Infant (outcome), 106b
Bottle Feeding Performance (outcome), 106–107b
Bowel Continence (outcome), 107–108b
Bowel Elimination (outcome), 108–109b
Bowel Incontinence (diagnosis), 575b
  definition of, 575
  outcomes, 575
Breast Milk, Insufficient (diagnosis), 576b
  definition of, 576
  outcomes, 576
Breastfeeding, Ineffective (diagnosis), 576b
  definition of, 576
  outcomes, 576
Breastfeeding, Interrupted (diagnosis), 577b
  definition of, 577
  outcomes, 577
Breastfeeding, Readiness for Enhanced (diagnosis), 682b
  definition of, 682
  outcomes, 682
Breastfeeding Establishment: Infant (outcome), 109–110b
Breastfeeding Establishment: Maternal (outcome), 110b
Breastfeeding Maintenance (outcome), 111b
Breastfeeding Weaning (outcome), 112b
Breathing Pattern, Ineffective (diagnosis), 577b
  definition of, 577
  outcomes, 577
Burn Healing (outcome), 113b
Burn Recovery (outcome), 114b

C

Cardiac Output, Decreased (diagnosis), 578b
  definition of, 578
  outcomes, 578
Cardiac Pump Effectiveness (outcome), 115b
Cardiac Rehabilitation outcomes, 702–703b
Cardiopulmonary outcomes
  class, 48–67t
  development across editions, 45–46t
Cardiopulmonary Status (outcome), 116b
Care recipient (term), 7
Caregiver (term), 7
Caregiver Adaptation to Patient Institutionalization (outcome), 117b
Caregiver Emotional Health (outcome), 118b
Caregiver Home Care Readiness (outcome), 119b
Caregiver Lifestyle Disruption (outcome), 120b
Caregiver-Patient Relationship (outcome), 121b
Caregiver Performance: Direct Care (outcome), 121–122b
Caregiver Performance: Indirect Care (outcome), 123b
Caregiver Physical Health (outcome), 124b
Caregiver Role Endurance (outcome), 125b
Caregiver Role Strain (diagnosis), 578–579b
  definition of, 578
  outcomes, 578, 579

Caregiver Role Strain, Risk for (diagnosis), 648b
  definition of, 648
  outcomes, 648
Caregiver Stressors (outcome), 126b
Caregiver Well-Being (outcome), 127b
Change in rating score (term), 7
Chemical Dependency outcomes, 703b
Chest bones, 105f
Child (term), 7
Child Adaptation to Hospitalization (outcome), 128b
Child Development: Adolescence (outcome), 137b
Child Development: Middle Childhood (outcome), 136b
Child Development: 1 Month (outcome), 129b
Child Development: 2 Months (outcome), 130b
Child Development: 2 Years (outcome), 133b
Child Development: 3 Years (outcome), 134b
Child Development: 4 Months (outcome), 130–131b
Child Development: 4 Years (outcome), 134–135b
Child Development: 5 Years (outcome), 135–136b
Child Development: 6 Months (outcome), 131–132b
Child Development: 12 Months (outcome), 132b
Childbearing Process, Ineffective (diagnosis), 579b
  definition of, 579
  outcomes, 579
Childbearing Process, Readiness for Enhanced (diagnosis), 683b
  definition of, 683
  outcomes, 683
Childbearing Process, Risk for Ineffective (diagnosis), 649b
  definition of, 649
  outcomes, 649
Childcare provider (term), 7
Childhood
  early, 7, 398–399b
  middle, 7, 136b, 398–399b, 402–403b
Circulation Status (outcome), 138–139b
Client (term), 6
Client Satisfaction (outcome), 139–140b
Client satisfaction (term), 6
Client Satisfaction: Access to Care Resources (outcome), 140b
Client Satisfaction: Caring (outcome), 141b
Client Satisfaction: Case Management (outcome), 142–143b
Client Satisfaction: Communication (outcome), 143–144b
Client Satisfaction: Continuity of Care (outcome), 144–145b
Client Satisfaction: Cultural Needs Fulfillment (outcome), 145–146b
Client Satisfaction: Functional Assistance (outcome), 146b
Client Satisfaction: Pain Management (outcome), 147b
Client Satisfaction: Physical Care (outcome), 148b
Client Satisfaction: Physical Environment (outcome), 149b
Client Satisfaction: Protection of Rights (outcome), 150b
Client Satisfaction: Psychological Care (outcome), 151b
Client Satisfaction: Safety (outcome), 152b
Client Satisfaction: Symptom Control (outcome), 153b
Client Satisfaction: Teaching (outcome), 154b
Client Satisfaction: Technical Aspects of Care (outcome), 155b
Clinical settings, 36–37
Coding, 47
Coding structure, 47t
Cognition (outcome), 156b
Cognitive Orientation (outcome), 157b
Cognitive-perceptual pattern outcomes, 566–567
  community-level, 567
  individual-level, 566–567
Combination measurement scales, 18–19, 20t

Comfort, Impaired (diagnosis), 580b
  definition of, 580
  outcomes, 580
Comfort, Readiness for Enhanced (diagnosis), 683b
  definition of, 683
  outcomes, 683
Comfort Status (outcome), 158b
Comfort Status: Environment (outcome), 158–159b
Comfort Status: Physical (outcome), 159–160b
Comfort Status: Psychospiritual (outcome), 160–161b
Comfort Status: Sociocultural (outcome), 161–162b
Comfortable Death (outcome), 162–163b
Communication (outcome), 163b
Communication: Expressive (outcome), 164b
Communication: Receptive (outcome), 164b
Communication, Impaired Verbal (diagnosis), 580b
  definition of, 580
  outcomes, 580
Communication, Readiness for Enhanced (diagnosis), 684b
  definition of, 684
  outcomes, 684
Community (term), 7
Community Competence (outcome), 165b
Community Coping, Ineffective (diagnosis), 581b
  definition of, 581
  outcomes, 581
Community Coping, Readiness for Enhanced (diagnosis), 684b
  definition of, 684
  outcomes, 684
Community Disaster Readiness (outcome), 166–167b
Community Disaster Response (outcome), 167–168b
Community Grief Response (outcome), 168–169b
Community Health outcomes, 703–704b
  development across editions, 45–46t
  domain, 48–67t
Community Health, Deficient (diagnosis), 581b
  definition of, 581
  outcomes, 581
Community Health Protection outcomes
  class, 48–67t
  development across editions, 45–46t
Community Health Screening Effectiveness (outcome), 169–170b
Community Health Status (outcome), 170–171b
Community Immune Status (outcome), 172b
Community Program Effectiveness (outcome), 173b
Community Resiliency (outcome), 174b
Community Risk Control: Chronic Disease (outcome), 175b
Community Risk Control: Communicable Disease (outcome), 176b
Community Risk Control: Lead Exposure (outcome), 177b
Community Risk Control: Obesity (outcome), 178b
Community Risk Control: Unhealthy Cultural Traditions (outcome), 179b
Community Risk Control: Violence (outcome), 180b
Community Violence Level (outcome), 180–181b
Community Well-Being outcomes
  class, 48–67t
  development across editions, 45–46t
Companion books, 736
Compliance (term), 7
Compliance Behavior (outcome), 181–182b
Compliance Behavior: Prescribed Activity (outcome), 182–183b
Compliance Behavior: Prescribed Diet (outcome), 183–184b
Compliance Behavior: Prescribed Medication (outcome), 185–186b
Concentration (outcome), 186b

Confidence (term), 7
Confusion, Acute (diagnosis), 582b
  definition of, 582
  outcomes, 582
Confusion, Chronic (diagnosis), 582b
  definition of, 582
  outcomes, 582
Confusion, Risk for Acute (diagnosis), 649b
  definition of, 649
  outcomes, 649
Constipation (diagnosis), 583b
  definition of, 583
  outcomes, 583
Constipation, Perceived (diagnosis), 583b
  definition of, 583
  outcomes, 583
Constipation, Risk for (diagnosis), 650b
  definition of, 650
  outcomes, 650
Consumer (term), 6
Contamination (diagnosis), 584b
  definition of, 584
  outcomes, 584
Contamination, Risk for (diagnosis), 650b
  definition of, 650
  outcomes, 650
Coordinated Movement (outcome), 187b
Coping (outcome), 188b
Coping, Defensive (diagnosis), 584b
  definition of, 584
  outcomes, 584
Coping, Ineffective (diagnosis), 585b
  definition of, 585
  outcomes, 585
Coping, Readiness for Enhanced (diagnosis), 684b
  definition of, 684
  outcomes, 684
Coping-stress-tolerance pattern outcomes, 569
  community-level, 569
  family-level, 569
  individual-level, 569
Core outcomes
  definition of, 7, 700
  efforts to identify, 700–729
  feedback on, 735
  for nursing specialties, 700
Critical Care outcomes, 704b
Critical paths, 10
Cup Feeding Establishment: Infant (outcome), 189b
Cup Feeding Performance (outcome), 190b
Curriculum development aids, 38

D
Data source (term), 7b
Death Anxiety (diagnosis), 586b
  definition of, 586
  outcomes, 586
Decision-Making (outcome), 191b
Decision-Making, Readiness for Enhanced (diagnosis), 685b
  definition of, 685
  outcomes, 685
Decisional Conflict (diagnosis), 586b
  definition of, 586
  outcomes, 586

Decreased (term), 7
Definition changes, 733–734
Delirium Level (outcome), 192b
Dementia Level (outcome), 193b
Denial, Ineffective (diagnosis), 587b
    definition of, 587
    outcomes, 587
Dentition, Impaired (diagnosis), 587b
    definition of, 587
    outcomes, 587
Depression Level (outcome), 194b
Depression Self-Control (outcome), 195b
Dermatology outcomes, 705b
Development: Late Adulthood (outcome), 196–197b
Development: Middle Adulthood (outcome), 198–199b
Development, Risk for Delayed (diagnosis), 651b
    definition of, 651
    outcomes, 651
Development: Young Adulthood (outcome), 199–200b
Diabetes outcomes, 705b
Diagnoses. *See also* Nursing diagnoses
    medical diagnoses, 32–33
Diarrhea (diagnosis), 588b
    definition of, 588
    outcomes, 588
Digestion & Nutrition outcomes
    class, 48–67t
    development across editions, 45–46t
Dignified Life Closure (outcome), 201b
Discharge Readiness: Independent Living (outcome), 202b
Discharge Readiness: Supported Living (outcome), 203b
Discomfort Level (outcome), 203–204b
Disease (term), 7
Distorted Thought Self-Control (outcome), 204–205b
Disuse Syndrome, Risk for (diagnosis), 652b
    definition of, 652
    outcomes, 652
Diversional Activity, Deficient (diagnosis), 588b
    definition of, 588
    outcomes, 588
Documentation, 10
Drug Abuse Cessation Behavior (outcome), 205–206b
Dry Eye, Risk for (diagnosis), 652b
    definition of, 652
    outcomes, 652
Dry Eye Severity (outcome), 207b

E
Early childhood
    definition of, 7
    Parenting Performance: Early/Middle Childhood Physical Safety
        (outcome), 398–399b
Eating Disorder Self-Control (outcome), 208–209b
Educational programs, 38
Effective (term), 7
Electrolyte, Risk for Imbalance (diagnosis), 653b
    definition of, 653
    outcomes, 653
Electrolyte & Acid/Base Balance (outcome), 209–210b
Electrolyte Balance (outcome), 211b
Electronic health records (EHRs), 37
Electronic systems, 37
Elimination outcomes
    class, 48–67t

Elimination outcomes *(Continued)*
    development across editions, 45–46t
Elimination pattern outcomes, 565
    individual-level, 565
Elopement Occurrence (outcome), 211–212b
Elopement Propensity Risk (outcome), 212b
Emergency Care outcomes, 705–706b
Endurance (outcome), 213b
Energy Conservation (outcome), 214b
Energy Field, Disturbed (diagnosis), 589b
    definition of, 589
    outcomes, 589
Energy Maintenance outcomes
    class, 48–67t
    development across editions, 45–46t
Environmental Interpretation Syndrome, Impaired (diagnosis), 589b
    definition of, 589
    outcomes, 589
Evaluation, 39–40
Exercise Participation (outcome), 214–215b

F
Failure to Thrive, Adult (diagnosis), 590b
    definition of, 590
    outcomes, 590
Fall Prevention Behavior (outcome), 216b
Falls, Risk for (diagnosis), 654b
    definition of, 654
    outcomes, 654
Falls Occurrence (outcome), 217b
Family (term), 7
Family Caregiver Performance outcomes
    class, 48–67t
    development across editions, 45–46t
Family Coping (outcome), 217–218b
Family Coping, Compromised (diagnosis), 590–591b
    definition of, 590
    outcomes, 590–591
Family Coping, Disabled (diagnosis), 591–592b
    definition of, 591
    outcomes, 591–592
Family Coping, Readiness for Enhanced (diagnosis), 686b
    definition of, 686
    outcomes, 686
Family Functioning (outcome), 218–219b
Family Health outcomes
    development across editions, 45–46t
    domain, 48–67t
Family Health Status (outcome), 219–220b
Family Integrity (outcome), 221b
Family Member Health Status outcomes
    class, 48–67t
    development across editions, 45–46t
Family Normalization (outcome), 222b
Family Participation in Professional Care (outcome), 223b
Family Processes, Dysfunctional (diagnosis), 592b
    definition of, 592
    outcomes, 592
Family Processes, Interrupted (diagnosis), 593b
    definition of, 593
    outcomes, 593
Family Processes, Readiness for Enhanced (diagnosis), 686b
    definition of, 686
    outcomes, 686

Family Resiliency (outcome), 224–225b
Family Risk Control: Obesity (outcome), 225–226b
Family Social Climate (outcome), 227b
Family Support During Treatment (outcome), 228b
Family Therapeutic Regimen Management, Ineffective (diagnosis), 593b
    definition of, 593
    outcomes, 593
Family Well-Being outcomes
    class, 48–67t
    development across editions, 45–46t
Fatigue (diagnosis), 594b
    definition of, 594
    outcomes, 594
Fatigue: Disruptive Effects (outcome), 229b
Fatigue Level (outcome), 230b
Fear (diagnosis), 594–595b
    definition of, 594
    outcomes, 594–595
Fear Level (outcome), 231b
Fear Level: Child (outcome), 232–233b
Fear Self-Control (outcome), 233–234b
Feedback
    on core outcomes, 735
    on linkages to NANDA-I nursing diagnoses, 735
    on measurement scales, 735
    on outcomes, 735
Fetal Status: Antepartum (outcome), 234–235b
Fetal Status: Intrapartum (outcome), 235b
Fluid Balance (outcome), 236b
Fluid Balance, Readiness for Enhanced (diagnosis), 686b
    definition of, 686
    outcomes, 686
Fluid & Electrolytes outcomes
    class, 48–67t
    development across editions, 45–46t
Fluid Overload Severity (outcome), 237b
Fluid Volume, Deficient (diagnosis), 595b
    definition of, 595
    outcomes, 595
Fluid Volume, Excess (diagnosis), 595b
    definition of, 595
    outcomes, 595
Fluid Volume, Risk for Deficient (diagnosis), 655b
    definition of, 655
    outcomes, 655
Fluid Volume, Risk for Imbalanced (diagnosis), 655b
    definition of, 655
    outcomes, 655
Frequently asked questions, 6–19
Function (term), 7
Functional Health outcomes
    development across editions, 45–46t
    domain, 48–67t
Functioning (term), 7
Future development, 22
The Future of Nursing: Leading Change, Advancing Health
    (IOM), 32

G

Gait (outcome), 238b
Gas Exchange, Impaired (diagnosis), 596b
    definition of, 596
    outcomes, 596
Gastroenterology outcomes, 706b

Gastrointestinal Function (outcome), 239b
Gastrointestinal Motility, Dysfunctional (diagnosis), 596b
    definition of, 596
    outcomes, 596
Gastrointestinal Motility, Risk for Dysfunctional (diagnosis), 656b
    definition of, 656
    outcomes, 656
Gastrointestinal Perfusion, Risk for Ineffective (diagnosis), 656b
    definition of, 656
    outcomes, 656
Genetics outcomes, 706b
Gerontology outcomes, 707b
Goals, 8–9
Grief Resolution (outcome), 240b
Grieving (diagnosis), 597b
    definition of, 597
    outcomes, 597
Grieving, Complicated (diagnosis), 597b
    definition of, 597
    outcomes, 597
Grieving, Complicated, Risk for (diagnosis), 657b
    definition of, 657
    outcomes, 657
Growth (outcome), 241b
Growth, Risk for Disproportionate (diagnosis), 657b
    definition of, 657
    outcomes, 657
Growth & Development outcomes
    class, 48–67t
    development across editions, 45–46t
Growth & Development, Delayed (diagnosis), 598b
    definition of, 598
    outcomes, 598
Guidelines for submission of outcomes, 735
Guilt Resolution (outcome), 241–242b

H

Head bones, 105f
Health (term), 7
Health Behavior outcomes
    class, 48–67t
    development across editions, 45–46t
Health Behavior, Risk-Prone (diagnosis), 599b
    definition of, 599
    outcomes, 599
Health Beliefs (outcome), 243b
Health Beliefs outcomes
    class, 48–67t
    development across editions, 45–46t
Health Beliefs: Perceived Ability to Perform (outcome),
    243–244b
Health Beliefs: Perceived Control (outcome), 244b
Health Beliefs: Perceived Resources (outcome), 245b
Health Beliefs: Perceived Threat (outcome), 245–246b
Health concerns, 32
Health Knowledge outcomes
    class, 48–67t
    development across editions, 45–46t
Health Knowledge & Behavior outcomes
    development across editions, 45–46t
    domain, 48–67t
Health & Life Quality outcomes
    class, 48–67t
    development across editions, 45–46t

Health Maintenance, Ineffective (diagnosis), 600–601b
   definition of, 600
   outcomes, 600, 601
Health Management outcomes
   class, 48–67t
   development across editions, 45–46t
Health Orientation (outcome), 246–247b
Health patterns, 561–570
Health-perception-health management pattern outcomes, 563–564
   community-level, 564
   family-level, 564
   individual-level, 563–564
Health professionals (term), 7
Health Promoting Behavior (outcome), 247–248b
Health-promotion nursing diagnoses, 682–698
Health providers (term), 7
Health Seeking Behavior (outcome), 248b
Hearing Compensation Behavior (outcome), 249b
Heedfulness of Affected Side (outcome), 250b
Hemodialysis Access (outcome), 251b
Historical development, 44
HIV/AIDS outcomes, 707–708b
Home Healthcare outcomes, 708–709b
Home Maintenance, Impaired (diagnosis), 601b
   definition of, 601
   outcomes, 601
Hope (outcome), 252b
Hope, Readiness for Enhanced (diagnosis), 687b
   definition of, 687
   outcomes, 687
Hopelessness (diagnosis), 601–602b
   definition of, 601
   outcomes, 601, 602
Hospice & Palliative Care outcomes, 709–710b
Human Dignity, Risk for Compromised (diagnosis), 658b
   definition of, 658
   outcomes, 658
Hydration (outcome), 253b
Hyperactivity Level (outcome), 254b
Hypercalcemia Severity (outcome), 255b
Hyperchloremia Severity (outcome), 256b
Hyperglycemia Severity (outcome), 256–257b
Hyperkalemia Severity (outcome), 257b
Hypermagnesemia Severity (outcome), 258b
Hypernatremia Severity (outcome), 258–259b
Hyperphosphatemia Severity (outcome), 259–260b
Hypertension Severity (outcome), 260b
Hyperthermia (diagnosis), 602b
   definition of, 602
   outcomes, 602
Hypocalcemia Severity (outcome), 261b
Hypochloremia Severity (outcome), 262b
Hypoglycemia Severity (outcome), 262–263b
Hypokalemia Severity (outcome), 263–264b
Hypomagnesemia Severity (outcome), 264–265b
Hyponatremia Severity (outcome), 265b
Hypophosphatemia Severity (outcome), 266b
Hypotension Severity (outcome), 266–267b
Hypothermia (diagnosis), 602b
   definition of, 602
   outcomes, 602

I

Identification of outcomes, 11
Identity (outcome), 268b

Immobility Consequences: Physiological (outcome), 269b
Immobility Consequences: Psycho-Cognitive (outcome), 270b
Immune Hypersensitivity Response (outcome), 270–271b
Immune Response outcomes
   class, 48–67t
   development across editions, 45–46t
Immune Status (outcome), 271–272b
Immunization Behavior (outcome), 272–273b
Immunization Status, Readiness for Enhanced (diagnosis), 688b
   definition of, 688
   outcomes, 688
Implementation
   in clinical settings, 36–37
   in educational programs, 38
   in electronic systems, 37
   steps for, 38
   strategies for, 38
Implementation planning, 36–37
Impulse Control, Ineffective (diagnosis), 603b
   definition of, 603
   outcomes, 603
Impulse Self-Control (outcome), 274b
Inappropriate (term), 7
Increased (term), 7
Indicator ratings, 35–36
Infant (term), 7
Infant Behavior, Disorganized (diagnosis), 603–604b
   definition of, 603
   outcomes, 603–604
Infant Behavior, Organized, Readiness for Enhanced (diagnosis), 688b
   definition of, 688
   outcomes, 688
Infant Behavior, Risk for Disorganized (diagnosis), 659b
   definition of, 659
   outcomes, 659
Infant Feeding Pattern, Ineffective (diagnosis), 604b
   definition of, 604
   outcomes, 604
Infant Nutritional Status (outcome), 275b
Infection, Risk for (diagnosis), 659b
   definition of, 659
   outcomes, 659
Infection Control & Epidemiological outcomes, 710–711b
Infection Severity (outcome), 276b
Infection Severity: Newborn (outcome), 277b
Information Processing (outcome), 278b
Injury, Risk for (diagnosis), 660b
   definition of, 660
   outcomes, 660
Insomnia (diagnosis), 604–605b
   definition of, 604
   outcomes, 604–605
Institute of Medicine (IOM), 32
Instrumental Activities of Daily Living (IADL), 469b
Intracranial Adaptive Capacity, Decreased (diagnosis), 605b
   definition of, 605
   outcomes, 605
Intravenous Therapy outcomes, 711b

J

Joint Movement (outcome), 279b
Joint Movement: Ankle (outcome), 279–280b
Joint Movement: Elbow (outcome), 280b
Joint Movement: Fingers (outcome), 281b
Joint Movement: Hip (outcome), 282b

Joint Movement: Knee (outcome), 283b
Joint Movement: Neck (outcome), 283b
Joint Movement: Passive (outcome), 284b
Joint Movement: Shoulder (outcome), 284–285b
Joint Movement: Spine (outcome), 285b
Joint Movement: Wrist (outcome), 286b

K

Kidney Function (outcome), 287b
Knowledge outcomes, 22–31t
Knowledge: Acute Illness Management (outcome)
    definition and indicators, 288b
    related performance outcomes, 22–31t
Knowledge: Anticoagulation Therapy Management (outcome)
    definition and indicators, 289–290b
    related performance outcomes, 22–31t
Knowledge: Arthritis Management (outcome)
    definition and indicators, 290–291b
    related performance outcomes, 22–31t
Knowledge: Asthma Management (outcome)
    definition and indicators, 292–293b
    related performance outcomes, 22–31t
Knowledge: Body Mechanics (outcome)
    definition and indicators, 293b
    related performance outcomes, 22–31t
Knowledge: Bottle Feeding (outcome)
    definition and indicators, 294b
    related performance outcomes, 22–31t
Knowledge: Breastfeeding (outcome)
    definition and indicators, 295b
    related performance outcomes, 22–31t
Knowledge: Cancer Management (outcome)
    definition and indicators, 296–297b
    related performance outcomes, 22–31t
Knowledge: Cancer Threat Reduction (outcome)
    definition and indicators, 297b
    related performance outcomes, 22–31t
Knowledge: Cardiac Disease Management (outcome)
    definition and indicators, 298–299b
    related performance outcomes, 22–31t
Knowledge: Child Physical Safety (outcome)
    definition and indicators, 299b
    related performance outcomes, 22–31t
Knowledge: Chronic Disease Management (outcome)
    definition and indicators, 300b
    related performance outcomes, 22–31t
Knowledge: Chronic Obstructive Pulmonary Disease Management
    (outcome)
    definition and indicators, 301–302b
    related performance outcomes, 22–31t
Knowledge: Conception Prevention (outcome)
    definition and indicators, 302b
    related performance outcomes, 22–31t
Knowledge: Coronary Artery Disease Management (outcome)
    definition and indicators, 303–304b
    related performance outcomes, 22–31t
Knowledge: Cup Feeding (outcome)
    definition and indicators, 304–305b
    related performance outcomes, 22–31t
Knowledge: Dementia Management (outcome)
    definition and indicators, 305b
    related performance outcomes, 22–31t
Knowledge: Depression Management (outcome)
    definition and indicators, 306b
    related performance outcomes, 22–31t

Knowledge: Diabetes Management (outcome)
    definition and indicators, 307–308b
    related performance outcomes, 22–31t
Knowledge: Disease Process (outcome)
    definition and indicators, 308b
    related performance outcomes, 22–31t
Knowledge: Dysrhythmia Management (outcome)
    definition and indicators, 309b
    related performance outcomes, 22–31t
Knowledge: Eating Disorder Management
    (outcome)
    definition and indicators, 310–311b
    related performance outcomes, 22–31t
Knowledge: Energy Conservation (outcome)
    definition and indicators, 311b
    related performance outcomes, 22–31t
Knowledge: Fall Prevention (outcome)
    definition and indicators, 312b
    related performance outcomes, 22–31t
Knowledge: Fertility Promotion (outcome)
    definition and indicators, 313b
    related performance outcomes, 22–31t
Knowledge: Health Behavior (outcome)
    definition and indicators, 314b
    related performance outcomes, 22–31t
Knowledge: Health Promotion (outcome)
    definition and indicators, 315b
    related performance outcomes, 22–31t
Knowledge: Health Resources (outcome)
    definition and indicators, 316b
    related performance outcomes, 22–31t
Knowledge: Healthy Diet (outcome)
    definition and indicators, 316–317b
    related performance outcomes, 22–31t
Knowledge: Healthy Lifestyle (outcome)
    definition and indicators, 317–318b
    related performance outcomes, 22–31t
Knowledge: Heart Failure Management (outcome)
    definition and indicators, 319–320b
    related performance outcomes, 22–31t
Knowledge: Hypertension Management (outcome)
    definition and indicators, 320–321b
    related performance outcomes, 22–31t
Knowledge: Infant Care (outcome)
    definition and indicators, 322b
    related performance outcomes, 22–31t
Knowledge: Infection Management (outcome)
    definition and indicators, 323b
    related performance outcomes, 22–31t
Knowledge: Inflammatory Bowel Disease Management
    (outcome)
    definition and indicators, 324b
    related performance outcomes, 22–31t
Knowledge: Kidney Disease Management (outcome)
    definition and indicators, 325–326b
    related performance outcomes, 22–31t
Knowledge: Labor & Delivery (outcome)
    definition and indicators, 326b
    related performance outcomes, 22–31t
Knowledge: Lipid Disorder Management (outcome)
    definition and indicators, 327b
    related performance outcomes, 22–31t
Knowledge: Medication (outcome)
    definition and indicators, 328b
    related performance outcomes, 22–31t

Knowledge: Multiple Sclerosis Management (outcome)
   definition and indicators, 329b
   related performance outcomes, 22–31t
Knowledge: Osteoporosis Management (outcome)
   definition and indicators, 330b
   related performance outcomes, 22–31t
Knowledge: Ostomy Care (outcome)
   definition and indicators, 331b
   related performance outcomes, 22–31t
Knowledge: Pain Management (outcome)
   definition and indicators, 331–332b
   related performance outcomes, 22–31t
Knowledge: Parenting (outcome)
   definition and indicators, 333b
   related performance outcomes, 22–31t
Knowledge: Peripheral Artery Disease Management
   (outcome)
   definition and indicators, 334b
   related performance outcomes, 22–31t
Knowledge: Personal Safety (outcome)
   definition and indicators, 335b
   related performance outcomes, 22–31t
Knowledge: Pneumonia Management (outcome)
   definition and indicators, 336b
   related performance outcomes, 22–31t
Knowledge: Postpartum Maternal Health (outcome)
   definition and indicators, 337b
   related performance outcomes, 22–31t
Knowledge: Preconception Maternal Health (outcome)
   definition and indicators, 338b
   related performance outcomes, 22–31t
Knowledge: Pregnancy (outcome)
   definition and indicators, 338–339b
   related performance outcomes, 22–31t
Knowledge: Pregnancy & Postpartum Sexual Functioning
   (outcome)
   definition and indicators, 340b
   related performance outcomes, 22–31t
Knowledge: Prescribed Activity (outcome)
   definition and indicators, 341b
   related performance outcomes, 22–31t
Knowledge: Prescribed Diet (outcome)
   definition and indicators, 342b
   related performance outcomes, 22–31t
Knowledge: Preterm Infant Care (outcome)
   definition and indicators, 343b
   related performance outcomes, 22–31t
Knowledge: Sexual Functioning (outcome)
   definition and indicators, 344b
   related performance outcomes, 22–31t
Knowledge: Stress Management (outcome)
   definition and indicators, 344–345b
   related performance outcomes, 22–31t
Knowledge: Stroke Management (outcome)
   definition and indicators, 345–346b
   related performance outcomes, 22–31t
Knowledge: Stroke Prevention (outcome)
   definition and indicators, 347b
   related performance outcomes, 22–31t
Knowledge: Substance Use Control (outcome)
   definition and indicators, 348b
   related performance outcomes, 22–31t
Knowledge: Thrombus Prevention (outcome)
   definition and indicators, 349b
   related performance outcomes, 22–31t

Knowledge: Time Management (outcome)
   definition and indicators, 350b
   related performance outcomes, 22–31t
Knowledge: Treatment Procedure (outcome)
   definition and indicators, 350–351b
   related performance outcomes, 22–31t
Knowledge: Treatment Regimen (outcome)
   definition and indicators, 351–352b
   related performance outcomes, 22–31t
Knowledge: Weight Management (outcome)
   definition and indicators, 352b
   related performance outcomes, 22–31t
Knowledge, Deficient (diagnosis), 606b
   definition of, 606
   outcomes, 606
Knowledge, Readiness for Enhanced (diagnosis), 689–690b
   definition of, 689
   outcomes, 689–690

L
Labels, 8, 11
Late adulthood
   definition of, 7
   Development: Late Adulthood (outcome), 196–197b
Latex Allergy Response (diagnosis), 607b
   definition of, 607
   outcomes, 607
Latex Allergy Response, Risk for (diagnosis), 661b
   definition of, 661
   outcomes, 661
Leg bones, 105f
Leisure Participation (outcome), 353b
Levels of abstraction, 3–4, 6–8, 8t
Licensing, 40
Lifestyle, Sedentary (diagnosis), 607b
   definition of, 607
   outcomes, 607
Lifestyle Balance (outcome), 354b
Liver Function (outcome), 355b
Liver Function, Risk for Impaired (diagnosis), 661b
   definition of, 661
   outcomes, 661
Loneliness, Risk for (diagnosis), 661b
   definition of, 661
   outcomes, 661
Loneliness Severity (outcome), 356b

M
Maternal-Fetal Dyad, Risk for Disturbed (diagnosis), 662b
   definition of, 662
   outcomes, 662
Maternal Status: Antepartum (outcome), 357b
Maternal Status: Intrapartum (outcome), 358b
Maternal Status: Postpartum (outcome), 359b
Measure (term), 7
Measurement of outcomes, 3, 10
Measurement scales
   and associated outcomes, 12–18t, 20t
   changes in, 734
   combination of, 18–19, 20t
   diversity of, 11
   example of, 40
   feedback on, 735
   single, 11, 12–18t
   using, 34, 36

Mechanical Ventilation Response: Adult (outcome), 360–361b
Mechanical Ventilation Weaning Response: Adult (outcome), 361–362b
Medical diagnoses, 32–33
Medical-Surgical outcomes, 711–712b
Medication Response (outcome), 363b
Memory (outcome), 364b
Memory, Impaired (diagnosis), 608b
    definition of, 608
    outcomes, 608
Mental (term), 7
Metabolic Acidosis Severity (outcome), 364–365b
Metabolic Alkalosis Severity (outcome), 365–366b
Metabolic Regulation outcomes
    class, 48–67t
    development across editions, 45–46t
Middle adulthood
    definition of, 7
    Development: Middle Adulthood (outcome), 198–199b
Middle childhood
    Child Development: Middle Childhood (outcome), 136b
    definition of, 7
    Parenting Performance: Early/Middle Childhood Physical Safety
        (outcome), 398–399b
    Parenting Performance: Middle Childhood (outcome),
        402–403b
Mobility (outcome), 366–367b
Mobility outcomes
    class, 48–67t
    development across editions, 45–46t
Mobility: Bed, Impaired (diagnosis), 608b
    definition of, 608
    outcomes, 608
Mobility: Physical, Impaired (diagnosis), 609b
    definition of, 609
    outcomes, 609
Mobility: Wheelchair, Impaired (diagnosis), 609b
    definition of, 609
    outcomes, 609
Mood Equilibrium (outcome), 367–368b
Moral Distress (diagnosis), 610b
    definition of, 610
    outcomes, 610
Motivation (outcome), 368–369b
Mutilation Self-Restraint (outcome), 369–370b

N

NANDA International (NANDA-I), 2
NANDA International (NANDA-I) diagnoses, 32–33, 571
    comparison with NOC outcomes, 5, 5t
    NOC linkages, 562, 735
Nausea (diagnosis), 611b
    definition of, 611
    outcomes, 611
Nausea & Vomiting: Disruptive Effects (outcome), 372b
Nausea & Vomiting Control (outcome), 371b
Nausea & Vomiting Severity (outcome), 373b
Neck bones, 105f
Neglect Cessation (outcome), 374b
Neglect Recovery (outcome), 374–375b
Neonatal Jaundice (diagnosis), 611b
    definition of, 611
    outcomes, 611
Neonatal Jaundice, Risk for (diagnosis), 663b
    definition of, 663
    outcomes, 663

Neonatology outcomes, 712b, 728–729b
Nephrology outcomes, 713b
Neurocognitive outcomes
    class, 48–67t
    development across editions, 45–46t
Neurological Status (outcome), 376b
Neurological Status: Autonomic (outcome), 377b
Neurological Status: Central Motor Control (outcome), 378b
Neurological Status: Consciousness (outcome), 378–379b
Neurological Status: Cranial Sensory/Motor Function (outcome),
    379–380b
Neurological Status: Peripheral (outcome), 380–382b
Neurological Status: Spinal Sensory/Motor Function
    (outcome), 382b
Neuroscience outcomes, 713–714b
New outcomes, 11
New specialty areas, 700
Newborn (term), 7
Newborn Adaptation (outcome), 383b
NIC. *See* Nursing Interventions Classification
NMDS. *See* Nursing Minimum Data Set
NOC. *See* Nursing Outcomes Classification
Noncompliance (diagnosis), 611–612b
    definition of, 611
    outcomes, 611, 612
Nurse Practitioner outcomes, 714–715b
Nursing diagnoses, 5, 32–33
    differences between NOC outcomes and, 9–10
    health-promotion nursing diagnoses, 682–698
    NANDA-I diagnoses, 32–33, 571
        comparison with NOC outcomes, 5, 5t
        NOC linkages, 562, 572–642, 643–698
    nursing-sensitive patient outcomes as resolution of, 9
    risk nursing diagnoses, 643–698
Nursing Interventions Classification (NIC), 2
Nursing Minimum Data Set (NMDS), 2
Nursing outcomes
    definition of, 2
    measurement of, 3
Nursing Outcomes Classification (NOC), 2
    classes, 44
    coding, 47
    coding structure, 47t
    completeness of, 4–5
    considerations when using in practice, 32–36
    current classification, 1–31
    definition of, 2–6
    development of, 22
        across editions, 45–46t
        future, 22
        historical, 44
    domains, 44
    fifth edition, 45–47
        label changes for, 733
        outcomes new to, 732–733
        outcomes revised for, 733–734
    fourth edition, 45
        label changes for fifth edition, 733
        outcomes retired for this edition, 734
    future development of, 22
    general comments about, 735
    guidelines for submission, 735
    implementation in clinical settings, 36–37
    implementation in educational programs, 38
    implementation in electronic systems, 37

Nursing Outcomes Classification *(Continued)*
   implementation planning, 36–37
   knowledge outcomes, 22–31t
   levels of abstraction, 3–4, 6–8, 8t
   linkages to health patterns, 561–570
   linkages to NANDA-I diagnoses, 562
   organized by health patterns, 563
   overview, 43–68
   performance outcomes, 22–31t
   previous editions, 736
   refinement of, 22
   in research, 39–40
   revisions, 44–47
   second edition, 44–45
   taxonomy, 7, 43–68
   third edition, 45
   translations, 736
Nursing Outcomes Classification (NOC) outcomes
   comparison with NANDA-I diagnoses, 5, 5t
   definition of, 2
   development of, 6–8, 735
   differences between nursing diagnoses and, 9–10
   feedback on, 735
   frequently asked questions, 6–19
   general principles for development of, 735
   guidelines for submission of, 735
   licensing, 40
   measurement of, 3
   as not assessments, 5–6
   as not diagnoses, 5
   as not goals, 8–9
   as not prescriptive, 5
   not within patterns, 570
   selecting, 32–34
   sensitivity of, 4
Nursing quality and effectiveness, 39–40
Nursing-sensitive outcomes
   rules for standardization of, 9b
   use by other disciplines, 4
Nursing-sensitive patient outcome indicators (term), 6
Nursing-sensitive patient outcomes
   definition of, 2, 6, 7
   identification of, 9
   as resolution of nursing diagnoses, 9
Nursing sensitivity, 9b
Nursing specialties
   core outcomes for, 700
   new specialty areas, 700
Nutrition: Imbalanced, Less than Body Requirements (diagnosis), 613b
   definition of, 613
   outcomes, 613
Nutrition: Imbalanced, More than Body Requirements (diagnosis), 613b
   definition of, 613
   outcomes, 613
Nutrition: Imbalanced, Risk for More than Body Requirements (diagnosis), 663b
   definition of, 663
   outcomes, 663
Nutrition, Readiness for Enhanced (diagnosis), 691b
   definition of, 691
   outcomes, 691
Nutrition-metabolic pattern outcomes, 564–565
   community-level, 565
   family-level, 565
   individual-level, 564–565

Nutritional Status (outcome), 384b
Nutritional Status: Biochemical Measures (outcome), 384–385b
Nutritional Status: Energy (outcome), 385b
Nutritional Status: Food & Fluid Intake (outcome), 386b
Nutritional Status: Nutrient Intake (outcome), 386b

O
Obstetrics outcomes, 728–729b
Obtains (term), 7
Occupational Health outcomes, 715–716b
Oncology outcomes, 716b
Operating Room outcomes, 717b
Ophthalmology outcomes, 717b
OPT. *See* Outcome-Present State-Test Model (OPT)
Oral Health (outcome), 387b
Oral Mucous Membrane, Impaired (diagnosis), 614b
   definition of, 614
   outcomes, 614
Orthopedics outcomes, 718b
Ostomy Self-Care (outcome), 388b
Otorhinolaryngology & Head-Neck outcomes, 718–719b
Outcome indicators
   definition of, 7
   using, 34
Outcome labels, 11
Outcome-Present State-Test Model (OPT), 2
Outcome ratings
   establishing, 34–35
   to evaluate care, 35
Outcomes. *See also* Nursing Outcomes Classification (NOC) outcomes; *specific outcomes*
   assessment of, 10–11
   development of, 11
   documentation of, 10
   identification for use in practice, 11
   new, 11
   new to fifth edition, 732–733
   nursing outcomes
      definition of, 2
      measurement of, 3
   patient outcomes, 6
      measurement of, 10
      nursing-sensitive, 2, 6, 7, 9
   personal lists of, 10
   rating of, 10
   retired for this edition, 734
   revised for fifth edition, 733–734
   selecting, 32–34
   standardization of, 11

P
Pain: Adverse Psychological Response (outcome), 389b
Pain: Disruptive Effects (outcome), 391b
Pain, Acute (diagnosis), 615b
   definition of, 615
   outcomes, 615
Pain, Chronic (diagnosis), 615–616b
   definition of, 615
   outcomes, 615–616
Pain Control (outcome), 390b
Pain Level (outcome), 392b
Pain Management outcomes, 719b
Parent (term), 7
Parent-Infant Attachment (outcome), 393b

Parental Role Conflict (diagnosis), 616b
  definition of, 616
  outcomes, 616
Parenting outcomes
  class, 48–67t
  development across editions, 45–46t
Parenting, Impaired (diagnosis), 617b
  definition of, 617
  outcomes, 617
Parenting, Readiness for Enhanced (diagnosis), 692b
  definition of, 692
  outcomes, 692
Parenting, Risk for Impaired (diagnosis), 664b
  definition of, 664
  outcomes, 664
Parenting Performance (outcome), 394b
Parenting Performance: Adolescent (outcome), 395–396b
Parenting Performance: Adolescent Physical Safety (outcome), 397–398b
Parenting Performance: Early/Middle Childhood Physical Safety (outcome), 398–399b
Parenting Performance: Infant (outcome), 399–400b
Parenting Performance: Infant/Toddler Physical Safety (outcome), 400–401b
Parenting Performance: Middle Childhood (outcome), 402–403b
Parenting Performance: Preschooler (outcome), 403–404b
Parenting Performance: Psychosocial Safety (outcome), 405b
Parenting Performance: Toddler (outcome), 406–407b
Parish Nursing outcomes, 719–720b
Participation in Health Care Decisions (outcome), 407b
Patient (term), 6
Patient characteristics, 33
Patient outcomes, 6
  measurement of, 10
  nursing-sensitive
    definition of, 2, 6, 7
    identification of, 9
    as resolution of nursing diagnoses, 9
Patient preferences, 33
Patient satisfaction (term), 6
Pediatric Oncology outcomes, 721b
Pediatrics outcomes, 720–721b
Perceived Health outcomes
  development across editions, 45–46t
  domain, 48–67t
Perception (term), 8
Performance outcomes, 22–31t
Perianesthesia outcomes, 722b
Perimenopause Symptom Severity (outcome), 408b
Perioperative Care outcomes, 722–723b
Perioperative Positioning Injury, Risk for (diagnosis), 665b
  definition of, 665
  outcomes, 665
Peripheral Artery Disease Severity (outcome), 408–409b
Peripheral Neurovascular Dysfunction, Risk for (diagnosis), 665b
  definition of, 665
  outcomes, 665
Personal actions (term), 8
Personal Autonomy (outcome), 409–410b
Personal Health Screening Behavior (outcome), 410–411b
Personal Health Status (outcome), 411–412b
Personal Identity, Disturbed (diagnosis), 618b
  definition of, 618
  outcomes, 618

Personal Identity, Risk for Disturbed (diagnosis), 666b
  definition of, 666
  outcomes, 666
Personal lists, 10
Personal Resiliency (outcome), 413–414b
Personal Safety Behavior (outcome), 414–415b
Personal Time Management (outcome), 415–416b
Personal Well-Being (outcome), 416b
Physical Aging (outcome), 417b
Physical Fitness (outcome), 418b
Physical Injury Severity (outcome), 418–419b
Physical Maturation: Female (outcome), 419b
Physical Maturation: Male (outcome), 420b
Physiologic Health outcomes
  development across editions, 45–46t
  domain, 48–67t
Physiological Well-Being outcomes, 45–46t
Planning for implementation, 36–37
Plastic Surgery outcomes, 724b
Play Participation (outcome), 420–421b
Poisoning, Risk for (diagnosis), 666b
  definition of, 666
  outcomes, 666
Population (term), 8
Post-Procedure Recovery (outcome), 422–423b
Post-Trauma Syndrome (diagnosis), 618–619b
  definition of, 618
  outcomes, 618, 619
Post-Trauma Syndrome, Risk for (diagnosis), 667b
  definition of, 667
  outcomes, 667
Postpartum Maternal Health Behavior (outcome), 421–422b
Power, Readiness for Enhanced (diagnosis), 692b
  definition of, 692
  outcomes, 692
Powerlessness (diagnosis), 619b
  definition of, 619
  outcomes, 619
Powerlessness, Risk for (diagnosis), 667b
  definition of, 667
  outcomes, 667
Pre-Procedure Readiness (outcome), 425b
Premenstrual Syndrome (PMS) Severity (outcome), 423b
Prenatal Health Behavior (outcome), 424b
Preschool (term), 8
Preterm Infant Organization (outcome), 426b
Previous editions, 736
Protection, Ineffective (diagnosis), 620b
  definition of, 620
  outcomes, 620
Psychiatric-Mental Health outcomes, 723b
Psychological Well-Being outcomes, 48–67t
Psychomotor Energy (outcome), 427b
Psychosocial Adaptation outcomes
  class, 48–67t
  development across editions, 45–46t
Psychosocial Adjustment: Life Change (outcome), 427–428b
Psychosocial Health outcomes
  development across editions, 45–46t
  domain, 48–67t

Q
Quality evaluation, 39–40
Quality of Life (outcome), 429b

R

Radiology outcomes, 724b
Rape-Trauma Syndrome (diagnosis), 621b
  definition of, 621
  outcomes, 621
Rating of outcomes, 10
Rating scales, 40. *See also* Measurement scales
Rating score changes, 7
Recommended (term), 8
Reference persons, 3, 8
Refinement, 22
Refrains (term), 8
Rehabilitation outcomes, 725b
Relationship, Ineffective (diagnosis), 621–622b
  definition of, 621
  outcomes, 621, 622
Relationship, Readiness for Enhanced (diagnosis), 693b
  definition of, 693
  outcomes, 693
Relationship, Risk for Ineffective (diagnosis), 668b
  definition of, 668
  outcomes, 668
Religiosity, Impaired (diagnosis), 622b
  definition of, 622
  outcomes, 622
Religiosity, Readiness for Enhanced (diagnosis), 693b
  definition of, 693
  outcomes, 693
Religiosity, Risk for Impaired (diagnosis), 668b
  definition of, 668
  outcomes, 668
Relocation Adaptation (outcome), 430–431b
Relocation Stress Syndrome (diagnosis), 623b
  definition of, 623
  outcomes, 623
Relocation Stress Syndrome, Risk for (diagnosis), 669b
  definition of, 669
  outcomes, 669
Renal Perfusion, Risk for Ineffective (diagnosis), 669b
  definition of, 669
  outcomes, 669
Reputable (term), 8
Research, 39–40
Research studies, 39
Resident (term), 6
Resilience, Impaired Individual (diagnosis), 623b
  definition of, 623
  outcomes, 623
Resilience, Readiness for Enhanced (diagnosis), 694b
  definition of, 694
  outcomes, 694
Resilience, Risk for Compromised (diagnosis), 670b
  definition of, 670
  outcomes, 670
Resources
  available, 33
  definition of, 8
Respiratory Status (outcome), 431–432b
Respiratory Status: Airway Patency (outcome), 432–433b
Respiratory Status: Gas Exchange (outcome), 433b
Respiratory Status: Ventilation (outcome), 434b
Rest (outcome), 435b
Risk Control (outcome), 435–436b
Risk Control: Alcohol Use (outcome), 436–437b

Risk Control: Cancer (outcome), 438b
Risk Control: Cardiovascular Disease (outcome), 439b
Risk Control: Drug Use (outcome), 440b
Risk Control: Dry Eye (outcome), 441–442b
Risk Control: Hearing Impairment (outcome), 442b
Risk Control: Hypertension (outcome), 443b
Risk Control: Hyperthermia (outcome), 444b
Risk Control: Hypotension (outcome), 445b
Risk Control: Hypothermia (outcome), 446b
Risk Control: Infectious Process (outcome), 447b
Risk Control: Lipid Disorder (outcome), 448b
Risk Control: Osteoporosis (outcome), 448–449b
Risk Control: Sexually Transmitted Diseases (STD) (outcome), 450b
Risk Control: Stroke (outcome), 451b
Risk Control: Sun Exposure (outcome), 452b
Risk Control: Thrombus (outcome), 453–454b
Risk Control: Tobacco Use (outcome), 454–455b
Risk Control: Unintended Pregnancy (outcome), 455–456b
Risk Control: Visual Impairment (outcome), 456b
Risk Control & Safety outcomes
  class, 48–67t
  development across editions, 45–46t
Risk Detection (outcome), 457b
Risk nursing diagnoses, 643–681
Role Performance (outcome), 458b
Role Performance, Ineffective (diagnosis), 624b
  definition of, 624
  outcomes, 624
Role-relationship pattern outcomes, 568
  community-level, 568
  family-level, 568
  individual-level, 568
Rules for standardization, 9b

S

Safe Health Care Environment (outcome), 459b
Safe Home Environment (outcome), 460–461b
Safe Wandering (outcome), 461–462b
Satisfaction with Care outcomes
  class, 48–67t
  development across editions, 45–46t
Scale changes, 734. *See also* Measurement scales
School Health outcomes, 725–726b
Seizure Self-Control (outcome), 462b
Selecting outcomes, 32–34
Self-Awareness (outcome), 463–464b
Self-Care outcomes
  class, 48–67t
  development across editions, 45–46t
Self-Care: Activities of Daily Living (ADL) (outcome), 465b
Self-Care: Bathing (outcome), 465–466b
Self-Care: Dressing (outcome), 466–467b
Self-Care: Eating (outcome), 467b
Self-Care: Hygiene (outcome), 468b
Self-Care: Instrumental Activities of Daily Living (IADL) (outcome), 469b
Self-Care: Non-Parenteral Medication (outcome), 470b
Self-Care: Oral Hygiene (outcome), 471b
Self-Care: Parenteral Medication (outcome), 471–472b
Self-Care: Toileting (outcome), 472–473b
Self-Care, Readiness for Enhanced (diagnosis), 695b
  definition of, 695
  outcomes, 695

Self-Care Deficit: Bathing (diagnosis), 625b
    definition of, 625
    outcomes, 625
Self-Care Deficit: Dressing (diagnosis), 625b
    definition of, 625
    outcomes, 625
Self-Care Deficit: Feeding (diagnosis), 626b
    definition of, 626
    outcomes, 626
Self-Care Deficit: Toileting (diagnosis), 626b
    definition of, 626
    outcomes, 626
Self-Care Status (outcome), 464b
Self-Concept, Readiness for Enhanced (diagnosis), 696b
    definition of, 696
    outcomes, 696
Self-Control outcomes
    class, 48–67t
    development across editions, 45–46t
Self-Direction of Care (outcome), 473b
Self-Esteem (outcome), 474b
Self-Esteem: Chronic Low (diagnosis), 627b
    definition of, 627
    outcomes, 627
Self-Esteem: Chronic Low, Risk for (diagnosis), 671b
    definition of, 671
    outcomes, 671
Self-Esteem: Situational Low (diagnosis), 627b
    definition of, 627
    outcomes, 627
Self-Esteem: Situational Low, Risk for (diagnosis), 671b
    definition of, 671
    outcomes, 671
Self-Health Management, Ineffective (diagnosis), 628b
    definition of, 628
    outcomes, 628
Self-Health Management, Readiness for Enhanced (diagnosis), 696–697b
    definition of, 696
    outcomes, 696–697
Self-Management: Acute Illness (outcome), 475b
Self-Management: Anticoagulation Therapy (outcome), 476–477b
Self-Management: Asthma (outcome), 477–478b
Self-Management: Cardiac Disease (outcome), 479–480b
Self-Management: Chronic Disease (outcome), 481–482b
Self-Management: Chronic Obstructive Pulmonary Disease (outcome), 483–484b
Self-Management: Coronary Artery Disease (outcome), 484–486b
Self-Management: Diabetes (outcome), 486–487b
Self-Management: Dysrhythmia (outcome), 488–489b
Self-Management: Heart Failure (outcome), 489–491b
Self-Management: Hypertension (outcome), 491–492b
Self-Management: Kidney Disease (outcome), 493–494b
Self-Management: Lipid Disorder (outcome), 494–495b
Self-Management: Multiple Sclerosis (outcome), 496–497b
Self-Management: Osteoporosis (outcome), 497–498b
Self-Management: Peripheral Artery Disease (outcome), 498–499b
Self-Mutilation (diagnosis), 629b
    definition of, 629
    outcomes, 629
Self-Mutilation, Risk for (diagnosis), 672b
    definition of, 672
    outcomes, 672
Self-Neglect (diagnosis), 629–630b
    definition of, 629
    outcomes, 629, 630

Self-perception-self concept pattern outcomes, 567–568
    community-level, 568
    family-level, 568
    individual-level, 567–568
Sensitivity, 4
    criteria for evaluating, 9b
    of outcomes, 4
Sensory Function (outcome), 500b
Sensory Function outcomes
    class, 48–67t
    development across editions, 45–46t
Sensory Function: Hearing (outcome), 500–501b
Sensory Function: Proprioception (outcome), 501–502b
Sensory Function: Tactile (outcome), 502b
Sensory Function: Taste & Smell (outcome), 503b
Sensory Function: Vision (outcome), 503–504b
Sexual Dysfunction (diagnosis), 630b
    definition of, 630
    outcomes, 630
Sexual Functioning (outcome), 504–505b
Sexual Identity (outcome), 506b
Sexuality Pattern, Ineffective (diagnosis), 630b
    definition of, 630
    outcomes, 630
Sexuality-reproductive pattern outcomes, 568–569
    individual-level, 569
Shock, Risk for (diagnosis), 672b
    definition of, 672
    outcomes, 672
Shock Severity: Anaphylactic (outcome), 507b
Shock Severity: Cardiogenic (outcome), 508b
Shock Severity: Hypovolemic (outcome), 509b
Shock Severity: Neurogenic (outcome), 510b
Shock Severity: Septic (outcome), 510–511b
Short-term stays, 35
Skeletal Function (outcome), 511–512b
Skin Integrity, Impaired (diagnosis), 631b
    definition of, 631
    outcomes, 631
Skin Integrity, Risk for Impaired (diagnosis), 673b
    definition of, 673
    outcomes, 673
Sleep (outcome), 512–513b
Sleep, Readiness for Enhanced (diagnosis), 697b
    definition of, 697
    outcomes, 697
Sleep Deprivation (diagnosis), 631b
    definition of, 631
    outcomes, 631
Sleep Pattern, Disturbed (diagnosis), 632b
    definition of, 632
    outcomes, 632
Sleep-rest pattern outcomes, 567
    individual-level, 567
Smoking Cessation Behavior (outcome), 513–514b
Social Anxiety Level (outcome), 515b
Social Interaction outcomes
    class, 48–67t
    development across editions, 45–46t
Social Interaction, Impaired (diagnosis), 632b
    definition of, 632
    outcomes, 632
Social Interaction Skills (outcome), 516b
Social Involvement (outcome), 517b

Social Isolation (diagnosis), 633b
   definition of, 633
   outcomes, 633
Social Support (outcome), 518b
Sorrow: Chronic (diagnosis), 633b
   definition of, 633
   outcomes, 633
Specialty areas
   core outcomes for, 700
   new specialty areas, 700
Spinal Cord Injury outcomes, 726b
Spiritual Distress (diagnosis), 634b
   definition of, 634
   outcomes, 634
Spiritual Distress, Risk for (diagnosis), 673b
   definition of, 673
   outcomes, 673
Spiritual Health (outcome), 519b
Spiritual Well-Being, Readiness for Enhanced (diagnosis), 697b
   definition of, 697
   outcomes, 697
Standardization of outcomes, 9b, 11
Standardized care plans/critical paths, 10
Standardized outcomes, 2
Status (term), 8
Step-by-Step NNN Teaching Strategy, 38
Stress Level (outcome), 520b
Stress Overload (diagnosis), 634b
   definition of, 634
   outcomes, 634
Student Health Status (outcome), 521–522b
Substance Addiction Consequences (outcome), 522–523b
Substance Withdrawal Severity (outcome), 523–524b
Sudden Infant Death Syndrome, Risk for (diagnosis), 674b
   definition of, 674
   outcomes, 674
Suffering Severity (outcome), 524–525b
Suffocation, Risk for (diagnosis), 674b
   definition of, 674
   outcomes, 674
Suicide, Risk for (diagnosis), 675b
   definition of, 675
   outcomes, 675
Suicide Self-Restraint (outcome), 525–526b
Surgical Recovery: Convalescence (outcome), 526–527b
Surgical Recovery, Delayed (diagnosis), 635b
   definition of, 635
   outcomes, 635
Surgical Recovery: Immediate Post-Operative (outcome), 528–529b
Swallowing, Impaired (diagnosis), 635b
   definition of, 635
   outcomes, 635
Swallowing Status (outcome), 529–530b
Swallowing Status: Esophageal Phase (outcome), 530b
Swallowing Status: Oral Phase (outcome), 531b
Swallowing Status: Pharyngeal Phase (outcome), 532b
Symptom Control (outcome), 533b
Symptom Severity (outcome), 534b
Symptom Status outcomes
   class, 48–67t
   development across editions, 45–46t
Systemic Toxin Clearance: Dialysis (outcome), 535b

T
Taxonomy, 43–68
Teaching aids, 38
Teaching strategy, 38
Terminology, 7–8b
Therapeutic Response outcomes
   class, 48–67t
   development across editions, 45–46t
Thermal Injury, Risk for (diagnosis), 676b
   definition of, 676
   outcomes, 676
Thermoregulation (outcome), 536b
Thermoregulation: Newborn (outcome), 537b
Thermoregulation, Ineffective (diagnosis), 636b
   definition of, 636
   outcomes, 636
Tissue Integrity outcomes
   class, 48–67t
   development across editions, 45–46t
Tissue Integrity: Skin & Mucous Membranes (outcome), 538b
Tissue Integrity, Impaired (diagnosis), 636b
   definition of, 636
   outcomes, 636
Tissue Perfusion (outcome), 539b
Tissue Perfusion: Abdominal Organs (outcome), 540b
Tissue Perfusion: Cardiac (outcome), 541b
Tissue Perfusion: Cardiac, Risk for Decreased (diagnosis), 676b
   definition of, 676
   outcomes, 676
Tissue Perfusion: Cellular (outcome), 542b
Tissue Perfusion: Cerebral (outcome), 543b
Tissue Perfusion: Cerebral, Risk for Ineffective (diagnosis), 677b
   definition of, 677
   outcomes, 677
Tissue Perfusion: Peripheral (outcome), 544b
Tissue Perfusion: Peripheral, Ineffective (diagnosis), 637b
   definition of, 637
   outcomes, 637
Tissue Perfusion: Peripheral, Risk for Ineffective (diagnosis), 677b
   definition of, 677
   outcomes, 677
Tissue Perfusion: Pulmonary (outcome), 545b
Toddler (term), 8
Transfer Ability, Impaired (diagnosis), 637b
   definition of, 637
   outcomes, 637
Transfer Performance (outcome), 546b
Translations, 736
Transplant outcomes, 726–727b
Trauma, Risk for (diagnosis), 678b
   definition of, 678
   outcomes, 678
Treatment potential, 33–34

U
Unilateral Neglect (diagnosis), 638b
   definition of, 638
   outcomes, 638
Urinary Continence (outcome), 547–548b
Urinary Elimination (outcome), 548b
Urinary Elimination, Impaired (diagnosis), 638b
   definition of, 638
   outcomes, 638

Urinary Elimination, Readiness for Enhanced (diagnosis), 698b
  definition of, 698
  outcomes, 698
Urinary Incontinence: Functional (diagnosis), 639b
  definition of, 639
  outcomes, 639
Urinary Incontinence: Overflow (diagnosis), 639b
  definition of, 639
  outcomes, 639
Urinary Incontinence: Reflex (diagnosis), 639b
  definition of, 639
  outcomes, 639
Urinary Incontinence: Stress (diagnosis), 640b
  definition of, 640
  outcomes, 640
Urinary Incontinence: Urge (diagnosis), 640b
  definition of, 640
  outcomes, 640
Urinary Incontinence: Urge, Risk for (diagnosis), 679b
  definition of, 679
  outcomes, 679
Urinary Retention (diagnosis), 640b
  definition of, 640
  outcomes, 640
Urology outcomes, 727–728b

V
Value-belief pattern outcomes, 569–570
  community-level, 569–570
  individual-level, 569
Vascular outcomes, 728b
Vascular Trauma, Risk for (diagnosis), 680b
  definition of, 680
  outcomes, 680
Ventilation, Impaired Spontaneous (diagnosis), 641b
  definition of, 641
  outcomes, 641

Ventilatory Weaning Response, Dysfunctional (diagnosis), 641b
  definition of, 641
  outcomes, 641
Violence: Other-Directed, Risk for (diagnosis), 680b
  definition of, 680
  outcomes, 680
Violence: Self-Directed, Risk for (diagnosis), 681b
  definition of, 681
  outcomes, 681
Vision Compensation Behavior (outcome), 549b
Vital Signs (outcome), 550b

W
Walking, Impaired (diagnosis), 642b
  definition of, 642
  outcomes, 642
Wandering (diagnosis), 642b
  definition of, 642
  outcomes, 642
Weight: Body Mass (outcome), 551b
Weight Gain Behavior (outcome), 552–553b
Weight Loss Behavior (outcome), 553–554b
Weight Maintenance Behavior (outcome), 555b
Well-being (term), 8
Will to Live (outcome), 556b
Women's Health, Obstetrics, & Neonatology outcomes, 728–729b
Wound Healing: Primary Intention (outcome), 557b
Wound Healing: Secondary Intention (outcome), 558–559b

Y
Young adulthood
  definition of, 8
  Development: Young Adulthood (outcome), 199–200b